Zen and the Brain

The MIT Press
Cambridge, Massachusetts
London, England

Zen and the Brain

Toward an Understanding of Meditation and Consciousness

James H. Austin, M.D.

First MIT Press paperback edition, 1999
© 1998 Massachusetts Institute of Technology

This book was set in Palatino by Graphic Composition, Inc. and was printed and bound in the United States of America.

Library of Congress Cataloging-in-Publication Data

Austin, James H., 1925–
    Zen and the brain : toward an understanding of meditation and consciousness / James H. Austin.
        p. cm.
    Includes bibliographical references and index.
    ISBN 0-262-01164-6 (hc: alk. paper), 0-262-51109-6 (pb)
    1. Meditation—Zen Buddhism—Physiological aspects. 2. Meditation—Zen Buddhism—Psychology. 3. Consciousness—Religious aspects—Zen Buddhism. 4. Zen Buddhism. I. Title.
BQ9288.A96   1998
294.3'422—DC21   97-24693
                                                                                    CIP

To my teachers Nanrei Kobori-roshi, Myokyo-ni, Joshu Sasaki-roshi, and to all those whose contributions to Zen, and to the brain, have been reviewed in this book.

Science without religion is lame,
religion without science is blind.

Albert Einstein (1879–1955)

With all your science can you tell
how it is, and whence it is
that light comes into the soul?

Henry David Thoreau (1817–1862)

Contents in Brief

Contents in Detail

Chapters Containing Testable Hypotheses

List of Figures

List of Tables

Preface

> . . . I don't know what you mean when you say Big Mind and Little Mind. First of all there is the brain.
>
> J. Krishnamurti (1895–1986)[1]

During rare, spontaneous moments, experiences of very special quality and great import emerge from the depths of the human brain. To each person, these awakenings seem awesomely new. What they convey is not. It is the simplest, oldest wisdom in the world. The message is that ultimate meaning is to be found in this present moment, infusing our everyday lives, here and now. But one can't predict such major peaks of enlightenment. Their insight-wisdom is next to impossible to describe. Even so, these fragile events inspired our major religions in ways that still shape our cultural development.

Aldous Huxley called mankind's basic trend toward spiritual growth the "perennial philosophy." Herein, I take a different perspective. To me, the trend implies a dynamic, intimate perennial *psychophysiology*. It is a series of processes, slowly evolving, that culminate in defining moments of an extraordinary character. What are such "peak" experiences? How could they both profoundly enhance, yet simplify, the workings of the brain? This book summarizes the latest evidence.

This is also a story of one neurologist's personal quest and professional search. These two paths converge in ways that lead to one straightforward thesis: awakening, enlightenment, occurs only because the human brain undergoes substantial changes. Does prior meditation help the brain to change in this direction? If so, how? This subject is explored throughout the book.

Is it taboo to discuss religion in a neurological context? It wasn't to William James, almost a century ago. We forget that back in 1901–02, he had already joined these two topics, using the title "Religion and Neurology" for the first of his twenty Edinburgh lectures.[2] Since then, knowledge has exploded within the neurosciences.

Neuroscientists have received most of the Nobel prizes in the fields of medicine and physiology during the past quarter-century. Even the United States Congress, in an inspired moment, voted to call the last ten years of this century "The Decade of the Brain."[3] I hope the reader feels at least equally inspired, and ready to take up the challenge of learning how your own brain functions.

I know this will not be easy, and I ask your forbearance. Our educational "system" has not yet really prepared us for such a task. And the blizzard of new research data, piling up each day, also makes it a formidable job for any writer to condense the information and to make sense of it. I take on two final sets of responsibilities. The first is to summarize the often-murky topic of Zen in order to make clear how vital are its interrelationships with the brain. The second is to express my personal views as one recent witness to Zen experience, while still preserving all those basic truths long held sacred no less to religion than to science. In so doing, it became clear that some chapters required the form of a personal narrative. Most other chapters could be expressed in the form of essays.

Don't be surprised when you encounter topics, some personal, others scientific, set next to each other in unconventional ways.

It may seem small comfort to hear this in advance, but the chapters' uneven textures also serve an illustrative function. Indeed, it has long been recognized that Zen itself displays a most uneven juxtaposition of forms.[4] These jostle our biases, keep us intellectually off balance, and postpone any premature, comfortable equipoise. Gradually our understanding ripens. Only slowly do our attitudes shift. Meanwhile, if we ever think we have Zen in our grasp, we are surely in error.

In part I, we consider what the elusive subject matter of Zen is, and what it is not. Part II examines meditation from the standpoint of its basic physiological mechanisms, not its epiphenomena. Respiration, yes. But perspiration, blood pressure, and superficial brain waves, no. These are *not* where this book is coming from. The next section, part III, summarizes the latest relevant developments in brain research. In part IV, we move on to define both the usual states of consciousness and their alternative expressions. This groundwork serves as the prelude to parts V through VII. Here we present specific examples of several alternate states of consciousness. Moreover, we then break new ground to consider how, where, and when they arise in the depths of the human brain. Finally, part VIII goes beyond transitory "experiences." Here, we clarify both the nature of the advanced *stage* of ongoing enlightenment and its social consequences. Chapters that contain testable hypotheses are listed on p. xvi.

All along, the approach is secular. No reader need fear being brainwashed. Zen enters not through words but through experience. Nor, I hope, will any expect an easy prescription for instant enlightenment. No pat answers are to be found here, no shortcuts. Shortcuts and one-dimensional approaches have already given us too many wishful, incoherent pictures of meditation, consciousness, and of enlightened states. But this situation has not relieved me from the responsibility of oversimplifying the subject. To this end, you are invited to use the glossary, figures, and tables, plus three question-and-answer summaries. Still, I invite the reader's caution: nothing about the brain, or Zen, is ever as simple as this book might suggest. What seems plausible today may be incorrect for reasons other than my errors of commission, omission, and interpretation. Important facts aren't yet known.

Acknowledgments

Much of this book evolved over three separate sabbatical years. Thanks to the arrangements most kindly made by Professor Shuji Takaori, I was fortunate to spend eight months of the first formative period, 1974–75, in the Department of Pharmacology at Kyoto University School of Medicine. In Kyoto, my crucial contacts with Nanrei Kobori-roshi at Ryoko-in stimulated much of the form and the content of this book. The other half of this sabbatical was spent in the Department of Histology at the Karolinska Institute in Stockholm, again thanks to the efforts of Professor Kjell Fuxe.

The second sabbatical period, 1981–82, was spent at the National Hospital, Queen Square, London, and was kindly arranged by Professor Roger Gilliatt. My frequent contacts with Myokyo-ni (Irmgard Schloegl) at the Zen Center in London, both then and subsequently, proved invaluable.

The third year, 1988–89, was also divided. The first portion was spent at the Research Institute for Brain and Blood Vessels in Akita, Japan. Here, the facilities were kindly placed at my disposal by Dr. Ken Nagata and Dean Takeshi Kutsuzawa. The second half was spent at the National Institute of Neurology and Psychiatry in Kodaira, Japan, thanks to the kind efforts of Dr. Eijiro Satoyoshi. My participation in several of Joshu Sasaki-roshi's long retreats at Bodhi Mandala in Jemez Springs, New Mexico, were most helpful, both before and after this year in Japan.

Many others helped bring this book into being. I am grateful both to Judith Austin for her support and helpful editorial comments on the manuscript, and to Frank Urbanowski for his vision of a completed book. Dr. Kionobu Katou and Mrs. Ikuyo Suzuki graciously offered to help with the translation of Kobori-roshi's calligraphy.

Special thanks also go to those secretaries who both deciphered and typed the manuscript through its several draft forms. Most of all to Marcia Conner, whose heroic efforts were invaluable. Also to Jeannine Coppage, Bella Dwyer, Mary Halliwell, Velma Parker, Fran Randolph, Kim Smith, and Melinda Washam. The simplified illustrations reflect the skill of Sara Gustafson. I am indebted to my teacher, Terayama Katsujo, for his gift of Zen-inspired brushwork: the ideogram for emptiness (*mu*), and the *enso* evoking the moon of enlightenment.

I should also like to express my appreciation in general to all those who organized the annual Winter Conference on Brain Research. They enabled me to learn about the brain in a unique multidisciplinary way.

By Way of Introduction

I should not talk so much about myself if there were anybody else whom I knew so well.

Henry Thoreau (1817–62)[1]

This book began as a personal quest for information. I had come on sabbatical leave to Kyoto, Japan. As soon as I engaged in Zen meditation, I became puzzled. Nothing in my previous medical or other training had prepared me for this encounter. My ignorance was abysmal in three major areas: (1) Zen—What *is* it? (2) The human brain—How does it *actually* function? (3) Meditation and enlightened states—What *really* goes on during these? Stimulated by these questions, I have gone on to try to answer some of them in this book, to make the conceptual framework a little easier for the next person on the path.

We expect scientists to be impersonal about their data. But suppose we wish to move toward that scientific goal which William James had predicted. To reach a "critical science of religions," he said, the basic material must come from "facts of personal experience."[2] In my case this could only mean extracting entries made in my journal. You will be reading material that describes an unusual interior world from the *inside*.

Neuroscientists in a university setting, myself included, tend to feel uncomfortable if invited to disclose their own varieties of religious experiences. Publicly to acknowledge that one follows an Eastern mystical tradition is awkward at best. It is viewed as "too far out," a frank abandonment of one's critical academic faculties. Is this true? It is no longer for me alone to say.

We expect serious scientists rigorously to challenge their biases and to reject any belief system that does not fit their data. In fact, Zen students face a not dissimilar task. They, too, must be keen enough to diagnose, and strong enough to pull out by the roots, the dysfunctional aspects of their own egocentric self. Moreover, at the same time, Zen encourages them to keep their critical distance and to challenge whichever of its aspects do not fit. If, in the process, students happen to introduce some of their own observer biases, this is not a problem unique to the study of "altered" states.[3] Even the subatomic physicist introduces uncertainty into each process of observation.

No neurologist overtaken by a major alternate state of consciousness is a "nerve doctor" at that very instant. No self-referent ego is there. No special discrimination scans the moment, biased by its years of training. Analysis isn't stunned. It simply *isn't there* for several seconds. Later, when the episode is over, a few persons might be able to drop such an experience. But what of others like myself, long immersed in the neurosciences, whose commitment to Zen is not so total as that of a monk? As the reader may have guessed by now, some of us might try to puzzle out such experiences. Indeed, one of my teachers recommended that I probe these intriguing experiences, using them as the focus for deeper questioning. Why was I surprised to hear this? After all, many Zen students incubate that other kind of riddle called a *koan*, and enter into a similar long-drawn-out process of concentrated inquiry.

So, in this book, the subject—neurologist—and investigator are one and the same person. It is rare today to find this kind of a clinical autobiography. Ideally, in the future, whoever writes such a book should be a fully enlightened Japanese master, fluent in English; a person who has both a doctorate degree in neurophysiology, hands-on experience in psychophysiological research, years of intercultural teaching experience; and also a physician whose training in both neurology and psychiatry has been doubly certified.

Herein, one student of the Way begins the daunting task of coordinating the facts in these same fields, bringing to the task his background in neuroscience research and a persistent curiosity. To flesh out the personal narrative, I add only those few autobiographical details that seem relevant.[4]

I owe both the stimulus for this work and much of my inspiration to Nanrei Kobori. Kobori-roshi was as open and as interested in learning about the brain as I was in trying to understand Zen. He afforded me a unique opportunity: to study Zen, in Kyoto, with an English-speaking Japanese master of exceptionally broad cultural interests. Unfortunately, such a special opportunity is now no longer readily available at most Zen temples in Japan. It is with his express permission that the substance of our Zen discussions is now open to a wider audience. The dialogue chapters, then, serve to preserve something of the flavor of an authentic Japanese Rinzai Zen master. He was the product of a swiftly vanishing past.

Such fully open dialogue is a trend of our time. It was not the style of previous generations. If the issue lingers of the proprieties of someone going public with private experience, then it, too, was already addressed in the last century by that pioneer American pragmatist, Charles Peirce, when he said: "What is utility, if it is confined to a single accidental person? Truth is public."[5]

Part I

Starting to Point toward Zen

None by his own knowledge, or by subtle consideration, will ever really understand these things. For all words and all that one can learn or understand in a creaturely way, are foreign to the truth that I mean and far below it.

John Van Ruysbroeck (1293–1381)

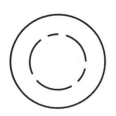

1

Is There Any Common Ground between Zen and the Brain?

> Ideologies, philosophies, religious doctrines, world-models, value systems, and the like will stand or fall depending on the kinds of answers that brain research eventually reveals. It all comes together in the brain.
>
> Roger Sperry (1913–94)[1]

The event is incredible: from grubby origins, a beautiful monarch butterfly emerges. Egg to caterpillar, yes. But how could a chrysalis transform itself into a fluttering butterfly? Unimaginable! It has to be seen twice to be believed.

There are plenty of reasons why we might also view with healthy skepticism the current crop of "born-again" humans. We have no clear idea *how* such an event might occur; why should we believe that it happens? Yet, long ago in a distant land, a man's brain abruptly changed. He too underwent a metamorphosis. His transformation was so complete, enduring, and influential that he is still remembered as the Enlightened One.

Most of us in the West already think we know what "enlightenment" is. To us, the Enlightenment was that long period of intellectual ferment in the sciences and arts during the eighteenth century. It received its impetus from Newton and other giants of thought who proved that, through reasoning, we could discover those "natural laws" which govern our physical universe. To us, thereafter, the word "enlightenment"—*Aufklärung* in German—would mean that truth became clear only when it had first passed through logical sequences and rational discourse. How could enlightenment have a second, *non*rational meaning? An insight-wisdom that preempts language and goes *beyond* reasoning? We have never quite accepted such a notion.

In fact, there never has been anything really convincing to be *said* about Zen. Only the same old soft evidence of the centuries. Only that it keeps conveying the same remarkable message: the human brain can be shaped, etched, and transformed by years of practice. To what end? To yield striking ongoing constellations of perception, insight, attitudes, and behavior. These flow spontaneously, blending conduct fully in harmony with whatever social setting prevails (see part VIII).

Even after he, too, was enlightened in this manner, the man they called the Buddha still viewed himself as a man. To himself, he remained only the most recent of many in the past who had become awakened. His now legendary accomplishment still serves as our prototype: Start by transforming only one person's brain, and whole societies may then undergo authentic change on a major scale. Indeed, the Japan of today still demonstrates how the Buddhist message has been woven into the cultural fabric of a nation for countless generations.[2]

Yet, Eastern religious themes leave us feeling uneasy. (Even the term *Buddhism* seems alien. Where else do we meet *ddh* in our own language?) We take for granted the Western icon of the bleeding, crucified Christ. Yet, curiously, we still find it strange that an Eastern approach could also accent the kinds of suffering in the world. Our image of God tends to conform to Michelangelo's theistic vision. He is that majestic, white-bearded patriarch, reaching down to create man in His own image with the mere touch of His right index finger. Always a white male, and always a capital *H*. True, it was our own culture that spawned the phrase, "God is dead." But atheism still feels uncomfortable. Something must be wrong with any foreign import that leaves out "God," the Creator.

Disquieted by anything mystical, we still might concede that mysticism was implicit in the lives of Jesus of Nazareth, St. John of the Cross, Plotinus, and others in our own culture. But who can know, without trying it, what it really means to meditate as the Buddha has been portrayed, sitting in his strange, cross-legged lotus posture? We are latecomers to meditation. In contrast, many centuries before Siddhartha Gautama, the East had already discovered a curious fact: a person who sat quietly in this manner, in full awareness, might finally awaken extraordinary states of consciousness. In Asia, this knowledge passed through the yogic traditions, then evolved through the newly developing Buddhist traditions in India, China, and Japan.

How could such quiet meditative sitting cultivate the arrival of insightful mental states? In this and subsequent chapters of this book, we shall begin to answer this question. And as we learn more about Zen's subtler mechanisms, we shall discover another curious fact: Its messages are not really so alien to the West after all. Indeed, as many of the opening quotations will illustrate, our own arts and literature have been saying the same things for centuries. Could it be that at their source, human brains everywhere gravitate toward the same kinds of natural messages?

Extraordinary states of consciousness are invested with special experiential qualities. Many lesser events, "quickenings," are also distinctive. We will single out experiences of both types, examine each for its form and content. Soon we will discover properties that are of fundamental neurological significance. In fact, the various examples selected are useful models, ready to teach us how our own brain functions. Why is this one book so ambitious as to review both Zen *and* neuroscience? *Because the two fields are so intimately interrelated that each illuminates the other.*

So Zen is more than an agency of personal change. In this book, the topic of Zen will evolve to become an avenue for creating potential scientific change as well. For, starting in part III, we will be deriving *testable* hypotheses. Each of the twenty-two chapters containing these theories is identified on page xvi. Whether today's hypotheses are later proved or disproved is less important than the fact that when they are tested later, unexpected new basic mechanisms may be discovered.

But to explore illumination is a demanding task. In this respect, Zen can serve us as did Newton's prism, helping to split light into its spectrum of components. However, as Westerners studying Zen, we must soon open up to alternative ways and axes of thinking. Neither topic—Zen, or the human brain—is understandable in one dimension, at one time, at one level. So a word of caution: Having now chosen to probe the complex interface between these two big subjects, we will be setting off to travel paths of incomprehension. The trip will take us along strange new planes that tilt away at improbable angles. Mental illumination resists being split.

We cannot monitor the discharge rate of every single nerve cell while it is in the act of helping to sponsor our intricate mental functions. Do the climatologists try to describe a major storm front by tracking each of its raindrops and every local current of air?[3] No, they do not predict the weather by plotting droplets. They study huge weather systems moving over large regions. So, too, do brain researchers reach out to use other descriptive techniques. This means that some of our levels of analysis will also employ units patterned on a much larger scale, systems which then depend on abstract psychological constructs. Let it be clear that each such step moves us farther away from Zen and from the simple direct experience of wet raindrops on the face.

It becomes necessary, then, to proceed in several ways. Pursuing a kind of bottom-up synthesis, we will draw on simpler examples to help understand higher functions. At other times, we will follow the top-down approach. This means observing complex brain functions, then working back toward those basic psychophysiological mechanisms from which they spring. No, we won't try to develop a complete neurochemistry of behavior. Behavior grows out of the interactions of the whole nervous system, whereas chemistry is best suited to the study of its smaller, simpler subparts, such as the single cell.[4]

The literature surveyed for the two major topics of this book is vast and very uneven. Half-blindfolded and with mittens on, researchers are working to assemble a giant, shifting, three-dimensional jigsaw puzzle. Many of the pieces out on the table don't yet fit. So we can hardly expect that the two general lines of evidence—Zen and the brain—will always join in an orthodox way that satisfies most religious tests for authenticity and most formal scientific tests for proof.

But others blazed this same trail, making the job easier. Among them was that pioneer explorer, William James. We shall meet James many times on our path. He warned us, decades ago, of our limitations. Were he living today, he would caution us to avoid what he might now call the "neurologists' fallacy." This is the naive notion that a brain perceives an apple the same way that a neurologist conceives of the whole process. He was already preparing us for the awesome, impossible simplicity of Zen insight: an apple is an apple—in *itself*—without our being in the picture.

Can the reductionist, who would rely solely on the fragile edge of intellect, even get near reason's antithesis in Zen? Not without venturing out on very thin ice. In fact, if we seem too openly to "neurologize" about internal events in part III it is only because we have already accepted the sobering Jamesian caveat: "In principle, intellectualism's edge is broken; it can only approximate to reality, and its logic is inapplicable to our inner life, which spurns its vetoes and mocks at its impossibilities."[5]

Anyone who would venture into that inner life, the interface between neuroscience and Zen, will also encounter the hostile crossfire of substantial misunderstandings from both sides. Two illustrations suffice, from major parties of international stature. Closing his last, fine work, Jacob Bronowski expressed sadness at what he saw was a failure of nerve in the West. He believed that the West was in full retreat from knowledge whenever it took up such matters as extrasensory perception, mystery, and Zen. Sadly, he chose to lump them all together. He held that none of these could lead humankind to reaffirm its destiny. For, he concluded, it would be only through the ascent of self-knowledge that we could finally make "rational intelligence prove itself sounder than the reflex."[6] The reader will soon find that "self"-knowledge is what Zen is all about.

Christmas Humphreys came from the other direction. He regarded any approach to "the supremely spiritual school of Zen" that would involve "examining the brain in relation to Zen experience was rather like examining the car in the street to understand the mind of the driver indoors."[7] In fact, neurobiologists still go on openly studying reflexes and looking under the hood, not huddling passively in the trenches. Many of them still keep wondering: how does the inner life arise? Ever puzzled, they oscillate between two major fictions: (1) The brain can be understood; (2) We will never come close. Meanwhile, they keep pursuing brain mechanisms, partly from habit, partly out of faith. Their premise: The brain is the organ of the mind. Clearly, this three-pound lump of tissue is the source of our "insight information" about our very being. Somewhere in it there might be a few hidden guidelines for better ways to lead our lives.

Zen doesn't get preoccupied with such scientific flappings of the mind. Instead, what matters in Zen is the way our brain expresses—in simple awareness and in everyday behavior—those instinctual depths of self-knowledge that lie beyond the shallow fictions of the egocentric self.

To some, Zen is an exotic butterfly, now grown old and frayed along its wing edges. Fluttering beyond reach, it is a sublimely living thing. It was never intended to be examined close up with a lens, certainly not to be dissected. To others, their neural sciences should remain forever "hard" if not rigid. On principle, they reject the notion that there can be any reputable common ground between molecules, membranes, and mysticism. In their view, any attempt to localize mysticism in the brain is too close to last century's discredited phrenology. Still others may feel that Siddhartha's seemingly mild (but revolutionary) teachings have little bearing on today's harsh social realities.

These attitudes have lived in me in the past. I know them. Yet my hope is that the reader will discover, in the rest of part I and in part VIII, how increasingly relevant the Zen approach is to the serious social issues we confront today. For Zen has something practical to contribute to today's science, religion, philosophy, politics, and ecology. All these do come together, with Zen, in the brain.

Some readers will understandably be discomforted by the reports of animal experiments. Lay and scientific readers may be interested to know that Japanese Buddhists have set aside a memorial day, *Ireisai*. It is a requiem devoted to animals who gave their lives to benefit mankind. Both in the United States and elsewhere, substantial protections increasingly ensure that the kinds of research cited in these pages will have been conducted following humane principles.[8]

Authentic Zen has long sponsored the utmost freedom of personal inquiry. No person need fear the questions we must ask here, or the imponderables that will emerge. As is so often the case, each new discovery in the neurosciences will only add more mysteries to the process.

At the end, whatever simple truths the reader will have distilled about Zen and the brain belong to no one narrow religious, scientific, or philosophical belief-system. The insights discussed in part VII are not cultural constructs. Their truths are natural ones, part of everyone's ancient, universal biological heritage.

2

A Brief Outline of Zen History

The nature of Zen does not lie in scholarship, philosophy, in the Buddhist Doctrine, and not even in zazen. . . . It lies in one thing alone, namely seeing into the Buddha nature that is in each person.

M. Trevor[1]

The power of true center must be the most frequently mislaid artifact of human wisdom. It is as if the same message keeps washing ashore, and no one breaks the bottles, much less the code.

Marilyn Ferguson[2]

When I first encountered Zen in Kyoto, I understood little about its origins. Buddhism goes back a long way, two and one-half millennia. Within its traditions, the approach most systematic yet most elusive, the clearest yet most paradoxical, the subtlest yet most dramatic is Zen. To know its history is to understand it better. When I dug into the story of its past, this is what I discovered.

The Zen of which we speak is an ancient sect within Mahayana Buddhism. Not some New Age variant or "beat" imitation in any distorted Kerouac sense, it is a formal, comprehensive Way of spiritual development. It is a Way which will so reshape awareness that it finally grasps the reality of things as they really are.

Embedded in the word *Zen* is the story of how it evolved over the centuries. Its meditative techniques stemmed from ancient yoga practices. At that time, in India, the Sanskrit word for meditation was *dhyana*. This evolved into the phrase *Ch'un-Na*, then into the Chinese word *Ch'an*. Later, Buddhist monks transplanted this Ch'an form of meditation to Japan, where the Japanese pronounced it *Zen*.[3] Zen, then, stands for the school of Buddhism that emphasized meditation and that evolved further as it spread from India, to China, and to Japan. *Zazen* is its system of meditation.

The word *buddha* means enlightened one. The man who would later be called the Buddha was born in what is now southern Nepal in 563 B.C.E. His original name was Siddhartha Gautama. Out of the 2500-year-old mists of antiquity, only legends come down to us now. They portray him as a privileged child who led a sheltered life as the son of the leader of the noble Shakya clan. Protected from reality, he learned nothing about that harsh world outside the gate of his compound. When he finally ventured out, he was shocked by the suffering he saw: a sick man, an old man, and a dead man. Among them was a half-naked, smiling beggar—a holy man. The sharp contrasts between their situations and his own lifestyle haunted him for years. So finally, when he was twenty-nine years old, he vowed to take up his own search for the meaning of existence. Following the prevailing custom of that era, this meant that he would live the austere life of a wanderer, and would leave his wife and young son behind.[4]

After six years of searching for the truth, depleted by the rigors of his ascetic life, Siddhartha finally rested near the city of Guaya in northeast India. Here he broke his fast, accepted some milk gruel, and resolved to meditate beneath a nearby pipal tree until he reached enlightenment. On the seventh day, as the morning star shone in the sky, he finally came to supreme enlightenment. He was thirty-five years old.

Thereafter, he traveled widely, teaching what he had learned, for another forty-five years. His disciples passed on the bulk of his teachings, emphasizing certain fundamental points in his dharma, or body of basic truths. For example, early in his career, at Sarnath near present-day Benares, he preached a key sermon. It stressed the Four Noble Truths: (1) Life is full of suffering and dissatisfaction. (2) Our passions and other worldly illusions cause these sorrows. (3) The way out of suffering is to extinguish self-centered desires and aversions. (4) There is a sensible, eightfold Path for doing this. It combines right understanding, thought, speech, conduct, vocation, effort, mindfulness, and meditation.[5]

The Buddha had learned the hard way that the ascetic life has limitations. Thereafter, he would advocate the middle way. It was an ethical, commonsense approach to living, a way of moderation. It was a way that avoided both fasting and indulgence, and steered clear of other physical or mental extremes. He believed that everyone had the potential to be awakened, saying: "Look within, thou art Buddha." He died in 483 B.C.E., at the age of eighty, at Kusinagara, India.

Some two centuries after he died, the Buddhist reformation had flourished to such a degree that it was officially recognized by Asoka, who became India's first Buddhist emperor. The movement then spread slowly north from India and east to China along the old Silk Road. Then, during the four centuries after 200 B.C.E., Buddhism split into two schools: Mahayana Buddhism, meaning the "greater vehicle," and Hinayana Buddhism, "the lesser vehicle." The latter, more ascetic southern school was also termed Theravada (the way of the elders). It went on to become the major religion of much of Southeast Asia.

Around the year 520, the Indian monk Bodhidharma traveled to China where he introduced what would evolve into the Chan sect of Mahayana Buddhism.[3] Four striking statements describing Chan date from this early period. The quatrain illustrates how different this particular meditation school was from the many other religious movements that had come before, existed then, or would follow:

1. A special transmission outside the scriptures

2. Not depending on words and letters

3. Direct pointing to the human soul

4. Seeing into one's own nature, to reach Buddhahood

In China, many early Buddhists were uncomfortable with the various practices of Indian Buddhism. To them, its expansive abstractions were incidental to Buddha's central message. The Chan school of reformers was especially iconoclastic. They simplified the advanced yoga practices, deemphasized scriptural studies, and gave up esoteric practices.[6] Knowing well the hazards of the proliferating intellect, Chan teachers avoided thought-forms and ideas. They chose to cultivate and celebrate in everyday living the essence of Siddhartha's original enlightenment. Among the early Chinese masters was the unlettered Hui-neng (638–713). Hui-neng stressed that enlightenment occurred instantaneously. Moreover, he served as a living example of the fact that a person need not be a literate monk in a formal institutional setting in order to undergo the flash of enlightenment.

China already had a number of "quietist" schools as early as around 400 to 300 B.C.E. But it was Taoism—the indigenous religion in China at the time—that would make the major Chinese contribution to early Chan. Its Way, the Tao, was nothing less than the basic, unchanging, motionless principle underlying and pervading the whole dynamic universe. Taoist philosophy was already so comfortable with paradox that it could fit in well with Buddhist enlightenment. Moreover, it had long emphasized a life lived simply and spontaneously within the oneness of nature.

We can appreciate Taoism's subtle, understated approach to living from the following statement attributed to its legendary sage, Lao-Tzu: "Acting without design, occupying oneself without making a business of it, finding the great in the small and the many in the few, repaying injury with kindness, effecting difficult things while they are easy, and managing great things in their beginnings: this is the method of Tao."[7] Chan also drew some of its ethical base from Confucianism. Thus, it gradually evolved into what Kobori-roshi would later describe as "a strange dragon with a Taoist torso, Confucian feet, and the Buddhist enlightenment-experience for its eyes."[8]

During its early centuries in China, and its first several patriarchs, early Chan did not appear to employ the riddle called a *koan* as a concentration device.[9] Later, Chan adopted vigorous methods, including shoutings and beatings. These techniques were practiced especially by the activist school which developed around the dynamic Chinese master, Lin-chi (J: Rinzai). Two other masters preferred a gentler, contrasting approach. They were Ts'ao-shan and Tung-shan, who jointly founded the Ts'ao-tung school. Pronounced *Soto* when it came to Japan, their school continued to emphasize gradual, incremental enlightenment and less activist methods (table 1).

It was during the Tang dynasty in China (618–907) that Chan became most influential. By then, the early Chinese masters had evolved techniques which created a living religion, and brought to it personal immediacy. They focused on direct, concrete, everyday life experience and used the simplest earthy examples to train their students. From then on, the basic Zen approach to religion would be far removed from lofty abstractions, secondhand hearsay, and sterile scholarship. The early masters also introduced walking meditation and hard work to the monastery, for too much sitting could reach the point of diminishing returns.

Table 1
The Two Major Zen Schools

	Soto	Rinzai
Chinese source	Ts'ao-tung school	Lin-chi school
Representative figures in China	Both Ts'ao-shan (840–901) and Tung-shan (807–869) The two, combined, are Ts'ao-tung (J: Soto)	Lin-chi (died 867) (J: Rinzai)
Emphasis	"Just sitting" in zazen Gradual enlightenment	Zazen, koan study, and personal interviews Sudden enlightenment
Temperaments	Less activist	More activist
Sitting	Facing wall; no koan	Facing out; concentrating on koan
General aura	Less austere, rigorous, and demanding	More austere, rigorous, and demanding
Representative figures in Japan	Dogen (1200–1253) Keizan (1268–1325)	Hakuin (1686–1769)
Present status in Japan	More adherents 6.7 million (1956)* 7.1 million (1984); 9% of total Buddhists†	Fewer adherents 2.9 million (1956)* 1.7 million (1984); 2% of total Buddhists†
Representative centers	Eihei-ji in Fukui Prefecture Soji-ji in Yokohama	Daitoku-ji in Kyoto Engaku-ji in Kamakura

*Survey dated 1956. D. Suzuki, *Zen and Japanese Buddhism,* Tokyo, Tuttle, 1958, 104–111.
†*Shykyo Nenkan* [*Religious Yearbook*]. Tokyo, Gyosei Press, 1985, 58, 59, 74–77.

From this distance, the early Zen we see in the Tang and Sung (960–1279) dynasties leaps forth as a vigorous, inspired human product. It had then, as it does now, its full share of cultural contributions, contradictions, confusing features, and firmly held doctrinal disputes.[3] What remains so special about it? Distinctive of Zen in any era is the way its leaders have (1) devised methods for cultivating enlightenment in their pupils, (2) validated its authenticity, (3) ensured that they and their students continually infused their awakened awareness into the art of living, and (4) carefully sanctioned each successive generation of teachers. The semilegendary Bodhidharma, for example, was already the twenty-eighth patriarch in a long succession of master teachers, a line which extended back to Buddha himself.[10]

When the Rinzai school was imported to Japan, it was adaptable enough to flourish both under the rule of the emperors in their capital of Kyoto and under the more militant shoguns in Kamakura. Zen's continued influence in medieval Japan was attributable to the way it appealed to more sophisticated leaders of samurai society, not to the rough, unlettered samurai themselves.[11] Moreover, the Zen approach was flexible enough to enter the arts of tea ceremony, calligraphy, and landscape gardening, as well as the martial arts. In Kyoto, the huge temple complex of Daitoku-ji (where I started to train) was founded in 1324. It exemplifies Zen's pivotal role in influencing Japanese cultural development. From such monasteries and temples, Zen spread its cultural aesthetic into the daily life of the community. There it coexisted with the indigenous Shinto religion and complemented it.

Stimulated by the many publications of Daisetz T. Suzuki (who lived to the ripe age of ninety-five years), Zen came increasingly to the West's attention after World War II. As other religions recognized its ecumenical message, and as meditation in general came to the fore, opinions have differed about what constitutes the basic core of Zen, and how best this core could be adapted to the religious pluralism of the twentieth century.[12–14]

Still, in every land, the familiar symbol of Buddhism remains. The icon is that of the Buddha in meditation. In each country, painters and sculptors adapted his facial features and garments to fit in with the conventions of their own regional culture at that time. As a result, the early Buddhas of the Ajanta caves in India look different from those in the Longmen caves near Lo-yang in northern China. The latter images also differ from the large Buddha at Kamakura, in Japan. In the Zen school of Buddhism especially, he is still regarded as a man, not a god. An inspiration to all other human beings, not a He.

Early Indian sculptors started to depict the Buddha with a rounded lump on the top of his head. This protrusion, the *ushnisha*, long anticipated the "bumps" of the Western phrenologists of the last century. It was designed to represent an upward extension of the contents of the cranial cavity. In this manner, successive artists symbolized the fact that enlightenment conferred an expansion of consciousness, an enlargement of insight-wisdom, and the enhancement of mental capacities in general. Only a superficial glance would confuse the outer ringlets of this cerebral protrusion with the bulge of a conventional topknot of hair. Another added symbol was the dot between the eyes, the *urna*. It stood for the levels of enhanced perception that were associated with insight.

Old iconographies, but pointing to something deeper. Herein, we are asking, What do these two symbols imply? How has the brain beneath them transformed its functions? For in our reading of the history of Zen, the message always comes down as follows: in the final analysis, Zen training means *brain* training.

3

But What Is Zen?

Asked to explain Zen—
my puppy with the same name
looks, and thumps his tail.

Jay Hackett[1]

So much, then, for the historical record. But in themselves, how can the words of the previous chapter explain a universal process, one that begins with the immediate perception of things as they really are, then flows seamlessly into inspired behavior? For Zen is *living* experience, not musty principles in the abstract. It is a special form of Buddhism in which precepts and practice fuse. What are some of its main teachings?

1. *Zen emphasizes meditation as a way to enlightenment.* This final *spiritual awakening* focuses on one thesis: we and the universe are coextensive. This central

theme is implied in the term *Maha-prajna-paramita*. *Maha* means great; *prajna* means insight-wisdom; *paramita* implies reaching that other shore, the place where there are neither attachments to living nor fears about dying. The term points to that profound insight which frees one from all suffering caused by selfish, egocentric concerns.

Atomic physicists can tell us in words that we are all derived from stardust. But Zen takes our interpenetration with the universe literally. Its insight strikes as a fact of *experience*. This deepest truth is not captured in words. Insight information, like a cool drink of water, has an impact at levels beyond reasoning.

To D. T. Suzuki, the kind of Zen enlightenment that took place back in the Sung and Tang dynasties of China was subtly different from other kinds of spiritual illumination. Zen masters then, he noted, aimed to bring their students so intimately in touch with the "Being of Life which animates all things" that they felt its own awareness vibrate within themselves.[2] An endpoint this advanced would seem to go beyond the usual spiritual goals that we ascribe to those who practice most religions today.

Zen enlightenment today is still somewhat different from the others. No, it does not descend from some greater power up above. Its aspirants view it as emanating from that within, which is all around. It means awakening to our fundamental unity with that eternal universe right under our noses. It does not imply adding some new and esoteric concepts from the outside. The potential for such insight-wisdom is latent in each of us, and will ripen under the proper set of circumstances. Fully ripened, it will greatly simplify, stabilize, and liberate the person. Opening up to anything and everything, the aspirant will drop off childish passions and rechannel his or her energies along more mature lines.

2. *The intellect is not at home in the province of Zen.* Zen withdraws before the intellect. Hides, if you will. In this, it resembles the elusive Japanese bush warbler, the uguisu. Never is this warbler perched on high, singing assertively for all to hear as do the Japanese grosbeak and the American cardinal. Instead, the uguisu blends naturally into the foliage of smaller trees and thickets. There, its lyrical notes begin with a low, soft uprising whistle, then end in a loud, incredibly beautiful liquid warble: "hot-kat-kyot!" One memorable day, I actually saw the bird while it was singing. Only then could I convince myself that a creature this small and unprepossessing could create such beautiful music.

Zen teachings emphasize the straightforward. They devalue the discursive intellect with its edifice of words and abstract theories. Lengthy, complicated philosophical discussions are scholastic mumbo jumbo. Less is more. As the Tao Te Ching puts it, "Those who know, do not speak; those who speak, do not know."

3. *Zen values the simple, concrete, living facts of everyday direct personal experience.* When our brain takes in a red rose, it doesn't need to think about the word "red," ponder its wavelength, or try to analyze what chemistry caused it to be this color. It perceives red *directly*. Zen training encourages this same instantaneous, uncluttered awareness throughout everything else in the here and now. The Zen point of view appreciates each moment's sacramental quality. Imbued with genuine ecological reverence toward nature in all its forms, Zen practitioners learn to look humbly, "livingly," at the way they use each day's food, clothing, shelter, and companionship.[3]

Zen, living in this present moment, concentrates upon *this* bird song, *this* falling cherry blossom. It brings together all these present moments of quiet clarity into the flow of its timeless, ongoing awareness. This Zen doesn't soar or proselytize. It will erect no cathedral spires high in the sky. It is utterly down-to-earth, matter-of-fact. In Zen, life's firsthand earthy experience is *the* living reality. The *un*reality is our usual hectic existence, the one full of swarming thoughts, clouded perceptions, and self-centered behavior.

Today's New Age spirituality, newly wedded to high technology, is already promoting a host of brain-tuning devices. Authentic Zen will not be drawn into such artificial "mind gyms." Zen requires no contrived "virtual reality." It is like an art appreciation course. Its message is to *look* at natural things; *see* into them. One day, you will finally see, beyond yourself, into their own sacred qualities. Then you will comprehend things as they really are, in keeping with the basic unity of all things. This illumination will remain, and thereafter you will act authentically in relation to all things.

4. *Zen is intensely pragmatic*, wary of moralistic judgments, of manmade distinctions between good and bad. Its security comes from knowing, as a result of long experience, how people act after they have become totally committed to its path of awakening. Go ahead, let them then encounter some ambiguous laissez-faire situation. Increasingly they will act in accord with the "natural, right way" of things. And meanwhile, why burden them with another superstructure of someone else's doctrines imposed from without? Their behavior is going to become increasingly selfless anyway, because it will be proceeding in harmony with this natural order of things.

A favorite Zen phrase is, "A finger pointing at the moon." Symbols are crucial in religion. In Zen the pale moon symbolizes enlightenment, at many metaphoric levels. The real moon up there will still go on existing, long after our fingers and words down on earth have ceased to point toward it. Similarly, anything *said* about Zen is, at best, no more than a finger vaguely pointing off in its general direction. Consider this book as another example. It has nothing to do *with* Zen. It is only *about* Zen. On its pages are words *about* what we think goes on inside the brain. A real book about Zen could just as well have a plain cover, empty pages, and no title, yet could still be worn out from use because you sat on it. Zen is like swimming; you don't learn swimming by reading *about* it in a book. You learn to swim by *doing* it, in the water.

5. *You learn about Zen in zazen*, Zen meditation. It is the essential, fundamental practice for ripening the brain's intuitive faculties. To the Zen master Dogen, the practice of zazen in itself constituted enlightenment. The Zen meditative approach has a simple, unstated premise: moods and attitudes shape—*determine*—what we think and perceive. If we feel happy, we tend to develop certain trains of thought. If we feel sad or angry, still others. But suppose, with training, we become nonattached to distractions and learn to dampen these wild, emotional swings on either side of equanimity. Then we can enter that serene awareness which is the natural soil for positive, spontaneous personal growth, often called spiritual growth.

Meditative practice does not set itself against all conscious thoughts or emotions. Rather it encourages those that are selfless and freed from unfruitful links with the passions. Zen shuns hallucinations and dogmatism, except, perhaps, that which may be implied by some of its rigorous training methods. Because such methods are regarded as the fruit of centuries of experience, in the Orient, at least, the novice is unlikely to brush them aside.

6. *You needn't sit on a pillow to practice Zen.* Zen practice extends itself into paying bare attention to all the events of daily life. If a goal is to be defined, then it is to learn the art of letting go while paying attention. Sitting in clear-minded, open-eyed zazen, one develops the capacity to let go, and this gradually flows on into all other activities of one's daily life practice. Aspirants flounder until they finally let go of their attitude that enlightenment is something to "achieve." Those who keep trying to "gain" enlightenment discover that becoming truly goalless and selfless is the most difficult of all the arts of living.

7. *Zen stresses self-reliance, self-discipline, and personal effort.* It's up to the individual to enlighten himself or herself. Zen deemphasizes, even-handedly, not only those behaviors that are self-centered from the inside but also any authoritarian doctrines from the outside that might interfere with self-realization.

"Look within." True. But still, the long, hard meditative path to awakening is best traversed with the aid of the master, the *roshi.* He has traveled the bumpy road before. He may not speak about its every height, but he knows its twists, turns, and pitfalls. However, the Zen master only acts as guide and exemplar. It is the aspirant's own self-discipline and tolerance which will prove critical. Positive interactions within a small group are strongly reinforcing, yet the journey is mostly private, interior. The final responsibility falls squarely on the aspirant.

8. *The inner journey is but a prelude to going out.* Insightful awakening will reunite the aspirant deeply with what is understood to be the mainstream of the life force, the full range of life's joys and sorrows. But these rare moments are not to be savored for themselves. They are to be actualized. This means putting precepts into practice. It implies an increasingly selfless, simplified spontaneous affirmation of life. Whether this is the dedicated life of a monk or lay aspirant, it then becomes one of introspection, humility, labor, and service. What does the herdsman do in the old Zen story after he finally becomes enlightened? He does not retreat from the world to become a hermit. Instead, he goes forth with joy and compassion to mingle in the world "with helping hands."[4]

4

Mysticism, Zen, Religion, and Neuroscience

In the whole wide range of that eminently challenging science, the history of ideas, there is no subject more enduringly provocative than mysticism.

E. O'Brien[1]

Of mysticism it has often been said that it begins in mist and ends in schism.

Robert Masters and Jean Houston[2]

By now the reader will have sensed that we're straying into the area of mysticism. The topic generates heated discussions. We had best begin with familiar Western words and ground rules. These will help clarify what mysticism is, what it is not, and whether Zen is a form of it. Then, we'll need to define religion. In the process, we can decide whether Zen Buddhism is a kind of religion. Finally, we ask: Does neuroscience bear any constructive relationship with mysticism, religion, or Zen?

Nowhere is mysticism always received kindly. It has been suspect for millennia, for in ancient times the mystic (*mystes*, one initiated) was one who was initiated into secret, and thus troubling, esoteric rites. The word still troubles us. It conjures up dark associations, occult beliefs, mysterious doings. The skeptical man in the street sides with Samuel Johnson who held that, "Where secrecy or mystery begins, vice or roguery is not far off."[3] Here, we define mysticism in the most general sense as the ongoing practice of reestablishing, by the deepest insights, one's direct relationship with the ultimate, universal reality principle.

Other versions abound. William James held that a "consciousness of illumination" was the essential mark of a mystical state.[4] To Underhill, mysticism was "the science of ultimates, the science of unions with the Absolute, and nothing else."[5] To Dumoulin, true mysticism signified "an immediate relationship to absolute spiritual reality." It included all of our efforts to elevate ourselves to that "super cosmic, super sensory sphere" which is experienced immediately.[6] To Keller, mysticism was "the search, proper to each religion and carried out within each religion by some of its adepts, after full apprehension of what that religion defines as the highest and most intimate knowledge available to its adherents."[7] When we discuss mysticism here, its scope will not include spiritualism, supernaturalism, or any other activities believed to bend spoons or to otherwise suspend the known physical laws of the universe.

Worldwide, the mystical traditions tend to fall into at least two categories. One school holds that the deity principle or creative force lies *outside* themselves. They have the sense of moving through stages leading *up and out* toward its divine presence. The Christian approach follows this general orientation. From its perspective, when a person has been granted this intuitive apprehension of reality, it is a gift of grace bestowed from above.

The schools of Buddhist mysticism, including that of Zen, reflect the second orientation. They teach that the universal principle, or Buddha nature, already exists not only within each person but everywhere else.

Some observers contend that there is a third category, that of the prophetic religions. It is exemplified by some forms of Judaism, Islam, and evangelical Christianity, which practice intense, devotional worship. Vigorous prophetic approaches tend to become highly inspirational and arousing. They lend a distinctive, *numinous*, interpretation to the religious experience. Here, "numinous" implies the sense of having encountered the sacred presence of divinity. The person has the impression of being affected significantly by something both totally different from anything else and wholly other than his or her previous self. In the Buddhist meditative context, the flash of a major mystical experience is less violent than is the impact of a typical revelation in the prophetic context, and its tone is decidedly impersonal.[8]

Johnston observes that Christian mysticism engages in a special kind of concentration. It is one in which worship is pressured by suppositions of love which arise out of faith.[9] In contrast, the Zen Buddhist approach is to let go of all suppositions. Once beyond them, Zen aspirants then heighten their one-pointed concentration during meditative retreats and by their efforts to solve the riddle of a koan. (For example, "What is the sound of one hand?") Christian and Buddhist approaches also start from different premises. When preached by fundamentalists, the Christian message may sound more like: "You're a sinner; you need to repent and be saved in Christ!" The Buddhist teachings tend to come out sounding like: "Everyone suffers, but if you lead the right life and meditate, your own efforts will lead you beyond this anguish."

Is Zen a form of mysticism? Eugen Herrigel believed there was indeed a Buddhist mysticism. Its distinctive feature was the emphasis it placed "on a *methodical* preparation for the mystical life."[10] On the other hand, it is instructive to trace the steps through which D. T. Suzuki's opinions about Zen evolved during his long, influential career. In the beginning, back in 1906, he wrote: "There is no doubt that [mysticism] is the soul of the religious life."[11] About Zen, he also went on to say that "its doctrines, broadly speaking, are those of a speculative mysticism."[12] Much later, in 1939, he would write, "I am not certain whether Zen can be identified with mysticism."[13] Further, "These Zen masters are not mystics, and their philosophy is not mysticism."[14] And "Zen is a radical realism rather than mysticism." However he may have phrased such earlier opinions, by 1939 Suzuki had come to believe that Zen was "an altogether unique product of the Oriental mind, refusing to be classified under any known heading, as either a philosophy, or a religion, or a form of mysticism as it is generally understood in the West."[15] My sense is that Zen falls not only within but near the core of the general definitions of mysticism noted earlier. Yet, Zen *is* difficult to pigeonhole, both by those inside and outside of it. Why this is so will become increasingly apparent.

Meanwhile, what definitions of the term *religion* can Westerners agree on? As we approach the third millennium of our Christian era, most persons acknowledge that a religion does not have to mimic every familiar ecclesiastical, doctrinal, or institutional form that we have developed so highly in the West. William James defined religion as "the feelings, acts, and experiences of individual men in their solitude, so far as they apprehend themselves to stand in relation to whatever they may consider the divine."[16] Luckmann and Geertz define religion as "a set of symbols that purport to provide a unique interpretive scheme to explain the ultimate reality."[17] Currently, our simplest dictionary definitions say that religion is a system of faith or worship professed or practiced by its adherents. Again, Zen Buddhism falls well within these definitions. But the Zen Way is certainly no religion for Sundays only. It places special emphasis on one's *practicing moment-to-moment awareness in daily life throughout every day* of the week. The serious Zen aspirant embarks on a continuous, lifelong journey in the direction of becoming a fully developed *humane* being.

Most people expect that a neuroscientist would approach mystical issues with more objectivity than does the mystic. In practice, such distinctions are not always sharp. Scientists are rarely totally analytic. Indeed, when starting to work, they frequently employ the most subjective of premises, then make their greatest creative advances through intuitive leaps.[18] But whatever the two may have in common, science tends to hold mysticism at arm's length. The mainstream scholarly tradition in the West doesn't feel at home in any setting it deems irrational. Moreover, it will contend that no brain can criticize mysticism with the requisite intellectual rigor once it has been compliant enough to bend to the mystical.

Some basic scientists also fear mysticism, and for good reasons. Feeling themselves truest to the quest for the scientific grail, they strive in the laboratory first to collect a body of valid data, then to interpret it logically, thoughtfully. So their goal is always to *resolve* paradox, certainly not deliberately to create it. No wonder these scientists instinctively shun mystics. Mystics do more than grow comfortable with paradox. Some talk about it. And when they do, they issue long strings of arcane metaphors from an occult world which no scientist can understand.

Past centuries viewed such mystics as wild-eyed recluses who wore their hair long and affected simple, sometimes shabby garb. We know today that mystical experiences occur commonly in otherwise sane "normal" persons. Moreover, increasing numbers of them follow one mystical tradition or another, meditate regularly, both by themselves and with others, and participate in occasional religious retreats.

So the issue is not whether the mystic goes to a formal church or professes any set doctrine. The critical point relates to what actually goes on—moment to moment—within that broad definition of religion developed above. In this we would fully agree with Andrew Greeley, a Catholic cleric whose Ph.D. degree is in sociology. Greeley concludes that the mystic becomes truly religious when he or she finally knows "the way things really are."[19] In Zen, this short phrase also describes the special knowing, that deepest *understanding*, which serves as a valid criterion for a person being "religious." "The way things really are" expresses the profound insight that Ultimate Reality, infused with the sacred, lives in the eternal here and now. (see chapter 132)

Albert Schweitzer was once struck by a similar insight. This deep "reverence for all life" went on to transform the way he lived and worked as a medical missionary in Africa. Schweitzer developed his own version of what a mystic was. The mystic, he suggested, was a person who did live among the temporal and earthly, yet who still belonged to the eternal and superearthly, having transcended any division between the two.[20] But semantic traps and assumptions lurk within such views. How do we *know* there is an "eternity?" What does "superearthly" really mean? Nor do the questions end there. Mysticism itself is wide-open to challenges on other grounds. Ontology will ask of it, What are the first principles of being, and how do they interrelate with the true nature of reality? Epistemology probes, How do we really come to know, and what limits do we place on that knowledge? Putting it another way, are mystical experiences "merely subjective?" Or are they accurate intuitions that reveal our deepest, basic existential nature? Only in the latter case would the experiences be valid windows into an "ultimate reality" in the absolute objective sense. No one settles such issues in print.

Meanwhile, the reader becomes aware of a vital omission: Whatever happened to God in such questions? Greeley suggests that the mystical experience does not necessarily imply any special divine intervention.[21] No God takes over, so to speak, when the subject becomes a passive witness within the experience. Instead, Greeley concludes that what does take over are "deep powers in the human personality, normally latent." These are the powers which "produce in us experiences of knowledge and insight that are simply not available in daily life."

The Judeo-Christian form of monotheism sets its overarching deity up on high. Ruth Fuller Sasaki describes the Zen Buddhist approach to the universal highest principle as coming from another direction.

> Zen holds that there is no god outside the universe that created it and created man. God—if I may borrow that word for a moment—the universe and man are one indivisible existence, one total whole. Only THIS—is. Anything and everything that appears to us as an individual entity or phenomenon, whether it be a planet or an atom, a mouse or a man, is but a temporary manifestation of THIS in form; every activity that takes place, whether it be birth or death, loving or eating breakfast, it is but a temporary manifestation of THIS in activity. Each one of us is but a cell, as it were, in the body of the Great Self. [Having come into being, this cell] performs its functions, and passes away, transformed into another manifestation.[22]

Put simply, the insight of Zen beholds this "Great Self," not God.

If so, then where does the experience of this Great Self come from? The premise of this book is that it must come from the brain, because the brain is the organ of the mind. The same perspective holds whether mystical or peak experiences arise spontaneously, are cultivated, or are drug-induced. Our thesis is that prior meditative training and daily life practice help release basic, preexisting neurophysiological functions. This thesis will lead to the following proposition: mystical experiences arise when normal functions reassemble in novel conjunctions.

From such a vantage point the brain comes first, its mental phenomena come second. R. W. Sperry is one articulate proponent of this kind of "top-down" perspective.[23] His sound opinions developed in the context of his Nobel prize–winning research on animals and patients whose hemispheres were divided, leaving them with what came to be called a split brain. Sperry takes over the interface between science and religion at the points where James left off. He begins his own thesis on an optimistic note. He believes that the neurosciences have already rejected reductionism and mechanistic determinism on the one side, and dualisms on the other. As a result, he finds that the way is now clear "for a rational approach to the theory and prescription of values and to a natural fusion of science and religion."

To reach his conclusions, Sperry does more than avoid those dualisms that would regard the brain and the mind as two separate entities. He also rejects pure physicalism. Why? Because it holds to the unacceptable thesis that "all higher level interactions, including those of the brain, are presumed to be reducible and accountable, in principle, in terms of the ultimate fundamental forces of physics." Many others besides Sperry have already found fault with similar physical and materialist determinisms. How does it help us to know only about quarks, molecules, or the brain's high water content? Quantum theory alone doesn't allow us to predict the way they all come together to enable a brain to function as the organ of the mind.

Instead, Sperry holds that our brain functions in ways that go beyond the elemental forces of physics. In a very real sense, we have personal quirks which go beyond our quarks. Such a view implies that our whole brain develops new properties, *emergent properties*. They are properties generated only by *interactions* within the larger system as a whole, not by the acts of any small single constituent. Emergent properties are always much more than the sum of their parts. Take the novel emergent properties of H_2O, for example. We could never imagine that water is a liquid if we knew only the properties of its two constituent gases, hydrogen and oxygen.

Moreover, at its higher physiological levels of emergent processing, our brain also develops remarkable new *causal* properties. These are higher-level properties which can operate in top-down fashion. They *cause things to change* at lower physico-chemical and physiological levels. Whether such properties emerge consciously or subconsciously, they act to transform events downstream, shaping our value systems and the ways we behave.

Sperry's thesis then expands on this general principle of "downward causation." From this vantage point, he then presents his alternative view of the way things really are. It means simply "that higher properties in any entity, whether a society or a molecule, invariably impose [their causal control] over the lower properties of their infrastructure." He conceives these higher entities as being "causal realities in their own right." Therefore, they too will never be determined completely by the causal properties of their components, or by the laws which govern their interactions, or by the random events of quantum mechanics. So what modern neuroscience finally reveals to Sperry is a different kind of hierarchical universe centered on the brain. It is one "controlled by a rich profusion of qualitatively diverse emergent powers that become increasingly complex and competent."

In the last two parts of this book, we discuss how our brain functions come together to create our sense of time and to shape such emergent qualities as eternity, meaning, being, and knowing. Meanwhile, it is necessary to begin by asking much more naive questions. In part IV, for example, we ask, What is ordinary consciousness? Once we better understand what constitutes the ordinary, then we will find that the so-called mystical experiences become less of a bewildering hodgepodge.

5

Western Perspectives on Mystical Experiences

> The mystical experience is a *natural* form of knowledge in the sense that one need postulate no special intervention of the deity to explain it. Nevertheless, in the mystic experience, the person makes *contact* with the Way Things Are.
>
> Andrew Greeley[1]

Experiencing things as they really are? Yes, this is the central fact of enlightenment: "awakening" to the unity pervading all things. But such profound insights are only one of many alternative states of consciousness. Representative examples of the varieties, and there are many, are found in the writings of James,[2] Underhill,[3] Johnson,[4] and Bucke,[5] among others. Taken as a whole, they are confusing. And, as if religious and philosophical speculations hadn't muddied the waters enough, our own language and traditions soon confuse us with ambiguities and misinformation. So, before we of the West try to come to grips with reports about the "Eastern" varieties of religious experiences, we had better take stock of our own confusions, get our own bearings.

Who in the West are those rare beings who "get" religious or mystical experiences? They number in the millions. They are men and women of all ages from all walks of life, educational levels, and religious backgrounds. In Gallup's 1977–78 survey, 31% of the adult population acknowledged having a sudden or dramatic religious or mystical experience at some time in their lives.[6] The largest single category was "an other-worldly kind of union with a Divine Being." It carried with it "the conviction of the forgiveness of sin and salvation." In Greeley's survey, between 33% and 43% of persons over the age of twenty reported having a mystical experience. It conformed to the definition of "being very close to a powerful spiritual force that seemed to lift you outside of yourself."[7]

Maslow, finding fewer people who did *not* have peak experiences, finally began to use the term "non-peakers."[8] He was not referring to persons *unable* to have peak experiences, but to those so afraid of mentioning the experiences that they suppressed, denied, or forgot them.

In Great Britain, of 1865 persons surveyed, 35% answered yes when asked the following delightfully open-ended question designed by Sir Alister Hardy: Had they ever been "aware of, or influenced by, a presence of power" different from their everyday *selves*, whether or not this was referred to as God? Moreover, the percentage was even higher among the more educated, of whom as many as 56% answered yes.[9] Clearly, we are considering experiences that are not only of great moment but ones that affect a sizeable (if sometimes silent) minority: perhaps a third of the general population.

Must the experiences occur in church, or in a formal meditative context? No. In Wilson's survey, the experiences occurred spontaneously in 31%, not prompted by any formal religious context.[10] In Greeley's survey, 45% were prompted by exposure to the beauties of nature.[7]

Demographic surveys depend heavily on language, and language is a slippery issue when assessing mystical experiences. Bourque and Back, in the course of 1553 interviews, noted that certain people used religious code words to describe their experiences, whereas others used an aesthetic language code.[11] What influenced the choice of code? It was the person's setting and social situation. Subjects who reported "religious" experiences (32%) tended to have them in relation to a church service, to prayer, religious conversion, or when their own life, or that of someone else, was threatened. These subjects tended to report having only a single experience. And if they did have more than one experience, the subsequent ones were considered to be "similar." Various fundamentalist Protestant denominations were heavily represented in this sample.

In contrast, other subjects had experiences which did not arise within a formal religious setting. They were triggered by a heightened appreciation of beauty or by aesthetic qualities. Accordingly, this second group of subjects used the aesthetic language code. They tended to have different kinds of "triggers," to have more than one experience, and to consider that each one was different. Still other subjects (22%) had both kinds of experiences, religious and aesthetic, but each on separate occasions. Interestingly, aesthetic experiences *alone* caused little subsequent change in either their religious orientation or interpersonal relations, nor did it enrich their lives. Who, then, tended to have experiences which did transform them? It was the group of subjects who had *repeated* experiences, *both* aesthetic and religious, and who reported that each one differed from the others.

So mystical experiences come in all sizes and depths. Let's begin near the shallow end. Here the word *epiphany* has come into common usage. Epiphanies now tend to mean lesser peak experiences, hillocks, so to speak. This can be confusing, because Epiphany also refers to the day on which Christians celebrate several events in the life of Jesus. One of the roots of this tradition goes back to earlier centuries. Then the Eastern Orthodox Church interpreted epiphany in relation to the revelation which occurred at the time Jesus was being baptized in the river Jordan. He was then about thirty years old, and was praying while he was being baptized. At that moment, according to the story in the fourth chapter of the New Testament, the heavens seemed to open and he heard the words, "Thou art my beloved son; in thee I am well pleased." It would be in the fullness of this manifestation of divinity that Jesus then entered the wilderness. There he fasted for forty days and was tempted by the devil. Something else must have happened during this period. For afterward, when he returned to Galilee to begin his ministry, his words bore a new authority, and he spoke in the "power of the Spirit."

James Joyce called popular attention to some of the lesser epiphanies. One resembles a strong aesthetic response. It occurs when perception grasps the intrinsic essence of something in the "luminous silent stasis of aesthetic pleasure."[12] It is worth noting that when such an "aesthetic arrest" reaches major proportions, it will lack the impulse to possess, to analyze, or to reject the object of its attention.

A mystical experience also evolves. Its time scale can extend from fractions of a second, to seconds or minutes, rarely to hours. Here, we draw attention to what one might call the "march of mystical experience." Many descriptions do not address this key point. A mishmash of reported experiences results. In fact, major episodes tend to unfold in a sequence which includes at least four different categories of experience. The subject's personal history contributes interpretations increasingly to the last three.[13,14]

1. *Raw experience.* These first features are not thought about, they *happen.* They are theologically neutral, and lie far outside any of the person's prior beliefs, expectations, or intentions.

2. *Reflexive interpretations.* These are original interpretations which the person formulates spontaneously either during the experience itself or immediately after.

3. *Incorporated interpretations.* These contain references to features of the experience influenced by that particular person's prior beliefs, expectations, and intentions.

4. *Retrospective interpretations.* These contain references to religious or other doctrinal-type interpretations not formulated until much later, after the experience ends.

We will return, in part VII, to a personal version of these four categories. But first, I need to declare my biases on another matter. The question is, Does everyone have the same kind(s) of mystical experience, per se? Do the reports differ only because people describe them differently? The literature supplies three types of answers.[14]

1. All mystical experiences are, indeed, the same. Moreover, they are all described the same way, irrespective of their cultural or religious setting. This is not so.
2. All mystical experiences are the same, but the reports about each experience are culture-bound. This is also not so; the early raw data of experiences do differ.
3. All mystical experience falls into a relatively small class of *subtypes.* These cut across all cultural boundaries. Whereas the several subtypes are not culture-bound, the language used to describe them *is* culture bound. I hold this interpretation.

Outside observers, each with different biases, certainly differ in the way they try to squeeze someone else's experience into each of the earlier four categories. Most would agree that after the initial raw data impacts, the rest of the experience can be shaped by that particular person's previous history, expectations, and religious background.

Alan Watts noted that devout orthodox believers have so automatically associated the imagery of a lifetime of icons with their emotions that these symbols then seem to lie at the core of their mystical experiences.[15] How might this occur? During religious worship, one draws repeatedly on such earlier images. Soon, these take the form of relatively state-specific associations which will be linked to subliminal memory traces. Loose threads of such linkages could then be woven into the fabric of a fresh major religious experience.

The world has an array of doctrines—ample proof that people in diverse cultures interpret their religions differently. Yet it is important to realize that different methods of meditation give rise to other variables. Zen emphasizes the training of attention and bare awareness, and it encourages its adherents to practice infusing them into everyday life. Certain types of Zen meditation encourage an "emptying of the mind," or a "no-mind" approach. Experientially, this appears to leave the brain *relatively* more "empty." The meditator feels relieved, free not only from the pollution of buzzing thoughts but also from the burden of their heavy emotional commitment. The cumulative effects of a major unburdening could begin to influence even the raw data of the later mystical experience.

For example, there is the critical matter of *self.* In the two subtypes of Zen states we will consider later, the self becomes increasingly absent from the scene all during the first raw data phase of the experience. The self begins to dissolve first during deep absorptions. Finally, it totally vanishes in kensho. This lack of self creates an extraordinary perspective, and it has far-reaching consequences.

The more the roots of self are absent from the first phase on, the more does the resulting *im*personality influence the interpretations that enter during later phases of the experience.

Listen to a cat or a horse sneeze. One can identify with what the animal is doing. Yet, different people sneeze differently. Moreover, the same person will muffle the sneeze when it must conform to the existing social setting. Still, the core of our sneeze reflex closely resembles that of other animals, and it also draws on *several* physiological levels of our nervous system.

In this paragraph above, we are drawing closer to Zen than you might think. Why? Because similar considerations apply to other *innate* kinds of experience. It means no disrespect to draw this kind of analogy when discussing mystical and religious experiences. We may value these moments more, but in one sense, they are nothing special. They are not necessarily any more elevated, or rarified, than a sneeze. So it will be from this brain-biased perspective that we would now preview, in two sentences, why we think peak moments will occur in a Zen meditative context. It is that they *happen*. And when they do happen, it is not because the person held any pure doctrinal beliefs or previous conceptualizations, but because prior meditation and daily life practice had already opened up a few physiological intervals in the brain, and that these crevices happen to have become wider than usual.

We will be applying the term *extraordinary states* to the psychophysiological events which then surge up through the fissures into consciousness. We will define none of these states as arcane or exotic. They are innate, existing brain functions, rearranged into new configurations. Their raw data anticipate all words, doctrines, and sacred texts, all theological, philosophical, and neurological interpretations.

To each person the peak moments are intimate, private. But suppose one looks at their major topographical features within a meditative context, and from the vantage point that spans decades. A series of themes then tends to unfold. These themes fall into universal categories. Moreover, their sequences also reflect how far along the aspirant has come in meditative training. Laski emphasized that many such experiences are not at all consistent with the person's prior dogmatic beliefs. It was her position that the mystical experiences of persons in earlier centuries had given rise to dogma, not that each person's current experience had been derived from that dogma.[16]

This is partly true. The first part seems more true of subjects whose intense approaches to religion had been inspired by the revelations of the early prophets. The statement less accurately describes the subtler Zen traditions. *These try to evade dogma at the outset.* Zen *de*emphasizes momentary isolated experiences, and is very wary about how they are to be viewed.[17] It prefers instead to address the way the person then goes on to live each day on a moment-to-moment basis.

Some authors try to draw a line between a numinous experience and a mystical experience in general.[17] As noted before, a numinous experience is enveloped by a sense of the holy. Its sacred quality seems to come wholly from *outside* the person, say from God.[18] This point of view sets up, by way of contrast, a second group of subjects who conclude that their mystical experience was not bestowed from without, but that it happened either spontaneously, or arose out of *their* own efforts, or was referred to the cosmos, or to nature.

So it is not easy to characterize *the* mystical experience. Indeed, several Western authors have now compiled lists of criteria in their attempts to do so. Their lists are useful for general reference purposes, and for one other reason. For the "mystical" lists presented here will *not* be the same as those lists, to be cited subsequently, which were drawn up by authors who were citing the features of "alternate states of consciousness" (see part IV).

Let us begin with William James's original list of four characteristics.[2] First he listed *ineffability*, followed by *noetic quality, transiency,* and *passivity*. What is ineffability? Is it a valid criterion?

Ineffability means inexpressibility. It means that the experience resists being described in ordinary language. This difficulty stems from at least five factors: (1) Specific communication problems exist. These stand in the way of transferring the raw data and the quality of perception out from an extraordinary state back into the levels of language readily at hand in our other ordinary states. (2) Words have their own limitations. They prevent us from satisfactorily communicating deeply felt emotions not only to others but to ourselves as well. We learn this as an empirical fact. Remember how it was to be deeply, brim-overflowing in love, and to have tried to communicate this to the other person? (3) Suppose the person uses metaphors to try to bridge the gap. Metaphors have too many other meanings, which soon mislead and confuse the listener. (4) The elements that coexist are too paradoxical. It seems embarrassing to mention their bizarre nature to unsympathetic listeners. (5) The experience overcomes the subject with its abrupt onset, speed, and complexity. This makes it difficult accurately to describe to another person everything that did happen, and harder still to find a conceptual framework which will fit it.

Kaufmann was wary of James's three other criteria. He argued that noetic quality, transiency, and passivity are not specific for a mystical experience. He observed that they are also attributes of ordinary, purely sensory experiences. These too yield knowledge, do not last, and can overcome a passive recipient with their flood of sensory data.[18]

This objection is only partly true. The definition we will be using for *insight-wisdom* is wordless comprehension of the most profound significance. It strikes in a way completely different from our ordinary sensate-based knowledge. Indeed James's word *noetic* already implies the presence of this special, extraordinary kind of cognition. Where does ordinary cognition stop? To understand, let us begin with the usual dictionary definitions of the term. Cognition traces its origins to the Latin *cognoscere*, to know. Cognition then becomes definable in terms of those thoughtful mental operations which lead us to "know" all about an apple, for example, and to be able to employ logic to explain why it differs from a pear. When we use reasoning to try to *explain* such distinctions, we begin to appreciate not only what such a thoughtful process "feels" like but also how very slowly it seems to move.

James knew this. He wished to emphasize something different. When he placed together the two words "noetic quality," he wanted to make clear three striking experiential facts: (1) *Profound insight strikes directly.* (2) *On contact, vast quantities of complex information are communicated.* (3) *But no intervening thoughts complete the transfer.* So his words "noetic quality" imply the impact of a novel kind of thoughtless comprehension. It happens automatically. It is much faster than our usual reasoning, and more complex than our usual intuitive skills.

Deikman compiled another list[19] containing the following major characteristics of mystical experiences:

1. Realness

2. Unusual percepts

3. Experience of unity

4. Ineffability

5. Cosmic insight

Deikman added another important distinction when he noted that the experiences could be shallower or deeper.[20] Often, a shallow experience was linked with the more familiar forms of sensate experience. It presented ideational material which the person could organize later into more conventional concepts. Shallower experiences drew on recognizable emotions. In contrast, deeper experiences had less of a sensate quality. Their insights struck in the form of a compelling wisdom. Having penetrated further into the depths of the affective realm, they also resonated in ways that seemed more extraordinary in retrospect.

Laski, in 1968, reported the results of an early survey of over fifty friends and acquaintances.[16] Their experiences fell into two different categories. In one category, her subjects lost their normal perceptions. These she called "*withdrawal* experiences." "Withdrawal" implied that a sensate *subtraction* was involved, not an accumulation. Withdrawal experiences took place more slowly. As they evolved, they might also carry the impression of an *outflowing* into something larger, or indeed infinitely large, in association with darkness. This category of experiences will be referred to, using the term "absorptions." (see part IV; table 10, columns VI-A and VI-B).

Her second category was called "*intensity* experiences." They were brief, and were frequently prompted by triggers which involved objects, events, or ideas. They might be associated with words suggesting feelings of upward thrust or of positive movement upward. Afterward, during an extended "afterglow," the experience was interpreted and appreciated. "Normal" faculties and perceptions then gradually returned.

Her intensity experiences included three separate subtypes:

1. *Adamic experiences.* These involved feelings of joyful purification, of renewal of life, and of loving kindness to all. While the world might seem transformed, the self was still not lost. She chose the term "adamic," because it reflected Adam's total happiness and innocence before the Fall.

2. *Knowledge-contact experiences.* Knowledge entered through some new "contact." The contact came either from sources within, from an undefinable source,

or from without. Laski believed that only her most creative or intellectual subjects had adamic or knowledge-contact experiences.

3. *Union experiences.* These were the most highly valued. They were characterized by feelings of union with something else, or with someone else. They conveyed the feeling, which came afterward, that this contact had been total.

Laski's subjects placed an extra, subjective gloss of interpretation on their intensity experiences. William James had earlier used the term "overbelief" to describe this same phenomenon. It implied that the person believed more than the evidence warranted. Laski's subjects frequently capitalized their words. It was an index of the degree of their extrarational ontological overbeliefs. So, earlier, had Aldous Huxley when he used terms like "Absolute Enlightenment."

Laski chose to lump together all these several varieties of experience. She used the general term, "ecstasy."[16] But the word ecstasy usually implies an exalted state, one charged with intense *emotion* and beyond the person's usual abilities to control. So when she started her questions with, "Do you know a sensation of transcendent ecstasy?," it may have introduced certain of her own observer biases into her subjects' reports. Words aside, she clearly separated experiences of sensate withdrawal from those others which might lead to higher forms of insight-knowledge. She also remained aware that the latter forms might sometimes begin with a degree of withdrawal experience.

In Laski's survey, which general features were distinctive of both types of experiences? Her final summary included the following:

1. Triggering events occurred.
2. Some things were lost. They included such things as distinctions, desires, self, time, place, etc.
3. Some things were gained. These included the sense of unity, release, new knowledge etc.
4. Quasi-physical feelings occurred: a penetrating warmth; an almost painful joy.
5. Other feelings occurred consistent with intensity or withdrawal. Intensity was like the building up to a climax; withdrawal was a kind of merging into the experience.

Greeley later drew on a more representative national sample.[7] He presented his survey population of 1467 Americans with several descriptive phrases. He then asked his subjects to decide, from memory, how closely each of his "descriptors" actually fit their own much earlier experiences. The phrases illustrate the premises of his study. It suffices to begin by listing the five leading phrases that were most often responded to, followed by the percentage of the 513 responding subjects who recalled that they had undergone one or more of such experiences.

1. A feeling of deep and profound peace (55 percent)
2. A certainty that all things would work out for the good (48 percent)

3. A sense of my own need to contribute to others (43 percent)

4. A conviction that love is at the center of everything (43 percent)

5. A sense of joy and laughter (43 percent)

Many readers may wonder at this point: don't these five phrases seem too tame to describe *major* complex experiences? Indeed, could they have been drawn from the "shallower" end of the spectrum, say from Laski's subtype of adamic experiences?

Parenthetically, Maslow had already commented elsewhere on somewhat similar experiences. He preferred to designate them as "plateau" experiences. To Maslow, plateau experiences were moments when a person underwent serene, contemplative cognitions of intrinsic values. These were still near the cognitive end of the spectrum, for they remained more voluntary and were also less intense than a major peak experience. They were epitomized by a mother sitting quietly and marveling at the way her baby is playing.[21] Feelings of *deep peace and joy* are indeed prominent in such experiences. However, there is no major sensate loss, nor is there a true loss of self. For these reasons, and because many of these episodes do seem to form a separate cluster, we will be referring to them later under a separate descriptive heading. They will be designated as the *state of heightened emotionalized awareness without sensate loss* (see part IV; table 10, column V).

Now, did some of Greeley's subjects report deeper experiences? Depth certainly seems to increase as we now examine items which occurred less frequently in his list.[7] Soon, phrases appear which take on the flavor of insight-wisdom. Eight of these major descriptors are as follows: an experience of great emotional intensity (38 percent); a great increase in my understanding and knowledge (32 percent); a sense of the unity of everything and my own part in it (29 percent); a sense of a new life or of living in a new world (27 percent); a confidence in my own personal survival (27 percent); a feeling that I could not possibly describe what was happening to me (26 percent); the sense that all the universe is alive (25 percent); the sensation that my personality has been taken over by something much more powerful than I (24 percent).

But wait. What about the phrase "confidence in my own personal survival"? If the subject's self *were* being preserved, this would seem to be an unlikely description of a major peak experience, because—as Zen makes clear—the experience of awakening wipes out the egocentric self. So why did this phrase draw so many responses? Perhaps because Greeley's subjects found that it described the *after*effects of their experience. That is, a major awakening does leave the person feeling more competent in the world. It is a world which now seems much better and less threatening. In support of this interpretation, Greeley's analysis suggested that those who expressed "confidence in their personal survival" tended to have a higher level of "psychological well-being." They also tended to be the subjects who had deeper experiences, states marked by such earlier "classical," Jamesian-type elements as passivity, ineffability, a sense of new life, and of being "bathed in light."

How long does a mystical experience last? Estimates vary widely. So widely that most of the variation would seem to depend on how much of the "afterglow" the person regards as an integral feature. In Greeley's survey, 37 percent estimated that they lasted only a few minutes or less; 13 percent estimated ten or fifteen minutes, and 6 percent estimated half an hour. But 5 percent estimated the duration to be as long as one hour, 9 percent several hours, 21 percent a day or more, and 8 percent gave no answer.[7]

Greeley's data led him to an important conclusion: "There are lots of mystics around, more than anyone ever thought. They are happy people who apparently had happy childhoods. They are neither prejudiced nor maladjusted nor narcotized. They claim to have had contact with the Ultimate, and it does not seem to have hurt them. On the contrary, it seems to have helped."[22]

Maslow, too, had gone out of his way to make a similar "explicit" statement. He found no unusual occupations among those of his subjects who lived at the level of "Being" and who had peak or plateau experiences. They could be businessmen, industrialists, managers, or educators. They were not only the professionally religious, or the artistic and intellectual types whom society might presuppose would be prone to have mystical experiences.[23]

Gimello defined a mystical experience as a state of mind, one commonly achieved through some sort of self-cultivation.[17] He believed it usually included the following features:

1. A feeling of oneness or unity, variously defined.
2. A strong confidence in the reality or objectivity of the experience; a conviction that it somehow reveals "the truth."
3. Ineffability
4. An unconventional, qualitatively different mode of intellectual perception. During it, conventional intellectual operations are suspended or substituted for.
5. A paradoxical sense that opposites, of various kinds, coincide.
6. An extraordinarily strong affective tone. This might include various kinds of emotion which coincided in unusual combinations, such as sublime joy along with utter serenity.

A recent survey suggests that as many as 9% of subjects are *not sure* whether they ever had a peak experience.[24] Kaufmann takes the point of view of such persons. After an episode of some kind, looking back, they will ask themselves: *was* this, or was this *not* a mystical experience?[18] If all four of the following *post hoc* criteria were satisfied, then the person will usually decide that it was:

1. The experience must seem to have been a sharp break with everyday perception.
2. It is valued at a much higher level than is everyday perception.
3. The person finds no single explanation for it in terms of his or her ordinary state of sleepiness, state of fasting, fever, or fervent prayer. If ordinary explanations sufficed, the person might decide this was not a "real" mystical experience, and that would be it.

4. The person does find some objective correlative or source for the experience, either within nature as a whole, or beyond nature.

While a few subjects may reject their experiences following Kaufmann's criteria, most people *overvalue* their extraordinary experiences. The Zen master counters this tendency. He supports the student, but invests the experience with as few words as possible, and moves on. Following his example, the Zen aspirant learns to regard mystical experiences not as places of arrival but as points of departure.

The lists above are not complete. It is useful to enumerate several other characteristics, because we will find later that each of them have physiological implications:

1. Occasionally, a subtle sense of anticipation may occur, a vague prelude usually lasting minutes rather than hours.

2. Experiences do not repeat themselves in exactly the same way. Over a period of years, the same person may have several experiences, even within the same general subtype. These are not stereotyped. They vary qualitatively, unlike most seizures.

3. In general, experiences, even within the same subtype, tend to evolve toward deeper insights, especially during prolonged training in a monastic tradition.

4. Subtypes occasionally become juxtaposed and slide into one another. These create unusual mixtures, difficult to classify. Psychedelic drugs enhance this tendency, as do overzealous, pressured meditative techniques.

5. Some extraordinary experiences cause an immediate behavioral change in the person. A trained observer, such as a Zen master, readily appreciates the transformation. However, these immediate physiological changes tend to wear off over the next several hours or days.

6. Few of the so-called peak experiences reported by subjects polled at random yield major transformations that will last long enough to change their lives. As few as 1 to 4 percent of such subjects undergo major changes.[24]

7. However, when experiences are repeated, they are more likely to bring about an enduring change.[7,11]

8. Details of a major experience are not lost. They can be clearly recalled. But *the person does lose certain other things:* the older, dysfunctional attributes of the personality. This particular pattern—a new psychological profile which contains *both* preservation and loss—is quite unusual. It excludes the operation of the more familiar kinds of memory disturbances. Indeed, these preferentially wipe out our most recent memory functions, not our oldest ones.

Gradually, the Western world has come to appreciate that mystical experiences serve several practical functions: (1) They tend to resolve anxieties at various levels and to promote a physiological sense of well-being. (2) They help to actualize potential abilities. (3) To the degree that others have similar experiences, they contribute to the social bond within a group. (4) They prompt people to become directed toward other values and goals beyond themselves, to reevaluate the way they view this everyday world, the universe at large, and their place within it. (5) They stimulate scientists of many kinds to try to explain them. In the process of doing so, we develop a better understanding of the mechanisms underlying both ordinary as well as extraordinary states of consciousness.

Given this overview of Western perspectives on mystical experiences, we will soon, in part II, be in a better position to clarify how the seemingly casual system of Zen training could contribute to their development.

6

Is Mysticism a Kind of Schizophrenia in Disguise?

> All power of fancy over reason is a degree of insanity.
> Samuel Johnson (1709–1784)[1]

True, the chapter title may seem to have put the question too bluntly. But laypersons and professionals will become concerned when Harry or Jane develops hallucinations and delusional preoccupations about religion. Yes, a few otherwise normal persons do forge useful insights during intense periods of psychic crisis, and they can go on later to adapt and to mature. But still other disturbed individuals descend into what William James called a *"diabolical* mysticism, a sort of religious mysticism turned upside down."[2] In these subjects, the religiosity is unstable, takes a delusional course, and leads downhill.

James held no illusions about either of these trends. He considered that both the classic religious mysticisms and their "diabolical" counterparts came from the same mental level: from that large "subliminal" region where "seraph and snake" abided side by side. And so it was that he warned, with regard to the usual "religious" experiences: "To come from thence is no infallible credential. What comes must be sifted and tested, and run the gauntlet of confrontation with the total context of experience, just like what comes from the outer world of sense."[2]

So let us now begin to do this sifting. For in the process we will find useful contrasts which illuminate both the nature of the mystical path and of its schizophrenic opposite. For example, the conditions called schizophrenia affect about 1% of the population. Early in their psychosis, certain schizophrenic patients develop a heightened sense of themselves, of others, and of the world. In paranoid schizophrenia, self-consciousness can reach such extreme levels that the patient takes every stimulus to be self-referable and of personal significance. But is this what occurs during the objective vision of insight-wisdom? No. True, perception also finds stimuli from the outside world resonating with meaning. Yet at the same time, insight has bleached them of every last personal connotation.

Some patients with schizophrenia, overcome by their enhanced perceptions and emotions, believe they have divined the ultimate essence of things. Some will conclude that such experiences happen *to* them. Others perceive that their experiences seem to be taking place along a kind of vibrant living membrane which used to be the interface between self and other, but which now has become highly porous in both directions.

Table 2
Comparisons between the Mystical Path and Schizophrenic Reactions

	Mystical Path	Schizophrenic Psychosis
General nature and duration	An ongoing, more orderly development	May be compressed, disorderly, and disorganized
Hallucinatory phenomena	In general, more visual; not threatening	In general, more auditory; can be threatening
Ideas of self-reference	Enlightenment cuts off the personal connotations of stimuli	Stimuli generate ideas of self reference, especially in paranoid schizophrenia
A gap is experienced which splits outer social reality from inner personal reality	1	3
Inhabiting only the inner world and being fearful of it	0–1	3
Degree of tolerance for inner experiences	Trained for and well-tolerated	May be overwhelmed by them
Simplification of lifestyle and renunciation of worldliness	More under conscious control	More under unconscious control
Dissolution of social attachments	1	3
Reentry into society, improved by the experience	The usual goal	Less common
Subsequent ongoing, fruitful, well-integrated contacts with society	2	1 or 0
Sense of unity with the environment	2 (partially cultivated)	Less commonly perceived
Driving by cravings and aversions	Reduced	May be enhanced
Continued conscious control	Usual	Less effective

0 = none; 5 = maximal

Nearing such an interface, we must sift with care. For William James noted that ostensibly normal people also generate similar phenomena during their religious conversions.[3] He emphasized that revelation is accompanied by a deep harmonious sense of assurance, and by perceptions which assign the appearance of newness to the external world. But such insights do not always lead to an adaptive outcome. Nor are persons truly "born-again" until they integrate their higher plateau of values into their previous personality structures. Only then does the final result become an ongoing one, realistic and capable of being projected into the future. In these respects, as in the others cited in table 2, the maladaptive psychotic patient will again differ strikingly from the healthy mystic. The psychotic patient tends to have "positive symptoms" such as hallucinations and delusions. Other, "negative symptoms" include a withdrawal, in which motivation is dissolved to the point of apathy (table 2).

Nonsense frequently occurs in the ancient form of Zen dialogue called *mondo* (see chapter 26). And at first glance, you might think that some of these historical dialogues in Zen resemble the way schizophrenic patients talk nowadays.[4] Why? Because in schizophrenia, many sentences are also ungoverned by convention. To clarify the differences, it helps to ask, Why is schizophrenic language so inappropriate and irrelevant? Among the theories are the following: (1) Perhaps their language is in the form of a code. In this case the verbal nonsense conforms to the underlying code, and does not mean absolute nonsense. (2) Perhaps the meaning of schizophrenic language lies in its incomprehensibility. The speaker may be trying to discourage the listener. (3) Certain words within language are especially vulnerable. In fact, particular words become pun-prone because they have multiple meanings which open up paths for many free associations. It may be relevant to note that the Chinese and Japanese languages do have many words with multiple meanings. This might have made it easier for Oriental speech to branch out into free-floating realms of polysymbolism.

So for perhaps multiple reasons, the speech of schizophrenic patients is full of loose abstractions. It is also obstructed by roadblocks, called "blocking." In contrast, classic Zen speech uses the simple, direct words of immediate experience. These express its sense of freedom and spontaneity (see chapter 48).

Recent research suggests that schizophrenia is an organic disease. It may reflect either a kind of fetal arrest of brain development, a delayed maturation, or a premature degeneration. Abnormalities of structure are common in the temporal lobe, limbic system, and frontal lobe.[5] In the early stages of schizophrenia, when the disease is less severe, some patients already show smaller temporal lobes. Other patients, more severely affected, may show enlarged fluid-filled cerebral ventricles.[6] Among identical twins, the twin who develops schizophrenia tends to have smaller hippocampi and a larger third ventricle centered in the hypothalamus.[7] One possible result of such structural lesions is that they could subtly disconnect, and derange, those circuits which carry messages back and forth between the limbic system, the hypothalamus, and the prefrontal cortex.

Although the brain waves may be asymmetrical, it is not clear how this electroencephalographic (EEG) finding relates to the schizophrenic disorder[8] (see chapter 20). It is more likely that schizophrenic symptoms represent an imbalance among various neurotransmitters than that they are caused by a simple "dopamine overactivity" (see chapter 44). True, many antipsychotic drugs acutely block the second type of dopamine receptors. Yet, when given chronically, these same drugs *enhance* dopamine metabolism in the frontal cortex.[9] Moreover, many of the current generation of antipsychotic drugs also have the ability to antagonize the effects of serotonin at its third type of receptors. Normally, these ST_3 receptors inhibit the firing of the next nerve cells. And among these cells which could be inhibited by their ST_3 receptors are those intrinsic to the medial prefrontal cortex.[10]

Enhanced perceptions are an early symptom in schizophrenia, a symptom consistent with the mental hyperactivity of someone in a state of hyperarousal. To Fischer, the similarities suggested the hypothesis of an arousal continuum. It was one in which he would place our conventional everyday "I" near the *midpoint* of an arc which represented an arousal scale.[11] Off at the lowest end of the scale, the person would be in the *hypo*arousal state exemplified by yogic samadhi, and would proceed next toward the relaxed meditative tranquility of zazen. Theoretically, as arousal then kept increasing, and passed beyond its normal midpoint at "I," the subject would then become increasingly activated both cognitively and behaviorally. Fisher proposed that such sequences proceeded first through periods of sensitivity, creativity, and then anxiety. Next on the ascending scale came the successive extensions of hyperarousal that were said to represent acute schizophrenia and catatonia. Finally, at the most extreme, *hyper*aroused end of this activity scale came the ecstasy which occurred in mystical rapture.

Fischer also ventured to explain why we usually perceive our outside world as being separate from ourselves. His hypothesis began with the arguable premise that usually our cortical interpretive states went on functioning more or less independently of those derived from our subcortical activities. Suppose, on the other hand, a person moved off in *either* direction, to the right or left, along the arousal spectrum cited above. Then, he speculated, the two activities—cortical *and* subcortical—would tend to come closer together and become more integrated. As the person proceeded farther out, toward *either* end of the arousal spectrum, the two processes would tend to merge. Thus, in Fischer's view, if one were to move off either beyond mystical rapture at the high end, or beyond yogic samadhi at the low end, one would finally come into contact with one and the same larger, universal reality.

It is open to question whether such maps and hypotheses are valid. Is it legitimate to position schizophrenia and catatonia on any scale, and to fit them somewhere between anxiety and the ecstasy of mystical rapture? And there are sound practical reasons why clinicians must have firmer criteria than this. For they must decide, *yes* or *no*, Am I dealing with the early religiosity of the truly schizophrenic patient? Or are these only the religious impulses of a normal person who is wandering a bit more than usual along the mystical path? Table 2 goes on to emphasize some of these important empirical distinctions. For example, when normal people are on the mystical path they develop more conscious control and learn how to tolerate their inner experience. They also become increasingly free from both cravings and aversions, and integrate their mystical experiences more successfully than do schizophrenics.[12]

The "arousal scale" hypothesis tends to sow confusion for several reasons. It could seem to imply that all zazen is the same, and that zazen and yogic samadhi belong near each other, paired off toward one *hypo*aroused end of some spectrum opposite from ecstasy. It glosses over the fact that heightened periods of awareness also occur within zazen. It also tends to invite another misconception. It suggests that a subject might proceed, in stepwise increments, to develop each of the several categories of states above, simply by turning up the amplitude on a continuum of arousal per se. In humans, arousal is but one of many relevant ongoing brain functions, not the sole driving mechanism.

Still, the hypothesis offers a useful point of departure for the different theses to be developed herein. For we are going to propose that (a) alternate states differ qualitatively, and very substantially, in the ways in which each of their many physiological aggregates falls into place; (b) when these do come together, it will be in a novel fashion, one in which many other functions also drop out; (c) a blanket distinction between cortical and subcortical events does not allow one to separate either ordinary states or extraordinary states into neat categories; (d) no arousal curve remains smooth and unbroken. It has open segments, transition periods.

These are pivotal moments of change; and (e) the particular states in which deep *insights* occur are key transforming aspects of the mystical path. These insightful states are relatively far removed—both semantically, physiologically, and temporally—from those other categories of states which we usually think of when we use such words as rapture, samadhi, schizophrenia, and ecstasy.

Will it come as a surprise to find that the first step proposed in our thesis is to take a serious look at the issue of self?

7

The Semantics of Self

> The central problem of understanding states of consciousness is understanding who or what experiences the state. Our theories evolve with the center missing; mainly the "I," the Witnesser.
>
> Arthur Deikman[1]

For centuries, Zen training has been transforming the maladaptive self. Some changes occur in rare dramatic moments. Others, equally impressive, evolve slowly, incrementally. But what could cause a growing brain to develop a dysfunctional self in the first place? And by what means could it later become constructively transformed? In several following sections we will be asking, Which words stand in the way of our understanding? How does one go about constructing a self? What are its unfruitful aspects? Finally, in part II we consider how the meditative dynamic fruitfully restructures the self.

Obviously, a self must exist. What else could make us consciously aware of events arising outside or within us, of factual knowledge, and of the way we act within the external world? Turn to the dictionary definitions of consciousness, and they will all refer back to that core of *self* in the center. Never do the definitions acknowledge a striking fact: some extraordinary forms of consciousness retain no subjective *I* inside them. Still they are witnessed. Dictionaries use the term *experient* to stand for the person who undergoes an experience. Herein, we will employ a variant spelling, whose sole purpose is to alert the reader to a key distinction. Let *experiant*—now spelled with an *a*—serve to convey whatever still goes on experiencing when this usual personal self is *absent*.

Yet, the very notion of an experiant invites disbelief. How could any brain modify its awareness so remarkably that it leaves no subjective *I* inside which does the attending? We struggle to comprehend. Meanwhile, common sense dictates both our premise and our biased conclusion: if someone who aspires is to be called an aspirant, then behind any experience must be some kind of egocentric experiant; something still in there having it, attending to it, and being the source responsible for it. Accordingly, we in the West adhere to Jung's interpretation: "If there is no ego, there is nobody to be conscious of anything. The ego is therefore indispensable to the conscious process . . . I cannot imagine a conscious mental state that does not relate to a subject, that is, to an ego."[2] Many familiar words like *ego* and *id* have now become a part of our doctrinaire Western psychological interpretations of self. Accepted uncritically, they leave us unprepared semantically to understand the dynamics both of ordinary everyday states of consciousness and of various extraordinary kinds of Zen experience. Let us now examine a small series of troublesome words, starting with *ego* and *id*.

Freud's notion of the ego served a useful purpose. Lending further support to it were the two other abstract domains which he built nearby. They formed the interlocking, complementary triad: superego, id, and ego. They are so interdependent that it would be perilous to try to extract or modify any of them. To Freud, the three were not mere conceptual abstractions—they were personality constructs based on the anatomy of the brain.[3] The *superego*, for example, was a "genuine structural entity." Functioning as an overall observer, the superego acted as the keeper of our conscience. It was the upholder of societal ideals, and seemed the least ambiguous of the three. Why? Because it took on and acted out all the familiar, straightforward roles of our parental authorities.

Borrowing the word *id* from Nietzsche, via Groddeck, Freud regarded it as the repository of the passionate instincts. Therefore, to Freud, the id held to no laws of logic. It lived with sharp contradictions, had no concept of time, and did not deal in negations. "Naturally, the id knows no values, no good and evil, no morality . . . Instinctual cathexes seeking discharge—that, in our view, is all that the id contains."

Finally, then, to Freud, the *ego* was the pragmatic executor. It was the agency needed to strike a workaday balance between the other two. "In popular language, we may say that the ego stands for reason and circumspection, while the id stands for the untamed passions."[4] The ego, modified from the id, organized our behavior along rationally effective lines. It drew on hard-won lessons of personal experience, constantly reminding the id: the real world has consequences. Freud viewed the ego, in a sense, as a rider who guided a horse, not yet tamed, toward a destination.

But later, in common parlance, the term ego came to imply something quite different. Then it was diluted to imply only the *selfish* pejorative self. It referred to someone we didn't like, someone who we said had an "inflated ego" and was "egocentric." Unfortunately, the word ego then came to have two quite different meanings. This situation is a barrier to our understanding Zen. For Zen strengthens the first, weakens the second.

Can Zen be in two places at the same time? Zen regards the ego as holding to its original meaning. The term still refers to each person's capacity to deal confidently with life in a mature, realistic, matter-of-fact way. *The I that Zen diminishes is not the pragmatic ego.* If Zen were to remove such an ego, it would leave its adherents in a helpless "identity crisis."[5] Rather, Zen training aims to strengthen the ego in its original Freudian sense.

This means that Zen training is targeted at the other, negative, distorted self: the selfish I. Note that this selfish self was not something that Freud attributed to the ego portion of his original triad. Instead, it would have been derived from the id-ridden self and would be driven by its ignorant, passionate instinctual desires and aversions. So *it is this selfish self* that Zen trainees first need to define, identify, and then work through. Not in ways that crush or deny their essential natural selves, but in ways that will simultaneously encourage the flow of their basic ethical, compassionate impulses.

Long before Freud put forth his theories about the id, Taoists and early Buddhists had developed an original "big picture." It was a perspective that, to the reader, may now begin to sound vaguely familiar. All around and interpenetrating us, said their teachings, was a natural open domain. Surprisingly, it unfolded into full view only when the person's natural self awakened. It, too, was governed by no laws of logic except its own. It, too, encompassed every possible sharp contradiction. Indeed, it knew neither good nor evil. It was even outside time. It had no function. It existed in its suchness or thusness. It was. It was so universal that it went far beyond the ken of earthlings. We could only guess about it within the limitations set by our newly acquired systems of human values and factual knowledge. Moreover, even when someone did "awaken" to the presence of this Ultimate Reality, it was not a very special event. It meant merely that he or she had reestablished the original connectedness with what had always been present anyway.

No, said Freud. This was not reality. It was *un*reality. Still, he acknowledged that mysticism had anticipated some of his own formulations. He admitted that "certain practices of mystics" could enable the "perceptual system . . . to grasp relations in the deeper layers in the ego and in the id which would otherwise be inaccessible to it." But, no person could grasp these deep relationships, he stated, unless their mystical practices (which he downgraded) had first upset "the normal relations between the different regions of the mind." Freud doubted that such abnormal procedures could ever put that person "in possession of ultimate truths, from which all good will flow." Yet, he continued, "All the same, we must admit that the therapeutic efforts of psychoanalysis have chosen much the same method of approach. For their object is to strengthen the ego, to make it more independent of the superego, to widen its field of vision, and so to extend its organization that it can take over new portions of the id. Where id was, there shall ego be. It is like reclamation work, like the draining of the Zuider Zee."[3]

Freud's psychoanalytical goals, if not his methods, came closer to Zen than is sometimes appreciated. Indeed, long before Freud, Zen training methods also encouraged the practical self to mature, to shed its excess psychic baggage and widen its field of vision. The training also helped to reclaim the passions from inappropriate conditioning, and to do so in a way that would rechannel their energies along other lines. To understand how such complex processes might unfold, we need to find a fresh conceptual framework. If it is to be a useful model, it should begin by returning us to our simpler origins, to the way our infant brains first built up our notion of self.

Is our society ready, today, to become familiar with some basic landmarks and vital functions of the young and growing human brain? Can we appreciate its functional anatomy as eagerly as we look forward to seeing the faces and hearing about the dysfunctions of the latest media personalities?

8

Constructing Our Self

> The person is a conglomerate of independently functioning mental systems that in the main reflect nonverbal processing systems in the brain.
>
> Michael Gazzaniga[1]

Listen in on the playground. Children are heard arguing. One boy says; "Oh yeah? Who says so?" The second, jaw thrust forward, asserts: "Me, myself, and I." Consider these three words. His language hints at the way each of us had built up our "self." Way back then, we might have uttered such words in a different order, but these are close enough.

We erected our self slowly, using nerve cells and circuits as building blocks. First we linked them at deeper subcortical levels, then at superficial cortical levels. They were almost Tinkertoy configurations, and it would take us years to assemble all of them. Now, each of our adult selves resides inside immense, distributed nerve networks. Together they code for a sensate physical body, feel visceral imperatives, think and know and act in this world, remembering the past and projecting it into an imaginary tomorrow.

It all happened slowly, but in a sequence of steps. We can glimpse part of the way the story unfolds by selecting some visible milestones early in development. Early on, when our outer brain layer, the cortex, finally begins to convolute, it declares its strong bias toward vision. In the fetus, the visual cortex in the *back* of the brain wrinkles first. Thereafter, it favors those visual pathways that lead up to it. The particular nerve fibers leading to the visual cortex will be the first ones that a three-month-old infant brain covers over with white layers of fatty insulation.

Only at eight months does the infant white matter mature farther forward in that central region between the parietal and frontal lobes (see figure 2). Not until one year of age will the myelin sheaths be mature in the white matter of the temporal lobes.[2] At that time, our proud parents may well praise us by saying we are a "big" one-year-old. Yet our brain still remains immature. Why can't it express more than the bare framework of our final personal identity? Because it still lacks the personal. And therefore, it can't yet possess things personally.

But wait until around eighteen months! Now the long subcortical association pathways finally link all our lobes together. Finally we start to make the vital elementary distinctions. Now we can distinguish between "me" and "you," between self and other. This enables lines to be drawn in no uncertain terms. At this point we firmly stake our claim to each possession: "Mine!" Its vigor is unmistakable.

Around this time our mental sets also develop other hard edges. We resist violently if asked suddenly to change our routine. It is as though we had been asked to climb up, or jump from, a sheer precipice. Parents know this as "negativism," but it seems to have more the flavor of self-preservation rather than of aggression.[3] Now that we are adults, could we learn to modify our rigid responses, become even more flexible?

Sometime between fifteen and twenty-four months of age we act self-consciously. Place the viewing child in front of a mirror and she or he will recognize that a dab of rouge on the nose is an imperfection of self.[4] The blemish obviously mars the expected image. *Whose* image? Revealed in such behavior is a person who by now has developed some kind of a larger "me" to be looked *at*. Moreover, an inner "I" has recognized that some dreadful "bad" spot is spoiling "my" nose.

Comparable pronouns then find their way into that complex behavior we call language. The words enter in a cluster around the start of the "terrible two's." The order in which they enter is informative. First comes "mine," "me," "you." Then "I."[3] Also around age two, we start projecting our own mental states *outward*, imputing them to other persons. Suppose mother pretends to be distressed. We will reach out to console her with budding empathy.[4] Yet we still won't have gone on to establish a firm sense of our own identity—of ourself as a presence which continues—until somewhere between six and nine years.[5] By the end of that first decade, most of the brain will have finally insulated over its bare wiring. It is now well insulated with myelin, fore and aft. Moreover, its messages are passing readily from one side to the other. They leap across the white bridge of the corpus callosum at their peak physiological efficiency in ways that unify the verbal and nonverbal capacities of our two hemispheres.[6]

What constitutes this personal imperative dwelling deep inside us, this insistent self whom we slowly become aware of as children? William James noted that this private self began with a physical nucleus. It arose from sensations referred from our head and throat. Surrounding them was a vague layer of the thoughts that originated in our central person and were referable back to it. Superimposed next were "self-feelings." These ranged from the heights of self-esteem to the most personal depths of despair. Linked with such emotions were our instinctive behaviors: self-seeking and self-preservation.[7] Did some outer boundary enclose our "inside" physical, mental, and psychic self? If so, it seemed to be our skin. "Other" began outside our skin. "Other" was everything external to us. As children, we had set up the barrier: self/other. It would prove to be a very thick barrier. Conceptually much thicker than our skin.

The barrier is still present. Even now, as adults, when you look at me and I look at you and we see the other person as "other," it is because we each perpetuate that ancient boundary on the surface of our own skin.[8] Meanwhile, a third person on the scene sees us both as "other." Clearly then, this distinction between self and other has some *relative* aspects to it. It is not something absolute, but rather an artificial, self-imposed mental construct.

Now then, suppose some fourth human observer arrives, one who happens to be graced with rare total, enlightened, universal awareness. This observer, *while still seeing different creatures,* goes beyond our fictional distinctions and now views all four of us as part of *one,* larger whole. No more thick skin barriers. After perspectives change, can experience itself change? Can starting with a different mental set really change experience?

You can demonstrate this to yourself at a far simpler level. Gently close your eyes. Then use one index finger to explore the skin of its counterpart. Start by moving the right finger, while letting the padded surface of the opposite index finger remain stationary. A sensation of shape arises. It is always referred to your *left* finger, the object. Your brain even projects this "fingerish" shape out to a nearby location in space. All the while, the skin of your right index finger seems to have become less sensitive when cast in its temporary role of being the active explorer. It develops merely the vague feeling of the formless rubbing process itself.[9]

Reverse, now, only the *role* of each finger. Let the skin areas rubbed together remain the same. This time, the left finger pad explores. Now, only the right finger takes shape. The whole perceptual experience "topples over" in the opposite direction. These two experiences cannot coexist. Perception switches from one set to the other as an either/or phenomenon. The brain came to a decision: one stationary finger is to be the *object*. It must therefore attend to it as an object, and will perceive it as a depersonalized "object," even though it was your very own, warm, attached finger.

Starting in childhood, other decisions made it obvious that our body contained some kind of a sensorimotor self. That is, we could feel our arm and see it in action when it stretched far off to grasp an apple out in this different world beyond our skin. But many other selves were not obvious; they were indeed invisible. Because, into each such extension, we were also thrusting and grasping with parts of our hidden conceptual and affective selves. Collectively, one may think of these as our various *psychic selves*. It is true that they go on acting covertly, but it would not be correct to regard their attachments as occult by any means. They are merely *incorporating* many notions sponsored by the rest of our corpus, our body.

What was the result? An elaborate possessive psychophysiology; a possessive self that went on to *incorporate* far more than we could ever imagine of the objects and people we've clutched, and of the emotional bonds and opinions we've attached to each of them. To some of these corporate selves, it will make a difference whether you are forced into handing over "your" apple to someone else, or offer it spontaneously as a gift expressing true compassion.

Another example, close to home, may help you to appreciate the psychic self. Suppose you and another teenager are now standing out on the sidewalk. You are both facing the same house. Imagine that, in your case, you have just returned here after a gap of five years. You are now looking at *your* home—at the very home where you grew up. On the other hand, you've just met the second teenager, and she had never lived in the house or seen it before. While standing there for several minutes, intimate reminiscences of your home start to fill your thoughts. But to this other teenager, it's just another house. She has no subjective ties to it. She sees it unsentimentally, objectively.

No child fortunate to grow up in one home can do so. We can't be impersonal, not when it's *our own* home. It grows on us, permeates us. Its elements become so near and dear they can make us homesick. Growing sentimental is an interactive physiological process. It is one in which we extend our personal self—building on countless memories and associations—not only into the rooms and people in our house, but out into every geographic detail of the yard and the neighborhood where we played with the other kids. All these become the stuff of our incorporating, possessive, reminiscencing selves. They become *my* house, *my* neighborhood! As William James noted, we extend this possessing "self" to include not only family and friends, but clothes, bank accounts, and other possessions.[7] So the infantile "mine" of eighteen months had now really grown up, though the true extent of its covert emotional bonds would remain largely invisible.

Let us now take stock of the Jamesian self to see what now makes up its core and layers. To do so is to be impressed. Already, this basic center of self contains (1) self-preservation behaviors; (2) sensations from the body, especially those from the head and throat; (3) thoughts and other possessions or recognitions; (4) self-feelings; and (5) instinctual self-seeking behaviors. Before the self can vanish, all this must drop out! Even so short a list defines a major psychophysiological agenda. *If, in a flash, an enlightened state of consciousness is to dissolve all such ties, it must extensively revise the way impulses usually flow in many circuits in the brain.* Where do these circuits lie? All over.

Toward a Psychophysiology of Self

Consider three simple examples of the issues that underlie our being "self-centered." Begin with a creature's first instinct, to preserve itself. Our survival imperatives arise from circuits hardwired into the stalk at the base of the brain, called the brain stem, (see figure 3), and from their extensions into the hypothalamus. Their survival functions are irresistible. If you're deeply submerged in water, running out of oxygen, these circuits will thrust you up to the surface, gasping for a lungful of air. Many of their instinctual drives and cravings seem almost as powerful as our basic need for oxygen.

Next comes defensive behavior. One major premise underlies it: a vulnerable creature must be protected. Is it really necessary to build a moat, battlements, or castle keep? Not unless there exists the threat that someone inside could be harmed, or their possessions stolen. To meet the threat, primates mobilize their defensive behaviors along an irregular perimeter that includes the central gray matter in the midbrain, the hypothalamus, and the amygdala (see figure 3; see also chapters 41, 43, and 52). These sites are like strongholds disposed along some archaic Maginot Line. None of our primal fears subside until their deep bunkers are vacated, neutralized, or bypassed.

Beyond self-preservation and defensive behaviors, the constructs of self become multilayered, emergent. Therefore, being self-centered is nothing to feel guilty about. It is everyone's lot, built in at many sentient levels that feed into the visceral core. Some of our self-centeredness began with that early strong neural bias toward the experience of seeing. When we spun around as a child, the world *did* move. Obviously, *we were the axis of a turning world.* Seeing it meant believing it.

And we have every reason to believe it still. Whenever our head and eyes move, the result is not a blur. Instead, the accessory optic system of the brain registers and adjusts instantly for the way each new visual image of the outside world keeps stimulating the retina.[10] Such hidden, automatic visual mechanisms reinforce our prevailing belief: we are definitely a physical self. Our vestibular apparatus complements this visual system. It sends us messages from the inner ear, telling us both about how we move and about the way gravity pulls on us. Normally, the above cues do more than stabilize the position of our head and eyes in space. We take them as proof that we exist.

So much of this early, unconscious, physical self-centering is first built up within our brain stem. The accessory optic system feeds into its highest level, the midbrain. The vestibular system directly informs the pons next below, while proprioceptive impulses from the head and neck muscles enter the brain stem at multiple levels. Finally, these hidden, axial elements of our sensate physical self begin to filter into consciousness, passing up through the midbrain,[11] thalamus, and cortex.

Here, higher up in the brain, other sensate messages code for increasingly subtle constructs of our physical self. To illustrate: certain nerve cells in the monkey's superior temporal region lie in wait to discharge their impulses. They are patterned to fire *only* when this monkey sees one particular external object, such as the head of another monkey. Moreover, these cells are also so highly selective that they will discharge *only* when this other head is being seen from a special perspective. It is that particular perspective which must refer back, for its line of sight, to the head of the *observing* monkey. So, these temporal nerve cells seem to have set up their own observing monkey's head as *the* "observation site" which serves as their standard point of reference for the construct of "other."[12]

At such higher levels, the brain will finally link many networks, synthesizing our notions of self into an "omniconnected anatomical structure." Within such resulting large distributed networks we finally integrate the facets of our sensorimotor self with those of our thinking, knowing, emotional, *psychic* self. Some have speculated that the brain represents these "selves" in a manner likened to that of a hologram, wherein separate bits of data distribute themselves throughout the whole image, and something of the whole image is contained in each bit as well.[13]

Who, as a child, escapes the limbic connections of their sensorimotor self? For shortly after that thorn prick is felt, and one's motoric self is seen to jerk the arm away, there occurs the wounded recollection that one has been stuck before. Now thorns become extra bad. And yet, this same "remembering self" was also capable of a stream of "good" memories. It could tap into pleasant autobiographical associations: the scent of roses or other memorable Proustian images, snapshots leaping out of the growing album of our personal history.[14]

Before long, we would have our well-developed—and often overused—capacity to label many things "good," or "bad." And some of these "bad" categories could hurt, almost like thorns.

As it matures, the front part of our brain brings a special executive focus into this self-oriented mixture.[15] Up in the frontal lobes, we begin to plan, to project, or to *restrain*, many of our body movements (see chapter 57; figure 2). Yet, among the many higher origins of one's omni-self, those coming from the crossroads of the temporal lobes are most intriguing (see chapter 56). Here, evolution would merge the functions of the old "smell brain" with those of both the larger limbic system and of the neocortex. And out of the resulting rich associative interplay would arise both instant recognition and deeper resonances of meaning.

It is within the temporal lobes that we match the tempo and pitch of primitive, internal bodily feelings against other messages coming in from the outside world. Here, we ask: Do their cadences correspond? Do the events jibe, or are they mismatched and out of phase? To "make sense" of such data, the temporal lobes must play various *interpretive* roles. This makes them especially suitable candidates for representing a crucial interface.[16] It is that common boundary between inner and outer. And it is at this interface, *where self meets other*, that events take place that will become vital to our understanding of Zen enlightenment (see chapter 142).

Yet the temporal lobes and their connections do more than erect thin conceptual barriers at this self/other interface. By merging both our recognition and affective functions, they help define each of us as a person who has very hard convictions. Indeed, our gut-level limbic emotions are poised, only one or more steps removed, to hyperpolarize each of our standard pairs of opposites. We have already mentioned two of the sets—those which constitute good or bad, self or other. Whatever additional sets of opposing issues we confront, including yes or no, we will soon address them from that private world which we have personally polarized into *yin* and *yang*.

Moreover, other novel functions emerge when we go on to link the temporal lobes with the rest of the brain. In these larger networks we begin to move well beyond the private constraints of our usual physical and psychic selves toward a larger domain of consciousness. Not that it is any better than the others, but it somehow seems qualified, as Williams points out, to draw the following conclusion: "'I am,' not simply as an isolated human organism but as a part of the whole population of surrounding events which are taking place at the time, and which have occurred in the past."[16] What constitutes this "I am," at such higher abstract levels? It is the larger, evolving consciousness that *we are part of the whole*. And yet it is only one of many facets of our self-awareness. As for the others, no Rosetta stone helps us translate from functional brain anatomy to those esoteric levels of cognition which allow us to look down our long interior hall of mirrors, and then believe it when we hear our thoughts murmur: "I am because I know."

This brief overview has suggested ways in which each young brain proceeds to construct its many-sided self. It will do so not in some psychological "epicenter," but by tapping into functions coded throughout many different physiological levels. How, then, could an edifice this vast disappear?

Later in this book, it will be clear that a knowledge of two major alternate states in particular can help resolve this question. Why? Because the person's constructions of self first drop off during deep absorptions (see part VI). And finally, they will be cut off completely during the flashing insights of awakening (see part VII).

But in these early chapters, it would be premature to venture theoretical answers to meet this challenging question. There are two major reasons why this is so. The first is that the brain is itself too complex, much too heterogeneous and interactive. So not until one approaches it in a comprehensive, interdisciplinary manner is it possible to advance even tentative explanations. The second reason stems from the fact that the investigators from our different tribal disciplines do not yet have a vocabulary which enables them to talk with one another using a common sign language. Misleading jargon stands in our way. Descriptive words are inadequate. It is time to return to simpler, basic words, those from cradle and playground.

9

Some ABCs of the I-Me-Mine

> To study the way of the Buddha is to study your own self. To study your own self is to forget yourself. To forget yourself is to have the objective world prevail in you.
>
> Master Dogen (1200–1253)[1]

> We have met the enemy, and it is us.
>
> Pogo[2]

Long before Pogo, Buddhism had also become very specific: our major problems and discontents arise from *within*. We start as fundamentally sound, and basically good. But in one sense, we become our own worst enemy. As soon as this notion gets personal, it becomes hard to accept. Notice how quickly people shift to the defensive whenever it is even hinted that their cherished personal self has caused some difficulty.

Reading this chapter may leave you, too, feeling uncomfortable. For our goal is to develop a seemingly naive system that describes some subtler aspects of this personal self.[3] Please do not think the system is too simple and childlike to apply to you. For this is not a new topic. Indeed, for many centuries the question Who am I? has been *the* central issue in Zen Buddhism. Obviously, we each have an explicit (but transient) physical self. To probe our sources of selfhood is not to ignore this basic fact. It is rather to define our sensitive *implicit* self in a way that comes to terms with its three different operational components. These three components themselves are not new. They are at least as old as each of us now is. We were just reintroduced to them at the start of the previous chapter. All we had to do was listen.

What we heard were older children who had been vocalizing them even before they started their terrible two's. Their operative words were *I*, *Me*, and *Mine*. In these three words lie clues as to how we constructed our invisible self. From here on, they are italicized with initial capitals. This is to emphasize how vital is their presence, and how telling is their absence. Following Pogo's lead, it serves our present purposes first to comment on their uncomfortable and unfruitful aspects. This could be misleading. For the point of Zen is not to crush or banish their powerful and "friendly" energies. It is to liberate, transform, and redirect them into their many other positive, constructive functions. The triad consists of the following:

1. The *I*. The *I* is. The *I* also acts. No one of us can appreciate how tall and strong our own *I is*. Nor can anyone know how threatening, say, the actions of the *I* might seem to others. But ask other persons. They know. They recognize our sovereign *I* instantly. They see it remain so proudly vertical that it never bows. They see it lean forward aggressively.

2. The *Me*. The *Me* reacts. Things happen *to* it. It is that part of the sentient self which, like any other object, is acted *upon*. Things can harm the *Me*. It is vulnerable. It can be harmed.

3. The *Mine*. The *Mine* possesses. Everything *I* possess is mine. It is the grasping self which clutches outward at material possessions or into other persons' lives. The *Mine* also has an inner turf. Inside, among its treasured intangibles, it holds tight to its cherished opinions and fixed habit patterns.

The three components interlock in a tight complex, each complementing the other. To keep the discussion simple, we may call this descriptive psychological construct the *I-Me-Mine*. No neuroanatomy or physiology textbook can localize all the nerve cells and circuitries which make up this emergent, widely distributed complex. But introspect for a long moment. Consider its premises, as outlined below in table 3. Then you may begin to appreciate the presence of a few of its negative and positive features in your everyday life experiences.

Further to clarify each aspect of the complex, let us expand upon the *I*. Usually, *I* is a noun. Then it stands for the person who at that particular moment imagines that he or she is a "self." Any dictionary contains so many attributes of the *I* that negative examples leap out even when we start to leaf randomly through the A's alone. How do they describe the pejorative *I*? In words such as *adamant, arbitrary, argumentative, arrogant*, and *autocratic*.

And it is virtually perfect, this *almighty I*. Can it ever, even rarely, fall into error? No. It makes excuses and shifts the blame. Always the fault must lie in unfortunate external circumstances, never in its own imperfections. Its vanity is constant. Observe how it monograms, grooms in the mirror, and polishes its self-image. It also gets indignant, which means that it is already so self-righteous that it can wax indignant. Highly personal biases determine its agenda. Attitudes filter what the *I* perceives, and distort what it then thinks is true. Some of these responses may begin to seem familiar.

But our *I* is not so simple. It carries many rigid masks in its repertoire. Each persona took many decades both to construct and to conceal. Where did we get the roles that our personas assume? They came not only from parents, siblings, friends, and teachers but increasingly from media personalities. Collectively, they

Table 3
Premises within the *I-Me-Mine*

I	*Me*	*Mine*
Exist physically. Feel. Am aware. Act. Know. Think. Personify roles.	Things happen *to* me, both physically and mentally.	All these thoughts and opinions, these body parts, are mine. These possessions are mine. Mine is the sole axis around which the rest of the world revolves.

now form the mosaic of our personal identity, our self-image. We shift our behavior from that of one role model to another depending on the situation.

For we also adopted the attitudes originating in each persona. These attitudes then shaped how each of our role model *I*'s *should* behave. The "good," most positive role models in the *I* are forever contending with their opposites, the "bad" personas, the shadow traits.[4] As a result, implicit in every *I* will be sharp contradictions, internal conflicts, and anxieties.

Next, the pronoun *Me*. It stands for our self as an object. What kinds of things can happen to the *Me*? Among the words in the B's, the dictionary includes *battered, besieged, blamed,* and *blushing.* So the *Me* suffers. It is *bothered* by all the "bad" events that must lurk in the jungle outside, things that go bump in the night. They threaten to harm, expose, or embarrass the *Me*. Mark Twain aptly exposed the *Me*'s tender underbelly when he observed: "Man is the only animal that blushes, or needs to." Moreover, the *Me* is also constantly on the receiving end of every self-inflicted, psychic wound that has been generated by the inappropriate activities of its two other partners, the *I* and the *Mine*. Hence, the more we hypertrophy these two partners the more they develop ways of coming back to embarrass or otherwise threaten the vulnerable *Me*. Beset by all its uncertainties, the *Me* likes to be praised, because flattery is comforting and feels "good" to it.

Finally, the adjective *Mine* stands for our grasping, greedy, possessive self. Even within the C's one can find many words that exemplify its negative attributes. The *Mine clutches*. But in every act of *clinging,* it winds up its own *captive.* It is self-indentured, because whatever is possessed also possesses. The more it grabs, the less satisfied it is, so it *covets* even more. Possessing more, it has more to lose. It will *cherish* the beauty of the outer physical self both in its mirror image and in the flesh. Inwardly, it *clasps* tightly to its pleasurable sensations, its thoughts and emotions.

Our *Mine* starts out in relatively simple fashion. It begins with the deceptive premise that there is a self/other split in perception. The simplicity is temporary. Because next, the *Mine* proceeds to enormously complicate its boundaries. As noted, it extends its invisible tentacles of self out through and beyond our skin. To the *Mine*, our skin surface is merely a porous envelope, never a barrier. Once in the outside world, the *Mine* attaches itself onto any other elements it desires. The large arrows in figure 1 illustrate, schematically, how the *Mine* thrusts in *two* directions; both in and out (figure 1).

The result is inevitable. Because the *Mine* becomes so tightly attached to things, anything it values must be defended. The cherished internal valuables include *my* biased thoughts and *my* strong opinions. Later on, they might also include *my over*valued spiritual insights. A *Mine* so easily threatened, fearing loss, leaves apprehension in its wake, and this psychic load shifts back and forth among the three partners.

Why do we remain so ignorant about the *Mine*? Because we never actually *see* its long insinuating arms. But they have the suction cups of an octopus, and the strength of their hold is beyond belief. Will the arms ever let go? Not until the flash of enlightenment cuts them off. Only then can the experiant appreciate

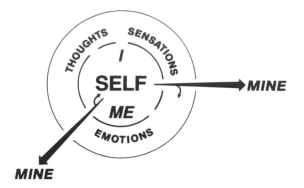

OUTER WORLD

Figure 1   The ordinary self/other world of the *I-Me-Mine*
A visual model for the way we construct the illusion of a self/other world. Our *I-Me-Mine* is a tightly knit triad. It consists of a complex of attributes which relate our sensate physical self to our thoughts and emotions. It includes a sovereign *I*, a vulnerable *Me*, and a possessive *Mine*. Note that the small, curved arrows of the *Mine* not only thrust out toward what we possess in the outer world. They also curve back to attach themselves to our several inner notions of selfhood.

how extensive were these arms and how intrusive was their grasp. Finally, at this moment, all the cut tentacles of the *Mine* lie exposed on either side, struck off by that cold, bloodless stroke of insight-wisdom.

Master Dogen was making a fundamental point in the quotation at the beginning of this chapter. Training in Zen boils down to studying the *self*. As a prelude to having it drop off. So the training begins with becoming intellectually aware that there is an *I-Me-Mine* complex, identifying its responses in one's everyday life, probing it and pruning it. But soon the real work must begin, that of redirecting its potential energies. And this means nothing less than abdicating the sovereign *I*, abandoning all the ramparts defending the *Me*, and abolishing each enslavement by the *Mine*.

No single flash of insight-wisdom accomplishes this. The *I-Me-Mine* had already set up its covert fantasy world and had gained its long head start when we were children. It is a triad expert at sabotage, camouflage, and denial. We underestimate both the vast circuitries dedicated to support it and the widespread problems they cause. As the *Hsin hsin ming* wryly understates it: "The Great Way is not difficult; just avoid picking and choosing."[5] Not difficult? Just try to eliminate one long-established habit! Try to surrender one firmly fortified opinion!

Beginners come to Zen no less innocent than do other novice monks and nuns come to their other monastic traditions. No one is aware how much their invisible *I-Me-Mine* fantasy world has monogrammed everything, and fitted it neatly into an airtight, subjective frame of reference. For the result seems like a plausible edifice. Yet it is as fictitious as was the old Ptolemaic concept of the astronomy of the universe. Back in the second century, such a concept had also seemed self-evident: we, on Earth, stood literally at the pivotal center of the whole world. Hence, as was taken for granted, every other planet, moon, and sun could only orbit around us.

Not until Copernicus (1473–1543) did we appreciate the true way our solar system exists. Finally, with the Sun placed at its center, the earth, moon, and planets fell into their correct relationships, rearranged *as they really were* and had been all along. Modern astronomy began when earthlings shifted into the Copernican way of looking at a heliocentric world. It wasn't easy. But it was the true, enlightened view. It finally enabled us to get beyond our egocentric-geocentric dogma, a doctrine which had once insisted that our two feet stood on private property, and were therefore always at the absolute center of everything. Now we could understand orbital realities from a valid universal perspective.

The paragraph above is a reasonably accurate analogy for the "awakening" spoken of in the meditative traditions. It arrives after a very long probing into the depths of space: the *inner* space of the subjective personal self. There, finally, when the shift occurs into full objectivity, it opens up into a new, enlightened paradigm, equally Copernican in scope.

After such awakenings, the italicized, initial uppercase personal pronouns of the old triad will never again be the same. Not gone entirely. Just reduced to a *lower profile* of manageable proportions, shrinking toward a smaller i-me-mine. Thereafter, these lowercase letters stand increasingly for someone whose basic energies are still being rechanneled through the same triad. Now, however, they emerge transformed, and function in salutary directions. These A-B-C attributes enable the person to become more *actualized, buoyant,* and *compassionate.*

As we move to the next chapter, our goal will be to address other misunderstandings and fears that arise about Zen practice. They center around the terms *narcissism, depersonalization,* and *derealization.*

10

The Zen Mirror: Beyond Narcissism and Depersonalization

> Human understanding is like an irregular mirror, which distorts and discolors the nature of things by mingling its own nature with it.
>
> Francis Bacon (1561–1626)[1]

> The wild geese do not intend to cast their reflection. The water has no mind to receive their message.
>
> Zenrin Kushu[2]

A mirror reflects. Water reflects the geese flying overhead. Instantly, unsentimentally. Reflection does not change the mirror, the water surface, or the geese. It is an optical process, a fact of life.

When waves no longer ripple the water's surface, it finally reflects the moon. Some day, some year, when the Zen aspirant finally drops into that same calm, unruffled state, the awesome lunar perspective will emerge (see chapter 138). As the brain instantly images reality, directly and clearly, it seems to act like the surface of a mirror. Zen frequently uses this analogy of the mirror to imply that one's perceptions register in the same way that still water accurately images the moon overhead. Nothing else enters in: no self-centered notions, no intellectual interpretations, no old emotionally loaded associations. So the reflecting mirror of Zen symbolizes the natural, immediate way the brain works preconsciously.

Thus, when Master Huai-hai (720–814) was asked, "What does right perception mean?," he would answer, "It means perceiving that there is nothing to perceive." But fortunately for all, the junior monk persisted, asking, "And what does that mean?," At this point, his Tang master finally became more explicit: "It means beholding all sorts of forms, but without being stained by them, because no thoughts of love or aversion arise in the mind."[3]

In contrast, we in the West find that our roots of the word *reflection* take a different turn. They mean a bending back. Francis Bacon understood that humans do bend and distort the true nature of things, discoloring them with our personal interpretations. Let us again specify precisely where these maladaptive distortions come from: it is from the *ignorant side* of our *I-Me-Mine* complex, not from its natural actualizing, buoyant, and compassionate functions.

Greek mythology gave us Narcissus. We still pay homage to him with every sidelong glance at our face in the mirror. And it would be another reflected face, also within our Western traditions, which would pose the rhetorical question, "Mirror, mirror on the wall, who is the fairest one of all?" The question seems to be the essence of *narcissism,* that value-laden word which suggests that the viewer is both neurotically absorbed in self and turned away from society. Some would say that when a meditator retreats into the posture of zazen it implies a similar inward turning, a mere preoccupation with what lies below one's own navel. So they ask: Don't meditative disciplines simply foster that other form of self-worship, the one already well-known under the term *narcissism?*

People who seem self-absorbed don't necessarily have a narcissistic personality disorder. A decisive question is, How do they see *other* persons? Healthy people see others existing as *separate* persons. In contrast, narcissistic people view others as only grandiose or devalued extensions of themselves.[4] By such criteria, narcissism represents one more example of that old inturned, Ptolemaic mode with which our *I-Me-Mine* bent the mirror and routinely distorted the image of other persons. True, Zen meditation does require plenty of self-discipline to escape from distractions and to make time for sitting. But does the whole process of Zen aim to magnify or adore the self? No; to dissolve its fictions.

So any notion that Zen might be narcissistic arises out of a profound misreading of both Zen and narcissism.[5] Zen meditative practice leads the person out of narcissism, not into it. For whatever reasons students begin Zen, their path thereafter is progressively humbling. Stunned by the way kensho's swift stroke has cut off all self-references, the residual diminutive i is doubly awestruck (a) by the enormity of what was lost, (b) by how much of it soon returns. Thereafter, the long meditative path leads increasingly outward, in the direction of selfless, compassionate service to others.

Another term, *depersonalization*, sounds more ominous. It describes the feeling that the near side has dropped out of the self/other boundary. In depersonalization, experience loses its usual, highly subjective, private affective content. In absorption and kensho the experiant also loses this inside, personal self-identity. If Zen sponsors such depersonalizations, doesn't this imply that Zen and depersonalizations are both pathological?

Depersonalization experiences occur spontaneously in many well-integrated normal subjects. The episodes last only a few seconds or minutes. Thirty-nine percent to 46 percent of college students reported having them in studies published during the 1960s. The same figure of 46 percent was also found in a study of exceptional high-school students.[6] Depersonalization episodes also occur nonspecifically in association with neuroses and psychoses, and with or without exposure to drugs or to loss of sleep.[7,8] Not unless they last longer, or are ongoing, are they classified as a "disorder" that falls among the dissociative disorders according to the latest *Diagnostic and Statistical Manual of Mental Disorders.*

In contrast, during *derealization*, the change takes place on the outside of the self/other boundary. On this instance, the environment is perceived to be unreal, estranged. Again, normal persons sometimes experience such brief feelings. Only when "everything" continues to feel like an ongoing "dream" is there cause for concern. Derealizations also lack specificity, and may even coincide with depersonalizations.

I vividly recall the only episode of derealization I ever had. I was seven or eight years old. My mother and I were walking downtown looking off to the right toward some dark, empty, store windows. Their panes were so angled that they converged with our path ahead. As a result, we saw ourselves walking in several reflections at once, each glass pane serving as a kind of large mirror. So here we were: walking in real life, shown to be walking in the image of one mirror pane, and also shown as walking in the reflection from another. A moment before, there had been only one, actual, "real-life," walking. Now I had two extra visual images, and they weren't congruous with my preexisting mental set. At this point, everything became highly unreal for a few seconds. I was troubled by the discrepancy, challenged by the deeper issues it raised. How "really real" *was* our ordinary life? How does one *know* which reality is the real one? The questioning still goes on.

People react differently when their perceptions of reality change on either side of the self/other boundary. Most normals who still preserve insight can adjust to an alteration of their inner or outer reality set. However, when depressed patients lose their warm sense of personal subjectivity, they feel that a profoundly unpleasant psychic gap has opened up. In their lack of feeling they perceive a worrisome distancing from other persons and things. It is a major loss.

Fortunately, the kinds of boundary changes that emerge from the meditative context are beneficially alloyed. Yes, the person's former implicit physical self does drop out in internal absorption. But the experiant is then taken up into the highly positive connotations of a vast, silent space suffused with bliss. Yes, during a major awakening, every last subjective root and branch is cut off. The Buddhist technical term for this is *annatta*, the state of non-*I*. But the event is not perceived as *loss*. It is perceived as being totally emancipated from every previous bond implicit in the *I-Me-Mine*. Moreover, this flash of insight brings the experiant into wordless contact with the sense of eternal Reality itself, in all its immanent perfection. So this event conveys the *finding* of true Realization, not its loss.

These other positive attributes bring to absorption and kensho a sense of awe and grace. They convey no uncomfortable sense of personal loss, no troubling sense of unreality. So the other two old psychological terms don't fit. Perhaps *im*personalization and *neo*realization might be closer to the mark. However worded, the two large categories of states we will encounter in Zen are certainly not "disorders" in any psychiatric sense. Very seldom does the experiant find these are unpleasant, either at the moment or in retrospect.

Japanese Zen imported its orthodox traditions of Chan from the mainland many centuries ago. Rigidities are built into its systems of ritual and custom. Such conservatism is not quick to respond with enthusiasm to the gamut of today's New-Age religions. But Zen's critics still go on accusing Zen of the same, age-old faults of narcissism, and worse. Ferguson rises eloquently to defend those in today's Aquarian cultures who have been similarly indicted. Yes, she replies, "Critics call them narcissistic, not knowing the thoughtful nature of their inward search; self-annihilating, not knowing the spaciousness of the Self they join; elitist, not knowing how desperately they want to share what they have seen; irrational, not realizing how much further their new world view goes toward resolving problems, how much more coherent it is with everyday experience."[9]

But Zen's critics seem undaunted. To them, Zen remains just one more obscure mystic way which leads into a series of fanciful delusions. Still, it is only fair to point out that Zen also cuts off other, major selfish illusions and delusions. These dysfunctions have consistently sabotaged those other salutary A-B-C attributes of our *I-Me-Mine* complex which can go on to create our better selves. Critics also claim Zen is radical nonsense, an attack on our hard-earned citadel of rationality. True, its assault is uncompromising. But its targets are again the old arrogant-vulnerable-indentured aspects of the *I-Me-Mine* complex. There, the method of Zen is to infiltrate ignorance and unreason, not to defeat rationality per se. Moreover, its usual assault does not need to be a frontal one, nor one which is ushered in with fanfare. Rather is its standard approach the silent one, acting through intuition and attrition.

Zen is patient. Indeed, as we bring out further in part II, it will be only very slowly that sitting meditation and mindful daily life practice disarticulate the *I-Me-Mine*. Only gradually does Zen training seem to infiltrate and whittle away at every nerve network which had trapped us inside our usual, ignorant fantasy world. One might visualize it as operating on each ignorant and deluded network using a long series of present participles, words which end in *-ing*. First, the training encourages a "loosening up," a process of easing. This dampens the brain's previous overdriven activities. Then, by slow erosive action, in brief quickenings, and in rare larger events, the approach becomes a process of "giving-up," of "letting go," of "opening up." In such ways does the training translate finally into processes that emerge as receptive, insightful, and transformative. These three processes enable adult brains to keep "growing up," and continuing to mature through longer intervals now called "passages." Some adult passages are no less impressive than the earlier phases we went through as children.

It does not suffice to prune only a few outwardly visible branches of the *I-Me-Mine* complex. Mere thoughts quickly regrow. What needs pulling out are all those deeper invisible side roots of longing and loathing. They mediate our strongest desires and aversions. They send out long covert extensions which invade—or recoil—at personal depths that we had never suspected were there. It then becomes apparent that something very curious and important is going on in Zen: its long-range training methods turn out to be remarkably selective and well-balanced. *What gets cut off are precisely those imaginings and emotional ties which have maladaptive overtones.* Therefore, it is no calamity to surrender the counterproductive aspects of the *I-Me-Mine*. The outcome is someone not less human, but more humane.

Beginners start off on the wrong foot. They reason as follows: I will *attain* enlightenment. I'll make a conscious commitment, by willing my "own" thought process. Invariably, they keep inserting their own *I* in there (for who else can do all the willing and the striving to "gain" enlightenment?). In fact, long months and years will pass—years of submitting, enduring, "letting go," accepting, and unlearning—before the aspirant realizes two astonishing facts. First, the world is, and always has been, right here to awaken to. Second, the moments of awakening arise *of themselves,* when the time is ripe. When nobody is around.

Nobody.

11

Where Does Zen Think It's Coming From?

Prior to the advent of brain, there was no *color* and no *sound* in the universe, nor was there any flavor or aroma and probably rather little sense and no feeling or emotion. Before brains the universe was also free of pain and anxiety.

Roger Sperry (1913–1994)[1]

Ah, if my brush could only catch
the faint
Scent of the white plum-blossoms
that I paint!

Shôha[2]

Brains brought pain and anxiety into the universe, along with other qualities. The Zen Buddhism we have been pointing toward throughout part I offers *teachings* about these matters. You don't have to believe them. Nor must you embrace doctrines that run counter to common sense. As novices continue their practice, they will discover on their own, the most effective way, how each experience validates the teachings. Successive awakenings then cut off each outmoded premise, whether it was rooted earlier in ignorance or in delusion. Thereafter, their old egocentric universe will never be the same.

Nervous systems arrived late on planet Earth. Only recently did the human brain evolve its many striking conscious properties. None of its convoluted sensibilities, and no part of any of the rest of the whole universe is extrinsic to the scope of Zen. So, in its larger universal context, Zen embraces all of life's natural dimensions. One of them is the sentient, experiential dimension.

Every brain still goes on informing its bearer about what it encounters in the everyday worlds of its personal experience.[3] There are at least four of these worlds, and they overlap. Start with the first, *perceptual* world. You might suppose that it would be the most familiar one. Yet, how rarely do we savor the miracle whereby impulses from our sense organs are transformed into the scent of plum blossoms, or into taste, sight, and touch! We feel the thrust of our second, *emotional*, realm. Its pulsing, visceral energies invade us with fear, love, desire, or anger. Next, using thoughts, ordinary mentation fumbles its way along in the third, *rational*, world. It uses the vehicle of language to help reason out what seems to be true. Less often do we catch—let alone hold on to—the glint of the fourth, complementary, world. It is our ordinary *intuitive* world. Its insights dart in, extracting and integrating knowledge otherwise hidden among countless networks within our brain.

Is there another dimension beyond all these—a fifth, *trans*personal world? The early masters thought so. Indeed, Huang-po believed that enlightenment was our open access into this "Universal Mind." Those less sure today may still find Siu's concept interesting.[3] He views this dimension as the universe of "sage" knowledge. No boundaries constrain this world. It extends infinitely beyond what a single brain can either imagine about itself or can project into nature. Instead, sage knowledge is intrinsic to *all* nature. It is nature's essence shared intimately by one and all. Some readers may be more comfortable thinking about this fifth dimension as a "Great Self," a kind of earthly Mother Nature projected on a cosmic scale. Still others use different words to describe it, such as Buddha Nature, or they conceive of it as the highest, universal principle.

Rational knowledge can bring us intellectually in tune with the facts of scientific mankind. And ordinary intuitive knowledge can then go a step further, so that we include in our scope the totality of mankind. But sage knowledge is the profound comprehension that all our atoms resonate in their oneness with all other forms of stardust everywhere in the universe.[3] Sage knowledge, then, is a kind of "self-articulation of the Ultimate Reality itself."[4] This is where Zen appears to be coming from. Within this fifth dimension, our levels of human awareness and those of the ontological unfolding of reality will correspond so intimately with each other, stage by stage, that they may be thought of as ultimately constituting one and the same process.

Zen training does in fact orient itself in this general direction. But Zen itself remains unadorned. Yes, it still encompasses all of the four earlier levels. But it will steer just as clear of all such abstract notions of "levels" as it does of every other entangling conceptualization. Negating itself, it withdraws before each step of the advancing intellect. Zen is more at home with "soft" things closest to poetry, with elusive scents of plum blossoms, with other experiential things that don't reduce well to numbers. Therefore, at first, it will seem far removed from our rigorous fields of science which are packed with coldly objective data and hair-splitting discriminations. On the other hand, when the Zen aspirant finally awakens in kensho, it will be to the coldest, clearest basic truths stripped of every soft personal sentimentality.

Yet, it is especially in such matters that Zen masters and orthodox neuroscientists tend to part company. Each group would prefer to hold fast to its own hard-won citizenship. In fact, each is trying to objectify experience. In practice, the two camps operate using the biases imposed by their own training. Each is hampered by the limitations imposed by their complex methods. Perhaps the most one might hope for is that neither group will go out of its way to avoid, to deny, or to suppress the other's field.

From its vantage point, Zen continues to invite us to look critically, objectively, into our sovereign, self-referent *I*. Slowly, we then discover the fictions that made it seem vulnerable. We find a self that had been indoctrinated by others, one currently assaulted by the senses, driven by emotions, beset by thought-forms, bound by long-fixed habit patterns of behavior. This discovery is more humbling than scary. Finally comes the major flash of insight. Only then, from the fresh new perspective of No-self, No-I, can sage wisdom spring.

Where is Zen going? Look for no well-intentioned but overemotional intrusions; no busybody mentality. Its province is the simple, deft, preventive measure. Its moves are the more effective low-profile actions. These anticipate future problems, and head them off. Forget about crusading impulses which must remake the world in one's own self-image. They are covert distortions of the creative process. Mature adults no longer need to carve their names into the bark of a living tree. First, let our self-indulgent, self-referent *I* drop out of the scene. *Then, in the long view of things, salutary behavior will flow freely along novel constructive lines.*

Meanwhile, newcomers approach Zen as if they were sitting down to sample an elegant, exotic, five-course meal. What could spoil such an otherwise splendid occasion? Only the attitudes that they bring with them. First, they try to translate each word on the menu into English, bringing a dictionary to the table. Then they strive to analyze each morsel of food solely in terms of the source of its unusual ingredients. Soon they wonder when the dessert will come, imagining how delicious it must be. And all along they worry about the size of the bill and the tip at the end.

Zen is the awareness of the whole setting, the simple tasting of each mouthful, and the enjoying of the company.

So far, we have begun by presenting some orthodox Zennist views about where Zen thinks it is coming from. But suppose we now ask, Where is Zen really coming from? Then we must do two things. First, get into the brain and repair our own ignorance. Second, strip off the heavy baggage of centuries of mystical, philosophical, and doctrinal speculations. So it will be to find out how the brain itself functions, both in meditation and in various specified states of consciousness, that we now turn in the next three parts.

Part II
Meditating

Yet, grace, if thou repent, thou
canst not lack, but who shall
give thee that grace to begin?

John Donne (1572–1631), *Holy Sonnets*

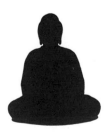

What Is Meditation?

It is like the pacification of turbulent waters by pouring oil over them: no waves are roaring, no foams are boiling, no splashes are spattering, but a smooth, glossy mirror of immense dimension, and it is in this perfect mirror of consciousness that myriads of reflections, as it were, come and go without ever disturbing its serenity.

Soyen Shaku[1]

A monk asked master Chi-Ch'en: "What is the way upward?" The master replied, "You will hit it by descending lower."

J. Wu[2]

When we were children, playing alongside railroad tracks, long freight trains of coal cars came thundering by a few feet away. It was too much. Every sense was assaulted. We were overcome by the earth trembling underfoot, by the noise and smoke, the flashing by of car after car. We learned to turn away, retreat, and cover our ears.

Meditation helps us retreat from all the wheels going around. It relieves us from self-inflicted trains of thought, trains driven by and loaded with the fossil fuel of ancient emotions. It returns us to the way we were, before the thundering trains came, back at play in the world, in that open, trackless landscape where life's distractions are less intrusive.

Zen meditation is a relaxed attentive state, a passive activity. Both aspects are important. So when Zen talks about "no mind," it does not mean complete mental blankness, as though one were asleep. It implies freedom from thought pollution. When the incessant chatter drops out, what remains are those few mental processes essential to the present moment. Nor does Zen meditation mean a voluntarily override of thoughts. Thoughts are as natural to the world as are clouds and trees. Rather does meditation pacify those pressures from the *I-Me-Mine* which drove the excesses of thought in the first place. Thoughts then drop off by themselves. As Shunryu Suzuki expressed it, "You yourself make the waves in your mind. If you leave your mind as it is, it will become calm."[3]

Sitting quietly for twenty minutes once or twice a day helps most people relax inside a kind of buffer zone. Within it, you begin to introspect and to get back in touch with the connections between your body and brain. But the recommended approach goes further than simple physical resting per se.[4] It means taking on a passive attitude and using a simple concentration device. This usually implies focusing on the breathing, or on repeating some simple word which is in keeping with the person's belief system.

Meditation then becomes several things other than a way to relax, physically and mentally. It becomes a way of not thinking, clearly, *and then of carrying this clear awareness into everyday living*. There, with senses enlivened, it sponsors an active, behavioral alternative to the statement, "Stop the world, I want to get off." Deeper levels of meditation also become the prelude that helps access still other states of extraordinary brain activity. If meditation has already clarified the brain and made it more receptive, personal growth is then more likely to occur after these states enter.

However, if meditation remains isolated from some larger religious context, it does not tend to provide the foundation for sustained spiritual growth. The Zen master provides the first, essential, supportive instruction in meditation. Both then and thereafter, he demonstrates by example his deep spiritual respect for the whole process. This respect is reinforced when the meditator practices in a group that shares the same authentic spirit.

Zen meditation is called *zazen*, from the Chinese, *tso-ch'an*. One enters into it with a seriousness of purpose befitting the posture which the Buddha himself used. Nor is it viewed casually as something in itself, as merely a means to an end. Instead, it is one vital part of a total training method. This training will gradually reshape brain and body, behavior and attitudes, consciousness itself.

The great Soto master Dogen said this about meditation centuries ago:

A quiet room is recommended for the practice of zazen, and food and drink are taken only in moderation. Free yourself from all attachments . . . think neither of good nor evil, and judge not right or wrong. Stop the operation of mind, of will, and of consciousness; bring to an end all desires, all concepts and judgements.

To sit in zazen, put down a thick pillow and on top of it add a second one. Thereafter, one may chose either a full– or half–cross-legged position. In the full (lotus) position, one places the right foot on the left thigh and the left foot on the right thigh. In the half (lotus) position, only the left foot is placed upon the right thigh. A robe and belt should be worn loosely, but in order. Next, the right hand rests on the left foot, while the back of the left hand rests in the palm of the right.

The two thumbs are placed end to end. The body must be maintained upright without inclining to either side or forward and backward. Ears and shoulders, nose and navel must be aligned. The tongue is kept against the palate, lips and teeth are firmly closed while the eyes are to be always opened. After the bodily position is in order, also regulate your breathing. If a thought arises, take note of it and then dismiss it. When you forget all attachments consistently, you will become zazen itself naturally. This is the art of zazen[5]

Before settling in, the meditator can loosen up by bending the trunk a few times to the right and left, moving the shoulders and trunk around. One initiates the tonic firmness of the trunk first by bending forward and thrusting the buttocks out in back, then slowly returning to the erect posture. Thereafter, the posture remains stable. The ears are back on a plane with the shoulders, and the nose is on a plane with the navel. Shoulders and arms hang naturally, the lower abdomen is released and everything above it is relaxed. This becomes possible because the lower trunk now provides most of the support for holding the body erect.[6]

So the zazen position is nothing mysterious. It sensibly distributes the body's weight evenly, using as its tripod the two knees and the base of the spine. The knees rest on a mat and the buttocks on a cushion. The head is held erect and the chin tucked in. Because muscles all along the spine keep it straight, the head then stays in line with the center of gravity. The mechanics of this erect posture are simplified, and one needs only the minimal amount of muscle tone to maintain it. The same erect posture tends to perpetuate itself after the sitting ends, contributing to the ongoing physical sensation that one is "centered." The relief of being "on-center" is well-known to every potter who starts with an eccentric lump of clay, every clothes washer who spins an off-balanced load.

The adept may come to view zazen as the universe expressing its own enlightened true nature. But the lay meditator struggles, for early practice is rigorous work, and hard on the legs. Formal Zen meditation periods vary in length, but they usually last between thirty and forty-five minutes, longer than the transcendental meditation (TM) sittings of twenty minutes. Attention lapses, the back and shoulders slump, the head droops, and one soon loses the appropriate physical and mental attitude. Meditation becomes boring.

Ken Wilber points out that the various approaches to spiritual practice each differ in their special conditions.[7] Zen's special condition involves sitting in zazen, becoming frustrated by it, discovering the sources of one's own resistances to it, and overcoming them. No pain, no gain. Indeed, it is in the very process of being frustrated that *one diagnoses oneself most clearly as the source of the resistances.* And also discovers ways to draw on one's inner resources against being distracted. Zazen's special conditions teach the body-brain in the most practical way, by the seat of one's pants. A nice, big, puffed-out cushion might seem ideal, but it cuts off the circulation to the legs; too thin a cushion offers little support. As in learning to follow the breath, and to place the hands comfortably, it takes many sittings before each person finds the golden mean. We are all built differently.

Last, but not least in these pages, we will discover that meditation is a vital probe for understanding how the brain works. But much sifting is required: one review of meditation cites close to one thousand articles[8]; the latest has a 124-page bibliography.[9] Indeed, my journey into zazen would turn out to be both an odyssey of professional enlightenment as well as one of self-discovery. It all began unexpectedly, in Kyoto, and in the following way . . .

13

Ryoko-in, Kyoto, 1974

> One thing is everything
> all things are One.
> If you know only this, then
> don't worry about attaining perfect knowledge.
>
> Master Seng-ts'an[1]

This summer, I have come to Kyoto on sabbatical leave. My project is to study the brain with my friend and colleague Professor Shuji Takaori. Shuji acquired his fluent English when he trained at the University of Michigan for his doctorate in neuropharmacology. His major research interest is the locus ceruleus. This fascinating group of nerve cells releases norepinephrine throughout the brain (see figure 9). The question we are asking seems straightforward: How does the cerebral cortex change when messages reach it from the locus ceruleus?[2]

My introduction to Zen begins as a happy accident, the way good things often do. My old friend and classmate in medical school Jock Cobb and his wife Holly, knowing we are leaving for Japan, have given me Herrigel's book, *Zen and the Art of Archery*. Now, living in Kyoto, it is easy to become immersed in its rich history and age-old expressions of Zen culture.

Kyoto is a place of beginnings. Lofty Mount Hiei looks down from afar at the front door of this small house where my wife and I now slip off our shoes and sleep inside on straw mats, Japanese style. High on Hiei's slopes, among the tall cedars, stands its ancient temple of Enryaku-ji. Here, the Tendai school of Buddhism had taken root after being transplanted from China. Three centuries later, near the end of the twelfth century, it would be the Tendai monk Eisai who came back to Kyoto to teach the more rigorous form of Chan Buddhism he had learned to practice in mainland China. And it was also on Mount Hiei that young Dogen was later ordained. After making his own pilgrimage to China, Dogen would return in 1227 to import the traditions of the Soto school of Chan into Japan. The Rinzai school of Buddhism went on to consolidate its influence in Kyoto in 1324. In that year, the monk Daito became the first abbot of its large new temple complex, called Daitoku-ji.

During these early centuries, Japan had no written language appropriate to greet the influx of Chinese culture. So the Japanese were obliged to write the word *Zen* (as they then pronounced *Chan*) in two of the imported Chinese characters (*kanji*).[3] The idiograph on the left conveyed meanings. Among them were some distant religious associations with the radiant well-being of spiritual power. The other character, on the right side, implied one only, and it suggested the way the word was to be pronounced.

Inspired by the cultural fabric of Kyoto, I have become even more curious to find out about this religious oneness. Why is it still so influential in Japan? A colleague, Dr. Yoshi Osumi, also a physician-investigator, has known other Americans who had received Zen training. They went to a small subtemple at this same Daitoku-ji, named Ryoko-in. He volunteers to telephone the temple and arranges for me to go there to meet its Zen master, Nanrei Kobori-roshi.

I had been stationed in Japan in 1950 and 1951 during the Korean episode. I had been impressed then by some of its larger Buddhist temples, in Kyoto, Nara, and Kamakura. Still, at Ryoko-in, I find myself unprepared for the tranquility that flows from the exquisite simplicity of its gardens and buildings. Nor am I prepared for the simple dignity, sophisticated interests, and conversational agility of the luminous, friendly man of steel who is its roshi. This is not the last time Zen will take me by surprise.

We meet on a typical sweltering hot July day. The roshi, head shaven, looking lean and fit, is enveloped by a thin white flowing garment. He smiles and is perfectly composed throughout the interview. He is not perspiring and does not otherwise appear to be affected by the heat. After bowings and greetings, we seat ourselves into low, comfortable wooden chairs. Our spacious antechamber looks out through open screens at a beautiful, simple Japanese garden. The distant buzz of locusts and the hum of other, nearby insects surrounds us. Soon I notice an interesting phenomenon. If a fly or mosquito enters the space around the roshi's face, a simple wave of his hand wafts it away, gently but effectively. He never blinks or turns his head to dodge the intruder. I am struck by this display of self-control. Even more impressive is its continuing success. His insects don't return. Mine do.

We quickly embark on a stimulating, free-flowing discussion for the next hour and a half. I take notes throughout the interview. In the following paragraphs, I directly quote, condense, or paraphrase the ways Kobori-roshi introduces me to Zen.

Early on, the roshi emphasizes that Zen is not a theology. It is a *living* system. It is oriented toward ego consciousness, not toward egocentricity. The sudden shift of consciousness that realizes this is called *prajna*. He defines prajna as the basic, central undivided knowledge-wisdom of enlightenment.

He notes that academic persons are driven by curiosity. They need to know about many things, to define them, and then to discriminate among them. In Zen, on the other hand, one simply accepts all things, taking a broad, compassionate interest in all of them. Be careful, he warns me. "Don't be confused by abstractions or by the word definition of an object or person. This is like confusing one's finger with the moon."

I miss the meaning, and ask him to explain. Pointing off into the air with his right index finger, he says, "Each language has a word for moon, but the word is not the *real* moon. The word is like a finger; it only points in the *direction* of the real moon. You should not mistake the one for the other." True reality, he continues, is not in the word. It is in the very object *itself*. Our human mind creates big problems. It always tends to take mental snapshots of real objects. "Remember," he says, "that all the words and all the concepts we invent are like snapshots. They are abstractions, not the *real* thing itself."

I speak about how my deepest sources of inspiration have come from time spent in the outdoors appreciating the workings of nature. Mountains were especially significant, whether looking up at them or enjoying the expansive view down from them. Zen, he observes, preserves that same "mountain view." It takes the natural view back and infuses it into daily life.

He then points to a piece of purple cloth nearby. "You can see that a rich purple dye was added. It made the fabric seem attractive. Zen is *not* like this. It is not some dye. It is not some new refinement that adds something esoteric from the outside. Zen is the return to the basic simplicity of the undyed fabric."

He then mentions that Zen training methods are strict and seems almost to be forewarning me. Do I know, he asks, why they are strict? I say no. "When the Zen master says NO!, this is the direct way he gradually conditions away years upon years of his students' unfruitful thinking and behavior."

By the end of this first interview I have formed several impressions. I very much like Kobori-roshi as a man. We interact well. I also sense he is telling me some unsettling things I really need to know. The first is that I, as a Westerner, have some basic attitudes that need changing. The second is that, because I am an academic person, Zen will be more difficult for me to grasp than it would be for someone else. Words will be especially troublesome. When we part, it is in a most friendly fashion, but he leaves no hint of an invitation to any subsequent meeting. From this, I am left to conclude that if there is ever to be any follow-up it will be entirely at my initiative.

I telephone the temple myself a week later, stumbling along in my newly acquired, halting Japanese. The roshi gives me a courteous, but formal reception. I feel like a foreigner, and it takes a concerted uphill conversational effort in English to make the next appointment a firm one.

This time, I arrive at Ryoko-in early. I pause inside to admire some simple pottery vases and teacups. I am fascinated to hear from the attendant that the roshi himself had made them, and that his brush had also turned out the striking, bold calligraphy hanging on the wall.

Our second interview takes place in another room of the subtemple. The roshi enters dressed in a light-brown, flowing garment. This time we are seated on cushions at a low table. Again, he is poised and comfortable; I must adjust my leg position frequently for comfort. (I thank him, silently, for having thoughtfully provided a chair the first time.) I begin by commenting on how effectively the design of the wall around the outside of Ryoko-in incorporates a series of very old roof tiles. He seems pleased that I have noticed. He mentions, in a self-effacing way, that he had designed it, preserving the aged tiles from former roofs in token of the way this temple's history had stretched back many centuries.

Buddhism itself goes back over two thousand years, he continues, and it expresses many cultures. Buddhism became associated with Taoism and Confucianism when it moved north from India into China. There it took on a distinctive Chinese character. During its early centuries in China, no separate Buddhist schools represented either the gradual awakening, which would be emphasized later in Soto Zen, or the immediate awakening stressed by Rinzai Zen. "Our way in this temple," he adds, "is to value both the gradual and the sudden types of enlightenment."

The Chinese preferred down-to-earth, tangible things. They never felt at home with the many abstractions of Indian theological thinking. "Take the question, What is truth? The Chinese answer is direct, concrete: 'That pine tree over there.' Zen respects what exists here and now. We don't chase abstract ideas or floating words."

Our conversation then comes to a long silent pause. I realize something basic. Much of my entire life consists in chasing abstractions. Each idea is linked to a whole set of other associations. How radically Zen departs from what I have known before!

Finally, in the silence, the roshi acts. He leans forward, and with one swift graceful movement sweeps up the small teacup from which he has been drinking. "This cup is 'round,'" he says. "Roundness is right here, in the cup in front of us. This roundness is not related to any distant concept of 'roundness,' nor is it to any other words we may have built up in our mind. Likewise, we may think that a Greek column is beautiful. But it, too, exists in the same way, in itself. It does so quite apart from us and from any architectural formulas that were used to design it."

Our discussion then meanders into the topic of creativity. He observes that creativity is a Western preoccupation, not an Eastern one. "Zen," he says, "doesn't try to add to nature. It doesn't try to create something new out of it. It is simply being at one with nature just as it already is." The early Chinese approach to nature had already taken the form of Taoism: the *Way*. But Westerners still have a hard time adopting the Taoist view of nature. First they must break out of their own language structure. This contrasts, he explains, with the culture and language of China and Japan. "Here, in the East, the free, personal self is already one with nature."

Indeed, the Japanese system of writing demonstrates this. "See how it expresses the word for nature." Here, he borrows my notebook, and draws the appropriate kanji symbols in it. "The word for nature is composed of two characters. The first of these also stands for 'self.' The second means 'being.' So the word, nature, already implies 'being itself.' It does so from the very first moment a child uses it." He then writes out the verb form, "to be free," using similar ideograms. Again the symbols represent not only self and nature but imply the way things exist in their essential selves. "From these examples of kanji characters you can see that the basic principle lies down deep in the very roots of comprehension itself. It is that all things exist in themselves, in *their* own, free natural state. They are their *own* manifestation. Not ours. They are free from any mental concepts that we humans have been conditioned to build around them.

"When you progress in Zen, you gradually shed your many abstractions, layer by layer. Each layer involves both language and psychological conditioning. You peel off many layers during meditation, which we call *zazen*. Then, when you go deeper into the meditative state, the process is not one of sleep or of unconsciousness. Instead, it is more of a kind of 'downing.'" Noticing my quizzical look, he then uses his whole hand to point far down toward the mat. "There are two aspects to this going down process," he continues. "One is psychological. In this state one becomes all clear and shining. Grateful. No doubts." Whereupon he pauses. His face lights up and his eyes close gently. After perhaps five seconds he tilts his head and continues. "Maybe in one sense it is a deepening; maybe in another it is like rising so far up in an airplane that you leave behind all the city's noise and smog. Then you are finally high up beyond all the clouds in the shining clear sky."

I grope for some analogy that might clarify this serenity from meditation which I have just witnessed in his face. I now know that the roshi is a potter. This same week, I made great progress in my own pottery lessons in night class. I *finally* centered my wobbly clay on the spinning pottery wheel. I venture this recent observation from personal experience. Is it like centering the clay?, I ask. He smiles and nods yes, that's the general idea.

"But no word describes the second factor in meditation," he continues. He apologizes in advance, saying that "metaphysical" is the closest he can come. "It seems to be the result of experience coming freely out of the unconscious. When it ripens, it comes in *un*conditioned form. No one else can do this for you," he emphasizes. "No teacher. It is your own self, turning on your own inner light."

He then explains what he means by the word *unconscious*. He does not use it in the Freudian sense. Nor does it refer in the Jungian sense to some collective unconscious. Instead he uses it to refer to the larger sense of the "universal unconscious."

We then take up the subject of the Japanese tea ceremony. He observes that it is pervaded by feeling tones of harmony, reverence, purity, and tranquility. He emphasizes that the participants enter into it in a spirit of equality. There, relationships each to the other are not conditioned by ideas of social rank, privilege, or gender. One's perceptions awaken in the tea ceremony, and everyone shares in this liberating experience. Each goes on to revere the others. "In the same way," he concludes, "wisdom, *prajna*, does not exist for itself. What it leads to ultimately is to sharing, to compassion, to love."

Another long, silent pause. Again, I gather that the initiative for entering Zen training will be up to me. When I ask Kobori-roshi if it might be possible to do so, he pauses. "The temple has firm rules," he says. "We think it is worthwhile to start only if the person can then continue for a minimum of six months."

Waves of uncertainty sweep over me. The first laboratory experiments were off to a slow start. There were already minor tremors from the culture shocks and aftershocks of living in Kyoto. Is this the time to enter Zen training, to commit oneself to even stranger ways of thinking and doing? On the other hand, didn't I seek out Japan to find new problems to solve? So, sensing an affinity with the man, his ideas, and his temple, I ask, "May I see you again?"

He agrees!

14

Zazen at Ryoko-in

Colored blossoms scatter and fall.
In this world of ours, who lasts forever?
Today let us cross the last mountain range of life's illusions,
No longer to dream shallow dreams nor succumb to stupor.

Iroha poem[1]

Our first two long interviews are highly stimulating. But the roshi has given no hint of an invitation to join the Zen group. Our third interview is blessed by the weather. It is such a beautiful, clear summer day that we dwell first on the seasons. Kobori-roshi explains that Japan has many seasons. Even if one starts with the four usual seasons, there will be four other transition periods in between them. So even in winter, the first green shoots of spring come thrusting up through the blanket of snow. Next, the spring plum and cherry blossoms unfold and fall off. Then, in late summer, the leaves of a few trees are already turning the colors that signal the arrival of fall.

Many Japanese poems, *haiku*, focus on just these interfaces between the seasons, he points out. I remark that the Japanese as a people seem extra sensitive to the seasons. He adds that they turn this same sensitivity toward internal events as well. Japanese children frequently ask, "How is your inner weather?"

With no further discussion, the roshi begins to show me the proper approach to meditation! I am enormously relieved. This is my first tangible evidence that I am being accepted as a lay student at the temple. Only later do I find that, in earlier centuries, it was routine to turn down all Zen aspirants at the temple gate. If they persisted—in spite of the closed temple gate—they were usually invited inside after nightfall.

"First," the roshi says, "our way follows some general principles. Life involves being open-eyed. There are many different ways to meditate. We prefer to sit in zazen open-eyed. Using this approach, a person more naturally carries Zen practice into the rest of everyday life. Other ways of sitting with eyes closed started in India. They involve separating oneself from ordinary life. Indian philosophy emphasized life as suffering. To close one's eyes may perhaps seem to be the easiest way to retreat from it temporarily. But the Chinese already had their own view of life. It was different. Life was affirmed; life was worthwhile. Therefore, our way is to practice zazen with open eyes. This means *active* sitting, not passive sitting. It is more difficult, but there are fewer transition problems."

He then demonstrates the correct sitting posture. In actual fact, it differs only slightly from the poised, erect way he has been sitting all during each interview. "First, you cross your legs, both legs if you can, one if you cannot. Place your left foot comfortably on your right thigh. Then you sit erect: backbone straight, chin down, head back. Think of a long, steel rod. [He gestures.] This rod goes straight down your spine into the center of the earth and then straight up again high into the sky." I get the picture.

"Rest your forearms on your upper thighs, not on your hips. Loosen the stiffness around your shoulders, place your left hand in your right palm and bring your thumbs up together, nail to nail." Looking down now at his fingers, I am astonished to discover what I had overlooked before: his fifth fingernails are long, Chinese style.

"Next, you let all the weight of your trunk settle down to your abdomen, still keeping your back straight. You keep the back end of your bottom elevated with two rolled cushions. This leaves both knees pressing gently on the floor. Now, your base is solid like a triangle. Your posture is like that when you sit on a horse. You sway a few times to either side, then you settle in. No moving. When you breathe, emphasize breathing out. Say the word, 'one,' to yourself at the same time you exhale. Breathe all the universe in; let it all slide back out. [At this point he utters a long steady, sustained exhalation: "O . . . n . . . e."] Then let your eyes become powerful so that they penetrate deeply into one spot. Keep your eyes on this one spot. Do you see that leaf out there in the garden? Look powerfully into that leaf, so that your vision goes directly into it. You must first learn to see into things and then through them.

"Your next step is to concentrate on some simple phrase that helps you relax, yet still keeps you focused. Many such phrases come down to us from the Han dynasty. For example: 'White clouds embrace mystical stone.' If you use any phrase like this, concentrate only on the general *feeling* of it. Forget the words, and do not try to visualize the scenery. When you finally reach that stage of practice when no thoughts are in your mind, you may take on a koan.

"You should do zazen as frequently as you can. Morning or evening sitting generally works best. We say that morning sitting is golden; evening is copper.

Sitting will be in the zendo here from nine to eleven every morning and on Sundays from ten to twelve. Wear comfortable, loose dark clothing. All other instructions will come from Robert, the American who leads the sitting.

"Always remember," he concludes, "to carry your sitting into the rest of your living. Doing this, zazen gradually works its way into your life. For regular Zen monks, the life in practice then becomes an endless book, composed of only three chapters. The first is this staying in the very core of our sitting, even when we move out of the sitting posture. The second is communicating this same core both to others and on into all things. The third is helping other people to develop their own core."

Leaving the temple that day, feeling enormously privileged, I bow more deeply than I could ever have imagined, in gratitude to the roshi.

The next day I start formal zazen at Ryoko-in. Shoes off at the main entrance to the temple; an admiring glance at the old well inside and at the interior gardens; walking on age-polished wooden floors; slipping on a tight pair of narrow sandals outside, shuffling over the smooth, flat rocks. Past the sliding door into the zendo. Very dim inside . . .

When my eyes accommodate, I make out the outlines of a large rectangular room. On a low platform, around its two nearest sides, sit several figures. They rest on cushions, cross-legged, looking down at the old tile floor out toward the center of the room. Finally extricating my large, Western-sized feet from the small sandals, I try to place the sandals neatly together, like the others, at the base of the platform. Up now on the squeaking wood platform onto a large, flat square mat. Under my buttocks goes another rolled cushion. Down finally, into the half-lotus posture. Other human outlines filter in, until nine cushions are occupied.

Shortly before 9:00 A.M. comes a sound. "Dock, dock, dock." The group leader, the *jikijitsu*, is tapping on wood. Next comes a solid *CRACK!* I *jump!* I find later that two hard wooden blocks have been struck together. Then a small bell tolls, in measured, beautiful notes. Its final ring carries on and on throughout the zendo, penetrating into my brain. Silence. Sitting has begun.

This first sitting in the *zendo* is very difficult. My practice yesterday, at home, lasted only a few minutes. It was no preparation for this thirty minutes at one stretch. The first ten minutes in the zendo are bearable, the next interval is unbearable; the final minutes are torture. Pains in the knees and thighs are the chief problem. (When I later tell Dr. Osumi about this, he smiles and says, "Zazen is good for the central nervous system, but bad for the peripheral nervous system.")

At long last, the bell rings again. Relief! At this signal, the other figures on the mats begin to stir. Detaching themselves from the platform, they stand up, put on their sandals, and file toward the second door leading outside.

But I have a big, practical problem: my left leg is numb from the knee on down. The leg is rendered powerless, as though I had sustained a stroke.

As the last sitter exits from the door, I stay on the platform massaging the feeling back into my leg. After a minute or so, function returns and I limp over to the door. Looking out, blinking, into the sunlight, I see a small courtyard. Around the inside of this enclosure, the other lay adherents are walking, clockwise, very deliberately, in single file. Their hands are held loosely in front of their chest, and they are looking down at the ground in front of them. This, I gather, is *kinhin*, walking zazen.

No sooner do I catch up with the tail end of the line than the group leader at its head reenters the zendo door, and we all go back inside to sit another round of zazen. At the close of this second period, the numbness affects only my left foot. When I join the group walking outside, I am faintly reassured to see that several others are now limping also. During the final thirty minutes, I don't try so hard. I avoid pushing my left foot far over on my right thigh. Without my forcing it, the sitting goes easier. After another bell, and some rhythmic chanting in Japanese, the morning sitting is over. After repeated bowing with the two hands placed together, we file silently out through the main zendo entrance.

I start talking, and the response is a finger over the lips. No loud talking, I find, is the general rule throughout Ryoko-in. Once outside, I introduce myself to the others. They are an interesting, diverse group: a world-class professional potter from Australia, a Japanese-American girl from Hawaii, and two Japanese male university students. The Americans include a widow traveling slowly around the world, a woman sociology teacher from a Midwestern university, a married couple from New York, each teaching English at a nearby Japanese university, and Robert, the leader. He has studied Zen in Japan for several years, and is semipermanently established at the temple.

Over the succeeding months, I settle into the temple's routine. *Its* strict Rinzai routine is not going to change. *Mine* has to. First, I learn to be on time. Once, misjudging travel times, I arrive late and disturb the others in the zendo. Afterward, I am soundly chewed out by the *jikijitsu*. Chastened, I learn to leave home early, allowing plenty of time to take the series of three trolley cars. This means I now have extra minutes to enjoy a leisurely walk through the rest of the large old temple complex at Daitoku-ji. When I arrive at the subtemple, I bow and walk slowly through its outer garden, feeling the soft crunch of freshly swept gravel underfoot around the flat rocks. I look deeply into its leaves and into the exquisite moss covering its carefully tended grounds. I inhale the beauty of its old, gnarled tree trunks, the mountains-in-miniature of its old rocks. It is a fine prelude to zazen . . .

I learn much from my fellow students in the Zen group, or *sangha*. The widow had also been a student at a different, Soto Zen temple. I ask her what was the most important thing she had learned from her previous roshi. "Let go," she says. "Let go of all your conditioned worries, the thoughts and ideas you hold onto." I find these two simple words very helpful.

On one other occasion I inquire naively: "What is the connection between going back to one's original self and becoming enlightened?" She replies that she, too, had been puzzled about this. When she had asked her previous roshi to clarify it, he replied as follows: "It isn't as some special earlier original self that you become enlightened. Enlightenment isn't something you add. It exists throughout the universe *all* the time. All you have to do is simply allow it to express itself. Then, when you plug into it, you cease to be a separate self and simply blend in with the rest of the enlightened universe." I find this is vaguely reassuring, but not yet comprehensible.

With practice, zazen becomes second nature. The zendo routines settle into place; legs and back adjust to the sitting posture; the three-ring circus of thoughts retreats sooner from my brain. Respirations quiet by themselves. Some days nothing flows easily. During others, kinhin merges more naturally into and out of sitting zazen. Indeed, it strengthens it and becomes less of a distracting interlude. As zazen ripens, I begin to experience longer periods of a steady, relaxed awareness. For a neurologist, these thought-free periods are a most unexpected experience. No thoughts? Who would believe that an attentive brain could focus lightly on *nothing!*

The more I learn to sustain my attention on the slow, rhythmic movements of my lower abdomen, the sooner my thought stream dries up. Whenever I become perfectly aware of these proprioceptive movements, during inhalation and exhalation, thinking fades away. Moreover, a curious sense sometimes unfolds: my physiological center of gravity seems to move down from my upper chest to the waist and lower abdomen. At such times, an upright bearing becomes almost automatic. I become the roshi's horseback rider.

Sutra chanting provides some other surprises. It complements zazen. Normally, when we chant or sing, we prolong the act of expiration. Chanting contributes to the overall focus of breathing down in the lower abdomen rather than up in the chest. The way I chant Japanese monosyllables, they need no translation and require no thinking. Something about their sound and rhythm then becomes comforting in itself. Among my favorite phrases are those at the close of the sutra of the Heart of Great Wisdom.[2] They can be rendered in English as

> Gone, gone beyond, gone altogether beyond.
> Awakening, fulfilled!
> Heart of Great Wisdom!

Working outside on the temple grounds, I pull weeds, split kindling, sweep, and keep the place clean. Is this menial work necessary? Or, like kinhin, is it Zen in motion? It takes longer to appreciate that no kind of work is "menial" unless I judge it to be, that any work takes place in the ongoing now, and is to be fully entered into as an integral part of my daily practice. It didn't take old master Pai-chang Huai-hai (720–814) this long to clarify what work should mean to his monks back in the Tang dynasty. "A day of no work," he said, "is a day of no eating."[3]

Vivid complementary colors enter my vision during zazen, particularly in hues of yellow-green, and of pink to reddish purple. Gradually, over the months, these occur less frequently. Solid, wooden feelings of body, lips, and tongue are also less evident. Sluggishness after sitting evolves increasingly into a sense of mental clarity and composure.

Slowly, feelings of calmness and clarity begin subtly to extend themselves out of the zendo, entering into life's everyday affairs. It becomes easier to accept unpleasant things. Even when irritated, I have a growing sense of *who* is becoming upset. This leaves more time to develop an objective remedy to improve the situation. Life's central issues assume a higher priority. In earlier years, on vacations in the mountains, I could perceive that this one person is a part of the larger whole in an ongoing now. Now, in the busy streets of Kyoto, I start to enlarge upon this perspective. In parallel, the former sense of being a private isolated self tends to diminish. But all this comes and goes, still mostly at the intellectual level.

Observing these changes, an old paradox starts to resolve itself. Back when I first started to read about Zen, the literature placed emphasis on *abrupt* forms of awakening. It was difficult to conceive what a "gradual" awakening meant. But now I observe definite changes taking place in my own mental topography. Attitudes seem to be undergoing a kind of deep, slow continental drift. "Policy" shifts seem to be evolving at depths which go on to affect the strategies and tactics of behavior. If this is a kind of very gradual awakening, then it appears to be taking place.

In years past, sudden insights sometimes flashed in to help solve problems in my laboratory research. I speculate: could *prajna's* intuitions be of a similar kind? Could such brief insights, by analogy, resemble a quick "spiritual earthquake?" Little do I know.

15

Attention

> The faculty of voluntarily bringing back a wandering attention, over and over again, is the very root of judgement, character, and will.
>
> William James[1]

James was correct. And training both attention and awareness is also absolutely central to Zen. Everyone knows what it *feels* like to "pay attention." What goes on, technically, is that we enhance the way we process information from a preselected location in space.[2] Attention seems like a simple matter, but within it is a whole series of interrelated phenomena. They include *awareness*, a word derived from being wary, watchful. Awareness implies perception, a purely sensate phase of receptivity. *Attention* reaches. It is awareness stretched *toward* something. It has executive, motoric implications. We attend *to* things.

We can be more or less attentive. The term *attentiveness* conveys how much intensity we devote to the act of paying attention. This intensive aspect of attention resembles in a sense the separate "volume" control function found on an older radio or TV set. But in those days you first had to turn on the separate off/on knob. Then, before anything else could happen, you had to wait for the set to warm up. The brain responds in a similar fashion. It reacts sluggishly when we first awaken. This fact reminds us that *arousal* is basic. First, we must be sufficiently aroused. *Then* we become generally aware enough so that we can attend. Arousal, awareness, attention.

Attention shifts. The process of shifting happens either voluntarily, or involuntarily. Recall what happens at a cocktail party. We can look in one direction, while still deploying attention elsewhere to eavesdrop on the nearby conversation. Moreover, we can also shift attention inward. Our thoughts can then range widely over a big interior field of personal topics. In Kyoto, I discovered that it is all too fertile a field. My mind wandered, and this interfered seriously with zazen.

Suppose a person chooses to direct attention outward, to one single item within extrapersonal space. Then, before the subject can shift from that one item to another, it will take a long time: almost half a second, averaging around 400 milliseconds.[3] In the very earliest phase of the processes that shift attention, the two brain hemispheres seem equally facile.[4] Yet, when they both generate what may seem to be a single so-called searchlight of attention, its beam is not a steady one. It flickers on and off each time we shift from one locus to another. In so shifting, we close an attention "gate" at the first spot, then quickly open it up again when we reach the second location. This is useful. It avoids the blur that would come if we had lighted up every intervening possibility.

Which stimulus do we select, if given a choice? A lifetime of motivations determines the choice.[5] Past chooses present. As it does so, it first uses gross selection factors which resemble the coarse scanning controls available on a multiband radio. When we use these on the radio we can decide first whether we wish to tune into shortwave, longwave, AM, FM, or the citizens' band.

The brain, too, has its own kinds of options and tuning controls. Some controls are coarse, others fine. Together they create what William James spoke of as the "clearness of all that we perceive or conceive."[6] This clarity will bring sharpness and precision to attention.

A child can learn a lot about practical optics by focusing through a lens. What one learns bears certain analogies to mental "focusing." For example, when we first peered through a thick convex lens, it was to discover that the spot in the very center of the field was clearly in focus, and also enlarged. But everything else, from the center on out, was increasingly blurred. Soon we found out how much fun it was to focus the sun's radiant energy through this lens to burn a spot through a leaf or a piece of paper. Years later we would encounter a different lens. This wide-angle lens brought in a very large area, more of which stayed in focus at any one time. Each item, however, was reduced in size.

In a similar manner, perception can "open up" to take in a whole larger field, as attention distributes itself over a large domain. Or, using *selective attention*, we can focus down on one item. There we can *persist*, holding our attentive focus fixed on but one element of a field. Then we can further *concentrate* such persistent attention. This usually implies intensifying it in a smaller area. Once attention is concentrated, it becomes less readily distracted by the entry of conflicting or irrelevant items. But if one begins with arousal alone, and *it* becomes too intensified, then the person does become easily distracted. This particular complication can be observed especially in the hyperactive behavior of agitated manic patients. Their attention span lasts but an instant on one item. A moment later, it is swept on like a wind-driven tumbleweed, bumping into a succession of other items at random.

What happens when too much noise and too many sights overstimulate the brain's primary sensory pathways? Normal persons tune down their responsiveness. But people differ widely in how readily they can tune down their responsiveness to excessive stimulation. And they also vary in how readily they can tune *up* their sensitivities to detect fainter stimuli at low intensity.[5] One wonders: are some meditators "oversensitive" to begin with? Do they tend to use meditation to withdraw from their environment in ways that could lessen the excessive intensity of their experience? (see chapter 29).

On the other hand, during rare moments, the same meditators may also make a major shift into an extraordinarily different mode. It is a shift that carries the properties of clarity, persistence, and concentration far beyond their ordinary limits. Now, as attention transforms itself, *involuntarily,* it reaches that state called *absorption.* Absorptions tend to occur after emotional or devotional aspects have come in to pressure and color an already heightened mode of ongoing attention. Absorptions convey the sense of being held, transfixed, and riveted. It is a process during which extra, concentrated energy involuntarily infuses the act of attention.

Sometimes, as children, after we had been keenly attentive to a movie, we found that a foot had gone to sleep. Later, we discovered that the usual sense of our body image might even fade out when we were drowsy or preoccupied. From such ordinary experiences we learned that, when our attention was diverted elsewhere, we might not notice things, ourselves included. More extensive degrees of this kind of "dropping out of self" also occur during absorptions.

How can we now, as adults, voluntarily bring back and refocus our wandering attention, that faculty which James believed was so critical? To sustain attention takes a steady, dynamic flow of impulses. Much of this tonic flow starts down in the brain stem in our ascending reticular formation[7] (see chapters 36 and 37). Suppose, for example, you start with a hungry monkey, and then observe how he responds when you place an apple on the shelf off to his left side. If a small lesion has previously cut off the *right* half of his reticular activating system, the hungry monkey ignores the apple when it is in his *left* field of vision. This monkey is not blind, but neither does he "see" the apple over on his left side for all practical purposes. Why? Because his lesion blocked the right side of his cerebrum from being activated by the right side of his reticular system. But now move the apple over to the shelf on his *right* side. Here he can process it because his left hemisphere still remains connected to an intact left reticular formation. Now, he quickly sees, grabs, and munches on the apple.[8]

The monkey's impaired attention is loosely called "neglect." It is accompanied by abnormally slow brain waves over the right hemisphere. These slow brain waves point to a sluggish, less aroused right hemisphere, the side wherein the reticular formation no longer reaches up normally to activate his higher mechanisms of attention.

We might be curious at this point: is there some process which is the reverse of neglect? Could it be a form of *hyper*attending? If so, which of the several aspects of attention just considered would become prominent when a person becomes hyperattentive? And what parts of that person's brain would be responsible?

16

The Attentive Art of Meditation

The whole point of Buddhism may be summed up as *living in the present.*

Dhiravamsa[1]

"Living in the present moment." This is a short working definition of *meditation.* A longer one is also useful: "a family of techniques which have in common a conscious attempt to focus attention in a non-analytical way, and an attempt not to dwell on discursive, ruminating thought."[2] Why does "conscious" belong in the definition? For two reasons. First, because it reminds us that, at its beginnings, meditation is self-initiated. Before meditators finally relinquish intention, they consciously use it to guide awareness in very subtle ways. Second, the word "conscious" paves the way for understanding some distinctions that later on will become increasingly important. For when we come to states of absorption and insight-wisdom we will discover how certain functions become directed *un*consciously—that is, automatically and *un*intentionally.

Candor insists that any working definition of meditation employ the word "attempt." It bears reemphasis: meditation is hard to understand, hard to arrive at, hard to maintain. An artful process, it takes much patience, practice, and skill.

With calm relaxation as its prelude, sustaining bare attention then becomes the keynote of meditation.[3] If we use bare attention both as its basic premise and its defining characteristic, meditation currently divides into two generic categories.

1. *Concentrative meditation* is sustained attention which focuses persistently on a single item until one tends to become more or less absorbed in it. The item could be a flower, a mantra, the movements of breathing, or a koan.

2. *Receptive meditation* is sustained attention, *unfocused.* It opens up to whatever experience is available, neither overreacting to it, nor associating to it, nor interpreting it.[4] This kind of openly receptive meditation encompasses the several meditative approaches which are translated as "mindfulness," "insight meditation," and "just sitting."

At this point, the process looks simple: calmness → bare attention → concentrative or receptive meditation.

Meditation in general is not this straightforward. Nor is it in Zen. It is difficult to classify the attentive art of meditation into only these two types. Why? Consider how many different ways we use a camera. We can begin with film of extra sensitivity, or with finer-grained or color film. We can expose many, or few, frames per minute. Our hands can aim the camera straight ahead, or they can turn it around, away from the outside world, and direct the camera so that it looks back at the handler. We can switch lenses, varying the field from regular to wide-angle, to telephoto, or to zoom. The shutter can be opened wide or narrowed to a slit to gain an extra depth of field in focus. Older cameras require much deliberate, conscious thought; newer versions handle most functions automatically. Similarly, each brain, sifting through its "family of meditative techniques," settles on what part of its repertoire happens to work best at the time.

In practice, Zen meditators will find themselves trying out different styles at different times, both while sitting on the mat and while attending to the events of the present moment in everyday life.[5] But disclaimers are in order, for none of the basic meditation techniques are unique to Zen. Figures on seals excavated from the Indus Valley culture depict classic seated yoga postures dating back to around 2000 B.C.E.[6] So many of the Zen approaches stem from methods long used in yogic traditions which were later taken over by the early Indian Buddhists.

Evolutionary neurobiologists might trace some of the basic receptive processes much further back. It was their hunting skills that enabled protohumans to survive. "The hunter is the alert man," says Ortega y Gassét.[7] The alert hunter knows that "the solution might spring from the least foreseeable spot on the great rotundity of the horizon." So the hunter deploys his "universal attention." It makes no presumptions, "does not inscribe itself on any one point and tries to be on all points." Receptive meditation resembles this kind of "universal attention."

Of course, meditation in our era has been refined. Now we conceive of it as a mode of attending to the wide range of aspects of living in general, not simply to hunting. And from out of its equanimity arises the potential for rectitude of action to flow, not mere spontaneity.[1] Along with this equanimity arises that same sense of genuine well-being which one recalls having experienced after a good long vacation. Remember? After a week or so away, the feeling arrived of being *with it*, mentally attuned and physiologically competent.

Once the meditator establishes this same firm foundation, in a retreat setting, the concentration approach can evolve into lesser absorptions, and the deeper levels of mindful awareness can begin to yield brief intuitions of various sizes. But meditators will usually have to wait until they have honed various skills over a period of many days or weeks in such a retreat. Only then, finally, will their increasing one-pointedness and serenity open up to access more advanced levels of alternate states.

17

Restraint and Renunciation

> Poverty is not the absence of goods, but rather the overabundance of desire.
>
> Plato (c. 427–347 B.C.E.)

> Most of the luxuries, and many of the so-called comforts, of life are not only not indispensable, but positive hindrances to the elevation of mankind.
>
> Henry David Thoreau[1] (1817–62)

It is time to emphasize what Plato and Thoreau had learned: meditation has a necessary prelude. It goes nowhere unless the requisite foundations are laid. The serious aspirant on the meditative path makes an *ongoing commitment* to follow a more restrained, simplified life. The essential practices involve nothing more, but nothing less, than cultivating ordinary common sense, morality, and ethics in everyday living. They imply a "letting go" of self-indulgence, without that nagging feeling of having sacrificed something vital. It is what every backpacker learned the hard way: the hike depends as much on what you leave behind as on what you carry.

The Buddhist meditative Way begins with right living. The aspirant voluntarily adopts sensible restraints, and renounces situations which could lead to unfruitful behavior. Given this background, zazen can then be conducted as an integral part of the daily practice of a wholesome life, not as a kind of head-in-the-sand isolation.

This restrained, moral, disciplined living is termed *shila* (in Sanscrit). It spills back into meditation and strengthens it correspondingly. The reasons are straightforward. The simpler life has fewer clinging attachments, cravings, and materialistic goals. Fewer distractions means fewer intrusions from discursive thoughts. The meditator finds it becoming easier to cultivate the "meditative mood,"[2] to enter meditation and to remain centered in it longer. This turns out to make it easier to exercise restraints and practice renunciations. Self-control is not as difficult when there is less self to control. It takes years to really learn this fact, decades to put it into practice.

The "beat Zen" of the "dharma bums," the pop psychologies, and amateur drug-induced psychedelic states are caricatures. Chief among the reasons why they fail is the fact that there are no substitutes for *shila*. It remains that bedrock foundation of daily life practice, the ethical guidelines that are so central to Buddhist and other religious disciplines.

Buddhist monks or nuns, like their Christian counterparts, renounce far more than we realize.[3] One obvious example: the cosmetic vanities that focus on long hair. These vanities are literally cut off, not once but every five to seven days, each time the head is shaven. The austere monastic life tends to discourage notions of rank among the younger monks at the entry levels. All become poor, and each performs the most menial of tasks. The monastic life is a planned withdrawal toward simplicity, away from our usual hassling "civilized" complexities. Because this detachment is voluntary, it has the quality of an opt-out, not of a cop-out. With time, many material and other unessential "needs" become less pressing. As St. John would observe: "Now that I least desire them, I have them all without desire."[4]

And over time, and with repeated cautioning by the roshi, the aspirant realizes the deeper level of wisdom in Dogen's old statement: "Cut off the mind that seeks, and do not cherish a desire to gain the fruits of Buddhahood."[5] The hot pursuit of enlightenment is seen to be but another form of grasping, spiritual materialism. From then on, the ongoing quest will become truer, steadier.

Buddhism, too, has its precepts and Ten Commandments.[6] The commandment against intoxicating liquor becomes less difficult to follow than one might think. I would find, over time, that my taste for liquor had simply dropped away. This was a natural development, and it was no sacrifice.

Zen Meditative Techniques and Skills

Each of us literally chooses, by his way of attending to things, what sort of a universe he shall appear to himself to inhabit.

William James[1]

What's the best way to meditate? Rodin provided the West with two bronze examples of how *not* to go about it. The more familiar one is his tense, muscular statue *The Thinker.* The other example is his standing statue. It is entitled *Meditation* (1885), but the head is hanging down, and the eyes are closed.

Zen meditation will train one's attention in unfamiliar ways. Novices to zazen get off to a shaky start. They have too much to remember. They are trying to pay attention to four items, all at once: (1) the eyes directed straight ahead and down on a small area; (2) the lids slightly lowered; (3) the inner sounds of numbers silently counted out from one up to ten, then starting again; (4) each number linked with each successive expiration. Even accomplished meditators may find it next to impossible to *maintain* attention on these simple, but arduous tasks. First, the incessant flow of thoughts has to trickle away and the daydreamings drop off. One must adjust to bodily aches, other sensate experiences, and to the ups and downs of affect, including boredom. After days, or weeks, the beginner goes beyond the number system and settles perhaps on some word like "one," again timed with breathing out. The visual focus softens, because attention is turning increasingly to the discrete movements of the lower abdomen during breathing. The mental focus softens further as pressured thought trains now drop out. *Awareness itself* then starts to become the content within awareness.

Finally, the silent repetition of "one" drops out, and after long practice, bare attention settles on breathing movements down in the lower abdomen, or *tanden.* Now the meditator no longer breathes, but *is breathed,* slowly and quietly. Then, breathing itself drops out of awareness. During a long retreat, the resulting still point extends into minutes, developing a force of its own that admits no distractions.

The approach to meditation outlined above starts with active bowing and other sitting rituals, becomes less willfully directed, then relatively effortless, and finally passive. The early phase of zazen is basically a letting go of thoughts while becoming aware of breathing out. Gradually, what started out as a shallow form of meditative "concentration" slides into a "passive," concentrated awareness.

No contemporary student, East or West, is likely to try to meditate for as many consecutive hours, and days, as did the semilegendary Bodhidharma or other early patriarchs in the Indian traditions. Farther to the north, Chan and Zen did not strive for the florid levels of absorption. Instead, they emphasized the Middle Way, attending to the events of daily life, steering between the sluggish quietude of the tortoise and the neuroticism of the hare.

Should meditation remain effortless and goalless, as it flows naturally into the basic experience of being? Or should some of it involve a more active, directed element of striving? If each factor has some role to play, then when and how much of each? The debate has gone on for centuries. Within Zen, the Soto school still emphasizes the goalless and effortless approach. Its form of zazen, *shikantaza*, implies "just sitting" quietly, in awareness, not working on any koan, or counting the breath. It is an alert condition, performed erect, with no trace of sluggishness or drowsiness.[2] During retreats in particular, shikantaza can be shifted, or shifts itself, into long moments of *extra*attentiveness. This means a kind of listening as though one were blind, of looking as though one were deaf, of feeling as though all one's pores were open and receptive. The senses seem to stretch out to close the gap between stimulus and perception, that interval which had once been occupied by the old judgmental barriers of interpretation. At such times, the meditator enters a state of high perceptual expectancy. It is the way one listens, knowing that a tiger lurks in the jungle nearby.

In the rigorous school of Rinzai Zen, one blow from a flat stick would quickly straighten out Rodin, and the second swat would straighten up his languid model. Moreover, this Rinzai school also takes on an extra degree of striving, because its adherents work toward resolving their koan. Not infrequently, progress ensues just after the moment when they can no longer sustain such pressures. Ideally, a student's breaking point is carefully calibrated.

There is a kind of attentiveness that develops late during the practice of the deeper, effortless mode of Zen meditation. To me, the phrase "opening-up" is the most descriptive, least confusing, term for this later development. It implies that the meditator has gone beyond thoughts, and has already passed through (a) the phase of preliminary, passive concentration, and (b) the more passive "emptying out" and "letting go" phases. So that finally, instead of the meditative focus narrowing down, the large attentive field then gently opens up to a reflective surface, like that of an immense mirror. Now, any and all stimuli enter softly. But they drop out from awareness as quickly as they enter, attracting no emotional response in the process.

A second style of deeper Zen meditation does narrow down the meditative focus. It gently drifts attention over to engage a single meditative object or theme to the exclusion of all others. Such an approach also implies that the meditator is now not only detached from the outside environment but is focusing on some mental item generated internally.

Living Zen

Let us now review the four major phases discussed in these last two chapters. They are (1) preliminary concentration, (2) letting go, (3) opening up, or (4) focusing down. It is during zazen that the meditator will learn these as *skills*, not merely as techniques. Practicing zazen twice a day makes it much easier to develop and maintain these skills. Having first defined their nuances on the cushion, one then slowly learns to adapt these same skills to the simplest acts of one's daily life. Zen training places a major emphasis on transferring sitting zazen into "living Zen."

Living Zen implies being attentive in each present moment. This, too, gets off to a shaky start. First the meditator tries to extend the same meditative mode that permeates sitting zazen into *kinhin*, or walking zazen. The approach is to become *one with walking*. No thinking of anything else; no daydreaming. *Just walking*. Each foot meeting the ground. Each footstep has already arrived where *it* belongs. It is not on its way to some final destination. Imagine you are balancing an antique Ming vase in the palm of one hand. One finally reaches a comparable degree of alertness, and becomes able to hold it for long minutes, during prolonged meditative retreats.

No one would mistake the total program of Zen training for quietism. Just as kinhin introduces the meditative mode into the act of walking, so does vigorous physical work around the monastery then introduce meditation into other activities. And quietism certainly does not describe that deep intense existential search, or the active excursions some trainees make into the martial arts. In these and other daily life practices, the meditator slowly learns to deploy attention wholeheartedly into the *now*. No ruminations. None of the ambivalence that could come from juggling six distracting things "in mind" at the same time.

When attention is fully deployed into behavior, it means, quite literally, that the person *leans into just one activity at a time*. It means that one's posture and attentiveness totally engage the moment, whether the act is eating, reading, or looking up at cloud formations. Such behavioral postures are not unique to Zen. Watch any well-trained sushi slicer. You'll see him lean forward into each piece in turn. Zen develops the same *single*-minded approach. It draws on the same single-minded skills already learned during quiet sitting and walking. And, because the meditator has already practiced doing this during zazen, undivided attention then becomes free to shift into whichever field is required, a broader or a more restricted field.

Most persons will find it easier to meditate in the morning before breakfast, in the late afternoon before supper, or late at night before retiring. Such times may reflect the implicit rhythms of our biological clock. It is difficult to fall asleep after splashing cold water on one's face in the morning, easier to stay awake before eating any meal, and easier to meditate in the evening after having left behind the echoes of the day's activities.

In traditional Zen meditation, the eyes remain partially open. A later chapter will clarify the physiological bases for this (see chapter 139). This approach differs from TM and from other forms of meditation that permit the eyes to close. Zen Master Dogen's teacher in China taught that the eyes could be closed during zazen, but only if the meditator had first practiced zazen for forty or fifty years and never dozed off![3]

Physiological Changes during Meditation

All that is clearly established by the data on autonomic-metabolic measurements during meditation is the hardly surprising conclusion that meditators are in a state of relaxation.

J. Davidson[1]

Many reviews have now clarified what kinds of changes meditation produces in the body.[1–8] The consensus: meditation causes *secondary* physiological and biochemical changes that are appropriate to how much relaxation is involved.[8,9]

Readers interested in the secondary changes can find a four-page list of them in Shapiro's summary.[4] Shapiro goes on to cite some eighteen hypotheses invoked to explain how meditation might cause such changes. He concludes that a multidimensional model will be necessary because no single explanation is satisfactory.[10] Woolfolk adds that the "findings reflect the influences of very complex sets of social, cognitive, perceptual and physiological variables."[2]

Herbert Benson began to simplify this situation. He emphasized that those who meditate in a quiet setting develop a *relaxation response* whenever they combine a mental device, a passive attitude, and a decrease in muscle tone.[5] His subjects practiced a "simple, non-cultic technique" of meditation. Sitting quietly and comfortably, they deeply relaxed all muscles, saying the word "one" silently during each expiration, maintaining an attitude of peace, and letting relaxation unfold at its own pace. The resemblance to "just sitting" in Zen meditation is clear.

After relaxing daily for weeks and months, his patients reduced their systolic and diastolic blood pressures, and had fewer premature ventricular heartbeats, both during sleep and while awake. When they then encountered stress-producing circumstances, his subjects *increased* their blood norepinephrine levels.[11] Despite the increase, they did not increase their heart rate or blood pressure. This led to the suggestion that the subjects had also developed measures to counter the stimulant action of norepinephrine. These mechanisms remain to be clarified.

In two other recent critical reviews, the heart rate, skin resistance, breathing rate, and blood pressure responses to meditation were contrasted with those obtained during simple resting.[6,7] In his critique of twenty-three studies of meditation, Holmes concluded that, *as opposed to simple resting*, meditators do not show *consistently* lower heart rates, skin resistance activity, respiratory rates, blood pressures, or biochemical changes.[7] It should not be surprising that Joe, Mary, Bob, and Betty have individually different responses. The fact is, we are much more mixed-up genetically than are laboratory rats.

Reviewing seven studies, Holmes further concluded that meditation did not help control the body's arousal response to threatening situations. In fact, meditators, if anything, appeared *more* physiologically arousable in response to stress than did controls. In contrast, advocates of the transcendental meditation technique believe that it is more effective than is simple rest with the eyes closed in reducing such indices of stress as the rate of breathing and plasma lactate levels. They point out that it may be of greater adaptive significance for a person to be able rapidly to recover from stress than to reduce arousal in the face of threatening circumstances.[12]

Meditators who practice intensively do feel that their senses become more acute. Those who practice mindfulness meditation intensively (sixteen hours a day for three months) show a measurable, slight increase in their visual sensitivity.[13] When tested with a tachistoscope they detect single brief flashes of light more readily than before. They also distinguish successive light flashes, each separated by a shorter interval. Advanced meditators appear more sensitive to their own mental and perceptual processes. Some report that each light flash has three components: its beginning, its lasting, and disappearing.[14]

Let us make the tentative assumption that meditative practices do, to varying degrees, help many people feel more relaxed.[15] And concede that the practices do so, whether they are from the East, or are the Western secular techniques such as progressive relaxation, autogenic training, and self-hypnosis. Let us further assume that many of the techniques are reasonably effective, but not consistently so, in improving such indices of relaxation as the slower rate of breathing, the increase of skin resistance, and the increase of alpha waves in the electroencephalogram. If so, why go further? Is there any advantage to choosing one method over another, at least as a *technique* for obtaining the initial relaxation response?

Boals would object to the very concept implied in this question. It implied that meditation was solely a relaxation technique. He believed that this was a limited view, one that had "outlived its usefulness." He concluded that meditation was instead a complex process of *learning how to deploy attention*.[16] Zen traditions over the centuries support this larger view.

In fact, both Zen and the other age-old meditative traditions also provide a supportive social and cultural framework. This appeals to many meditators, helps them meditate longer, more often, and more intensively. Once they begin, many of the more persistent Zen meditators, moreover, will develop inclinations to follow the Way, going well beyond their initial "relaxation response" in the quest for different values.

Meditation is difficult to evaluate physiologically, much more so than you might suppose. For example, early research suggested that Zen masters and monks who had practiced for ten to twenty years would show, during their zazen, a large drop in basal metabolic rate.[17] More recent research yields a different interpretation. When TM meditators were studied, it was found that they were relatively tense to begin with during the control period. This initial "tension response" was prompted by the mental stress of their entering the artificial experimental situation itself. Thereafter, although their metabolic rate did fall during meditation, most of this drop could be attributed to their subsequently becoming more at ease and reducing their muscle tension. This, in turn, could be explained by the relaxation and improved body posture associated with the period of meditation.[18] Even among experienced meditators, who self-rated themselves as generally "tense," meditation coincided with a 13.5 percent drop in oxygen consumption.

Several artifacts are implicit in studying meditation in a laboratory setting. Indeed, anyone who consents to be a subject for an experiment changes even before the electrodes, tubes, or other connections are attached. Some pituitary hormones may show a brief phasic increase fifteen minutes *before* meditation starts, a rise which has been attributed to learned behavioral conditioning.[19] Meditators also respond to other so-called, demand characteristics of the experiment. This phrase refers to all the clues that let them know what the experimenters want and what their hypothesis is. Now, a goal, an expectation, is set. The meditators may think to themselves: "I will try to be a 'good' subject. I will try hard so that my recordings will be valid and will help advance scientific knowledge." Or, "I can't relate to this experimenter. Why should I cooperate so much?" Similar expectations, nuances shared by subject and investigator alike, are diametrically opposed to the goalless, passive, open state conducive to deeper levels of meditation. The more vigorously this desired state is sought, the more it eludes the grasp. Werner Heisenberg's general principle is true no less in meditation research than it is in physics: attempts to measure meditative states introduce new inaccuracies and uncertainties.

Existing research on meditation has other limitations. One is crucial: *no physiological or biochemical measurements can define the precise subjective quality of the meditator's private state of awareness at any one moment, let alone sequentially.* Many reports are pilot studies containing brief "one-shot" samples. Most experiments are not repeated using sufficient numbers of reliable subjects, studied over many years. This means that we still lack the requisite longitudinal view. And meditation is but a prelude to certain brief extraordinary alternate states. Their nature cannot be communicated exactly at that very moment without some kind of interruption of the internal flow of events.

"Meditation" is not monolithic. We have emphasized that several different meditative styles coexist today. This is another reason why research on "meditation" does not lend itself to simple generalizations. TM and yogic traditions prefer closed-eye techniques. Zen traditions emphasize the half–open-eyed approach. Even within Zen itself there are several meditative practices and styles of living, quite apart from the issue of whether the meditator also "works" on a koan. Not surprisingly, when Pekala recently reviewed the phenomenology of meditation he found that none of the twenty-eight studies was adequate methodologically. None fulfilled the key criteria of reliability, validity, and comprehensiveness. None was adequately controlled either for the demand characteristics of the experiment, or for a meditator's tendency to develop symptoms during introspection.[20]

Meditation and Sleep Cycles

The relationships between meditation and sleep cycles are very important. For one thing, *meditators take naps,* as do people in general. In fact, as many as 61 percent of normal people nap more than once a week and for over an hour.[21] People tend to take naps at either of two times: when the body temperatures are higher, or between 2 and 4 P.M.[22] Naps are physiologically restorative. For example, healthy male college students were studied who habitually took naps lasting from half an hour up to two hours. They increased their efficiency, their alertness, their EEG frequencies, heart rates, and body temperatures. They also shortened their reaction times and increased the frequency of their spontaneous skin resistance responses.[23]

Naps have implications for meditation research that tend to be overlooked. Morning naps may contain elements of REM (rapid eye movement) sleep. These morning REM episodes can slip into each nap earlier than usual.[21] Moreover, any studies purporting to show that meditators (who may also take catnaps) will improve in physiological categories such as those cited above must also have appropriate controls. These should include subjects whose nap habits are also observed longitudinally. Otherwise, one cannot exclude the possibility that whatever benefit may have occurred is attributable simply to repeated naps alone.

Firm evidence shows that meditators fall asleep. One study was performed on five TM meditators, four of whom were teachers. They spent 19 percent of their time in stage 1 drowsiness, 23 percent in stage 2 sleep, and 17 percent in stage 3 or 4 sleep. Even during their first twenty minutes, over 40 percent of their time was spent in stages 2 to 4 of sleep.[24,25] The fact that no REM sleep episodes were observed may be explained by the fact that the studies were performed in the afternoon when the pressures to enter REM are lower.

Some have suggested that meditation of various kinds is nothing more than a prolonged drowsiness, a kind of partial sleep. This view overlooks three facts. One is that meditation is also associated with very long-range, positive changes in attitude. Another is that meditation increases the frequency of absorptions and deep insights. Third, everyone sleeps at night, and some will nap during the day, but these do not create new attitudes, or lead to absorptions or kensho. So something about meditative training is different. Wherein lies the difference?

1. Meditation encourages a finely held awareness and attentiveness for relatively long intervals, even though the person sometimes lapses into other periods of drowsiness.

2. When practiced as zazen, it holds the person in one erect posture. This cuts down not only on movements but on sensations feeding back from them. Zazen becomes long intervals of sensorimotor deprivation. These intervals are so timed that they intrude into what had formerly been the day's usual waking cycle, not its sleep cycle.

3. Meditation permits the panorama of thoughts to be observed repeatedly as they enter and drop off. There is no more convincing demonstration of the fact that our thoughts and their attachments are transitory.

4. It sets up a quiet period, a retreat during which larger issues can be mulled over dispassionately.

5. Ideally, it takes place in the context of a meditative mood. This usually implies that the person has already made some kind of spiritual commitment and renunciation.

Many claims are made that meditation improves personal health, well-being, and performance. Even twenty-minute TM meditation periods are said to improve the condition of hospitalized psychiatric patients.[26] Relatively short periods are also purported to show beneficial effects on health, perceptual ability, athletic performance, learning abilities, academic performance, anxiety, creativity, and substance abuse.[27,28]

As a generalization, Zen moves "out" toward a flexible interrelatedness and away from a rigid, in-turned frame of self-reference. From the many reports, suffice it here to extract one study which illustrates a way to investigate some of these issues. It is based on measurements of subtle differences in the ways humans perceive their visual environment.[29] The subjects were forty unpaid normal volunteers, selected from those who attended a public introductory lecture on TM. The twenty men and twenty women were divided into two groups. One group meditated. Their control group did not. These non-meditators had expressed a wish to learn TM, but had agreed to postpone their instruction for three months. This selection procedure controlled to some degree for the motivational aspect of the experiment, because all subjects in both groups had demonstrated their desire to learn TM. The meditators then practiced TM for twenty minutes, both morning and evening, for three months; the non-meditating controls sat quietly for twenty minutes each morning (only) for three months.

Two psychological tests were used to measure all subjects. In the Rod-and-Frame Test, the subject must correctly orient a rod to a truly vertical position even when the rod has been placed in the center of a square frame which itself has been rotated out of a perfect vertical alignment. So the goal is to place the rod in a truly vertical position and not to be distracted by the frame that surrounds it. The error, expressed in degrees, is the difference between the true vertical and the position the subject has placed the rod in. Subjects who did not meditate did not improve their performance. In contrast, the meditators became more accurate after three months. In the males, the average pretest error of 3.3 degrees dropped to only 2.0 degrees. Female meditators also became more accurate, their error falling from 3.7 to 2.3 degrees. The slight differences between the meditators and the non-meditators were considered to be statistically significant.

In the Embedded-Figures Test, simple black-and-white figures are obscured by a veil of twenty-four complex overlying colored patterns. The goal is to see through all this camouflage and rapidly discern the hidden black-and-white figures embedded underneath. The meditators, after three months, took less time to detect the figures. The men dropped from an average of 48 seconds initially to 43 seconds, and the women dropped from 69 seconds to 63 seconds. Again, the results were statistically significant.

These two tasks were originally designed to test the way people deploy their visual perception. The subjects are usually not aware of the skills involved. Moreover, performance on these tasks normally changes rather little over time, if at all. So the study implied that regular meditation had improved the subjects' abilities to focus on the essence of a visual problem and to avoid distractions.

Critics can rightly find flaws in the experimental design. The flaws illustrate the kinds of problems plaguing meditation research. For example, the control group had not rested in the evenings; the meditators might have felt the subtle demand characteristics of the situation to do better; and more subjects are required than a mere twenty in each group.

Schuman emphasizes what researchers should be focusing on. It is on those primary processes in the *central* nervous system which underlie alternate states themselves.[3] Otherwise, investigators will keep on being sidetracked by all the secondary physiological changes in the body and the brain which accompany the "low arousal" meditative states. It is true that the skeletal muscles of the spine do hold the central nervous system erect during meditation. And it is also true that the brain, as part of the body, has important interactions with the cardiovascular,[30] pulmonary, digestive, and endocrine[31] systems. Yet here we will not be preoccupied by such bodily changes. Our plan is to go well beyond the phase of relaxation. Our goal is to discover which salient changes—primary in the *brain*—underlie alternate states of consciousness. This means penetrating the phenomenology, the semantics, the claims and counterclaims. Our focus will remain on the brain, for therein lies the psychophysiological basis of extraordinary states.

The early investigators were hoping that "brain waves" might clarify what went on in the "higher centers" during meditation. Do brain waves tell us something useful about a person's state of consciousness?

20

Brain Waves and Their Limitations

> Concluding anything about alpha is perilous.
>
> Barbara Brown[1]

During our experiments in Kyoto, we monitored "brain waves" arising from the cat brain. It is an old technique. [In 1929, Hans Berger coined the term electroencephalogram to describe the recording of the human brain's spontaneous electrical potentials.] Since then, electrodes attached to the scalp or to the coverings of the brain have been used to follow, mostly at a distance, the electrical activity of the brain beneath.

The brain is no power plant. Even when researchers amplify its faint potentials up to 50 microvolts (μV), its output amounts to only 50 millionths of a volt. For comparison, a flashlight battery puts out 1.5 volts. Moreover, estimates are that the whole brain generates only enough total current to light a 25-watt light bulb.

Nor is the brain's electrical activity constant. It pulses up and down from one fraction of a second to the next. Its rapid pulses take the form of rhythmic waves. If you are out at a shoreline, you might see waves of water arriving perhaps once every several seconds or so. EEG waveforms cycle much faster. They rise and fall from one to fifty times *each second*. Waves of excitation create the crests; waves of inhibition, the troughs.

The several major categories of EEG waves cycle at different frequencies. For purposes of this discussion, we will concentrate on the four faster frequencies seen during the waking state. *Alpha* rhythms cycle up and down eight to twelve times per second. Slightly slower rhythms, *theta* rhythms, occur four to seven times per second. Much faster rhythms occur at lower amplitude and are more irregular. They are the *beta* rhythms at fourteen to thirty cycles per second (cps) and the *gamma* rhythms at thirty to fifty cps.

Alpha Rhythms

Alpha activity is a phrase often shortened to alpha, for the sake of simplicity. It is seen most readily over the occipital cortex, but alpha varies remarkably from person to person.[2] In one study, alpha waves were associated with pleasant, relaxed states in only fourteen of twenty six subjects who were monitored during different subjective states. During alpha, another seven subjects were more aware of their own internal ongoing thoughts and feelings, as opposed to stimuli from the outside world. But two were thinking about past experiences, and three reported no feelings or thoughts of note.[1] So if you had only EEG alpha waves to look at, you could not accurately predict either the form or the content of that person's "inner weather" or their "mental landscape."

Alpha changes. More alpha activity occurs during "thinking" per se, especially during *non*visual thinking. Alpha waves tend to drop out as soon as visual components enter during daydreaming. But later on, once the person becomes drowsy, alpha remains even though visual experiences are going on. During that still later drowsy period just on the brink of sleep, alpha slows or disappears. This event may last 1.5 seconds or so, in association with a sense of "floating."[3]

Alpha responds. Especially pertinent to meditation is the fact that *persistent attention facilitates alpha*. Indeed, requesting the person to keep paying attention to what is being seen produces more alpha than does simple viewing alone.[4] So an easy way to bring out alpha rhythms is to induce a state of readiness, attentiveness, or heightened awareness. This fact, long known, is periodically rediscovered.[5] Alpha also increases when attention shifts away from visual stimuli to auditory stimuli.[6] Subjects who listen intently to hear a faint sound develop impressive, regular high amplitude alpha bursts. These can run for more than a minute.[5] Questions that evoke some personal impact also enhance alpha. For example, one subject had an EEG showing only 5 to 10 percent alpha rhythms to begin with. Then the subject laughed in response to a question. Following this, alpha activity increased, to occupy almost 100 percent of the recording for the next half minute.[5]

A "simple" mathematical problem may not interrupt alpha. But alpha does disappear when it becomes difficult to think about a problem. For Einstein, even the most intricate mathematical operations were so routine that his brain still generated alpha rhythms. Yet, on one occasion, Einstein's alpha activities suddenly dropped out. He appeared restless. He had discovered that he had made a mistake in his own calculations the previous day![7]

Alpha also drops out after subjects quickly attend to some brief *external* signal, such as a sudden, startling noise. But, as noted above, alpha is enhanced when subjects *voluntarily decide to shift* their attention into an alerted but untroubled mode. For all these reasons, investigators who would wish fully to evaluate alpha waves during meditation must monitor and carefully specify what *kind* of attention is going on, and on a moment-to-moment basis.[4] This is rarely done. As a result, many inferences about meditation based on whether alpha is present or absent have not been substantiated.

Alpha shows regional differences. Up to one third of subjects increase their alpha rhythms in the occipital region during mental tasks. Another third show decreases.[8] If the eyes stay open during various *motor* tasks, alpha can increase over the temporo-occipital region, but it decreases over the frontal and central regions whether the eyes are opened or closed.[9]

Given the above complexities, we can appreciate Brown's caveat that it is perilous to conclude anything about alpha.[1] Still, the standard biofeedback techniques have long been used to train people to relax. And these methods have usually been directed toward enhancing their alpha rhythms and reducing their beta rhythms. When patients who are severely and chronically anxious do learn to facilitate their alpha rhythms, they gain a global feeling of increased well-being. Their alpha increases even before their inner feelings show marked improvement. However, the symptoms stay relatively unchanged in that other group of patients who cannot learn to increase their alpha.[10]

Pertinent to our understanding of zazen are three simple biofeedback techniques which help subjects develop more alpha: (1) The subject's eyes remain *open*. This technique engages relaxation skills which can be more easily transferred to the stressful situations in ordinary daily life. (2) A light is used as a feedback target. This stabilizes visual fixation, and dampens random eye movements. (3) The subject is encouraged to maintain a passive attitude.[10]

It helps to keep the eyes open for another reason while learning to control alpha activity.[1] At first, when the eyes stay open, and the subject is relaxed, alpha rhythms normally occupy only 2 to 25 percent of the recording. Suppose, theoretically, one could then train alpha to increase well beyond these figures, say up to 100 percent of the time. Then the implication would be that normal subjects could still have another 75 to 98 percent "more room in which to learn." In contrast, if the eyes stay *closed*, then three quarters of the subjects easily develop alpha rhythms, and they soon occupy some 85 percent of the recording. But this would leave only another 15 percent of the time in which to learn to produce more alpha rhythms. At least for biofeedback purposes, this 15 percent is not enough "room" in which to learn to train one's abilities to relax.

Theta Rhythms

Theta rhythms of 4 to 7 cps are not conspicuous in the alert EEG of normal subjects. Theta rhythms edge in as we become drowsy, when our alpha rhythms fade, when the external world recedes even more, and when daydreams and fantasies take over.[1] Then theta activity is most easily identified from the parietotemporal region. Because theta varies, its mental correlates are also difficult to pin down. During mental tasks, a distinctive theta rhythm can be detected from the scalp over the midline of the frontal region. It appears more often in extroverts who begin with a low anxiety level, and in other subjects after their anxieties and arousal levels have been reduced by drugs such as diazepam (Valium).[11]

Persons highly experienced in self-hypnosis tend to show more theta activity both during hypnosis and while awake.[12] Astronauts also show increased theta when they become weightless during orbital flights. This finding is attributed to the fact that fewer vestibular stimuli reach the brain stem in a weightless environment.[13] Some patients fall asleep excessively during the daytime. They show synchronized theta bursts during their repeated "microsleep" episodes.[14]

Beta and Gamma Rhythms

Beta activity is also difficult to link with one specific, discrete subjective state.[1] During beta activity, nine of twenty-six subjects reported feeling tense and anxious. Another five reported some degree of excitement, concentration, and alertness. One felt hungry, and eight others identified no particular feeling state. Still, three reported that they felt loving, warm, and content during beta rhythms. This finding, that a positive affect can occur during beta activity, could be germane to the phenomena of bliss experienced in internal absorption.

Beta rhythms increase temporarily during states of vigilant attention. But beta then drops off when attempts are made to maintain vigilance for as long as two hours on a radar monitoring task. At this time detection performance also drops, and alpha and theta frequencies increase.[15]

Recently, interest has focused on gamma activity, a term applied to rhythms faster than 30 cps. Waves that oscillate forty times a second are ubiquitous. They can be detected both in single nerve cells and from larger constellations of neurons. This fact hinders current efforts to be sure where they arise, and what they imply in relation to states of consciousness. In normal humans, modern research techniques have now uncovered a set of different changes in 40 cps EEG activity which can be correlated with attentive responses to auditory clicks.[16] Moreover, such changes distinguish one group of "fast-reactors" from another group of "slow-reactors." The findings are noteworthy, because similar methods could be applied to clarify why Zen adepts act quickly (see chapter 154).

*   *   *

Four key terms imply important physiological distinctions. We will use these words frequently. *Synchronized* waveforms are those which recur regularly and smoothly. They include the regular, very rhythmic alpha and theta waves which rise to higher amplitudes. The contrasting term is *desynchronized*. (Historically, the word has referred to the *irregular* fast and low-voltage frequencies in the beta and gamma range. More recently, it has been acknowledged that some of these fast frequencies do have regular wave forms.) When any of these four basic EEG or other physiological rhythms persist over time, it can be called a *tonic* rhythm. However, if the rhythms go through phases, shifting on and off quickly, they are then called *phasic*.[17]

How does a brain generate the rhythms picked up by an EEG? What the EEG electrodes do, up on the scalp, is pick up and pool huge numbers of the faint potentials produced by each nerve cell's luxuriant tree of dendrites (see figure 4). To these, the EEG also adds other potentials picked up from countless cell bodies. When pooled, the potentials then take the usual form of much larger and slower waves.[18]

The alpha rhythm is a basic rhythm. Even a small cylinder of cortex, isolated far from the rest of the brain, can still generate its own independent ten-per-second alpha rhythm. Each single wave within this train of ten waves reflects two phenomena. The crest is the moment when most of the dendritic excitation comes in phase all at the same time. The trough that follows is the interval when dendritic activity is more inhibited and relatively quiet. In this sense, the electrical peaks and valleys are like the penetrating rhythms of the temple drums. Silence on either side augments the impact of each beat.

Still, only about 20 to 50 percent of the EEG reflects those brain activities generated directly under a large electrode recording from the surface. The rest seeps in from sites more distant. Recent sophisticated techniques increase the spatial resolution of the EEG, deploying arrays of 120 electrodes over the scalp. Some still conclude that "EEGs represent neither signal nor noise but [are] chaotic carriers of brain information."[19]

Deeper structures like the thalamus (see figure 3) generate their own rhythmic activities. They also export trains of impulses up to reach the dendrites of cortical nerve cells. Now, the crests of alpha waves recorded in the human thalamus peak just before those in the cortex. Moreover, electrical stimuli delivered slowly to thalamic nuclei also *evoke* a series of prominent waves up in the cortical EEG. These findings suggest that the thalamus acts as a pacemaker which sets some of the rhythms for the cortex.[20] After successive thalamic stimulations, the amplitude of the cortical waves keeps getting higher and higher. Finally, as the thalamus recruits a critical number of cortical cells, the cortex becomes overexcited. At this point, it fires back down to the thalamus and other subcortical regions. Out of such studies has grown the concept that the brain has "reverberating circuits." This means that rhythmic firings in one part of the brain go on to influence the excitability of other nerve cells some distance away, and are then influenced in return.

Certain leaves are sensitive to the faintest breeze. For instance, bamboo leaves (like those of the aspen) are the first to rustle, long before their larger limbs bend. As I was about to leave Kyoto, Kobori-roshi presented me with one of his own ink paintings. It was a bamboo stalk, with leaves, skillfully rendered. The inscription read: "Only the bamboo knows the pure breeze." In the brain, ripples of excitation sweep back and forth over dendrites. Many rustling excitations stop here, destined never to pass farther down over the nerve cell body itself. And few indeed will ever help set off the actual nerve impulse which fires down through the body of the cell, then out through the long trunk which is its axon. (see Figure 4) In fact, only a small part of our EEG is made up of those few spike discharges which finally do issue out from the long axons of cortical nerve cells.

It is just as well that this is so. Suppose that every time a dendrite got excited it *did* trigger off its entire nerve cell. Then our brain might be involved in continuous convulsive seizures.

And when similar considerations are applied to other levels, they may help explain why vast gaps remain between what our EEG displays at a given moment, what we sense is going on within our current state of consciousness, and what our overt acts of behavior are at the same time. With this caveat, we now turn to consider how the EEG evolves during meditation.

21

The EEG in Meditation

One might conclude either the process of meditation is unique to the meditator or that the essential information is not carried by the frequency component of the EEG.
C. Brown and colleagues[1]

We know that people's EEGs differ, that an individual's EEGs vary, and that meditation is not one state but a series of dynamic physiological changes. So it comes as no surprise to find that many different EEG changes have been recorded during meditation, and that most studies are open to criticism.[2,3] Griffith concluded, from data on yogic meditation, that it was all "rather confusing, taken as a whole."[4]

One can make a few soft generalizations. At least from the standpoint of brain waves, the zazen that is performed in full concentration while sitting in a chair yields probably about the same EEG as that performed when the subject is sitting on a cushion in the usual half–cross-legged lotus position.[5] Early during meditation, the EEG tends to show increased amounts, or amplitudes, of alpha activity. Next, theta activity increases, even though some of these theta waves may be consistent with drowsiness. Other theta patterns occur in short bursts, and still others occur for longer periods at higher amplitudes. Interestingly, Buddhist meditative chants are themselves associated with enhanced, rhythmic, synchronous theta activity.[6] Finally, in meditation, low-voltage fast beta ripples may sometimes be superimposed on still slower waves.

First we will expand upon these alpha, theta, and beta wave generalizations. Then we can address the controversies that have grown up around the issues of drowsiness, sleep, and "right brain vs. left brain" functions.

Alpha Activity

When more alpha activity occurs during the early phases of meditation, it does not mean that the subjects are merely "idling" mentally. Nor are they otherwise deferring their attention. In fact the reverse is true, for attention does facilitate alpha rhythms. Subjects can increase their alpha rhythms by concentrating on the sounds of a metronome or on a visual stimulus.[7]

We noted that alpha persists during tasks that can be performed easily or automatically. Accordingly, alpha waves occupy some 50 percent of the record when experienced Soto Zen monks are engaged in their walking meditation, kinhin. In contrast, alpha waves occur only about 20 percent of the time in inexperienced practitioners. Moreover, the control group of graduate students generates no alpha waves during the act of walking.[8]

Devout Protestants who pray regularly for thirty minutes a day increase their alpha frequency from 9 to 11 cps. One person who frequently shed tears during her everyday prayer practice increased her EEG frequency the most. Another subject, who had engaged in Sufi meditation for eighteen years, also experienced a free flow of tears during meditation. At this time the alpha frequency increased from 11 to 12 cps. Such observations suggest that emotional arousal can generate faster alpha frequencies. Alpha feedback techniques were used during a sixteen-day meditative retreat, and they did increase the amount of alpha rhythms. However, biofeedback did not make it any more likely for kensho to occur.[9]

The EEG differs in one other respect besides frequency and amplitude during various forms and stages of meditation. This third characteristic is *coherence*. The word describes how *uniform* the EEG activity is over the whole cerebral surface. Coherence is a measure of how many of the EEG peaks and valleys are all in synchrony at many different electrode sites. For example, there would be *no* coherence if the left frontal lead were to show ten-per-second alpha waves while the left central lead recorded only five-per-second theta activity.

Several TM studies have emphasized that meditation leads to periods of EEG coherence. These can last for over forty seconds and involve the alpha, theta, and beta frequencies. The increased alpha coherence is more evident frontally, and it tends to correlate with both the clarity of ongoing experience and with a suspension of respiration.[10] The strong and sustained alpha coherence which can occur during meditation distinguishes it from the way non-meditating subjects *lose* EEG coherence when they start to drop off into normal sleep.[11]

Theta Activity

It will be the rare circumstance when a meditating subject develops a major alternate state in the laboratory, and is already so "wired up" that all the EEG and other aspects of this state can be studied carefully as they evolve. Banquet addressed some of these issues in his early study of TM meditators.[12] A push button was an important feature. By pressing this button, his subjects could indicate what they were experiencing, using a prearranged code of five signals. Theta activity predominated during their "second" stage of meditation. Later, the initial short theta bursts were followed by longer, rhythmic theta trains. These lasted ten seconds to several minutes. Next, increasingly rhythmic theta trains became synchronized in both the anterior and posterior EEG leads. While they were meditating, the EEG of these TM subjects showed a *rhythmic* theta pattern. So this was not exactly the same theta pattern as are those more irregular forms of theta activity which occur during ordinary drowsiness. Moreover, theta sometimes kept on *after* the subjects stopped meditation, even when their eyes were then open.

Topographic EEG mapping methods confirm that theta predominates during zazen. In one experienced Soto Zen monk who entered a deeper stage after thirty-two minutes of zazen, alpha and theta activity predominated throughout the frontal and parietal regions. Moreover, alpha activity still occurred diffusely throughout the occipital and temporal areas even when the monk's eyes were open.[13]

Beta Activity

In their pioneering study in 1955, Das and Gastaut reported an EEG pattern that contained still faster frequencies. It appeared when their Indian yogic meditators were under the impression they were entering what they called "samadhi."[14] However, Anand and his colleagues could not confirm this finding that faster frequencies were linked to the samadhi of other subjects.[15,16] What explained the faster frequencies in the first report? The possibility was raised that they were only an artifact caused by excess tension in scalp muscles, picked up by the surface EEG electrodes.[3]

Banquet's meditators showed definite evidence of faster EEG activity in the beta range. It developed at a certain time: after they had passed beyond their "second," rhythmic theta stage of meditation.[12] At this point, his meditators pushed the button to signal that they were in the presence of their "third" stage. It was one said to be of "deep meditation or even transcendence." During this stage, their EEGs then showed beta activity at 20 cps. At first, their fast activity took the form of intermittent spindle-like bursts of beta activity interspersed between alpha or theta rhythms. Then, beta activities continuously rippled over the surface of the larger slower waves which took over and became the slow ongoing background activity.

The amplitude of this beta activity fluctuated, reaching the relatively high levels of 30 to 60 μV. It tended to appear first over the left hemisphere. Predominating anteriorly, it extended back to include all leads. A special method of computerized analysis, called compressed spectral array, showed that even faster activities were also present. These reached gamma frequencies of 40 cps. In contrast, if control subjects developed faster frequencies, they occurred at several different rates and were not as rhythmic or regular.

During this third, deeper meditative level, muscle activity recorded from the subjects' chins tended to disappear. Relaxation of the chin muscles is one important characteristic of desynchronized REM sleep. However, these subjects showed none of the typical rapid eye movements found in dreaming sleep. And it was of interest that the meditating subjects could still readily, and correctly, respond to questions by pushing their button. None of these actions changed their EEG activity during this stage.

Now, it is a noteworthy fact that these meditating subjects could send messages out of their third, deep state. This capacity resembles the way that one other group of subjects can also communicate signals to the investigator. These particular subjects are the so-called lucid dreamers. (In chapter 73 we shall find that these lucid dreamers also remain alert enough to signal their responses to the world outside even while dreaming.) Banquet's subjects showed one other important finding while in their third, deeper meditative stage. Stimuli from the outside were not "getting all the way in." An external light flash or click stimulus did not "penetrate" far enough to change their ongoing EEG. The EEG continued, as before, to show a mixture of slow and fast frequencies.

To summarize, when Banquet's subjects were in their third meditative stage they showed a distinctive pattern: (a) a particular subjective state; (b) prominent, fluctuating beta EEG activities, (c) no chin muscle activity, (d) reduced EEG responses to sensate stimuli from the outside, and (e) the ability to remain alert enough to signal out. We will find later that two of these same features correspond in key details with the present writer's experience of internal absorption (see part VI). Moreover, these same features will help us clarify the physiological mechanisms of absorption.

But not all faster EEG frequencies in the beta and gamma range need to have the same significance. One recent special EEG study of TM meditators showed that they, too, had an abrupt onset of more desynchronized EEG activity. It occurred when they thought about their mantra, and this EEG episode could last for one to two minutes.[17] Nor are increased beta frequencies specific either for some states called samadhi or for the interval when a subject concentrates on a mantra. During "touch healing," the "healer" also shows faster EEG frequencies while in the act of focusing attention of an unusual degree or kind upon the patient.[1] At this time the healer's beta rhythms increase in amplitude and have frequencies falling in the range of 25 to 33 cps. Slower beta frequencies may also increase to between 13 and 25 cps. Finally, *non*-meditators also show episodes of beta spindling when they become drowsy enough to drop off into stage 1 sleep.[3] This important point does not dilute the importance of faster frequencies. Instead, it emphasizes that there exists in the brain a natural tendency to insert moments of fast spindling activity. One of them happens to be revealed briefly during that especially dynamic interval when drowsiness yields to stage 1 sleep.

Meditation and Sleep Cycles (Continued)

Some meditators fall into deeper levels of sleep, especially when they are sleep-deprived, tired, or bored. In one study, a third of the EEG samples showed the characteristic stages of sleep 1, 2, and 3.[18] These meditators slept overtly and in brief "microsleep" episodes. One other study followed the EEG in subjects who had practiced the Jacobson form of progressive relaxation for six years. They spent 52 percent of their time in stage 1 (transitional) sleep and in stage 2 (light) sleep. In contrast, trainees who were still novices in the Jacobson method spent only 23 percent of their time in sleep, and TM meditators (with three years of experience) spent 29% of their time in sleep.[19]

In Fenwick's laboratory, almost all meditators showed the slow, rolling eye movements diagnostic of drowsiness. Many also had gross jerkings. These jerks were comparable with those seen in transitional periods when other persons are descending into sleep. These findings led the authors to suggest an important point: meditators seemed able to hold themselves at the transitional level, a level at which they were neither entirely awake nor entirely asleep.[20] Other EEG studies confirm that some experienced meditators do learn to enter and remain in a stable EEG condition, a phase intermediate between wakefulness and drowsiness, yet one during which they do not actually fall asleep.[21]

Some yogic meditators also maintain a relatively stable mixture of alpha and theta activity during meditation. They "hold on" to this mixture for as much as 80 percent of the time during a forty-minute meditation period. This led to the speculation that regular meditation was a kind of practice in developing a special skill. The skill lay in repeatedly "freezing the hypnagogic process at later and later stages (first in the predominantly alpha wave stage, later in the predominantly theta wave ranges)."[22]

But how to interpret the frequent sleep episodes? To some researchers they suggest only that meditation is simply a "low arousal state." Others would dismiss meditation as being no more effective than taking an extra nap during the day. This book will propose several alternative explanations for the fruits of meditation. Some of these proposals will cast the cyclic events of sleep in a much more creative role. Meanwhile, we can make the following plausible case for meditative training: *it is teaching the person how to reach—and hold onto—one of several abilities to attend.* Even so, the most highly trained meditators will still slip up occasionally and drift off into sleep.

The EEG and Other Tests for Lateralization of Function

Some suggest that meditation is a "right hemisphere experience." Others find no evidence, either from the EEG or from tests of performance, which would confirm such a theory.[3,23] One study reported that TM meditators activated their left hemisphere more during analytic tasks and their right hemisphere more on spatial tasks. However, simple relaxation with the eyes closed gave similar findings.[24] Moreover, long-term meditators showed no evidence that meditation had improved either their performance on tasks of a kind usually assigned to the right hemisphere, or that it had interfered with their performance on "left hemisphere tasks."[25] Reviewing the evidence available, Pagano and Warrenburg concluded that meditation does *not* shift the way the brain processes information from a mode that is primarily "linear" and left-hemispheric into an approach that is more "holistic" and right-hemispheric.[23]

Other EEG findings are also of interest. Within a period of extended meditation, the surface EEG findings can become dissociated from behavior. When such moments of noncorrespondence occur, they are significant for several reasons. Chiefly they suggest that behavior has other correlates of its own, and that these mechanisms lie much deeper in the brain than the surface EEG can reach. Noncorrespondence also provides hints about how the surface EEG might miss moments when meditation opens up quickly into brief, alternate states of consciousness. For example, one subject who fell sound asleep during meditation then showed the usual, extraslow delta EEG waves of deep sleep. But next he lost this delta activity, awakened, looked at his watch, and once again closed his eyes. Following this, his delta waves promptly reappeared. True, he had gone directly from sleep, to waking, to sleep again. On the other hand, he had not shown the usual *stepwise surface* EEG findings one expects the average subject to show when passing through the several lighter intervening stages of sleep.[18] (These successive sleep stages are pictured in figure 14.)

Similar episodes of "microawakening" and microsleep are not uncommon during meditation. In a person's topography of awareness, such micro events set up sharp cliffs or plunge into deep valleys. Their steep sides inform us that the meditator tends to rise up abruptly, or drop down, through many physiological layers. Ordinarily, the cliff edges are rounded off, and such transitions evolve relatively slowly during intervals that last for many seconds or minutes. But suppose the brain passes suddenly through its transition periods. This could open up more opportunities for the shearing off, as it were, of adjacent aggregates of functions. During meditation, some unstable fragments of physiological mechanisms seem to be briefly "loosened," and are then available to recombine in new, unexpected ways.

22

Breathing In; Breathing Out

> One of the basic tenets of meditation is the notion that passive awareness is a natural, elementary, and direct form of experience that is ordinarily overwhelmed and obscured by the activity of the mind. The purpose of meditation, therefore, is to allow the mind to become quiet and thereby uncover the capacity for this experience.
>
> M. Schuman[1]

Can breathing help uncover our capacity for direct experience? You might not think so. After all, breathing is automatic. We constantly inhale and exhale. Yet this whole chapter will be devoted to breathing. Why? Because breathing is an excellent example of the intimate relationships between psyche and soma, brain and body. The way we breathe not only becomes a central focus in zazen, it also gives us a sensitive, reliable index of how our emotional life influences the rhythmic workings of our brain stem.[2,3]

The brain stem is that stalk at the base of the brain made up of medulla, pons, and midbrain (see figures 2 and 3). The medulla is its lowest segment. Here we keep track of those chemical signals in the bloodstream—low oxygen and high carbon dioxide—that drive us to breathe more. From the medulla, impulses flow down the spinal cord and out through peripheral nerves to contract the muscles of the rib cage and diaphragm. The chest expands, the diaphragm descends. All this translates into breathing *in*.

Then, as the lungs expand, their stretch receptors become increasingly taut. This sends signals up the vagus nerves to inform the brain stem. There they generate a flurry of inhibition, which turns inhalation off. Finally, as we start to breathe out, much of our exhalation proceeds passively, driven by the elastic recoil from the chest and abdomen.

One other factor dampens inspiration: the proprioceptive messages that return from our lower abdominal muscles. We are not consciously aware of most of these impulses, yet they too ascend to inhibit the medulla and to turn off inspiration.[4] Note what happens in zazen. The meditator trains bare conscious attention to focus on these faint up-and-down breathing movements in the lower abdomen, the *tanden*.

The boatman times his "yo ho heave ho!" cry. Its end coincides with his strongest pull. Martial arts trainees also exhale and shout during their most vigorous movements. But singing tends to be overlooked. We forget how *chanting—* that great prolonged communal exhalation—also brings exhalation into the formal practice of group meditation. Chanting and other breathing techniques prolong expiration, and they create slightly higher pressures within the lungs and abdomen. In this manner such practices may further increase the inhibitory tone of the vagus nerves, and do so in subtle ways that further reduce respiratory drive within the brain stem.

Using respiration as our model, we will examine changes in respiration that illustrate three basic ways in which local physiological functions can be changed in the brain. In simple terms, these involve (1) excitation or stimulation; (2) inhibition, cooling, or damage; and (3) release of excitation from prior inhibition.

It turns out that very small regions in the medulla serve specific respiratory functions. In animals, one can cause shallow inspirations by cooling the upper ventral medulla. The inhibition from this cooling reduces its local functions.[5] In contrast, expiration is prolonged by cooling only one side of the *lower* ventral medulla. Inhibiting this lower region does not change the depth of inspiration, nor does it suspend breathing. However, it is not unusual for neurologists to find that strokes which damage the mid to lower part of the pons also stop their patients' breathing for many seconds at a time. Indeed, a small stroke sometimes markedly reduces respiration, even though it may seem to involve only one side of the lower brain stem.[6]

Once when I was in the laboratory in Kyoto, and not at all mindful of such facts about breathing, I observed a curious phenomenon. At the time, I was performing pharmacology experiments on cats and was monitoring the field potentials of several larger groups of nerve cells throughout the brain. As I looked at all these discharges, I became puzzled. Every few seconds, the firing waxed, then waned. The resulting wave forms were a series of peaks and troughs. Why did they follow a regular rhythm? Why were the rhythmical firings at sites higher in the limbic system synchronous with those of other cell groups down in the brain stem? Further observation provided a simple explanation. Every time the cat breathed *in*, its nerve cells fired much more. Every time the cat breathed *out*, these discharges slacked off. *Breathing out was quieting the brain.* Lesser degrees of this same phenomenon have since been observed in the human amygdala and hippocampus.[7]

The human pupil is another index of similar rhythmic changes. Again, *inspiration is the activating mode.* Breathe in and your pupil dilates slightly; breathe out and it constricts. If you inhale deeper and exhale further, you will create extra wide swings in the dilatation and constriction of your pupils.[8] Still other rhythms are superimposed on the intrinsic beat of respiration itself. We tend to breathe faster every ninety minutes or so, and some lesser rhythms recur every thirty to sixty minutes or so.[9]

Well-trained meditators dampen their breathing in several ways. Some will slow their respirations to as low as four or six per minute. They also reduce the overall volume of air they breathe, lengthen their exhalations, and increase the extent of their abdominal breathing. Akishige found this out when he studied six Rinzai Zen monks who had meditated an average of eleven years. During ordinary quiet sitting they averaged only six breaths a minute. At rest, most of us breathe two to three times faster. During zazen, his monks did breathe slightly faster: eight per minute. Four Soto Zen monks, who averaged twenty-one years of practice, started with an average resting respiratory rate of nineteen. Their rate fell to sixteen during zazen.[10]

Normally, we spend slightly less time breathing in (43 percent) than breathing out. When the monks merely sat quietly, they spent less time than this in their inspiratory phase. But during zazen, their time in inspiration fell even further. Now it consumed a mere one-quarter of the whole breathing cycle.

So, the major change during formal zazen was that the monks now spent much more time breathing *out*—about three-quarters of their respiratory cycle. Indeed, the distinctive finding was that these monks were always prolonging their expiratory phase, both during the simple act of sitting quietly and during their formal periods of sitting in meditation.

Why did the two groups of monks breathe at different *rates?* It was speculated that they had used different techniques to train their breathing. These particular Rinzai monks had been trained to breathe softly—so softly that they did not ruffle a single hair in a tuft of rabbit fur attached to their nose(!). Monks of the Soto sect had it easier. They had allowed respiration to take its own course. However, neither group of monks appeared to have prolonged their expiratory phase solely on the basis of conscious training efforts. Rather, their introspective reports suggested that these longer expirations had evolved naturally during zazen.[11]

The expiratory pause is the final phase at the end of one cycle of breathing in and out. In this pause, no expiratory movements take place. Which of our basic human emotions shows an increase during this pause? Only tenderness. In contrast, fear lengthens the phase of inspiration and increases the amplitude of breathing.[2] In general, states of tension increase chest breathing; relaxation favors abdominal breathing. Akishige's subjects found that abdominal breathing was easier to perform in the half-lotus position. Abdominal breathing was less successful if the meditator, say, sat cross-legged with the buttocks resting on the floor, or sat upright on folded knees with the buttocks resting on the heels.[12]

When both brain and body quiet down, less oxygen is needed. When monks slow their breathing rates to only four breaths a minute, each of these breaths contains an increased tidal volume of air, for a total volume of 3.2 to 4.4 liters per minute. Even so, this total volume is still substantially less than the volume of air that normal controls breathe at rest: around 6 liters a minute.

Parenthetically, not only monks, but cats too can be trained to prolong their expiration. In the cat, each prolonged expiration inhibits not only many of the single inspiratory nerve cells in the medulla which are influenced by respiration but other nerve cells there as well.[13] The flow of air along the nasal passages also influences the brain, because air flow stimulates nasal nerve endings. These stimuli go on to induce a rhythmical 40 CPS activity up in the olfactory bulb, which is the higher extension of the central nervous system overlying the nasal passages.[14] When slow meditative breathing reduces the volume of air flow, it also reduces the discharges of nerve cells in the bulb. In summary, then, *whenever we breathe more quietly and prolong the phase of expiration, we are probably quieting the firing activity of many nerve cells, both in the medulla and above.*

Several meditative traditions refer to periods during which thoughts drop out of consciousness. In the TM tradition, some of these episodes are described using such terms as "pure consciousness" or "transcendental consciousness." They are also viewed as being concrete experiences of pure abstraction having no mental boundaries. In recent decades, these brief moments of clarity were found to coincide with periods of apnea, in which breathing stops. In 1982, a study of forty TM subjects yielded a total of 565 such episodes.[15] These subjects also breathed relatively slowly, even when they were not experiencing pure consciousness. Yet, why should their breathing *stop?*

Breathing stopped abruptly, and these temporary episodes were not followed by compensatory over-breathing. In actual fact, all air flow did *not* cease. A little flow continued, at a very low amplitude, fluttering between two and seven times per second. Some episodes ended with breathing in, others with breathing out. In this report, an average episode of breath suspension lasted nineteen seconds; the longest, thirty-one seconds.

Subjects who were most experienced in TM had more episodes of breath suspension. Some, but not all, of these episodes coincided with the experience termed "pure consciousness." In one accomplished subject, breathing paused during the expiratory phase. The pause was at a point midway between the usual two peak tides of inhalation and exhalation. In this subject, episodes of pure consciousness then lasted an average of eighteen seconds. They occurred frequently: about every fifty-two seconds.

Scalp EEG recordings have been performed. In the TM subjects reported in 1982, the amplitudes of theta waves increased. Theta peaked sharply at the *start* of the periods of breath suspension, and then decreased quickly at the offset of each episode. Fast EEG activity might also occur occasionally before the episode but not during it. In contrast, frequent bursts of faster beta activity might occur *after* the end of the period of pure consciousness. At this later time the faster waves often coincided with a subtle instability in the peripheral autonomic nervous system. Then, the phasic skin resistance became unstable and basal skin resistance fell abruptly.

However, just before these subjects entered the episodes of pure consciousness, the measured levels of most other *peripheral* physiological functions were about the same as they were during the episode itself. So, what caused the episodes? Some covert events—not yet identified—must have converged in the *central* nervous system. These events appeared to have set the stage for that kind of early mental experience which in Zen might be called moments of "no-thought." In the 1982 report, the external reflections of these covert internal events included a high degree of coherence in the EEG, mostly in theta and alpha frequencies; a high amplitude of theta activity; a low amplitude of delta and beta EEG activities; a stable phasic skin resistance; and a high basal skin resistance. Later during each episode, several of these indices started to reverse themselves.

Some different findings were observed in the recent (1997) study of sixteen TM students.[16] Their breathing was suspended for an average of only eight seconds. Moreover, in this group, the most reliable correlates were a decrease in heart rate and an increase in skin conductance responses. In contrast, the EEG changes in these subjects were less consistent and were evident chiefly as alpha activity presenting throughout the frontal-central-parietal leads.

Note: such brief, clear, and quietly aware moments are not merely the typical normal drowsy prelude to sleep. Instead, when we are drowsy, the signs are shallow abdominal breathing, slow mentation and reaction times, and flatter alpha waves in our EEG.[17] Nor can anyone produce such moments of mental clarity *voluntarily* by choosing to hold the breath.[18]

These studies of TM subjects link clear, thought-free consciousness with two quite different sets of physiological evidence. The most impressive of these events suspends respiratory drive and causes a relative hypoventilation. The second cluster of associated findings are more subtle and variable. They include peripheral autonomic changes and tendencies toward increased EEG coherence. It is of interest that coherence can extend over a broad area and might involve a range of alpha-theta (and later beta) frequencies. These observations hint that no single tiny, sharply localized spot is generating the thought-free episodes.

Instead, the moments of clarity appear to stem from a series of linked physiological changes. To help explain both their quality and the widespread EEG correlates, we will begin by dropping a suggestion here, the evidence for which will be developed further in part III. Simply stated, this no-thought clarity is what might be expected to occur when a person shifts certain functions within the deep and *centrally located* recesses of the brain.

Most studies of meditation have approached the less fruitful edges of the larger central problem. Not so these TM studies of breath suppression and no-thought clarity. These pioneering studies, while not yet completed, focus our attention on a core issue: meditation opens up surprising gaps in thought, intervals that might last a quarter of a minute or so. Obviously, they invite hypotheses and stimulate further research.

For example: suppose that further training could enable such moments to become longer and deeper. Would they then help create the kind of larger gap through which major absorptions—even insights—could surge? And this is not to overlook the remarkable paradox: how could a person's brain *do* these two things at the same time? How could it (1) suspend so vital a function as breathing? Yet (2) leave the subject still able to perceive—in clear awareness—a mental landscape free of thoughts? It suffices here to introduce four mechanisms and to cite other potential contributions as well.

The first mechanism centers around the fact that respiration *stops*. This implies that the sensitivities are greatly reduced in those basic circuits, first mentioned above, that normally drive our respirations. It suggests that the brain stem may itself have become relatively unresponsive to its usual sources of stimulation (either neural or chemical). In fact, other studies have found that TM meditators were *less* stimulated than were average subjects by the very strenuous respiratory stimulus of breathing extra carbon dioxide. This result helps explain why the subjects whose breathing stopped did not then engage in compensatory over-breathing. And incidentally, it provides further confirmation that meditation does reduce central respiratory drive.[19]

Is respiration suspended during each successive state encountered in Zen training? (See tables 10 and 11.) We don't know. If it were, it would be difficult to pinpoint any particular site as solely responsible for this suspension. Because, in the brain stem alone, each breath—in and out—reflects a series of oscillating rhythms. Countless cells are integrating their discharges, acting at different levels. During any single respiratory cycle, inspiration and expiration are so well-coordinated that each component of the pair phases in and out at precisely the right time.[20,21] Moreover, respiratory impulses are subject to a variety of influences as they descend from the lower medulla into the spinal cord.[22]

The second mechanism also begins with the medulla. But it focuses on the ways the medulla's ascending pathways rise to change still other functions at higher levels. The lesson I learned from observing cat brains in Kyoto was that their rhythms of breathing go on to resonate through many higher regions. Among them is the central nucleus of the amygdala (see figure 3). Here, nerve cells fire measurably *less* whenever breathing is quieter and when expiration is prolonged.[23] This reduced firing in the amygdala could itself contribute to physiological calming.[24] We will see in part III how pivotal is the role of the amygdala in generating emotional valences within the limbic system. So, what happens when well-trained meditators not only breathe quietly but also prolong expiration? These two factors may contribute to those long moments when their thoughts and emotions, either positive or negative, become much less resonant.

A third mechanism may enter in. An average person can learn to dampen emotions by paying mindful attention to slow respirations. In one experiment, male college students were placed under the imminent threat of receiving an electric shock to the hand. One group was instructed to self-regulate their breathing. Their goal was to pay specific attention to their breathing in order to maintain it at the slow rate of only eight breaths per minute. Despite their being placed under psychological duress, this mindful group stayed at a lower arousal level than did their controls. The evidence for this was threefold: they reported lower levels of subjective anxiety, and they had correspondingly less change in their skin resistance and finger pulse volume.[25]

A fourth set of mechanisms might contribute to change, simultaneously, both breathing and consciousness. The factors involved also reflect inhibitory events, *first* taking place lower in the brain stem, but going on *secondarily* to release awareness functions at still higher levels. For example, many studies show that morphine and its related opioids also dampen respirations.[26] Some aspects of a brief slowing might, therefore, reflect a selective, local inhibitory pulse of the brain's own opioids.[27] (See chapter 47.) Moreover, a pulse of serotonin can also suppress respiration when released at the terminals of ST cells of the raphe magnus in the upper medulla.[28] Could similar transient inhibitions (whatever caused them) occurring at local sites in the mid pons or lower pons, also enhance awareness by releasing acetylcholine from *its* nerve cells still higher in the pons? (See chapter 38.)

All the evidence required to support this particular mechanism for heightened awareness is not yet in. (See chapters 37 and 71.) However, it appears that parts of the medulla and lower pons normally hold in check certain of our higher mechanisms of arousal and awareness. So, as meditation increasingly inhibits the respiratory drive, and as other brief local inhibitory pulses are superimposed on its own localized calming effects, this combination could overcome the usual restraints imposed from lower levels, releasing awareness circuitries at successively higher levels. Perhaps such an abrupt release from prior inhibition might help explain why some of the autonomic correlates of breath suppression[16] resemble those seen when the brain orients to significant stimuli. (See chapter 36.)

Stimulating the midbrain reticular formation itself causes alerting. However, it also produces other changes of the kind that occur in anxiety. The stimulated animal breathes faster and shortens its expiratory phase.[29] So it does not seem likely that activating the *whole* midbrain reticular formation would prompt a human meditator to go into episodes of *no* breathing plus a quiet, thought-free hyperawareness. Even if only certain of its parts were stimulated selectively, the rest of the midbrain would still need to be uncoupled from these usual excitatory influences which normally tend to drive the breathing cycle.

This discussion emphasizes that quiet meditation sometimes releases remarkable levels of clear awareness, coupled with breath suspension. But several paradoxes remain. For instance, if we are to regard some brief moments of breath and thought suspension as shallow preludes to absorptions, then we must also clarify how still deeper absorptions could shift past this awareness into a major *hyper*awareness.

So, it is not too soon to begin to ask: could one further source of such heightened levels of awareness begin up somewhere near the "ergotropic triangle"? (This energizing region, to be discussed in chapter 43, lies just above the midbrain.) The triangle becomes of more than general interest to us now, because next to it lie several other noteworthy sites. And these are well-known to *suppress* breathing when they are stimulated. For example, Hess could slow the rate of breathing and produce shallow breathing when he stimulated the local region where the hypothalamus receives the fornix.[30] Brief stimuli delivered to the anterior thalamic nucleus in humans also markedly reduces the amplitude of their breathing for a minute or more.[31] Moreover, patients who receive deep electrical stimulation at other intriguing sites also stop breathing, and for long periods. These other higher regions include the orbital prefrontal cortex, the limbic system sites it interconnects with, and the ventral lateral thalamus (see figure 3). In these stimulated patients, breathing stops during the inspiratory phase and is held there.[32] One may hope that future research might be directed toward meditating subjects who, fortuitously, have had depth electrodes already in place for some unrelated medical indication. Depth recordings could help clarify which levels interact to cause these intriguing links between no-thoughts, clear consciousness, and breath suppression.

Meanwhile, we go on breathing. How casually we assume that one breath follows another! But this present chapter on how we breathe will have alerted us. Likewise, many other basic aspects of Zen experience will soon begin to interrelate in intriguing ways with psychophysiological events, again in regions deep along the central axis of the brain.

The Effects of Sensorimotor Deprivation

> When the senses and thought are annihilated, all the passages to Mind are blocked, and no entrance then becomes possible. The original mind is to be recognized along with the working of the senses and thoughts, only it does not belong to them, nor is it independent of them. Do not build up your views on your senses and thoughts . . . but at the same time do not seek the Mind away from your senses and thoughts.
>
> Master Huang-po (d. 850 A.D.)[1]

These early words of caution from Huang-po are not doubletalk. Back in the Tang dynasty, he was already stressing the critical point as clearly as translation allows: you don't become enlightened by closing off your senses and by blotting out all thinking processes. Still, we have just noted that meditative training does seem to "quiet" at least some of the brain. So couldn't meditation "simply" be a kind of sensory deprivation?

Yes and no. For one thing, "sensory" deprivation is not simple. Nor is it all sensory. But Zen meditative training does point toward a major simplification: you let go of your busy cognitive landscape, and limit your attention to the breathing movements of the lower abdomen. The result? Now you're minimizing the future-oriented cerebrations of the frontal lobes. Disappearing along with them are the corollary impulses from your sensory association and limbic motivational systems. Visual input falls when your eyelids are half-closed and the eyes are positioned slightly downward. A silent environment reduces auditory input as well. When these factors combine, your meditative awareness becomes free to shift toward simpler perceptions, into those contributed more directly by your brainstem, thalamic, and parietal lobe circuitry.

Then, too, you don't move in zazen. And the added muscle relaxation itself goes on to have secondary effects. The drug gallamine triethiodide (Flaxedil) stops muscles from contracting. As a result, the EEG becomes more synchronized, and the level of vigilance falls.[2] In other animal experiments, curare has been used to paralyze the calf muscles. Even so, some stretch receptors still function within this lax muscle. These receptors continue to send signals if the paralyzed leg is stretched. And these muscle stretch signals are then strong enough to cause cortical EEG arousal. This set of studies suggests that the brain's arousal level depends to some degree on how much stimulation it keeps receiving from the tonic proprioceptive (self-informing) messages which flow back up into it when the muscles, joints, and tendons move. So whenever you stop moving, and stretching, it contributes further to the total sensate deficit. As a result of this mechanism, both sensory deprivation and meditation cause a noteworthy drop in the feedback of proprioceptive signals that can enter the brain. This implies that less stimulation enters from the eyes, face, tongue, jaw, neck, trunk, and all four limbs.

So there is more to zazen meditation than sensory deprivation. Sitting without moving means *both sensory and motor deprivation*. Restless energies build up, urges previously discharged in various movements. To clarify the mechanisms of meditation, it helps to review how much has been learned from studying the other, experimental forms of what we will here call sensorimotor deprivation, or SMD. The analogies prove useful even though SMD differs from zazen.

To cite one example of the differences: during Zen meditative retreats, one interrupts the relatively short periods of zazen and inserts periods of motor *activity*. These interruptions differ from the way researchers conduct their typical long, so-called sensory deprivation experiments.[3] However, zazen and SMD are similar in the way each provides a "depatterning" environment. This means a setting that cuts down both the amount of incoming stimuli and the patterns by which the brain lends significance to them.[4]

In SMD experiments, the subjects lie quietly. Their vision and hearing are blocked. Padded cuffs about the hands and feet reduce their joint movements and the tactile stimuli to the skin. Clearly, it is "unphysiological" to be so confined, let alone to have to sit or lie down for many hours. Not surprisingly, many persons find SMD painfully boring. Their thoughts skip around, and they can't stick to any one topic. They can vividly recall the visual aspects of their memories, but their intellectual performance drops.[5] When they finally get up to move around, they are sluggish, speak slowly, can't actively manipulate ideas or readily invent short stories.

But suppose these SMD subjects are allowed intermittent exercise and are provided with meaningful information. Now they suffer fewer cognitive defects from being physically immobilized. Again, *perceptual* deprivation (in which the sensate input is limited to diffused light and to white noise) reduces their test performance more so than does simple sensory deprivation (silence and darkness). The major drop in task performance occurs during the first twenty-four hours if the experiments last for several days. Thereafter, the subjects learn to adapt. Over the course of repeated sessions, their performance improves slightly.

Certain other functions improve during SMD, not decline. In one study, for example, SMD subjects were perceptually deprived for only fifty minutes, an interval comparable with some extra long zazen periods. In this instance, as words flashed by, they recognized more words than did control subjects, even though they had been exposed to the words for a shorter time.[6] After seventy-two hours of SMD, hearing becomes more sensitive. The subjects react faster to signals on vigilance tasks and miss fewer of them. Long hours of sensory deprivation also enhance touch, pain, and taste sensitivities. Even visual deprivation *alone* improves touch and pain sensitivities. It also increases auditory discrimination and heightens the sensitivities to smell and taste. These improvements continue for as long as a day *after* the deprivation ends. There is no truth in claims implying that meditation itself confers unique benefits in this regard.

During certain types of SMD experiments, the subjects can request bits of information. The longer they had been deprived of stimuli, the more fresh information they request. What do they seek out? *Meaningful* sequences of stimuli. They don't want simple words or mere noises. The nature of this search helps understand something crucial about the changes that evolve during long meditative retreats. For retreats and SMD share one other phenomenon. *Both extend the same general search for meaning in ways which probe topics at deeper existential levels.*

The universal search for existential meaning asserts itself gradually. The way the search phenomenon evolves is well illustrated in a recent study of SMD subjects. They had volunteered to be immersed in the quiet warmth of water tanks.[7] Tank isolation isolates subjects comfortably from most external stimuli. After repeated sessions the subjects finally drop off notions about their physical self-image and its relationships. Their thinking then evolves. They start to think about new ways they can relate to other persons. They develop new orientations toward larger issues of context, not content. They discover how inherently ambiguous it is to define "self" in terms of the usual, fixed, physical boundaries of self/other, inside/outside. Continuing to focus on this ambiguity, they then recognize how artificial was the manner in which they had earlier defined their self-identity. At this point they start seeing things afresh—"not new landscapes, but with new eyes . . ."

After having undergone many prolonged courses of profound isolation in the tank, a few persons will then go on to "gradual learning, slow conceptual drift, durable long-term change, and an occasional surprising revelation."[7] Along the way, they also experience many sensate phenomena and affective responses. To these, no special religious significance can be attached.[6] Likewise, Zen deemphasizes the hallucinations and other side effects that occur in association with zazen.

In general, several kinds of visual phenomena arise during SMD. Sometimes they intrude when the subject is alert, at other times during drowsiness. After SMD experiments that last only eight hours, vision becomes distorted more when the subjects are deprived of *patterned* stimuli than when all sensory stimuli are cut off per se. Some positive visual images pop in which represent "luminous dust," "idioretinal sensations," or "phosphenes." These indicate that nerve cells in our large visual brain still go on actively generating spontaneous lights, patterns, shapes, and forms, even in complete darkness.

"Luminous dust" can account for a few vague visual phenomena that enter during SMD or during drowsiness. But it will not explain the highly organized, formed, visual hallucinations that suddenly appear in SMD already full-blown. Some researchers soften this word. They refer to their subjects' hallucinations under the generic phrase "reported visual sensations." (This catchall term is reminiscent of another noncommittal phrase, "unidentified flying objects" or UFOs.)

Most hallucinations are brief, impersonal, and have no psychodynamic significance.[6] Others start with simple, unstructured, meaningless sensations that then evolve in a more complex, structured, meaningful way. After five to eight hours of SMD, many images show vivid colors and striking details. These seem compatible with the kinds of "quickenings" described as typical hypnagogic or hypnopompic hallucinations (see part V). SMD will release, for the first time, otherwise typical hypnagogic images in subjects who never have seen them before.[8] It will also provoke more of them in subjects who had experienced them before.[9] In keeping with the way hallucinations tend to enter during transition periods, the SMD subjects frequently cannot decide whether they are awake or asleep at the time.

The research in SMD was furthered by two concerns that arose during the Cold War. One concern was prompted by the methods used to isolate prisoners before they "confessed" during the Communist purge trials in the USSR. The other concern grew out of the brainwashing techniques that the Chinese military employed on prisoners during the Korean War. These left the impression that solitary confinement plus drugs could cause almost anyone to "change their mind" and "confess." But sensory deprivation is *not* the same as brainwashing. The techniques of brainwashing that interrogators used during the Korean War hinged on degrees of *over*stimulation. Many prisoners never submitted. Those who did often recanted when it was safe to do so.

Meditative situations differ strikingly from SMD experiments and from brainwashing. In zazen, solitude is sought out voluntarily, in a religious context, and in the company of other like-minded persons. True, SMD can make the person more suggestible to perceptions of external influences. It can also make some persons, of relatively low intelligence, more susceptible to propaganda. However, in *normals*, SMD techniques do not reinforce a message that these subjects are better persons.

How does SMD exert its effects? No major changes appear in standard EEG leads once the subjects have already become adapted to their earlier SMD experiences.[10] Still, subjects respond differently. Some of them will normally have depended more on the presence of outside visual cues, using such cues to tell themselves precisely which position they occupied in three-dimensional space. These particular subjects will show more EEG arousal, tending to have relatively more beta and relatively less alpha activities. Others will have relied more heavily on interoceptive cues, meaning those entering from muscle, joint, tendon, and vestibular systems. These subjects will become less aroused. Short-term SMD studies show no consistent pattern of circulatory, respiratory, or muscular changes. However, the data vary among different laboratories, not unlike those from studies performed on meditating subjects.

Human subjects must also lie very quietly during their neuroimaging studies to make it possible to measure brain metabolism. In a sense, they are undergoing a short-term variation on the theme of SMD. One such imaging technique is called PET scanning   positron emission tomography.[11] (The color plate presents a sample PET scan.) PET studies show that brain metabolism stays relatively higher in the frontal regions when normal subjects are in their usual so-called "resting" states. And, when both eyes and ears remain open, metabolism is approximately equal in the two hemispheres.[12] When the eyes alone are open, metabolism increases more in the deeper occipital cortex next to the midline than it does over the lateral cortex. Blocking either the eyes or the ears reduces the brain's local metabolic rate. When both are covered, metabolism drops still further. Typically, this drop occurs more in the *right* cerebral hemisphere than in the left.[13]

SMD blunts the way humans respond to drugs. Even two hours of preparatory SMD minimizes LSD's effects. It reduces both the subjective symptoms and the changes which LSD would otherwise produce in standard physiological measures such as heart rate, respiration, or EEG. When subjects are first isolated and then given the powerful drug phencyclidine ("angel dust"), their subjective responses to it are greatly reduced or absent.[10] On the other hand, some persons who had already used LSD previously will report that they respond to it more during SMD. Given the population sampled, it is not clear how much their comments might reflect primary personality and other physiological variables or some acquired sense of freedom in reporting unusual experiences.[14]

Some persons withdraw prematurely from SMD because they find the conditions too stressful. These subjects, during their baseline studies, tend to be the ones who excrete abnormally low levels of epinephrine in their urine. Therefore, persons who can't stick it out for the duration of SMD may begin by differing biochemically—and perhaps in other constitutional ways—from those who do.

When animals are placed in solitary confinement, isolated for weeks and months, their situation bears a remote resemblance to that of hermits. There are secondary consequences to this less active, less stimulating social life. The brain changes biochemically. Young rats isolated from one another for thirteen weeks remain behaviorally active. However, biogenic amine levels fall in the limbic system. Norepinephrine levels and norepinephrine turnover drop both in the hippocampus and in the central amygdaloid nucleus. Dopamine also falls in the central amygdala.[15]

In conclusion, sensorimotor deprivation changes the brain experientially, physiologically, and biochemically. It does so in ways germane to meditation and meditative states, but it does not provide an exact model for meditation.

24

Monks and Clicks: Habituation

Although the many psychophysiological studies have drawn a fairly consistent portrait of the physiology during some meditative states, in our opinion they have contributed relatively little to a meaningful understanding of states of consciousness during meditation.

David Becker and David Shapiro[1]

The statement above is an accurate interpretation of the literature. Why do we still know so little about meditative states? To understand, it helps to begin with a specific issue in research: the way normal subjects respond when they listen to the recurring sound stimulus of a click. At first, each click causes them to drop out their alpha waves. This is a temporary phenomenon known as "alpha blocking." But suppose you keep repeating the same clicks monotonously. Soon, each repeated stimulus no longer causes alpha blocking. The brain has finally "gotten used to" the stimulus. This phenomenon is called *habituation*. It implies that an organism will tune out any habitual stimulus found not to have important consequences.

It might seem that the meditative approach called mindfulness or "opening up" meditation would be just the reverse of habituation. For it implies staying so sensitized, so receptive, that each stimulus seems new, fresh, and important. Theoretically, meditators who practiced mindfulness meditation would keep reacting to each click. Theoretically, each stimulus would keep blocking alpha, and they would not habituate.

At first, this theory gathered impressive supporting evidence. Hirai reported that experienced Soto Zen monks did not tune out repeated clicks during meditation.[2] Instead, their alpha waves kept on being repeatedly blocked by the click. This implied that the monks did not habituate. In addition, the monks reported afterward that, though they clearly perceived each click stimulus, the simulus did not appear to disturb them.

But artificial clicks, pure tones, or modulated tones are poor substitutes for natural physiological stimuli.[3] A way around this is to test subjects by letting them hear meaningful names. Names of their spouse or of their children are distracting stimuli, and stop their alpha waves at first. Gradually, however, normals also habituate to each distracting name, just as they do to clicks. In contrast, Hirai reported that when some Zen monks were meditating they did not habituate their alpha waves to names. Names repeatedly blocked their alpha waves. Again, afterward, the monks reported that they heard each name during meditation. Moreover, they correctly identified each name precisely, but they then made no further associations to it.

It seemed, therefore, that while they were meditating, these Zen monks retained both their keen perception and their EEG responsiveness. They registered auditory stimuli briefly, but the stimuli did not set off further trains of associations. Hirai summarized this meditative state as one of "relaxed awareness with steady responsiveness." The monks seemed to be reacting quickly, reflexly, not referring a stimulus on for whatever "judgment" of cogency or of affective valence would lead them finally to tune it out when it was repeated. Such an interpretation evoked the image of a brain which had become physiologically open, nonjudgmental. It was just the kind of continuous alpha blocking one might have expected after long training in a no-minded form of bare awareness.

But earlier studies of Raja Yoga meditators[45] and of TM meditators[6] had reported that *no* alpha blocking occurred after stimuli were repeated. These other reports of no alpha blocking during other forms of meditation raised two important possibilities. Perhaps sensory stimuli did not get in to block alpha waves during yogic meditation, because the sensate messages had stopped somewhere below the cortical level (if not lower).[7] Perhaps, on the other hand, the particular Zen monks Hirai had studied were deploying their attention in a different way. Perhaps they were in a special meditative mode that enabled sensate messages from the outside environment still to register, but thereafter not to go on to be reacted to *emotionally*. It will turn out subsequently, in part VI, that the first of these possibilities does afford a plausible explanation for the sensate loss during the internal absorption of samadhi. In contrast, the second mechanism may be relevant to those more advanced levels of training which allow meditation either to plumb deeper levels or to influence stages which represent the residues of an ongoing enlightenment (see part VIII).

The Japanese Zen monks studied in Hirai's research had undergone many years of monastic practice.[2] The fact that they also meditated with their eyes open and had been studied with certain of the earlier EEG techniques qualifies how readily one can generalize such findings to other meditators studied elsewhere. Indeed, it had already become clear that what kind of stimulus was used and how it was presented would critically alter the results when humans and animals were tested for habituation.[8]

One noteworthy finding was that, while sleeping, subjects reduced habituation to the sound of a tone. Hence, hypotheses derived from studies of normal waking subjects could not be transferred to the way they might respond to stimuli when they had entered slow-wave sleep or were dreaming.[9] Of particular note was the evidence that subjects who had entered REM sleep made no clear EEG response to the stimuli used, nor did stimuli presented during REM sleep cause habituation of either their heart rate response or their finger pulse response. Moreover, habituation studies in general gave inconsistent results, even when the stimulus parameters were well defined.

Later, Becker and Shapiro performed a carefully controlled study of how meditators responded physiologically to clicks during meditation.[1] It turned out that the way control subjects habituated was about the same as that of *eyes-closed* Zen meditators (who averaged seven and a half years of practice), of yoga meditators (averaging five years), and of TM meditators (averaging seven years). Instead of showing differences from controls, each group of meditating subjects habituated their alpha EEG rhythms and skin conductance responses at about the same rate. The Soto Zen meditators were engaged in "just sitting" while they meditated for 30 minutes. The subjects in one control group were asked to attend to the click stimuli; those in the other were asked to ignore them.

Such a major failure to replicate previous studies is important. It poses a problem for those who would otherwise prefer to think that something very special goes on when an advanced trainee meditates, something which enables repeated stimuli not to cause habituation of the alpha blocking response. On the other hand, when some meditators are surrounded by technically sophisticated equipment in a laboratory, they may find it difficult to reach the depths of meditation. So even this 1981, eyes-closed, report[1] does not fully address the hypothesis to be developed further in this book: when meditation *does* shift into the rarer moments of *internal absorption,* clicks should not then interrupt the EEG. The explanation to be proposed is that the brain will have blocked these and other external stimuli from having entered at the subcortical level.

One can only look forward to some future study of monks in Japan who (a) have clearly passed all criteria for an advanced degree of ongoing enlightenment; (b) have maintained their zazen practice, with eyes partially open, at a very high level for more than a decade; (c) are thoroughly adapted to the highly artificial conditions of the experiment; and (d) can be studied while they reliably and reproducibly enter states of deep absorption.

One might think that studies of evoked potentials would help clarify meditation (see chapter 64). Indeed they would, if the potentials happened to drop out during a period of internal absorption while recordings were being continuously monitored. However, varying levels of attention and distraction themselves change the height of evoked potentials. So, too, does sleep. This creates problems in interpreting evoked potentials. In one study of TM practitioners who had two to four years of experience, the evoked potentials varied only slightly. However, they did vary substantially from one meditative session to another and were independent of whatever stage the EEG was in at the time. Meanwhile, one is left nodding in full agreement with Paty and colleagues who concluded that "The relationships between changes of consciousness and electrocortical activities must, therefore, be interpreted with much prudence."[10,11]

25

The Koan and Sanzen: Kyoto, 1974

Unwilling to disregard greed and anger,
You trouble yourself in vain to read the
Buddhist Teachings.
You see the prescription, but don't take the medicine—
How then can you do away with your illness!

Layman P'ang (740–808)[1]

My only fear is that a little gain will suffice you.

Master Hakuin (1685–1768)[2]

It is now a few weeks after I began formal sitting in the meditation hall at Ryoko-in. The roshi is starting to conduct his brief private interviews, called *sanzen* in the Rinzai tradition. These take place during the second of the three morning meditation periods. They are devoted mostly to problems the trainee is having in practice. Just before entering his chamber, you kneel and pick up a small wooden mallet. Your next task is not easy. It is to announce your presence by striking two authentic notes on a small bronze bell. The roshi, having listened to the bell and observed your subsequent bowings, prostrations, and behavior, knows only too well exactly where you are in your practice. He conducts the interview with all seriousness, and with gradually increasing formality and firmness, especially during the meditative retreats called *sesshin*.

At my first sanzen, he focuses on breathing correctly. "Are you breathing down in your lower abdomen? Are you breathing *out* on 'one'? Are you really *concentrating* on 'one'? Not on the idea of 'one,' but on the *total* reality of it?" I have not consistently done any of these. Heal thyself, physician, I mutter to myself on the way out.

By the second sanzen things are better. Thoughts are much less of a problem, and so it is with misplaced optimism that I now ask for a koan to work on. I have no idea what to expect. He says, "When every phenomenon is reduced to one, then where is that one reduced to?"

My brain reels! My gaze shifts away. What on *earth* did this mean? He waits until my gaze returns, and then looks at me directly, saying, "Not what, not why or how. Not when, but *where* is that one?" I am utterly baffled.

Seeing my bewilderment, he rephrases it slightly: "When all things return to the one, *where* is the one returned to?" This sounds vaguely better, but it still means absolutely nothing. "Because you are a scholar," he continues, "you will try to concentrate on this koan using your mind and your knowledge. It won't work. You must take the koan inside yourself and penetrate it. This is no small thing; it is a major undertaking. You must concentrate on your koan everywhere, but take care not to do so near automobiles. Once when I was a young monk concentrating on my koan—which, by the way, took years—a passing automobile almost struck me down. This story tells you how deep your concentration must be."

At the next sanzen he begins by asking gently, "Where is 'one'?" I shake my head, saying "I really can't get anywhere *near* this koan." He replies, "Your problem is that you've encapsulated your 'one' inside layers of ideas and ten thousand other conditioned things. You must strike through these layers, break away from any philosophical approach. Finally you will get down to the deeply religious insight. Then it will be no separate matter. It will be something that you will find totally and consciously acceptable."

"But," I reply, "I am still having trouble even defining what 'one' means." He says, "If you find that unity is a better word, use unity." This helps not at all. "Be clear about one thing: the answer to 'where' will not be 'everywhere,' and it will not be 'nowhere.' Such answers are things out of the conscious, conditioned mind. When you finally reach your answer, it must be *clear, definite.* Your answer cannot be shaken by *anyone.*"

Another sanzen. He begins with a firm question: "If all ideas are melted into one, *where* does that one come from?" No answer from me. I am learning. I am sitting more and talking less. He continues, saying, "The koan is contradictory; you cannot find the answer by logic. Head and body working *together.* That's what you need to penetrate the koan. You will finally find this union of mind and body inside Zen."

In the following months, head and body do not come together. I cannot crack this koan. Reading about Zen is not supposed to be helpful. I read, anyway. In one place, I find that this "Where is one?" koan was attributed to Master Chao-chou (778–897) back in the early Tang dynasty. Reading elsewhere, I come across a vague but potential word answer to the koan. It dates back to the time of Seng-t'san, the third Zen patriarch, who lived even earlier. There, in the *Hsin hsin ming,* I find the statement: "When all things are viewed in their oneness, we return to our original nature." I'm confused. Could this be the answer? If so, how could an answer precede a question? For if Seng-t'san's statement were to be regarded as an answer at all, then it had arisen almost two centuries *before* Chao-chou had posed his question. So I keep wondering: Does "one" mean "oneness"? Does "oneness" mean "unity"? And, by the way, what *is* my original nature?

All my word problems are self-inflicted, and they multiply. At another sanzen, still perplexed, I bring up yet another puzzling paradox. "How is it," I ask, "that emptiness—this central Buddhist concept—can exist if supposedly, at the same time, everything in the universe is all linked together? Doesn't the latter imply that there is a very high degree of fullness?" "You are getting diverted," he answers. "You have to *know* emptiness," he replies. "You must stop splashing along the surface with all your words and concepts. You cannot understand emptiness with words or with ideas. You must dive down deep into zazen. There, forget about emptiness. Forget about fullness. Get back to working on your koan, on 'one'. Keep on thinking; 'where' does that 'one' come from? This is your problem; keep to it." Trying to help, he then closes by saying, "If you continue your zazen, 'one' will finally become itself, and others, and everything else in the universe." I continue sitting, but nothing like this happens.

Next we begin a short, three-day retreat. It involves sitting several times in the morning and evening of each day. Maybe I can't pierce this koan, but I have been developing an almost palpable perception of being "in touch" with everything going on. By the third day, perception is becoming clear, immediate. The word "now" seems to symbolize this immediacy.

Sanzen again. No preliminaries. As soon as I enter, the roshi demands, "Where is 'one'!" "Now!," I blurt out. He raises his eyes, looks at me sharply. I meet his gaze. He nods slightly. "A little better," he says. "But much too logical. You must get inside the koan, immerse yourself in it like it was a tub of warm water."

December arrives all too soon. I have come to see him for my last, long farewell interview before leaving Kyoto. "I'm disappointed", I say, "that I didn't make more progress with the koan." He reassures me, replying, "I worked over a six-year period on my first koan, with four years taken up during the war." I mention, lamely, that the term, "original nature" might seem to be a kind of "word answer" to the koan. He dismisses this casually, saying, "Of course, no word answer is relevant. Stay with the koan itself. Break down through the where of the koan, and then it will open up."

He illustrates. He points down and in, extending both arms into a long V. But at the bottom, he leaves a gap of three inches or so between the tips of his outstretched fingers on both sides. "A deep valley of the mind will open up like this," he explains. "Once you've gone through one of the experiences, a valley is cut in the mind, and it will stay open. Go into that opening.

"When you get back to Denver," he continues, "keep up the same discipline there, even though you sit by yourself, that you did here in Kyoto where you sat formally in the zendo with the other people. Keep on going like a train in a tunnel, and you will finally reach the daylight at the other end. Don't stop in the tunnel." I resolve to follow his advice.

*   *   *

The years pass quickly. It is always refreshing to come back to Ryoko-in to see Kobori-roshi. Two years later, on one of many such visits, I mention that my koan is still "Where is 'one'?" and that I am still asking questions of it. He replies, "Where, what, when—they are all adverbs. Finally you will stop asking your questions. Remember, you weren't asking questions at the moment when you were born. And at the moment of your death you will not be asking questions. Get back there. This koan, 'Where is one?' is a big block of conceptual ice. It has sharp edges. First you must melt all the edges, finally the block itself."

My problem is that I lack the intense mental heat and the large segments of time required to melt this big block of ice. In order to keep up my research and other professional activities in the world of full-time academic medicine it has become necessary to compromise. Mine becomes a persistent, but partial commitment, far less than that of a monk. Yet this first impenetrable koan may have helped in subtle ways. Perhaps it contributed to the set of conditions underlying the deep absorption which had arrived earlier during that first December in Kyoto. We will come to that episode in part VI.

And the roshi's earlier comment about having to *know* emptiness would prove prophetic. I would not know emptiness for another eight years, not until the next sabbatical in London (as will be discussed in part VII).

26

A Quest for Non-Answers: Mondo and Koan

The greater the doubt, the greater the awakening; the smaller the doubt, the smaller the awakening. No doubt, no awakening.

C. -C. Chang[1]

The koan is not given as an object to understand. It is given to you to solve your own problem . . . to manifest yourself as a perfect being. If you are completely free from everything, you don't need the koan.

Joshu Sasaki-roshi[2]

Ancient Chinese masters emphasized a quality which came later to be called the "great doubt." The phrase causes confusion. This doubt does not involve hesitation. Nor will it lead to irresolute action. Instead, the great doubt is that natural desire, now grown urgent and persistent, to resolve life's nagging existential questions.[3] It is the primal ontological questioning, the same questioning which still drives humankind everywhere to ask, Where did I come from? What am I? Is there any deeper meaning to all this? The great mass of doubt, then, focuses our personal *I-Me-Mine* problems back on those fundamental issues: life, death, and our small presence in the vast universe.

The probing attitude begins as a simple wondering, then evolves into a quest for answers. After that, the quest becomes fruitful to the degree that the aspirants develop enough faith in themselves, in their roshi, and in the Zen training program to put forth a resolute effort. For, as Kaufmann observes, it is the essence of religion "to claim authority and impose some obligation: it asks for a commitment."[4] Zen certainly requires an intense personal commitment: a formal enrolling in a long program that will retrain consciousness. This is no passive auditing of some casual teacher's snap course for a semester. There will be quizzes, exams, internal audits, discomfort. Total commitment to such a quest becomes a serious matter. It resembles the way your attention would focus when you first discover you had locked your car keys, your dog, your glasses, your lunch, and your wallet inside your car.

The Mondo

Meanwhile, one reads about the old masters' many bizarre answers and behaviors. We encounter the story about the earnest young monk who asks old Joshu about the real meaning of Buddhism. And promptly hears this non sequitur: "The cyprus tree in the courtyard." What is one to make of these old, incomprehensible replies? Such questions, and answers, are termed *mondo*. If we permit them to, they can help us interpret where the masters of old and the roshi of today are coming from. One begins by realizing the limitations of logical concepts. Overall *form* is key, not content. So, it is no use trying to read literal meaning into the words of the Zen mondo. If you insist, you will be baffled and disappointed, if not intellectually offended.

Does every mondo handed down from the Tang dynasty describe a totally spontaneous exchange? No one in our own century knows this for a fact. Nor do we know what the whole context was, or whether the translation is still accurate. It is unfortunate today that we still find mondo quoted, without explanation, in ways which almost flaunt their incomprehensibility. What they exemplify, instead, is how much freedom the master's enlightenment experiences had opened up to him, and how this freedom then flowed into the conduct of his everyday teaching activities.

Suppose you are a busy roshi. Your monk asks a question. The question discloses an attitude, a mental posture, which will block his progress in Zen. Why bother to parry such a question, let alone to answer it in kind? In such instances, many old mondo provide good examples of how an enlightened Zen master used to operate. How did he deflect a concept-laden question? By responding simply and with free-floating spontaneity. No, the old masters were not usually trying to put anything over on their monks,—nothing intellectual, that is. Nor were they behaving irresponsibly by their own cultural frames of reference. Instead, one finds preserved in the old mondo the flavor of the ways in which the roshi once felt free to respond with perfect liberty in all actions—including speech.

So it will be useful to recall this interpretation of the old dialogues when we begin, in the next chapter, to describe a roshi operationally. For, in any era, he will be a person whose responses actualize "that perfect freedom which is a potentiality for all human beings. He exists freely in the fullness of his whole being. The flow of his consciousness is not the fixed repetitive patterns of our usual self-centered consciousness, but rather arises spontaneously and naturally from the actual circumstances of the present."[5] Can we maintain such a point of view?

The Koan

Matters of life, death, and the universe are awesome in scope. Some aspirants find it helpful systematically to narrow the focus of all their questioning down to one issue, their *koan*. A koan is the distillate of a verbal exchange long ago in a distant land and in a much different culture. The word *koan* started as an old Chinese legal term. It referred to a public document of a case so significant that it set a legal precedent. In like manner, the old classical Zen koan still endure. Many of them, having begun as mondo, would set precedents that would be handed down for centuries.

In any century, students who truly concentrated on their koan could shut off the flow of other distracting ideas and channel themselves toward one central focus of inquiry. Yet a koan in itself has no literal meaning. It is an artificial concentration device, a metaphor which stands for the great unanswered questions. Each of two koan I have worked on had a cryptic enigmatic quality. The first koan grew out of an ancient dialogue between a monk and his Chan master. The monk had asked Chao-chou (778–896): "All things are reducible to the one, but where does the one return to?" The old master (again, Joshu in Japanese) replied: "When I was in the district of Ching, I had a robe made that weighed nine pounds."[6]

Presumably, the monk was puzzled by his master's response. What stunned me was the question itself. In Kyoto, when Kobori-roshi first uttered the words of this koan—the one I would be expected to use—I became a child. It was as though I had been led to believe my schoolteacher would be speaking to me in English. But now I heard instead, in *French*, "Explain the phrase 'An army marches on its stomach.'" Even to approach such a sentence, one first has to understand some French. It might help if one could recall a bit of old military history, and knew what a long march implies. Then one would also need to drop out standard thought patterns and develop some new, culturally flexible, idiomatic, metaphoric ways of thinking. But it is a different matter to address a Zen koan. You must take off your thinking cap and shift toward direct experience. Students learn this the hard way. Not until much later in their practice will they discover that the koan, like a mondo, is not a question that has a wordy answer. It is a *procedure* for exploring life's deepest existential issues.

I did not resolve the first koan I received. It distills into three words, "Where is One?" Such summary words are called the *hua tou*, and they are a useful shorthand way to address the full koan.[7] But, again, they do not pose a specific question. So, neither they nor the full koan can be "solved," and certainly not by an answer which makes sense in conventional terms. Once, to Kobori-roshi, I did venture an intellectually correct answer. Stiffening, he responded vigorously: "Show me your *deep* understanding!" *Show* me. He couldn't have been more explicit.

Still, the student inside everyone casts about, looking for rational answers, word answers. So ingrained is our habit of solving all problems by analytic thought that we keep throwing thoughts "at" the koan even though it has no logical solution. This leaves us baffled, because a koan cuts across every previous assumption we've been programmed to believe is true about ourselves and about the world we live in. Yes, it does serve as a kind of loose metaphor for the principles of existence. But no aspirant knows the basis for this metaphor when starting to work on the koan.[8] Moreover, so long as you harbor intellectual notions of what the "correct" answer is, they will block your access into the deeper levels of consciousness, the ground from which intuitions will spring.

What *does* resolve the koan? Only the flash of profound insight. *Prajna* cleaves the layers of unconscious and preconscious mental processes, makes direct sense out of apparent nonsense. Down at such deeper physiological levels, no conventional thought structure imposes its formal, logical constraints. No discursive intellect laden with hair-splitting distinctions makes its home among such circuitries. Nor is the nature of the koan such that it can be resolved through analogies, symbols, or anything said about symbols. These, too, add cognitive and affective layers which can only deflect the immediate thrust of insight.[9]

Accordingly, it is hard to find a toehold on the sheer wall of a koan, let alone to hang on and keep working on it. One measure of a Zen master is how well he can keep convincing his students that their koan is vital to their existence, charged with the deepest significance. The better the master and the student work as a team, the more the student feels that resolving the koan is itself a matter of life and death. Later, we will see that life and death issues sometimes evolve into alternate states of consciousness (see chapter 104).

Beginners are frequently assigned the koan *Mu*. It stems from a monk's question, again to venerable master Chao-chou: "Does a dog have Buddha nature?" Old Chao-chou's answer: "Mu." The "Mu" is interpretable at many levels. A basic implication is emptiness. For present purposes, let us regard the old master's response as an exclamation, one which briskly negates the monk's question. On what grounds? On the grounds that it is as empty of meaning as all things are empty of distinctions. Notwithstanding, one first addresses a koan such as "Mu" as though it were not "empty." Indeed, it may convey the vague feeling of having some distant, covert meaning, if one could only fathom it. Starting as a mere preoccupation, the koan then grows into a kind of obsession. In the persistent student, what finally evolves is a process of *becoming one* with the koan. The student assimilates it, and becomes absorbed in it to a degree that excludes other thoughts and activities.[9]

Daisetz Suzuki held that "To solve a koan one must be standing at an extremity, with no possibility of choice confronting one."[10] Many stories from the old days illustrate how focusing on a koan could *drive* the student to such an extremity. When Hakuin was twenty-four, he was concentrating so intensely on his koan, "Mu," that he could not sleep. Having also forgotten to eat and to rest, he commented later that "it was as though I were frozen solid in the midst of an ice sheet extending tens of thousands of miles . . . To all intents and purposes I was out of my mind and the *Mu* alone remained."[11] *That* is concentration!

Nowadays, a prudent roshi is unlikely to let things go quite this far. Having sensed such obsessive preoccupation, he would also have warned the student to look both ways when venturing out in traffic. Nevertheless, while still applying lesser degrees of pressure, the roshi will never accept a rational answer. The student is on the spot: an answer is expected; no *conceivable* answer is ever accepted! It is a Catch-22 situation.

Still the roshi keeps prodding and encouraging. He watches and waits. Sometimes for years. He accepts nothing until he senses that the aspirant has gone deeply enough in meditation so as to have become fully immersed in the koan. Having finally spotted this level of behavior, he may then choose to deliver a well-timed shock. Sometimes even a light touch will do. It acts like the peck of a mother hen on the outside of an egg, a stimulus which arrives at the precise moment that the maturing chick is also hard at work, pecking away on the inside.[12] Maybe this particular shock will trigger awakening; maybe not.

In a very real sense, no person then "resolves" the koan. At least, no egocentric *I-Me-Mine* self remains around at that moment. Where, then, do the issues linked to the koan resolve themselves? In those deeper brain circuitries which have suddenly become *un*conditioned. The more intense the previous quest for answers, the more widespread had it been embedded in the psychophysiological operations of the brain, the greater will be the relief when kensho arrives. Great doubt; great *release*.

But only a special kind of insight—a major alternate state of consciousness—will illuminate so meaningful a resolution. Prior to this event, no word answer would ever suffice. Thereafter, no roshi would conclude that such a state was valid until he sees his pupil's behavior confirm it. Again, how does he know? At the instant of insight, the resolution is both so transforming and so energizing that the student can demonstrate its validity in *spontaneous, fluid action*. This implies two things. First, that the scope and depth of the insight have released the student into a major degree of freedom. Second, that the freedom has entered deeply enough so as to be held onto thereafter in a form that is recoverable.

The more profound and complete the resolution, the longer it infuses the student's spontaneity, no matter how vigorously the roshi presses his challenges during their next critical interview. Subsequently, the remaining traces of this same liberated behavior may enable some students to recall parts of it almost at will.[9] Another approach is to offer students a much less convincing, secondhand way of demonstrating their progress. They may be asked to select certain metaphoric "capping phrases," called *jakugo*. These are parts of old oriental poems and literary passages which seem best suited to suggest that the student's insight has grasped something of the implications of the koan.[13]

It suffices merely to note that some people have collected other "answers" to a koan, responses that are unlikely to prove convincing. Before 1916, in Japan, such contrived answers were kept private. Whether they should ever later have been made available to the public is still vigorously debated. Misleading, so-called answers to various koan have since been printed in English.[14] Could any such crib sheets be further from the point? Indeed, the fact that these versions do exist illustrates how profoundly the koan has been misunderstood over the centuries.

Take, for example, the demand of Hakuin's memorable koan: "Show me the sound of one hand!" The ersatz "answer books" would suggest that the student display action—thrust forth one hand. Or the challenging question, "What does Mu look like from the back?" To this, the pupil who might wish to seem to be identifying with the koan would turn around and present her back to the master. And to the challenging question, "What is a stone called?," the pupil could give his own name, thereupon seeming to demonstrate that all distinctions had been lost between subject and object.[14] No hard-nosed roshi who knows his students will be fooled by any such rehearsed, pretend answers. Nor is the serious insightful student likely to try.

What special qualities, then, enter the kinds of responses that are acceptable? They resemble a pun expressed in the playful pantomime of a charade. They escape from ordinary abstractions. They are responses that condense swift *action* into the question's key words. Their spontaneity briskly engages all those fresh, fluid elements of mime and demeanor that can't be faked. Here, the roshi is in his element. An expert diagnostician, he is already familiar with each student's body English.

An old story from the Tang dynasty reveals how master Pai-chang (J:Hyakujo) once challenged his monks.[15] He set a water bottle on the floor. Then he asked, "If this isn't a water bottle, what do you call it?" One monk spoke up, saying "It cannot be called a piece of wood!" Far too intellectual. Whose response did the master accept? That of Wei Shan, the monk who stepped up and simply overturned the bottle with his foot.

This kind of novel behavior is fully in keeping with the way the insight-wisdom of kensho overturns each old bottled-up preconception, and at every level. Now, let the roshi exercise his quality-control function. What happens when he challenges the student? Only authentic, spur-of-the-moment, responses emerge. To each of the roshi's fresh challenges, the student's reactions prove highly inventive, so creative that they overturn both conventional explanations and magical explanations as well[16] (see chapter 154). Some responses do take highly "unorthodox" forms. Still others fall into patterns that illustrate more orderly themes. For instance:

1. The student's response bypasses the question as it stands. It sidesteps all of the question's tacit assumptions. The response pays no attention to any of its absurdities, nor to any of its potential metaphysical aspects.

2. The student's behavior centers on a concrete element in the question. On the water bottle, for example.

3. The student's response emphasizes action. It speaks louder than words.

4. The action shifts the student's identity away from the usual self and toward something else that is not the usual self.

5. When the response is not a "real" action, it displays a kind of lighthearted, playful pretending. After all, what *is* a water bottle? Something to be overturned.

6. The student's response quickly bypasses so many cultural layers that it might seem to suggest some disrespect. Thus, in one act, the action may dethrone both the pretensions of the intellect and the master's elevated social position. To whatever degree this act reduces the master to the position of having ordinary feet of clay, the student then directly engages these feet. Because now the teacher and pupil stand on the same level playing field, sharing the same common ground: earthy, everyday reality.

An apocryphal story exemplifies some of the points above. The master says, "If it's that easy for *you* to hear the sound of one hand, let *me* hear it too!" Whereupon the pupil slaps the master's face. Previously, no such action was thinkable, certainly not in the East. But this is Zen. A domain of no-thought. What makes the slap uniquely Zen? The way it condenses several complex possibilities into one simplified act, and does so in a new context. For it answers the roshi, devalues any excessive social height he had before, and temporarily puts the pupil on a par with him.[16]

Besides Mu, the novice is frequently assigned simpler "breakthrough" koans such as Hakuin's "Sound of One Hand," or "Original Face." Then, after the first episode of *kensho*, a different koan can be assigned to encourage some five successively deeper layers of insights beyond those at the entry level. The following two examples suffice to suggest the elusive quality of these remaining levels. For instance, a koan for the next level is: "Empty-handed, yet holding a hoe; walking, yet riding a water buffalo." Reasoning won't help. There's nothing of substance to work with. Only the shift into insight will clarify this statement. At which point the sudden comprehension is just as convincing as when you "meet a close relative face to face at a busy crossroads and recognize him beyond question of a doubt."[17]

After that, the next level of koan is said to help the student understand the so-called realm of differentiation. Again, there is the example of the monk who wants to know what is the essence of Buddhism. So he asks his master, "What is the meaning of Bodhidharma's coming from the West?" At which point, old Chao-chou comes up with that classically oblique answer: "The cyprus tree in the courtyard."[18]

No firm evidence indicates that koan-like questions were a formal part of the process of Zen training before the advent of the sixth patriarch in China, Hui-neng (638–713). But on one occasion during his tenure he was said to have asked Nan-yueh the following question: "Who comes toward me?"[18,19] Nan-yueh could not answer his master's question and withdrew. And the issue was not resolved until this monk had wrestled with his "great mass of doubt" for another eight long years.[20] By the time of the late Sung dynasty (960–1279), the view came to be held that it would be especially from the soil of such great doubt, tilled vigorously with the aid of a koan, that great enlightenment would spring.

Meanwhile, Chan masters Chao-chou and Ta-hui (1089–1163) were among many who kept emphasizing that meditators should subject their koan to concentrated introspection only at depths far beyond the reach of the intellect.[21] Today, because we lack a more accurate term, we talk about such a long quest proceeding at levels we call "the subconscious." As yet, we have not clarified the psychophysiology of the subconscious. But we are familiar with another version of the long subconscious phase. It corresponds closely with that sustained period, termed "incubation," which is one of the several stages of the creative process.[22] Nowadays, we use the familiar words "intuition" or "insight" to describe the generic process which, by piercing a large mental logjam, finally yields the simple solution to a major puzzle.

In Zen, the brain resolves an *existential* impasse. In this context, one calls it "enlightenment" or "awakening," *kensho* or *satori*. It is also termed "insight-wisdom" or "seeing into one's true nature." The two intuitive processes are similar in form if not in content and degree.

Because many years usually elapse before awakening, the koan serves several useful interim purposes. It helps sustain the aspirant through long dry periods. The roshi keeps bringing it up during interviews, helping to preserve its sense of urgency long after the initial heat of passion subsides.[13] But many people in the old days found that it was too stressful to maintain the urgency of a koan for long periods. Realism took over, at least by Bukko's time in the thirteenth century. The view circulated that a koan should be dropped if the student did not progress to kensho within three to five years.[8] Then, after the koan was dropped, a cooling down period would ensue. Finally, in due time, kensho could still emerge spontaneously. Indeed, as Leggett observes, "many people come to success if they first have the experience of wrestling with the koan and later reduce the effort, but few come to success at the time when they are putting out exceptional effort."[23] I can verify this from personal experience. Again there is the resemblance to the creative process: intuition finally strikes after long preparation and incubation. During such an interval mere intellect is thwarted.

One fact is important to appreciate. *Kensho can occur in association with the general concentration and incubation fostered by a given koan, but not yet resolve the salient issue embedded in that particular koan.* D. T. Suzuki illustrates this key point using the story of Kao-feng (J:Koho; 1238–1285), a Chinese master who lived in the later Sung dynasty.[24] When Kao-feng was still a young monk, his tough master gave him the difficult question: "Who is it that carries for you this lifeless corpse of yours?" He could not penetrate this question. Still later, he took on the different koan: "All things return to the one; where is the one returned to?" Six days after having fixed this "Where is One" koan at the very center of his consciousness, he abruptly realized enlightenment. It was triggered by seeing a verse on a portrait. But note what his insight had resolved at that instant. It was the much *earlier* issue embedded in the first koan about "Who Carries." Unresolved by this awakening were those current issues, the ones he had been trying to address with the aid of his latest "Where is One" koan.

In China, the artificialities implicit in koan studies gave rise to a split which persists to this day. One school strongly favored them, another abhorred using them, and the rest remained lukewarm. Still, in Kyoto, Daito Kokushi (1282–1338) went on to inaugurate a systematic program of koan study. Four centuries later, Hakuin further advanced serial koan studies as part of his overall activist approach in revivifying the traditions of Rinzai Zen in Japan.[11] He warned vigorously against a "dead Zen," one in which the pupil might have attained perfect tranquility of mind, but still lived only an inactive life.[25] We can still feel the heat of the fire that committed Hakuin to probe his own koan. It emanates from his statement that "You must closely examine yourself with the same urgency that you would devote to saving your own head if it were ablaze."[26]

In Hakuin's era, as in China earlier, monks often moved from one school to another. Even some Soto Zen temples also prescribed koan studies to a lesser degree.[8] Dogen himself thought koan were neither nonsensical nor meaningless. Rather, he viewed them as parables, allegories, metaphors for the critical question of life and death. Those students today who persist, and who resolve their koan, will finally have come to a similar perspective. For they, too, will finally have discovered the critical distinction. *A koan is realized, not solved.*[27] This realization arrives not at the level of mere thought, but as a result of direct experience.

Objections aside, koan studies have continued to be used for several other reasons. First, it gives the aspirants a welcome sense of continuity. They are participating in a tradition. Their koan is time-tested. Through it, they become a kind of living link with that long chain of historical persons whose strenuous efforts extend far back into the mist of ancient China.

Second, the students who take on the burden of a koan are already demonstrating great faith in the Zen way in general, and in their roshi. Finally, the koan helps the roshi. It serves him both as a useful teaching function and as a way of testing. He knows it intimately. Like a trained psychologist, he has become well-versed in fielding its standardized "inkblot" responses. But in a sense, he shares the same kind of educational problems as does a one-room schoolteacher: his students vary greatly in age and level of ability. Accordingly, the koan makes it easier for the busy roshi in a large monastery, or one confronted by many new faces at a large sesshin, quickly to discern and keep track of how far along each student is.

In the tradition of the Soto school of Zen, zazen usually implies "just sitting meditation" with no koan. In the Rinzai tradition, one may probe the koan both during the depths of formal meditation practice and at any other time. During zazen, what effect does it have on one's brain waves to concentrate on a koan? Preliminary EEG studies have explored this question in a limited way.[28] During zazen only, the subject's alpha waves fluctuated considerably. In contrast, his alpha activity became higher and more integrated when he also focused on a koan during zazen. Concentrating on his koan enhanced alpha activity more so when he meditated in the standard zazen posture with legs crossed than when he merely sat at ease, or was lying down.

As this meditating subject focused attention on the koan, his external visual awareness waned markedly, even though his eyes were still open. This observation suggested that, in general, a meditator could become less distracted by visual events taking place in the external environment by turning attention internally to concentrate on a koan. On the other hand, while this meditating subject was focusing on his koan, his alpha activity did *not* increase if he merely proceeded to close his eyes. Nor did his alpha activity increase if the room itself was dark.

A koan provides something to work on, push against, strain toward. It takes effort. In humans, mental effort does increase blood flow to the brain. Yet cerebral blood flow reaches its optimal levels when the person's mental effort is accompanied by *medium* anxiety levels, not by low levels or by high levels of anxiety. Earlier studies of normal subjects, using psychological tests, had given results which helped anticipate such findings. These prior test results showed that we also solve problems most creatively in general, and solve standard *verbal* analogy problems most effectively, when we work under only medium levels of anxiety. And it will be at such moderate levels that we increase the blood flow to the brain, chiefly over its *outer, cortical surface.*[29]

Of course, the research just cited on cortical blood flow shows only what happens when our *ordinary* mental processes function under various degrees of stressful circumstances. So studies of this kind, sampling mostly surface blood flow, will not help us understand all that a koan contributes. For a koan is not a conventional verbal analogy problem. A koan requires a *non*verbal approach to concentration, degrees of introspection that go beyond linguistics. Most standard blood flow techniques do not yet provide a useful way to sample accurately the many deeper, and more subtle brain activities that may be involved.

So everything about a koan seems to have become rather complicated. Can what the koan adds to Zen be summarized? A koan is indeed a concentration device, but a nonspecific one. It helps keep the meditator focused, undistracted, and unified on one central theme for a relatively long period. It serves as a means to an end. In this sense, it may help to consider the analogy of the long pole, and of how it functions in relation to the pole-vaulter. When placed in the right spot, and when thrust against in the right manner for the right length of time, the pole provides a dynamic element for that leap which will leave conventional mentation far behind. At the zenith, the vaulter reaches a new, selfless perspective. Then, once having crossed over that high bar, the vaulter lets go of that particular pole. Having served its purpose, it drops away. Later, the trainee might wish to take on a longer pole—address a more difficult koan still farther beyond reach—and attempt to repeat the process. Viewed weightlessly, from the peak of the arc, the elevated perspectives remain unforgettable thereafter.

Back when the beginner first heard the koan, it was an enigma. But this was only from an *outside* perspective. Then, so it seemed, by wielding the intellect as usual, one might somehow crack its hidden code. No. This can't happen. Only after having been bone-tired, cold, wet, and hungry—and then becoming mobilized by a steaming hot meal—does the mountain climber's body and visceral brain grasp the essential truth. Then it becomes clear what is meant by the statement "an army marches on its stomach." And it will be, likewise, only through an equivalence of tasting—through direct, penetrating personal experience—that the student finally realizes an astonishing fact. At its core, the koan is no more, and nothing less, than "a simple and clear statement made from the state of consciousness which it has helped to awaken."[30]

To the reader, this last quotation may seem as obscure as a koan itself. If so, the writer's personal experience working on a second koan will later be of some assistance (see chapter 129).

27

The Roshi

The sailor cannot see the North, but knows the needle can.

Emily Dickinson (1830–1886)[1]

A Zen teacher cannot help others unless he himself possesses the discerning Dharma-eye . . . he is able to know someone to his very marrow just by observing his face . . . It is in this essential point, the possession of the Dharma-eye, that our sect surpasses all others . . . Look at the Buddha-patriarchs. . . They could all tell the black from the white in less time than it takes a spark to jump from a flint. They grasped the essentials with lightning speed.

Master Bankei (1622–1693)[2]

Suppose you are a music student, and you wish to become a concert pianist. You will need to practice for years under the watchful eyes and ears of a respected, inspiring teacher. Zen Buddhism is the same. The novice will take years to learn how to interact with the keyboard and pedals of a human brain, the most complex organ in the known universe. How soon, if ever, will Zen aspirants come to a true awakening, to enlightenment? Much of this hinges on the quality of their interactions with the master, the *roshi*.

But Carl Jung held that we in the West didn't have the right background of "mental education" necessary for Zen. "Who among us would place such implicit trust in a superior Master and his incomprehensible ways? This respect for the greater human personality is found only in the East."[3] At the outset, let us take a critical look at Jung's twin preconceptions, superiority and incomprehensibility. They raise issues which lead every skeptic to ask: Does Zen Buddhism have valid messages? If so, do they ever arrive in a form that an average person can decipher?

Let us focus on the rare Zen master who is fully enlightened. He would satisfy most of Jung's criteria for being a "greater human personality." His superiority would be evident in many ways, both in his context and in ours. Only after long years of rigorous training did his own master certify him to train others, both Zen monks and laypersons. Each successive teacher in his long teaching lineage was also certified. The written documentation can usually be traced far back in old Japan and sometimes even to China. Indeed, the word *roshi* is itself a token of this fact. It arose, as have other r/l transpositions, from the way Japanese lips and tongue pronounced the name of Lao-tzu, the Taoist sage of ancient Chinese legend.

Zen masters continued down through the ages to transmit what was called the "lamp of enlightenment." True, the lamp of illumination did pass from hand to hand. But what constituted the illumination from such a lamp? Nothing that originated in scriptures, said Bodhidharma. No form of didactic teaching that anyone could impose on students from without. Rather it was a form of education in the original sense of that word: a leading forth—from the interior—of something already there. In Zen, it is a slow process to tease out what is "in there." It is one-on-one, very intensive and time-consuming.

Harsh military realities penetrated the culture back in olden times. Moreover, it was already appreciated that each personality would have set up barricades to protect itself against change. So then, as now, it came to be accepted that rigorous discipline would be the way to train a monk to assault these well-defended battlements of his inner space. Young head-shaven monks were sometimes treated like recruits in a Marine boot camp.

But could there ever be justification for a Zen master striking his monks? It may help to interpret such early behavior in the light not only of the turbulent cultural setting of those early days but of the roshi's top priorities. For he began with many raw, young trainees. His task was twofold: (1) to help them shake off their cultural indoctrinations and routine ways of thinking; and (2) to so sharpen their attentive powers that they could start directly experiencing the real world—that world right under their noses.

We in the West also have a hard-nosed military history. Out of the First World War has come an apocryphal story which helps bring home the point. It concerns a young second lieutenant who had failed to get his stubborn army mule to move. He asked for help from his sergeant, a veteran mule trainer. The trainer picked up a plank of wood. Without changing his expression he crashed it down on the mule's head, right between his ears. The astonished officer remonstrated, saying "That's no way to teach a mule!" The sergeant replied casually, "I haven't started to *teach* him yet. That was just to get his attention!"

The roshi gets his students' attention early. He sometimes uses audacious means. Like any wise teacher, he enlivens the complexities of the subject with pithy examples and humor. But no doubt remains about the most vital matter: it is the student who bears the final responsibility for progress. As Joshu Sasaki-roshi phrases it, "If you have a dependent mind, you better go to other religious that treat you kindly, but not to Zen. You are not children anymore. I'll never be kind to you. You should walk all alone and come to realization by yourself."[4]

The roshi in the Japanese tradition trains students mostly by example and by indirection. He communicates two of his subtler points by example. One is his calm alertness. The other is the fine art of examining life's troubling events with utmost objectivity. As her roshi said to Irmgard Schloegl, "Look at getting mad from this perspective. If you had but five more minutes left to live, and it would still be worth getting mad over, then by all means do so."[5]

But much of the rest of the Zen a roshi transmits is allusive. Does he specify what he is searching for? No, nor what his students' response should be. This is frustrating. It leaves his students groping, stumbling. But as a consequence, they will be discovering Zen *for* themselves, and *in* themselves, on their own terms of reference. It will be a long, slow process of trial and error.

So how accurate is the charge that the roshi's subtle ways are incomprehensible? The word fits none of the contemporary roshi I have known. Quite the reverse; they are all down-to-earth, matter-of-fact communicators. But their methods can appear devious. For what they still do, in common with the old masters, is steer clear of responding with words or by deeds which will only stimulate more abstractions in the minds of those who question them. Frequently this means directing the student's attention to the simplest of examples. Tangible objects are readily at hand in the space in front of them: a bell, a stick, a flower. In this way do roshi train their students constantly *to be aware of explicit sensory experience.*

Nothing abstract, nothing elaborate. Just concrete encounters with everyday perceptions. "This cup is round," says Kobori-roshi, having focused us both on his empty tea cup. Right *here.* Right *now,* in this present moment. Initially, this approach seems so elementary as to appear naive. But how long does it take before one begins to really practice this fine art of immediate, ongoing mindful perception in everyday living?

In the opening quotation, Bankei was emphasizing an important point: a Zen master grasps the essence of a situation with lightning-like speed. Why? Perhaps it was Bankei's way of defining how a master behaves. *This is what finally happens when a person becomes free of discriminations between self and non-self.* It is not a matter of similes, not of being "like" something. This is what it actually *is* when a genuine master finally resonates in natural, selfless harmony with things as they really are. The result is a person who perceives, understands, and verbalizes in quick, seemingly unorthodox ways, unconstrained by the usual formal, logical structures of language and behavior.

Do many old Zen mondo and behaviors continue, at our usual cognitive level, to express sheer nonsense? Yes, but much of this evaporates when we finally step back and stop trying to force them into *our* own logical frames of reference. Customs were much different back in the Tang dynasty (618–907). It was then more acceptable for a Zen master—somewhat as we now expect of a modern jazz musician—to be at liberty to take off on brief, impromptu, freewheeling flights of improvisation. We can hardly demand today that the artistry of either man must adhere to every strict rule of standard composition. From such a charitable perspective we can begin to glimpse method in the madness, and start viewing it as an expression of the roshi's enlightened, blithe spirit.

In today's large classrooms, teachers examine students using questions which are true/false, multiple choice, and of the essay type. Nothing like this for Zen masters. Never any wordy discourse. Nothing to encourage any legalistic judgments about "good" or "bad." Instead, their methods pointed the way to lively perceptions, encouraged quick insights that pierced quibbles, cut off attachments. Intuitively, they had diagnosed a basic human problem: our brain's association networks are already jam-packed with fine discriminating thoughts. Is something really true? Or only partly true? Or mostly false? Each such decision calls up one more hair-splitting deliberation. These resonate way back to old affective circuits, to attitudes which had imprinted us since childhood with sticky notions about "right" or "wrong." So let us regard the older exchanges between master and monk as an open demonstration of another basic Zen theme: *direct, simple, responses quickly bypass all this mental clutter.*

A roshi engages in many lighthearted behaviors. They, too, are less incomprehensible than might first appear. A pixie humor jars students out of fixed ways of looking at things. It serves to counterbalance a sober student's tendencies to heavy thinking. Sometimes the way a roshi responds to boring verbal questions may even resemble the technique used by Peter Ustinov, who once said, "I find that a most effective way of quelling bores is simply to say, suddenly and irrelevantly: 'Now, Singapore—does that mean anything to you?'"[6]

But the roshi has a much more serious role. He is the quality control. In this function, he is a stern taskmaster. He is compass needle in more ways than one. He punctures old belief systems. He denies spiritual significance to hallucinations and to brief affective responses. He insists that spiritual insights—of whatever depth—are but an early milestone on a long, long journey. Moreover, he stresses that his students' insights will remain sterile until they are infused into everyday life behaviors. Any novice, reaching out to a roshi for some quick spiritual face-lift, soon learns that the Way is never finished. No superficial cosmetic surgery for Zen. The overhaul arises deep from within, from pulling on one's own bootstraps.

One of the roshi's crucial functions, then, is to say "no." His role is to afflict the comfortable. He dispenses tough love. Whether he does so gently or firmly, no student remains complacent, certainly not in rigorous Rinzai Zen. His private interviews, *sanzen*, can build up residues of frustration. As I sit before Sasaki-roshi, he says: "Show me how you look at this flower." No matter what behavior I engage in, it doesn't seem to satisfy him. What *does* he want? He is waiting for me to act from deep meditative levels or from the flashing insight of *kensho* itself. It will be years before I fully appreciate this fact and understand the basic reasons for it.

All the while, every roshi has become expert at judging his student's levels of functioning. Having repeatedly demanded that the student *show* him the true understanding of the koan, the roshi now has a vast backlog of data. He knows how inept the struggling student is. His "Dharma-eye" penetrates the response of the overconfident student, discerning how little is genuine. The roshi of old did not suffer fools kindly. Contemporary roshi are relatively patient. More like midwives than remote psychoanalysts, they just keep things moving along. Why do they remain so supremely confident that their students can enlist interior processes which will transform consciousness? Because they have seen it happen many times: their pupils proceed, through various quickenings, until finally their intuition ripens into awakening.

In the interim, the roshi remains the exemplar. He knows where true north is. He needles, prods, nudges, and encourages the student in this general direction. *The roshi himself is a concentration device.* He creates suspense out of silence. Students pay very close attention to him. Bankei described how a master's every word and action then goes on to strike right into the core of his students' affliction "like a sharp gimlet, dissolving their attachments, breaking off their shackles, ushering them into a realm of wonderful freedom and blissful joy . . ."[7] Then, as soon as his students finally do enter the realm of kensho, their sudden transformation affects every expression, word, and gesture. Each act is newly inspired. It is this freedom that the roshi has been looking for. He knows it, exemplifies it.

The roshi has help in the monastery. The general disciplinarian is the *jikijitsu*. This monk wields the stick, literally and figuratively. He plays the role of the "bad cop," especially during meditative retreats. His unsmiling countenance will be balanced by that of the kindly *shoji*, the "good cop" who organizes the work and the kitchen details. This is not all playacting. Some personalities fit better into one role than the other. Yet when the two of them switch jobs, they alternate their roles as well.

At some point, the student will be ready to give up, discouraged both by lack of progress and by what seems like the unfeeling authoritarian figures of the roshi and the jikijitsu. Now, the situation softens, temporarily. The roshi and the shoji deftly reach in to comfort the afflicted. The student now finds the carrot at the other end of the stick: a warmly sympathetic mentor who not only makes helpful suggestions about how best to practice but who is strongly supportive at every other human level. As our frosty breaths mingle in *sanzen* at 5 A.M. on a frigid Rohatsu sesshin, the warm humanity of that twinkling 82-year-old fellow being, Joshu Sasaki-roshi, is comforting indeed.

A roshi contributes anecdotes about his own long journey. These help develop a common bond and sense of purpose. Their relationship, at first an uneasy one for the student, then evolves into a more realistic, sharing one. The student finds increasing compassion in the roshi and slowly begins to understand his methods. Gradually, the roshi becomes a model for that mature compassion which lies at the heart of Buddhism.

Whereas the roshi in my experience have been extraordinary human personalities, none of them have been truly eccentric. As monks, all were the survivors of an arduous obstacle course. Otherwise, they could not have been selected to be abbots in charge of a training monastery. Tempered by their earlier training, roshi grow wiser. They have learned where their former egocentric selves were coming from, so to speak. In the clarity of mindfulness, they have observed how they interacted with many different persons, and analyzed why. Cut from human cloth, flawed like the rest of us, their Zen exposure improved them far beyond their original baseline.

Did each of them "master" Zen? Not fully. Nor did it automatically transform them into 100 percent perfect, living Buddhas, even though their Western students of this century still expect as much. Nowadays, it would invoke much controversy if roshi were to try to assume the same kind of rigorous roles as did those masters who proved so effective back in the Tang dynasty. Contemporary pupils anticipate receiving far more from their leaders, and expect to give less in return, than did many other acolytes in earlier centuries.

Yet, in every era, roshi have openly displayed their differences as individuals. Their basic personality types have shined through in the kind of living Zen they practiced and taught. In temperament, some will have started out at the gentler and more flexible end of the spectrum.[8] The Zen practiced by Bankei, in the seventeenth century, for example, expressed his own basic outflowing personality in a way quite different from the tougher approach of Hakuin, who was soon to follow (1686–1769). Bankei simplified Zen and popularized it. He objected to the use of the koan, even though he had been trained in the Rinzai tradition. He believed that it was a "mistaken business" first to use such riddles to heighten some "great wall of doubt" and then to try later to break through this wall. He, like many others, was aware that back when Zen was in its golden age in China—during that 140-year period starting in the early eighth century—masters had not yet been using the koan as a standard concentration device.[9]

Zen has always left wide latitude for personal expression among its roshi. Consider the sharp contrasts between these two later Japanese masters, Bankei and Hakuin, and those differences that much earlier would have separated a ninth-century iconoclast like Lin-chi (J: Rinzai) from the softer approach of Dogen (1200–1253). Dogen held the liberal view that each student should recognize "that there might be superior views to his, and should visit good masters widely and also examine the sayings of old masters. However, he must not cling even to the sayings of the old masters. Thinking that they too may be wrong, and that he should be cautious while believing them, he is to follow better views as he encounters them."[10]

Fortunate students will seek out and find one similarly mature roshi who leads a group of fellow students all of whom share a strong affinity yet still preserve their religious independence. However, other aspirants may not be able, for personal or other reasons, to resonate positively with the messages from a particular teacher and *sangha*. They will probably not progress at an appropriate rate, and will be best advised to seek more fruitful relationships elsewhere.

Today, we have inherited some idealized if not romanticized views about Zen masters. Pioneers they were, and legends treasured through many past centuries have made them larger than life-size. In recent years, many sincere seekers on the spiritual path have paid a heavy price for taking, "on faith," another kind of "leader," one who merely preaches authentic living but who cannot put its basic principles into selfless practice. Newspaper articles cite some leaders' sexual involvements with disciples, mention their ninety-three Rolls-Royces, note the federal charges against them, cartoon them sitting on mountaintops uttering inane "truths." The well-documented story of the Rajneeshee in Oregon[11] has now become only one of the milder episodes illustrating how hazardous it is to follow uncritically a charismatic guru into a malignant cult. The general public is increasingly aware that absolute power corrupts, whether the seeker meditates in a temple in Japan, an ashram in India, or in some religious community in the West. Little wonder the public distrusts gurus and evangelists of any stripe.

Is a religious leader authentic? Or is it all smoke and mirrors? For each aspirant, authenticity becomes of the utmost practical importance. The people, the setting, must *be* genuine, not merely appear so. Maslow, among many others, warned that religion becomes the institutionalized enemy of true mystical experience whenever it is led by bureaucratic, power-hungry people.[12] One does well to remember that Buddha himself led a reform movement against the Hinduism of his era.

Strong antiauthoritarian trends also exist today. But they will have swung much too far if they go on to lump all Zen masters with "gurus" in general. Looking back over all the centuries, authentic Zen stands erect on very high ground. The vast majority of its roshi have been highly selected exemplars who were tempered by a demanding apprenticeship. Slowly they matured into truer, simpler persons. Not power-seeking. Empowered from within. Perfected beings? No, but conducting themselves in ways that would lift them beyond both their personal limitations and whatever cultural distortions occurred during their particular historical era. The same can be said of Irmgard Schloegl, and of the other remarkable women late in our century, compassionate mentors who have increasingly stepped into the challenging role of leading a *sangha* in the West.[13]

28

The Mindful, Introspective Path toward Insight

> In fact, we do not need to make conscious efforts to look into the mind. If you can be passive and very objective, then you as the subject will be absorbed into the action, the looking itself, and then it becomes easier to look, because the looking has no obstructions or resistances.
>
> Dhiravamsa[1]

We learn it as children: just trying to be better isn't enough. No one can will him- or herself into moral purity. Nor can calmness plus heightened powers of concentration alone prompt more than transient moments of absorption. But meditative practice does something else. It helps you pause and examine your mental processes dispassionately. Soon, you identify self-centered behaviors and distractions. After that, a series of small insights then enables you to let go of them. Letting go paves the way for being able to focus on items in the next agenda, one at a time, in a sustained way.

Slowly, the aspirant who follows the Zen Buddhist path learns to merge the practices of meditative concentration with restraint (*shila*) and insight (*prajna*). The triad functions as an interactive unit, much as do lungs, heart, and brain. Reinforcing one another, they gradually bring their *coordinated* impact into thoughts, attitudes and behavior. *Together, they help one sort things out, observe which options work better, arrive at constructive solutions, keep one's best intentions on-line.* The result can be nothing less than a spiritual renaissance.

The early Indian Buddhists summarized their meditative approach back in the fifth century.[2] One general pathway was the direct route of insight meditation, *vipassana*. The other was the route of calming meditation, *samatha*. The latter began with a calm serenity, developed into one-pointed concentration, and finally shifted into the full meditative absorptions of samadhi. When later Christians described the first, direct route to insight, they called it the path of "dry-visioned sainthood."[3] They, too, drew the same distinction. This path of piercing insights differed from that other route which could lead to the blissful tears and moist-eyed contemplation of the absorptions in all their splendor.

The Chinese schools of Chan went on to develop along the lines of the northern Buddhist tradition. They further refined the art of taking the basic, clear awareness that arises during sitting meditation and extending it into natural interactions during everyday life. In this manner, the Chinese believed they were cultivating the path toward insight-wisdom, *prajna*. But they used different words to describe the first direct path of discernment. Among them was *kuan;* the Japanese would later call it *kan*.[4] Later, the techniques of the Zen schools were translated into English. And somewhere along the line, words with these implications tended to be left behind. Sometimes nothing was said, in Zen, about the specific phrase "insight meditation" as such. The term seemed almost to have dropped out. What happened to it? Does Zen really practice insight meditation? If so, what is this style of meditation? And how exactly does it help one develop insight? Neither question has a simple answer.

Zen tends to be vague on these matters. In contrast, many persons in the West now freely use the terms "mindfulness," or "insight meditation" to describe the meditative practices used by the southern Buddhist schools of southeast Asia which follow in the Theravada tradition.[1] Is the Zen way really so different? Or is this another semantic problem?

It seems to be largely a matter of words and emphasis, for in most respects the northern and southern practices are fundamentally similar. Whatever names attach to Buddhist mindfulness, it still starts out the same way: as a *nonreactive, bare awareness open to anything.*[5] Indeed, the same basic "meditative" approach is available to almost anyone. "All" you must do is set aside mental space, then dedicate it fully to the here and now. The task is formidable. Only slowly does its outcome open up awareness, nonjudgmentally, so that awareness can take in the natural ongoing changing sequences of direct experience.

The mindfulness of which we speak begins by applying itself gently to any of the following four general areas:

1. To activities of the body, including the rise and fall of the movements of breathing.

2. To feelings and sensations. Emotions and sensations are noted to arise, and to pass away.

3. To various states of the mind. Anger and pleasure, greed and the absence of greed, are registered, recognized, and seen to be transient ripples atop the deeper, mental seascape.

4. To other mental contents or concepts. Sensual desires are noted, traced back to their origin, and then seen to pass away.

Mindfulness in Zen also begins as a relaxed mental posture. Its awareness observes the eating of food, notes its chewing, tasting, and swallowing. Mindfulness during walking in kinhin means paying gentle attention to the lifting of the feet, the stepping forward, the feel of the weight being placed on the heel and the ball of each foot.

Mindfulness involves attending to the processes of dressing and undressing. It is a steady, persistent returning to a simple mental focus, time after time. Try it. You'll find that you must first set aside a lifetime of mind-wandering habits.[6] Only slowly does the background noise level fall, both internally and externally. With long practice, the advanced meditator develops enough clear mental space to be conscious of each percept individually. With no thoughts.

Only then does mindfulness register the bare perception, observe with detachment, notice without elaboration. After a long while, the brain finally seems emptied of all save the first, fresh entry of raw sensory data and that open, mirror-like receptivity which greets it.

Up to now, we have been describing how mindfulness meditation *begins*. But from here on it will evolve. Rarely does this point receive the emphasis it deserves. As it evolves, it proceeds in both external and internal dimensions along lines that are increasingly intuitive. So, on some brief occasions, paying bare attention will turn into an *out*flowing: a totally appreciative, sacramental approach to the wondrous commonplace events of the present moment. At other times, bare attention turns *in*ward. Now, its functions expand to include *introspection and self-analysis*. Personal matters rise into it spontaneously to become grist for the mill of intuition. Indeed, it then resembles psychoanalysis[7] in the way it observes the topics it submits to intensive introspection. For now, though thoughts do occur, they are observed *non*judgmentally.

Freud himself once commented on the nature of the process in general. At the time, he was addressing physicians who wished to practice psychoanalysis. He advised them to keep their unconscious processes open. To be nonjudgmental about the figurative implications of what their patients were saying. Physicians should maintain, he said, a measure of "calm, quiet attentiveness—of evenly hovering attention."[8] It remains for meditators to adopt similar measures of calm attentiveness and introspection. Then they too can begin to self-diagnose whatever may rise up into consciousness. Here, in their own mental field of the moment, they will discover their own fixed ideas, attachments, fears, and unfruitful social traditions.[1] Deploying this same "evenly hovering attention" they will discern which of their old false attitudes are standing in the way of their new efforts at self-restraint.[9] Introspection is a natural phenomenon. It requires no postgraduate degree. But you do have to pay attention. And to one thing at a time.

In the earlier phases of insight meditation, feeling states become more readily identified: "You're getting angry," "You're feeling happy," "You're feeling sad." In later phases, insight meditation probes more deeply into the *root* causes of such emotions. Quietly, it asks, *Why* do you get angry? *Why* are you afraid? When deeper motivations are laid bare, they disclose the root cause of our discomforts: the clinging attachments of the *I-Me-Mine*.

Why, then, is it so difficult to become enlightened? Wilber diagnoses our problem as *diffuseness*.[10] We scatter our awareness. It isn't focused on the present. We improvise a rich fantasy life, fill our own home videos with it, mingle past memories with scenarios for the future. However, bare, mindful awareness sees *nothing permanent* in this mishmash that passes for consciousness.

Earlier, in order to survive in the everyday world, we had constructed set after set of perceptual biases which functioned automatically. They helped us filter out most incoming stimuli. Suppose one were to give the name "automatization" to this usual process. Then the reverse of it would correspond to that process of opening up which takes place during the early perceptual awareness phase of mindfulness.[11] This discrete, mindful attentiveness "reinvests actions and percepts with attention." Focusing lightly on one item at a time, it becomes the "undoing of automatization." Neither neglect nor scattering occurs. Most current Zen approaches steer away from the kind of compulsive labeling of events practiced during some Theravada forms of insight meditation. And they also deemphasize the kinds of highly pressured, emotionalized extremes that can occur in concentrative meditation.

On the other hand, some Zen writings tend to overemphasize the major flash of *prajna*. At least, they say rather little about the important silent, interior dialogue that goes on when the aspirant looks inside with increasing objectivity. The omission causes confusion. Until the record is set straight, beginners may fall all too easily into the belief that their sole aim is to pay attention with "no mind" and "no thinking."

Zazen is not this empty-headed, either on or off the sitting cushion. In Zen, the introspective dialogue happens by itself. Feeling and thoughts meet, in the open. Quietly, critically. It might seem, at an interface so soft and wide, that this process is gentle. But the questions do penetrate, deeper and deeper. Introspection implies inspecting far inside, ruthlessly exposing the source of one's own errors. Much later, it will evolve into *dis*passion, the process that allows one to make light of the errors of others.

Zen itself hasn't truly overlooked the slower, lower-level intuitive processes. Indeed, the classics of Zen literature provide ample historical precedents for acknowledging their existence. One of these legends dates back to the very beginnings of Chan.[12] Then, a monk asked the sixth patriarch, "Master, when you sit in meditation, do you see or not?" His master, Hui-neng, arose, and—in order to demonstrate the point—was said to have struck him three times. He then asked the monk, "When I hit you, did it hurt? Or didn't it?" The monk answered, "It did, and it didn't."

The Master said, "Likewise, I see, and I also do not see." The monk said, "Please explain." Hui-neng answered, "My seeing is always to see my own errors; my non-seeing is to not see the evils of people in the world." Introspection. Dispassion.

And a second story originates with master Hakuin. We tend to remember him for his strong emphasis on koan studies. But Hakuin also cited other mental activity of the more personal introspective kind, for he said: "He who wishes to seek Buddha must first of all look into his own mind . . . you yourself must examine closely."[13] In such ways does the meditator—who begins by practicing awareness—gradually "look into his own mind" and begin to encourage that natural discerning art we call intuition. How all this goes on to facilitate the major flash of insight-wisdom is something we will finally take up again in part VII.

29

Inkblots, Blind Spots, and High Spots

> We must get at the Eastern values from within and not from without, seeking them in ourselves, in the unconscious. We shall then discover how great is our fear of the unconscious and how formidable are our resistances.
>
> Carl Jung[1]

> Illusions commend themselves to us because they save us pain and allow us to enjoy pleasure instead. We must therefore accept it without complaint when they sometimes collide with a bit of reality against which they are dashed to pieces.
>
> Sigmund Freud[2]

Inkblots

Often, we can trace back the source of a major religion to a personal meditative retreat of one kind or another. One of them took place under a bo tree near Bodh Gaya. Others took place in the desert of Judea, and in a hill cave near Mecca. In each instance, a historical person suffered in the process of overcoming his fears, illusions, and resistances to change. But suppose we try, thereafter, to clarify some general psychological principles that apply to the spiritual path. Soon the path becomes soft and slippery. We encounter words like "introversion" and "individuation," "rebirth" and "regression," "actualization" and "altruism." In order to highlight such topics, it will prove useful straightaway to pose two basic questions. First, *who* starts meditating nowadays? Next, why do so few stick to it?

In a sense, meditators select themselves. For the Way is a long, hard spiritual struggle. Those who persist on its rigorous path appear to have started out with some distinctive attributes. For example, they seem more readily able to become absorbed in a nonverbal mode of mental activity.[3] This capacity to shift one's attentional focus into absorption has an interesting correlate. It goes along with the person's being able to remember a four- to six-note pattern of musical tones. And that particular musical function appears to be lateralized more to the right temporal lobe of the brain.[4]

Among those who begin the transcendental meditation program, those who persist will have found its rationale credible and appealing.[5] They also are inclined to be interested in their own mental processes, more anxious but reserved, as well as more detached and impersonal. In general, those persons who persist in meditation may have been disposed to practice self-criticism and to have considered undergoing psychotherapy in the past. Moreover, the more introspective subjects—those varying relatively little in mood and behavior—tend both to continue *and* to go on to a successful outcome.

Other evidence also suggests that being introverted may help a person on the spiritual path. Or at least assist to the degree that introversion is a trait associated with the ability to maintain one's degree of arousal at a more steady, tonic level. Even when children are only two years old, the ones who are destined later to be shy and introverted will already dilate their pupils more and develop a faster pulse when they respond to stress than do their socially outgoing counterparts.[6] During vigilance tasks, introverts tend to prefer silence. In contrast, extroverts prefer settings where the amount of auditory stimulation varies. When the background noise does vary, these changes seem to keep extroverts on their toes. Extroverts, perhaps because they are less readily aroused to begin with, perform best when they seek out extra stimuli.[7]

In one EEG study, the baseline brain waves of subjects classified as extroverts were higher in amplitude than those of the introverts.[8] The two groups differed further when they responded to psilocybin. This psychotropic drug is the active agent of the "magic mushroom" which the native tribes of Central America use in their religious ceremonies to induce alternate states of consciousness. After psilocybin, the introverts showed relatively little EEG change from their originally lower baseline level. In contrast, the extroverts proceeded to flatten their EEG patterns toward lower voltages (in keeping with enhanced arousal), and showed more variable alpha activity. One subset of extroverts scored high on a creativity test and had a variable style of handwriting with low handwriting pressure. These extroverts turned out to be the ones more affected when they took psilocybin, and they also became more sluggish at the peak of their drug experience.

The authors of a different study first performed a battery of psychological tests on a group of fifty subjects.[9] The tests defined six different types of personality. It then turned out that each type thereafter responded in a different way to the drug LSD. When human fingerprints, faces, and personalities are so distinctive, we should no longer be surprised to find that our individual brains show different psychophysiological responses, or that religious experiences affect individuals in subtly different ways.

A given range of stimuli does arouse some persons more than others. Could it be that the subjects who gravitate toward certain kinds of meditation, and who persist, are seeking to *lower* their level of stimulation to some range that seems more optimal for them? Do introverts, who are higher-strung to begin with (but who have lower voltage EEGs), then go on both to seek out and to tolerate the quieter meditative disciplines? To avoid the effects of sampling artifacts on the answers to such questions, we still need many more well-controlled, long-range, multidisciplinary studies. Meanwhile, it would be of interest to keep following into adult life those young introverted children who have started with higher levels of arousal responses to see how many of them might tend to gravitate toward the quieter meditative disciplines.

The nature of the family setting may help determine the outcome among meditators. In Andrew Greeley's survey, those subjects who later tended to have mystical experiences had grown up having closer ties with the kinds of parents who themselves had a more joyous religious approach.[10] But given the fact of a favorable family setting, by what means could it go on to create such differences among groups of meditators? Let us consider two options at the extremes. Suppose the way we, as children, perceived our two parents over the generation gap was as follows: they were the all-powerful and dominant ones; they would beckon but remain mostly unapproachable. Thereafter, would we be influenced to keep looking up, *outside* ourselves, for the highest governing principle?

Or suppose, on the other hand, that our parents made no claim to be final authorities. Instead, they encouraged us early to develop a pervasive sense of individual self-worth, confidence, and independence. Would that particular kind of approach encourage another attitude? Would it then make it easier for us to realize that the central principles governing the universe were not always "way up there," not out of reach, but perhaps down closer to what was in front of us? Whichever way our early home life had first oriented us toward such issues, our encounters with the world will soon bring in other cultural biases and religious traditions. In my own instance, having three sympathetic, and effective teacher-examples also proved to be a major impetus to continue on the rigorous way of Zen Buddhist practice.

Maupin's study revealed individual differences among his subjects even after even after as short a period of meditative practice as two weeks.[11] The subjects were twenty-eight male students who concentrated on their breathing for only forty-five minutes a day. Even so, six of the group reported having briefly entered a state of clear awareness with calm detachment and a nonstriving attitude. It turned out that these six, during the course of their inkblot (Rorschach) tests, were the same individuals who also generated more free thoughts, had more visual imagery, and proved to be better at tolerating unrealistic experiences.

What do people experience, *subjectively*, when they meditate? Subjective levels are almost as difficult to define as to study. Semantic problems and archaic notions prevail. Effects based on expectations further compound the situation. Indeed, both the investigator and the subject insert biases into any study projected from their own traditions and systems of belief.

But let us make due allowances for such problems. Then, what does tend to unfold is *a sequence of experiences*. In many persons it proceeds in a relatively orderly manner, stretched out over months and years of their meditative training.

When Brown and Engler studied some of these stages, they used the inkblot test, finding that the results provided a useful index of the changes, both cognitive and perceptual, that had taken place.[12]

These authors studied three groups of meditating subjects, mostly from our Western culture. To avoid confusion, it will help first to specify what level of expertise each group had already reached. Group 1 was composed of thirty relative beginners. These novices were followed during a three-months' retreat involving continual, intensive daily practice. During this period they pursued the standard concentration-mindfulness meditative approach typical of the southern (Theravada) Buddhist tradition. They made slow progress. Still, half of them developed some skill in concentrating. But only three subjects accessed a higher level of concentration and progressed to notable insights. And of these, only one reached a level of equanimity, still short of enlightenment.

Group 2 was composed of eight subjects. They participated in the same retreat. These eight were already further along in their practice. Indeed, all had previously come to insights, and half of them had realized deeper insights.

Group 3 was even more advanced. It was made up of ten Southeast Asian subjects, eight women and two men, all middle-aged, and two masters were included. In this last group, all but one had reached final enlightenment during an earlier retreat of short duration. Before that prior awakening, they had also practiced for periods varying from six days to three years. In general, their prior enlightenment episodes were considered to have transformed all the members of this last group of meditators. Why? Because their experiences had permanently affected both their ongoing *traits* of perception and their approach to life.

What happened in the inkblot tests? In group 1, the novices, it turned out that only about half of them showed changes that differed from their baseline Rorschach tests. The changes were slight, even though the subjects had meditated intensively for three months. But the skills of thirteen of the other beginners had progressed to the level called "samadhi." And in this latter subgroup of beginners, the inkblot responses became distinctly different. Parenthetically, it should be pointed out that when these thirteen other novices were in the act of being tested they were obviously not then sitting in the depths of a completely quiet total meditative absorption. Instead, they were actively looking at the test cards and talking. However, the investigators still considered that this subgroup of subjects had at least partially maintained their state of "samadhi" during the actual testing.

The novice "samadhi subjects" made fairly concrete responses to an inkblot. They did not generate many associative elaborations to its shapes, edges, and outlines. To them, inkblots were perceptions of color and form which frequently shifted. Their responses suggested that "samadhi," so defined, was a distinctive state. It was one in which perception did continue, but without its being further elaborated upon—as we do usually—into a flurry of loose associations or interpretations.

In sharp contrast were the Rorschach test results among subjects in the more advanced group 2. Four of these eight meditators had previously reached the level of some real but shallow insights. Let us begin with this particular subgroup of four. Their inkblot tests proved interesting, for reasons both quantitative and quantitative. Each of the four subjects made many responses to each card, revealing that they were widely open to the flow of their internal associations. The result was a rich cultural diversity of associative elaborations, an intensity of affect, and an abundant metaphoric use of color. Whereas the subjects did make original associations, these were not loose but tended to fit into a certain outline. The general trend was toward flexible responses rich in content. Moreover, even though the subjects' previous insights had struck an impersonal note, their current Rorschach tests proved to be "deeply human and fraught with the richness of the living process . . . we are dealing with a very unusual quality and richness of life experience."[13]

How impressed were the authors by the way these four subjects performed on their inkblot tests? The reader may judge from the authors' summary description: the "experience may be likened to the extemporaneous music of a jazz musician."

We now take up the second *sub*group, the remaining four subjects within group 2. These were the most advanced Western meditators who had already come to deep additional insights. During their moments of major insight they were said to have experienced a perfect, pure awareness of *stillness* and *vastness*, "the Supreme Silence." At that instant, they considered that their consciousness had "expanded" into a new, major understanding of the ground nature of reality. After this period of mental silence and deep peace, they had gradually emerged from their brief experience, feeling detached, light, and elated for the next hours to several days.

But the inkblot tests had not been performed on these four more advanced subjects until long after this particular meditative retreat was over. Tests performed weeks and months later would not be timed to reveal the immediate effects of brief changes in mental *state* which had occurred during the retreat itself. Instead, the subjects' responses at such a late date would be reflecting the nature of their own underlying *traits*. Why? Because it is the working assumption that one's traits remain the most enduring and ongoing "structural" elements of one's personality. Still, these delayed test results remain of interest, because they might suggest to what degree the subjects' much *earlier* major insights—the insights even *before* the retreat—had subsequently transformed their ongoing perceptions and attitudes.

A case could be made for this interpretation. Because these four subjects perceived inkblots as interactions between form and energy, or between form and space. Indeed, they tended to view their own internal imageries, in response to the inkblots, as being manifestations of energy or space. And it was from this particular perspective that the four subjects developed a unique, dynamic approach to their inkblots even while they were making seemingly ordinary responses. For example, they seemed to be witnessing "energy/space in the moment-by-moment process as it arose and organized into forms and images," following which it then dissolved back into "energy/space" again.

Frequently, the inkblot responses made by the members of this second advanced subgroup referred to the spinal column and to the sex organs. Their responses also displayed various themes of conflict, but the subjects were open and not defensive about these conflicts. Personal interviews later on supported the findings of the inkblot tests. The four subjects interviewed were direct and matter-of-fact. They tended to see their personal drives and psychodynamic states as intense mind states. They could experience and act upon these states with awareness, but not necessarily invest them with emotion to any great degree.

In group 3, the last study group, only one Rorschach test was obtained. It was from a Southeast Asian Buddhist master who was regarded as having already passed through most, if not all, of the four levels of enlightenment. As such, he was considered to be all-wise, compassionate, and emancipated from personal suffering. To appreciate how unusual his Rorschach responses were, it helps to review how *we* react when we first look at an inkblot. We accept the premise that the blot exists. It is *real*. We believe that we *project* our imaginings onto it. Not so, from this master's perspective. He viewed the inkblot itself as a projection of the mind. He also approached the test cards in a most unusual way: he used them to instruct the examiner toward a larger view of the world within a cosmic perspective. In doing so, he integrated this "cosmic" view and his mind into one single associative theme consistent with Buddhist doctrine.

Such Rorschach results, obtained from different groups and cultures, are certainly intriguing. But when so few persons make progress out of any large group at entry, it begs the original question: what selection factors entered, and how did they operate? So this stimulating pioneering study emphasizes how much more data we would still like to have: correlated physiological and psychological measurements, performed on culturally well-defined groups by multiple outside observers, observers who are *blinded* to each subject's stage of development; both *baseline* tests and interviews which will then be repeated at prescribed intervals as the same subjects are followed for periods of many months and years. William James would contend that issues this critical at the interface between science and religion merit nothing less than a major coordinated effort.

Blind Spots

Psychoanalytical psychiatry left many blind spots in its turbulent wake. Contemporary psychiatrists are reexamining them. Freud never had a peak experience so far as is known. He held a dim view of religion's illusions and delusions, believing that they were comparable with a childhood neurosis. Many still share his skepticism. No one is easily impressed merely by reading, secondhand, that other persons have been "reborn" by their religious experiences.[14]

Some orthodox psychoanalysts who follow Freud still cling to the earlier word-formulations. These old phrases would have us continue to interpret mystical experiences as being "regressions to an infantile mode," as acts performed "in the service of the ego." Others would interpret them as regressions further back to experiences in the womb, or in the passage from the womb, or as expressing feelings the infant had when nursing at its mother's breast. Hunt expresses the opposite view: mystical experiences are not regressive. Instead, they are the ultimate expressions of human creative capacities, because they fully integrate the brain's metaphoric symbolic functions with those of the special senses.[15]

One can be misled by the term "born again." It does not imply regression. For adult brains undergo highly adaptive psychophysiological transformations during major enlightenment experiences. Indeed, long before these brief moments occur, the networks of any mature adult's brain will already have gone on to function in a highly complex manner, and in ways far more advanced than those that a baby's immature nervous system is capable of experiencing, remembering, or acting upon.

Jung took a much more open, balanced view of religion's assets than did Freud. He concluded that his older patients became mentally ill because they had lost what religion basically had to offer them. Moreover, none of his older patients got well until they had regained their religious outlook.[16] Yet a singular fact remains. Even when Jung had his heart attack, and went through his striking episode in the hospital of looking at the world most objectively, he did not describe actually *losing* his own personal self (see chapter 138). Moreover, even when he spoke of the ways in which normal persons reach their full psychic development, he chose words which still tended to refer back to a self that was omnipresent. The descriptions of this self were cast in standard Occidental terms. Thus, one reads: "The goal of psychic development is the self. There is no linear evolution: there is only a circumambulation of the self. Uniform development exists, at most, only at the beginning; later everything points to the center."[17]

Jung also used the term *individuation*. By this he meant the process of "self-realization" through which the individual person became "whole." Nevertheless, even mature individuation, he said, still "gathers the world to itself" despite the fact that it was not egocentric and did "not shut one out from the world."[18]

From his experience with his Western clientele, Jung would be led to conclude that anyone who attempted to become detached was merely trying to break free from moral considerations.[19] This point has given rise to a common misconception. Is it true that the mystical path toward detachment—best termed "nonattachment"—is solely a form of escapism? Some psychoanalysts now believe that modern mysticism is much more specific. Yes, they say, it *does* move away. From aggression. Then, in the process of moving away from aggression, they speculate that mystical experiences take on a different form. At this point, so the current theory goes, those earlier psychic energies which had once sought out instinctual sexual and material gratifications can be liberated from their earlier aggressive ties. Finally they can be transformed into something more blissful.[20]

Some psychiatrists are criticizing their colleagues for having tried to force Buddhist enlightenment experiences to fit into such old diagnostic categories as depersonalization, dissociation, or conversion. Shimano and Douglas believe that their psychiatric colleagues commit a grave error if they try to classify enlightenment as a form of psychopathology. Instead, having practiced meditation themselves, these authors arrive at a different conclusion: "Personal experience through the adequate practice of meditation is essential to the proper interpretation of the irreducible Zen experience of reality."[21] What does it *mean* to experience reality?

We take up again the kind of episode that many persons enter for a fleeting instant: an experience which confers at least the surface layer of such a major insight into reality. After this, relatively few go on to fully *actualize* this moment of insight-wisdom. Actualizing means putting one's insight-wisdom *consistently* into practice in everyday life. Maslow interviewed several dozen well-known "self-actualizing" people, conducting what he called a "Pre-scientific, freewheeling reconnaissance."[22] He wondered: were those actualizers who *did* have peak and/or plateau experiences any different from the others?

They were. He called them "transcenders." How did transcenders view their earlier peak experiences? As the precious "high spots" of life. As the moments which had transformed the way they subsequently looked at the world and themselves. Only on occasion did some transcenders later go on to manifest their brand-new perspective. But the others did so in an ongoing manner "as a usual thing." In either instance, the subjects appeared to be living at what Maslow would call the "level of Being." This phrase meant that they were directing their life toward intrinsic values, toward ends, not means.

His *non*transcending self-actualizers were different. They inhabited a hard-nosed, competitive world. It was the all-too-familiar one in which each of us asks, of other people and of things: do they have what I need? Existence at this level means quickly using up the useful, discarding the useless.

In sharp contrast, the real transcenders appreciated the sacred in the secular. Nevertheless, they still kept their firm practical grip on reality. Maslow believed this latter pragmatic quality was like a traditional Zen attitude. It was the perspective that fully accepted all things as "nothing special." Transcenders also used the language of "Being" in a natural way. They would quickly recognize one another, communicating readily on first meeting. They responded more to beauty; to holistic, cosmic viewpoints; moved more readily beyond self; were more innovative. The more they knew, the more awed and humbled they were by the increasing mystery of the universe. Being more objective about their own talents, they regarded themselves as instruments. Still aware of evil, they remained objective about it, striking out swiftly to stop it, and with less ambivalence. These transcenders tended to regard everyone as fellow members of the same sacred human family. It was an attitude that helped them interact more effectively with other people who did not perform well. It enabled them to punish transgressors for the sake of the greater good, yet still treat fools kindly.

But Maslow's transcenders had their downside as well. They were not as happy as his other, healthy self-actualizers. They seemed prone to a kind of "cosmic-sadness." This arose out of "the stupidity of people, their self-defeat, their blindness, their cruelty to each other, their short sightedness." So his transcenders had not yet become 100 percent emancipated. They were still troubled by that large gap between the ideal and the actual—by that gulf between what "should" be or "ought" to be possible and the sad conditions which do in fact exist in the real world. Long ago, Siddhartha had started out on his own quest, having been greatly troubled by that same gap, and he would not become fully emancipated from it until he was thirty-five years old.

Soon we will examine where such "shoulds" and "oughts" come from. In the process, we will observe how Zen training keeps addressing this very gap, itself the source of so many of our downside attitudes. Then we will discover why such strongly prejudiced opinions take us so many decades to reconcile. And to go beyond.

30

Sesshin and Teisho at Ryoko-in, 1974

> Buddhist philosophy tells us that man must return to his own real self, namely to non-ego. He must awaken to the fact that the self he normally considers to be his self or ego is a false self, full of ignorance and subject to suffering.
>
> Nanrei Kobori (1918–1992)[1]

A sesshin is a Buddhist religious retreat. Practice intensifies during this week. Like the other lay aspirants, I sleep at home and come to the temple for more frequent meditation periods during the rest of the day. The roshi holds daily private interviews with us and gives several lectures, called *teisho*.

He begins: "In ancient times, the purpose of meditation was to relieve the mind from being influenced by material conditions. Back then, the historical Buddha was only one of many awakened persons. Everyone is capable of being awakened; each one of you here has the potential to become a Buddha.

"Everyone speaks about going on to Nirvana. Words! The etymological roots of the word Nirvana mean being extinguished or blown out. These roots might lead you to think it is all a negative condition. However, at least one interpretation is that it is only the undesirable passions that are extinguished. They are like fires, and when they are blown out, our original purity still remains.

"Buddhism has a deep compassion for others. It deemphasizes our desires to keep on being our separate single self in the endless chain of love, birth, suffering, and death. Instead, it teaches us to share freedom and purity with others, and to go on to Nirvana with others. The *yahna* of Mahayana Buddhism means a big boat. One uses it to cross the river and to arrive at the other shore. It is no small boat, because everyone else in the universe is there sharing this passage!

"Zen as a religion does have a certain philosophical base. These ideas may help to understand it, and to begin to put it in practice. But Zen is more." At this point, he takes off his glasses and says: "Here, I hold my glasses. It is one thing for me to know that these glasses have a frame. It is still another to understand scientifically how the lens focuses." Then he looks directly at me and smiles, saying, "But *using glasses* is to know what glasses *really* are." I feel I have been delivered a personal message.

At another teisho, he says, "Politicians and sociologists develop ideas about freedom. But these ideas are all rice cakes painted on rice paper. No real rice is there to satisfy a hungry stomach! No laws give us our basic freedom. Freedom comes only from being liberated from all other kinds of conditioning. Freedom is to *be* in the here and now. Thus, we teach being free *internally*. This is different from all these other external freedoms.

"Ordinarily, we think *this* way. But thinking *this* way implies there can also be a *that* way. *This* opinion implies *that* one. Beginning implies end. The essence that is expressed out of zazen is a lack of these discriminations. Zazen removes all such relative, comparative thinking. If you make everything exist in the immediate now, you will not become concerned with past or future. *Now* is.

"The Western world depends on using words to transmit information. But in Japan, the strongest, deepest truth is that which passes unsaid from master to student. A student recognizes the greatness of his teacher by the way he stands in the rain, holding up an umbrella. No words are necessary.

"What about samadhi? This old Sanskrit term has taken on many different meanings. And it, too, is not the final purpose of zazen. Samadhi involves a kind of non-distinction, but you must break through it, go beyond it. Zen is concerned with the essence of the moment of true enlightenment, *prajna*. Not with rituals, not with words. This essence is closer to the feeling of poetry, art, and other inexpressible things. No words. The more things are spoken about, the less of their truth remains, for words separate them from their basic selves. In the monastery, particularly in earlier days, the monks communicated not with words but with sounds on wood or with bells.

"For seven years, I was the monk responsible for each sesshin, the *jikijitsu*. In sesshin, we sat from early morning into the night. After three or four days, no distinctions remained between being asleep and being awake, none between day or night. The seed of enlightenment springs out of this soil of nondistinction. But bear in mind that nondistinction alone is not what you are looking for. It is not the final product. What you are looking for is the wisdom of prajna. Bear in mind that no drug will plant this seed, nor can a drug be the soil of enlightenment."

31

Sesshin

Question: Sesshin has a very strong form. Is that form essential?

Joshu Sasaki-roshi: Form or rules are very important. We are not trying to keep you inside of them but to cut off your ego. This is very important as a way of teaching. To cut off your ego is the first step in Zen practice.

Joshu Sasaki-roshi[1]

Many religious traditions hold periodic retreats. Retreats do more than afford time for solitude. They make it possible to reorder priorities so that one can then rededicate oneself to the central purposes of life. A *sesshin,* from the Chinese *che-hsin,* literally means the joining of mind to mind. It is a Zen religious retreat during which the sangha unites for extended periods of meditation. In a monastic setting, a sesshin frequently lasts five to seven days and may recur as often as once a month for up to ten months a year.

The retreat is usually held in the shelter of a temple or other secluded place. Now the aspirant becomes relatively free from worldly distractions. Moreover, when minds join in a group effort, the participants become team members. This sense of community makes for an intensified, sustained effort not possible to reach by acting alone. During sesshin, daily personal interviews, *sanzen*, are held especially in the Rinzai tradition. In the roshi's daily lectures to the group, he comments on the sayings of previous Zen masters, draws from his own experience, and applies Zen principles to the events of everyday life much as does any good minister who delivers a practical sermon.

First, the biological clock is reset. We will later clarify why this is so important. Days start at 4 to 5 A.M., and end at 9 or 10 P.M., or later if the meditator so chooses. Commonsense rules are in force. Discipline is strict during the formal zazen periods, which may total some six hours or so each day. Soon, leg, shoulder, and back complaints become a major problem, and mental side effects, *makyo*, may become prominent. A sesshin, then, meshes some of the physical hurdles of an Outward Bound experience with rigorous inward-bound challenges. Zazen provides ample opportunities to encounter both kinds. One must endure, and learns to do so.

Zazen periods of twenty-five to forty minutes are interspersed with periods of walking meditation, chanting, work, exercise, rest, and light meals. During all of these, the aspirant minds his or her own "business." This means not talking, reading, or telephoning. Most lay students need at least the first half of the sesshin merely to settle down, and to become free from distractions. Gradually, one becomes steady, utterly single-minded, and concentrated in the meditative mode.

Zazen periods are not uniform in texture. They vary substantially within, and among themselves. The beginner tends to subject them to "good" or "bad" value judgments. The variability reflects more than the meditator's fluctuating ability to relax and to concentrate, because unpredictable physiological currents also swirl in to shift one's inner weather. Changes blow hot or cold quickly, sometimes ranging from elation to despair over five to ten minutes. Periods of arousal can be permeated with energy and a positive affective tone, or with feelings of tension and pessimism. Brisk walks during kinhin for only five to ten minutes can lift mood for an hour or so.[2] After several sesshin, one becomes less judgmental, learns to take what comes.

Communications with others take place mostly through gestures, in writing, or in brief whispers. Seeing oneself in a mirror is avoided. The trainee talks only with the roshi. The roshi is increasingly supportive during his personal interviews once or twice a day. He blends a mixture of advice, encouragement, expectation, and demand, keeping the student pointed in the direction of the koan. The roshi exhorts the student to take the koan deeper into the lower abdomen, the *hara*, to incorporate it and sometimes to roar it out. A time may come when "Mu," or "One" feels as though it were on a hair trigger, ready to be roared out at the slightest tap or sound. When this condition arrives naturally, it may prompt quick vocal utterances that take one by surprise.[3]

Increasingly, insights of various sizes flash in during the simplified routine and clarity of a sesshin. They are empowered by a reflective mode which seems to scan the whole range of the meditator's personal life history. One's foibles rise up for especially close inspection. Observed in the power of silence, recurring behavior patterns stick out like a sore thumb. But now they are examined at a distance, more objectively, and are less threatening to self-esteem. Decisions then flow spontaneously about how to improve oneself. Smaller-sized, more ordinary intuitions, which resolve life's lesser problems, seem to be followed by better sitting posture, fewer muscle achings, and better concentration. At night, dream scenarios become clear and more inventive than usual. Personal growth during a sesshin is incremental, as the Soto tradition has long emphasized.

Most sesshin end on an upbeat note. Is this more than simple relief from suffering? Yes. The aspirant who before had been plugging along in life now has a palpable sense of being revitalized and rehumanized for a few days after it ends. The effect surpasses the way one is refreshed by a two-weeks' vacation. Such positive experiences are not unique to the Buddhist tradition, for they occur commonly in other forms of religious retreat.

The term "deepening" conveys some of these more profoundly resonating affective levels. Deepening is coming back into close, steady, compassionate touch with a world that has taken on a freshened, sacramental quality. What we know about neurotransmitters and other messenger molecules (see part III) affords one plausible explanation for some of its aspects. Rinsed free of the attachments of self, the meditator now feels more intimately and empathetically aware within this larger world. Before the retreat, a blur of perceptions had taken in an ordinary world, as though it had been seen with but one eye and listened to with only one ear. Now, perception is both sensitized and subtly transformed: two eyes and both ears are wide open. A very wide-awake brain is taking in the world afresh. Deepening goes beyond this. The person not only sees and hears more but seems to see stereoscopically, into novel phases of life, and to comprehend more in every new dimension disclosed. With one's perceptions open and expanded, thoughts and actions also take on a lively, efficient quality. When problems enter from the inside or outside they now meet composed responses, and simpler solutions suggest themselves.

Unfortunately, for most part-time lay students, such changes fade after several days. Still, some residues persist. So, too, do the memories of "what it felt like to be *really* living." More fortunate are those serious students and monks who practice for months and years in a full-time monastic setting. They enter each sesshin having had a solid backlog of their intensified practice in daily living. They also attend more than one or two sesshin a year. Even then, it will take them years of steady practice, relatively sheltered from the blizzard of worldly distractions, before each sesshin can exert its major cumulative effects.

Converging into a sesshin are many factors which help generate alternate states of consciousness.[4] These include (1) sleep loss, (2) relative isolation, (3) reduced feelings of personal responsibility, (4) prolonged zazen with sensorimotor deprivation, (5) the increasingly open release of previously repressed thoughts and behaviors, (6) prolonged immersion in the meditative mode, (7) stress from the pains of sitting and from the self-imposed pressures to resolve the koan, and (8) powerful reinforcements that come from being in the group effort with other people who share the same earnest commitments.

How do all these affect the brain? This will be our subject in parts III through VI.

The Meditative Approach to the Dissolution of the Self

> The Buddhist Way, the training in Buddhism consists mainly of breaking up I into its component parts and reassembling them in a manner that comes closer to what is truly human.
>
> Irmgard Schloegl[1]

> I sat there and forgot and forgot, until what remained was the river that went by and I who watched . . . Eventually the watcher joined the river and then there was only one of us. I believe it was the river.
>
> Norman Maclean[2]

Like pages piled into a thick hospital chart, our daily newspapers document society's major ills. Shrill headlines vie with advertisements. Which will dominate: angst, or a status-conscious consumerism? "I'm looking out for Number One" seems to be the prevailing slogan. Successive *Me* generations are swept up in the cult of never growing old. Greed is the creed, as each person grasps for *Mine.* We have grown up in this contagion of the *I-Me-Mine,* caught a full share of its insidious attitudes and lifestyles (see figure 1). We are culturally imprinted, conditioned to respond in set ways to the turmoil of life's daily issues.

All this poorly used circuitry wastes much energy. Its dysfunctional parts need to be redirected, neutralized, or bypassed. Rarely does the flashing grace of kensho help to get rid of them. Meanwhile, the dysfunctions yield, but only slowly, to three approaches: to daily life practice, *shugyo;* to renunciation, *shila;* and to meditation, *zazen.*

Wise teachers like Schloegl get right to the point: the old I must be transformed. The process is endless. Zen uses various approaches to reshape the input to the *I-Me-Mine,* to defuse it, and to redeploy its output. In summary here, it suffices to specify nine methods. The first three are now obvious. The remaining six are subtler and tend not to be put into words that stray into print. Others could be added. One encounters their origins in commonplace observations. Sometimes, while totally relaxing by a river, the self just vanishes . . .

1. The beginner to zazen soon discovers what ordinary thinking is: an agitated, Brownian motion of proliferating abstractions and associations. Each sets off a chain reaction. This incessant chatter of thoughts swirls around the axis of self/other concerns. It leaves little spare time for completely clear, calm reasoning. In contrast, meditation dispenses with discursive thoughts. It finally develops an awareness so clear that it goes not only beyond reasoning but beyond unreasoning fears and other concerns.

When Descartes observed himself think, he took Western rationality to what one may paraphrase as its logical conclusion: To think is to be. Zen meditation drops this emphasis on thinking. It substitutes *being* in its place. It turns the statement around into: *Not* to think is to be. Zen emphasizes an open, *no-thinking* awareness. It is this approach which will point ultimately toward the state of no-I, the major step in dissolving the *I-Me-Mine* complex.

2. Meditation teaches both brain and body its personal nuances, ways that seem to help their mutual processes of relaxation flow back "there" again spontaneously. One of zazen's functions is to ease the meditator so many times into the states approaching pure awareness that moving back and forth through this interface then becomes the natural, habitual, neurophysiological response. So natural, in fact, that the meditator no longer struggles to maintain a toehold back in that old subjective maelstrom, the state we call ordinary consciousness.

But the aspirant's great dilemma keeps returning: how do I still attend to what is going on without willfully engaging my *I-Me-Mine* in this very act of paying attention? The riverbank attitude helps. It is a letting go of oneself, of letting things happen, of *not* striving. This means *not trying* to do something. It also means not trying *not* to do something. Finally, a state beyond trying arrives. Then, awareness just *is*, a simple matter-of-fact awareness of awareness. But, before the usual turbulent stream of thought finally settles down into this deep calm millpond, zazen will have exposed the meditator's every mental ripple, eddy, and crosscurrent. They come . . . and go.

3. Meditation's third obvious role is to reduce sensory input and feedback. Normally, these enter both from the special senses which confer vision, hearing, and balance, and from various proprioceptive systems. Proprioceptive impulses are those sensate messages which arrive from nerve endings out in muscles, joints, and tendons. Coding for one's physical self, they tell us where one's own head, arms, legs, and trunk are positioned in space. This incoming sensory traffic quiets down when movements stop. Learning to relax, to sit quietly without wobbling or fidgeting, goes on to create a condition of sensori*motor* deprivation. Prolonged meditative sitting does even more. It dampens the notion that one must always be a doer, an acting-out, motoric self. Once all those impulses fade so far away that you don't *feel where* you are, you begin to forget *that* you are, and no longer feel the impulse that you *must keep doing* something.

Ordinarily, it's hard to forget that we exist. We constantly reinforce this sense of self. We answer the ever-ringing telephone, hear ourselves speak, see how other people react to us socially, keep looking at the clock. Meditative retreats shut down these avenues of sensory distraction. Retreats enable meditators to forget about clock time, to remain silent, to keep interpersonal contacts to a minimum, even to avoid observing their reflections in the mirror.

In what follows next, we try to put into words six slower, subtle processes. These also serve to erode the dysfunctional self. Less often enunciated, meditators know these as facts of experience, especially during sesshin.

4. Formerly, each like and dislike generated a sticky web of thoughts. As renunciation and zazen cut back on these desires and aversions, the meditator is less often entrapped in their net. Zazen now becomes less distracted, plumbing deeper levels of no-thought, remaining there longer and more effectively.

5. Previously, it was difficult to engage in direct, unconditioned experiences. What stood in the way of genuine relationships with oneself, with other persons, and with material possessions? That old backlog of ignorance, passionate longings, and loathings. When these distortions recede, the mental landscape expands. Within its expansion, a more mature introspective self emerges. It starts

asking discrete questions: "How did I get this way? How do I stop?" Now intro-spection has the time, and the mental space, to keep the dialogue "on-line." Its self-scrutiny operates silently, penetrating the camouflage of the *I-Me-Mine*. Pre-viously, the process yielded only a few brief, almost subliminal insights. Now the insights dart in and stay longer, exposing the litany of one's defects with unspar-ing, clinical objectivity.

Washburn draws a useful analogy to this process. It is the way we behave after we return to our own country, having recently lived in a foreign land long enough to have learned to appreciate how its culture developed.[3] Now we go beyond merely looking *at* our own country. From a fresh perspective, we really start to *see into* it, clearly, deeply, objectively, for the first time.

6. Meditators start getting much more critical about themselves. Off come the halos. They discover how strongly they resist not only zazen but push against most forms of outside structure and against self-discipline in general. Illuminat-ing disclosures come from observing these struggles. They learn to diagnose their willful selves, their restless, finger-tapping selves, to "see themselves as others see them." They catch themselves flushing deeply when they are embarrassed. They discover that anger is the other side of fear—fear that the *Me* will be injured, fear that the *Mine* will be robbed of its precious possessions. They realize why they scold themselves after having done something foolish. From such clues they learn how much extraneous authoritarian input they have incorporated. Slowly, they become able to forgive themselves.

They also learn to penetrate the sham of their own pernicious "spiritual materialism," that impure "spiritual self-seeking" which William James cautioned against.[4] The remedy comes from encountering a hard nosed Zen. Its rules permit no indulgences. It allows no trainee the misplaced luxury of being proud of—and thus becoming attached to—any major experience which had dissolved the *I-Me-Mine*. Instead, Zen sees each surrender of self as but one fleeting milestone on an endless pilgrimage.

7. Given the luxury of bare attention, and of quiet time in which to reflect, trainees at more advanced levels of meditation learn to take the long view. Experi-entially, it becomes clear what is meant by the phrase, "This, too, shall pass away." Things are seen to be impermanent in practice, not merely in theory. Major events strike hard. But they fade. They come and go. What is, *is*. What *might* happen is not yet here. Finally comes the realization that to try to "gain enlightenment" is the antithesis of the Zen approach.

8. Other realizations encourage the meditator: it is a relief first to distance the self, then to lose it. *It feels good to do so.* The first of these surprising facts of experience comes to the beginner in zazen. Thoughts actually do drop off, the bodily self fades, yet clear awareness persists! Other episodes later, during sa-madhi and kensho, convincingly dissolve the self. And during each state, you don't let go of *your* self. You are let go *of*. Having finally lost the self in these three different ways, having lived safely through the realities of being "there," and of coming back, the aspirant no longer fears the outcome. In fact, there enters a mild amusement at the old sophistry which had once contended, within all ordinary logic, you can't have an "experience" unless an "I" is there to have it.

9. At first, sitting is something to "do." When true clarity finally arrives later during sesshin, the meditator realizes what sustained attentiveness is. Still later comes the fresh perspective: zazen is not doing but *being*—being in a way that extends beyond the context of the mat to enter into the appreciation of the miracle of everyday living. Finally, the meditator comes to appreciate that just sitting, in full quiet awareness, is in itself the receptive appreciation that constitutes enlightenment. It is a natural way to celebrate that simple awareness of the now, the one which Dogen long emphasized.

Along the way, as one's grasping self-interest shrinks, fewer situations then arise to conflict with one's basic ethical values. Observation then confirms the foregoing points. Daily life does flow more harmoniously whenever the meditator lowers the flapping flag of the sovereign I, shortens the defensive perimeter, and lets go of the clutching tentacles of personalized attachments.

*　　　*　　　*

The closing pages of this section on meditation are an appropriate place to confront another deceptive word: *zero.* Arab scholars discovered the concept of zero. But only after they had finally gotten past the number *one.* At this point mathematics could take a quantum leap.

From the beginning, we have all been programmed to, as we say, "look out for Number One." Gradually, each trainee moves past this old, selfish Number One, keeps going back through a neutral equanimity, and finally on in the direction toward zero. But isn't this a dangerous thing to do? We can almost hear our own protests welling up: "Give up *myself* to a mindless oblivion? Become a *zero*? No way!" Reasonable objections. In theory, someone who just "lets go" might fall into a careless, unfeeling, zombie-like state, become an aimless dropout, drifting with the prevailing winds and currents.

But remember, no one engaged in authentic Buddhist training relinquishes either moral compass, anchor, or rudder. Early Indian Buddhists already had in place their own right-minded ethical code, the eightfold path. In China, Chan was further grounded in both the strong, family-based social ethic of Confucianism and in the deep Taoist respect for the natural order of things. Moreover, another foundation for meditative training is the sangha. It exemplifies hard work, and its fellowship of lay students and monks provides a cohesive support group.

So whenever we have spoken of the direction toward "zero" it has been as a very temporary and imperfect metaphor. In the Zen context, it *always stands for losing only the unfruitful part of the self, not for a totally vacuous personality.* Zen training does not wipe out all personality structure, to leave only a nobody. It spares the pragmatic ego in Freud's original sense. It leaves intact all those vital functions that help us manage situations in real life. Indeed, this maturing ego grows increasingly flexible and practical, finding new ways to navigate both life's vicissitudes and the rigors of the Zen training process. Who, then, are the best candidates for meditative training? Not zeros, but persons already tough-minded to begin with, reasonably well-integrated, mature, differentiated, and autonomous. As Engler aptly notes: "You have to be somebody before you can be nobody."[5]

Zen training is an agency of personal change. And it contributes a distinctive, fourfold creative encounter that shapes the process of change. What it provides, first, is a setting so rigorous that it soon exposes how much the meditator has been distorted by the *I-Me-Mine* triad; second, so open and free of distractions that the trainee's own insights then disclose how insubstantial and lacking in continuity these distortions are; third, so interactive that it provides ways to work off these dysfunctions in daily life practice; and finally, a setting so intrinsically appealing that the aspirant tends to stay the course no matter what happens.

In such dynamic ways do persistent practice and rare insights help shrink the once almighty *I*, the vulnerable *Me*, and the intrusive *Mine*. Not gone entirely. Just reduced to manageable proportions. Just i-me-mine. Something more considerate of the *you*, the *we*, the *ours*, and the rest of the biosphere. Being diminutive, this new i-me-mine carries a very low profile. Smaller and streamlined, it no longer sticks up high to trip the positive functions of the mature ego. Neither is it windblown by every shifting, hot or cold breeze from the old instinctual self. Nor will it be overloaded by distortions imposed by others' guilt-ridden consciences.

In fact, some of its shrinking is only apparent. Look beneath the i-me-mine. There, at its base, we find that its' many positive attributes have substantially expanded.[6] Especially does its living taproot, always spared, now probe deeper, grounded in ways that perceive life's deeper rhythms. Now we recall, its lower-case letters stand for the a-b-c's of someone revitalized, more *actualized, buoyant,* and *compassionate.* Where did the hitherto partisan self of the Me generation go? Into a simpler generic member who belongs to the We generation. To this person, it will seem only natural to celebrate Earth Day every day. Delusional? It hardly feels that way. It seems like a return toward one's original state in the eternal scheme of things.

Still, any meditator's progress is uneven at best. Backsliding occurs. Let strong passions arise, and the old italics and capital letters rear back up. Aspirants relearn during every such sobering reencounter why so few persons have ever become perfectly evolved, selfless beings. Yet, endured decade by patient decade, the unfruitful parts of the complex grow smaller, their wasted energies subside sooner, to be put to better use. Each kensho deepens, leaves less protruding.

From these perspectives, the Zen approach is a glacial, erosive process of *unlearning* and personal restructuring. It operates on what seems almost a geological time scale. Very few earthquakes are thrown in to shake things up. Any novice expecting a permanent quick fix is soon disappointed. The trainee, it turns out, was first learning simply how to unlearn. Then the receptive process of relearning opens up. As it unfolds on its own, it seems to reconnect the person with what are now new and vital relationships. Yet they are the ones which have always been there: life's ageless immanent, everyday miracles.

Part III

Neurologizing

You must be familiar with the very groundwork of science before you try to climb the heights.

Ivan Pavlov (1849–1936)

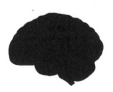

Brain in Overview: The Large of It

Only those contents of consciousness can be developed that correspond to the organization of the brain.

Walter R. Hess (1881–1973)[1]

Must one learn strange words like zazen? Can one remember everything about the frontal lobe? No. But this is the way Zen is. And if you're anything like me, you'll become fascinated by the latest discoveries about the human brain, the center of our being. How do its different regions function, individually and in concert? We begin to answer this question in part III, always heeding Pavlov's advice: first, become familiar with the groundwork of neuroscience, the better later to climb its heights.

For many readers, this is uphill hiking. Most of us will have been short-changed by the educational system, and will have previously found the brain impenetrable. But that old black box of Pavlov's era is no longer terra incognita. The first three chapters permit you to review the major features of the terrain ahead. Thereafter, you can browse and skip around. Gradually, the relationships between Zen and the different brain regions will become clear. Cross-references will help you return to specific chapters in part III and to reinterpret their contents.

Let us first look at the outside of the brain, starting at the top with the *cerebrum*. Its outer layer, our wrinkled *cerebral cortex*, is called the gray matter. Its gray color comes from many billions of nerve cells. It interconnects with subcortical regions using bundles of white, insulated fibers: white matter. Fissures and arbitrary lines divide the cerebrum into four pairs of lobes: frontal, parietal, temporal, and occipital (figure 2).

What did evolution keep adding to hominid brains? Mostly association cortex. Humans now devote 80 percent of the volume of the entire brain to their convoluted cortex. In monkeys, this outer rind of cortex occupies only two thirds of the brain. The association cortex in the front part of our *frontal lobes* helps us to generate goals that are personally desirable, to consider how socially appropriate they are, and then to decide which behaviors will project best into the future. Many other higher-order executive functions arise in the frontal lobes, including those which direct speech and other precise, willed movements.

Behind lie the *parietal lobes*. In the parietal lobes we not only receive sensations but reach fine discriminations among them. Here, attention engages perception at its higher abstract levels. Which of those several keys in our pocket is the car key? This one, our fingers tell us. As the parietal lobe makes covert "representations," it relates our fingers' sensate image to the shape of each key.

Below each parietal lobe, deep to our temple on either side, lie the *temporal lobes*. They decode and interpret what we hear and see, and process other more elaborate, patterned sensory messages. The left temporal lobe is especially important in understanding language-related concepts.

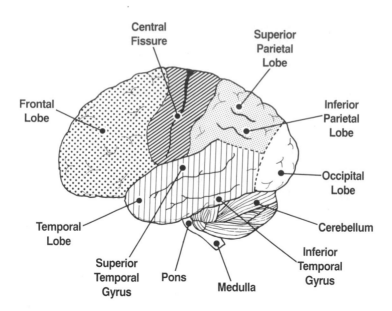

Figure 2 The left cerebral hemisphere
This lateral view shows its principal lobes. At the base of the cerebrum are the pons, medulla, and cerebellum. The prefrontal cortex occupies most of the convex, dotted surface of the frontal lobe. The crosshatched area in front of the central fissure represents the primary motor cortex; that behind it represents the primary somatosensory cortex. In back, the dotted lines suggest the approximate boundaries between the temporal, parietal, and occipital lobes. (Not shown is a band of premotor cortex which lies just in front of the motor cortex. Within the whole parietal lobe, the upper and lower portions are also known as the superior and inferior parietal *lobules,* respectively. (Redrawn and modified with reference to several standard texts, including figure 1-2 in *The Human Nervous System,* 3rd Ed. C. Noback and R. Demarest, New York, McGraw-Hill, 1981.)

The *occipital lobes* at the back of the brain register impulses concerned with vision. Next, they pattern them into streams of visual messages that relay forward through both temporal and parietal lobes. Throughout this complex mosaic we will generate, and regenerate, those mental images which we call our "mind's eye." Growing up, we have developed certain patterns of expectation within the temporal-parietal-occipital regions. These serve as mental templates. They help us both to recognize and to inject meanings into what we see.

Now let us view the other half of the cerebrum, this time from the inside (figure 3). At the base of the brain is its enlarged stalk, the *brain stem.* Its lowest level is the *medulla,* which rises up from the *spinal cord.* Its intermediate level is the *pons;* its highest level, the *midbrain.* The *reticular activating system* extends through the core of the brain stem. This system alerts us and orients us toward important external stimuli. Other brain stem mechanisms help us slide into and out of the stages of sleep. Behind the brain stem lies the *cerebellum,* which helps coordinate our movements and equilibrium.

The bulbous, enlarged *thalamus* extends out of the isthmus at the top of the brain stem. It processes sensory messages arising from our head and body. The *basal ganglia* are distributed around it, especially in front. They pattern our motor

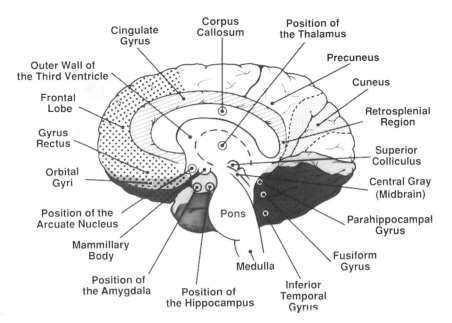

Figure 3 The right cerebral hemisphere, viewed from the inner surface
This shows its inner, medial surface looking up at it from below. The view also depicts the brain stem as still attached. However, the cerebellum behind it has been removed. The lowest part of the brain stem is the medulla. The pons and midbrain lie successively above.

Note that major parts of the limbic system lie disposed in the form of a large oval around the midline of the brain. They include the cingulate gyrus and parahippocampal gyrus, the hippocampus and amygdala buried within the medial temporal lobe, and the hypothalamus.

The position of the thalamus is merely suggested by longer dotted lines. However, its mediodorsal thalamic nucleus projects extensively over the whole prefrontal cortex. The large dotted stippling emphasizes this fact. The faint stippling indicates other thalamic input to cortex: the pulvinar projects up to the cuneus, whereas the lateral posterior nucleus projects up to the precuneus. The long cingulate gyrus (diagonal lines) receives extensive thalamic projections from the anterior thalamic nucleus (not indicated). Below it, the corpus callosum is shown sectioned in half as occurs after so-called split-brain surgery. The fusiform and nearby lingual gyri are the color-responsive regions of cortex. (Redrawn and modified with reference to several standard texts, including figure 1–8 in *The Human Nervous System*, 3rd Ed. C. Noback and R. Demarest, New York, McGraw-Hill 1981.)

responses. Centered deep beneath the thalamus lies the small *hypothalamus*. It coordinates an array of instinctive visceral and endocrine functions. These help us to seek food when we hunger and drink when we thirst. They also help increase our pulse rate and blood pressure in response to a threat.

Sweeping up from the hypothalamus on both sides are several other structures connected to it. These have become known collectively as the *limbic system*. Limbic connections infuse emotional overtones into our experience and into our affective responses. One limbic component, the *hippocampus*, also helps us process data and relay them to be stored in various memory circuits.

The basic functional units within each of the brain regions above are the *nerve cells*, the *neurons*. These we take up next.

Brain in Overview: The Small of It

> No response is determined solely by one structure or even one system, and responses are not based on simple yes-no decisions but on the interactions of numerous yes-no decisions.
>
> W. Waters and D. Wright[1]

The nervous system is basically simple: it receives information, then translates it into appropriate action. Things get more complicated when one asks, What goes on between these two events?

At its receiving end, each single nerve cell thrusts out its many *dendrites*. They reach out for stimuli, almost like tree branches searching for the sun's energy (figure 4). Their twigs swarm with tiny *receptors*. Receptors are sites tuned in to receive the specific chemical messages released by the previous nerve cell. Activate a receptor and it adjusts the flow of ions that pass in and out through the membrane of the underlying nerve cell. At a critical point, this cell membrane loses its previously charged, polar electrical properties. Instantly, the whole *depolarized cell fires*, generating the nerve impulse. This impulse skips quickly down the nerve fiber, the *axon*, to exit through its *nerve terminals*.

As each nerve impulse reaches the end of its nerve terminal, it releases specific chemical substances. These molecules pour out of tiny round storage packets called vesicles, and deliver their chemical messages into the gap between the two nerve cells. This dynamic zone is the *synapse*.

In general, when the first, primary chemical messengers reach their receptors, they then change the next cell in one of three different ways.[2-4]

1. *Chemical messengers can act as transmitters.* In this instance, the chemical messenger acts directly, and is the prime mover. It transfers the signal from the near side of the synapse, the *pre*synaptic side, quickly over to the far side, the *post*synaptic side. To transmit its *fast* excitatory messages, the brain usually uses molecules either of acetylcholine or of glutamate. They *increase* the excitability of the next cell by *de*polarizing it.

On the other hand, other primary transmitters *decrease* the next cell's excitability. For example, GABA excels in this latter inhibitory role. It acts by *hyper*polarizing the next cell.

Back, now, to that first nerve cell, the cell that released its transmitter into the synapse. Having once fired, it recovers quickly to fire again. All along, it recaptures most of its transmitter molecules, takes them back up again into their storage vesicles, and recycles them. It is a remarkable sequence of events. Many nerve cells fire as fast as the wingbeat of the honeybee, generating impulses up to an incredible several hundred times a second!

2. *Chemical messengers can act as modulators.* In this case, the chemicals are not the prime movers. They merely modify, secondarily, the way the other primary transmitters are already acting. They nudge whatever excitation, or inhibition, is already underway, and do so *to a lesser* degree. For example, one typical modula-

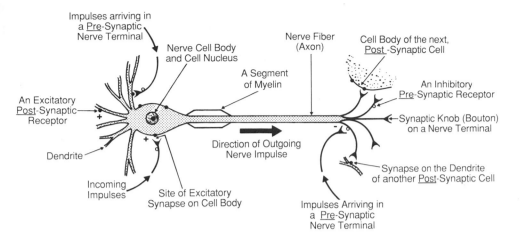

Figure 4   A simplified diagram of a prototype nerve cell
Impulses come to it from other neurons off to the left, and exit from it off to the right. At left, fine *pre*synaptic nerve terminals deliver these incoming nerve impulses. When they release a chemical neurotransmitter, it travels across the gap of the synapse. There, on the far side of the synapse, it activates its special excitatory *pos*tsynaptic receptors. These are shown as small black dots. After enough receptors are excited, as indicated by positive (+) signs, the neuron fires its impulse down the axon toward its own presynaptic terminals, indicated by the large arrow. The process repeats itself when the message reaches the dendrites and spreads down into the cell body of the next, *post*synaptic cells, suggested off to the far right. Small open circles represent inhibitory *pre*synaptic receptors. When these are activated, they shut down the amount of transmitter released. This process is indicated by negative (−) signs.

tor is norepinephrine (NE). Some NE receptors cover the terminal endings of acetylcholine nerve cells. Acting here, NE stops them from releasing their acetylcholine. Broadly generalizing among the biogenic amines, one may say that norepinephrine enhances sensate responses, including those to noxious stimuli, whereas dopamine energizes, and serotonin enters into mood-related behaviors.

3. *Chemical messengers can act as neurohormones.* When a hormone is released into tissue fluids by a nerve cell, it may diffuse a relatively long distance before it can find its specific receptors. Moreover, this hormonal messenger needs no synapse to act.

Every day, people talk with each other in ways that find their counterparts in these three modes of cell-to-cell communication.[3] Neuro*transmission* resembles a private telephone line. Two people on this line are conducting a brisk, efficient business conversation. Theirs is a hardwired connection, and its private link corresponds to the synapse. Neuro*modulators,* on the other hand, superimpose a "gain" control. Given an ongoing conversation, they can either amplify the conversation or mute it. Finally, neuro*hormonal* communication resembles the way a public radio station widely broadcasts its programs. The messages are widely diffused, but only those radio sets tuned in to the specific wavelength can receive them.[5]

The brain has countless trillions of the receptors mentioned earlier. They stud its dendrites, cell bodies, and axon terminals. Think of their outside rim as a tiny receiving station. Its shape is exquisitely designed: it will bind only one particular kind of "first" chemical messenger.[6] A balance is struck between excitation or inhibition when many different receptors are activated on a given cell. The balance decides whether the cell fires, determines how frequently it fires, and influences how long the burst of firing will last.

Suppose now that one presynaptic nerve cell *changes* its routine patterns of firing. How does the next cell downstream, its postsynaptic target cell, detect the message? Perhaps the simplest analogy is the way a scanner reads bar codes at the checkout counter. It takes only a few bars (bursts) of different width, spaced at different intervals, to represent every item in the supermarket. The bar code on the jacket of this book is an example.

Such easy generalizations have limits. Each chemical messenger is used in different circuits throughout the brain. Therefore, no one modulator, no single transmitter molecule or receptor can be said to be the sole "cause" of any one behavior, be it eating, walking, or dreaming. Instead, it turns out that a given chemical messenger does two major things. First, it subtly influences *many* behaviors by acting at several levels in the brain. Second, it also increases or decreases the functional contributions made by its fellow chemical messengers and their receptor systems.[7] As a result of these interactions, the brain is gifted with an immense array of functions, each one subject to multiple variations and gradations.

Does a human brain have enough nerve cells to allow it to do all its work? Anatomists come up with different estimates every year or so. Some years the optimists estimate as many as a trillion. In other years, the conservatives say that the brain holds "only" 300 billion nerve cells. The latter figure is still about the same number of neurons as there are stars in our own galaxy, the Milky Way. To begin to bring such abstract numbers down to earth, it may help to recall that each earthling now shares the planet with over five billion other people. Already, the number seems unmanageable. Still, we have only to reflect back to the example of our English alphabet. Although limited to a mere 26 letters, these letters can still be arranged in groups which will express all the works of Shakespeare— aided, of course, by suitable pauses, punctuations, and capitalizations.

Therein lies the key. It is the pauses and other notable events that permit messages to cluster, to be organized and reorganized. In the brain, the situation is somewhat similar to the ways in which individual citizens become more effective when they organize into larger units. Once people drop their differences and leverage their numbers, they discover new ways to operate. Empowered at successive local and regional levels, they may go on to restructure events in a national arena.

In this book, we will be asking of each reader a much more private question: can one person's behavior change in like manner? And the answer will be yes. How can this happen? By reconfiguring the flow of impulses throughout a sufficient number of networks in the brain[8] (see chapters 74 and 75).

35

Brain in Overview: Coordinated Networks Synthesizing Higher Functions

> The brain and the mind constitute a unity, and we may leave to the philosophers,
> who have separated them in thought, the task of putting them together again.
>
> Sir Russell Brain (1895–1966)[1]

The task is not only for the philosophers. Neuroscientists also reduce the brain to smaller manageable units as we have just done. But no one is reduced to being a reductionist except as a temporary measure. In the interactive brain, no part exists in isolation.

Given its billions of interacting nerve cells, how does any brain the size of a grapefruit manage to blend them all together harmoniously? How can it pattern global assemblies of cells so that they generate what we so loosely call "the mind?" Will we ever be able to specify the huge circuitry that accomplishes even one of its miracles: our higher order perceptions, thoughts, emotions, and insights?

Not in "The Decade of the Brain." But research has long outdated the old fixed maps of the brain that I studied back in medical school. Neuroscientists now envision brain cells as parts of a *dynamic meganetwork*. Its relays link many widely distributed systems. They operate most often with their circuitries arranged in parallel. Such circuitries are multidimensional and polytopographic. They stretch not only up from the brain stem to cortex and back down again, but interconnect each side of the brain with the other and enlist the cerebellum as well.[2]

Think one small thought. It resonates through many areas of cortex. These are not fixed into some rigid design, as though they were a checkerboard mosaic of black-and-white tiles cemented onto a flat floor. Rather, our cortex resembles a kind of fluid kaleidoscope. How can it shift into so many different patterns of shapes and colors? First, because the thalamus, limbic system, and basal ganglia stand poised to give its excitabilities a new twist every so often. Second, because these interacting regions develop unusual properties as they engage the cortex in oscillatory behaviors.

Undergo the simplest experience. It draws on widely represented systems of *neural networks*. In texture, each experience differs from the others based on differences in the size, shape, and temporal patterning within its regional networks. Moreover, these regional configurations will differ further depending on how many other connections they make with still larger looping circuits.[3] Such loops are elastic; they vary with the situation.

Our lives depend on those deep, critical circuits which generate our life-support systems and basic housekeeping functions. They include such brain stem functions as swallowing, breathing, and regulating blood pressure. We were born with them. They *are* fixed. We call them "hardwired," because they reflect our basic "nature," so to speak. Other circuits are more flexible, "softer-wired." They reflect the way we were brought up, our "nurture." And the circuits that were used to condition us will become especially important in Zen (see chapter 74).

Nerve cells continue to fire spontaneously, day and night. This produces a lot of ongoing background noise. How can one *new* message get in, register its signal, make that large blip which creates a lasting impression? It will happen only when many messages converge, high in signal impact, that relate to the same general theme. To serve this purpose the brain has extra, *reinforcing* nerve cells standing by, ready to contribute their extra input. What they contribute depends also on our nurture. Did mother smile and nod with approval when we finally swallowed those first spoonfuls of distasteful pablum? If so, our modulating circuits then added their positive reinforcement. Did she frown when she instructed us, in no uncertain terms, "Never cross the street before you look both ways!" A negative reinforcement.

In such ways did our growing brain learn to modulate its messages. Its soft-wiring provided a dynamic architecture, one that now far outstrips the capabilities of the usual computer. A computer also starts out in a vaguely similar way (having first been programmed by human brains). That is, it too begins with only two possible states. Not excitation or inhibition, but the two digital states: 0 and 1. These the computer arranges in bits which contain either 0 or 1. It then collects eight such bits of information to form a byte. Each such byte becomes the building block that computers manipulate when they convey concrete types of data.

Basically, our simpler computers today still remain rigid machines. Speaking only machine language, they are constrained to act within certain robotlike limitations of stimulus and response. From then on, more sophisticated computers do achieve artificial intelligence, but only to the degree that they have been designed to mimic the flexibilities inherent within the wiring patterns of the brain.

Among the first artificial capabilities to be added were patterns that could interact to yield higher-order, abstract functions. Then, more recently, computer designers followed the lead of their own human parents. They began to add specialized "smiles and frowns," connections that could be "strengthened" or "weakened" so as to give their offspring more flexibility. Now, the latest programming also reinforces positively. It retains in its memory only those "decisions" that had recognized a correct pattern. *Better yet, it erases incorrect decisions.* Erasure was a second major step.

Is there, then, some other secret basis for human *biological* intelligence? If so, it would seem to lie in the enormous *range* of our brains' capacities, their seemingly endless arrays of flexible, graded options for perception, mentation, and behavior. Staying aware of this range, we will avoid the trap of invoking supernatural "outside forces." Such a course can only further mystify mysticism.

No, our goal in part III is to highlight a series of basic mechanisms. For it will be when these mechanisms line up that they cause the brain's set-points to change. Then a whole array of its linked functions can suddenly shift from one state into another. To know what different parts and interconnections of the brain *can* do is especially important for understanding Zen. Because in Zen we will be exploring two of the brain's more inconceivable options. And we will find that while one of them shifts into higher-order comprehension, the other has shifted into *erasing* functions. Put simply, Zen may seem to add some things, but others drop out simultaneously.

Ancient sky watchers had fertile imaginations. They invented constellations in the night sky. To do so, they had to draw artificial lines linking a small number of stars. These creations still go by the names Orion's "belt" and Cassiopeia's "chair." The first watchers had no way to know that many points on their "star lines" were located countless light-years farther away from Earth than were others. So they remained comfortable with these fictitious outlines on their sky maps, maps as flat as the surface of their two-dimensional Earth.

Our situation presents a different challenge. We're asking, How do the states of kensho and internal absorption take over the internal universe of a person's brain? For these states, too, begin by "lighting up," and linking what are probably widely scattered active neuronal clusters. But our neuroscientists now have a *three*-dimensional perspective. They know how far apart such groups of nerve cells are, both in millimeters *and* in milliseconds. Moreover, they can arrive at more informed guesses about what kinds of actual functions might emerge when assemblies of such cells are truly linked together. Yet, even when the resulting brain networks do light up, as it were, we will find that these luminous states of consciousness also contain very black holes among their intrinsic features (see chapter 112).

These same two intriguing attributes, light and dark, additions and subtractions, will then turn out in parts VI and VII to have even more remarkable experiential correlates.

36

The Orienting Reflex and Activation

> All the quadrupeds emphasize their direct forward gaze by a corresponding movement of the ears, as if to supplement and aid one sense with another.
>
> John Burroughs (1837–1921)[1]

Our spaniel dozes on the rug, muzzle between forepaws. A footstep falls outside, and his head lifts. Pointing toward the noise, his eyes open wide, his nostrils flare, and his ears prick up. Watching his own dogs orient, Pavlov discerned that this reflex went beyond the simple act of being startled. He thought the brain was asking a more basic question: What is the *nature* of this thing? For this reason, Pavlov called it the "What *is* it?" reflex. In this respect, Zen master Bankei may already have anticipated him two centuries earlier, for Bankei had commented on the way the human orienting reflex had dual, "reacting-plus-inquiring" features.[2]

The orienting reaction does involve *arousal*.[3] Arousal in its simplest form is a brief, phasic reaction to input.[4] Arousal includes both a low voltage fast-wave component in the EEG, an energizing of behavior, a subjective dimension (often overlooked), and complicated responses within the autonomic nervous system.[5] Arousal is not a unitary state. Indeed, one can split off the increases in heart rate, respiratory rate, and blood pressure, the behavioral and EEG arousal.[6] Moreover, we will remember something longer if we have been moderately aroused. So arousal also serves as a foundation for memory and for other higher functions. In this particular role it helps determine how much and what kinds of information we process.

Once our spaniel has descended further into deep sleep, another faint footstep won't stir him. Only when he is "lighter" will the stimulus rouse him. Only when his brain is operating near this more elevated plane of *tonic* arousal will the next noise prompt him into a brief *phasic* arousal, one strong enough to cause his ears to prick up. Arousal carried to its furthest extreme could cause him to become hyperexcitable and develop seizures. At the opposite, low end of his scale of arousal, he might not respond because he had been deeply anesthetized or was in coma. Note what we have been doing. We have been using how quickly our dog responds to a weak sensory stimulus to gauge what his basic level of arousal is.

Beyond arousal lies *activation*. It implies an extra *tonic readiness for action*. To be effective, activation must be superimposed on arousal. It is a "let's-do-what-needs-to-be-*done*" process. It expresses the potential to act quickly. In humans, activation typically *slows* the heart rate. Moreover, during vigilance, as part of the tonic readiness to act, the heart rate also slows, and the blood pressure also tends to go lower.[6] In contrast, brief *phasic* arousals speed up the heart rate.

In knee-jerk situations, at the most primitive level, each response is tightly yoked to its stimulus. Theoretically, under such robotlike conditions, a brain's input determines its output. This invariability leaves no extra room for arousal or activation to intervene to yield their higher-level gradations of response.[3] But emotions change this situation. When brains are made irritable, defensive, or fearful, they draw upon the limbic system for their extra reserves of both activation and arousal. For example, today's breeds of house cats have evolved to become so "civilized" that many older cats won't even bite a mouse. But gently pinch their tails, or otherwise provoke them. Now their instinctive mouse-attacking behavior leaps forth, swept along on the crest of their higher levels of activation and arousal.[7]

Arousal begets arousal. We used catnip in the laboratory in Kyoto, observing cats before and after they smelled it. As soon as most cats sniff the odor, their brain waves speed up. Becoming increasingly excited, their pupils dilate and they seem transported into another state. There they relate with increasing intimacy to the catnip through a scale that includes biting, nuzzling, fondling, and even mating attempts.

A major reason why arousal is not a unitary state is that many mechanisms blend as they enter into it and issue from it. What are some of their pathways?

Arousal Pathways in the Reticular Formation and Beyond

EEG changes seemingly identical with those in the physiological arousal reactions can be produced by direct stimulation of the reticular formation of the brain stem.

G. Moruzzi and H. Magoun[1]

What did Moruzzi and Magoun observe when they stimulated the cat's brain stem? Instantly, the cat behaved like our dog does when he hears a noise. It pricked up its ears, opened its eyelids widely, and assumed an alert posture. Its cortical EEG lost its alpha waves and shifted into low voltage fast-wave activity.

But the researchers could also cause the same cat to doze off. How? By making a small lesion that destroyed the identical region which they had previously stimulated with electricity. The lesioned cat's EEG now showed slow, synchronized activity. So the midbrain reticular formation was a crucial region, one that seemed capable of generating our own arousal, alertness, and desynchronized EEG activity. Soon, in lecture halls, broad arrows of chalk would be drawn on blackboards. As they thrust up from the brain stem below, they symbolized how impulses rose up from this reticular formation to activate the cerebrum.

Nothing about the brain remains this simple. By 1967, the Scheibels had drawn attention to the reticular formation's several other functions.[2] It could set operational modes, filter the sensory influx, modulate and monitor cortical function, and help vary the motor output. Yes, it had networks of smaller cells that relayed impulses slowly across many synapses. But it also had large cells with long axons. These quickly extended their potent influence out of the brain stem, both up and down. And many reticular nerve cells spread out their dendrites, espalier fashion, in a plane at right angles to the long axis of the brain stem. Set this way, their synapses easily intercepted signals in transit from other fibers which were passing through their dendrites like arrows piercing a Japanese fan.

Physiologically, many reticular cells turned out to respond to *all kinds* of these incoming signal "arrows," not just to stimuli of one kind. In such a system, the original stimulus properties of a message get diluted. A signal which might start as a specific "sound," for example, would soon become lost in the hum of the whole reticular pool. So it seemed that the reticular core would function not to convey "the pageantry and color of the passing parade, but the loudness of the shouting that accompanies it."[2]

Another surprise came in the *lower* reticular formation. This part, down in the medulla, turned out to play a *strong net inhibitory role*. Both human subjects and animals showed the same puzzling phenomenon. For, as everyone knows, barbiturates are "sleeping pills." Why, then, didn't patients fall asleep, especially when a strong barbiturate drug was being injected into the artery that supplied their brain stem? Indeed, these patients remained conscious and responsive even though sufficient amobarbital had entered their brain stem to paralyze the nerve cells supplying their jaw and eye muscles.[3] And furthermore, why did this barbiturate shift their EEG into its low voltage, fast-wave alerting response, instead of into a sleep pattern?

Cats behaved much the same way. Suppose you had cooled the lower brain stem of a sleeping cat, inhibiting its stem up as far as the mid-pons. This cat would then awaken and develop fast cortical EEG activity.[4,5] Very curious! But a fact of particular relevance to Zen. For it suggested that—lower down in the part you had just cooled—the normal reticular formation must contain a covert *inhibitory* region. Such a region could be the source of a normal tonic braking action. And its usual function would be to actively suppress the arousal mechanisms at higher levels.

Exactly where are these higher mechanisms? They enter at several successively higher levels. If we follow in the pioneering footsteps of Moruzzi and Magoun, we can at least begin in the midbrain, and defer some of the arousal mechanisms of large cells to the next chapter.

The Role of the Midbrain and Its Connections in Arousal

The midbrain, at the top of the brain stem, is a potent source of arousal.[6,7] Suppose you now inactivate the midbrain reticular formation by cooling it on both sides. The cerebral EEG activity then becomes slow and synchronized, especially up in the frontal and parietal regions.[8] This finding illustrates another intriguing point: some of the normal relays from the midbrain reticular formation *preferentially activate the frontoparietal region*.

But the midbrain is no wider than the tip of your little finger. How could so small a region cause any large brain to sit up and take notice? As we will soon discover many more times, in the nervous system there is no single answer. In general, there are *two* basic answers: some parts are excited, others are inhibited. Midbrain stimulation strikingly increases the metabolic activity of other, vitalizing regions. These include the intralaminar nuclei up in the thalamus, especially its central median nucleus (see figure 11). Moreover, other thalamic nuclei also show major increases. They include the anterior ventral nucleus and the anterior part of the thalamic reticular nucleus.[9]

Yet, in sharp contrast, this same midbrain stimulation also *suppresses* metabolism elsewhere. In a rat's brain, reticular stimulation *reduces* the net firing of other cells, including those in the cerebral cortex and the limbic system. Recent metabolic studies of amphetamine, in normal human subjects, confirm these interesting results. This "stimulant" drug causes a surprising *drop* in cerebral metabolism, especially frontally.[10]

The metabolic studies pose a paradox. Paradoxes hold our most important lessons. For decades, a convenient line of reasoning went as follows: When you stimulate the midbrain it activates the cortex. And the cortex expresses this by developing much faster EEG activity. Given the latest evidence that the cortex was metabolically *suppressed*, how could one reconcile this fact with cortical EEG *arousal*?

For years, it had also been known that arousal released more acetylcholine (ACH) in cortex. The ACH levels increased in cortex whether the animal was arousing naturally or did so as the result of midbrain stimulation.[11] Only later did physiologists discover that the primary role of ACH in cortex was largely *inhibitory*. Indeed, what ACH did was suppress the firing of vast numbers of *short interneurons* in cortex.

But ACH also had one other role to play. ACH also excited the *large* cortical nerve cells. These—while much fewer in number—are the *output* neurons, so-called because they have long axons that quickly export their cortical messages out to distant sites. So yes, arousal does *reduce* metabolism in cortex. But it does so as the *net* effect of two processes. The first one slows the firing of the many small, short inhibitory cells within cortex. This causes the major drop in *their* local metabolism. This drop outweighs the small increase referable to the excitation of the few output cells.

Implicit in the foregoing account is an important message. *Excitation is not the sole mechanism that causes our major activations, whether in cortex, thalamus, or elsewhere.*[12] When the brain shifts its functional state in any major way *it has deployed whole arrays of excitations and inhibitions in dynamic interactions.* In fact, we now know that at least *four* different factors are responsible when cortical or thalamic functions become activated: (1) The few large cortical output cells fire faster, and send out volleys of their impulses through long axons. (2) Their large cell bodies also respond more to incoming excitatory stimuli. (3) Secondary opposing synaptic processes stop. (This reverses the prior trend toward those slow, synchronized spindle-shaped waves which are the physiological opposite of low-voltage fast activities). (4) The small, short, cortical inhibitory interneurons not only fire more slowly, but they also respond less to incoming stimuli.[12]

Many of the fast excitatory pathways, rising indeed like arrows from the midbrain, employ excitatory amino acids to activate higher levels. And if one were to inject analogues of these excitatory amino acids into the midbrain reticular formation itself, they would also cause a prompt local overstimulation.[13] The injected cat then becomes so intensely hyperexcitable that it can no longer carry out any purposeful or goal-directed behavior. Its EEG continues to show impressive low voltage fast-wave activity for as long as twelve to fourteen hours.

During this long first phase, the cat seems "in-turned." It does not orient, even toward loud noises from its outside environment. Then, twenty-four hours later, what does the cat look like after many of its midbrain reticular nerve cells have been either permanently etched out or otherwise deactivated? It appears transformed. In this late phase, it is a calm, docile single-minded animal. It shows "a certain indifference" to its environment. That is, while fully engaged in one activity, other stimuli from the outside won't distract it into displaying its normal orienting responses. One may wonder: could such simplifications of behavior have anything remotely to do with Zen? (see chapter 152).

Severe hunger and fear are stressful states. They increase excitability in the midbrain reticular formation, in the cortex, and in those two geniculate nuclei concerned with vision and hearing.[14] And one can also increase the firing rates of reticular nerve cells in the brain stem by injecting various excitant drugs into the peripheral bloodstream, *not* directly into the brain stem.[15] Yet even so, these excitant drugs—which include LSD, mescaline, and pentylenetetrazol

(Metrazol)—produce *fewer direct changes within the reticular formation itself than one might expect.*

But the drugs do affect other circuits elsewhere, and the EEG offers one index of these events. For as the animal becomes increasingly excited, its EEG evolves from low-voltage, fast into high-voltage, hypersynchronized *slow* activities. So as the brain moves toward its most hyperexcitable states, many *other* parts of the nervous system—not only the brainstem reticular cells—are being swept into complex interactive responses. Similarly, enhanced degrees of hyperactivity may be relevant to some trance states that occur in the revivalist's tent. These extremes will not become part of our explanation for quiet, conventional meditative states.

Yet, when a pulse of norepinephrine enters the midbrain reticular formation, it also causes behavioral alerting and a low-voltage fast desynchronized EEG.[16] Norepinephrine causes even more arousal when additional sensory stimuli are entering, such as extra noise in the laboratory. Other studies suggest that norepinephrine and dopamine cause *prolonged* EEG arousal when they are released together from their synapses around the lower end of the central gray matter and the midbrain reticular formation.[17] Moreover, after you give reserpine (to deplete the brain of its biogenic amines), even very small doses of lerodopa will replenish the functional levels of both amines. At this point, the reenergized brain undergoes a striking behavioral and EEG arousal.[18]

Hypothalamic, Thalamic, and Subthalamic Mechanisms

After the small upper end of the midbrain is severed, highly specialized postoperative care allows researchers to study the animals for many weeks thereafter.[19] The surgical section divides the brain into two parts. The large upper portion contains the hemispheres: the cerebral cortex and its related subcortical structures (see figure 3). The small lower part consists of the brain stem (midbrain, pons, and medulla) still connected with the spinal cord.

The brain is now uncoupled. Its two parts each reveal their own basic sleep-waking mechanisms. The isolated forebrain can now stay "awake" even when the brain stem falls "asleep." Smelling food or catnip, this forebrain develops its own low-voltage, fast-wave, cortical EEG arousal activity and its associated theta EEG activity in the hippocampus. How could catnip rouse this isolated forebrain if those upward-directed shafts of its lower reticular "arrows" had all been cut?

There must be other routes. The leading candidates are pathways to, and through, the hypothalamus (see figure 3 legend). Patients go into deep coma if their hypothalamus is damaged. One small but critical region is back where the posterior hypothalamus and adjacent subthalamus join the midbrain.[20] Here, the circuits passing *through* the hypothalamus play a key role in generating ongoing, tonic forms of behavioral arousal.[21,22] In cats, surgical lesions here cause coma *if* they cut axons. However, the cats still stay awake if only small *chemical* lesions are made here, for these destroy only the local cell bodies of the hypothalamus itself.[23]

Farther on is the *ventral medial nucleus* of the hypothalamus. Some studies suggest that it is among the brain's most sensitive sites for generating both EEG arousal and behavioral arousal.[24] Here, minimal electrical stimuli prompt the cat to rouse out of deep sleep.

Other nerve cells in each side of the *lateral hypothalamus* send many fibers up to innervate the whole cerebral cortex on the same side.[25,26] Why, then, do monkeys show a *generalized* EEG arousal on *both* sides if only one side of their lateral hypothalamus is being stimulated electrically? Because the effects of the stimulation *descend* to the brain stem, enter the reticular activating system there, and then relay back up on both sides.[27] Certain nerve cells in the back of this lateral hypothalamus will be noteworthy when we consider the mechanisms of concentrative meditation and absorption. These posterior cells broadcast their influence up to the outer cortex, to the cingulate cortex, and to the hippocampal formation.

The brain stem exports a stream of impulses up to this lateral hypothalamus. Smaller lesions that cut these normal pathways, if placed just below the hypothalamus, will indeed slow the EEG, but it stays slow for only a few weeks or months. However, human patients go into deep coma when lesions occur still farther forward that destroy both the hypothalamus itself *and* the fiber pathways going through it in both directions.[26] And from this deepest coma, the patients do not waken.

On the other hand, when the ventral anterior nucleus of the *thalamus* is being stimulated in comatose human patients, their EEG desynchronizes and they go into a brief behavioral arousal for the next ten to twenty seconds.[28] Moreover, brain-damaged patients who had remained in relatively shallow comatose states may lighten after they are stimulated in the *intralaminar nuclei of the thalamus* over a period of many months.[29]

Cortical and Other Limbic Mechanisms in Arousal

Sometimes, a meditator's mental content seems to trigger the flash of spiritual awakening. Why? As we search for reasons, one potential source might reside in those networks that elaborate upon our mental functions at higher, cortical levels. In our ordinary activities, we can *decide* to be aware, to orient and be attentive. So a few arousal mechanisms do seem to flow down from above, as it were. Indeed, decades ago, Segundo and colleagues made an interesting observation about what happened when certain parts of the cortex were stimulated. The animal's drowsing or sleeping EEG was immediately transformed into the low-voltage fast-wave tracing of wakefulness.[30] These arrows pointed *down*.

Which special regions of cortex can activate lower regions in the rest of the brain? In the monkey they include the superior temporal region, the inferior frontal region, and the cingulate gyrus. These are relatively small regions. Yet when any one site is stimulated electrically on only *one* side, it too transmits the message farther down. But following this event, they bounce back up. When the messages return, they arouse large regions of the cortex on *both* sides. At this point, the parts of cortex that are now *bilaterally* aroused include the cingulate gyrus, superior temporal gyrus, and the tip of the temporal lobe, as well as the lateral frontal regions, and the sensorimotor cortex.

Now we understand how the cortex can arouse itself. And on both sides. Yet its capacity to do so does not depend solely on using pathways that must descend *all* the way down to the midbrain.[31] It has other shortcuts to self-arousal. They are the routes that interconnect the cortex with the several arousal mechanisms we have just cited in the preceding section: in the hypothalamus and limbic system,[32] the subthalamus, and in the diffusely projecting nuclei of the thalamus.

What do we experience when impulses descend from the cortex and limbic system to be relayed through our arousal mechanisms? Normally, such descending impulses may help us to be stimulated by our own internally generated thoughts and images. But such pathways may also become overactive. And at these times they can yield less fruitful results. We lead hectic lives, in a cultural hyperbole. Given this constant information overload, periods of quiet meditation can enable us to slow down and to arrive at more optimal baseline levels of awareness and arousal.

In summary, decades of research have now shown that this state we call "waking" arises from the interplay among several hierarchical levels. The relays which generate our arousal and activation functions do not only ascend from the brain stem to stop in the hypothalamus. They go on—up to the thalamus, cortex, limbic system—*and back down again.* Arousal is heightened when more norepinephrine, dopamine, and excitatory amino acids are released into the midbrain. But acetylcholine plays a pivotal role in determining the quantity and the qualities of our consciousness. How much acetylcholine contributes will become clear in the next chapter.

38

Acetylcholine Systems

It is easy to ascribe a cholinergic basis to just about any CNS phenomenon.

A. Karczmar[1]

The ponto-mesencephalic cholinergic system, via its widespread connections with the diencephalon and cholinergic basal forebrain, is anatomically and electrophysiologically suited to modulate the cognitive processing of sensory information.

N. Woolf, J. Harrison, and J. Buchwald[2]

One could not chose a more appropriate transmitter than acetylcholine to start the discussion of messenger systems. It was the first neurotransmitter to be identified, by Loewi, seventy years ago. Since then, the roles of ACH have continued to grow in importance—as they will in this book—even though other messenger molecules have entered the scene.

The nerve cells that release ACH are called cholinergic. They are both widespread and very influential, for ACH is implicated in alertness, arousal, and memory functions, plus the usual forms of fast brain waves which occur in the EEG during waking and REM sleep. It turns out that ACH is the salient transmitter in many of the arousal and activation mechanisms cited in the previous two chapters. Much of what researchers have recently discovered about ACH in the brain keeps falling into two major categories. There are two ACH cell clusters, lower and upper; two classes of ACH receptors; and two separate pathways, already noted and to be expanded upon later.

Lower and Upper ACH Cell Clusters

The lowermost grouping of ACH nerve cells extends throughout the brain stem. It is called the *caudal ACH column* (figure 5).[3-7] In a book about Zen, there are several reasons for considering it first, even though it is lower anatomically. For these ACH cells of the brain stem, through their long axons, play vital roles in governing our levels of consciousness and in shaping our sensory perceptions.[7]

The top of this lower ACH cell column begins where the midbrain joins the pons.[2] Here, in one compact nucleus, primates concentrate most of their local ACH nerve cells. The result is the *parabrachial nucleus*. Its medial part supplies ACH to the pulvinar of the thalamus. Axons from its lateral part deliver ACH to the mediodorsal thalamic nucleus.[7] These are two very important thalamic nuclei, as we will soon discover.

What happens when you excite this key parabrachial region? A discrete electrical stimulus markedly activates the thalamus: (1) it directly excites (depolarizes)

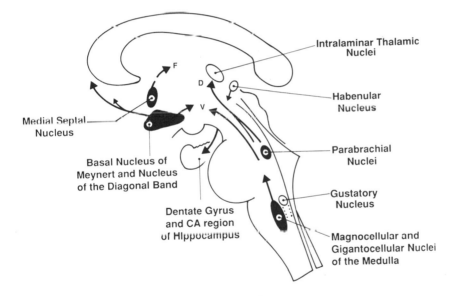

Figure 5 Major acetylcholine systems
The *upper cluster* of acetylcholine (ACH) nerve cells centers in the basal forebrain region. It includes the basal nucleus of Meynert which projects up widely to the neocortex. This basal forebrain region also supplies ACH back to the habenular nucleus which relays down to the midbrain. The medial septal nucleus releases its ACH down in the hippocampus via fibers which travel in the curved fornix (F).

In primates, the lower ACH cell column is concentrated in the parabrachial nuclei. It supplies ACH to the thalamus. Farther down, the lower column also includes the especially large ACH cells of the medulla. These deliver ACH to the midbrain reticular nerve cells, to the thalamus, and to the hypothalamus. D, dorsal cholinergic pathway; V, ventral cholinergic pathway. The position of the gustatory nucleus is also shown. The dots below it show the location of the nucleus of the solitary tract.

the particular thalamic cells that project up to cortex; (2) it shortens their former, long-lasting inhibitory periods; (3) it helps them fire more in response to other incoming excitatory volleys.

As part of their response, some animals also generate large electrical potentials, called ponto-geniculo-occipital (PGO) waves, which first arise in their pons. These PGO waves in animals have been interpreted as "a physiological correlate of the hallucinoid imagery" that humans visualize when they dream.[8] When ACH is released from the terminals of the parabrachial nucleus and of its neighbor, the *dorsolateral tegmental pontine nucleus,* it helps spread these pontine excitabilities beyond the visual system.[9,10] Indeed, when you stimulate these same two pontine ACH nuclei, the result triggers PGO waves both during the transition period which leads into REM sleep and during REM sleep itself.

A separate mixed population of cells in the midbrain suppresses the firing of these ACH cells of the parabrachial nucleus. But then, when the parabrachial cells are finally released, they discharge in a burst of spikes. Following this, some 70 to 200 milliseconds later, a PGO wave peaks in the thalamus.[11] This phenomenon becomes of special interest in relation to the ways that a sudden stimulus can trigger an alternate state, yet do so unpredictably (see chapter 105).

The ACH nerve cells within the dorsolateral pontine region are intriguing for other reasons. They contain two coexisting messengers: not only the opioid dynorphin B[12] but also nitric oxide, the unstable gas which enhances excitatory transmission.[13–15] Some ACH cells with these extra capabilities also project as far as the mediofrontal cortex. Here, the release of ACH itself, plus the effects of its comessenger(s), could relay an unfamiliar excitatory jolt all the way up from the brain stem to the frontal lobe.[11]

The same caudal column of ACH cells continues down into the pons and medulla. Here it includes two groups of especially large ACH cells. These constitute the *gigantocellular* and *magnocellular* nuclei. One learns to respect large nerve cells. Evolution assigns them roles commensurate with their size. Most cells in these nuclei release their ACH to activate either the midbrain reticular formation or the medial and intralaminar thalamic nuclei[16] (see figure 11).

Some of the extralarge cells in the gigantocellular formation tend to fire in brief (phasic) spike clusters. In contrast, the magnocellular neurons tend to fire in sustained (tonic) discharges. Moreover, *these magnocellular cells take the lead* when the brain begins to ascend from states of sleep. They start to fire even while the rest of the brain still slumbers. Only a long *thirty to sixty seconds later* do their distant effects become visible as fast ripples in the EEG waves up on the surface of the cortex. By then, other events down in the deep trench of the brain stem have already shifted the brain from slow-wave S-sleep up into its highly active form of dreaming sleep (REM sleep).

However, some of these large lower ACH nerve cells have been creating their excitation indirectly. Because, first, they have excited the smaller cells up in the midbrain reticular formation, as discussed in the previous chapter. Then, some of these midbrain cells will go on to release their own ACH up into the lateral geniculate nucleus on both sides[17] (see figure 11). Still other axons supply ACH directly to the posterior hypothalamus and to the intralaminar nuclei of the thalamus.[18]

We turn now to the cell bodies of the *upper ACH system*. They cluster much higher, occupying a deep region technically called the *basal forebrain*. It lies in front of the hypothalamus, on the undersurface of the frontal lobes (see figure 5). Here, there are two major clusters of larger ACH cells. They are grouped into the *basal nucleus of Meynert* and the *nuclei of the diagonal band*. They supply their ACH to the cerebral cortex through long, slender axons.

It has been speculated that these ACH cells of the upper system are among the few "network" neurons whose functions might be malleable enough to contribute to cognition.[19] Some of them also contain the coexisting peptide vasopressin.[20] The *medial septal nucleus* holds one other important deep, midline group of ACH cells. Soon, we will find these cells releasing their ACH into the hippocampus via the fornix (see figure 5).

The basal nucleus of Meynert also engages in an extensive two-way dialogue with limbic regions. So one of its major functions could be to process limbic signals, encode them, and then relay their motivational significance up to inform the neocortex. Some cells in this basal nucleus fire five times faster during any kind of low voltage fast-wave EEG arousal. Accordingly, the ACH from these particular cells is one likely source for the higher levels of ACH that are released into the cortex during arousal.[21] Moreover, the several cell types in the basal nucleus also send ACH (and other) messages to the reticular nucleus of the thalamus. The *net* effect of this may be to sponsor greater degrees of excitation.[22]

One other cholinergic pathway delivers ACH down and back to the medial *habenular nucleus* (see figure 5). This nucleus serves as a nodal point. It relays messages from forebrain regions to various sites in the brain stem.[23] When the habenular nucleus is stimulated, one of the results is to activate local inhibitory (GABA) mechanisms downstream. These inhibitory functions markedly slow the firing of serotonin nerve cells in the midbrain raphe.[24] But the major habenular projection site is to the interpeduncular nucleus in the midbrain.[25,26] We still have much to learn about how each of these two relays influences consciousness.

Two Classes of ACH Receptors

Will the molecules of ACH excite the next nerve cell or inhibit it? The result depends on which kind of ACH receptors are activated. There are two large classes of ACH receptors. One class is called *muscarinic*. In general, we will be noting chiefly the excitatory responses of the muscarinic receptors to ACH. *Muscarinic* is an old term. Back in the nineteenth century, the alkaloid drug called muscarine was isolated from a mushroom. Subsequently, it was discovered that its pharmacologic actions and molecular configuration were similar to those of ACH. The story illustrates a general principle. When a potent drug molecule arrives—whether it has been synthesized by a plant or a biochemist—its shape usually fits into a receptor site as a key fits into a particular lock.

Many receptors of the muscarinic type are waiting to be activated by the brain's own ACH in such diverse regions as the caudate nucleus, the hippocampus, the two geniculates, and parts of the thalamus. These muscarinic receptors begin to excite the next nerve cell *relatively slowly*.[27,28] Consider for example, the responses of the thalamic cells referred to in the section above. Many thalamic cells won't fire faster until a long 1.2 seconds after their incoming ACH nerve cells had been stimulated down in the brain stem. But once they start, muscarinic responses then develop momentum, and the thalamic cells continue to discharge for as long as twenty-one seconds. During this same period, groups of thalamic cells now become increasingly excited and develop fast, thirty-five- to forty-five-per-second gamma rhythms. Some of these oscillating rhythms may then be transmitted up to the cortex, for the cortex then shows its typical low voltage EEG pattern at similar fast frequencies.[10,29] Later we will pursue the obvious question: could these muscarinic responses, set off out at the terminal end of ACH networks, be the source of the longer phases of some alternate states, especially when these states continue for many seconds? (see chapter 142).

Because muscarine mimics the effect of ACH, it is called an ACH *a*gonist. Its opposing drug is atropine. Atropine is an *ant*agonist; it blocks the muscarinic effects of ACH. Suppose you give humans a modest blocking dose of atropine (1.25 milligrams) intravenously. What happens when this antagonist enters the brain and prevents the brain's own ACH from activating its muscarinic receptors?[30] The subjects don't think as clearly. They become less attentive, and can't focus their attention in a sustained manner on a specific task.[31] To meditators, ever struggling to maintain attention on the present moment, several of these *in*attentional symptoms may seem familiar. Some of the antagonistic effects of atropine may reflect the fact that it blocks the normal effects of ACH on the particular, M_3, subtype of muscarinic receptors which are concentrated in the hippocampus and cortex.[32]

Suppose, once again, you stimulate the ACH nerve cells down in the dorsolateral region of the brain stem. The stimuli also cause other cells to be more excitable, cells as high up as in the anterior thalamic nucleus. Now, *they go on responding for several minutes* when they receive stimuli entering from other sites in the cortex and subcortex. The prefrontal cortex itself projects back down to these same dorsolateral ACH nerve cells of the caudal ACH column. This circuitry has led to an intriguing speculation. Could we be using long loops like this—which include segments of the frontal cortex—to insert elements of "will" into our cognitive processing?[33] But if so, note that an advanced Zen trainee gradually develops something quite different: *the capacity to disengage,* to *let go selectively,* particularly of those willful impulses which have strong egocentric attachments.

We come finally to the second, very much faster, category of ACH excitations. In this instance, ACH is activating a different class of receptors, called *nicotinic.* Nicotine is the familiar addictive stimulant of the tobacco plant. Again, the older pharmacologic term, *nicotinic,* remains in use. Why? Because the nicotine of tobacco origin turned out later to be one more agonist that was capable of mimicking the fast excitatory effect of the brain's own ACH.

Deliver nicotine to its receptors on thalamic nerve cells and they fire instantly. Moreover, these thalamic cells also fire a mere 140 milliseconds (0.14 second) after you deliver electrical stimuli to the relevant ACH cell bodies down in the parabrachial region. This is a quick discharge, but a brief one: it lasts only 1.3 seconds.[29] Which nerve cells have many nicotinic receptors and are prone to discharge quickly? They reside not only in the medulla, hypothalamus, and thalamus but also in cerebellum, and to a lesser degree in cerebral cortex.

The low-voltage fast activity increases in the EEG when either nicotine, or ACH itself, acts on nicotinic receptors. This stimulating effect of nicotine in humans peaks within one minute after intravenous injection. It then wears off a few minutes later. When given to animals, nicotine increases the metabolism of glucose in a number of other brain regions well supplied with nicotinic receptors. These "hot spots" include the medial habenula, the anteroventral nucleus of the thalamus, the interpeduncular nucleus, the superior colliculus, and the lateral geniculate body. This list also includes one other intriguing region, the retrosplenial cortex buried just behind the back end of the corpus callosum.

It is hard to quench the glowing embers of such hot spots. Former smokers know the pangs of nicotine withdrawal. In belated recognition of nicotine's stimulant properties, the U.S. Surgeon General's office finally declared in 1988 that it was addictive. Human subjects do "like it" when they receive nicotine intravenously. It is a curious fact that these subjects cannot distinguish between the euphoriant effect of nicotine and that of morphine or amphetamine.[34] Why is this so? Could some of the similarity imply that when we activate our nicotinic ACH receptors it can cause a secondary release of other messengers? Could these messengers include brain opioids or amines? This latter hypothesis is testable and needs to be resolved.

Meanwhile, the first part of the hypothesis has just been tested. When nicotine activates its *pre*synaptic receptors, it causes a major enhancement of fast excitatory transmission.[35] So it appears that some of the "smoker's kick" reflects the way these nicotine receptors are opening up the "nozzle" on other incoming terminals. This allows the other terminals to release much more of their fast-acting ACH or glutamate transmitters into the synapse.

Even this brief survey illustrates how impressive are the potentials of the ACH systems. Quickly, for many seconds, or in a more sustained manner, ACH receptors are enhancing and shaping the contents of our consciousness at many levels from the medulla up to the cortex.

39

The Septum and Pleasure

> With septal stimulation, the patients brightened, looked more alert, and seemed to be more attentive to their environment during, and at least for a few minutes after the period of stimulation. With this basic affective change, most subjects spoke more rapidly, and content was more productive; changes in content of thought were often striking, the most dramatic shifts occurring when prestimulation associations were pervaded with depressive affect.
>
> R. Heath[1]

The septal region is a convenient place to begin to sample the emotional overtures of the limbic system. As early as 1878, Paul Broca had called part of this larger system the "grand limbic lobe." But back then, what he was referring to was only the large elongated, C-shaped region which lay at the inside margin, or *limbus*, of the old cortex deep in the brain. Residing next to the midline, this inner margin extended back from the cingulate and parahippocampal gyri down around, and into, the hippocampus[2] (see figure 3). Then Papez, in 1937, proposed that the closures within the loops of limbic circuits were the basis for emotion. He also emphasized the way these circuits engaged the hypothalamus. More recently, MacLean, now calling it a limbic *system*, placed emphasis on its various links with the amygdala as well.[3,4]

In the working shorthand that behaviorists use, limbic operations tend quickly to translate into "emotional-affective." They are, of course, much more complex. So if shortcuts are to be used, it may be appropriate to mention one of the (more printable) memory devices which medical students use. It would summarize seven limbic functions with "the four M's and the three F's": *m*ating, *m*emory, *m*ood, *m*otivation; *f*ear, *f*ighting, *f*ood.

Front and center lies the septal region. It is the midline gray matter above and in front of the third ventricle. It includes both the medial septal nucleus (see figure 5), the lateral septal nucleus, and the *ventral striatum*[5] (see figure 7).

MacLean views the septal region as involved in those "feeling and expressive states conducive to sociability and the procreation of the species."[3] But the individual functions within this region have remained difficult to tease apart. Many passing fibers pierce the region, and it has Byzantine interconnections with many other limbic and brain stem regions.[3,6] For example, in animals, if opioids are injected into the septum, they stop the medial septal nucleus from releasing its ACH into the hippocampus.[7]

What does septal stimulation do in man? It is prudent to begin with Delgado's caveat. "Electrical stimulation of the brain is a rather crude procedure, and to explain the finesse, coordination and drive of many of the evoked reactions, it is necessary to assume the activation of physiologic mechanisms."[8] Which mechanisms might be activated?

For a sample at least, one must turn to the report of Heath and his group at Tulane. They described the symptoms reported by fifty-four patients whose septal region was being stimulated.[19] The stimulations consistently induced "a pleasurable response." They also immediately relieved the severe intractable pain and anguish associated with advanced cancer. Stimulations were repeated twice a day, or once every three days, for a lengthy period. They left the patients relaxing "in comfort and pleasure." And there were other important findings: increased alertness and attentiveness; enhanced abilities to calculate; acceleration in all movements, including speech; and rapid shifts from depression to optimism. Moreover, these changes persisted for minutes *after* the stimulation ended.[10] However unconventional were some of the other procedures cited below, these early observations are worth noting, given that we are searching for the sources that enhance the functions of the human brain and relieve suffering.

The patients were not told exactly when the electrical stimuli were being delivered. And they usually could not explain why they underwent their striking shifts in mental content. For example, one patient had been on the verge of tears, condemning himself as responsible for his father's near-fatal illness. But then, "When the septal region was stimulated, he immediately terminated this conversation and within 15 seconds he exhibited a broad grin as he discussed plans to date and seduce a girlfriend." Asked why he had so abruptly changed the direction of his conversation, he could reply only that "the plans concerning the girl suddenly came to him."[1]

Electrical stimulations did produce sexual *thoughts*, but did not lead to objective evidence of sexual arousal. However, in later studies, gross chemical stimulations were used. These *gradually* led both to sexual arousal and to a state of general hyperarousal.[11] One female patient received either acetylcholine (400 micrograms) or norepinephrine (140 micrograms), injected into the septal region on both sides. On most occasions, either ACH or NE began to raise her mood within one or two minutes. Moods peaked after ten to fifteen minutes evolving through a mild euphoria, an increased awareness, a more rapid and more accurate response to questions, and a "sexual motive" state. After another five to ten minutes this sexual state culminated in repetitive orgasms.

Before these drug injections, wires recording from the septal region showed only the subject's usual baseline low amplitude, fast-wave activity. Soon, as her mood then was elevated, she added more twelve-per-second activity. This then spread to the other septal leads and developed into high amplitude spindle-shaped waves. Later, while the patient was having orgasms, a striking and consistent finding was spike and large slow-wave activity. This had an overlay of low voltage fast-wave activity (see chapter 37). Between orgasms, high amplitude spindling reappeared. None of this deep activity down in the septal region showed up in conventional scalp EEGs.

Large amounts of ACH or of NE were always injected on both sides. So we don't know how many of these primary messenger molecules had spread out to stimulate their receptors at sites *outside* the septum per se. Still, the high amplitude septal spindlelike activity at 12 cps, found in human subjects, is a noteworthy deep accompaniment of excess arousal. Moreover, the authors considered that the later, deep septal spike and slow-wave activity with its ripples of fast activity was similar in appearance to the usual EEG findings shown in the *scalp* EEGs of other patients with epilepsy while they were actually having their major epileptic seizures.

During pleasurable, positive emotions, spindle waves consistently appeared in the septal leads. Occasionally they spread to the amygdala as well. In contrast, at other times when the patients were experiencing negative emotions like fear and rage, high amplitude spindling developed in both the amygdala and hippocampus.

These earlier human studies suggest that powerful hyperarousal states are accompanied by evolving EEG changes in deeper limbic structures. *Only depth electrodes detect such changes.* The patients' sexual overtones may be relevant to the semierotic flavor which some other persons report during their states of mystical ecstacy. It is of incidental interest that, in patients who have genuine epileptic seizures, erotic feelings occur only rarely as initial phenomena. But when a sexual aura then does occur, the patients are usually women, and their seizure discharges begin in deep limbic structures on the right side.[12] So on the basis of gender, it is possible that women might experience certain erotic resonances of their mystical states in ways subtly different from men.

40

The Attachments of the Cingulate Gyrus

If you would make a man happy, add not to his wants, but subtract from the sum of his desires.

Seneca (4 B.C.E.–65 A.C.E.)

Gently spread apart the right and left hemispheres at the top of the brain. Then peer down into the cleft between them. Now you will see the two cingulate gyri. Lying just above the corpus callosum, these gyri stretch out from front to back like an elongated letter C (see figure 3). Each is girdled along its waist, as its Latin name suggests. Running through the core of the gyrus in both directions is a cablelike bundle of association fibers, the *cingulum.*

The cingulate gyrus interconnects with many key sites. The regions include the anterior thalamic nucleus, septum, hippocampus, and subiculum, plus the neocortex of the frontal, parietal, and temporal lobes (see figure 6). Its anterior portion also projects down to the large cells of the basal lateral amygdala.[1]

In the early years of research in animals, strong electrical stimuli to the cingulate gyrus prompted many visceral and behavioral responses. Or large lesions damaged the gyrus on the two sides and produced varieties of tameness. Most studies were too gross to decide which effects were attributable to the cingulate cortex per se, and which were due to disconnecting the cingulum bundle which coursed through it.

In human studies, stimulating the cingulum region produced brief negative responses. One fifth of the patients became anxious and tense. But there were no changes in heart rate, respiration, or skin resistance. However, "positive" responses did occur if the cingulate *cortex* was stimulated much farther forward. And among these responses were *relief* from anxiety and tension, plus feelings of well-being and relaxation. These positive experiences could last for a half a minute to two minutes. They were elicited repeatedly by stimulating sixty times a second.[2] Again, as in the septal region, one observes that when the brain is stimulated in certain more anterior and midline regions, there occurs a relief from anxiety and a sense of well-being.

But this is hardly the whole story. Surgical operations which *remove* the anterior cingulate region improve symptoms in only certain psychiatric patients: those who suffer from major affective disorders, major anxiety problems, and especially from obsessive-compulsive behaviors.[3] Two findings from animal research become of interest in this regard. One is that an increased release of dopamine also causes repetitive, stereotyped behaviors. The other is that stimulating the anterior cingulate region causes dopamine nerve cells back in the midbrain to fire in bursts.[4]

Patients suffering from intractable pain have had their cingulum sectioned on both sides. Thereafter, they speak less often, initiating only one-third as many spontaneous utterances as before.[5] Monkeys also lose certain of their normal vocalizations which arise at a higher behavioral level after having had cingulate gyrus lesions on both sides, although they still utter their spontaneous, socializing "cooing" noises.[6]

Throughout this book, our quest will be to discover how the human brain creates—*and relieves*—its self-inflicted sorrows and sufferings. Drug addiction affords one striking example of the way attachments generate anguish. No bondage exceeds being enthralled by drugs. Few lusts, few cravings drive behavior as intensely as do those that afflict the addict. The addictions to morphine and meperidine (Demerol) are well-known examples. Addicts who abruptly stop their drug habit suffer a severe cold-turkey withdrawal. Remarkably, their symptoms and signs can be relieved surgically. The procedure interrupts both cingulum bundles.[7] Each lesion is small: the size of a large pea.

Postoperatively, the former addicts show two striking changes as soon as they recover from anesthesia. First, they display "intense euphoria and self-confidence." They now refuse their former addictive drugs. Secondly, they do *not* undergo withdrawal symptoms, despite having been on hard drugs before the operation. When three addicts received a "sham" operation, it did not relieve their drug addiction. This excluded the possibility that just any kind of surgery directed to the head might have caused their symptoms to disappear as a kind of placebo effect. However, cutting the cingulum did not benefit everyone; a few patients relapsed and resumed their drug habit after a few days or within the first six months.

In a subsequent report, an impressive success rate of over 80 percent was reported in a group of hard-drug addicts.[8] (Addicts who had primarily sociopathic disorders were excluded.) In this study, the patients stayed on their addicting drugs until the day of surgery, then received lesions in the front part of the cingulum. Again, drug craving was relieved, and most patients suffered no withdrawal symptoms. Psychometric tests performed later suggested that the cingulumotomy had not caused significant cognitive side effects.

Norepinephrine fibers sweep back through the cingulum, pursuing their long journey up from the brain stem to reach the parahippocampal and hippocampal region (see chapter 44). But many other circuits also travel through the cingulum, in both directions. It seems likely that human subjects who benefit from cutting the cingulum will have had an interruption of various fibers serving several kinds of circuits. Why? Because the patients have cut so *many* psychophysiological attachments. The addicts have done more than escape from having a few days of severe, acute withdrawal symptoms and signs. They have also broken free from the grip of their long-established habits of severe substance abuse.

A patient of mine had an unusual first symptom referable to a small, invasive tumor of his right midcingulate gyrus. He neglected shaving over the left side of his lower face, neck, and chin. This neglect continued, despite the fact that he could still see the excess growth of his own beard and that his relatives pointedly called it to his attention.

The *retrosplenial cortex* begins back where the cingulate gyrus leaves off (see figure 3). Surely, this region will turn out to have many more intriguing functions than the few cited here that have been revealed thus far (see figure 12). Perhaps it helps enliven perceptions. For example, lesions here reduce the usual habituation which occurs after various sensory stimuli enter from the opposite side of the environment[9] (see chapter 49). Moreover, the potent hallucinogen phencyclidine ("angel dust") selectively damages nerve cells in this retrosplenial region.[10]

Meanwhile, to generalize, one may say that the cingulate gyrus and its limbic connections are interactive links in a larger integrated network. It is one which normally helps us to personally animate our attention and to attach it to things in external space.[11] So, whatever process cuts down on the flow of nerve impulses throughout this network on one side of the brain could dissolve the way a person melds affect and higher functions. And the result could lead the subject to "de-value" emotionally—and so to depersonalize—events which are taking place in the opposite half of space.

Suppose we now look further into this concept of "devaluation." Let's turn it around to ask, how do we normally attach positive values to things? Opioids are among the many possible candidates. It is noteworthy that the cingulate cortex is relatively high in enkephalin cell bodies and in mu and sigma opioid receptors (see chapter 47). Could these local opioid systems, interacting with other input entering the cingulate, help to create some of the limbic contours of our value systems? Is this one of several ways that our brains become hostages, held captive in the firm grip of their own desires? It is an interesting sidelight to observe that one region of cingulate cortex is involved in the initiation of grasping. And it is also involved in the release of the handgrip once grasping has occurred.[12]

But before one starts to grasp at, or let go of, the above questions, it would be very helpful if brain research could settle on why anterior cingulumotomy cuts off the addict's craving for opiates. What makes pea-sized lesions so very effective here? Have they sliced that output pathway that links this anterior part of the cingulate gyrus with the amygdala? Or have they severed the ACH fibers curving up from the basal forebrain?[13] Or are the lesions so situated anteriorly that they have blocked the input which the cingulate receives from the subiculum, both directly and indirectly?[14] (see figure 6).

Yet other lines of questioning will still go on. For, with regard to our own quest, at how many sites within the above circuitries does meditation itself gently act? Because meditation too, will gradually dampen everyday lusts and cravings. And there remains the critical issue, to be taken up in part VII: how does the nonsurgical penetrating thrust of insight swiftly cut off these two emotions at their very roots?

The Amygdala and Fear

Rage, rage against the dying of the light . . .

Dylan Thomas (1914–1953)[1]

No man is free if he fears death.

Martin Luther King, Jr. (1929–1968)[2]

In the two previous chapters, we began to make loose and qualified associations, relating certain deep anterior midline regions to some of our positive, energized, pleasurable states. Now, the amygdala introduces us to our brain's *negative* valences. These are the sources of our burning, raging fear of death. The amygdala, too, gets its name from its shape: like an almond. Each amygdala is an extended ovoid mass of gray matter buried near the inside tip of the temporal lobe. Collectively, its several nuclei are now called the amygdaloid complex. An accurate term, in view of its other complexities.

A brief survey of its anatomy helps us understand what the amygdala does. Vital subcortical input comes over to it from the mediodorsal nucleus of the thalamus and speeds up from the ventromedial hypothalamus. Impulses descend to it from the cortex of the anterior cingulate gyrus, the prefrontal, orbitofrontal, and the temporal regions. The amygdala then gives rise to two major outflow paths. Its upper path leads back to the ventromedial hypothalamus. The lower pathway curves down to inform the brain stem and the base of the brain.

As hominids evolved, they left us many legacies. One was an amygdala whose basal and lateral nuclei had become very large, but whose corticomedial and central nuclei had become relatively small.[3] Many kinds of peptide nerve endings funnel into these smaller nuclei, but the *opioid* peptide terminals are dispersed more evenly.[4]

Sensate messages filter down to the amygdala from the association cortex only after they have been highly processed. And as these cortical messages descend, they pass at each step through a series of synapses increasingly invested with acetylcholine terminals and opioid receptors.[5] So the closer our layers of sensory associations draw to the limbic system, the more they can be influenced by cholinergic and opioid receptors.

The amygdala itself contains sophisticated wiring patterns. These add critical physiological implications to all the other cited architectural features at the interface between the temporal lobe and the limbic system. For example, the circuitries of its large basolateral nuclei already resemble those of a cerebral cortex in miniature. This suggests that the amygdala could be competent to insert emotional resonances, either positive or negative, which further color the meaning of our higher-order associations.

Consider further the interesting findings in certain cats who happen to have been born defensive and easily frightened. What makes them different when they encounter threatening stimuli? These timid cats generate the most activity in the pathway connecting the amygdala to the hypothalamus.[6] Moreover, the normal basolateral amygdala has options for relaying another set of messages to both the dorsal and ventral striatum. Over these other output pathways the amygdala can instantly insert its bias into our affective behavior.[7-9]

The amygdaloid complex is relatively small. Are we so sure it contributes to behavior? Could it really be helping us smile or frown? Such questions prompt us to reflect on Herbert's caveat: "We must overhaul our methods of studying behavior if we are to make functional sense of the new knowledge about the structure and organization of the limbic system."[10]

True, earlier electrical stimulations of the amygdala in animals did cause different kinds of behaviors. They included fearful, ragelike, and defensive reactions, autonomic and endocrine responses, plus simpler arousal responses. But the stimuli were gross, and so once again one must discount the results of most of the earlier stimulation research. Moreover, when lesions were made they were too large. They also cut fibers passing through the amygdala on their way elsewhere. In contrast, the newer generations of smaller lesions yield results much more interpretable. They are made by injecting local excitotoxins. These chemical lesions *selectively* destroy intrinsic nerve cells, but they spare the extrinsic axons on their way to and from other regions.[11] Excitotoxic lesions have interesting implications (see chapter 152).

Meanwhile, we still need to overhaul the ways we study behavior. First, how shall we define it? Always in terms of action? Sometimes *in*action is an impressive form of behavior. To explore such possibilities, let us begin by observing a dominant rat who regards his home cage as his castle. He possesses it and marks it. He defends *his* cage as though it were a part of himself. On the biological high ground of his very own turf, he is action personified. This owner rat is a "winner." He always defeats a normal intruder rat. Let us then turn our sympathies to the intruder rat, as one does to an underdog. How does this second rat behave, after being defeated, when we return him to *his* own home cage next door? There he stays quiet, "frozen" in his corner. This vanquished intruder is "once bitten, twice shy." Never will he venture over even to sniff at, let alone to challenge, the victor who goes on patrolling the boundary of his own nearby castle-cage.[12]

Now, suppose we bring in a third rat. He too, will be cast in the role of the intruder. But one small aspect of his behavior has been modified. A very discrete lesion has already been made in this third rat's *corticomedial* amygdala. At first, he seems normal. Indeed, he still fights just as hard, because this tiny lesion won't change his gross combative behavior either before, or during, his inevitable defeat. But observe how he behaves *after* being defeated. Now one sees that this latest, *lesioned* intruder differs strikingly from the normal intruder. He moves freely about his own cage. He even thrusts his muzzle out though the wire of his cage, sniffing incautiously toward the victorious rat. Had this third rat really been in, and lost, the battle? You'd never guess it. He seems oblivious of the proprieties, of his expected social boundaries. He hasn't learned his lesson.

No naivete of this degree will help any creature adapt to surroundings that are always hostile and competitive. But taking this experiment as a clue, we might simplify one aspect of the normal functions of the medial amygdala as follows:

it contributes to survival skills, to behaviors that in the inner city one might call "street-smarts." Taken together, the smaller corticomedial and central amygdala also participate in those systems mediating basic drives. What enables them to do so? Note again those outflow paths projecting messages into the hypothalamus, striatum, and the brain stem.[13,14]

Earlier generations relied on the active practice known as "spare the rod and spoil the child." Did the amygdala enter into this adage? Probably. For the amygdala does seem to be a major factor in *aversive* learning experiences. These are the kinds of learning which depend on negative, highly arousing, stressful, or otherwise unpleasant circumstances. Did the amygdala even take on the contrasting role, the one implicit in the old "carrot-and-stick" approach? Probably, even if it is a lesser one. For it also fosters *positive* learning experiences. These are the kinds that occur when appetitive, food-and-drink reinforcements are added. These are the "carrots" that enhance learning.[15]

When researchers use the "stick" approach, they can aversively condition rats to fear a pure tone. They begin by delivering this tone along with a mild foot shock. Soon, just the tone alone causes the rats to "freeze," and it increases their heart rate and blood pressure. Suppose, however, that lesions had been made earlier in the *lateral amygdaloid* nucleus. They prevent these fearful autonomic and behavioral responses. So this lateral nucleus is an essential earlier interface in conditioning.

When sound stimuli arrive at the lateral nucleus, it then relays its signals on to the central nucleus. The central nucleus then becomes the next link in the chain of "emotionalizing" circuitry that underlies aversive conditioning.[16] Finally, when the central nucleus exports such messages, it will be preparing the animal to respond to the impending stressful event.[14]

Suppose you place lesions at a much higher level, far up in the conditioned rats' auditory cortex. Do lesions this high stop the sound from entering, and stop the tone from causing fearful behavior?[17] No. Already the brain will have shunted in, lower down, those pivotal sensory signals crucial for comfort or survival. Indeed, it will have mobilized them into its behavior long before.[18] Everyone knows by now that mere high-minded thoughts won't banish deep fear and rage.

Up to now, we have been observing how *learning* takes place in *adult* rats. These adults have learned to fear through the process of conditioning. But the amygdala had been primed long before. It was already genetically programmed to help generate *primal* fear. A normal rat innately fears a cat. Seeing a cat, it freezes. However, rats lose this instinctive fearful behavior after they have had lesions of the amygdala. They will even climb up on the back of a sleeping cat after you have rendered the cat harmless with a hypnotic drug.[19]

Can one create a *functional* block in the amygdala, banish fear without actually destroying nerve cells? Yes, researchers can inject two kinds of drugs *directly* into the amygdala to reduce a rat's anxiety behaviors. This approach takes advantage of an important fact: the normal amygdala is loaded with receptors sensitive to opioid drugs and to other antianxiety drugs. When we humans tune down and resolve many of our own anxious fears, it seems likely that we will be using these same two kinds of receptors.[19]

Rats are paranoid about new tastes and smells. Rats not suspicious about what they might eat dropped out of the gene pool long ago. Today's survivors have hardwired such phobias into their brains. The *basolateral amygdala* normally contributes to this innate tendency to fear any new taste. It also helps the rat further condition its already keen aversion to certain odors. But after having small lesions made in their amygdala, the rats no longer recoil from a novel food in a novel environment.[11] In primates, too, novel stimuli prompt many nerve cells in the amygdala to fire vigorously.[20]

Then what about the "carrot" approach? Now, the amygdala responds "positively." Its small central nucleus seems to lend "seasoning" to some of these positive resonances, flavoring the brain's appetitive memories for food.[13] On the other hand, studies in cats show that the central nucleus can also enter into the visceral counterparts of fear. For cats can be conditioned to become fearful by using a variety of techniques that follow the "stick" approach. Their blood pressures rise, and they breathe faster. However, these elevated blood pressures fall and breathing rates slow after their central nucleus has been inactivated.[21,22] In fact, an effective way to suppress a fearful cat's brief "hair-on-end" reaction is to inject an enkephalin opioid into the amygdala's upper output pathway.[23,24]

When an awake animal breathes *in*, many of its amygdala nerve cells discharge. In contrast, while *exhaling*, only half that number fire. Fewer still fire when the animal enters quiet sleep or REM sleep.[25] Such findings reemphasize an important point cited back in chapter 22. Not only does meditation affect breathing; breathing can go on to influence meditative experience. More specifically, *expiration quiets down the firing of the central amygdala*.

Different Kinds of Aggressive and Fearful Behaviors

A poet, sensitive to the ultimate roots of rage, is only one illustration of the broad scope of aggression. Aggression takes many other forms, and the early years of meditative training can modify only some of these.

As noted earlier, cats can be prompted into a very aggressive attack when electrical stimuli are directed into the hypothalamus.[26] Suppose, however, the researcher first destroys the amygdala on both sides. Now, despite the stimuli to the hypothalamus, it becomes more difficult to drive these various kinds of attack behaviors. Yet, even though these lesioned animals do become calmer, they have arrived at only a temporary serenity. How can one bring back their attack behavior? By stimulating them with a dopamine agonist.[27] Such relapses imply that aggressive behavior is not going to stop if one merely reduces the relevant functions of the amygdala per se. At a minimum, one also needs to reduce certain dopamine and hypothalamic mechanisms as well.

Most of the evidence presented so far has come from research models in lower animals. What about the heart-pounding rush of fear in primates more like ourselves? When Brown and Schafer studied primates, over a century ago, they discovered a surprising fact. They could tame wild monkeys if they removed the temporal lobes on both sides.[28] Today we know that one critical feature responsible for this "gentling" process is the loss of the amygdala. Indeed, monkeys do become "strikingly fearless" after both their right and left amygdalae have been removed. So naive, in fact, that they will approach and handle a snake! No normal monkey comes near a snake.[29] These monkeys' fearless, incautious behavior resembles that of the lesioned rats and cats.

Even so, the lesioned monkeys still show a few lingering traces of fear behavior. Suppose you place them in different, fear-provoking situations. Then, a few of their facial expressions and postures still reveal fearful or submissive behaviors. Where might these come from? Some of the responsible visual messages normally enter from the nearby inferotemporal cortex.[30] Elsewhere, on the output side, such lingering fearful behaviors might also reflect the way that dopamine systems keep exerting their same persistent influence, noted above, when DA activates the nearby motor circuits of the striatum.

Clinical studies of humans confirm that the amygdala is a major primary nodal point when we consciously experience fear. When it is stimulated selectively, the subjects experience mental tension and behave in a tense manner.[31] In one such patient, stimulation immediately induced fear. Fear later came back when the afterdischarges spread back into the amygdala on return from the hippocampus.[32] Moreover, one other patient had recurrent episodes of spontaneous fear lasting minutes to hours. These fears were prompted by an epileptic focus that was discharging into the right anterior temporal region. The fearful episodes ceased when the amygdala was removed along with adjacent parts of the medial temporal lobe.[33]

As is also true of lower animals, the evidence that would link the human amygdala with aggression is less consistent. "There can be both aggressive behavior without limbic lesions and limbic lesions without aggressive behavior."[33] Neurosurgical lesions aimed at the human amygdala sometimes relieve excessively aggressive behavior, but sometimes they do not.[34]

Recent studies suggest that human subjects employ several different anatomical pathways as they proceed to channel various kinds of emotions out into the autonomic nervous system.[35,36] Future research may tease out many subtly different shadings of diverse human social interactions that can be influenced by the subdivisions of our amygdala.[37] Consider, as but one of these possibilities, the effect that small lesions have on male rats. Corticomedial lesions reduce their heterosexual behavior, but do not change they way they act aggressively toward other males. In contrast, lesions of the basolateral amygdala reduce aggressive interactions among male rats, but do not affect their sexual behavior toward females.[38]

To summarize: Our amygdala enters early into a vital "loop" of incoming signals. It comes instantly to conclusions about their survival or reinforcement value. It then relays its biased affective valences on to other circuits. They, in turn, will orchestrate the appropriate behavioral responses both instinctual and learned, somatic and visceral. In addition, the amygdala is a nodal point for many circuits linked to our primary experience of fear.

The findings reviewed above will later become of critical importance. They will help us understand how a person could briefly lose all fear, both during kensho and during the spectrum of near-death experiences (see chapters 136 and 104, respectively).

42

Remembrances and the Hippocampus

> At least some of the structural correlates of memory are vested in a widespread series of cortical association projections that converge onto the para-hippocampal gyrus and hippocampal formation, and a series of hippocampal output pathways that diverge from these structures and largely reciprocate them.
>
> G. VanHoesen[1]

It curls up to resemble a sea horse's tail. This is how it came to be named the hippocampus. Years ago the same curl of the hippocampus also reminded some anatomists of the ram's horn, or cornu, associated with Ammon, a mythological figure from ancient Egypt. Today, we perpetuate this quaint legend. We still label subdivisions of the hippocampus starting with the two letters *CA*, where *C* stands for *cornu* and *A* for *Ammon*.[2] Yet in spite of decades of studies using newer technologies, we ourselves still remain at sea about many of the things the hippocampus does. And, we still postulate other semimythological formulations about how it accomplishes its missions, whatever they are.

We humans relegate our small hippocampus to the innermost part of the temporal lobe. Here, a long fold, the parahippocampal gyrus, rolls up into the larger *hippocampal formation* (see figure 3). This hippocampal formation includes the dentate gyrus, the hippocampus itself, the subiculum, and the entorhinal cortex. Evolution carved their intricate neuroanatomy as though they were made of clay. Useful parts were added to, other portions shaved away. In the small mouse brain, the hippocampus remains so large that its upper and lower divisions make up 45 percent of the cortex. However, in humans, the hippocampus occupies less than 1 percent of the volume of the cortex.[3] Even our immediate primate relatives use different transmitters within the dentate gyrus in strikingly different ways.[4] These facts invite caution whenever we use findings from animal research to speculate about how the human hippocampal region functions. We not only don't think like Peter Rabbit or Bambi, we can't even be sure we use our hippocampus exactly the same way as do our closest primate relatives.

In humans, the major input to the hippocampus comes down the *parahippocampal gyrus*[1] (see figure 3). This large neocortical gyrus curves down along the lower inside edge of each temporal lobe. Posteriorly, it includes the entorhinal cortex, and it extends back along the midline to the foremost tip of the occipital region. The parahippocampal gyrus is unique: it intercommunicates with *all* areas of cortex. Major projections come into it from the limbic system, from sensory cortex, and from polysensory association cortex.[1] This means that most of the messages entering our hippocampus have already been highly processed by the time they funnel down the *perforant pathway* and into that old, archicortical structure, our hippocampal formation.

Broadly stated, we learn by repetition; "practice makes perfect." It has long been assumed that we "strengthen" synaptic connections by using them more. In fact, repetition does enable the limbic system to respond more efficiently.[5] It is almost like priming a pump. Once the hippocampus has been primed by stimuli that come down the perforant pathway, its own subsequent responses are greatly enhanced. This important phenomenon is called *long-term potentiation*. Three seconds after granule cells down in the hippocampus receive their first priming burst from above, they open up the gates. Now they transmit impulses much more efficiently across their synapses. This enhancing effect rises to its peak fifteen to twenty seconds later.[6]

What is the most effective rate at which to deliver these brief trains of potentiating stimuli? Stimulating at the natural theta frequency: five to seven times per second.[7] Why is the result called *long*-term potentiation? Because transmission remains increased for as long as one to three *weeks* after the stimulation.[8] This is a long time. The way long-term potentiation resembles memory processes has not gone unnoticed.[9]

Where does this theta rate come from? Chiefly from the *medial septal region*, the second major source of hippocampal input.[10] Medial septal cells are "pacemaker" cells. Their acetylcholine drives theta rhythms throughout the hippocampal formation. What has driven the medial septum, in turn? Mostly the impulses rising up to it have come from the midbrain reticular formation.[11] (These, by the way, are not diagrammed in figure 6.)

Many animals show striking, high-amplitude hippocampal theta activity. Their theta waves are impressively synchronized. The peaks and valleys are almost sinusoidal in their regularity. Yet it has been hard to pin down what all this means.[12,13] Moreover, it requires special techniques to correlate the hippocampal theta activity with arousal or attention in primates, including man.[14-16]

In contrast, hippocampal *de*synchronization has attracted rather little attention. Its low-voltage fast-wave activity is flatter and less eye-catching.[17] Still, even the cat spends some 14 percent of its usual time in EEG periods of low-voltage hippocampal desynchrony. And when a cat is highly aroused, it develops an obviously fast desynchronized hippocampal EEG.[18]

What causes such *de*synchrony in the hippocampus? One mechanism resides in the midbrain. Indeed, if you stimulate here at higher voltage, two interesting things happen. One is the fast EEG activity. The other is an "arrest of ongoing activity and the attentive fixation of gaze."[19] Moreover, *both* the hippocampus and the neocortex desynchronize if you stimulate the caudal reticular nucleus of the pons[20] or the median raphe nucleus.[21] A recent speculation is that these hippocampal fast rhythms relate to fine-grained information processing within small parts of the hippocampus itself, as local circuits resonate with many other regions in a larger functional loop of circuitry.[22]

Decades earlier, it had been discovered that stimuli *new* to an animal also desynchronize the EEG both in the hippocampus and in the cortex.[23] Introduce such extraneous novel stimuli during deep sleep and they still desynchronize the hippocampus. This occurs even though the stimuli are too faint to rouse the animal. Moreover, the hippocampus can respond early during those transition periods when sleep is giving way and the brain starts ascending normally to the waking state. In this instance, the hippocampus desynchronizes six seconds *before* the cortex.[24] So further studies of early hippocampal *de*synchronization seem warranted. We very much need to clarify two issues: how transition periods admit alternate states of consciousness, and how novel events trigger these states. The particular ACH pathways rising up from the brain stem to activate the *medial septal* region would be a logical place to begin.

No EEG leads placed on the scalp alone can monitor deep limbic regions.[25] However, depth recordings have been made from electrodes in the human hippocampus. These show both slow (delta) and fast (beta) waves during quiet waking and more activated behaviors.[26] Suppose the patient engages in repeated emotionally charged discussions. Now bursts lasting twenty seconds can recur for up to the next half hour.[25] In responding to music, our left hippocampus seems more sensitive to the musical dissonances (say, of a Charles Ives). The right is attuned to resonate with the harmonies of a barbershop quartet.[27]

A Transcendent Hippocampus?

The hippocampus has become of further interest to Zen, because "transcendent" states of consciousness have been ascribed to discrete changes postulated to take place in certain of its CA cells.[28] Is the hypothesis valid? To begin to evaluate it further takes some persistence. We will need to pick up the trail of the impulses we have just seen enter the hippocampus, then stick with them on their way out through the rest of its circuitry.

The spoor is somewhat easier to follow, because the major flow of information tends to proceed in one general direction.[29] The arrows in figure 6 represent this oversimplification of flow. Once messages have come down the parahippocampal gyrus, they then enter cells of the perforant pathway in the entorhinal cortex. These nerve cells then transmit their impulses to granule cells down in the dentate gyrus. After 400 or so perforant path fibers have discharged, they will have released enough glutamate to fire *one* granule cell in the hippocampus.[30]

These small granule cells issue axons called "mossy" fibers. Something of a misnomer. They certainly gather *no* moss. In fact, they speed messages on to the next, larger CA3 pyramidal cells. Moreover, when mossy fibers fire frequently, they can potentiate the responses of their CA3 target cells for the next fifteen to thirty minutes.[31] Some mossy fibers also release the opioid dynorphin, along with their own glutamate.[32] In this region, dynorphin has three intriguing actions: (1) it enhances the spontaneous bursts of CA3 cells[33]; (2) it promotes *long*-term potentiation[34]; (3) in minute doses, dynorphin is reinforcing, and it prompts a rat into self-stimulation behaviors.[35,36] Why do some of our remembrances become especially memorable? It is reasonable to speculate: some memories could be enhanced by virtue of the ways that both glutamate and opioids excite CA3 cells.

Consider the pivotal position of these larger CA3 pyramidal cells. They lie at an obvious crossroads in the limbic system.[37] Here they could provide a single association matrix, one which could affix the stamp of a specific event onto that particular framework supplied by its context. But what enables one CA3 cell to send its message in two directions, both to prefrontal regions and to midline limbic structures? Its cell body issues *two* axons. Each pursues a different outflow path. The two resemble the split, upper limbs of the letter Y. One branch projects

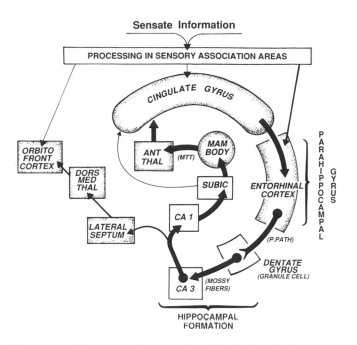

Sensate Information

Figure 6 A hippocampal crossroad and the limbic circuitry
Impulses undergo much processing on their way down to CA3 cells (bottom square). From CA3 cells, they are shunted to CA1 cells, to the subiculum, and to the mammillary body via the fornix. The mamillary body then sends a strong projection to the anterior thalamic nucleus via the mamillothalamic tract (MTT). From the anterior thalamic nucleus impulses flow to the cingulate gyrus, then down to the entorhinal cortex of the parahippocampal gyrus, and finally down the perforant path (P. PATH) to the granule cells of the dentate gyrus, and over to the CA3 cells. This completes the Papez circuit, shown in thicker black arrows.

The CA3 cell also sends off a second branch. Its pathway leads through the lateral septum on to the mediodorsal nucleus of the thalamus, and thence to the orbitofrontal cortex. The relay from granule cells to CA3 cells is via axons called mossy fibers. Some of these release dynorphin. Many axons of the perforant path use glutamate, an excitatory amino acid.

The few arrows shown on this and other wiring diagrams are oversimplifications. The situation is more like a haystack, for countless pathways go in many—and frequently reciprocal—directions. The diagram is therefore highly selective and schematic. (Adapted and modified from several sources, such as: from J. Eccles.: An instruction-selection hypothesis of cerebral learning. In *Cerebral Correlates of Conscious Experience*, eds. P. Buser and A. Rougeul-Buser, A. Amsterdam, North-Holland, 1978; M. Carpenter.: *Human Neuroanatomy*, 7th ed. Baltimore, Williams & Wilkins, 1976; and A. Brodal. *Neurological Anatomy*, 3rd ed. New York, Oxford University Press, 1981.)

to the lateral septal nucleus. It then relays its CA3 influences to the mediodorsal thalamus; and so on, up to the prefrontal orbital cortex. The second branch peels off the CA3 cell and goes back to excite its neighbors, the smaller CA1 cells (figure 6).

What do these latter CA1 cells contribute? Are they merely a conduit for data that will be further stored and consolidated elsewhere? Maybe not. Perhaps they too add to the general sense of context: that conjunction between an event, its occurrence in time, its place in space, and the lively coloration it receives from its emotionalized limbic correlates. In any event, messages coded with some potentials for context then flow on from these CA1 cells over to the nearby subiculum. From the subiculum, they have the options to go (1) on to the mammillary region and up the anterior thalamic-cingulate pathway; or (2) back up to the entorhinal cortex. From here they can be recycled through some of their circuits of origin.

What would happen if a person stopped that stream of messages which normally flows from CA3 cells on to CA1 cells? As part of his theory, Mandell postulates that a person's "inside world" would dominate.[28] His hypothesis further predicts that such a deficit of messages might cause the comparator functions of the hippocampus to fail. As a result, the theory goes on to propose that (1) the feeling of "I" would be lost, and (2) "transcendent" consciousness would arise.

At this point, it will help to recall the earlier discussion of the cingulate gyrus in chapter 40. For this subiculum path finally leads on up to the cingulate gyrus. And *if* any one of its several synapses were, indeed, to *under*function, then clearly the cingulate would be deprived of some of its usual input (see figure 6). A predictable result would be to diminish whatever contributions this entire multisynaptic CA1-cingulate pathway might already have been making into the limbic resonances of the self. Conversely, if the sequences along the long CA1-cingulate pathway were to *over*function, and to keep cycling, then the reverse might occur: these facets of the self could become more intrusive.

Further to evaluate the hypothesis that "transcendence" represents a block at this local CA3 to CA1 site,[28] it also helps to turn back the clock. Over a hundred years ago, Sommer discovered an important fact: epileptic patients lost nerve cells in one special part of their hippocampus. This vulnerable region is called Sommer's sector, and it corresponds with the CA1 field of nerve cells.[38] Later, when researchers were looking for a model to mimic epileptic seizures, they found that intense electrical stimulation of the rat hippocampus also caused its CA1 cells to die.[39]

Recent human studies have documented the mental capacities *during life* of a patient whose nerve cells in the CA1 region were later found, at autopsy, to have previously been destroyed on both sides. During life, the patient suffered *a severe, ongoing amnesia*. Despite this, his other cognitive functions remained intact. Moreover, he did *not* lose his "I" functions. He possessed a sturdy fund of older autobiographical information. These personal facts he could still recall. Yes, he soon forgot immediate events. But he still knew who *he* was, and he knew *about* himself in the past. He also recognized the faces of famous persons.[38] Such evidence would not substantiate the claim that the "I" is lost selectively when there is a discrete failure of CA1 cell function. Nor does the theory receive support from the many patients who, in spite of their having recurrent epileptic seizures, neither lose the "I" nor access a "transcendent" consciousness.

As we noted in part I, the ingredients which make up the self fuse into a tenacious construct. Nothing so deeply rooted and widely distributed easily gives up its old self-centered personal memories. In parts VI and VII we will take up what happens when meditators do lose the "I." At that point, we will consider alternative mechanisms for losing the egocentric self. These explanations need not be accompanied by a host of other severe amnesias, either transiently or ongoing.

Messenger Molecules

Not specified in figure 6 are the transmitter pathways that enter the hippocampal formation. Here, acetylcholine (ACH) plays a complex role,[13] though its net effects are largely excitatory. When it acts on its own inhibitory *pre*synaptic receptors, ACH releases the next cell. Now, this cell can fire repetitively when other excitatory inputs impinge upon it.[40] As a result, CA1 and CA3 cells are stimulated to fire more when they receive impulses from both the distant medial septal nucleus and from the entorhinal cortex.[41]

Opioid axons are included among the fibers descending from the entorhinal cortex. At high rates of stimulation these fibers release some of their enkephalin close enough to CA3 cells to excite them relatively quickly.[42–44] Opioids also excite CA3 cells indirectly by inhibiting the local GABA neurons which had once held them in check (see chapter 45).

Release norepinephrine locally, and it inhibits the *spontaneous* firing of hippocampal cells for over a minute.[45] On the other hand, norepinephrine gives an extra boost to the discharge rate of CA cells after their firing has already been stimulated by glutamate.[46] Humans and other primates invest their dentate gyrus and CA3 regions with many norepinephrine receptors of the alpha$_1$ type.[47] And when their beta norepinephrine receptors are activated, CA1 cells become more excitable for a lengthy period. Long-term potentiation further increases this effect.[48]

Clearly, the hippocampus is a responsive site in general. It is not only a sensitive region that reacts early in response to arousal and to novelty. Well supplied by all this rich, varied input, hippocampal cells have many occasions to vary their firing rates during the day.[49] If you add the same amount of serotonin to them locally, but at different times, the cells go on to vary their firing rates over a twofold range. Indeed, when rats are most active, they raise their hippocampal norepinephrine and serotonin to levels 40 percent higher than at rest. Stress and pain increase norepinephrine levels immediately. However, *serotonin does not reach its peak until fifteen minutes after the pain ends.*[50] The implication is important: during stressful situations, norepinephrine mechanisms could be engaged before those of serotonin (see chapter 53).

Remembrances and Allocentric Functions

Given all its complexities, the hippocampus has now prepared us to believe that it performs more than one function. What could they be? Earlier, to Penfield, the hippocampus seemed "to store keys-of-access to the record of the stream of consciousness."[51] Torda later viewed it as "an active filter and a distributor of information." It was "continuously engaged in a match-mismatch activity which helped it detect the novelty of signals and the adequacy of a remembered response plan."[52]

Then came other studies showing that the hippocampus has "place cells" which play a role in *spatial mapping*.[53] Place cells act like a kind of "internal compass." When they discharge, they probably help set up a large constellation of coded coordinates. The brain refers to this map when it reconstructs its version of three-dimensional space.[54] For example, when a monkey sees a visual stimulus and keeps track of its position, it fires perhaps one out of every eight of its hippocampal cells. Most of these cells (69%) respond to that specific site where the stimulus originated in *outside* space. Because cells with these sensitivities are *other*-centered, they are called *allo*centric.

In a very different category are another 10 percent of the cells. They fire *only* if the visual stimulus arises in that particular spot in outside space that will relate back to *the head and long axis of the monkey's body.* Because these cells use head-body coordinates and are self-centered, they are called *ego*centric. Clearly, such brain cells are coding for different sides of the self/other boundary. Only 2 percent of the place cells respond with regard to where the outside stimulus is positioned in absolute space.[55] Serotonin tends to inhibit the allo- and egocentric spatial processing functions of the hippocampus, and it is likely that other messenger molecules do so as well.[56]

Despite its many attributes, our small hippocampus remains only one of several modules contributing to those "central representations" which collectively make up our memories. Indeed, as we shall soon see, *cortical* circuits are also critical to our remembrances. Especially to those that lead into, and out from, the perirhinal cortex and the other adjacent areas of cortex. These regions are near the anterior tip of the temporal lobe.[57,58]

Hippocampal lesions prevent humans from *thinking about* the ongoing present and the recent past. In contrast, the lesions *spare the procedural motor skills* learned in the past.[30,59] The now-classic patient, H.M., was studied for years after having had much of his hippocampus, amygdala, and overlying temporal cortex removed on both sides. H.M. showed two kinds of memory gaps. They merged as they overlapped. His massive loss involved one particular long segment of *retrograde memories.* He had lost two or three years' worth of these memories.

When had these particular events occurred? They took place during the two years or so leading up to the day of his operation. In addition, H.M. had a severe *ongoing anterograde amnesia.* This means he couldn't remember events that had just taken place, those of the most immediate present. Then, which of his memories *had* survived? The old memories. He had spared most of his old childhood and earlier adult remembrances.

From such observations has come the following rule of thumb: let an event take place, and after two years or so it will normally have gone on to leave its memory traces scattered widely throughout the brain. From then on, these older "engrams" will have become so dispersed, stabilized, and consolidated that they will be relatively invulnerable to any recent damage localized to any one spot. Such a generalization would help explain why patients like H.M. preserve their very old memories even after they sustain a new lesion in the hippocampus on both sides.

The chronic dementia called Alzheimer's disease produces a similar checkered pattern both of memory sparing and of memory defects. The patients reminisce accurately about their earlier years. What perplexes them is where they just (mis)placed their glasses. Nor can they recall the article they read moments before in the paper. *Again, it is the recent and ongoing memories that are most sensitive to loss.* Among the reasons that patients with Alzheimer's disease develop such a devastating memory loss is that they have a series of lesions. These cut off the hippocampal formation from the rest of the brain.[60]

It is an old clinical observation that the brunt of memory loss falls heavily on the recent memories but much more lightly on the remote memories. Ribot noted this back in 1881. Since then, as a general rule, almost all patients seen in the throes of an acute dementia secondary to diffuse head trauma or to toxic-metabolic disease will have tended to bear out the dictum: *ongoing, anterograde memories are more vulnerable to loss than are retrograde memories.*[61]

Recent case reports suggest that there are exceptions to this general rule.[62] In each case, the distinctive point is that *localized* trauma—to the polar *cortex* around the tip of the temporal lobe—appears to be responsible for the unusual outcome. One patient was a young woman in whom a severe closed-head injury had caused such a marked, persistent retrograde memory loss that she couldn't even recall facts about public events or events in which she had personally participated. The paradox: in the acute phase, her memories for recent and ongoing events had been relatively intact, and they remained so. Her radiologic studies showed no abnormalities of the usual memory-related structures. Where were the major defects? In the cortex of the anterior poles of both temporal lobes.

In a second case, trauma had also damaged the cortex of both temporal tips and the right lateral prefrontal region. Again, what this second patient had lost were his old autobiographical memories for personal events. And once again, there had occurred this distinctive relative sparing of general information functions and of recent memories. These two clinical reports lend support to the results of recent studies of memory loss in animals.[57] So when the anterior temporal cortex and its connections are impaired on both sides, the usual proportions of memory loss need not follow the familiar Ribot rule, but can reverse themselves. In this singular instance, the old, autobiographical and other self-related memories bear the brunt of the process, whereas the most recent memory functions remain relatively spared.

Now let us return to reexamine the previous CA3 to CA1 synapse hypothesis for the flash of enlightenment.[28] As its *primary* event, does it strike *only* those particular synapses and circuits *confined within the hippocampus on both sides*? Were this to be the case, then Ribot's general rule would lead us to anticipate the usual two corollary postulates. First, that the flash of enlightenment would then have blotted out both the subject's ongoing immediate memories, plus those most recent retrograde memory traces that had been laid down only moments before the flash took place. Second, that these two losses of memory would follow the standard pattern: not only would memories of events during the present moment be lost but even more severely lost would be retrograde memories. In brief enlightened states, neither postulate occurs.

As we shall find in part VII, enlightened transformation implies the reverse pattern. What happens, instead, is that (a) the *earlier* maladaptive associations drop out. These involve one's personal roots that can be dated far back, into one's childhood and adolescence. (b) The subject accurately registers fresh *ongoing* perceptions. (c) These acute impressions of the present moment are preserved indelibly along with other immediate memory functions. (d) The brain retains, subliminally, the impact and clarity of the peak moment. (e) The changes occurring during this peak moment leave traces that the person can later access to transform behavior along new lines of procedure.

So if enlightenment is going to transform a person's old behavior patterns in a practical way, *it must subtract only certain brain functions, and subtract these highly selectively*. It follows that the flash of insight-wisdom (a) will have to operate in quite a different way than occurs in the known disorders causing focal changes solely or primarily, within the human hippocampus itself; and (b) will need to change several other brain regions, including at least the more anterior regions of temporal cortex, as in the recent case of the young woman patient just cited. These other regions of human cortex lie far outside the narrow limits of the hippocampal CA3 to CA1 synapse.

Certain other patients can also teach us about the way we lay down memories. They suffer an *acute* memory loss, but fortunately recover from it after a few hours. Their memory disorder is called *transient global amnesia*.[63] While they are actually in its throes, the patients' own words accurately describe their amnesia. The words point to a process that is severe, telescoped, and which wipes out immediate memories as fast as each new event presents itself. Repeatedly the patients ask, "Where am I? . . . What day is it? . . . What year is it?" Even when you supply them with the correct answer repeatedly, it won't sink in for more than a few seconds or be impressive long enough to be recalled.

During this amnesia, in most instances, the current generation of tests detect no obvious structural lesion in their brains. When sensitive tests do disclose small areas of structural damage, some of these lesions may localize in the *medial* aspect of one or both temporal lobes, yet at sites that need *not* have directly damaged the hippocampus itself. The implication is that these patients have been suffering from a transient disorder of brain *function*, not structure.

Can one envision a positive mental state the reverse of such a brief global disorder? If so, its physiological antonym has not yet been named. Perhaps if it were, it might be called something akin to "transient global supermnesia."[64] What would it be like? An abrupt onset and brief surge of vastly enhanced mentation. A mental field focused on the immediate present. A present moment *found*, not lost. A moment reinterpreted unforgettably. Each of its novel events entering into a coherent whole, a unity that could be impregnated with the generic essence of eternity. In chapter 142, we will be considering the possibility that several striking interpretive features of such a state could be the result of both highly selective *hyper*functionings and *hypo*functionings within various sites, both in the temporal lobes *and* elsewhere.

Suppose, meanwhile, you were still curious about the hippocampus. What does it really accomplish with all these CA cells, place cells, potentiations, memory filters, and so on? If you happened to be a postmaster, several of its functions might seem vaguely familiar. Maybe both your post office and the hippocampus do occupy only 1 percent of the large space at hand. But operationally, their activities add something vital to the rest of the neighborhood, for they are much more than simple ordinary way stations. Yes, to begin with, they both sort messages in reasonably orderly fashion, noting how they have been stamped with various urgencies, destinations, zip codes, and postage, before using this information to route them to sites near and far. This is only their usual humdrum routine.

But then a few special messages come along which are also *registered*. They attract more attention than others. Beyond these singular messages, at certain times each year, the processing volume in each of the two operations undergoes a marked increase, whether of mail or of impulses. One of these occasions is during circumstances of special urgency, general stress, and anxiety. These are the moments when an incoming message reflects the needs for an extraspeedy express delivery. The other big increase occurs around the time when each aged year is drawing to its close. Nights grow cold and dark. Now the thankful community draws together to celebrate its shared humanity along with close family and friends. And out of this period of cold dark nights and inclement weather will emerge those ageless themes, so deeply familiar to Christianity and Buddhism alike: the themes of gratitude, of being born and reborn in innocence.

43

Visceral Drives and the Hypothalamus

In winter, a bonfire spells delight
but when summertime arrives what a nuisance it becomes!

Master Bankei[1]

Conflicts between longing and loathing are a disease of the mind.
Gain and loss, right and wrong, away with them once and for all!

Master Seng-ts'an[2]

The hypothalamus, weighing in at only four grams, might seem to be a trifling flyweight in any contest with a heavy human brain weighing 1400 grams.[3] But it rivals the newer computer chips in its complexity. And, like the old Ponte Vecchio which bridges the Arno river in Florence, the hypothalamus serves two kinds of functions. It carries on essential local business and housekeeping activities in its own bustling side compartments. At the same time, it acts as a bridge that conducts a two-way traffic, and carries enough exotic raw materials to stimulate a kind of renaissance on both sides.

Our hypothalamus is centered at the base of the brain, below the thalamus (see figure 3). Here, it is strategically placed to integrate our primitive instinctual drives. The words we attach to them include sexual longing, hunger, thirst, fear, anger, and aggression. It can participate in these drives, because it links the limbic system, brain stem, and forebrain areas with many vital endocrine functions of that master gland just below it, the pituitary.[4] In the process, it governs our internal environment—its water and salt balance, temperature, cycles, and hormones.

Originally, instinctive behaviors evolved in ways that helped preserve the self and perpetuate the species. They are legacies hardwired eons ago into the base of our brain and brain stem. But today, overworked parts of our ancient hypothalamic circuitry keep raising intractable problems for man, the social animal. Consider how you got "hot under the collar" during your last heated argument. Zen masters have always been very clever at reminding us how hot-tempered we are. They know how to provoke us, allowing us to *feel* how longings and loathings consume us in the fires of passion.

It could be worse. In fact, among all animals, the human hypothalamus has become the shortest in relation to the length of the rest of the cerebrum. This anatomical fact has two major implications. First, as we grow up and mature, the rest of our brain develops functional pathways which will subordinate the hypothalamus if not subdue it. The general term for this is *conditioning*. Conditioning helps us learn to civilize our basic, inborn elements of behavior (see chapter 74).

But something else is needed, something crucial: the capacity to *unlearn*. It is in this second arena that the Zen approach becomes of great interest. *Zen sponsors a systematic unlearning in human beings.* Now, if you were to remove almost everything above the midbrain from rats, they will still go on learning. That is to say, they can still be conditioned into learning if you *leave only the lateral hypothalamus,* and deliver reinforcing electrical stimuli into it.[5] And rats still manifest their other conditioned behaviors, even after you have selectively removed the cortex, hippocampus, striatum, and septum.

However, after these forebrain regions are gone, there is a major difference in the properties of the conditioned behaviors that the rats can then develop. What is so different? *Now these same behaviors do not disappear readily.* Rats with no forebrain cannot *un*learn. Many experiments have suggested that "higher" regions normally send down to the hypothalamus certain critical kinds of negative feedback information. These negative messages from above normally help the hypothalamus and other parts of the brain *dampen* their more reflexive behavioral responses. And, as a result of its being negatively reinforced (or of no longer being reinforced), a stimulus that had once been so exciting now loses its salience.

Walter Hess's careful observations showed that an animal's behavior could change markedly when parts of its brain were stimulated.[6] For these studies, he received the Nobel prize in 1949. Since Hess's work, a simplified way to summarize the functional anatomy of the hypothalamus has been to separate it into several parcels. In general, its more *lateral* and *posterior regions* serve to integrate those functions of the rest of the brain that are energy-expending. These functions find expression in the body through the sympathetic nervous system (see figure 9). In contrast, the more *anterior and medial hypothalamic regions* help direct energy-conserving, parasympathetic activities.

Lateral Regions

Each lateral region contains two elements: nerve cells, and fibers which pass through in both directions. Hunger is one of several natural kinds of stimuli that cause these lateral cells to fire. Place an apple in front of a monkey, and the fruit now triggers the firing of as many nerve cells as had discharged at other times when the monkey had become very highly aroused in general.[7]

Certain brain circuitries respond to desirable stimuli which, like food, have positive "rewarding" properties. Others respond to stimuli that have unpleasant, negative, aversive qualities.[4,8] In either instance, the lateral hypothalamus serves as one nodal region that helps us develop these polarized responses. We underestimate their strength if we think of them, in the abstract, as having "merely" a positive or negative sign. *For, when relayed further, these polarized visceral responses end up being firmly attached to our notions of good or bad, right or wrong, gain or loss.* These notions are hard to let go of. Zen goes to work on them.

Stimulate a monkey's lateral hypothalamus, and only three milliseconds later the impulses will have activated nerve cells up in the motor cortex. Responses this fast may help explain why self-stimulation here is such an effective way to enhance voluntary movements and make them goal-oriented.[9] Researchers can deliver an ongoing series of stimuli after wires have been permanently implanted in the lateral hypothalamus. The stimuli will activate the lateral hypothalamic nerve cells or the fibers passing through the region, or both. Behavior changes in either event. The changes are both short-term and long-term. For example, if you stimulate a number of rats chronically, it turns out that their behavior falls into two categories. One group of rats happens to eat more; the other group drinks more. Once the drinking rats have gotten firmly into their habit of drinking in response to hypothalamic stimuli, they resist any attempts to bait them over into the other, eating, pattern. They can't break the habit. Their rigid drinking behavior persists.[10] Lateral hypothalamic stimulation does enhance certain kinds of approach functions. Weak stimuli here will orient an animal more forcibly toward an attractive odor.

Why do we find it so hard to break our own compulsive patterns of behavior such as drinking or eating? Because our appetitive habits have gone on to enlist more components than the primitive "drive" systems within the hypothalamus and its immediate connections. We recruited extra layers of *acquired* patterned responses from high and low. Larger "loops" of these circuitries have gone on to entangle the hypothalamus in extensive reinforcing networks. Consider the implications for anyone who would wish to diminish cravings, extinguish desires. A smoker who wishes to kick the habit of nicotine will need to unlearn many fixed behavior patterns. Most of these added repertoires—lighting up, mouth movements, and inhaling—are imbedded at reaches beyond the mere prescription of a nicotine patch. So if the intent is to transform behavior, *as it is in Zen,* then the brain must be modified in at least three sets of ways: (1) the way it perceives stimuli, (2) the way it responds to stimuli at basic visceromotor levels, and (3) the way its many other layered systems *reinforce* the interactions between the first two.

Stimuli to the lateral hypothalamus also change short-term behaviors. Again, the results are relevant to Zen. Why? Because they resemble some of the events during brief states of absorption in humans. In cat experiments, one reads with interest the following account: "Stimulation of the lateral hypothalamic system, which induces desynchronization of hippocampal electrical activity, causes mainly *fixation of gaze* and an *attentive posture*" (italics in original). The cat shows "arrest of ongoing behavior, the assumption of fixed posture and gaze, postural and ocular fixation, sometimes preceded by a brief alerting or orienting response, steady fixation of gaze."[11]

Let us assume in this experiment that the stimuli have been delivered to the cat's *right* lateral hypothalamic region. It will then be on this same right side that the stimuli induce discrete low-voltage fast-wave EEG activity, especially in the right *visual area* and right hippocampus. Is it important that both visual and hippocampal regions desynchronize on the *same* side as the stimulation? Yes. It suggests the possibility that humans might sometimes extract a lateralized visual image as a memory trace from past experience—along with a fixed gaze and posture—when their lateral hypothalamus is excited more on one side than the other. These last points become relevant to what caused several early features during my experience of absorption (see chapter 111).

Lateral hypothalamic stimulation does excite the visual cortex itself. However, it also goes on to *reduce* the response of this visual cortex to *external* visual stimulation. This result indicates that visual messages *from the outside world* are being shut down.[12] We can now relate this visual shutdown to inhibition that occurs at the level of the thalamus. This sequence of events will also be relevant to what caused the visual blackness during my state of absorption (see chapter 112).

Stimulating the lateral hypothalamus does other things. It makes nerve cells of the septal region fire faster and more continuously.[13] Moreover, at the same time, greater degrees of stimulation can stop all active behavior for the next thirty seconds.[14] Hypothalamic stimulation can also reduce the responses to painful stimuli delivered to the foot or the nose, suppress startle responses to loud noises, and dampen other complex behaviors that involve higher circuitry.[15]

Posterior Regions

Hess believed that the *posterior hypothalamus* as a whole sponsored energy-expending functions. These he called "ergotropic." Recent studies of single nerve cells in this region suggest, in fact, that many cells are involved more with movement than with tonic EEG arousal per se.[16] In man, this energizing region forms a triangular zone called the "ergotropic triangle." Looked at from the side, its apex lies under the superior colliculus, and its sides extend over to the front border of the mammillary body[17] (see figure 3).

In Japan, decades ago, some patients who had suffered uncontrollably violent rage attacks were quieted after lesions were made in the posteromedial hypothalamus. Before making their electrolytic lesions, the neurosurgeons first delivered weaker stimuli to help define the exact boundaries of this triangle. Weak stimuli within the triangle caused a widespread sympathetic nervous system discharge: increased blood pressure and heart rate, flushing of the face, and dilated pupils.[18] These lasted for two minutes after the stimuli stopped. Higher-frequency stimulation also desynchronized the hippocampus, other limbic regions, and the cerebral cortex.

During stimulation, these highly aggressive patients reported being "obsessed by extreme horror." After sites in the triangle had been destroyed, their personalities changed. They became markedly calm, passive, and tractable. Their decreased spontaneity returned toward normal within a month. They were sleepy for only the first few days, presumably because the lesions were small.

The surgeons believed that the lesions had cut "overactive" connections that otherwise would be carrying a normal flow of impulses between the triangle, parts of the limbic system, and the neocortex.[18,19] It was also postulated that the weak stimuli had excited, and that the lesions had destroyed, a part of the fiber bundle which conveys messages down from the posterior hypothalamus to the central gray region and adjacent parts of the nearby midbrain.

When painful stimuli are delivered to a person's leg or arm, a slight delay occurs before the signal arrives up in the same general region of the posteromedial hypothalamus. The lag indicates that some impulses, those related to "slow pain," are indeed conducted slowly, but finally do reach this region. Following this lead, neurosurgeons made small electrolytic lesions at the site. This time their goal was to relieve severe pain states caused by cancer on the opposite side of the body.[20] Again, during stimulations made to locate the correct spot, the patients reported a "very unpleasant sensation of fear or horror." After the lesions, they too became more placid, and specifically replied "No" when asked if they still had pain. In contrast, after frontal lobe lesions made to treat pain, other patients will say, "Yes, I still feel pain, but it doesn't bother me so."

Such studies indicate that excessive stimulation to the posteromedial hypothalamus can spread to give rise to a major dysphoric experience of fear or horror. We are, therefore, in the presence of deep circuitries that can *tap into, if not subserve, the sources of human suffering and anguish*. Zen goes to work on these sources.

A sheaf of many nerve cells containing *histamine* lies in the posterior hypothalamus near the mammillary bodies. Their terminal fibers supply histamine widely to the hypothalamus and limbic forebrain.[21] Many persons may recall having been made sleepy by the earlier antihistaminic drugs. It was not surprising, then, to find that histamine itself is an agonist which has many energizing actions. Indeed, it excites most hypothalamic cells when it acts on its H_1 receptors. Histamine also has relatively weak inhibitory actions elsewhere, and its H_2 receptors generate cyclic adenosine monophosphate (cAMP). In these respects histamine resembles the other biogenic amine systems to be discussed in the next chapter. The details of how it functions in our arousal mechanisms still need to be worked out.[22,23]

An overarching pathway called the *fornix* carries the impulses down into each mammillary region which begin within the hippocampal formation, cingulate gyrus, and parahippocampal gyri. In return, the mammillary body sends its major projection bundle, the *mammillothalamic tract*, up to the anterior thalamic nucleus. This anterior nucleus then relays impulses on up to the cingulate gyrus and down to the midbrain.

Anterior Regions

Stimulating the posterior ergotropic triangle prompts cats to go into ragelike behavior.[19] But this excessive behavior can be held in check. The way to block it is to stimulate a little faster in and around the *anterior hypothalamus* at the same time.

This experiment suggested that the two regions, anterior and posterior, were in a precarious, seesaw balance. And it lent support to Hess's idea that the anterior hypothalamic region had energy-conserving, "trophotropic" functions. He observed, furthermore, that when the normal braking action of the anterior region was removed, the cats became so ferocious and hyperactive that they reached the point of insomnia and exhaustion.

In the anterior hypothalamic region lie the preoptic nuclei. They act as a kind of central thermostat in regulating body temperature.[24,25] Moreover, electrical stimuli inhibit various motor functions and cause sleep when delivered into this anterior hypothalamus and into the basal forebrain.[26]

Yet it is the tiny suprachiasmatic nucleus that plays a key role in setting our biological clock in its daily rhythms of sleep-wakefulness. It is a light-sensitive pacemaker. It monitors light impulses from its perch just above the crossing point of fibers in the optic pathway. The nucleus has a very dense network of serotonin terminals,[26] and other nearby nuclei have many opioid receptors.[27] Damage to this small region disorganizes the brain's light/dark activity cycle.

I never fully appreciated how important this cycle was. Then I entered a "rat room." Here, hundreds of rats were being maintained in racks of cages. The lights were turned on for twelve hours, and were off for twelve hours. Rats, unlike humans, are highly active in the dark. The lights were on when I first visited the rat room at the Karolinska Institute. All was quiet. Not a rustle. Every rat was asleep. The next time, I entered the room during their dark cycle. Now, the noise was deafening. Hundreds of rats were scurrying around and scuffling in their cages.

One hypothalamic nucleus, curved like an arc, merits special attention. It is a vital nodal point for regulating the release of hypothalamic hormones.[28] This *arcuate nucleus* lies in front of the mammillary bodies (see figure 3). Its multiple functions are difficult to clarify, because it packs together many different nerve cells that respond to many different chemical messengers.[29] The reader has an objective index of how complex the arcuate nucleus is: *twenty* authors from fourteen different laboratories contributed to *one* recent article![30] Let one brief example serve to illustrate how important it is. A profound loss of pain occurs when you stimulate the arcuate nucleus, either electrically or with the transmitter glutamate. In fact, this arcuate nucleus appears to mediate the long-lasting opioid type of analgesia produced when the leg is stimulated by electroacupuncture.[31,32] Can the pain and tingling from a meditator's left leg ascend to influence not only the right hypothalamus but the arcuate region? This point will become of interest when we consider which mechanisms converged in my brain and led to the state of absorption (see chapter 122).

The lie detector test is a familiar technique. It is based on a simple-minded premise: human subjects know that truth differs from falsehood. Sensing this gap—this "mismatch"—between real truth and their false statement, subjects increase their pulse rate, blood pressure, respiratory rate, and perspire more. But in order for the hypothalamus to *integrate* all these effects, it must first receive information from many other circuits. Consider what kinds of instruction it needs to respond in such a test. One type of input recognizes what is usually true;

another registers what is in the act of being said. Finally, some kind of "conscience" must oversee each of the above. This monitor then discerns what gap, if any, lies between truth and utterance. Later we will come to an intriguing application of the lie detector test (see chapter 142).

Meanwhile, how could you establish that, during more *ordinary* events of the day, the hypothalamus itself can integrate emotional valences into such visceral reflexes as heart rates and blood pressures? First, you might set up a conditioned response in animals, resorting to a brief electric shock as the standard aversive training procedure. Then you might make a lesion only one millimeter in diameter on both sides of the hypothalamus at the point where the fornix enters it. These small lesions would stop all the emotionally conditioned rises in heart rate and blood pressure which the animals had developed earlier.[33]

Advance this way, pleads longing. Retreat, says fear, as it pulls in the opposite direction. Emotion *moves* us. Motion is in the word itself, as Sir Charles Sherrington pointed out.[18] In this respect, the hypothalamus is a whole *yin-yang* land crammed with potentials for sharply opposing patterns of behavior. Here, lion and lamb lie next to each other. Close nearby, both the amygdala and the central gray region contribute to the circuits mediating aggression or tameness.

Will the human species survive? Only if it begins to strike a better balance between its powerful aggressive traits and its gentler nurturing instincts. Obviously, men and women behave differently. But starting from the gonadotrophic systems up in the hypothalamic-pituitary complex, how do the different masculinizing and feminizing hormones—hormones made down in our different endocrine glands—return to act "upstream," as it were? Where do our bodies' androgens and estrogens, having entered the bloodstream, act to modify these tough or gentle behavioral options back up inside our brains?

The nuclei just in front of the mammillary region illustrate this important point. Nerve cells here have many androgen-binding sites ready to receive testosterone. In contrast, other regions nearby are endowed with a surprising *dual competence.* Here lie the potentials for behavior to shift either way. For both the ventromedial nucleus and the amygdala can convert a masculinizing hormone like testosterone into other, feminizing hormones which activate *estrogen-binding sites.*[34]

After testosterone and estrogen from the body exert their effects on their many target nerve cells in the medial regions of the hypothalamus and preoptic area, these hormonally responsive regions then relay messages down to the midbrain. Here, their signals influence a variety of behaviors. Some are reproductive in nature. Some are aggressive, others playful.[35]

To help modulate its responses, the hypothalamus receives a very rich supply of two biogenic amines, norepinephrine (NE) and serotonin (ST).[36] Serotonin inhibits the release of gonadotropin releasing hormone. In humans, the hypothalamus also has many alpha NE receptors which serve chiefly excitatory functions.[37] Some of the reduced drive associated with the aging process could reflect the major drop in NE that occurs in the aging hypothalamus.[38] But probably the fast transmitter, GABA, plays the major role in harnessing our instinctual drives under normal circumstances. For GABA nerve endings account for half of the synapses in the hypothalamus.[39] When a GABA-active drug (muscimol) is delivered locally, it inhibits the anterior hypothalamus and preoptic region. Soon, the cat becomes extravigilant and develops insomnia. In contrast, when this same GABA agonist inhibits the posterior hypothalamic region, the cat now falls asleep.[40] (In a sense, this GABA agonist has acted as does local cooling.)

The Zona Incerta

The zona incerta is a separate region, located under the thalamus but lying off to each side. Its nerve cells, too, are a kind of specialized continuation of those coming up from the midbrain reticular core below. Stimulating the zona incerta in animals quickly transforms their EEG into low-voltage fast-wave activity. Cooling it produces sleep. The zona incerta probably contributes to our higher-level, reticular-like activating functions, especially to those keyed to frontal lobe and limbic activities.[41] It is one obvious candidate among the regions that could help add to expanded states of consciousness.

For example, some research suggests that the zona incerta contributes to the appreciation of the intensity of light. After lesions destroy the zona incerta, rats who had learned earlier to make visual distinctions between black and white cannot change their behavior in response to such visual cues.[42] Perhaps the zona incerta receives some input of relevant messages about how intense light is from the lateral geniculate nucleus nearby. And if this zona incerta also contributes to our own normal light intensity functions, it might play a role in the brief, unusual experience that people have when they sense they are being enveloped by an especially bright light (see chapter 85).

*   *   *

Suppose the reader could now actually enter the brain. Imagine that you were perched up in the posterior hypothalamic region and could peer about. You could then see many of the crucial regions of the midbrain and diencephalon soon to be discussed. The supposition is not a novel one. In the seventeenth century, Descartes ventured to suggest that our pineal gland, which does look down on this same key junction, served as the seat of the "soul." Not too wild a guess, considering what was then known. In the present century, Penfield would postulate that the region of central gray matter within this same midbrain-diencephalic junction constituted the "highest brain-mechanism."

If you now chose to descend toward the brain stem itself, your steps would take you toward those several key nuclei that give rise to its biogenic amines. And you would be passing two other important nearby sites which we will return to discuss later on. These are the central gray substance and the superior colliculus.

Biogenic Amines: Three Systems

> Our ability to predict and explain short- or long-term changes in central nervous system neural function depends largely on our basic knowledge of the specific dynamic interactions within and among the various neural circuits and their individual components.
>
> Karen Gale[1]

An exciting era began when Swedish anatomists made amines fluoresce inside nerve cells. Now one could actually see and localize the nerve cells that made these potent amines, and could map the pathways that released them into the rest of the brain. But these small cells are greatly outnumbered. Our brain holds only a million or so of them.[2] Can they exert much influence over the fifteen *billion* other nerve cells in human cerebral cortex alone?

They can. Because each aminergic nerve cell spreads out a huge network of terminals. Trace one slender axon downstream after it exits from its dopamine nerve cell. You can see its fluorescent branches fanning out like the Mississippi delta. Indeed, they may go on to divide into 500,000 or so nerve endings, reaching many hundreds of other distant nerve cells.[2] This is but one of many remarkable features of the three systems which deploy the major amines: dopamine, norepinephrine, and serotonin.

Dopamine Systems

The supply of dopamine (DA) stems from two major sources in the midbrain (figure 7). The first DA source is called the *substantia nigra*. The name refers to its darkly pigmented cell bodies. Its outflow path supplies DA higher up to the deep motoric nuclei called the basal ganglia. Humans concentrate more DA in one of them, the putamen, than anywhere else: 5740 nanograms per gram.[3] The putamen and its outer partner, the caudate nucleus, are together known as the *dorsal striatum*. Normally, when we release DA at this top end of the *nigrostriatal* pathway, it helps us quickly execute the full range of our motor patterns and associated movements. What happens if DA drops to very low levels on only one side of this system? The Parkinson syndrome. The patient slows down, hampered by the sluggish arm and leg movements on the opposite side of the body.

The second DA source is the *ventral tegmental* DA system. In humans, its cells send much of their DA up to supply the nucleus accumbens in the *ventral* striatum. A separate DA pathway supplies the limbic system. Two other branches supply DA to the cortex in the prefrontal and cingulate regions.[4] There, an especially dense network of DA fibers covers the inner part of the prefrontal region. The mediodorsal nucleus of the thalamus also sends its major input into this same region of medial cortex.

This is a remarkable convergence. The way these two pathways, DA and thalamic, blanket the frontal cortex remains one of the brain's anatomically

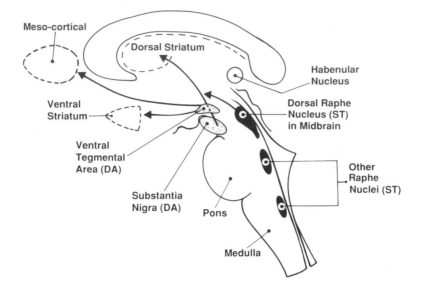

Figure 7 Dopamine and serotonin systems
The substantia nigra and the ventral tegmental area (stippled) provide the most dopamine-containing nerve cells. The dorsal raphe nucleus (black), in the midline of the midbrain, contributes most of its serotonin to the cerebrum, while other lower raphe nuclei supply regions lower down.

constant features.[5] Dating as far back as the tree shrew, it reminds us of our arboreal origins.

Other regions of the primate cortex also show dense DA terminals. They include the motor cortex, the inferior parietal lobe (area 7), and the association cortex. Relatively few terminals supply the primary visual, auditory, or somatosensory cortex.[6]

How can we tell what functions all these different DA nerve cells perform? One way is to monitor them, using fine wires, while observing which everyday activities prompt them to fire more briskly. It turns out that DA cells are not especially active when animals are responding to many stressful stimuli nor when they are waking up from the low arousal state of sleeping.[7,8] And even when a cat is awake and active, the DA cells in its substantia nigra are firing only 20 percent faster than when it is quiet.[9] Certain of a cat's DA cells even fire *less* at a time when a noxious pinch is being delivered to the skin of its hind leg or foreleg.[10] Moreover, DA cells also *slow* their firing rate for up to ten seconds at times when the cat orients toward an interesting event. For a laboratory cat, an interesting event occurs when you open its cage door.[9]

Yet, those other DA cells in the ventral tegmental area are more sensitive. They fire a short three-second burst if a sound occurs or if the face is touched. And these burst firings do not habituate.[11] In Zen, we will be asking, How do sudden sensory stimuli trigger the brain? One answer is that they might prompt certain DA cells into bursts of firing, more likely the DA cells in the ventral tegmental DA system.

Suppose you reduce the social stimuli to an otherwise gregarious animal so as to make it a kind of a hermit in an opaque cage. In a sense, the prolonged isolation then becomes a kind of sensorimotor deprivation. The several DA systems then react in different ways.[12] In rats, this slows the metabolic activity of the DA nerve cells that supply the frontal region. However, isolation *increases* the metabolic activity of those other DA neurons that project up to the dorsal and ventral striatum. And at this time, even though the isolated rats have quieted down and show few *spontaneous* behaviors, they jump more when an electrical stimulus is delivered to the foot. These studies suggest that, after extensive social isolation, a sensate stress is able to trigger a surge of impulses through DA motor systems. In such ways may very prolonged forms of meditative isolation go on later to heighten a subject's responsivities.

It is one thing to measure how fast a nerve cell itself fires when one is recording from the body of that cell. But what is happening out at its terminals far downstream? Could they have been "shut off" at that time? Or could they have been "opened up," thus releasing more of their chemical messenger molecules into the synapse? In fact, the brain has an array of tiny receptors, poised to accomplish either feat. They operate, like nozzles, on *pre*synaptic nerve endings. When they act, more DA, or less DA, is released into the next synapse. Some presynaptic receptors are *self*-regulating, and are called autoreceptors. Sensitive to DA themselves, their net effect will be to reduce the release of DA. But other major transmitters can open up DA terminals and release more DA.[13,14] Acetylcholine, glutamate, and GABA act in this manner.

Suppose the next cell is a *post*synaptic neuron, one which belongs to the caudate nucleus. Covering its cell body are a subtype of receptors called the DA_1 receptors. They convey DA's *inhibitory* responses, and slow the firing rate of this caudate cell.[15] However, elsewhere in the brain, when still more DA is released on other DA_1 receptors, the net result is behavioral arousal and EEG desynchronization.[16,17] Why? Because these other DA_1 receptors go on to inhibit GABA systems. In this instance, DA inhibition stops GABA from exerting its own usual local inhibitory role on arousal mechanisms.

Some DA_2 receptors afford a direct contrast. They more directly mediate excitatory responses. Studding the dendrites on the next neuron, they respond to low DA concentrations.[18] Each year, as more receptor genes are cloned, research adds a daunting array of new receptors. It now takes a new kind of specialist just to keep track of all the new subtypes within receptor families and to assign functions to each of them. One of the more recent subtypes is the DA_3 receptor. It is prominent in the ventral striatum and elsewhere in the limbic system.

Does each person's brain contain the same number of DA receptors, distributed in the same pattern? No. Early in life, the brain responds to whichever levels of hormones prevail: either male (androgen) or female (estrogen). Maleness starts early. Only a few days after male rats are born, having now responded to their own androgen levels, these males already show more evidence of DA receptors in their cortex and amygdala than do females.[19]

Receptors are now assuming importance in disease, not only in health. For example, some evidence indicates that DA_2 receptor levels increase in three conditions. One is in schizophrenia, in those patients who have "positive" symptoms such as delusions, hallucinations, and thought disorders.[20] Another is in a

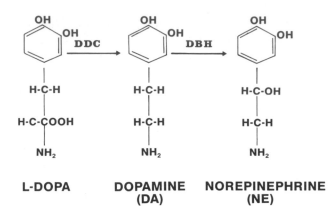

Figure 8 Dopamine and norepinephrine metabolism
Levodopa is the precursor molecule. It evolves first to dopamine (DA). In nerve cells of the locus ceruleus, the DA is then converted to norepinephrine (NE). DDC, dopa decarboxylase; DBH, dopamine beta-hydroxylase. NE is further converted into epinephrine (Adrenalin).

subgroup of Parkinson disease patients who are prone to show abnormal movements, motor fluctuations, and tendencies to psychosis.[21] A third condition is narcolepsy.[22]

Many DA nerve cells have dual potentials. They also make the peptide cholecystokinin (CCK).[23] CCK is excitatory. This means that it could functionally antagonize some of the local inhibitory effects of DA.[24,25] These doubly competent cells supply the limbic system and the prefrontal cortex. In these crucial regions, DA and CCK having an impact together might lend complex and unusual qualities to a person's experience.

How, then, can one summarize the major functional role of DA systems in the human brain? First, that they yield prominent *motoric* effects. When patients with the Parkinson syndrome receive levodopa by mouth, they convert it to DA in the brain (figure 8). There, DA strikingly energizes their slow movements and remobilizes them. Decades of animal research on rats and mice have shown that DA *energizes* when it enters the ventral or dorsal striatum. More than that, *any drug that indirectly releases DA* into their nucleus accumbens precipitates rodents into a distinctive motor sequence: they move around more, sniff more, and engage in repetitive grooming behaviors.[26] So in the accumbens, the drug does not have to be DA itself. It could be an opiate, alcohol, or a barbiturate. But DA contributes something more than a general mobilizing effect. This became clear when animals pressed on a lever, "working" to receive food as a "reward."[27] The animals became more selective and efficient, suggesting that DA was helping to sustain *goal-directed* behaviors.[28]

Physiological studies confirm that DA has other effects beyond those which are purely motoric. One can observe this most clearly in those Parkinson disease patients whose sluggish arm and leg movements occur only on *one* side. When these patients are exposed to visual stimuli, it will be the opposite hemisphere, the side low in DA, which has below-normal amplitudes of *sensory* evoked potentials. What happens after the patients are treated with levodopa? It restores the lower sensory potentials on their DA-deficient side toward a more normal height.[29] But, even before levodopa is given, any task that requires keen attention will also heighten the amplitude of the patients' visual potentials. Out of such evidence comes the suggestion *that DA can normally enter in to influence our several mechanisms of attention, and does so in subtle ways that enhance the impact of sensory stimuli.*

"Extroversion" is a shorthand label for some of our outward-directed behaviors. It has other correlates. Extroverted persons tend to show higher spinal fluid levels of DA breakdown products.[30] Spinal fluid samples from aggressive patients also show the same evidence of higher DA turnover, namely, an increase in homovanillic acid.[31] However, after the same aggressive patients had practiced yoga meditation for six months, their levels of DA breakdown products fell, from the initial fifty-one down to forty-one nanograms per milliliter, a statistically significant reduction. In contrast, yoga meditation did not reduce the metabolic by products of norepinephrine (NE) in their spinal fluid.

Cocaine jolts the brain into a briefly energized, twenty-minute "high." Before they "crash," those who abuse cocaine or amphetamines experience major psychic stimulatory effects, chiefly because the drugs increase the synaptic levels of DA and NE. But such drug highs have no firm cultural foundation, and are not supported by long spiritual training and restraint. So their brief peaks represent one more drive toward self-indulgence. And they leave in their wake additional cravings for stimuli at multiple receptors, plus a host of other problems at the personal and societal levels.

Norepinephrine Systems

The second group of biogenic amine nerve cells makes norepinephrine. Most NE cells cluster in that pair of nuclei called the *locus ceruleus*, literally a "blue place" (figure 9). Each human locus ceruleus is a long, tube-shaped aggregate of pigmented NE neurons. It extends for some sixteen millimeters along each side of the pons and midbrain. The two nuclei together comprise only a mere 15,000 to 60,000 nerve cells.[32,33] Yet, again, each one of their slender *dorsal* bundles of NE fibers fans out to supply a huge terminal field. A second group of amine fibers, those in the *ventral* NE bundles, comes up mostly from other NE cells farther down in the medulla. It delivers its NE more to the hypothalamus, and it also conveys axons from the nearby epinephrine nerve cells which also lie down in the medulla.

The primate brain has a dense network supplying NE to the cortex of area 7 in the posterior parietal lobe, to the pulvinar-lateral posterior nuclei of the thalamus, and to the outer layers of the superior colliculus in the midbrain. In contrast, relatively little NE goes into the temporal and inferior temporal cortex.[6] Already, one can make out a distinctive feature of the NE system: it has a generally *sensate* distribution. Therefore, when we are overtaken by a physiological surge of NE, it seems likely that it could influence the way we process spatial data and respond with appropriate visuomotor reflexes. Yet humans still resemble other animals: we too reserve for the hypothalamus our highest concentration of NE: 1150

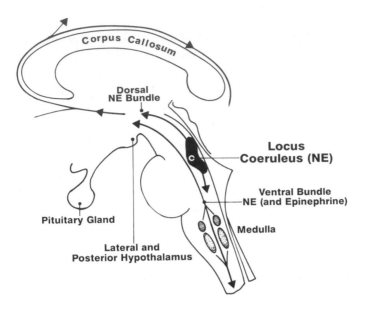

Figure 9 Norepinephrine systems
The locus ceruleus (in black) contains the major cluster of norepinephrine (NE) cells. Its bundles of axons project up and down as do those of other nearby NE and epinephrine-containing cells.

nanograms per gram.[3] This chemical fact of life underlines how important NE continues to be for the vital instinctual functions of our hypothalamus.

The meditative path is a long spiritual struggle. Aspirants undergo suffering before suffering is relieved. In this regard, NE cells in the locus ceruleus are noteworthy: they fire especially in response to *noxious, painful, stressful stimuli*.[8] In the rat, they fire faster for up to thirty seconds after noxious pressure on the toe.[34] In the cat, locus NE cells also fire faster during a conditioned response. But they do so *only* if the conditioning had been performed earlier with a *noxious* stimulus, not with food or some other rewarding stimulus. When a simple stimulus is strong enough to arouse a cat, it will prompt a brief discharge from NE cells. But this response dwindles as the stimuli are repeated.[35]

In monkeys, too, painful or stressful stimuli make NE cells fire faster. The cells also discharge more during various non-noxious visual or other stimuli, and during spontaneous arousal. But monkeys are not cats, and what really sets the monkey off is fruit juice, its favorite nourishment. Now its NE cells fire at their highest rates: seven to fifteen times a second. In brief, the NE cells of the primate brain are especially turned on by noxious stimuli *and* by certain attractive stimuli. In contrast, their firing slows markedly both in the presence of opioids like morphine and during desynchronized (REM) sleep.[34]

Most input to the locus ceruleus comes up from one small part of the medulla. This nucleus is the lateral paragigantocellular nucleus. It is continually engaged in regulating breathing, blood pressure, heart rate, and pain responses.[36] Therefore, most of the messages that will enter the NE system from below have already been highly processed.[37] So it seems possible that one result of the regular, slower breathing and physiologically calming effects of meditation is to quiet down the firing of the locus ceruleus. This could occur chiefly because its cells received fewer excitatory impulses from the paragigantocellular nucleus. Even so, a sudden painful stimulus could cause NE cells to discharge.

What happens when such an NE cell does fire more frequently? One way to find out is to deliver tiny amounts of extra NE, through micropipettes, on another distant cell supplied by NE nerve endings and covered with NE receptors. Then microelectrodes recording from that second cell will detect changes in its firing rate. Researchers were surprised by what happened next. For NE turned out to have rather few *direct* effects on these postsynaptic cells. What it does is *modulate*. For example, NE does very little to change the slow, background firing of CA cells in the hippocampus. But once these larger hippocampal cells have already been excited by added glutamate, then NE further boosts their firing rate.

NE also makes hippocampal cells fire more when they are already being excited by *natural* visual and auditory stimuli coming from the outside. Moreover, in this instance, it reduces the cells' spontaneous background activities at the same time. So, with the level of static reduced, the signal-to-noise ratio is enhanced. Now each new incoming blip stands out as a much sharper, higher peak.[38]

Of course, NE won't always affect every postsynaptic cell the same way. The result hinges on whether NE is activating its alpha$_1$, alpha$_2$, or beta NE receptors on the next cell. In general, when the next cell's alpha$_1$ receptors are activated they broaden the width of the bands open to incoming signals, and they generally increase this cell's tendency to become more excited.[39] The brain then goes into a more aroused state.[40] Suppose, on the other hand, *beta* NE receptors are activated. They potentiate the stimulus signal, narrow its bandwidth, and allow it to last longer. Indeed, this beta receptor effect can render hippocampal cells more excitable for as long as several hours.[41] A point to remember when we observe how consciousness changes during long rigorous meditative retreats.

Other effects of NE also depend on what state the brain is in at the time. During arousal more NE is released in the thalamus. Here, by acting primarily on its alpha$_1$ receptors, NE contributes to the overall excitatory effect. However, during lower arousal states and states of light sleep, NE may act more on its postsynaptic alpha$_2$ receptors. Now comes the paradox: at this particular time *NE can promote slow-wave, synchronized sleep.*[42] This paradox tends to be overlooked. However, these observations may be relevant to the earliest prelude which can usher in a major internal absorption. They suggest that a single but extended NE surge could go on to help create two different states in tandem. Suppose the NE surge were to begin when the thalamus already happens to be in a drowsy phase. Then NE might first prompt a "blank" period of sleep, having activated its alpha$_2$ receptors. Next, an exaggerated excitatory phase might occur, one of rebound arousal. In this second phase, NE could be activating more of its alpha$_1$ receptors. As a result, the first moment of enhanced sleep might then rebound into a second state of strikingly enhanced alertness (see chapter 111).

Another way to understand what locus ceruleus nerve cells do is to stimulate them directly.[38] Then researchers monitor what effect the brief pulse of NE has when it reaches the hippocampus or cerebral cortex. It turns out that the influence of NE starts slowly, but lasts a relatively long time. For example, single responses are delayed for 50 milliseconds or so after the stimulus. However, they last for at least 350 milliseconds.

Once NE receptors are activated on the outside of the next nerve cell, they set off a cascade of secondary *metabolic* consequences *inside* this postsynaptic cell. NE receptors of the beta type are especially effective in generating the second messenger molecule, cyclic AMP. CAMP then greatly prolongs the actions of NE in subtle ways that we shall soon take up in chapter 48. In much of cortex, those particular NE systems that are linked to second messengers are concentrated in the superficial layers. There they stand poised to exert their early tuning, biasing function on incoming signals.[5]

Some alpha$_2$ NE receptors are located on locus ceruleus nerve cells themselves. Certain drugs that mimic the effect of NE can activate these autoreceptors and slow the cells' firing rate. One such NE agonist is the drug clonidine. Clonidine markedly relieves the suffering of human addicts while they are undergoing their agonizing withdrawal from opiates. It reduces such severe symptoms as anxiety, restlessness, and aching in muscles and joints.[43] This clinical observation strengthens the evidence that links excessive activity within the NE systems of the locus ceruleus with states of anxiety and tension. Other preliminary studies, made on patients who suffer bouts of panic, suggest that they, too, may not be able to dampen an excessive activity of their NE systems. Perhaps, the speculation goes, certain panic-prone persons lack those normal central mechanisms that would otherwise hold their NE systems in check.[44]

So, briefly to summarize the foregoing, it seems clear that noxious or painful stimuli readily engage NE cells. We would expect them to fire more during long, rigorous stressful meditative retreats, when aching muscles and joints are prominent symptoms. Moreover, when NE is first released on cells of parietal cortex, pulvinar, and superior colliculus, it could set the stage for the next excitatory stimulus which reaches them. Now the next stimulus can become a greatly enhanced signal, impacting within that large volume of space which these same regions represent to visual and other sensory experience.

Norepinephrine also helps focus attention. It helps attention pick out the more explicit sensory cues from the environment, as opposed to messages of a more neutral kind which convey only general context.[45] Moreover, the framework of attention could be enhanced in more enduring ways after NE impulses go on to make more second chemical messengers. Beyond that, NE mechanisms interrelate in so many ways with other systems[46] that it is a formidable task to identify which NE subsystems per se enter into a specific *human* behavior.

Until now, we have spoken of NE only in the context of the brain and spinal cord, that is, the *central* nervous system. But back in 1946, Ulf von Euler had already shown that NE was the chemical mediator released by *peripheral* sympathetic nerves when they innervated tissues in the rest of the body. Since then, it has been found that when locus ceruleus nerve cells do slow their firing rate up in the brain stem, a similar message to "slow down" gets relayed downstream to these other distant sympathetic nerve cells and their fibers. These distant cells also slow their own firing rate and release less NE. As a result, less NE leaks out into the bloodstream.[47]

Serotonin Systems

The third group of biogenic amine nerve cells releases serotonin (ST). These ST cells are buried deep along the midline core of the brain stem. Here, they cluster into a series of structures known as the *raphe nuclei* (see figure 7). Raphe cells synthesize ST using the following reactions:

Tryptophan → 5-hydroxytryptophan → 5-hydroxytryptamine (serotonin)

In the brief account that follows, we will discover how ST subtly influences functions as vital as sleep, vision, mood, social behaviors, pain, and the response to stress.

Most raphe cells up in the midbrain supply their ST both to the thalamus and to the limbic system. The largest group of these cells forms the median raphe nucleus. It sends relatively thick axons to supply both the septal region and the CA cells of the hippocampus. Cells in the dorsal raphe nucleus deliver their ST through more slender fibers. These reach the frontal lobes, the caudate, and putamen. Still other raphe nerve cells reside farther down in the midline of pons and medulla. Their ST supplies the hypothalamus, thalamus, lower regions of the brain stem, and spinal cord.[48]

Raphe cells start to fire slowly, and their firing also tapers off slowly. Again, this pattern speaks for a system designed to modulate our slower state-dependent or tonic pacemaker functions, not for one which serves those brisk, stimulus-response reactions which help us adjust quickly to external events on a moment-to-moment basis.[49,50]

In primates, many ST terminals end down in the fourth layer of the primary visual cortex. Here they can also influence visual reception. In fact, they do so at an even earlier cortical stage than do most of the NE terminals which happen to lie deeper in this particular visual region.[51] Moreover, a rich supply of ST nerve endings covers parts of the temporal lobe. This ST is poised to influence the stream of visual interpretations and associations through which sensation evolves at its later stages.[6] In general, up in cortex, ST plays an inhibitory role when it reduces the excitatory responses evoked by other incoming sensory stimuli. Yet, ST can enhance excitability indirectly—and for as long as several *minutes*. It does this by reducing the inhibitory influences of GABA. Serotonin tends to *preserve* the general noise level of spontaneous firing in the background. This means that serotonin's net effect is to *reduce* the signal-to-noise ratio, unlike the way NE acts.

Serotonin cells of the dorsal raphe are distinctive in other respects. Simple outside stimuli, such as auditory clicks or visual flashes of light, make them fire four to five times faster. This particular increase is short-lived, and does not habituate. Properties of this kind suggest that dorsal raphe cells are among those which may remain active and responsive during quiet meditative wakefulness when discrete stimuli are repeated. However, during a generalized arousal response, the same ST cells can also be swept up into the more widespread longer-lasting firing patterns. This latter increase in ST firing is nonspecific, and it does habituate.

Serotonin cells of the dorsal raphe are excited directly by input from the lateral hypothalamus,[52] and indirectly after local NE blocks their nearby GABA neurons.[53] In contrast, these ST cells are inhibited whenever input coming down from the habenula increases the effects of local GABA.[50]

Noxious stimuli do not cause nerve cells to discharge in the raphe magnus nucleus. Nor does morphine slow the firing of ST cells, even in doses that produce analgesia.[54] These are sharp contrasts with the responses of NE cells. *Sleep is what causes ST cells to fire much less.* Their firing rate falls to especially low levels in REM sleep.

Down in the medulla, most ST cells lie in the nucleus raphe obscurus or pallidus.[55] Many of their descending fibers also release substance P or thyrotropin-releasing hormone (TRH) or both. These two excitatory peptides stimulate large motor cells of the spinal cord.[56] Accordingly, when the flow of impulses increases in this descending spinal ST system, the result could enhance the reflex tone of the extensor muscles along the neck and the back. This phenomenon might contribute to the erect posture which I experienced after a major absorption (see chapter 120). Serotonin, like NE, also modulates the excitability of many other motor nerve cells in the spinal cord and brain stem. The net result is to increase the startle response to a sudden sound.[50]

The ST systems engage in countless reciprocal interactions with the NE and DA systems. Because each amine system can affect the others unpredictably,[57] and because most drugs are only semiselective, researchers cannot tease out the contributions of one system if they give drugs which act widely in the brain. But certain drugs do seem to heighten the influence of both ST and DA systems in the same direction. In humans, these DA and ST interactions may combine to create feelings of well-being and empathy which are remarkably enhanced.[58]

Stressful circumstances cause major changes in ST levels in the hypothalamus.[59] The way the levels fluctuate can be clearly observed when rats are stressed by ether. First, they show a *fall* in ST levels in the hypothalamus. The lowest levels are not reached until some twenty to thirty minutes later. Next comes the *rebound.* It brings ST levels to their peak a long sixty to ninety minutes *after* the ether stress. Finally, ST levels slowly return to normal after two hours.

Such findings illustrate why we need to pay very close attention to the *time relationships* of a precipitating event. This caveat is true whether one is trying to understand what causes the sequence of mental phenomena during "ether dreams" or near-death experiences, during absorptions or kensho. Of course, some of the initial depletion of the ST levels could reflect the fact that ST had been released from its terminals. Perhaps it had been "used up" faster than it could be replenished. Another factor could be that the incoming flow of ST had been shut down at its presynaptic terminals. Could NE have been involved in this process? Whatever the explanations, the major changes in ST levels hint that ST does enter into the responses of the stressed hypothalamus. And more ACTH is released into the bloodstream from the pituitary gland after ST falls in the hypothalamus (see chapter 53).

Serotonin affects sleep. Humans undergo a marked, prolonged *drop* in their REM sleep when they take PCPA, a drug that lowers ST by blocking its synthesis. Then, later, researchers can replenish serotonin by providing their subjects with more of its natural chemical precursor, 5-hydroxytryptophan. At this point, the effects of the natural precursor drug will restore sleep in general, including both desynchronized and slow-wave sleep.[60,61]

The ST systems include at least three *major* families of receptors: ST_1, ST_2, and ST_3.[62] Again, the list of families and subtypes keeps growing. The receptors interact in complex ways when they enter into such human behavioral states as depression, obsessive-compulsive disorders, and anxiety.[63,64] Our own cortex, including the cingulate cortex, contains many ST_2 receptors.[52] They reside both on *post*synaptic sites and on *pre*synaptic terminals. To activate the *post*synaptic ST_2 receptors is usually to *inhibit* the firing of the next nerve cell. However, the net result of activating *pre*synaptic ST_2 receptors in prefrontal cortex will be to *reverse* ST's usual local inhibitory role.

These ST_2 receptors have intriguing potentials, because it seems likely that they play a key role in generating hallucinations. Indeed, many hallucinogens do act as agonists on ST_2 receptor sites. This list includes both LSD and psilocybin. The evidence suggests that this action hinges on the way the drugs mimic the effect of the brain's own ST.[68] When ST_3 receptors are stimulated, they subserve more brisk excitatory responses (similar to those of ACH nicotinic receptors).[66] Cannabinoids reduce these excitatory actions.[67] ST_{1A} receptors also increase the excitability of the next nerve cell.[68]

In humans, low ST levels correlate with states of depression. Some patients have fewer periods of depression when they are treated with the same sleep-promoting ST precursor cited above, 5-hydroxytryptophan.[69] This finding becomes even more interesting when correlated with three other findings. One is that the brain *normally* has a dense concentration of postsynaptic ST_2 receptors in the intermediate layers of prefrontal cortex.[70] Another is that these same ST_2 receptors increase in number in the tip of the prefrontal region in patients who have had a major affective disorder.[71] The speculation is that these patients do not have a primary increase in ST_2 receptors, but a *secondary* one. That is, it represents a so-called upregulation in the number of postsynaptic ST_2 receptors. In this manner, by increasing the numbers of its ST receptors, the patient's brain could "compensate," so to speak, for some earlier primary process which had caused less ST to be released from ST terminals up in frontal cortex. The third finding is confirmatory. It is that ST levels are in fact reduced in the brain stems of depressed persons who have committed suicide.[72]

Then what happens when ST tone *increases?* Certain drugs do have the effect of heightening ST tone. Now the results go in the opposite direction, toward the outwardly turned "socialization" behaviors. In monkeys, these ST agonist drugs especially increase the approaching, grooming, resting, and eating activities of the dominant males. And the ST-active drugs do more than increase the kinds of behaviors that promote social dominance. They also reduce in-turned solitary, vigilant, and avoiding behaviors.[73,74]

Over a thirty-year period, certain strains of wild silver foxes have been bred selectively to produce tame behavior. At present, the tame foxes behave almost like domestic dogs. Metabolic studies suggest that these foxes have enhanced ST tone in the midbrain and hypothalamus. In contrast, these tame foxes have fewer ST_{1A} receptors in their hypothalamus.[75] Because this ST_{1A} receptor subtype usually conveys an excitatory message,[68] foxes that have fewer such receptors in their hypothalamus might tend to be tamer. Other supporting evidence comes from a study of monkeys. Those who are the most aggressive and combative tend to show evidence of having the lowest ST turnover (in their spinal fluid samples).[76] In the future, studies that correlate brain amines and their receptors with social behavior should help us better understand why we humans, and pet animals, display such a wide range of temperaments. Of course, I would not think of volunteering our latest family member—a golden retriever whose temperament is exemplary—for any of this research.[77]

In brief, the human studies suggest that having normal to slightly higher levels of ST function may tend to translate into a number of socially useful, salutary effects on mood and behavior.[78] In contrast, low ST levels correlate with depressions, and stimulating ST_2 receptors excessively contributes to hallucinations.

Any writer would now be hard-pressed to condense into one short sentence all the ways that DA, NE, and ST have been shown in this chapter to play their modulating roles. But perhaps one might close by drawing an analogy somewhat as follows. These three amine systems further emphasize the brain's basic response functions, inserting suitable pauses, occasional italics, and sometimes multiple exclamation points.

45

GABA and Inhibition

> There is hardly a behavior that does not involve GABA. One is tempted to conclude that for just about every function of the central nervous system—sensory-motor activities, vigilance, memory, and emotion—a well-balanced, yet adjustable, gabaergic activity, "specialized" for the various networks, is a *necessary condition.*
>
> W. Koella[1]

Nerve cells are designed to fire repetitively. They are also subjected to a barrage of stimuli. How do we cope with this situation? Only by filtering most stimuli out by *inhibition*. If it were not for the ways inhibition filters and turns down the gain, our brain would keep discharging us into hyperexcitable behavior of one kind or another.

A major solution is GABA, the brain's inhibitory workhorse. The acronym stands for gamma aminobutyric acid. Remarkably, the brain makes it from glutamate, its major excitatory amino acid transmitter (figure 10). It is awesome to see how Nature arranged, in this one efficient chemical reaction, for excitation to be followed by a corresponding capacity for inhibition. Not that inhibition would

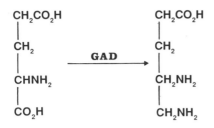

CH$_2$CO$_2$H   CH$_2$CO$_2$H
|
CH$_2$ GAD   →   CH$_2$
|
CHNH$_2$ CH$_2$NH$_2$
|
CO$_2$H   CH$_2$NH$_2$

GLUTAMATE   **GAMMA-AMINOBUTYRIC ACID**
(GABA)

Figure 10   Glutamate and GABA
Glutamate is a key excitatory amino acid transmitter. It is converted to gamma-aminobutyric acid (GABA), an inhibitory transmitter, with the aid of the enzyme glutamic acid decarboxylase (GAD).

be some afterthought. For here is the simple demonstration that unity prevails whenever two naturally opposing processes each depend on, and counterbalance, the other. How do GABA and glutamate serve the nervous system? As yin and yang.

Some would estimate that GABA is involved in one third of all the transmission at synapses.[2] Others suggest that GABA nerve cells alone make up 40 percent of the total population of nerve cells, and that glutamate nerve cells add perhaps another 30 percent.[3] In broad perspective, the brain applies its fast-acting GABA circuits at all levels to hold in check its various local excitatory processes. Most GABA nerve cells are small, inconspicuous interneurons. Deploying short axons, they inhibit their close neighbors either presynaptically or postsynaptically. A typical example are those many small local GABA neurons which suppress the outer layer of the superior colliculus[45] (see figure 3). GABA pathways, diverging rather little from their cells of origin, present a striking contrast with the fibers from biogenic amine nerve cells.[1]

GABA holds local visual responses in check at several other levels. High densities of GABA receptors occur in the lateral geniculate nucleus[6] (see figure 11). How effective is GABA inhibition? This can best be appreciated after you apply a drug that stops its inhibiting role. When you apply this drug, bicuculline, to the nerve cells over the surface of the visual cortex, it *expands, some three- to fivefold*, the receptive area of the visual fields. As part of meditative experience, it is common to encounter expansions of perception and of other mental functions to at least this degree (see part V).

Some GABA cells inhibit the brain's pivotal nerve cells, the larger ones that directly command other essential nerve cell populations. To the degree that GABA normally holds them in check, then reducing this negative GABA influence will promptly unleash these command nerve cells. This process frees them to enter into other major types of behavior.[7] GABA mechanisms do hold aggressive behavior in check in several animal species.[8] Indeed, if one first makes rats hyperactive by injecting dopamine into their nucleus accumbens, they will quiet down quickly after GABA is injected into this same nucleus.[1]

As might be anticipated, antagonist drugs that reduce GABA activity too much can unleash enough hyperexcitability to cause convulsions. In contrast, the GABA *agonist* drugs mimic or enhance GABA's inhibitory functions. Some of them have become widely known because they are prescribed, all too often, for their tranquilizing, "antianxiety," or sleep-producing properties. Among such drugs are those in the benzodiazepine class (e.g., diazepam). They enhance GABA transmission by acting on that large receptor complex which includes receptor sites responding both to GABA and to benzodiazepine drug molecules. Travelers may undergo a brief, ongoing amnesia when short-acting benzodiazepine drugs like triazolam (Halcion), prescribed for sleep, are superimposed on the physiological stresses of travel.[9] This clinical side effect emphasizes that, when GABA systems become overactive, they can block the way a person accesses recently acquired memories.

Clearly, GABA influences mentation, and its effects are not limited to the inhibition of simpler sensory or motor functions.[10] Indeed, the GABA-active drugs like diazepam and alprazolam (Xanax) go on to relieve more than the ordinary levels of "civilized" anxieties. They also relieve those deep primal anxieties which infant monkeys undergo when they become separated from their mothers. Diazepam stops their agitated behavior and their cries of distress. It also reduces their high brain levels of dopamine, as well as the high blood levels of ACTH and adrenal cortisol which are linked to their stress reaction.[11]

In such ways do molecules of GABA become pivotal messengers for the kinds of excitatory and inhibitory events in the brain that will be important in Zen experience.

46

Peptides

> Peptide hormones in the brain may exert a modulating effect on neural activity by determining or influencing the background or "climate" on which the specific actions are projected.
>
> Ulf von Euler[1]

Peptides are proteins made up of short amino acids linked into a long chain. The brain makes a bewildering variety of them. The major ones are concentrated in nerve cells of the hypothalamus or in its downward extension toward the pituitary gland.[2] Moreover, at least eight distinct types of peptide nerve cells project their subtle messages from hypothalamus up to influence the thalamus.

Brain peptides exploded only recently on the research scene, but they have been around for a very long time. Even invertebrates as far down as the earthworm and snail make beta-endorphin, prolactin, and adrenocorticotrophic hormone (ACTH). Obviously, each such peptide does not now exercise the same function in the human brain as it did in the earthworm. New species devised new uses for their old peptides. What role do peptides play in humans?

Speculation has gotten out of hand. It is a time for regaining perspective and for emphasizing caveats. The seven cited below are especially applicable to peptide research, but they remain valid whenever we try to assess the functional role of other transmitter-modulators.

1. *The same peptide can exert two, or more, different effects on behavior.* Behavior varies with the dose, and whether the peptide is injected into the brain itself (intracerebral), into the brain's cavities (intraventricular), or into other sites in the rest of the body such as the veins (intravenous) or the abdominal cavity (intraperitoneal). Moreover, behaviors can switch remarkably, depending on how much time elapses between the moment the peptide is injected and when the behavior is first measured.

2. *None of the above artificial routes used in research exactly duplicates the way peptides are released naturally in the brain.* There, peptides may also be released from endings other than synapses, especially during high-frequency burst firing.

3. *Peptides coexist with other messenger molecules.* Both may be coreleased simultaneously from the same nerve cell and then modify each other's actions.

4. *In research studies, we don't really know what dose of peptide to give.* Normal peptide levels in the brain are very low, several orders of magnitude less than those of the well-known neurotransmitters. At low doses, peptides might act preferentially on some of their presynaptic receptor sites; at high doses they might activate postsynaptic receptor sites.[3]

5. *A few peptides, even in minute doses, go on to influence posture and behavior for a very long time.* For example, only twenty nanograms of LH-RH, luteinizing hormone–releasing hormone, causes lordosis when injected into the hypothalamus of a female rat. This sexually receptive posture persists for eight hours.[4]

6. *Much earlier work was too crude to clarify exactly where, when, and how peptides changed behavior.* Moreover, most tests are still performed using rats and mice, placing them in artificial situations, and then describing the complex results using a complicated jargon. Thus, "negatively reinforced conditioned behavior" translates into a rat who gradually discovers, each time it sees a light go on in his cage, that it can then avoid getting shocked if it quickly jumps off an electrified grid onto a safe place. Integral features in such "behaviors" are vision, lower-level "decisions" about moving or not moving, the ability to jump, and so forth. Because these are highly complex behaviors, we cannot conclude that when rats are given a peptide intravenously they do something for the same reasons that humans might do when we respond to our own native peptides released in our own brains.

7. *Until defined peptide cell clusters can be discretely stimulated and then clearly correlated with well-defined physiological functions, we won't know whether their peptide is only a evolutionary remnant, a "silent passenger" like our appendix, or whether it is indeed a vocal member of the increasingly large chorus of chemical messengers in the brain.*[5] This said, a select few of the peptides are worth noting briefly, to give some idea of what they add to the general climate of the brain. Among them is substance P, discovered by von Euler.[1] It is an excitatory peptide made up of a chain of eleven amino acids. It appears to have some neurotransmitter functions when

slender pain fibers release it onto the sensory nerve cells of the spinal cord and of the trigeminal nerve. Substance P also stimulates behavior when injected into the dopamine region of the ventral tegmental area. Nerve cells that contain both substance P and dynorphin lie in the preoptic area and in adjacent limbic regions. They may help drive sexual behavior.[6]

Cholecystokinin (CCK) levels are relatively high in human frontotemporal cortex, where CCK coexists with dopamine.[7] Nerve cells making vasoactive intestinal peptide (VIP) also reside in cortex. Here, VIP enhances the inhibitory effect of norepinephrine, and each of these two systems inhibits those cortical nerve cells which use cyclic adenosine monophosphate as a second messenger.[8] Neurotensin also excites most pyramidal cells in the prefrontal cortex, and it could be coreleased here along with dopamine.[9] Vasopressin richly supplies the limbic system, and excites hippocampal CA1 nerve cells at low concentration.[10] Normal subjects who have been injected with vasopressin intravenously recall more efficiently what they had listened to earlier in a narrative text of prose.[11]

Several peptides injected by these and other very artificial routes have the potential to transform more complex animal behaviors and to enhance attention. They appear to help rats "learn" in tasks of active avoidance or of passive avoidance. Many, too, can help rats "unlearn" when they need to revise old behaviors in order to cope with new tasks. In such experiments, the avoidance behavior that was previously useful tends to drop out or be unlearned after it is no longer reinforced.[12]

Peptides Associated with Stress Responses

Three of these—ACTH, corticotropin-releasing factor (CRF), and beta-endorphin—will be considered many times in subsequent chapters. ACTH nerve cells are prominent in the arcuate nucleus of the hypothalamus and in the pituitary gland. In general, human studies suggest that when ACTH-like molecules are given by the artificial intravenous route they increase attention and motivation in normal persons if the subjects are already bored or mentally fatigued.[13–15]

CRF has excitatory properties when it is injected into the fluid of the cerebral ventricles. It increases wakefulness in animals by 70 percent and doubles the length of desynchronized REM sleep.[16] CRF nerve cells are concentrated in the paraventricular nucleus of the hypothalamus. There, CRF coexists with the kind of opioids called enkephalins.[17] If these two peptides were coreleased on targets in the human brain, they could yield an intriguing medley of excitatory and inhibitory effects.[18]

As yet, researchers have identified no single peptide as the sole primary cause of mental illness in man. This does not rule out future discoveries of merit, for ample room remains to discover, and to be confused by, the wealth of data about existing and additional peptides.

With this preamble, we now turn to some especially intriguing peptides. They are called *endogenous opioids* for two reasons. First, because the brain itself makes them, and second because their properties resemble those of opiates.

47

The Brain's Own Opioids

Among the remedies which it has pleased Almighty God to give to man to relieve his sufferings, none is so universal and so efficacious as opium.

Thomas Sydenham, 1680[1]

In Russia religion is the opium of the people; in China opium is the religion of the people.

Edgar Snow[2]

Consider three items. Opiates have relieved suffering for ages. Marx is passé, but his dictum lingers: religion is "the opium of the people." Finally, the Buddha's central message, as summed up in the key phrase, "Suffering do I teach, and the way out of suffering."

Are these items separate? Or could this message—the relief of suffering—be connected with the opiate-like substances found recently in our own brains?

I learned about opiates firsthand from two inadvertent, personal experiences as a patient in the hospital. The first time, I was having minor surgery to remove a small, deep benign tumor. The preliminary was a small dose of morphine, slipped in as the routine preoperative medication. I still vividly recall the result. All worldly tensions melted away, and I was riding on a cloud in a totally blissful experience. I was only a first-year medical student at the time, but I found this state so delicious, so compelling—so full of obvious addictive potential—that I resolved never to take narcotics again.

Years later, another minor surgical repair required hospitalization. It was early in the morning, and I was still half-asleep when the nurse quickly gave me an injection. Again, it turned out to be the all-too-casual, routine pre-op order of morphine. By the time I figured this out, all annoying dissonances had melted away. Once again I rode high on a cloud in a wonderfully relaxed, carefree blissful state. And something else happened. I saw everything suffused with a pink color. I was literally looking at the world through rose-colored glasses.

Between these two impressive experiences, I also observed how opiates act on animals in the pharmacology laboratory. There, as second-year medical students, our assignment was to inject rats with morphine and observe their strange behavior. A lapse of several minutes occurs between the time one injects a drug like morphine into the body's *general systemic circulation* and the time that it seeps into the nervous system. At first, the concentration of the drug in the brain is still low. During this early phase, the drug may tend to act on its *pre*synaptic receptors. Later, when more drug reaches the brain, the higher drug levels then tend to act more on *post*synaptic receptors. We did not know about such possible drug mechanisms at the time.

But we could witness the remarkable phenomenology of the rat's motor response. First, the injected rat became quiet. Then it went into a curious waxy immobility, termed cataplexy. The rat stiffened and remained fixed into whichever posture we set it in. Decades later, it would be discovered that other drugs, the dopamine *agonists*, could prevent these early motor phenomena. The agonists stimulate DA receptors, mimic the effect of DA itself, and reverse the stiffening.[3] Hence, many of morphine's early actions on the motor system are now attributed to the way opiates temporarily *reduce* the release of DA from its presynaptic DA terminals. This is the reason why the first phase is treatable with DA agonists.

Some minutes later in our laboratory experiments, we watched the injected rat enter the second phase of its response to morphine. This was a *hyperactive* phase. Now the rat repeatedly washed its face with its paws and showed other energized stereotyped behaviors. Again, only recently came an explanation for this delayed opiate phase. It turned out to be the reverse of the previous one. Now the rat brain shows *increased* DA turnover. Its DA levels increase 55 percent in the nucleus accumbens.[4] Moreover, in this instance, it will take a DA *antagonist* to block the rat's resulting hyperactivity. Clearly, when a single pulse of an opiate spills into the nervous system, *it causes biphasic indirect effects in other systems*. First it shuts off DA functions, then it reenergizes them. Early inhibition, later rebound. We will find this see-saw principle illustrated many times in this book.

Opioid Types and Their Receptors

Why do poppy plants make opiates? Who knows? But many simple creatures were also manufacturing opioids and using them to their advantage millions of years before humans learned how to extract opium from poppies. The brain's own opioids are called *endogenous opioids*. Even as far back as the earthworm, nerve cells were making two different classes of them.[5] They are the two peptides called beta-endorphin and leu-enkephalin. Perhaps, it is speculated, these opioids were released during times of painful injury. They might then have served an adaptive function, allowing a wounded creature to blot out distracting pain and so to escape more readily.

Humans and other higher animal species now use three separate intrinsic systems to make opioids within the brain. First are the *beta-endorphin* nerve cells. Their cell bodies center mostly in the arcuate nucleus of the hypothalamus (see figure 3) and in the lower part of the solitary tract nucleus in the medulla. From the hypothalamus, a fountain of their axons sweeps out to innervate the subcortical depths of the brain. This endorphin network supplies our primitive brain regions, the nuclei close to the midline and near the fluid-filled ventricular cavities. Yet three key regions are conspicuously lacking in beta-endorphin: hippocampus, cerebral cortex, and striatum.[6]

The second opioid system makes *enkephalins*. Its cell bodies are much more widely distributed. They release their two opioids into the other key cortical and subcortical structures. These particular opioids are named leuenkephalin and metenkephalin. They are short molecules, only five amino acids linked together. Metenkephalin is so named because it ends in the amino acid, *met*hionine; leu-enkephalin ends in *leu*cine. Especially high enkephalin levels exist in the globus pallidus, caudate nucleus, and nucleus accumbens. The high levels in the globus pallidus are attributable to enkephalin out in the far terminals of those enkephalin cell bodies that lie still higher up in the caudate nucleus and putamen.

Suppose a nurse gives you an injection of *exo*genous morphine. It activates the same receptors inside your brain as do your own two enkephalins. Only it does so artificially, from the outside. This means that your experiences on morphine, and mine, have this in common with the rats' behaviors on morphine: they reflect the way the drug acted on opioid receptors that were already in our brains, waiting to receive our natural enkephalins instead.

The third opioid system makes the *dynorphins.* They, like the first two, start as large precursor molecules. They then split off into their own family of smaller peptide molecules. The few dynorphin nerve cells issue both short and long axons. These resemble those of the enkephalin systems, and they pursue a somewhat parallel course.[6]

Two places in the brain synthesize all three opioids: the arcuate nucleus and the nucleus of the solitary tract. Moreover, in the arcuate nucleus, the separate enkephalin and dynorphin cells each make DA.[7] This intriguing feature is termed "coexistence." It has potentially important implications.

Opioids differ from the other neuromodulators in two key respects. First, like other peptides, they are synthesized only up in the nerve cell body, not out in its terminal endings. So once a single surge of opioids has passed out of the nerve ending, the nerve cell body takes a relatively long time to replenish them. Second, opioid nerve terminals do not recapture their peptide molecules. This means that opioids act for only a short time, because enzymes outside their nerve endings quickly break them down. Still, beta-endorphins do tend to act longer than enkephalins.[8]

After opioids are released from nerve endings, they tend to travel a relatively long distance before they encounter their receptors. This implies that many opioid effects are not only slightly delayed in onset but build up slowly.[9] Major events, prompting opioid nerve cells to fire trains of stimuli, will release them, but single stimuli may not. Once released, metenkephalins and beta-endorphin *inhibit* most of the next nerve cells they contact. One noteworthy exception is in the hippocampus. Here, the net effect is to excite some CA1 cells and make them fire faster.[10,11] The several facts cited above suggest that unusual experiential overtones could occur at the peak of a major surge of endogenous opioids. Blended into such a moment might be generalized inhibition, local hippocampal excitation, plus other effects produced by the corelease of DA. Equally important, the inside "fix" could directly affect the brain's cortical, subcortical, and central core functions, have biphasic effects, and subtle indirect effects as well.

Opioid receptors themselves are of several types and subtypes[12] (table 4). In rat brain, mu and kappa receptors reach their highest levels in thalamus and midbrain, and frontal cortex shows the most leuenkephalin receptors.[13] In humans, mu receptors reach high levels in thalamus and temporal cortex, and high kappa receptor levels also occur in the temporal cortex and regions nearby.[14]

Several chapters later we will find how the brain makes associations as it channels sensate messages forward from the occipital into the temporal regions. In primates, mu receptors show a striking parallel distribution: they too become much more concentrated at each step further along in these same processing hierarchies.[15] Many mu opioid receptors not only cover the region around the amygdala but are concentrated as far forward as the medial orbital cortex of the

Table 4
Opioids and Their Receptors

Opiate, or Endogenous Opioid	Acts Preferentially on This Receptor Type*	Comment on Actions
Opiates, enkephalins	mu_1	Contribute to analgesia at sites above the spinal cord; induce catalepsy; release prolactin; increase ACH turnover in the hippocampus
Morphine	mu_2	Slows breathing in particular
Enkephalins	delta	Create analgesia from local sites in the spinal cord
β-Endorphins	epsilon	Released, together with ACTH, into the brain
Dynorphins	kappa	May also sedate

ACH, acetylcholine; ACTH, adrenocorticotropic hormone.
*Opioids tend to act on more than one receptor type.

frontal lobe.[16] The auditory association pathway also shows a similar increasing gradient of opioid receptors. Many lines of evidence, converging on these key regions, suggest an important conclusion: *here, in these key frontotemporal regions, the brain takes what it sees and hears, then colors and shapes it into complex interpretations.*

Another interesting fact about morphine in humans is that it reduces the *net* metabolism of the cerebral cortex. This alone does not tell us much, because various stimulant and depressant drugs do the same.[17] But morphine exemplifies the way drugs turn out to have many different actions when pharmacologists study them long enough.[18] Even at present, our review has turned up eight topic areas which are influenced by morphine and other model opioids. And each of these will be shown to be of great importance to Zen. They include breathing, fear, pain and suffering, mood, novelty, motoric activity and motivational drive, conditioned responses, and muscle tone.

1. *Breathing.* A woman, overdosed with morphine, arrives comatose in the emergency room. She isn't breathing. The antidote? An opiate antagonist. Within minutes after the drug, naloxone, is injected intravenously, the patient starts to breathe spontaneously and moves around. Animal research shows how the naloxone acts. It quickly seeks out opioid receptors, inserts itself, and pushes away a morphine molecule so that it can no longer act on the same receptor.[19] Naloxone blocks opioid receptors so effectively that it can even precipitate an addict who had been taking a steady dose of opiates into an opiate withdrawal syndrome.

In a normal person, morphine's most striking effect is the way it slows respiration. Would an antagonist like naloxone block the bliss that occurs in internal absorption along with any associated respiratory slowing? Some day, it may be possible to test such hypotheses.

2. *Fear.* Morphine abolishes fear. Anyone who has ever been lost, or who has observed a lost child, knows how deeply distressing is the anguish of separation. Infant monkeys separated from their mothers cry out their fear in anguished "cooing" vocalizations. Opioid agonist drugs are an especially effective remedy

for this profound separation distress. They promptly relieve the infants' loud cries and other anxious behaviors.[20]

3. *Pain and suffering.* For centuries, the balm of opiates has relieved not only the sensation we call pain but the suffering that goes with it (see chapters 80 and 81). It is less well appreciated that prior stress, and then release from this stress, can make a given dose of morphine more effective. During World War II, Beecher made an interesting observation. He noted that as soon as severely wounded soldiers found out that they would not have to return to battle, they needed less morphine postoperatively than did other patients in civilian life who had suffered pain from comparable surgical problems.[21,22] Throughout the sequences of first being stressed by battle, of then being hurt, and finally of being relieved from hazardous duty, the soldiers underwent what was called in those days "psychic processing." In fact, the extreme psychic and physical stresses they had gone through had rendered them extraresponsive to low doses of morphine. After prolonged stress, certain stress hormones do drop to low levels.[23] At this point, beta-endorphin levels increase and opioid receptor activity is heightened. For instance, a drop in the levels of adrenal glucocorticoids increases by 80 percent the brain's abilities to bind opioids to its receptors,[24] and low testosterone levels increase the binding by 60 percent.[25]

Many similar examples have established the principle: a given dose of a drug becomes more effective depending on the person's set and setting, attitude, and mood. In one sense, it makes little difference whether it is a packaged drug like morphine, one that becomes widely dispersed when it is first injected into the body, or is an endogenous opioid which we release by natural means into our own brain in discrete locations. In either circumstance, a host of factors critically influences how the circuitries respond when each molecule acts upon them. So many of our brain's responses to opiates and opioids are not immutable. They change, depending on how prior stress has gone on to modify the "processing" within its frontal-temporal-limbic regions.

In animals, even a tiny amount of morphine also blocks pain when it is microinjected into certain key brainstem regions. These special regions include the central gray substance, the locus ceruleus, and the raphe magnus.[26] A different way to relieve pain in humans is to stimulate, electrically, a small region two to three millimeters outside the wall of the third ventricle. Among the structures represented here is a part of the parafascicular nucleus. This deep relay station sits astride the ancient pain pathway ascending from the spinal cord. Two striking events occur when this region is stimulated. One is that pain stops. The second is that a cozy feeling ensues. The patients report a generally comfortable, relaxed feeling as if after a good meal, a feeling of generalized warmth, pleasure, relaxation or well-being.[27]

Do these words elicit a sense of déjà vu in relation to a similar cozy feeling described earlier in this chapter? What happens during such deep stimulations? There will be another occasion to ponder these questions in chapter 119, which describes the bliss that pervades the later phases of internal absorption.

Meanwhile, we do know something about what happens when electrical stimuli are delivered to sites deep in the human brain near that long pathway that endorphin fibers take next to the midline. A little beta-endorphin then seeps out of the brain and enters the brain's fluid-filled ventricular cavities.[28] But this doesn't count. For what the stimulation did *first* was to release endogenous opioids out from their nerve endings and *into the brain itself.* Then, having already acted briefly on their local opioid receptors within the brain itself, a very few of these surviving opioid molecules would finally leak out of the brain, seep into its internal cavities, and be detected in the fluid samples obtained from them. Human subjects are also relieved of their pain when substantial amounts of beta-endorphin (200–400 micrograms) are injected directly into the fluid cavities of their cerebral ventricles. This does not cause euphoria, nor does it change blood pressure, pulse, respiratory rate, or other obvious neurological functions.[29,30]

Stimulating the central gray substance in humans, high up behind the third ventricle, also relieves chronic pain. These stimulations also increase, by some 35 to 600 percent, the levels of beta-endorphin that seep into the ventricular fluid. At the same time, they also double the levels of ACTH in the same fluid. The finding that both beta-endorphin and ACTH are released *together* reflects back on their common nerve cell of origin in the hypothalamus. Both coexist in the same arcuate nerve cell, where they had once been split off from the same large precursor molecule.[31]

Beta-endorphin has also been injected directly into the central gray substance in the rat.[32] Here, in the midbrain, only a minute amount (1.2 nanomoles) produces profound catatonia, apparent sedation, and analgesia. During this state, metabolic functions drop elsewhere, in both the medial and lateral geniculate bodies and in the superior colliculus. This evidence suggests that when beta-endorphin is released in the central gray substance, the distant effects could include a reduction of vision, of hearing, and an increase of muscle tone as well. Again, such findings may be pertinent to some of the exceptional depth reached by that black pervasive silence which envelops the person during a major internal absorption (see part VI).

Having now seen that stimulation releases, together, the two coexisting peptides, ACTH and beta-endorphin, we await future studies that will test what happens when both are delivered *together, in the brain directly.* Only in this way can researchers mimic their normal dual interactions deep within the vital central regions of the brain.[18] Brain metabolism does increase when animals are injected with a single small, potent analog of the ACTH molecule (ACTH 4–9) in the abdominal cavity of the body over a period of ten days. Activity increases especially along the links of that limbic circuit which flows up from the hippocampus, parasubiculum, mammillary body, and anterior nucleus of the thalamus to link with the anterior cingulate gyrus[33] (see figure 5). However, such metabolic experiments go only halfway. They need to be extended to deliver brief pulses of beta-endorphin and ACTH at discrete sites in the brain itself.

4. *Mood.* We know little about what the particular beta-endorphins do that arise, separately, in the *pituitary* gland, after they go on to enter the bloodstream.[34] But this unsettled state of affairs has left room for many cocktail party anecdotes about the "runner's high." Research suggests that only one part of this delayed "high" is attributable to the release of endogenous opioids—from one source or another—and that only this part is blocked by naloxone. One study focused on

twelve long-distance runners who regularly ran more than forty miles a week. Their usual feelings of joy and euphoria didn't arrive until some thirty to forty minutes *after they ended* each run.[35] Immediately after they had run six miles, the runners were first rated psychologically for their baseline levels of "joy, euphoria, cooperation and conscientiousness." Then they received *either* (a) two intravenous injections of naloxone, 0.8 milligram each, spaced twenty minutes apart; or (b) two separate injections of saline as a placebo control. The ratings then continued. Naloxone did more than reduce their delayed joy and euphoria. It increased the runners' reports of deep ischemic leg pain.

Other human studies suggest that the brain itself undergoes tides in the release of beta-endorphin. Levels rise in the morning and fall in the evening. Beta-endorphin levels normally peak in spinal fluid around 6 to 7 A.M., and in blood plasma at around 9:30 A.M. They then fall, reaching their lowest levels around 8 P.M.[36] The presence of such tides opens up two interpretations: (a) If an overshoot were to occur, the momentum of the morning tidal rise might carry endorphin to even higher levels during the morning hours. (b) But if a brief pulse were to occur at "low tide"—that is, in the evening—it might stand out against a low background and be most effective physiologically.

Most of the early morning increase in the spinal fluid is attributable to beta-endorphins coming from the brain itself, not from the pituitary. Sometimes, children develop an abnormal elevation of beta-endorphin in their spinal fluid. In such instances, these high levels may indicate that the opioid release is reaching concentrations high enough *in the brain* to cause the child to stop breathing.[37] As we have just seen in the example of the overdosed adult patient, treating the child with the opiate blocker naloxone also improves breathing. When this treatment begins, some children then develop symptoms of the opiate withdrawal syndrome. This makes it even more likely that the elevated endorphins had, indeed, been the cause of their prior episodes of respiratory arrest.

5. *Novelty.* Novelty releases beta-endorphin into the brain. If humans respond anything like rats, beta-endorphin would begin to increase after only two minutes in the new environment.[38] This fascinating link between novelty and brain endorphin has very practical applications. One reason is that *beta-endorphin appears to "mark" with some sense of salience a current task that might be put to use in the future.*[39] No old, mundane, overlearned task will do. To increase beta-endorphin will take something special—the challenge of a new training situation or a modification in the existing one. Another practical point is that when some new situation does present itself, it will usually require the brain to invent a new kind of response. In this respect, the release of endorphin and ACTH *together* may, in a sense, be a way to clear the decks, a means of getting rid of the old behavior in preparation for the new.

The cause of this particular surge of beta-endorphin can be narrowed down to the element of novelty per se in the test situation. For, in this instance, the rise is not due to pain, stress, or to associated arousal. Then, as soon as the rat senses this out-of-the-ordinary event, it releases a brief pulse of beta-endorphin into its hypothalamus. *The whole surge is over in less than three minutes.* Thereafter, the beta-endorphin level falls in the hypothalamus. It will take the rat the next three to six hours to resynthesize fresh endorphin molecules. In rats, novelty affects enkephalins less consistently.[40] However, in other brain sites, and in primates, including ourselves, it would seem reasonable to search for evidence that enkephalins and dynorphins may also play roles of their own in shaping those unique climates of salience that highlight special moments of consciousness.

In the studies cited above, both a *brief rise of brain beta-endorphin and a fall to low levels appear to be significant events.* Why? Because once a task has regularly prompted the release of the opioid, the rat will then need an extra pulse of beta-endorphin in order later to retrieve and perform this very same task again at its peak efficiency. This means that its task performance has become "dependent" on beta-endorphin. This condition is called "state dependence." It occurs with various other drugs as well.[39]

So once a rat's learning of a task has been linked with additional beta-endorphin, it will retrieve and perform this task more readily whenever some novel circumstance arises in the future, one that again prompts another release of endorphin. It is worth pausing to consider the important long-range implications of this finding. In such ways does novelty act to provide both the original setting and the later stimulus, each of which subtly changes the climate of the moment and encourages the subsequent search for novel stimuli.

In the broadest context, one might trace some of the biological roots of novelty back to the hippocampus and its connections (see chapter 42). One of the functions proposed for this larger hippocampal formation was that of comparing present events with those of the past. If the events corresponded, it would signal "match." And, if they did not, it would signal "mismatch," that is, something *new* that had not been encountered before. Now, normally the subiculum exports most of the messages from this hippocampal formation over to the mammillary body (see figure 6). These messages travel to the hypothalamus along the major pathway called the fornix. And it is along this very same arched path that the particular impulses travel which enable novel events to release beta-endorphin into the brain. For if the rat's fornix is interrupted, then novelty no longer causes its beta-endorphin to surge.[40] This experiment suggests that as soon as impulses within limbic circuits confer some kind of "recognition of novelty," the brain relays this information on to the arcuate nucleus of the hypothalamus. This nucleus then releases its beta-endorphin (and ACTH).

6. *Motoric activity and motivational drive.* It is easy to be reinforced and motivated by opiates. Too easy. Any brain, human or animal, can finally get so hooked that it will go to great motoric lengths to work for an addictive drug if you keep supplying this drug from the outside. For example, monkeys will press a lever switch up to 12,800 times to obtain a single major intravenous shot of morphine or cocaine.[41] But much smaller doses are also effective. Monkeys still learn to press a lever even though it delivers them only a minute intravenous dose of morphine, 10 micrograms per kilogram. This tiny dose is an effective way to motivate them, even though it is still too low to hook them, and it is too low to cause withdrawal signs when the morphine is withdrawn.[42]

Opioids have indirect effects on motor systems. Many of its actions are caused by the way opioids interact with DA and other biogenic amines. DA and opioid terminals mesh together in the dorsal and ventral striatum and limbic system.[43] Especially in the ventral tegmental area do opioid terminals end on DA nerve cell bodies (see figure 7). Here, when the two join forces, the results are striking. Minute doses of opioids injected into this ventral tegmental region activate mu and kappa opioid receptors. This translates into *faster* firing of the local DA cells, into more DA released up in the ventral striatum, and finally into rats that become highly mobilized for the next hour or so.[44-46] Some of their hyperactivity resembles that which we students had observed in our rats during the second phase of their response to morphine.

Impulses converging into this lower mesolimbic DA pathway provide one important way to influence motivational drive at a basic motoric appetitive level.[46] A rat is a quick learner. Before long, it will press repeatedly on a lever that delivers electrical self-stimulation through wires implanted into its own ventral tegmental area. And, as just described, the rat can be energized by a single opioid injection into this very same spot. But can you addict the rat by *continually* infusing opioids into this area? No. (The rat does not develop withdrawal signs after the opioid infusion is finally stopped.)

Where *can* you inject morphine to cause addiction? One sensitive spot, higher in the midbrain, is the central gray substance (see chapter 52). Here, the animal does develop the usual withdrawal signs as soon as you stop the opiate. So the topic we have so glibly introduced by calling it "motivational drive" soon becomes a complex issue. It is one that opioids influence in different ways and at levels high and low. Of course, we humans pride ourselves on being different from rats. We believe rats are motivated relatively more by the "lower" appetitive stimuli. We think that rats are driven by food, drink, or sex, whereas *we* are influenced more by "higher" cognitive factors.

True, rats do move much more after opioids are injected down low, into their ventral tegmental region. But these rats can't talk to us. And we need to know, *in terms of human experience*, the answers to several important questions. When opioids are released locally in our ventral tegmental region, do *our* DA cells then release more DA from their terminals up in the *frontal cortex and limbic system?* (see figure 7). If so, then how would more DA in these regions translate into our cognitive and affective functions? Would it energize, awaken, and enhance our mental processes?

Then, too, what kind of balance is struck when enkephalins are separately released at a site farther downstream in the nucleus accumbens itself? For here, in the *ventral* striatum, enkephalins *shut off* the local reinforcing functions of DA and other messengers.[47] So, wouldn't this have the opposite effect? Wouldn't it quickly block goal-seeking attitudes and behaviors?[3] Because we cannot view in isolation these two opioid-DA mechanisms, set at opposite ends of the ventral tegmental DA system. Normally, they exist in an intricate balance, each capable of offsetting the other. Indeed, even as pharmacology students we had observed how, in the same rat, the motor aspects of the DA-opioid balance could be tipped in strikingly different directions.

This is a convenient place briefly to take up several other features of the enkephalin system. The reason is that enkephalin receptors are also poised to modify the effects of biogenic amines at many other presynaptic and postsynaptic sites.[48,49] Moreover, in the locus ceruleus, enkephalin may coexist with NE inside a number of NE cell bodies.[50] Many of the ST cells that descend to the spinal cord also contain enkephalin.[51] So, when NE and ST nerve cells fire in strong bursts, this surge could carry into experience some resonances of enkephalins as well.

One enkephalin pathway, curving down from the entorhinal cortex, releases enkephalins near CA3 cells of the hippocampus. Here, metenkephalin has two actions. It causes the hippocampus to respond more to stimulation of the perforant path. It also decreases the spontaneous activity of granule cells. The resulting combination increases the signal-to-noise ratio in a manner resembling the action of NE. So the result makes it much easier for the hippocampus to drop what it had been doing in its previous mode and to shift into the processing of new information.[52]

A separate enkephalin pathway runs up from the mammillary body region to reach the anterior ventral nucleus of the thalamus.[53] Another relays back down to the ventral tegmental nucleus of the midbrain.[54] These circuits provide additional pathways by which limbic functions could influence distant sites. And farther down in the spinal cord are the cell bodies of still other enkephalin neurons which inhibit incoming pain fiber activity from an arm or a leg by as much as 50 percent.[55]

7. *Conditioned responses.* Opiates abolish conditioned responses when fear and noxious stimuli had been used as the agents of aversive conditioning.[56,57] Earlier, it was noted that one nodal point in such aversive learning experiments is the central nucleus of the amygdala (see chapter 41). Manipulating opiate receptor tone in this nucleus does two things. It profoundly influences how long it takes to acquire *aversive* training responses. It also determines whether or not such trained responses will remain. The medial septum enters into conditioning in a different way. Its opiate-sensitive mechanisms do *not* depend on situations that are unpleasant or fear-producing. For in the septum, opiates inhibit conditioned responses only when *neutral* stimuli had been used as agents during the training process.

How relevant are these two sets of results to the way our own opioid system functions? They suggest that opioids could be brought to bear in the amygdala to reduce our conditioning if the prior conditioning events in the environment had taken on a strong negative valence. At this point, some of the tough-but-gentle, yin-yang aspects of Zen, and of its roshi, could start falling into place. In contrast, opioids may become more involved in functions of the medial septum–hippocampal system when neutral stimulus events had been linked together during our prior associative processing.

8. *Muscle tone.* Opiate agonists increase the tone of certain muscles that straighten the spinal column. Extension of the spine is most prominent after *dynorphins*, the third category of intrinsic opioids. This dynorphin family acts especially at kappa but also at mu receptors (see table 4). When dynorphin is injected into the ventricular fluid inside the brain of a rat, it produces a striking rigidity of the rat's neck and back muscles. A high-amplitude, slow-wave activity also develops in the EEG.[57,58] The rat's neck and trunk muscles contract in a distinctive

manner: they become stiff enough to suspend the rigid animal across a gap between two platforms, a rat-length apart. This phenomenon has given rise to the term "platform catalepsy."[59] Platform catalepsy peaks ten minutes after dynorphin is injected into the fluid, then fades off within an hour. In contrast, morphine and beta-endorphin develop their peak of stiffness more slowly, after about an hour. It will take several hours before this increased tone fades.

Dynorphin fibers are among the mossy fibers in the hippocampus. This means that dynorphin is released on the CA3 cells of the hippocampus (see figure 6). When dynorphin is injected selectively into the hippocampus, it flattens the hippocampal EEG temporarily. Unlike enkephalin, it depresses both the spontaneous firing of CA1 and CA3 cells, and dampens their firing in response to glutamate. But the firing rebounds after this first phase of depression. Dynorphin also excites a few cells in these regions, as does leu-enkephalin.[11] In the spinal cord, low doses of dynorphin will increase glutamate transmission, and higher doses go on to have local neurotoxic effects.[60]

In summary, the brain's own opioids have brief but striking properties. They are poised to slow respirations, block suffering, enter into novel and positive affective responses, confer salience, and act in many other intriguing ways that bear directly on Zen experience.

48

Ripples in the Next Cell: Second and Third Messengers

> The degree to which an adrenergically innervated structure can be stimulated is inversely related to the degree to which it had been previously stimulated.
>
> B. Weiss, L. Greenberg, and M. Clark[1]

Translation: next week, the same nerve cell may respond differently. Neurons are not like lightbulbs. After a cell fires, it keeps changing chemically. So next week, even though an identical stimulus arrives, the cell may fire a different way. What gives it this extra flexibility, and what does it have to do with Zen?

In broad outline, the process begins with the "first messengers." They are the usual neurotransmitters, modulators, and hormones. We have just seen how they activate their receptors on the *outside* of the nerve cell. Here the fast transmitters instantly trigger the flux of ions which sets off the nerve impulse. But metabolic events are far slower. They come into play when receptors trigger "second-messenger" systems within the cell membrane. These second systems relay the chemical signal into metabolic sequences farther inside the cell.[2,3] There, several "third messengers" take over, called protein kinases.[2,4] They relay the signal still farther, on into the very nucleus of the cell. In the nucleus, the message is further translated. As a result, the cell receives instructions to express its genetic code in a different way. Then, some 24 to 48 hours later, the nerve cell starts to make more enzymes or different kinds of enzymes. These become the basis for the cell's later, more prolonged change in excitability.[5]

It is this delayed metabolic cascade which grants a nerve cell the special capacity to reshape its own chemical structure and transform its responses. These later messengers promise the neuron a future different from its past. And in their ripple effect one begins to see the subtle ways that Zen could transform the brain.

But how do these crucial second-messenger systems actually operate? An instructive model is the system which generates cyclic adenosine monophosphate (cAMP).[6] Called the adenyl cyclase system, it creates a special phosphate bond of extrahigh energy within each molecule of cAMP. Thus empowered, cAMP then becomes a second messenger, capable of relaying its energy-rich phosphate group to activate certain protein kinases. They, in turn, will attach phosphate to still other proteins. To what end? The final goal will be to change the number of free calcium ions which the cell membrane will allow to rush inside the cell.

For meanwhile the cell has also been slowly restructuring the pores and ion channels of its surface membrane. Once modified, these pores and channels will open and close differently from before. Now a different flux of ions can pass through them, enabling the nerve cell to change its previous firing responses. By virtue of the pores and the long ion channels that tunnel through its membrane, the nerve cell has gained a remarkable adjustability.

A self-adjustable excitability is the "light" at the end of each such tunnel, the nuances of which go far beyond any lightbulb Edison could ever have dreamed of. The way a nerve cell finetunes its own response has become a key area of research. For their pioneering studies of these tunnel-like ion passageways, Neher and Sakmann received the Nobel prize in medicine in 1991. And only three years later, Rodbell and Gilman would be awarded the prize for their work on the special kind of receptor proteins now known as G proteins.[2]

What happens physiologically to the nerve cell as a result of all this? It strikes a new balance between being excited and inhibited. One can observe this in the simpler systems of the mollusk. In order to sensitize its responses, the mollusk starts with serotonin. This first messenger sets off a cascade of molecular dominos. The net effect will be to increase the cAMP levels out in the nerve cell's presynaptic terminals. More calcium ions then flow in, and the active zone of the sensory terminal itself finally changes. Now, as this nerve ending releases even more of its neurotransmitter into the synapse, it stimulates the next cell into firing faster than before.

Norepinephrine also turns up the response of the adenyl cyclase system. First it acts on its beta-receptors. Then, once the system has been primed, the stimulation of alpha receptors will enhance it even further. However, continued stress keeps releasing more of the adrenal hormone corticosterone. This cuts back on the added alpha receptor effect, and reduces the total cAMP response.[7]

But what does the next, postsynaptic cell do if *less* NE reaches it? The cell compensates. It makes more of the beta NE receptors.[1] Has less become a prelude to more? Yes, because these added beta receptors now upregulate the cell, making it extrasensitive to NE, even though fewer pulses of NE may now be reaching it. In brief, *un*used receptors multiply. This creates an extra sensitivity on the far side of *un*used synapses. The reverse also holds true. If a synapse is used excessively, it tends to be downregulated. This means that fewer receptors are available on the next, postsynaptic cell, and that less cAMP is being generated. Clearly, one nerve cell has remarkable flexibilities. And in its range of options is the implication that a whole brain can be affected whenever its messenger systems change, either acutely or in a more prolonged manner.

Now, human subjects do *feel* that an initial quieting takes place during the more relaxing forms of meditation. If their "relaxation response" does "calm" the brain, could it also be slowing the otherwise heavy NE traffic impinging on many of its NE receptors? And could meditation then enter a phase of enhanced sensibilities, one consistent with a kind of upregulation?

Probably not until many days later. Certainly not until genuine, total relaxation had occurred under truly nonstressful situations. For it is first necessary to have a rather long "quiet" period before postsynaptic NE receptors do become so sensitized that NE can then prompt them to produce more cAMP. Indeed, the brain's cAMP systems do not become supersensitive to NE until two to four days *after* the drug reserpine has been used to deplete its biogenic amines. But at that point, the supersensitivity becomes such that one pulse of NE can make more cAMP for a week or more.[8] It is interesting to note in this regard, that the hypothalamus and hippocampus are the most effective sites for upregulating the responses to NE.

At present, we still await final *proof* that cAMP *itself* can subtly affect a well-defined behavior of the *mammalian* nervous system.[9] On the other hand, recent evidence[10] suggests that certain of the special receptors for glutamate (called "metabotropic") can enhance excitation relatively quickly, and that this action lasts for as long as two minutes.[6] Metabotropic receptors responding to acetylcholine, NE, DA, and ST might also be able to enhance excitation by similar mechanisms. But meanwhile, let us look further into the elegant studies performed earlier on the mollusk, our simpler invertebrate cousin. These model experiments by Kandel and colleagues, next to be described, have proved that second messengers do cause nerve cells to "behave" differently. Moreover, their studies provide us with a glimpse, in stunning detail, of how a specific nerve cell works, and of how it adjusts to change, all in a behavioral context.

49

The Aplysia *Withdraws*

The art of being wise is the art of knowing what to overlook.

William James (1842–1910)[1]

"Wisdom" has rudimentary origins. Consider the sea mollusk *Aplysia*. True, it has only a few nerve cells. But some of them are huge: 1 mm in diameter, the size of a large period! And not only big, but "smart." How do we know? Because one of them can be singled out and monitored while it is in the act of performing tasks. These tasks provide us with simplified models for memory and learning.[2]

The resting mollusk seems to exude *aequinimitas*. This vanishes as soon as some researcher squirts seawater on its siphon. Threatened by this noxious stimulus, *Aplysia* sensibly retracts both its siphon and its gill. Researchers have now mapped out the whole circuitry which leads to this act of defensive withdrawal.

Within the wiring diagram are a mere twenty-four sensory neurons, six motor neurons, plus several excitatory and inhibitory interneurons which interconnect them. A minor constellation indeed. Can so elementary a reflex yield clues to the ways nerve cells learn and remember?

Yes. Gradually, each *Aplysia* "gets used to" the ill-behaved scientist, finds that mild squirts of water are not really causing it bodily harm. It *learns* to overlook the stimulus, to ignore it. *Aplysia* "habituates." In a sense, its simple form of habituation is a kind of "remembering to ignore." Or, as James put it, of "knowing what to overlook."

This memory occurs at a sharply localized site. It centers on specific *presynaptic* nerve endings. Here, sensory terminals had been poised to take their incoming signal about the noxious squirt, and relay this message across the synapse to the next set of motor nerve cells or interneurons (see figure 4). *It is at this precise spot, where the incoming sensory impulse pauses, that presynaptic inhibition causes habituation.* What does it do? It reduces the flow of calcium ions. Less calcium, less neurotransmitter released into the synapse. Less neurotransmitter, in turn, means less firing of the next, postsynaptic nerve cell.

Note that up to this point, each noxious squirt still evokes its sensory signal. But now the sensory message gets "hung up." It no longer leaps on into its next synapse. The result: *Aplysia* doesn't shift into its defensive mode. But the mollusk underwent more than a mere "functional" change in the process of reducing its defenses and blunting its usual motor withdrawal response. Its *nerve cells changed their structure!* Looking at the critical synapse with the aid of an electron microscope, one sees fewer and smaller active zones on the membranes of its *pre*synaptic side. These are the visible expression of the "nozzle" on a sensory terminal that had shut down.

In a sense, long-term habituation in *Aplysia* does mean "overlooking" the stimulus. It has a physiological opposite, called *sensitization*. Sensitization proceeds in accord with the wary principle "once bitten, twice shy." The smart mollusk "catches on" after stronger noxious stimuli keep repeatedly irritating its head or tail. Once sensitized, it goes into a vigorous reflex withdrawal as soon as it feels even the faintest ripple of water. This "twice-shy" reaction lasts for the next several weeks. Sensitization alters the very same presynaptic terminal as does habituation. But it does so in the opposite way: now transmission has free access to pulse through the critical synapse. Again, the incoming sensory nerve ending shows a corresponding structural change. This time there are *more* active zones on the terminal end, and they are larger.

Like humans, *Aplysia* also "forgets." Suppose the researchers had limited its training period merely to one short session of ten noxious squirts. In this instance, its "memory" trace will fade after only a few minutes. But if they subject it to four rigorous training sessions, *Aplysia* becomes suitably impressed. These repetitions enable it to "remember" for up to three weeks.

Aplysia is not the ultimate microcosm. It is not the perfect model which allows us to predict how one of our human circuits will operate during our higher levels of behavior. But this mollusk still gives us intriguing, metaphoric glimpses of how the links within some circuits may operate. And in such studies are very general hints about how Zen training experiences might influence the synapses of the brain. In brief, *Aplysia* shows us *that defensive reactions can drop out, be inactivated, deprogrammed, and no longer operate automatically.* Moreover, the *Aplysia* model also illustrates the principle in reverse: some experiences will sensitize nerve cells by invoking metabolic mechanisms. These, too, can hyperactivate a synapse by pulsing more transmitter into it. Finally, *Aplysia* reminds us how science itself breaks free of its own outworn conceptual boundaries once they prove to be no longer valid. For the previous century or more, we had built up sharp distinctions between "structural change" and "functional change." Now, the newer electron microscopic techniques could show, at high levels of resolution, that nerve cells changed their membrane structure at the same time that their *function* changed. Once more, an old distinction was no longer tenable.

Habituation and Sensitization in Humans

In simpler systems, whether those of mollusk or rabbit, habituation means that repeated stimuli yield a decreasing response. Sensitization implies that responses increase when stronger stimuli are repeated.[3] While the simple models are excellent examples, they can only tell us about the elementary categories of learning.

Higher forms of learning require more than several dozen neurons in a special reflex arc. Higher-order learning needs a very large network of *associative* nerve cells. Only such a network, interposed between the early sensory stimulus and the later motor response of the reflex arc, can form the basis of *associative* learning.[2] So how do these networks enable the large mammalian brain to respond to stimuli? Here, we include both artificial electrical stimuli, and those which enter naturally from the outside world.

It makes a very big difference *where* one stimulates. Stimulating certain spots, electrically, causes the arousal response and sets off its typical low voltage fast EEG activity. However, this initial response then also rapidly falls off, habituates, *if* you continue to deliver the same stimuli to such various sites as the amygdala or sensory cortex,[4] or to the roof of the midbrain and the central gray substance,[5] or to the caudal reticular nucleus of the pons.[6]

In contrast, stimulating certain other parts of the brain causes either a slight initial sensitization, or the stimulation goes on to produce a sustained increase in the response. Among the sites which remain sensitive and do *not* habituate are other parts of the midbrain[4,7] the midline intralaminar nuclei of the thalamus,[7,8] the lateral hypothalamus,[7] and the septal and habenular regions.[5]

There could be a message in the way these latter regions *sustain* their responsivities. One begins to wonder: when a person continues to perceive the fresh quality of outside stimuli, could more of these latter kinds of sites be included in the active circuitry of the moment? The issue is critical. For in the regions exemplified by these five sensitive sites, we are addressing the basis of the freshness of vision of the artist or poet; focusing on possible ways to relieve the depressed person held in the grip of a dreary gray world. And approaching the essence of Zen.

Suppose one delivers to the brain more *natural* stimuli coming from the outside, not artificial electrical stimuli coming from internal wires. Then, as we observed in the case of the monks and the clicks, the situation can become more complicated (see chapter 24). At first, the design of such experiments might appear simple enough: provide repeated stimuli from the outside, such as sound clicks or flashes of light; then see how rapidly the response habituates. Next, after it does habituate, make a subtle change: vary either the intensity of the stimuli or their timing. This minor change quickly restores the brain's ability to respond as it did before. So it is clear that the brain detected the slight change you made. How? Presumably, it matched your latest stimulus against a whole series of earlier patterns of expectation that it had already set up.[4,9]

But questions arise. Are clicks and flashes really meaningful and adequate stimuli? Which stimuli are best, and which responses *are* the best ones to measure when testing for habituation in humans?[10–12] One reason the results have been confusing is that different aspects of the arousal response—such as the EEG and heart rate—do *not* correlate with each other. Nor do they habituate at the same rate during various tests.[11,13] Moreover, some people habituate consistently; others do not.[10]

Interestingly, when subjects are in desynchronized (REM) sleep, they show *no* significant habituation of their heart rates and finger pulse responses. Nor does the human EEG response habituate if researchers deliver sensory stimuli to the brain during either REM sleep or stage 2 sleep.[10] These findings invite the following speculations: could the fact that stimuli sometimes do take on a very freshly rinsed perceptual quality suggest that they were entering during physiologically comparable substates? (Even if, at such moments, a meditator couldn't recognize that these substates had merely been displaced out of their usual location within conventional REM sleep or stage 2 sleep?)

From the foregoing, it becomes clear that none of the previous studies of habituation or sensitization permit us to make a facile leap from *Aplysia* to human associative learning. The major research effort required would need not only many appropriately selected subjects but meticulous attention to what their level of arousal is, to the kinds of stimuli that will be meaningful, as well as to which parameters of response should be measured. Until researchers agree on such matters, we can still marvel at the inherent powers of the presynaptic terminal, while withholding final judgment on the conflicting evidence that meditation does or does not influence habituation[14] (see chapter 24).

50

Matters of Taste

Seeing is deceiving. It's eating that's believing.

James Thurber (1894–1961)[1]

The Zen Way plumbs depths that code for our strongest convictions. We can learn about these processes from our sense of taste. For taste, gustation, is our primordial special sense. To taste is to *know* directly, by way of the primitive visceral responsitivities in our brain stem. Thereafter, at higher levels, taste compounds with our sense of smell. This we discover during a severe sinus infection. Then, as smell drops out, we also lose our sense of taste.

Taste was designed to be acted upon immediately. Taste messages from the tongue buds arrive first in the *gustatory nucleus* in the medulla (see figure 5). Yes, its impulses are then ready to relay up to the thalamus. There they can start to filter into our more refined, conscious perception of taste.[2] But other impulses can quickly descend into that larger nucleus just below it: the *nucleus of the solitary tract*. This solitary nucleus does more than receive other sensory impulses arising from the viscera. It also coordinates many cardiovascular, respiratory, *and vomiting* reflexes. This arrangement is no accident. It ensures that any vile-tasting stimulus will be vigorously expelled as soon as it arrives. Do you take a strong "visceral" dislike to some things, find some persons' actions distasteful or disgusting? The links of taste-related circuitries may be compounding over more networks than you realize.

Animals once poisoned are twice shy. They have learned to avoid what made them sick. In experimental jargon, they developed a "conditioned aversion" to the offending substance. This means they actively reject it. Humans also learn, as we say, from "bitter" experience. The word speaks volumes. Because we, too, reject certain things that we've learned, by *association*, have unpleasant consequences. How does the rest of the brain learn about noxious tastes and start to correlate them with thorns and other "bad" stimuli? One route centers around the nearby acetylcholine cells of the parabrachial nucleus (see figure 5). Earlier, we saw how this cholinergic relay then leads up to the amygdala, thalamus, zona incerta, and the hypothalamus.[3] However, when both the right and left parabrachial nuclei are blocked, rats no longer can be conditioned to develop their otherwise robust taste aversion.[4,5]

As everyone knows, taste has a positive side. Sweets and chocolate taste *good!* Opioids and opioid receptors appear to have helped one develop an early taste preference for Heath bars. Normal mice already possess an inborn preference for sweets, and it is easy to encourage their original sweet-tooth. However, some inbred mice lack opioid receptors. These mice can't be tempted by sweets.[6]

The average rat is almost as susceptible to the lure of chocolate as you and I are. Give it chocolate milk or sweet candies, and it promptly releases beta-endorphin within the hypothalamus.[7] Some of the nerve cells in the lateral hypothalamus then project back down to supply the gustatory nucleus and the parabrachial region.[8] Just below, in that same nucleus of the solitary tract just cited, beta-endorphin must play another prominent role in visceral functions. For inside it is the brain's second major cluster of beta-endorphin nerve cells. Moreover, this solitary nucleus receives further reinforcements of beta-endorphin sent down by fibers from the arcuate nucleus of the hypothalamus. And it also receives many biogenic amines, for good measure.[9]

One taste of a small rich sponge-cake sent Proust's brain spinning off into a rush of memories. But a head full of nostalgia is not what kensho is all about.

Precisely the opposite. It cuts off all those personalized remembrances. And so one is now led to consider a curious exemption. Because taste stimuli are *not* a trigger for kensho, unlike sounds, sights, and other sensory avenues (see chapter 105). Why not?

Perhaps an explanation begins with the fact that taste came first in evolution. Later, when our other refined *special* senses arrived—those of smell, sight, and hearing—their functions were added later, and at higher anatomical levels. So the primal role that taste played in survival determined the early placement of a gustatory nucleus at a site far down in the medulla. And here it resides still, positioned relatively far below those key cholinergic sites up in the midbrain and pons which effectively activate the brain. Are equivalent taste stimuli less effective than other sensory stimuli in setting off those cholinergic peaks of ponto-geniculo-occipital activity? Experiments have not yet clarified whether such taste stimuli are less effective in prompting PGO waves in animals, let alone in humans. Lacking these studies, one is left to speculate that what exempts taste from being a sensate trigger for kensho may be related to its basically much lower and more primitive connections.

You taste something on your tongue. Do your taste buds signal something so palatable that it could fuel appetitive drives? Or is it distasteful? The amygdala is one other part of that higher circuitry which "decides" if a stimulus event will become either rewarding or aversive.[10] Amygdala cells soon learn to respond differently, and their relay circuits are already hard-wired at birth. Even newborn babies smile when a sweet stimulus reaches their tongue. Their body English leaves no doubt about what they find distasteful: they pucker to a sour stimulus, and grimace when recoiling from a bitter stimulus.[11] Moreover, when babies taste a sweet solution of sugar, their EEG becomes more activated in the left frontoparietal region. After this, the plain taste of ordinary water is an obvious letdown. Now, their expression shifts to one of disgust, and their EEG shows a greater right frontoparietal activation.[12]

The foregoing lines of evidence make clear that it is not the wisps of a few abstract thoughts which make us feel delighted or disgusted. The visceral roots of longings and loathings start very deep, even though they go on later to have extensive upward ramifications.

51

The Mouse in Victory and Defeat

> Not in the shouts and plaudits of the throng,
> but in ourselves, are triumph and defeat.
>
> Henry Longfellow (1807–1882)[1]

Mice, like rats, also defend their home cage. On its own turf, the resident mouse always wins. No intruder mouse has a chance. Again, let's look in, afterward, at the vanquished interloper when he has been returned to the safety of his own cage. We observe something curious. He appears more than chastened. He retreats into a distinctive "defeat posture." Sitting upright, his forepaws are folded passively against his chest; his head is extended, nose pointing up and out, ears flattened back.[2–4] Does something about this posture seem familiar?

What interests us mostly is another fact: this defeated mouse has become insensitive to pain. Much of his analgesia is caused by overactive opioid mechanisms. Certain mouse strains are most sensitive to the analgesic effect of a morphine injection, and these mice lose pain the most after they are defeated.[5] If this analgesia after defeat is caused by opioids, would the opioid antagonist naloxone block it? Indeed it does—whether it is injected into the central gray substance or in the region of the arcuate nucleus of the hypothalamus. So the analgesia of defeat appears to relate to stressful events which have stimulated the brain to release extra amounts of its own opioids into these two central sites. The control experiments excluded the possibility that the loss of pain was caused either by opioids released elsewhere in the body, or by pituitary or adrenal hormones which had entered the bloodstream during the stress of combat.

Other lines of evidence confirm that endogenous opioids play a pivotal role in this defeat behavior. One is the finding that beta-endorphins fall to low levels in the forebrain of the vanquished mice, to levels 40 percent lower than in the victors. This suggests that the defeated mice had first released most of their preexisting beta-endorphins into the brain. There they would soon be broken down and disappear faster than new endorphins could be synthesized.

After mice have been defeated daily, several times, they show successively less analgesia. Finally, they develop a *very high tolerance* to the extra release of their own opioids. At this point, one can give them even high doses of morphine (5 mg/kg) but cause no analgesia. Why not? Give a dose of naloxone to these repeatedly defeated mice, and the explanation soon emerges: this antagonist causes them to undergo opioid *withdrawal* behaviors. So the evidence lines up in one direction: *during defeat, the brain releases enough of its endogenous opioids to make an animal physically dependent.*[4] In one sense, the loser might seem to have come out ahead.

One need not conclude that brain opioids are a consolation prize, Nature's benevolent compensation to soften the loser's sting of defeat. Instead, the loser's recently acquired submissiveness has long served more adaptive ends. It is the kind of basic yielding to harsh realities which can go on to stabilize the social order. In humans, no less than in mice, yieldings might gradually help lower the flag of the sovereign *I*, "gentle" the person, and reduce interpersonal conflicts.

Within twenty minutes after the stress of battle, the defeated mouse has also increased the binding functions of the benzodiazepine receptors in its brain (see chapter 45). However, this increase affords no more than a short-term relief from the anxiety associated with stress, for it resolves within an hour.[6]

When male mice are housed together in large, interacting, social groups, they also enter into behaviors that fall into aggressive/submissive categories. Soon, it becomes clear where each mouse ranks in the so-called pecking order.[7] After the mice have established this social hierarchy, is there anything distinctive about opioids in the brains of those mice who have been the more dominant and aggressive? These males turn out to be the ones who show lower baseline levels of enkephalin. Indeed, *met*enkephalin levels in their brain stems are only one-fourth as high as those of the subordinate mice. Moreover, their enkephalin levels are only one-half as high as their subordinates in the rest of the brain above.

So what? It seems possible that some of the relatively lower enkephalin levels in this dominant-aggressive type of forebrain may have found expression in the basic preexisting motoric tendencies which these mice have to enter into more dominating forms of behavior. In contrast, in the other group of nonaggressive mice (these are mice who had not fought, even once), some of the relatively higher levels of enkephalin may be associated with their innate submissive tendencies. The fact that, *normally*, enkephalin concentrations are high in three motor nuclei now becomes of special interest in this regard[8] (see chapter 47). It suggests that enkephalins could play a role in helping to restrain aggression.

The mouse experiments could be pointing in the direction of Zen. For each year of monastic Zen training is long and hard. Every week presents the mindful aspirant with countless new opportunities to wrestle with the *I-Me-Mine;* to suffer from it; to subordinate and vanquish the self; to watch it fall off. What is involved when a person bows to harsh realities, learns to knuckle under, to suffer in silence? To make all these a part of oneself is to develop the patience necessary to survive any rigorous endurance training. The word itself, patient, comes from the Latin *pati,* to suffer. Today, we are still on the threshold of understanding how the human brain changes its messengers and receptors during the rare moments—and long decades—of such arduous training. Clearly, it will be important to test the foregoing hypotheses that, when the brain releases its own opioids, they will play several increasingly well-defined roles in shaping these processes of adaptation.

52

The Central Gray: Offense, Defense, and Loss of Pain

Let not the sun go down upon your wrath.

Ephesians 4:26

It was wartime. Humans—not mice—were locked in combat, consumed in the emotional fires of another world conflict. In neutral Switzerland, during this Second World War, Walter Hess was pressing a button, wondering what would happen when he briefly stimulated the medial hypothalamus of a nice, tame cat. What occurred next was in keeping with the times.

Instantly, the gentle tabby cat turned violently aggressive. And it *stayed* mad, consumed by its own "angry or aggressive mood," for several minutes thereafter. Not only that—stimulating the lateral hypothalamus seemed to call forth the cat's instinct for committing a more calculated act, a kind of murder in the first degree.[1] At first, the cat had responded with only a cool, quiet biting attack. But then its whole *attitudinal set* changed. Why would it now go through all the trouble to learn a whole new maze? Because the rat at the end of the maze had become a target that the cat now seemed motivated to search out and attack.[2]

Cats have other behavioral options. Like the mollusk, they can react defensively. Take the familiar Halloween cat posture. Threatened by a dog, the cat adopts its "defense reaction": turned broadside to look larger, back arched, hair erect, pupils dilated, ears flattened, *hiss!*

Some of these defense reactions have now been shown to be organized by a small core of the midbrain below the hypothalamus.[3] Its technical name is the *central gray substance*, often shortened to the *central gray* (see figure 3). Here the defensive behavior is hard-wired. The familiar threatening stimulus is a strange dog. However, the immediate internal stimulus could be a local pulse of electricity into the central gray[4] or even an excitatory amino acid, microinjected into the same spot. The cat's defensive display begins fifteen seconds after the chemical transmitter is injected, and it lasts for up to a minute and a half. Moreover, if one injects a more powerful excitatory analog, kainic acid, the cat's repertoire now expands. The result is a fierce, tooth-and-claw attack on any nearby target. Watch out! The tabby has become a tiger!

The central gray doesn't do all this by itself. Like the hypothalamus, it helps *orchestrate* such behaviors by virtue of its connections. It, too, seems trivial and inconspicuous, merely a thin column of nerve cells whose ancient lineage is long, forgotten. Buried in the center of the midbrain, it surrounds the aqueduct, that slender tube which drains fluid down from the third to the fourth ventricle. But when you stimulate the dorsal* half of this column of periaqueductal gray matter, it prompts the cat into its hissing, hair-on-end, affective defense. This dorsal part, working in concert with the medial hypothalamus and amygdala, contributes to a sense of fear and of other unpleasant states. Together, they integrate their results into the appropriate patterns of defensive behavior. On the other hand, if one stimulates the *ventral* part of the central gray, it brings out the cat's less emotional, quiet, biting attack. Now it becomes the cool predator that stalks its prey.[5]

The central gray offers more than the two behavioral options of offense and defense.[6] Surprisingly, stimulation of its rostral-dorsal region *blocks* that kind of affective attack which comes from stimulating the hypothalamus. Enkephalin cell bodies, and terminals, lie in this part of the central gray, and beta-endorphin fibers are also nearby.[7] Therefore, one theory ventured to explain this behavioral inhibition is that the local electrical stimulation of the central gray has released these opioids. The opioids, in turn, could then go on locally to restrain aggression by inhibiting this same region or some closely related one. The theory is supported by the finding that if you inject an opioid *agonist* into the central gray, it also blocks the same attack response that was being generated, separately, by stimulating the hypothalamus. The fact that opioids do wipe out aggressive instincts will come as no surprise, once you have been a patient and have observed all your own motivations dissolved by an injection of morphine.

A third set of recent observations also becomes of major interest to Zen. When mu opioid receptors are activated in the central gray, they bring about a remarkable, *secondary*, release of more opioids into the cerebrum. This was discovered when morphine was injected into the central gray. The surprise was that this

---

* In what follows, three of the terms are like the fins on a fish: *dorsal* generally means along the back; *ventral* implies in front; *caudal* implies toward the lower end. *Rostral* means toward the upper end.

injection caused an *extra release* of substantial amounts of both enkephalin and beta-endorphin. Moreover, these two opioids were released *a very long distance away;* notably into the nucleus accumbens of the ventral striatum, but also into the amygdala.[8]

So, once the central gray has been primed by the release of opioids into it, a complex network seems poised to release more opioids at other very important distant sites. Where could the original opioid priming be coming from? Obviously, the pathway descending from the arcuate nucleus is the most direct way to release beta-endorphin on mu opioid receptors in the central gray. And this beta-endorphin could be released during the natural response to novel or painful stimuli, or to other kinds of stressful circumstances. Researchers now need carefully to define the whole circuitry responsible for this primary and secondary release of opioids.[8]

Certain parts of the central gray, then, play several opposing roles, because they can either start, or stop, what are generally called *aversive* responses. Aversive responses are defined as those caused by a noxious, unpleasant stimulus.[9] They range from aggressive attack to defense reactions, and include efforts to escape. Local opioids are not the only ways to stop aversive responses. They can also be inhibited locally by injecting GABA$_A$ or serotonin agonists.[10–12] When humans are stimulated in the *lateral* aspect of the central gray, they are overcome by a "fearful, frightful or terrible" emotional response, and suffer agonizing diffuse sensations referred into the very core of the body.[13]

A fourth set of observations is of interest to Zen, because the evidence suggests that opioids associated with the central gray may help explain the natural ways we *relieve* pain and suffering. Again, different regions of the central gray respond differently.[14] Ventral stimulations *stop pain,* yet only for as long as the stimulus lasts.[15] But this analgesia is profound. Indeed, while being stimulated, a rat can undergo major abdominal surgery without recourse to any other anesthesia.[16] In contrast, brief dorsal stimulations are less effective, but this analgesia lasts for as long as twenty minutes.[6] Once again, a likely primary source for some of the loss of pain is the local release of opioids.[7] Opioids could be discharged from beta-endorphin nerve endings. Or they could also leak out of the cell bodies of those enkephalin and dynorphin nerve cells which are also located inside the central gray itself. In either instance, the analgesia develops only as part of a long cascade of events.[17]

The central gray enters into two more discrete motor mechanisms: those which govern head posture and vocalization. A series of motor relays normally holds our head extended on our neck. These pathways either go through the central gray or arise near the midline around it.[18] After a major episode of internal absorption, my head posture was held unusually erect. (see chapter 120). In contrast, a patient's head drops forward if small lesions destroy both sides along the midline of this same general region.

Animals vocalize when their central gray is activated.[19] Conversely, dogs who have been in pain will stop their nervous barking and no longer whine after large lesions remove both sides of the central gray.[20] Sometimes during a stressful sesshin, meditators utter spontaneous vocalizations. One may speculate that these sudden articulations reflect a momentary overflow of impulses reverberating between the limbic system and the central gray.

In summary, a vital part of our human legacy is this central core of ancient gray matter. Its intrinsic circuitries and connections can set in motion patterns of behavior likely to be aggressive or defensive. Release opioids into it, and it starts a sequence of events which can *suppress* aggression and obliterate pain. Moreover, once opioids have primed it, other circuits go on to release opioids into two key distant sites: the amygdala and the ventral striatum.

53

The Third Route: Stress Responses within the Brain

A pearl is produced only through the pearl-oyster's enduring the pain of having a grain of sand bore into its flesh, fighting against it, and protecting itself against it. We, also, by fighting all kinds of difficulties and overcoming them, strive to develop the jewel of spiritual cultivation.

Isshu-roshi[1]

Pearls were rare in past centuries. Then the Japanese perfected a systematic method for cultivating them. Cultured pearls are now within reach of the general population. Is there a message here? Does adversity—engaged in systematically—have a role in Zen? For during arduous meditative retreats, Zen resembles a contact sport, not a spectator sport. The participants encounter a variety of physical and psychophysiological stressors. Brain and body strain to respond, in a series of adjustments that we may call stress responses.

The traditional stress responses activate two systems in the body. Many readers may already be familiar with them. One route is hormonal, and relatively slow. It starts in the hypothalamus, moves down to the pituitary gland, where pituitary hormones—now entering the bloodstream—carry their message to the adrenal *cortex*, down in the abdomen. The second is neural, fast. Its signals speed down nerve fibers from the hypothalamus into the spinal cord. From there, the messages of the neural route exit via the fibers of the sympathetic nervous system. They finally release amines both from their own nerve endings and from cells in the adrenal *medulla*.[2]

Researchers have now studied the way we respond physiologically to a variety of stressors: immobilization, restraint, anesthesia, noxious stimuli, sleep loss, and prolonged sensorimotor deprivation. When human subjects are placed in such model stressful situations they use these two familiar stress systems—hormonal and neural—to respond in predictable ways.

Not until recently have the studies begun to clarify a third route. It is the avenue through which *stress responses directly change our brain itself*, not only our body. It turns out that our brain changes physiologically and biochemically. Moreover, it does so in ways that will clarify how we shift into alternate states of consciousness. Let us begin with several physiological examples.

You may have noticed that your mental performance drops off when you undergo psychic stress or lose sleep. Losing sleep for twenty-four hours destabilizes the electrical activity of the brain. It can cause a highly abnormal, paroxysmal EEG to develop in a third of the patients who have epilepsy. And these paroxysmal changes can occur even though the subjects may previously have had a baseline EEG that was either normal or only borderline. Losing sleep also precipitates some otherwise seizure-free patients into overt epileptic seizures.[3]

Normally, our heart rates vary and our performance skills go up and down. The cycles repeat every ninety minutes or so. But suppose one loses sleep while staying vigilant. Then these two indices change much more. In one study, normal subjects were asked to stay awake for as long as possible. Meanwhile, they needed to press a button which would signal that they were correctly responding to a task. Strained to the limit, all subjects finally came to the end of their rope. They stopped, unable to go on, after 21 to 44 hours. As they neared this climax, they went through wild swings of their usual up-and-down cycles in heart beat and performance.[4] Put simply, their stress responses had stretched, in *both* directions, the normal range of their physiological fluctuations.

As an integral part of this third route of stress responses, the brain also amplifies its usual biochemical fluctuations. One kind of stressor which illustrates this point is physical restraint. Animals, like humans, find it very stressful to be restrained. Rats restrained for one hour release more glutamate in their hippocampus, septum, and frontal cortex.[5] Physical restraint also increases the turnover of dopamine and serotonin some 40 to 60 percent for up to an hour *after* the restraint ends.[6] Rats restrained for one half to three hours bind more acetylcholine at their muscarinic ACH receptors.[7] This increased ACH binding is delayed. It only becomes evident—in the septum, striatum, hippocampus, and lower brain stem—ninety minutes *after* the restraint begins.

Pharmacologists have some new ways to determine which new drug is most effective in preventing anxiety. They focus on certain regional biochemical responses. One useful index is the release of DA. Stressful circumstances release DA both in the mediofrontal cortex and in the nucleus accumbens of the ventral striatum.[8] As one representative example, noxious pinches to a rat's tail over an eight-minute period will enhance DA metabolism for the next two hours in the nucleus accumbens. But an effective antianxiety drug, such as diazepam, will block this increase of DA. Moreover, the drug does so at doses too low to sedate the animal.[9]

Meditators experience a variety of "quickenings" and more overt alternate states during stressful meditative retreats (see part V). In this regard, it is of interest that rats do *not* become sleepy after they have been both stressed and sleep-deprived for 72 hours. Instead, they enter a phase when, for the next half hour, they become *hyper*alert and react excessively to stimuli. Their hyperalert state is distinctive for two reasons. First, their brains now show an increased number of DA_1 receptors. Second, certain drugs can prolong this state and will further enhance their alertness. Opioids are one class of these drugs, and drugs which act on DA_1 receptors are the other.[10,11]

The effects of a stressful event are very long-lasting. Suppose you introduce a second stressful episode as much as ten days later. This second event increases DA turnover in the frontal cortex even more so than did the first.[12] And, for as long as one *month after* a single episode of immobilization stress, diazepam still won't have regained its original effectiveness in reducing DA levels in the frontal lobe.[13,14]

Some things you never forget. I still remember the first time I explored an electric outlet with my finger, at the age of five. I was shocked by electricity. Rats are also impressed by similar noxious events. Electric shocks to their paws cause them to release more norepinephrine in the hypothalamus, hippocampus, and cortex.[15] Fortunately, however, inhibitory GABA receptors blanket the NE nerve endings in the hypothalamus. And by acting on these same presynaptic GABA receptors, antianxiety drugs like diazepam can shut off the release of NE and dampen the stress responses of the hypothalamus.[16]

How can a brain adjust to other stressful situations which involve "psychic conflict?" In the laboratory, researchers create model conflicts by using standard operant conditioning techniques. Put simply, this means that the investigator reinforces a *natural* behavior with food or water, so as to encourage it to recur more readily. Conflict ensues later however, when these rules are changed. Each natural response which had previously been reinforced will now be followed by an aversive consequence. So now the rat receives a brief electric shock to the foot.[17] The rat's dilemma: to act or not to act?

As we have just seen, it is no problem to calm this nervous rat by giving it the same diazepam-like drugs prescribed to relieve anxiety in humans. The conflict situation remains. But now the rat *endures* the conflict. Calmed, it now goes back to making as many of its earlier behavioral responses as it did before. Where in the brain do such GABA-like drugs act? And act not only to relieve such anxieties, but also act so discretely as to *maintain performance?* To determine this, researchers again use the technique of injecting tiny doses of these drugs *locally* at different test sites. Among the most effective sites are such limbic circuits as the amygdala and mammillary body, and the serotonin nuclei of the raphe. Moreover, an intact frontal cortex also contributes to the stressful impact of this conflict situation. Remove this "fretful" frontal cortex, and the rat endures the shocks. Seemingly "relieved" of one source of its anxieties, it again returns to its earlier high level of behavioral responses.

We come now to an essential aspect of stress responses *within* the brain. During general anesthesia, the brain demonstrates this finding in a major way. Earlier, we noted that the hypothalamus makes corticotropin-releasing factor (CRF) (see chapter 46). Normally, it issues little pulses of this CRF peptide every 45 minutes or so. But after ether is inhaled for only two minutes, the hypothalamus now develops a striking, sixfold increase of CRF. This ether-induced surge of CRF lasts up to 45 minutes,[18] and it goes on to trigger the release of ACTH. What interests us *now* about this particular increase of ACTH? *It is released inside the brain itself,* not only from the pituitary gland into the bloodstream, as had first been mentioned above.

Where in the hypothalamus does this CRF come from? Mostly from CRF nerve cells in the paraventricular nuclei.[19] And when NE is released here, it prompts these cells to discharge their CRF.[20] Once again, one finds that NE from the locus ceruleus is cast in its standard role: it enables the brain to respond to noxious, stressful stimuli. If, by way of contrast, we were to return briefly to that long-familiar pituitary-adrenal axis cited above, we would find that NE was also entering into those hormonal sequences early, and in the following manner:

Stressful stimuli → NE → CRF → pituitary ACTH → release of adrenal cortical hormones into the *blood*stream

But the peptide that the pituitary gland releases into the blood is only one small part of the larger CRF and ACTH story. Because the *third route* supplies CRF from the paraventricular nuclei to other parts of the *brain*. And while such CRF fibers remain distinct from the other axons that convey ACTH, yet both fibers fan out from the hypothalamus to release their CRF and ACTH widely throughout the diencephalon and the upper brain stem. Within these regions, CRF plays a separate *excitatory* role. It excites by potentiating the excitatory effects which glutamate has on other circuits.[21]

In chapter 47, we found where most of the ACTH in the brain itself is made. It is synthesized inside the very same arcuate nerve cells in the hypothalamus where much of the brain's beta-endorphin has also been made. This is the critical point of distinction: *stressful circumstances can release both beta-endorphin and ACTH together into the brain, through the same axons, and throughout the same deep midline regions.* Moreover, if there has been prior stress, this beta-endorphin contribution will have an even greater impact. Once again, using the example of morphine, one can observe that stress greatly enhances the effect of opioids. Primed by the effects of the prior release of DA, NE, and ST, morphine becomes significantly more potent when injected into the brain of an animal that had previously been agitated by physical restraint.[22]

In the context of Zen, these three peptides—and the brain's intrinsic avenues for releasing them—take on special importance. One may now summarize this third route as follows:

Stressful stimuli → NE → release into the *brain* of CRF, ACTH, and beta-endorphin

Why do patients have such prominent "ether dreams" under ether anesthesia? Several mechanisms may contribute.[23] We began by describing wide fluctuations in serotonin induced by breathing ether for only two minutes.[24] Indeed, during the next twenty minutes, rats will lose half of their hypothalamic levels of ST. After plummeting, ST then rebounds, overshooting to reach above normal levels at one hour.

Adrenal Cortical Hormones and the Brain

The adrenal cortical hormone corticosterone also rises to a sharp, four- to fivefold peak in the blood as part of its stress response to the ether. After reaching its apex at thirty minutes, corticosterone then falls back to normal levels an hour and a half later. Very high concentrations of steroid receptors stand poised in the hippocampus, septum, and amygdala to bind the *salt-regulating* hormones like corticosterone.[25] One factor contributing to the processes which cause stressed animals to forget their previously learned conditioned avoidance responses,[26] could be this release of steroids from the adrenal which then goes on to act on steroid receptors in limbic regions. Pavlov would have been very interested in these recent hormonal findings, having seen how remarkably his dogs' behaviors changed after they survived the stress of the flood.

When stress responses are prolonged, the adrenal cortex releases a second group of steroid hormones, called *gluco*corticoids, into the bloodstream. Once this second wave of steroids enters the brain, it has two intriguing side effects. It upregulates ST_2 receptors in the cerebral cortex. This particular action could contribute to the mechanisms that cause hallucinations. Moreover, glucocorticoids further enhance the loss of nerve cells in the hippocampus initiated by excitotoxins[27] (see chapter 152).

In humans, cortisol is the major glucocorticoid secreted by the adrenal cortex. Cortisol normally falls to its lowest blood levels in the late evening. At this time the low cortisol levels will be exerting *less* of their usual suppressant effect on ACTH. Accordingly, the late evening hours could be one time when a suddenly stressed brain might tend to release more of its ACTH, and perhaps beta-endorphin as well.[19] Could this combination of events, acting via the third route, help make the late evening hours an optimal period for evoking certain alternate states?

On the other hand, when do human cortisol levels normally rise to their peak in the blood? Not until dawn beckons. These are the hours, at the opposite end of the night, when we begin to awaken from sleep. Now is the time, during our first few waking hours of the morning, when the peak levels of adrenal cortisol will be most readily entering the brain, enhancing long-term potentiation in the hippocampus,[25] and increasing ST turnover in the hypothalamus and midbrain.

The foregoing experiments, in which ether was used, have not been cited to leave the impression that anesthetic drugs, including nitrous oxide, are *the* way to enlightened states. Anesthesia, after all, *reduces* the functions of many regions vital to our full conscious awareness. Neither the drugged brain nor the brain in deep sleep is in the most optimal state. For an optimal state implies the following fourfold capacity: (1) to *generate* valid insights, (2) to *register* them intimately in context, (3) to *remember* them, and (4) to *incorporate* their positive benefits into daily life. Dr. Oliver Wendell Holmes (1809–1894) learned this the hard way having experimented on himself by breathing ether. On one occasion, Holmes reached what he felt was an all-embracing truth. He hastened, while still under the influence of the ether, to distill its essence into writing. Later, he returned to find the words he had written. They turned out to be: "a strong smell of turpentine prevails throughout."[28]

Zen training means changing the brain. It implies remaining fully aware, open to introspection, enduring whatever happens. Then, is it worthwhile to lose so much sleep that consciousness becomes clouded and sluggish, or to resort to drugs that deprive consciousness of its clarity? These might sometimes create shifts into brief alternate states. Yet if one hopes to cultivate comprehensive insights that will remain "on-line"—meaning readily accessible to recall—such approaches would not seem to be optimal.

Still, the truism is well-founded: no strain, no gain. But Holmes came to appreciate that there are diminishing returns. It remains moot how close to the end of the rope the Zen aspirant should venture during a stressful sesshin. Meanwhile, for most persons, it will probably be safer to amplify to only modest degrees these stress responses of the brain's third route. This implies a kind of well-calibrated and well-prepared for disequilibrium. Enough to jostle the brain's natural cycles. Following which, they will rejoin as they may, in due course. For most persons, the optimum approach still means following the prudent Middle Way advocated later by the Buddha himself, and avoiding the extremes.

54

The Large Visual Brain

> The dragonfly:
> His face
> Is almost all eye!
>
> Chisoku[1]

> The things we see are the mind's best bet as to what is out in front.
> Adelbert Ames (1835–1933)[2]

A large compound eye nicely serves the dragonfly's modest visual needs. We have a relatively small eye. Social animals that we are, what humans need is a very large visual brain. Without it, how could we possibly make sense of all the complex situations we register visually? In Japan for example, a high-school student must recognize a minimum of 1800 separate idiographic *kanji* characters on sight even to become barely literate. This is only the beginning, because many characters change their meaning depending on the nuances of their context.

Vision changes in three distinctly different ways during hallucinations, absorptions, and the awakenings of insight-wisdom (see parts V, VI, and VII). Here, to lay the groundwork for why each of these changes occurs, it will help to look at an apple, and then travel along with the impulses associated with it as they move on through our large visual brain. Nerve impulses from the retina proceed back through the lateral geniculate nuclei (see figure 11) and the optic radiations to the visual cortex. Back there, one might casually say that each occipital lobe does "see" the opposite half of the environment. But along the way, many impulses had crossed sides and all had undergone countless transformations.

For the brain had to contend with that large nose separating our two eyes. Then there was the matter of the lens. Each lens had first turned the apple and the rest of the outside world upside down, switching left for right. So, only the "gift" of sight back in the brain will ignore the nose, unite the separate images, straighten out our topsy-turvy world, register each image at just the right moment, and then quickly *let go*. This gift doesn't stop there. It goes on to create the impression that our visual perception flows smoothly, like a rapidly played film-strip. An even more remarkable gift is still to come: we attach dimensions of meaning to the apple, and we relate ourselves to it.

In fact, it has now taken all four lobes of our brain on each side, and much of our subcortex and brain stem, to gather, represent, and vivify that apple lying on the table. Some of these processes involved our "first visual system." It is the one, glossed over above, which paused in the lateral geniculate nucleus before it relayed impulses up to the visual cortex (table 5). This first system will translate the data from the retina into a high-resolution image of the apple that can become a *conscious* visual percept.[3-6]

The "second visual system" began more as an early warning system. It appeared early in evolution, being better developed in the earlier simians than in higher monkeys.[7] This second system bypasses the lateral geniculate. It shunts its retinal data directly back to the *superior colliculus* in the midbrain (see figure 3). From here, messages are relayed up to the pulvinar and related thalamic nuclei, then farther up to the cortex. This system was designed to detect events, to locate them in space, and then to relay their coordinates elsewhere so that one could engage them in greater detail." In this second system, the midbrain is the entry point for our first quick grasp of space that will process spatial data *unconsciously*.

See how it works when you are walking in the dark. A light flashes off to the left. Instantly your head snaps to the left, thanks largely to your right superior colliculus. Or you duck to escape a low tree branch faint against the skyline. Both superior colliculi enter into this reflex "avoidance behavior." *No thinking*, in either instance. Urgency, not thoughts, dictates the functions of the second system. This is one reason why primates send so many norepinephrine terminals to the posterior parietal lobes, the pulvinar, and to the outer layers of the superior colliculus.[9]

The Colliculi

Our two superior colliculi are indeed "little hills," as their Latin name suggests. Of ancient lineage, their "bumps" serve as vantage points, surveying the scene with great sophistication, if unconsciously. For the superior colliculus represents

Table 5
"First" and "Second" Visual Systems*

Aspect	First System	Second System
Major connections	Lateral geniculate → visual cortex (geniculostriate)	Superior colliculus → pulvinar → posterior parietal lobe (tecto-pulvinar-parietal)
Major functions	More conscious visual perception	More reflexive visual responses in relation to orientations in space; unconscious perception; the basis for blind sight.

*The "systems" are generalizations. Primates, for example, also send important input down from the visual cortex both to the pulvinar and to the superior colliculus.[14]

more than what our eyes alone are seeing. It constructs an orderly visual envelope of space enlivened by our hearing, touch, and other sensory modalities.[10] How can it do all this? Because its single, so-called visual cells are not exclusively visual. Many of them also respond to the auditory *and* somatic sensory stimuli which enter from that very same region of space. They are *poly*modal, synesthetic.

So, in the colliculus, hearing, feeling, and seeing come together. One typical collicular nerve cell might respond both to touch *and* to pain stimuli coming from an animal's left rear foot. In addition, this same cell's auditory receptive field has also been tuned. Like a sonar system, it detects noises arising from just around that rear foot.[11] A barn owl has so highly integrated its visual and auditory maps of space that it can pinpoint the sound of a mouse squeak to within one or two degrees of the actual source.[12]

The superior colliculus promotes less to become more. Suppose its cells receive a single sensory stimulus, and they make only a relatively weak initial response. The colliculus then "turns up the gain." Its circuits amplify the interactions among incoming stimuli. The result is to *multiply*, not merely to add, the physiological impact from each successive stimulus.[13] In this manner, collicular nerve cells boost their responses enormously.

How do sudden stimuli "trigger" the rest of the brain? (see chapter 105). These striking leveraged amplification properties of the colliculi have interesting implications. Suppose, for example, that prior meditative training had finally created a lengthy quiet pause, a pause which happened to tune down the collicular responses to single stimuli. Then, if several sensory stimuli were suddenly to strike concurrently, they might have a great impact, totally unexpected in degree and in kind.

Blindsight

Normally, we integrate so intimately our first and second visual systems that we can never isolate the particular role each one plays in our everyday visual processing.[14] But strip away the cognitive luster of our first system. Now the second pathway reveals itself. The phenomenon is called *blindsight*. It can be best appreciated in those patients who have lost the function of their first, conscious visual pathway on *one* side.[15] Afterward, the patients seem "blind" to events that take place in their visual fields on the opposite side.[16]

This is no ordinary blindness. It is not the absolute visual loss that occurs when one entire eye is lost or when an optic nerve is severed. The blindness is *relative*. This fact emerges when you carefully test the patients' vision. Deliver a moving stimulus to their blind field. *They point at the target*, even though they can't *consciously* see it! It is worth noting that, in one respect, they behave like the rest of us. They perform best when they are relieved from tension. Free from the fear of making errors, their second visual system now works *intuitively*.[17] Zen exemplifies the same fact: behavior flows and intuitive functions work best when they are freed from self-concerns (see chapter 155).

Hughlings Jackson (1835–1911) would have been delighted to study blindsight. This Lincolnesque son of a Yorkshire farmer was to become the preeminent neurologist of his day at the National Hospital, Queen Square, London. Careful bedside observations of patients taught him that our normal functions were distributed throughout a vertical hierarchy up and down the nervous system. We can understand Jackson's thesis when we observe, as he did, how a stroke patient slowly recovers the lost motor functions of a leg that, at first, seemed completely paralyzed. Suppose it was the *right* leg, paralyzed because a clot had cut off all the blood supply to the large cells of the *left* motor cortex. At first, one might have been misled into thinking that this same leg region of cortex had been the *only* region which could have previously moved the leg normally.

But it wasn't. For the patient gradually begins to move his right leg better and better during the next few weeks. Why did his leg improve? Not because he had recovered the function of that hypothetical leg "center" up in the cortex. It had been destroyed. But because his nervous system had other options, described loosely under the term "plasticity." These now allowed him to access other motor patterns built in long ago at levels successively lower in the motor hierarchy. Blind sight operates in like manner. It also unveils the other pathways. In this instance, it reveals those sensory pathways within the visual realm. Nothing esoteric here. Blindsight merely uncovers the more ancient visual functions which had been buried in our second visual system.

Let us now take up the apple again, at the point in the occipital lobe where we left off with the topic of the first visual pathway. Here, in the primary visual cortex, nerve cells have several remarkable properties. Some translate impulses into the form of images in the finest-grained detail[18] and depth.[19] Some cells are so tuned that they will "see" only a horizontal line; others discharge only if the line is oriented vertically.[20]

If you overstimulate this primary visual cortex repeatedly, it feeds more impulses back down to the lateral geniculate nucleus. There, at once, a negative feedback mechanism shuts down what the geniculate "sees." In fact, it produces a circular zone of dense inhibition, shaped rather like a doughnut. Its purpose: to surround and to contain the spread of excessive excitatory discharges coming out of the "hole" in the center of the field. This inhibitory process acts to sharpen the contrast sensitivities of the *next* series of visual messages while they are passing through the geniculate on their way up to the cortex.[21,22]

To travel further with the apple, one would need a special guidebook. Currently, thirty or more cortical regions function as visual association areas, even in the monkey.[23] When anatomists try to plot out their intricate interconnections, their diagrams resemble the map of the Tokyo subway system.[24] Some areas function more as feature detectors. Others go on to process representations of images. Out of this mosaic emerges that grand perceptual synthesis we so casually take for granted: the miracle of vision.

However, there is a way to simplify how the brain reconstructs its visual image of an apple. One can suggest, to begin with, that the brain now employs two other interactive pathways. Put simply, one of them will be asking the general question: *What* is seen? The other will be inquiring: *Where* is it in space? In the next chapters, as we follow these two visual streams farther forward, it will be to discover that their flows mingle and are elaborated upon. Soon there emerges a representation invoking something far more subtle than the image of a round object, "out there," which they have simply recognized is a fruit.[25] In fact, all along an intimate *self-referent construct* will have been inserting its presence into the scene. So that from this point on, the fruit will become invested with very private meanings. And out of such covert constructs will spring a series of further questions. Initially, What does this apple mean to *me*? Next, What am *I* going to *do* about it? (see table 6, in the next chapter).

55

Where Is It? The Parietal Lobe Pathway

> We are as much as we see. Faith is sight and knowledge. The hands only serve the eyes.
>
> Henry Thoreau (1817–1862)[1]

Where is that apple I want to set my hand on? Is it high, low, near, far? Our "where" type of vision spots the target, relates it to other things. This process engages the upper visual function stream.[2,3] It is summarized on the right side of table 6. The upper stream draws heavily on the associations of our posterior parieto-occipital cortex. (see figure 2). The result is a sensory construct: a spherical object set in three-dimensional space. Something one can grasp.

We depend on these sophisticated constructs to represent very specific localizations within space. Suppose a patient develops a very slight degree of dysfunction of the *right* parietal association cortex. What happens? He still sees the fruit, but mislocalizes its image. The fruit is "displaced." He'll grasp at the wrong spot in space.[4]

The lower part of our parietal cortex is called the *inferior parietal lobule*.[5] There is nothing "inferior" about it, nor could it be more strategically placed. Here is another region where visual scene comes together with body scheme. Here, our *viewer*-centered representations *relate the self of our own physical body to the world outside it*. Perhaps in a sense, this is where we start to feel certain that the apple lies inside or outside the clutch of *our own* grasping hands. Do we know how far our arm can reach? We know exactly how far. Because every day, for years, we have made deposits of such representations into our autobiographical memory bank. Each entry in this personal account documented where the axis of our physical self and the length of our arm resided in space at that very moment.

The parietal lobe makes special contributions both to attention and to detecting events in motion at the outer edge of vision.[6,7] To perform these visual tasks, its nerve cells use extralarge receptive fields, and many of them fire when they detect events in either the right or left fields of vision. Moreover, some also "see" the central region directly ahead; others exclude it.[7–9]

The blind person has refined the sense of touch to read Braille. Finger touch alone defines its minute heights, depths, and patterns. The rest of us use the special sensitivities of our own *visual* brains to define topographic contrasts in visual space. These enable us to see images with sharply defined details, like

Table 6
Subsequent Visual Function Streams*

Aspect	Lower Occipitotemporal Pathways	Upper Occipitoparietal Pathways
Initial summary question	*What* is it?	*Where* is it?
Later questions	*What could* it mean? What *does* it mean? What does it mean to *me?*	What *could* it mean? What *does* it mean? What does it mean to *me?*
General trajectory	Lower (occipital → temporal)	Upper (occipital → parietal)
Major functions	More cognitively focused feature analysis (which includes using color); making affective associations	More general selective attention to the visual periphery, to movements, and to spatial constructs
Further interconnections	Limbic (amygdala, hippocampal formation), inferior frontal association cortex	"Second visual system"; cingulate gyrus and its extensions; dorsolateral frontal cortex
Representative regions in primates	V-4, V-P, infero-temporal, TE	Inferior parietal lobule and along superior temporal sulcus
Visual receptive fields	Continue to retain their more central focus while progressively expanding; some include regions on both sides	Continue to be more peripherally oriented while progressively expanding; some include regions on both sides
Other functions	Inhibitory surrounds (V-4)	
Damage in humans causes	Lack of recognition of what is seen (various agnosias)	Displacement, inattention, loss of spatial constructs, insensitivity to spatial contrasts, simultagnosia
Ultimate questions pending	What should I do about it? What am I going to do about it? (intention)	What should I do about it? What am I going to do about it? (intention)

*The "streams" are generalizations, and are each heavily interconnected at cortical and subcortical levels. The questions are "neurologized" abstractions.

those which have undergone fine-grained development in an Ansel Adams photograph.[10] In such ways we, whose gift is sight, resolve that blur on the skyline into a flock of snow geese flying south.

But suppose a lesion damages the right parieto-occipital cortex. The patient loses these unique spatial contrast sensitivities. On the other hand, what would be the shape and texture of an experience if the normal brain were to *augment* certain of these everyday functions of the parieto-occipital cortex? Could the person become more sensitive to visuospatial contrasts, and see images at extrahigh resolutions? (see chapter 113).

Attention as a Parietal Lobe Function?

A deficit of attention is typical of the patient who has suffered parietal lobe damage. Does it follow that the parietal cortex *itself* has "directed" our own attention?

Would attentiveness, per se, be enhanced if parietal functions *alone* were augmented? Probably not. Relatively few connections link the inferior parietal cortex with the inferotemporal cortex. Instead, we direct our attention with the aid of a much larger integrated network (see chapter 62). The circutry embraces more than that visual mosaic up in the temporal-parietal-occipital cortex. It also includes subcortical regions such as the pulvinar, the rest of the second visual system, and the brainstem reticular formation.[8] *Both cortical and subcortical levels interact when we pay attention.*

Space will later become an important topic in itself (see chapter 114). And so will what we hallucinate into it (see chapter 87). But here we can introduce these two key subjects by inquiring, How do we *envision* space? Bisiach began to clarify the process.[11,12] He conducted a classic experiment based on the topography of his own city, Milan, Italy. Its major landmark is the spire-tipped cathedral and the long plaza lying in front of it. Most of Milan's citizens know their plaza intimately. What helps anchor their memories of where the various shops are located as they stroll along the right and left sides of the plaza? That impressive cathedral at its one end.

Two of Bisiach's Milanese patients had lesions which damaged their right temporal-parietal region. As expected, both patients showed a defect in their left visual fields, were inattentive of their own left sides, and had impaired sensation over the left side of their body. Each patient was asked to *imagine* a familiar scene. First, they were to imagine they were standing at the *far* end of their plaza. This meant they would be looking way back down the plaza toward the now distant steps of the opposite cathedral. What, they were asked, did they envision in their "mind's eye?" Try putting yourself in the patients' shoes. You might be able to imagine some kind of a large distant building, with two lines of shops converging toward it.

Next, they were asked to imagine themselves standing on the front steps of the cathedral itself. This meant they would now be looking out down the same long plaza, but in the opposite direction. This time they would be looking back toward that spot they had imagined they had been standing on just a moment before. In each of the two instances, the researchers kept a record of what the patients reported as having "seen" in their imagination.

The descriptions from their first mental perspective were half-correct. That is, their "mind's eye" could conjure up the major shops which lay off to their *right side* of the plaza. They missed those off to their other side. In contrast, when they imagined that they now stood on the steps of the cathedral, they were again half-correct. Yes, they could still imagine half of the shops, those which again would be on their *right* side.

Now clearly, the patients had not *permanently* forgotten all those familiar buildings which would be lying off to their left side. For these same shops became available as soon as they had to be imagined within that perspective which would set them in their place off in the right side of space. The conclusion: the patients could not use spatial constructs to organize and to revisualize the *left* half of a familiar scene.

One patient was also asked to describe his own studio. It was an indoor studio where he had spent much of his life. Again he showed a similar deficit. He could not revisualize his studio furnishings off to the left. On those rare occasions when he did recall left-sided items, he spoke about them with a kind of absent-minded annoyance. In contrast, he talked in an interested, lively manner when he was recalling items which would have been located off to the right side in his studio.[11]

The Milan study suggests that we use our normal parietal and temporal connections to do more than represent the bare outside world as it exists now, at this present moment. We also employ their circuitries, along with temporal-limbic and other networks, to reconstruct and to revitalize images of this outside world. And these vital additions will help us localize, animate, and deploy those memories we pull up from out of our past (see chapter 89).

56

What Is It? The Temporal Lobe Pathway

While with an eye made quiet by the power of harmony, and the deep power of joy, we see into the life of things.

William Wordsworth (1770–1850)

That spherical object over there—*What* is it? A fruit? Much of our answer springs from the frames of reference within our lower visual pathway[1] (see table 6, at left). Its impulses stream forward from the occipital cortex to reach the tip of the temporal lobe[2,3] (see figure 2). Along the way, its channels interact with the limbic cortex, the parietal and orbitofrontal cortex, and the opposite hemisphere. In order to identify that fruit, the central zone of this lower visual function stream must process a sharply focused image. Then its algorithms must access frames of reference such as, What do various fruits look like? And, not incidentally, it will be inserting psychic reference points, specific for the observer.

These statements imply that even if a visual stimulus has first registered as motivationally "neutral" back in the primary visual cortex, its visual representations will then take on diverse subjective qualities. For example, some impulses can move down into the basolateral nucleus of the amygdala. Having already been colored there by an emotional valence, they can relay back up to influence other visual associations. Indeed, messages from the amygdala increasingly bias our visual associations the farther they travel toward the tip of the temporal lobe.[4]

This sounds familiar. Once before, we encountered this same pattern of increasing convergence toward the temporal tip. Then it characterized the way enkephalins and acetylcholine could increasingly influence the processing stream. Now the amygdala participates in this concentrated flow. Implicit in such a design is a plausible outcome: our affective states will increasingly shape the higher-order functions of our temporal lobe. On the other hand, suppose you wished to expunge all your personal, sentimental, psychic frames of reference. Suppose you wanted to drop the observer and develop only the objective, photographic image of a scene itself. One good place to start would be the "delete buttons" that take out egocentric messages as they flow forward through your temporal lobe.

What color is this round fruit? Several parts of the temporal lobe analyze for form and color. They include the fourth visual area, V4; the ventral posterior area, VP; and the inferior temporal cortex along the undersurface of the temporal lobe. These color-sensitive nerve cells in a monkey's V4 area are quite remarkable. Ready to detect both white light *and* differences in color, their specialized properties could help discriminate a camouflaged object from its background.[5] They are most sensitive to blue, green, and orange-red colors,[6] especially when these colors are intense.[7] They do even more. *They also fire more when the monkey is alert and paying attention.*[8]

Again, within this region lurk large rounded zones of inhibition. These "silent, suppressive surrounds" blanket a visual area thirty degrees or more in diameter. They prevent other neighboring cells from being excited by extraneous visual stimuli.

Like the monkey, humans respond instantly to a color. We fuse its several attributes long before the words arrive. But then human beings also have this *need* to define color further. So we have set up our intellectual prisms to go on—very un-Zen-like in this instance—to split color into three attributes. In doing so, we have now devised concepts employing such terms as *hue* (the degree of redness, greenness, etc.), *brightness* (luminance, intensity), and *saturation* (that scale which extends from whiteness through grayness to blackness). Patients lose the "redness" of an apple in the opposite visual field after damage within the lower visual association pathway.[9] And when it comes to perceiving both the hue and the saturation of an apple, the *right* side of our visual brain is better.[10]

The temporal lobes are also noteworthy in their gestalt processing capabilities. They help us flesh out the overall configuration of things we see, filling in the vacant spaces between a few specific local features.[11] The right posterior temporal cortex is better at helping us fill in these missing gaps. It lends a sense of "visual closure" to an otherwise incomplete picture.[12]

The Inferior Temporal Region

We began with an unknown fruitlike object out there in front. We then decoded its impulses in terms of their color and form. Our next visual relays run forward along the undersurface of the temporal lobe. This *inferior temporal* region has a ready supply of frames of reference. Its nerve cells are selective for the shape of certain fruits, for their color or texture, or for combinations of their stimulus properties. Moreover, many cells here have two talents. They respond to stimuli from the epicenter of the field where one's visual acuity is the keenest. And they also maintain extralarge peripheral receptive fields.[13] One such nerve cell might take in not only the center of gaze but also have a visually responsive field which encompasses an area over 625 degrees square.[5] This is a lot for one single cell to "see." It is equivalent to "seeing" a circle with a diameter of twenty degrees which could take in one ninth of the horizon in front!

Some inferior temporal nerve cells have fields so expansive that they even spill over across the vertical midline. What does this mean? Only that they are linked into circuits which have crossed over to tap into the visual field taken in by cells on the opposite side of the brain. What good is a cell with a visual field this large? Not to pinpoint the coordinates of a visual stimulus in space. Instead, it might be designed to insert subtle shades of meaning throughout a whole scene, *climates of feeling which interpret the visual message in some larger context.* For by virtue of having now represented the center of vision, and parts of *both* visual half-fields, this inferior temporal region has become tuned to represent the kind of high-level issues which make up "the big picture." Indeed, it has finally unified the visual space in front of the viewer "for the first time in the receptive field of a single cell."[14] Later, we will find out how such a sense of unification could become one constituent of sudden awakening (see chapter 133).

Suppose you were a monkey, learning a task. You have just discovered that only when you spot a *red* color will you then be rewarded with your favorite orange juice. How can you hang on to this critical learning contingency, this association link which you forged only seconds before? Certain inferior temporal nerve cells do participate in pivotal "memories" which hinge on this kind of colored association. And these cells discharge as soon as V4 cells send them "red color" messages.[15] The inferior temporal region has various other links with the amygdala and lateral hypothalamus. These circuits help monkeys select only those particular kinds of visual stimuli which they had previously learned were high—or low—in in reward value.[16] So within such networks meaningful distinctions could begin to take shape: notions about priority, of gain and loss.

Our environment presents an incredibly confusing mishmash.[17] To sort it out, each brain requires "shorthand" symbols. It needs jottings that will pass quickly back and forth within our normal memory and thought processes. The inferior temporal region seems able to extract these brief symbolic messages and then to translate them into forms suitable for other networks to manipulate. However, many of these symbolic functions are lost after area TE is damaged. This TE region of cortex lies near the temporal pole of the inferior temporal region. It in easily bruised when humans suffer trauma to the head. These patients then lose the same basic kinds of functions that lesioned monkeys also lose. In each instance, the subjects can't instantly answer a simple question: Is an object *new*? Or is it an old familiar one? So this anterior and inferior part of the temporal lobe is not some never-to-be-opened storehouse of musty, long-term visual memories. It takes objects seen in the present moment, compares them with templates of their *prototypes,* makes sharp distinctions, and then actively pigeonholes the items into distinct categories.[2,5,18,19] *Here, sharp distinctions are made.* Zen awakening, we recall, means *no* distinctions.

Another Look at Psychic Blindness

What happens in monkeys when lesions disconnect each temporal pole from its respective amygdala? They lose such critical discriminations. Superficially, they "see." Their visual acuity does seem "normal." But they don't infuse affective connotations into *what* they see. Gone are the useful notions they learned as infants. Lost are those street-smarts which helped them decide what was good or bad, threatening or nonthreatening. The lesioned monkeys will put anything into their mouth, whether it tastes good or bad, is edible or not. And they no longer fear that once-dreaded net which was used to capture them in their cage in the past. Other stimuli also lose their old affective qualities and their social implications. For instance, the lesioned monkeys seem indifferent to their former close social group, and are inattentive to their children. They don't visually explore their surroundings. Nor can they go on to learn the new associations which could help them correct this dire situation with the aid of new, adaptive behaviors.[20]

The term "psychic blindness" describes such negative phenomena. In context, that term is highly appropriate. Indeed, nothing about the lesioned monkeys' altered personal and social behavior provides any survival value in that particular setting. But psychic blindness, like blind sight, is worth a closer look. Does it remain applicable to *all* human situations? Does it apply to all of our excess emotional baggage? What about the extraheavy load our emotions place on the way we live?

At this point, it may be useful to suspend a final, pejorative judgment on some of these "negative signs of psychic deficit" which our primate relatives show after they have temporal lobe lesions. Suppose we step back and continue to pursue this same line of questioning into our own human world. What about the present human conditions, those social ills which cause the psyche to suffer—not too little, but too *much*—from what it sees? Our psychiatric counselors and social workers are already swamped by epidemics of drug abuse and violence. Why are their patients in such constant "psychic" turmoil? Is not their condition a reflection of "overloaded" frontal-temporal-limbic circuitries? Incalculable personal sufferings are the first result (see chapter 81), followed by behaviors so counterproductive that societies worldwide are undergoing major disruptions.

Zen inquires, Can we become not only more open but at the same time respond more selectively? Can we dampen only *certain* causes of our suffering, yet still emerge more compassionate in the process? It is a big, daunting agenda. The introspective meditator begins by thinking small.

Because one doesn't need to fixate on the obvious social problems "out there." One can begin at home. Every day, each of us is likely to be the unwitting subject to some overindulgent materialistic desire, to a strong aversion, or to some other personal "psychic" factor that operates disadvantageously. Consider the commonplace: how many of us eat or drink too much, nurture prejudices, or slide into debt charging on credit cards?

Monkeys provide one more model for such basic human problems. Their behavior is well known in India, where the villagers trap wild monkeys by taking advantage of their greedy desires. The villagers make a hole in a tethered coconut just large enough to admit the monkey's exploring paw. But this then makes the hole a size too small to permit the paw to exit, *if* that paw still keeps its firm grasp on the sweets inside. Consumed by its instinctual drives, *the monkey can't let go.* It traps *itself.* It becomes prisoner to its own self-inflicted desires.

To our Western way of thinking, freedom implies indulging in all the sweets of the world while still escaping from its constraints. In Zen, as Kobori-roshi said, our freedom arises from within. It comes from shedding ignorance and from learning to *let go*. Of what? Of two big, all-consuming passions: greed and hatred.

Temporal Lobe Discriminations

High up in the grooves of a monkey's superior temporal sulcus are other sets of discriminating nerve cells. They fire only when they receive a glimpse of those distinctive facial patterns which distinguish one monkey's features from another's.[21] But then, too, the superior temporal region also contains those other kinds of nerve cells which have large, bilaterally receptive visual fields, as well as poly-sensory cells.[22] Farther down in the middle temporal gyrus, the temporal lobe again enters into many other interactions with the amygdala. Here is another region where high-level frames of spatial reference seem to construct perspectives on the basis that there is some kind of "viewer" in the center. Such constructs could subtly mingle our physical self and our psychic selves (see chapter 8).

These few samples of temporal lobe functions hint at the realms of meaning with which it flavors our private experiences. Moreover, when the human temporal cortex is stimulated electrically, the subject goes on to make comparative interpretations about whatever event had then popped into experience. These interpretations are based on many subtle distinctions,[23] and their nuances would be impossible to detect if researchers had been limited to studying only monkeys.

For many of these interpretations refer back to that larger time frame which contains the human patient's own private world of psychic experience. And here we come to a fact of central importance: The stimulated patient draws conclusions based on two vital frames of reference. The two sets are *now/then* and *self/other*. The diagonal marks between these words reflect boundaries. Each diagonal mark represents an interface which will later become crucial to our understanding of Zen and the brain (see chapter 142).

The Use of the Question: When?

To explore the first issue, the now/then boundary, we do not have to limit ourselves to patients. Many normal people commonly experience memory quirks which reflect minor fluctuations in the functions of their temporal lobe. These include our brief episodes of *déjà vu* (French, "already seen"). Déjà vu episodes are inaccurate impressions. They carry the sense that the present *visual* moment resembles another one in an undefined past.[24] When I was an intern, I had déjà vu episodes only when I was short on sleep.

Less common among normals are episodes of *jamais vu* ("never seen"). Up to now, these two "time warp" phenomena have tended to be regarded as trivial symptoms, and of no consequence. Here, we propose them as useful models. For, in fact, they illuminate that very special quality which our temporal-limbic connections inject into all of our perceptions. Previously, we had asked "what?" as a way to simplify many of the recognition functions of the temporal lobe. But to better appreciate one of the lobe's other special functions we now need to ask, of each of the French-phrased experiences above, a *time*-related, rhetorical question: "When?"

Pose this question—"When?" Immediately, the answer is known. It comes as a snap judgment, the distillate of quick, comparative interpretations. No reasoning takes place.

For if you ask "When?" of a déjà vu experience, the instant answer is "Already." The implication is that I have already seen it before. And if you go on to ask "When?" of a jamais vu experience, the basic reply is "Never." Each answer is known directly. No thinking.

Normally, in our large visually organized brain, the process of seeing has become the major avenue that enables us to know. But it is not the only one. How do I *know* I went to the circus when I was a very young child? The visual details I've forgotten. But I do remember the repeated impact of the deep drum, each beat throbbing against my abdomen.

So, other interpretive avenues also add flesh and bones to an experience. These physical sensations round out our two simpler, seeing (*vu*) states, and animate them by infusing other, deeper nonverbal feelings. The French employ a different term, *vécu*, to describe such fleshed-out moments. *Vécu* means *experience*. It embraces all the deeper experiential aspects which reinforce our sense of what we have merely seen. All these sensibilities make the whole experience expand into a much larger reality. On the basis of this larger sense of reality, we decide— yes or no—that we participated in an event such as a circus, long ago.

So, once again, let us ask the "when?" question. Again, we receive the same quick answers: "already" or "never." If pressed to explain, déjà vécu might reply: I've already been personally involved once before in this same experience. Or, jamais vécu might say: I have never been personally involved in it. Already/never.

The issue of personal familiarity vs. a sense of estrangement returns us to the origins of the sense of self. The earlier discussion (see chapters 8 and 9) served, of course, to introduce one obvious point. There must be a "witness" at the core of the decision between these two types of vécu feelings. This witness is someone—actual or implied—who has all the experiential facts at hand to reach a decision. The decision "already" or "never"—pivots on one fundamental premise: *some kind of an ongoing, self-referent observer presides as the central, personal frame of reference.* Absent this central frame of reference, no basis exists for comparison.

Therefore, simply by asking "when?" of these four related kinds of temporal lobe phenomena, we uncover the first of our two implicit frames of reference. It is that old personal construct, *the self.* This witnessing self either has, or has not, seen an event or experienced it.

Many networks of this self interact within the temporal lobe and its connections. An important, controlled PET scan study shows that blood flow increases in certain temporal lobe regions—especially on the *right* side—when auditory messages reactivate personal memories.[25] These key "autobiographical" regions include the medial and lateral temporal cortex, as well as related sites chiefly in the limbic system. For example, when one evokes this personal self, among the other "satellite" regions involved are the amygdala, hippocampus, parahippo-campus, posterior cingulate, insula, and prefrontal cortex.

Now, before this witnessing self can answer the "when" question, it must also consult its own private construct of time. So, the second implicit reference— that related to *time*—is corollary to the first reference to *self*. The self now needs to scan a very long checklist of prior entries in its own personal data bank. Only then can it decide: yes, this event in the present moment *is* the same as that one which had come to my attention in time past. Or no, it is different, strange. Not part of *my* past history.

No psychophysiological theories about consciousness will approach completion until we appreciate that the brain has constructed these two fundamental interacting dimensions of meaning: self and time. Does this same understanding—of self and time—then make it any easier to appreciate Zen? Yes. Because it is part of the essence of awakening to dissolve the old boundaries between *self/other*, and between *now/then* (as we shall discover in part VII).

57

What Should I Do About It? The Frontal Lobes

Do not craze yourself with thinking, but go about your business anywhere. Life is not intellectual and critical, but sturdy.

Ralph Waldo Emerson (1803–1882)[1]

A genuine spiritual life is not one consisting of a series of disconnected and undefined experiences occurring at random; it is a constant dynamic process incorporating every element of our being.

Steven Batchelor[2]

In our journey so far, we have been tracking sentient impulses. We saw them first flow up into the back half of the brain. There, their patterns were recognized, their spatial percepts were developed, and meanings got attached to them.

Something different will happen in the front half. Here, we'll discover that potential scenarios have already been anticipating the arrival of these latest sensory elaborations.[3] For what lies in wait up front is a kind of subtle but dynamic matrix. Here, some things run in a fast-forward mode, helping to create a life of abstractions for an intellect that can be sharply critical. But here, too, are resources for our other more elemental activities. They will help life remain grounded, practical, sturdy.

Are these two processes incongruous? If so, their functions still come together in the *prefrontal cortex*. Long ago, to paraphrase the well-known soliloquy, many of its basic missions might have been summed up as: to *do* or not to do? Evolution then transformed its convolutions into the most distinguishing feature of the human brain. What was added? And how did it enable us now not only to socialize our instinctual drives but to go on to solve practical matters "intelligently?"

To begin with, the prefrontal region functions as an *association* cortex, as part of a consortium (see figure 2). Successive waves of excitation and inhibition cycle back and forth along its connections to the mediodorsal nucleus of the thalamus.[4] It also receives heavy contributions from the limbic system: direct projections from the amygdala, plus indirect projections from the amygdala by way of this same mediodorsal nucleus. It has extensive connections with the septal region, among many others. Checks and balances are built in everywhere. For example, what happens if you stimulate either the prefrontal cortex or the amygdala? Each of them inhibits the mediodorsal nucleus.

To simplify the functions of the prefrontal cortex, it helps to categorize them in terms of three major regions: orbital, medial, and dorsolateral cortex (table 7).

1. *Orbital prefrontal cortex*. This region spreads out along the undersurfaces of both frontal lobes. Its name comes from the way it extends horizontally above those bony orbits which contain our eyes. Normally, it helps control those impulses and vigorous primitive drives which could prove socially undesirable if carried to extremes. It seems to weigh the pros and cons, and to project cause-and-effect relationships. What makes it so sensitive to consequences? Note those extensive limbic interconnections.

Suppose patients lose the function of their orbital cortex. It takes only a trivial stimulus from the external world to release unusual impulsive behaviors. Place an object in front of them, and they can't resist grasping it. Having lost their own inhibitions, they can also be swept up into imitating the gestures of other persons. One dramatic example illustrates the point.[5] In this instance, the patient's

Table 7
Differing Prefrontal Lobe Attributes

Aspects	Orbital Cortex	Dorsolateral Cortex	Medial Cortex
Major roles	1. Helps inhibit socially undesirable, basic, primitive, internal drives	1. Helps extract and reconstruct sequences of meaning from ongoing experience	Helps engage the motoric aspects of motivational drives
	2. Helps inhibit impulsive behaviors prompted by irrelevant, ongoing, external stimuli	2. Helps organize associations simultaneously, at multiple cognitive and behavioral levels 3. Helps change mental sets	
Limbic interconnections	More	Less	More
Parietal association interconnections	Less	More	Less
Thalamic nucleus interconnections	Mediodorsal	Mediodorsal	Mediodorsal
Major biogenic amine input	DA	DA NE	DA

DA, dopamine; NE, norepinephrine.

abnormal behavior was prompted by the slender cues afforded when she glimpsed the usual medical instruments in a doctor's office. First she couldn't resist picking them up. Following this, her behavioral momentum was so unrestrained that she used the instruments to perform a physical examination on her startled neurologist!

Is such bizarre behavior relevant to Zen? Yes. For it certainly demonstrates *how the rest of the brain functions when it is freed from its weighty inhibitory constraints* (see chapter 142). Having considered earlier the change that occurs when only a single nerve cell is disinhibited, one now sees what happens to behavior when a patient's vastly larger brain systems are released. In this instance, the *behavioral release* is also spoken of as *dis*inhibition, for again it represents what happens after inhibition is removed.[6]

2. *Medial prefrontal cortex* (see figure 3). Lying inside, next to the vertical midline, this interior cortex normally contributes to drive, to motivation, and to other forward-leaning, active behaviors. (How handy it is to have the orbital regions nearby to hold in check the vigor of our more medial regions.) Sometimes, when a patient's seizures begin here, we neurologists get a few positive hints about what these midline regions might contribute to our normal functions.[7] One patient's seizures started with laughter, shouting, running, and other vigorous automatisms. Yet even so, all during this, the patient still remained aware and continued to react to external stimuli. Note how this contrasts with other patients whose epileptic seizures start elsewhere in the brain. They will usually have become unconscious or confused by the time their seizures have spread so far as to cause movements on both sides of the body.

Clearly, our own normal movements proceed in an exquisitely graded and more orderly manner.[6] But given our vast range of behavioral options, how do we stay goal-directed? Only by continually infusing each phase of the process with a frontal lobe variety of attention. To do so, to "actualize" in this manner, our frontal executive mode shifts into an ongoing corollary function called *intention* (see table 6, bottom). And now something subtle enters in; a property which keeps nudging this intention, repeatedly, into various facets of our ongoing activity. A commitment called *will*. The right hemisphere appears to process more quickly many of the external cues that enter into our more willed forms of *in*tention.[8]

Consider the onerous delight of mowing the lawn. Of course, I have only the best of intentions. Perhaps I'll mow the lawn when it's cooler. But, I won't actually *do* so unless I also *keep willing myself* to persist and to carry out my intention. My self-governing initiatives are soft, but crucial. When they drop out, after frontal lobe damage, good intentions can't stay "on-line." No initiatives are monitored. Inertia prevails. Unmown, the lawn . . .

3. *Dorsolateral prefrontal cortex* (see figure 2). This region is the largest. Its convex outer surface lies in front of the motor and premotor cortex. This dorsolateral convexity has major interconnections with the parietal lobes, less so with the limbic system (see table 7). Some of its higher-level "executive" functions are capable of placing one bare fact in its larger meaningful context. Still others proceed to organize such associations and direct them along lines that are appropriate, both cognitively and behaviorally.[9]

Taken as a whole, the curved prefrontal cortex might be said to "distance" us from the pull of our environment. In contrast, its parietal lobe counterpart tends more to foster behaviors that respond to the "pull" of the world outside.[6] Accordingly, as these two lobes keep striking new balances, some frontal contributions may nourish our more inner-directed, *egocentric* attitudes. To then describe the parietal influences as more *allocentric* is only to suggest the obvious role that other kinds of outside influences might play in helping to attract us toward the sensate world outside.[10]

Tap the knee tendon: the patient's leg jerks forward. Knee jerks spring from simpler circuits at lower, reflexive levels. Here, stimulus is rigidly time-locked to response. But up higher, among the networks of the prefrontal cortex, are circuits which engage the underlying caudate nuclei in very sophisticated levels of integration. In its higher-order functions, the mature human brain can blend three kinds of operations. First, of course, is that key element of *will*. The other two functions are *judgment* and *foresight*. They also contribute something important. They inject an open pause into what would otherwise be a headlong reflex pattern of stimulus-response. Then, into this gap, they insert some flexible behavioral options, chosen on the basis of hard-won practical experience, even reason.

So the prefrontal cortex does more than keep tabs on things that happened to work—or to fail—in the past. It projects fresh options into the future. And having weighed how practical and proper each act is, it keeps monitoring our ongoing behavior and fine-tuning it on a moment-to-moment basis. Can those two prefrontal extensions really do *all* this? Not without help. Let's examine what is involved.

To begin with, the prefrontal lobes execute four basic functional steps. These extract the relevant data, sequence them, form various sets, and then integrate them into concepts at still higher levels.[11] The second step, ordering the data into the correct sequence, is fully as important as any of the others. Cart comes *before* horse. You hang a Venetian blind, not a blind Venetian. Only after sets are assembled in some meaningful pattern can they be synthesized into concepts that are valid at higher abstract levels. These four functional steps describe the normal, facile "associative fluency" of the frontal lobes, and the ways they orchestrate the resources of the rest of our brain.

Patients slow down and become inattentive after frontal lobe lesions on both sides. They lose their intuitive skills, their sense of curiosity and concern, are distractible and apathetic, show blunted emotions. Turning these negative signs around, one may wonder: which positive qualities are the reverse of these deficits? Could the positive counterparts of such functions be experienced as enhanced insights and attentiveness, heightened interests, sharper mental focusing, and deepened emotional resonances?

In this regard, an interesting point has been largely overlooked: stimulating the frontal lobes brings out many positive feeling tones. Indeed, positive changes in mood occurred in approximately one quarter of the 2514 electrical stimulations in one large study, most of which were delivered to the patient's frontal lobes.[12] Moreover, several other observations on these stimulated patients illustrated the special flavor that their frontal lobes contributed. Their moods fluctuated from moment to moment. Their responses began with relaxation and feelings of well-being, smiling, and euphoria. Next, they developed a further extension of the euphoria, with outbursts of emotion either in a positive or negative direction. Finally, there occurred an abrupt sudden positive emotional response. This was followed by a satisfaction so sudden and complete that it precluded further attempts at stimulation. Many of these responses, noteworthy in themselves, resemble those fluctuations in mood and content commonly experienced during an intensive meditative retreat.

Let's examine the implications of the observation that frontal stimulation can *shift* a patient's experiential overtones. It illustrates how many of our normal frontal connections are "soft-wired." In other words, they hinge on very subtle associations derived from previous experiences.[6] It is precisely this dynamic, quicksilver quality which makes it so difficult to specify where our intimate subjectivities come from each time our frontal lobes inject them into everyday experience.[13]

But clearly the frontal regions can now subject the distant origins of some of them to higher executive analysis. For it is within the capacities of the frontal lobes to not only start to ask but to answer their own bottom-line question: Given all this information from the back of the brain, *what should I do about it?*

For years, they have been keeping track of incidental—but highly practical—trivia. Now, as a result, they can't treat a noun, like "hammer," as a mere word in the abstract. They seem to have been struck by the fact that hammer has a practical meaning. A hammer is *something to use,* to pound with. When a word inspires *this kind of active meaning* it activates the left prefrontal region preferentially.[14] And this same region also becomes activated as soon as the subject encounters a dangerous name, like "tiger," on a long list of benign animals. So the frontal lobes seem to be inserting a sturdy, *pragmatic note* into that large semantic network which we use to attach real meaning to sounds.

Our sense of novelty relates to the prefrontal cortex in an intriguing way. When normal subjects are surprised by novel stimuli, they generate a brain potential called a P300 wave (see chapter 64). It is most prominent over the frontal regions. Humans lose their P300 potential after prefrontal damage.[15] During kensho, the experiment is also struck by something completely new. When mental processes flash toward insight-wisdom, it is conceivable that relevant parts of the prefrontal cortex might both help generate the extra flavor of novelty and participate in it secondarily.

But wait. Don't some of the behavioral features commonly associated with Zen resemble some of the deficits found in patients after frontal lesions? Take, for example, the way anterior prefrontal lesions also reduce the amount of spontaneous speech, leaving it concrete and constricted in its narrative form.[16] And then, what about the patients who have both limbic *and* medial frontal lesions? They also dissolve the normal boundaries which had sharply separated some of their spheres of consciousness. As a result, they may not know whether they are at home or at their workplace.[17]

True enough, so far. That is why it is essential to consider the several other deficits in patients who have prefrontal lesions. For these patients can't change sets quickly. They are handicapped by other dysfunctions: behaviors which are sluggish and stereotyped. True, they do stay concrete and remain anchored firmly in the present. But *they aren't flexible*. These disabilities make it clear that the patients' behavior is precisely the opposite of that quick, wide-open freedom which occurs in kensho (see chapter 142).

And suppose, in the manner of a roshi, you were to challenge such patients with a new situation. They would be stumped, reduced to a narrow range of rigid behaviors. Their deficits contrast strikingly with the fluid adaptability so characteristic both of the brief awakenings and of the ongoing enlightened stage of Zen (see chapter 147). Advanced Zen training will finally free up brisk, highly creative behaviors, not stereotyped acts. And these liberated behaviors will be more appropriate to the whole social setting than is picking up a throat stick in some doctor's office, and thrusting it toward the surprised physician.

There remains the issue of time. For time does dissolve at the instant of kensho (see chapter 135). Superficially, this might resemble the problems with "time" found in patients who have frontal lobe lesions. But their abnormality resides in *sequencing* time. These patients can't arrange a series of words or events in the correct temporal sequence.[18]

Normally, our frontal lobes do help us to be forward-looking. But they also project past anxieties into this future. The outcome can be serious. For the present becomes *dis*-eased when it is preoccupied with neurotic worries. You can't drive forward safely in a car if you're always watching the rear-view mirror, worrying about getting a whiplash injury.

When a pig is overstressed, its frontal cortex *over*participates in the stress responses. As a result, the pig develops a fatal rapid heart action (ventricular fibrillation) when its coronary artery is occluded. This doesn't happen if the prefrontal cortex is cut off from its fatal connections with the brain stem.[19]

Humankind keeps searching for measures to reduce the anguish of its own stress responses. Surely we need to be cut free of some of the nagging messages which reverberate between our frontal cortex, the amygdala, and other limbic connections downstream.[20] Meditative techniques provide a useful remedy. First, a way to briefly let go of those crazed, worrisome messages. Finally, a way to be cut loose from them, and to go about our business anywhere.

The dopamine system plays a distinctive role in innervating *frontal* association cortex, less so the cortex elsewhere (see table 7). In contrast, the norepinephrine and serotonin systems more diffusely innervate the whole forebrain. Consequently, if a dopaminergic discharge were to surge through cortex, it would *preferentially* impact the associative functions of the frontal lobe.[21,22]

Mental sets do change faster when dopamine is released over the dorsolateral prefrontal cortex.[23] There, by acting on its DA_1 receptors, dopamine increases the firing of those prefrontal nerve cells which integrate recent visual cues into motor performance.[24] It is noteworthy that many parkinsonian patients, deficient in dopamine, can't shift mental sets into the new kinds of perspectives which create relevance out of irrelevance.[25]

A few pages above, we mentioned the frontal lobe contributions to our more subtle, *internally* directed mental attributes. These are our sense of self-awareness, our self-consciousness, and that pervasive notion which informs each one of us that we are indeed a stable continuing entity, still capable of change.[11,26] Moreover, superimposed on all our "self-continuity"[26] is yet another higher-level capacity: the special human attribute of being able to turn awareness around and *to look far back into ourselves*. Those persons who learn to do so, and who make a habit of doing so, can become the recipients of *insights* about themselves. Could this be one reason why the deeper levels of the mindful, introspective path are also called "insight meditation?" (see chapter 28).

Research has not yet clarified exactly how the brain generates all our inward-turned levels of self-awareness. The reasons are several. They seem to enter as emergent properties. And, in the normal population at large, there are big differences among individuals in how well they can—or wish to—turn inward to scrutinize themselves objectively. Moreover, by the time patients with severe frontal lobe damage have finally lost *their* self-awareness, too many other deficits will have obscured the clinical picture. So doctors can't then define and pinpoint any single discrete dysfunction as the cause for each aspect of their disability of self-awareness.

Perhaps this is one of the reasons why behavioral neuroscientists have yet to come to grips with the human brain's most unique property. This is the way it intuits *beyond self*. Only when graced by that gift which penetrates beyond self can the brain grasp the most simplifying of all megaconcepts, the principle of Ultimate Reality (see chapter 142).

If such self-negating forms of insight-wisdom are to issue from a three-pound brain, they must draw *selectively* on more than the frontal lobes' organizational abilities alone. They must access only *certain* of the temporal lobes' skills at comparative interpretations. They must register only some of the ways that the parietooccipital lobes perceive personal and extrapersonal space. In fact, awakening will imply that only *certain parts of the whole brain are now associating*, and in a most extraordinary way. The resulting experience will be one of the brain's most striking emergent properties (see part VII).

In the interim, we will do well if we keep on-line the two opening quotations, taken from Emerson and Batchelor. Because genuine spiritual behavior is indeed a constant dynamic process. It is one that incorporates every element of our being.[2] True, random mystical experiences can become influential. But transformative? Only to the degree that the person then goes on to incorporate them into the sturdy processes of everyday living.

58

Ripples in Larger Systems: Laying Down and Retrieving Memories

> All is not over when an impulse flashes across a synapse and onto its destination. It leaves behind ripples in the state of the system.
>
> Ralph Gerard[1]

How can light waves, as they "ripple" from a red maple leaf, come to be stored as an image-trace in the brain? And what causes this leaf-image to suddenly "pop out" weeks later? (see chapter 109). Put simply, our first step is to *encode* memories, then to *consolidate* them, and later to *recall* them.[2]

Some memory traces linger for a moment. Others endure for a lifetime. This implies that we have a few options for "storing" these traces, either in the form of (1) an immediate memory, (2) a short-term memory, or (3) a long-term memory. Immediate memory registers sensory percepts only for a moment. Our short-term memory lumps the incoming sensate stimuli into only a few conceptual units, called "chunks." For example, one chunk might constitute an entire verse of familiar poetry. Still, our short-term memory has a relatively limited capacity. It can only handle a mere seven to ten such chunks of information, and we forget these relatively quickly.

But long-term memory handles a huge number of chunks. Within its compartments, we represent memory traces in a much more stable form.[3] A chess master uses this kind of memory to scan some fifty thousand or more chunks in long-term memory, and relies on it to provide the best solution for his next move.

Earlier we touched on the key roles in memory played both by the medial temporal regions and by their adjacent temporal cortex on *both* sides. Before midcentury, scant attention was paid to the memory contributions made by the hippocampus, amygdala, and parahippocampal gyrus (see figure 3). Then, in 1953, the patient H.M. had both his right and left medial temporal regions excised surgically. Afterward, he had two major types of memory problems. One was an "absent-minded-professor" type of forgetting. He couldn't remember such *ongoing events* as what food he had just finished eating for breakfast. His other problem was a severe *retrograde amnesia*. The key point was that brain surgery had wiped out his memories for those last two or three years *just before* his operation. Yet it had spared his older memories for events during those earlier decades between 1920 and 1950. This was more than a dense amnesia. His memory deficit had a distinctive profile.[4] It suggested that, for the first few years immediately after an event took place, normal persons would be relying on the medial temporal region to help encode, maintain, and recall their memory traces.

This theory received support when researchers delivered brief stimuli to the medial temporal region in humans. During this disturbance, and for as long as the local afterdischarges lasted, the patients could not accurately recall their most recent visual memories.[5] Under normal circumstances, this same medial temporal region also helps us build up our general fund of *factual* information about a specific event, documenting when and where it occurred.[4]

Several other circuits in the limbic system, thalamus, and basal forebrain also help us remember. Avenues for such messages run up through the mammillothalamic tract to the anterior thalamic nucleus. Others pass between the amygdala and the thalamus.[6] After large lesions of the medial dorsal nucleus of the thalamus, patients suffer a memory impairment for both verbal and nonverbal material.[7] In one such patient, studies showed that the major disturbance was in the earlier, encoding phase of memory. Even though the patient could not lay down fresh memories, the process of memory retrieval remained relatively spared.[8]

Ways to Influence Memory

Specialists who study memory need a thicket of complicated wiring diagrams even to begin to "explain" ordinary memories.[9] The more so if one insists that their diagrams must also account for four sets of observations such as the following: (1) Certain drugs, higher arousal levels, novelty, and motivational factors can be used to enhance the laying down and retrieval of memories. (2) One can replay memories at will. (3) Memories also retrieve themselves spontaneously. This occurs either during dreams, during hallucinations, or when triggered by some sensory event. (4) Spontaneous alternate states remain vividly etched in memory. Let us consider these four observations further.

We remember items better if they had been processed during a condition of high arousal.[10] The degree of arousal is critical for one other reason: experiences tend to be "state-bound." What does this term imply? It means that we will recall an earlier experience best when the same arousal conditions prevail during this retrieval phase as had been in effect during the original experience.[11]

We sense that our level of consciousness varies throughout the day. So, during these natural fluctuations—and also when arousal levels fluctuate during meditation—we are neither learning nor recalling in a uniform manner.[12] Yes, we can still process some information and can store it during "lower" states of arousal; this still goes on even when we are asleep or in an hypnotic drugged state. And we can later recall much of these data *if* these two similar states of somnolence are recreated. But suppose such "low arousal" information has become entirely state-dependent. Then we will *not* be able to retrieve it once we have gone on later to enter a "high" state of arousal.

So our process of state-bound retrieval has an important property: recall goes best *downhill,* not uphill. Items that were first laid down in memory at the time when we were most fully awake and aware will later be remembered the best even as we descend through successively lower levels of awareness. *This downhill phenomenon helps us understand why alternate states remain vivid in memory.* And it also helps explain why we recall dream details better when they arise out of the activities of REM sleep as opposed to slow-wave sleep.

In general, the research in state-dependent learning suggests that once *outside* information has been learned under the influence of a certain drug, it will later be most readily retrieved *if* this very same drugged state is recreated. Then, what about information from the *inside*—the generic kind known as insight? Is it also subject to the same general phenomena? This hypothesis has yet to be tested. But given the other aspects of the downhill phenomenon, it is reasonable to think that a meditator who is fully awake when insight strikes could be most prone to remember the details and incorporate the resonances of this peak experience.

The novelty of an event also helps etch it into memory. Moreover, there is a carryover effect. It turns out that memory improves for a few *hours after* a single novel event.[13] This particular kind of anterograde improved memory in humans appears to be due to the quality of novelty per se, not to whatever additional arousal might have occurred. Under certain experimental conditions, a rat remembers its previous training better after it has received morphine or enkephalin[14] (see chapter 47).

Indeed, the particular set of conditions that prevails during an experiment is crucial in every study of memory, both in humans and in animals. *Whether opioids reduce memories, or facilitate them, depends on where, how, and when they are given.* Humans might undergo a localized or generalized surge of *endogenous* opioids. Either could release some potent and highly unusual blends of experience. One may speculate that the subject could encounter an experiential paradox. For example, within one mental field there might occur a combination of effects: some that were amnestic, others that were memory-enhancing. Certain older behaviors and attitudes might be forgotten; the very newest ones might be reinforced and long remembered. Are we open to consider what extraordinary kinds of new memory paradigms might then present themselves? (see chapter 143).

In conventional doses, several drugs do enhance memory even though they have widely differing actions. And they work even if they are given later, *after* the person is first trying to remember. These drugs include alcohol, diazepam, nitrous oxide, and so on.[2] How could drugs like these possibly *enhance* memory? One theory is that they act on systems linked to reward or reinforcement in ways that release "precognitive" brain functions. The results can be striking. Memory can improve as much as fourfold when drugs are used to manipulate its early encoding phase. These enhancing effects can be long-lasting. Moreover, the facilitated memories retain their original conceptual structure, and novel items are remembered in particular.[2] We do possess vast memory resources, but they need to be studied with great care, demystified, and tapped into appropriately.

Let us consider these resources. How does our brain normally nudge its circuits so that they can gain access to vast "memory banks" at subconscious levels? Many of these very subtle, higher overall "supervisory" functions appear to arise from connections of the prefrontal cortex. Given its intimate connections with the thalamus, this observation serves to introduce not only the general topic of the thalamus but that of its *medial dorsal nucleus* in particular (see table 7 and figure 11).

Novel stimuli, or arousing stimuli, can each release this medial dorsal nucleus from its GABA inhibition.[15] This allows the nucleus to go on to further stimulate the prefrontal cortex.[16] Moreover, at this point, it so happens that more dopamine is also released into this same prefrontal cortex.[8] So a dual excitatory surge can take place, both mediodorsal *and* dopaminergic, and both can enter the frontal neocortex at the same time. This event might have intriguing consequences. It might substantially enhance the usual ways information is processed. It could also shift processing into its most effortless parallel mode.[17] Many long-forgotten bytes of subliminal data might become instantly accessible. These bytes, retrieved into the foreground of consciousness in large integrated chunks, can be astonishing in their form, scope, and content. A person's ability to manipulate long verses with ease is only one of several possible results (see chapter 92).

We have now come to the end of a cursory survey of how the cortex functions. It is time to become familiar with the other nuclei of its close partner, the thalamus.

The Thalamus

> Experience is never limited . . . it is an immense sensibility, a kind of huge spider-web of the finest silken threads suspended in the chamber of consciousness, and catching every air-borne particle in its tissue.
>
> Henry James (1843–1916)[1]

Thalamus is an old word. It arose from ancient Egyptian or Greek roots which referred variously to an anteroom or to a bridal chamber. When the early anatomists traced the optic tracts back into it, they came to the correct conclusion: its large gray masses were the "chambers" which received visual messages sent from the eye.[2]

Research in this century informs us that the thalamus does much more: it actively contributes to our immense sensibilities, helps to resolve their incoming messages both in space and in time.[3] And another notion has developed: it functions as a kind of sensory "gate." For, indeed, we are most frugal about allowing visual and other sensory signals to pass through the thalamus.[4] Which sensate messages does this thalamic gate permit to rise up to the cortex? *It varies. It is highly state-dependent; it depends on our state of consciousness.*[5] What happens to a person's vision and hearing when the entrance chamber is blocked? The answers will come when we encounter the absorptions of internal samadhi (see chapter 111). Our explanations then will hinge on what we have learned about how the gates operate in the thalamus.

The thalamus is intricate in both its anatomy and its physiology (figure 11). It serves our purposes here to select examples from three categories of its nuclei:

1. The *specific sensory relay nuclei* are a good place to begin. They are the crucial gateways to the specific parts of cortex which yield our well-localized higher sensibilities. One typical example is the *ventral posterior lateral* nucleus. Into it are arriving all those basic sensory impulses from our *body* which will be refined into our discrete senses of position, of pain, and of touch. Just medial lies the *ventral posterior medial* nucleus. Here we perceive these same qualities of sensation when they enter from our *head.*

The two geniculate nuclei are the other key sensory relay nuclei. The outer one, the *lateral geniculate nucleus,* helps us see. It processes visual messages as they come back from the retina via the optic nerve and tract. The *medial geniculate nucleus* helps us hear, relaying auditory information up from the brain stem. These relay nuclei, in turn, then package their own axons into "bundles" that export their messages up to specific regions of the cerebral cortex.[6]

In cortex, we go on to refine sensation into higher-order forms that discriminate between a house key and a car key. However, a person would lose almost all of the *primary* forms of sensation if incoming sensate messages were blocked down in these four relay nuclei (two on each side).[7] The exception: our sense of smell. It enters the limbic system directly.

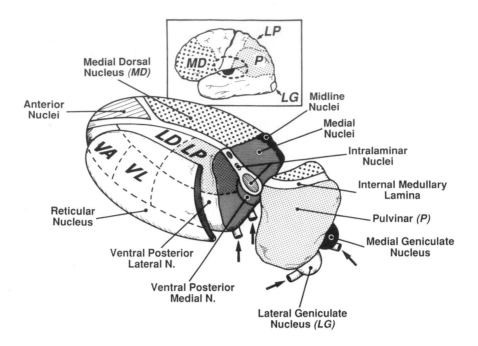

Figure 11   The thalamus

The small rectangle at top, above, encloses a side view of the whole left cerebral hemisphere. It is similar to that in figure 2, but now the thick dotted lines outline an oval region. This represents the deep central location of the thalamus. Off to the left, the large dots cover the prefrontal cortex. They represent the large projection area of the mediodorsal nucleus (MD) of the thalamus. Farther back, the parieto-occipital cortex is also covered by major projections coming from the pulvinar (P) and lateral posterior (LP) nuclei. Note, however, that the rest of the outer and inferior temporal cortex receives little direct input from the thalamus. It is "athalmic," aside from its small primary auditory cortex. This is Heschl's gyrus, shown as a dark-black ovoid.

Below is a much expanded view of a section across the left thalamus. The viewer is looking down at it from behind. Four small arrows suggest the ways our sensate information enters the specific sensory nuclei: (a) visual messages from the optic tract enter the lateral geniculate nucleus; (b) auditory messages enter the medial geniculate nucleus; (c) somatosensory messages from the head enter the ventral posterior medial nucleus; (d) somatosensory messages from the rest of the body enter the ventral posterior lateral nucleus.

The thin, curved cap is the reticular nucleus. It is shown, artificially detached from the several other nuclei that it inhibits. Dotted lines indicate their borders. They include the ventral anterior (VA), ventral lateral (VL), lateral dorsal (LD), and lateral posterior (LP) nuclei. The small intralaminar nuclei nestle like hummingbird eggs in the white meshwork of fibers of the internal medullary lamina. This same layer of white matter splits the thalamus into its three groups of nuclei: medial, lateral, and anterior. The parafascicular nucleus (not shown) relays pain messages ascending via the old medial, spinothalamic pain system. (Redrawn and modified from several texts sources, chiefly with reference to F. Netter. The *Ciba Collection of Medical Illustrations*. Vol. 1., *Nervous System*, Ciba. West Caldwell, New Jersey, 1983, 193. Novartis, with permission.)

How do the four specific sensory relay nuclei function? The lateral geniculate nucleus serves as a prototype. It is, indeed, the antechamber for most visual impulses entering our brain. Here, it can impose a gate on vision. But this is not a barrier of its own making. In fact, most synapses within it are not *directly* involved in conveying visual signals from the eye back to the primary visual cortex. Most synapses here originate in countless other *nonseeing* nerve cells. Yet this *non*retinal input is critical. It still *modifies* vision.[8] How? It cuts down on the volume of visual transmission passing through the lateral geniculate nucleus as soon as an alert monkey (or meditator) becomes drowsy or inattentive.

But suppose this same drowsy monkey is now touched, or hears a faint sound, or is given a mild electrical stimulation in its midbrain reticular formation. In each instance, the message is arousing. And the brain, reaching in with its *non*retinal, *non*visual input, now "opens the gate." Abruptly, a renewed flow of visual impulses surges through the lateral geniculate nucleus. In fact, the maximum transmission comes just during this particular sequence, the one which first became drowsy, then was suddenly alerted. It is a *permissive sequence*. It would allow (if unopposed) a manyfold increase in the volume of visual impulses to pass on into the rest of the large visual brain.

This surge of increased excitability through the geniculate nucleus is a basic physiological response. The gate starts to open no matter whether slow-wave sleep gives way to (a) the EEG desynchrony of natural spontaneous waking, (b) that of REM sleep, or (c) the frank arousal which comes from stimulating the midbrain reticular formation. The result, in each instance, releases the geniculate nucleus from its previous inhibitory restraints.

Yet the "gate closes" if one delivers electrical stimulation to the other *non*specific thalamic nuclei. And slow-wave sleep itself also greatly reduces the flow of visual impulses through the lateral geniculate nucleus. However, as if to compensate, sleep also renders the primary visual cortex itself much more excitable to direct electrical stimuli.[9] Aside from local GABA circuits, can the local input of biogenic amines also vary the flow of visual impulses?

Primates supply the lateral geniculate nucleus with dense networks of serotonin terminals (similar to the way ST nerve endings also supply the primary visual cortex of area 17, the inferior temporal region, and the superior colliculus.) And the ST fibers from the dorsal raphe nucleus can effectively inhibit *one third* of the relay cells in the lateral geniculate nucleus.[10] So changes in ST tone could be one explanation for some of the transient visual phenomena which occur during mediative states and quickenings (see part V).

Certain other meditative phenomena might reflect changes in norepinephrine tone. For example, the NE levels in many other thalamic regions tend to be higher on the right side. Among these nuclei are the several specific *sensory* nuclei of the ventral thalamus and two of the intralaminar nuclei.[11] But in sharp contrast to the potential *visual* effects which ST could have, cited above, few NE terminals supply the visual pathway after it leaves the lateral geniculate nucleus and flows on into the primary visual cortex. Moreover, NE nerve endings are also sparse in the inferior temporal region.[12]

2. The *association nuclei*. Two of these thalamic nuclei were introduced earlier. Each was singled out because it processes limbic messages, exports them up to cortex, and plays a role in memory. The larger, the *medial dorsal thalamic nucleus*, consults back and forth with the basal-lateral amygdala. Poised to catch each limbic vibration in its network, it then relays its own versions of their themes forward over much of the prefrontal cortex. It is a noteworthy point that its larger cells will direct their limbic overtones into the orbital frontal cortex.[13] What will

be the net effect of such interactions? Perhaps they infuse the "vibes" of potential consequences—pleasant or unpleasant—into our frontal lobes in ways that bias their behavioral scenarios. As noted earlier, most of the dopamine inflow to cortex is also being directed toward the frontal regions of cortex. In this way, DA could be an accessory to the larger impact of this medial dorsal nucleus[14] (see table 7).

The *anterior thalamic nucleus* is smaller. Much of its input arrives from the hippocampal formation, having first passed through the mammillary body. The anterior nucleus then relays its impulses up to the cingulate cortex (see figure 6). Humans suffer amnesia if lesions disconnect the pathways into either the medial dorsal or the anterior thalamic nuclei.[15] A third association nucleus, the *pulvinar,* is so remarkable that it merits a separate chapter.

3. The several *intralaminar nuclei* nestle like hummingbird eggs within the bands of white matter that split the thalamus. These nuclei are part of the *non*specific system. This means that they exert a more general influence, broadcasting *diffusely* both up to the cortex and forward to the striatum. Projections from one of them, the deep parafascicular nucleus, cover the front and sides of the frontal lobe, whereas the central lateral nucleus broadly influences parietal functions.[6] If one stimulates the intralaminar nuclei slowly, at rates between six and twelve times a second, they diffusely affect the cortex and increasingly *recruit* its responses.[16] This means that each successive stimulus to the thalamus calls forth an increasing cortical response. Recruiting takes place because cortical dendrites in these frontal regions become increasingly excitable. Soon, many of the outer layers of cortex will depolarize. Which regions does the thalamus recruit first? Those in *the front of the brain*, the frontal and motor cortex.

Long ago, Jasper made an observation which begs to be confirmed with modern methods: he could recruit all areas of the *sensory* cortex more readily after he had first removed the influences of their respective *specific* thalamic relay nuclei.[16] This finding—that recruiting functions increase when other sensory *relay* systems are shut down—is important for two reasons.[17] First, it emphasizes that the *diffuse* system, the one through which the *non*specific nuclei project, can interact *physiologically* with those other sensory nuclei whose functions are more specifically focused. Second, it suggests a mechanism which could help to heighten our consciousness as it turns inward. During internal absorption, for example, this could be one way that some cortical responsivities might become amplified even further (see chapter 118). Why? Because sensate gates appear then to close, a process which also shuts down the usual sensory input from entering via these specific thalamic nuclei.[18]

Currently, interest has revived in the "global" functions of the intralaminar nuclei. They are again being viewed as the major avenue through which the acetylcholine neurons of the brain stem widely activate the cortex during heightened states of attention.[19] Moreover, their larger nerve cells have intriguing properties. Some of them are capable of enhancing their basic 40-cps spike bursts and of firing at very high frequencies. In fact, their 40-cps bursts apparently resonate along with comparable rhythms arising from their cortical counterparts.[20] And the same generalized 40-cps activities, as they cycle within the *non*specific loops from thalamus to cortex, might also go on to resonate with other key networks.

Which ones? Those namely, which link the *specific* thalamic nuclei with their own particular regions of cortex, as was described first under (1) above.

Now, what could such a confluence of 40-cps resonances contribute to the brain? One theory, of interest to Zen, is that this coalition could engender a *kind of contextual unity within conscious experience.*[21] The intralaminar nuclei could be blending in some vague background sense of form. And the specific nuclei could be contributing to the specific content of the foreground.[4] That apple, out there on the table, would then be emerging into one's larger personal field of awareness.

Having mentioned, several times, that there exist "gates" *within* the thalamus, we turn next to the most important gate of all: the *reticular nucleus.* It might seem to envelop only the *outside* of the thalamus. But watch. It drops down like a portcullis, shutting off the further passage of sensate information.

60

The Reticular Nucleus

> The whole of the dorsal thalamus appears to be surrounded by a sheet of acetylcholine inhibited neurons
>
> R. Dingledine and J. Kelly[1]

It did not even look like a nucleus. At first, it seemed to be merely a thin, inconspicuous sheet of nerve cells that capped the contours of the thalamus (see figure 11). And so, because these nerve cells formed an interlacing network, the earlier anatomists called it "reticular," meaning netlike.* But looks were deceiving. It took a long time to realize which kind of nerve cells were in there, and what they did.

The cap contains large, potent GABA nerve cells. Their information comes from a gauze meshwork of long dendrites draped all over the outer surface of the thalamus. This network is designed to sample the signals which pass to and fro between thalamus and cortex. Suppose too many impulses are flowing in and out. Now the GABA cells become more excited. What happens next can be likened to the way a drawstring tightens on a monk's hood. The reticular nucleus then shuts down the flow of messages which would otherwise be streaming into the sensory relay cells of the underlying thalamus.

Most reticular nucleus nerve cells have *average* firing rates varying somewhere between five and thirty-four times a second.[2,3] Some are able to fire much faster, say 200 to 350 times a second, and can do so for as long as 1.5 seconds. When they fire, they "close the gate" within the thalamus and block sensate messages from relaying up to cortex.[4] After this burst they may pause. *The pause lasts for as long as three or four seconds.*[2]

The conventional belief is that the reticular nucleus does not actually, so to speak, "slam" the sensory gate within the thalamus. Rather, it helps the brain

---

* A note of caution. The reticular nucleus of the thalamus is completely different in structure and function from the reticular formation of the *brain stem,* with which it has an inverse, seesaw relationship.

generate complex, rhythmic oscillations. First, these shift in the direction of hyperpolarization. Next, they rebound toward greater degrees of *de*polarization, that tendency toward excitation which is its functional opposite. As these oscillations shimmer in thalamocortical circuits, their waves take the form of rhythmic spindle activity in the EEG.[5–7]

Suppose that an underlying specific thalamic nerve cell happens to be in its usual act of relaying sensate messages. Assume that it is firing at its customary rates of 20 to 100 times a second. Then, say, that a GABA cell in the reticular nucleus briefly inhibits it for only 80 to 250 milliseconds. At this point, the normal burst-pause capabilities of those GABA cells in the reticular cap open up some remarkable possibilities. Why? Because as soon as the sensory relay cell breaks free from its GABA inhibition it fires much faster than usual. During this long rebound phase, it can then fire as fast as 300 times a second. Moreover, when the *next* sensory impulses arrive at this same sensory relay cell, they find it hyperexcitable to the extreme. Now they can stimulate it into a three- to fifteen*fold* surge in its firing rate![8]

The interesting properties of the reticular nucleus have led to much speculation about what it does when we remain in our conventional awake state and pay selective, conscious attention.[8,9] But the interactive, burst-pause properties of thalamic nerve cells are noteworthy for another reason. They suggest hypotheses for two sets of meditative phenomena. The first is that the brain could shut off sensation during internal absorption by prolonging its *burst* phase of GABA activity. The second is that prolonging the *pause* phase could help sponsor the entry into consciousness of several kinds of "quickenings." At the sensate end of the spectrum, these events could include visual episodes perceived as blinding white lights (see chapter 85). At the mental end, brief "illuminations" of other kinds might be added to (see chapter 141).

The arrows in the lower right of figure 11 illustrate how sensate input enters the back part of the human thalamus. Overlying this region are the particular GABA cells that can inhibit a person's incoming facial, visual, and auditory sensation. Beyond that, each GABA neuron also tends to service a relatively large peripheral sensory field.[10]

In operation, the reticular cap covering the thalamus of one hemisphere blocks sensory impulses coming in from the opposite side of the body and the environment.[11] So how, in a major internal absorption, could vision, hearing, head, and body sensations be blocked on *both* sides? The answer is that much of the corresponding sensate regions of both reticular nuclei would need to be excited.

The brain already has far too many nuclei to keep track of. Why does this book single out the reticular cap at all? *Because its functions are the most relevant and strategically placed to stop or to enhance transmission through the thalamus.* But still, its cells undergo bursts or pauses for only a few seconds—this is not a very long time. Could larger regions of the nucleus become so excited that they would close the sensory gate for periods *longer* than several seconds?

One way to do so is to introduce events that first cause excessive excitability *of the cerebral cortex.* In fact, if you stimulate the cerebral cortex, it strongly excites most GABA cells downstream in the reticular nucleus. Now they fire in long inhibitory bursts.[12] Even if you restrict the zone of electrical stimulation to the small face region up in the sensory cortex, it increases the metabolic activity of cells down in the reticular cap and causes a corresponding *decrease* in activity of its nearby sensory relay nucleus.[13]

Stimulation in the front part of the cortex also causes prolonged effects on the reticular nucleus. The mechanism in this instance reflects the pathways which normally bring impulses—*non*sensory in nature—into the nucleus from the frontal and subfrontal regions. Several kinds of cells here, in the basal forebrain, serve also to excite the reticular nucleus, heighten its GABA inhibitory tone, and close the thalamic sensory gate.[14,15] On the other hand, selective local cooling will block this usual excitatory input from the frontal regions. And once this happens, a flood of enhanced visual transmission now surges through the lateral geniculate nucleus. It is followed by an increase in auditory transmission through the medial geniculate nucleus.

Can you also open the sensory gate, using *other* normal mechanisms? Yes. You can deliver (1) novel outside stimuli which arouse, or (2) direct electrical stimuli to the midbrain reticular formation.[16,17] Even a brief electrical stimulus to the midbrain inhibits some nerve cells up in the reticular nucleus. This lasts for a long *twenty seconds or more*. The mechanism is straightforward: when ACH is released by impulses coming up from the brain stem, this ACH stops the reticular nucleus nerve cells from firing.[14,17] In short, reticular *formation* excitation translates into reticular *nucleus* inhibition. And when the reticular nucleus pauses, more sensate messages flow through the thalamus.[11] On the other hand, both norepinephrine and glutamate can create faster tonic firing rates in reticular nucleus nerve cells.[18]

So, to sum up thus far, (1) *cortical excitatory states descend to excite the reticular nucleus and block sensation;* (2) *brainstem excitatory states ascend to inhibit the nucleus and allow more sensate messages to flow through the thalamus into consciousness.*

Changes in mentation are much more difficult to study than are changes in sensation.[10] Researchers have barely begun to inquire how the on/off properties of the reticular nucleus express themselves in the functions of the front part of the brain. As noted before, when the reticular nucleus does stop inhibiting the medial dorsal nucleus of the thalamus, the result translates into an increase in dopamine turnover up in the prefrontal cortex.[19] This implies that if one were suddenly to stop this reticular nucleus inhibition (by sending up an inhibitory pulse of ACH from the brain stem, for example), the result might cause a surge of dopamine activity to play over the medial frontal lobe. In this indirect, unexpected manner might an ACH pulse, perhaps when combined with a surge of DA, ST, and NE, create a long pause in reticular nucleus functions. Such a pause could last long enough to generate novel, secondary fluctuations of cognitive functions as high up as the frontal lobe.

Still, the reticular cap has one gaping "hole." The *anterior* thalamic nucleus escapes the cast of its inhibitory net. As a result, the anterior nucleus goes about its usual operations relatively independently. It avoids the processes of EEG spindling, and evades the usual, synchronizing effects which drowsiness and sleep exert on other brain regions.[6] Moreover, the anterior nucleus does not reach its peak of excitation by ACH for as long as fifty seconds *after* the ACH cells have fired down in the lateral dorsal tegmental region. But once the anterior nucleus is stimulated, its momentum carries it for as long as three minutes.[6] These observations suggest that when ACH from the brain stem finally does excite this anterior thalamic segment of the limbic circuit, its initial influence on a person's experience would lag behind the others, but would also last for a longer period (see figure 6).

How else, through several of its other related functions, could the reticular nucleus itself influence the range of meditative experience? Consider the ways it generates EEG spindles of hyperpolarization and rebound widely over the whole neocortex.[6] One might expect that such spindling (and the drowsiness which is its behavioral counterpart) would be the prevailing EEG theme *if* meditation had but a single relevant physiological mechanism, namely, always to "hold" drowsiness at one constantly fixed level. But several more subtle things may be going on. During prolonged meditative retreats, experienced meditators repeatedly pass up and down through many rapid, dynamic shifts in the spectrum between waking and sleeping. And, with practice, it is not mere drowsiness that they learn increasingly to hold on to. Rather it is a narrow or wide-open, one-pointed or global window of awareness and attention.

The distinction is important. For it is the *window of awareness* that meditators are training to keep open. Awareness remains paramount in importance, irrespective of whatever other physiological events may be going on that might tend to close or open the gates in the thalamus. So when meditators become increasingly skilled at holding on to states of awareness and attention, they may be gradually learning to uncouple these states, at least partially and experientially, from many of the brain's other recurring cycles and circuits.

Finally, after a long meditative prelude of weeks and months, a meditator's set-points change enough to shift into moments of deep absorption. Now an extraordinarily enhanced alerting takes over. Attention rises to new heights (see chapter 118). At such moments of attentional overload, the drawstring could close, and impulses from the bodily self would no longer be able to enter at the thalamic level.

At first, what this thin GABA nucleus seems to be preparing us for is a relatively novel concept: *a high-level blockade* caused by strong afferent inhibition. Even so, outside of it—*creating it* in fact—are other layers of extra excitation, still going on elsewhere. Suppose you were a subject who remained fully awake while these curious events were taking place. How would you experience such a state? This is what would drop *out* of your consciousness:

1. Vision

2. Hearing

3. Reference points for knowing where the head and eyes were positioned in three-dimensional space

4. Other proprioceptive, vestibular, and somatosensory input from the rest of the body (position sense and touch in particular)

Under these circumstances, some of your parietal lobe networks would be sensory-deprived. Shut off from their usual incoming data, they would have no sensate basis for embodying the usual coherent sense that you existed as a physical self. Nor could they help construct a concept about where this "no-self" was placed. Why not? Because no higher-order space existed that was defined by its more elaborate three-dimensional properties (see chapter 114).

The state described above could be envisioned as what happens when the reticular cap becomes exceptionally "tight." True, it would be shielding sensate messages from entering the higher matrix of consciousness, but *only those kinds that had usually coalesced at and above the thalamic level.*[20] For note where the block is placed. Its level is too high to interfere with all your usual *lower* primary and collateral sensory functions. These would still continue to operate normally all the way on up to the lower tier of thalamic nuclei. This means that useful position and touch information would still be entering into the operations of your spinal cord and brain stem. Moreover, visual reflex and reflex hearing functions would still continue in the superior and inferior colliculi.

Note that these more reflexive, lower-level sensate functions are the kind which normally go on *automatically* all the time. Normally, they do not rise into the foreground of consciousness and take the form of discrete "perceptions."[21] During absorption, furthermore, other unconscious proprioceptive functions would also be spared, those coming from the cerebellum and its vestibular connections. So even though you were a meditator who had been briefly "deafferented" up above, at the thalamic level, many of your basic circuits lower down would still be in operation. They would enable you to maintain normal tone, balance, and other reflex functions.[22]

Soon, in part IV, we will find that the four features of this sensate blockade cited above are commonplace, not novel. Indeed, they reflect only the garden-variety missions of the reticular nucleus: to shield our recumbent brain, as it rests, from the world of frenetic distractions coming in to it from both sides of our body and head.[20]

And later, in part VI, we return to this key nucleus further to clarify what happens to a fully alert person, one *not* sound asleep, whose window of awareness has just been thrown wide open.

61

The Pulvinar

> The seemingly simple and immediate perception of spatial relations conceals in fact a complex array of processes involved in the selection, assembly, and execution of visual routines.
>
> J. Allman[1]

The higher one ascends on the mammalian tree, the larger becomes the back of the thalamus. Finally it puffs out so much that anatomists gave it the Latin name *pulvinar* meaning "cushion." In present-day humans, a massive pulvinar now occupies one quarter of the thalamus[2] (see figure 11). Anything this size usually contributes something important. Another broad hint that our "higher functions" don't come from cortex alone but from cortex working in concert with its deep thalamic partners. In fact, the pulvinar is *the* essential thalamic counterpart for that vast sensate association cortex which covers the back of our brain.

So the pulvinar is not to be relegated to some lower-level functions which remain buried down in the "second" visual system (see table 5). In fact, its lateral nucleus also enters high up into an active dialogue with the posterior parietal cortex. Jointly, these regions sift critical data from a cluttered visual panorama, preparing it to enter into complex behaviors a few synapses later.[3] Because many other reciprocal connections exist between the pulvinar and the various visual areas, Allman and colleagues suggested that it functions as part of a "directing mechanism."[1] In this way, attention's "processing focus" could be shifted from one site to another, automatically, including shifts from internal to external loci. Indeed, recent human PET scan studies are in agreement with this theory. They show that the pulvinar becomes activated when we focus attention selectively on a central target in a otherwise "busy" visual field.[4] The medial pulvinar may also play a subtle role in memory circuits, because it shares many of the same connections as does the medial dorsal nucleus of the thalamus.[5]

After terminals from the pulvinar reach the visual cortex, they link up with the systems of long horizontal fibers which are interconnecting different regions of the cortex.[6] This architectural feature, common to the thalamus as a whole, enables it to integrate its functions into those that arise from the vertical cell columns stacked throughout the cortex.

The EEG reflects this intimate thalamocortical partnership. Recordings from the human pulvinar reveal that it emits its own prominent, spontaneous bursts of alpha waves. During such bursts, a subject who appears drowsy will still continue to perform his or her visual tasks adequately, although giving "the appearance of being an automaton."[7] And electrical stimulation of the pulvinar does evoke large amplitude alpha waves up in the cortex on both sides. But this doesn't occur until a long five to eight seconds later. Clearly, no stimuli this crude will enlighten us about the finer details of thalamocortical circuitry. Instead, the stimuli cause a disorderly, unphysiological discharge, one which jams most circuits. As a result, patients lose some of their visual functions for a few seconds after their right pulvinar has been stimulated. They can't discriminate patterns or develop an immediate visual memory, nor can they recognize random visual designs.

Stimulating the left pulvinar impairs speech. This suggests that the left pulvinar is semispecialized for language, as is its left cortical partner. Left-sided stimulation also interferes with a subject's finding the words to name objects. The disturbance erases even the names of objects which had been easily identified just before the stimulation began. Such findings may be relevant to the inexpressibility of brief mystical states. For when a person finds it difficult to describe things, or has a problem naming items, one cannot exclude the general possibility that some explanations might begin at *subcortical* sites. When the other thalamic nuclei are subjected to such stimulation or jamming, they are less likely to cause the same kinds of problems involving language, perception, or memory. So the pulvinar seems to play a distinctive role in *co*-operating and in *co*-sponsoring some of our "higher" associated functions related to vision and speech.

Arousal enhances the pulvinar's responses. It is when a monkey becomes aroused enough to show beta wave EEG activity that visual stimuli are most likely to cause the pulvinar's nerve cells to fire.[18] In the monkey's ventral lateral pulvinar, the average nerve cell will respond to any outside visual stimulus that enters within a field about 70 degrees square. But still other pulvinar neurons have huge response fields encompassing 1600 degrees square.[8] And the pulvinar has a few cells which deploy giant response fields. *These encompass a visual stimulus that enters from anywhere in the visual panorama of space.* Obviously, these neurons will not convey point-to-point visual representations. Most other pulvinar cells deploy their visual response fields to both sides of the outside visual environment, or to either the right or left side. Yet, some cells are also tuned to respond to visual stimuli that arrive from the very center of focused vision. In this respect, their properties resemble those we have noted in nerve cells of the inferior temporal cortex.[9]

Of interest to humans who meditate in subdued light are cells in the lateral pulvinar. They change their firing rates whenever a monkey is exposed to light—or to darkness—for sustained periods. These properties might assist other cells in the inferior temporal cortex to recognize visual patterns—even through the background lighting was dim—by increasing the contrast and by sharpening up salient features in the foreground.[9]

The visual cortex uses its fast glutamate pathways to excite the pulvinar.[10] Acetylcholine coming up from the parabrachial nuclei provides another source of stimulation. This ACH "presets" the pulvinar's threshold at a lower level. Now, with its set-point changed, the pulvinar fires more in response to all the other input it receives from the colliculi and surrounding regions.[11,12]

In humans, the left pulvinar has norepinephrine levels half-again higher than on the right.[13] Norepinephrine probably brings its subtle influence to bear on momentary sensory and perceptual processes and on the thalamoreticular ongoing traffic which flows tonically between the thalamus and cortex.[14] However, biogenic amines and other modulators might still exert their special kinds of "synaptic leverage" on thalamocortical functions. That is, if their messages arrived at just the right time, they might allow both cortex and thalamus to reinforce each other neurophysiologically.[15] Suppose, for example, that NE were to block certain GABA circuits, locally, in the pulvinar. The result could not only help attention shift quickly but it might also help to infuse other lively and direct qualities into perception.[16] Clearly, we need to know more about how the amine systems might go on to influence mentation when their effects are leveraged simultaneously at several levels.

Human beings have inherited a very large pulvinar. To what end? Increasingly, researchers are awakening to the implications of this encompassing, thalamic cushion. The pulvinar and its connections appear to make an initial contribution to *salience*. Salience is the process which automatically grasps items in our visual and auditory space, holds onto them, and permits them to be transformed into subjects of particular, meaningful interest. But the collective heads of the neuroscientists have thus far barely indented this soft thalamic cushion. We need now to define precisely how the pulvinar functions in our daily, waking lives.[17] Then its role in Zen will be increasingly obvious.

It is time now to move on to consider our higher levels of attention. Before doing so, it will be useful to sum up the major themes of the thalamus and its nuclei. As a simple aid to memory, it may help to use a few words that all start with the letter *S*. *Salience*, then, would be what the pulvinar inserts into our sensate world. The medial dorsal nucleus helps influence frontal *scenarios*. The anterior nucleus infuses *sensual* gratifications. The intralaminar nuclei *stimulate*. The lateral geniculate nucleus *sees*. And the reticular nucleus acts as a *shield*.

62

Higher Mechanisms of Attention

> Time flies like an arrow, so be careful not to waste energy on trivial matters. Be attentive! Be attentive!
>
> Master Daito Kokushi (1283–1337)[1]

To focus a camera on a maple leaf seems a simple act. Yet it sets in motion a hierarchy of circuitries. These transform attention, literally, into an "associative function."[2,3] Pivotal to Zen are the networks of attention which interact in the regions we have just finished discussing. These are the prefrontal cortex, the posterior parietal cortex, the cingulate gyrus, and the thalamus. Especially on the right side.

For example, normal subjects increase the metabolic activity in their *right* midfrontal cortex when they stay attentive to a simple auditory task.[4] In agreement with this finding, patients who have sustained damage to their *right* frontal lobe cannot pay attention during a monotonous, repetitive task.[5,6] One wonders, does this same asymmetry occur as the result of meditative practices which train attention? When I was following my own breathing movements, was this the kind of focused act that could be a subtle "training exercise" for some distant attentional networks that chiefly involved my right frontal lobe? (see chapter 64). Large-scale, controlled studies of meditation that employ neuroimaging techniques similar to those used for the PET scan in figure 12 may help answer such questions.

The prefrontal regions also seem to take part in our more *willed* forms of anticipatory focusing. No sharp dividing line separates these higher-order, more "strategic" and willfully intended mechanisms from the lower, more tactical decisions which automatically fix our attention. Normal subjects use the upper *inner* parts of their prefrontal cortex when they perform the more automatic types of motor tasks which have been so "overlearned" that they are habitual.[7]

The word "neglect" is used to imply the opposite of paying attention. It describes the way a lesioned subject *won't* respond to visual or touch stimuli coming from the opposite side of its environment (see chapter 15). Lesions at several hierarchial levels cause neglect. Among them, in the monkey, are lesions which damage the prefrontal cortex on either side. Metabolic studies clarify why this inattentive monkey doesn't respond. The results show that *other distant regions have also been disabled. These regions are, in a sense, "downstream" from the frontal region itself.*[8] Consider what happens clinically to a monkey who has had a *right* frontal lesion. He neglects the apple and other stimuli off to the left side of his environment. In his brain, the metabolic activity drops one third in the *right* basal ganglia, and it also drops 12 to 22 percent far down in the *right* superior colliculus. Yes, one may speak loosely of "frontal lobe" neglect. But the fact is that frontal lesions go on to cause secondary hypofunctions within several related *sub*cortical circuits. And the net result is that many kinds of functions linked to attention drop out downstream. Clearly, our frontal circuits normally exert their influence through other widely distributed systems.

Earlier, we asked, could those mechanisms which—in neglect—are *under*functioning go on to *hyper*function during a state of hyperattention? (see chapter 15). It now becomes easier to envision how this might occur. Both frontal and parietal circuits—linked as usual, hand in glove—could have their attentive functions amplified. Their networks in the *right* hemisphere in particular could help activate and direct visual attention not only straight ahead but off to the periphery as well.[9] Indeed, normally, it is these same two *right*-sided frontoparietal partners which will yield the larger evoked responses when they are responding to visual and other sensory stimuli.[10]

Electrical potential studies of the brain show that, normally, we bring our right parietal attention systems into play as soon as one-tenth of a second after a visual stimulus appears off in the periphery of space.[11] And during a generalized *bilateral* increase in attention, the right parietal region again shows the greater additional increase in its visual evoked responses.[12] In contrast, our left hemisphere directs its attention primarily to the right side of space, not to both sides.

Moreover, studies of human reaction times suggest that it is our right cerebral hemisphere which chiefly engages in the kinds of "premotoric" functions that prepare *both* sides of our body to respond behaviorally. It is this kind of normal deliberate, anticipatory preparation for action which goes by the term *intention.*[13,14] And when extensive right-sided lesions damage these functions, the patients neglect events that are taking place on *both* sides of their extrapersonal environment. This means they have lost the ability to direct attention *globally.*

Seven centuries ago, Daito Kokushi reemphasized how vital attention was to Zen. Recently, researchers have learned much about attention's finer details, basing their studies on a series of single parietal nerve cells in trained monkeys. The monkey sits quietly. It has learned that it will be rewarded when it actively directs its attention to fix on a central visual target.[15] Its parietal cells then become extraexcitable during this attentive fixation behavior, firing rapidly for up to five seconds. Note that this particular attentive process is a step above and beyond the monkey's preexisting, basic level of arousal or vigilance. For at this point the monkey is superimposing *an extra, independent, higher level of state control.*

The easiest way to test an animal's visual responses is to use a moving stimulus. So when researchers first tested parietal nerve cells to find out if they had "visual" properties, they began by asking, Do these cells fire when they "see" an outside stimulus which *moves* within their visual field? They made sure that the monkey remained in its "ready" state of "interested fixation," with its visual attention directed straight ahead. Soon, they found that the monkey's parietal cells were attentive to moving stimuli at the *outside edge of its visual fields*, on both sides. Indeed, these were the cells which yielded an outer, rounded "halo of very high visual sensitivity." It was not those other cells occupied with the central fixation point.[15]

Some parietal cells also fire vigorously if the monkey focuses on some object, like an apple, which it finds motivationally important. Others fire even when *attention itself*, not gaze, is directed off toward something merely glimpsed "out of the corner of the eye."[16] Researchers discovered these latter, "pure attention" cells when they trained the monkey further. Now, though it still needed to keep *looking* straight ahead, its main task was to deploy its *attention* off to a *secondary* visual target. This secondary target was a light off to the side. Now the monkey's job was to detect when this side light was being dimmed.[17]

We don't have to look far for a human analogy. Consider the classic "cocktail party phenomenon." We too have evolved skills that enable us to look in one direction while still tuning in, covertly, to monitor a different conversation off to the side. So this monkey experiment showed that some parietal nerve cells have this capacity to shift into a *higher level of directed spatial attention*. In chapter 116, we discuss the unique kind of visual attention, in humans, which looks far out into space. In that chapter, the more global aspects of this kind of spatial attention will become especially relevant. And so too will some physiological findings discussed in the next section below.

The parietal nerve cells, which possess visual properties, have extralarge visual fields. As many as 68 percent of the cells tested in one study could even "see" stimuli entering from *both* sides of their outside world.[16] Some cells also extended their response area to include the slender "temporal crescent." Where is this C-shaped responsive zone? It is the outermost rim of each visual field. It is, for example, the farthest crescent-shaped edge, off to the left, that can be seen with the left eye.

Area PG and Area V4

We have much to learn from the special visual properties of two groups of cortical cells. Each is a critical nodal point in the brain's widely distributed system of attention. One cluster lies in the inferior parietal lobule, in an area called PG (see figure 2). The other group of cells is in an area called V4. V4 is part of the visual association cortex, several synapses removed from the primary visual cortex.[18]

The monkeys in the experiments now cited are trained to fixate attentively on a small, centrally placed target light. They are rewarded each time they correctly signal that this *central* light has dimmed. So their task now requires two overlapping skills: (1) persistent, centrally directed attentive fixation; (2) keen, *central* visual discrimination. When would you use skills of this type? When you needed to focus your camera on the fine details of a leaf. And when the monkey performs *its* central fixation task, both PG cells and V4 cells greatly increase their firing rate, three- to fourfold. What might help stimulate them into doing so? Both the upper relays of the reticular activating system and the pulvinar.[18]

The monkey also takes time off, resting quietly between its formal task periods. Even so, he remains alert, anticipating the next task yet to come. And during this quiet, alert interval, only the V4 cells remain "on-line." Only *they* keep firing three to four times as much as before. They seem to have—and to keep—their "intentional" properties.

These V4 cells are not simply a relay site between the primary visual cortex and the inferior temporal lobe.[19] V4 cells are also *very color-sensitive*. Color turns them on. The fact that they discharge in response to color will help us understand how a hallucinated leaf could be so vividly colored (see chapter 113).

The nerve cells in the other visual area, PG, are different. When the monkey rests, they rest. However, once PG nerve cells are actively firing during their task of attentive fixation, they *seem to be registering the precise spot where the visual stimulus lies in the coordinates of external space.* Moreover, when they do so, *they refer back to that same egocentric perspective* which long ago had set up the physical self of this observing monkey as their central point of reference.[20]

Now, PG cells also base their internal standards of reference on the position of the monkey's eyes, not only on where its head is located.[21] Moreover, these head and eye reference systems interact in a dynamic way. When do some PG cells respond best? When the origin of the incoming visual stimulus lies 20 degrees *below* the horizontal in *head*-centered space; and *if*, at the same time, the *eyes* are also directed 20 degrees *down* from *their* horizontal position. These positions meet the optimum requirements for attention. It will not have escaped the attentive reader's notice how closely they resemble the position of gaze, with the eyes open and lowered, during zazen meditation.

Some neurological diseases derange attention, and in distinctive ways. After lesions of the thalamus, patients have problems *engaging* their attention. In addition, they can't efficiently process the visual information which is coming from the opposite side of their environment.[22] In contrast, after parietal lesions, patients are slow to *dis*engage their attention. Farther down, still other patients—those who have midbrain damage—are basically *slow* to *move* their visual attention. Herein, at these several levels, may lie clues to why our normal perceptions sometimes take on a quickened, direct, immediate quality. Could it be that at such moments we are experiencing extrafast processing speeds throughout these very same attentional circuits?

Looking, and Seeing Preattentively

You observe a lot by watching.

Yogi Berra[1]

Most "looking" goes on automatically. It expresses our strong, innate tendency to gaze at an object, a kind of "visual grasp reflex." Much of this reflex stems from the superior colliculus of the midbrain[2] (see figure 3). Yet we can choose where we want to look. Our higher frontal lobe "gaze centers" can override our reflex eye movements, using circuits that descend to the midbrain and pons.[3]

On the sensory side, we have just noted that the inferior parietal lobule has special "eye-position" nerve cells.[4] They register, subliminally, where the eyes are positioned *within the orbits* when they fix on a target. A distinctive sensation rises into awareness during the state of internal absorption. It feels as though one's eyes and vision itself are being *held* fixed on whatever is being perceived (see chapter 108). It suggests that the above gaze mechanisms have been amplified and have now taken a firm grip on the motoric act of looking.

We look at much more than we "see." Each second, by gross estimates, somewhere between 10^7 and 10^{11} bits of afferent information smite our various sensory end organs.[5] To shelter us from this barrage, the normal brain engages in an enormous filtering operation.[6] Only the rare stimulus, murmuring the right password, manages to pass through. As a result, consciousness finally registers and perceives only a mere sixteen to twenty bits of information each second.

These striking exclusionary properties of the brain require no formal act of attention on our part. They are *preattentive*. They go on automatically (table 8).

Table 8
Contrasts between Preattentive and Willed Processing

Aspect	Preattentive Processing	Willed Attentive Processing
Speed	Fast	Slow
General level	Automatic; preconscious	Volitional, controlled; more conscious
Amount of previous training	Considerable	Less
Conscious attention	Not a prerequisite	A prerequisite
Modifiable	Less easily	More easily
Capacity	Unlimited	Limited by short-term storage requirements
Type of processing	More parallel	More serial
Field	Large	Small
Degree of effort	Effortless	More effortful
Time frame	Less than one-twentieth of a second	Linked sequences of perceptual windows, each about one-twentieth of a second

Preattentive processing is fast, effortless, not constrained within the limited capacity of short-term memory. Nor are such preconscious functions easily learned, through deliberate efforts at training. But once acquired they are very difficult to change.[7]

Contrast this with our familiar type of willed attentive processing. We *control* it. We pay a price for consciously focusing our attention. Its capacity is very limited, and it is far slower. Suppose, for example, you decide to focus your conscious attention on a visuospatial task. It will take as long as 80 to 130 milliseconds before its associated electrical potential shows up in the brain.[8] Yet this willed attentive processing has advantages: you can adopt it quickly and can modify it more readily.

Preattentive vision effortlessly scans a wide area.[9] Within a mere one-twentieth of a second it (a) detects conspicuous features, (b) transforms them into the sets which represent the "figure," and (c) relegates irrelevant items to the "background." All this seem instantaneous. But only because it takes place four times faster than gaze mechanisms move our eyes. Well-trained monkeys do even better. It takes them only eight to fifteen milliseconds of retinal exposure to differentiate a square from a triangle.[10] So, at most, the monkey performs this act of preattentive discrimination in a mere one-sixty-seventh of a second.

In contrast, our willed attentive vision feels more effortful, yet it too collects several items during relatively small, successive, apertures of time. Each of these "windows" of serial attention lasts only about fifty milliseconds (one-twentieth of a second). Our thread of conscious attention pulls together a number of these brief sequences, and strings them together like rosary beads.

Recent experiments illustrate how very different these fast and slow processes are. Suppose you look at a sheet of paper, finding it covered with several letters of the alphabet. Most letters have *straight* lines: either green **X**'s or brown **T**'s. A rare letter curves. It is an **S**, also either brown or green. These **S**'s pop out from the mixture. Their shape makes them leap out immediately. This *happens*. This is preattentive processing. No thinking. *When an item pops out instantly like this, it suggests that parallel processes are operating* (see chapter 91).

Try looking at another sample of test paper. There, you will instantly spot the green **X**. It stands out clearly from among the many brown **X**'s. But where is a *green* **T?** You must hunt a long time to detect that rare **T**, hiding among those many **X**'s which it resembles. Why does it take so long? Because in this instance you are engaging in a two-step procedure, using both color *and* shape as conjunctive features. This means that you must shift toward *serial*, step-by-step processing. *In the serial mode, everything slows down.*[11]

There is an earlier and a later phase of selection even within preattention itself. The first step is more global, and is designed to admit stimuli only if they are more probable. The second step processes more details. It considers their context, notes any unpleasant implications, and engages in higher elaborations of probability.[6]

Suppose you volunteer to be the subject in an even simpler experiment. This time, all you need to do is come to a snap decision about a boundary.[12] It is an either/or decision. Your task is to look quickly at a closed, curving line, then conclude: Does a small x lie inside this curved line or outside? Inside outside? Instantly, in less than fifty milliseconds, you have your answer. No effort is involved.

Is preattention relevant to Zen? Yes, for three reasons. First, it illustrates how automatically we make distinctions between self (read inside) and other (outside). And we probably resolve such self/other decisions even faster than those distinctions you made about where the small x was placed in this experiment. After all, years of practice have firmly established the deep physiological premises which are the basis for our self/other distinctions. We call the surface layer "self-consciousness." The phrase acknowledges the sense that we are each grounded in an *I*, *Me*, and *Mine* (see chapter 9, figure 1).

The second reason is that similar ultrafast properties also characterize consciousness during the state of insight-wisdom (see part VII). This peak experience goes on to blend extraordinary perceptive, associative, and global discriminitive abilities. Again, such attributes speak for enhanced parallel processing.

The third reason is that, during internal absorption, the experiant arrives at an entirely new definition of heightened awareness. True, it has "expanded" far beyond its usual spatial boundaries. Yet in the process, response time seems to have *contracted*. The sense is that, with the leading edge of awareness having now shifted forward, *stimuli are contacting it earlier than usual.* This feeling is well described by the term *immediacy* (see chapter 118). Stimuli seem to be striking, and becoming percepts milliseconds sooner than usual, out in what was previously the domain of the *pre*attentive. Moreover, within the present moment, the stimuli are instantly absorbed as soon as they strike. The final blend makes for a heightened, quickened NOW. It fuses two remarkable qualities: immediacy and direct perception.

At ordinary levels of living, we keep paying another hidden price to be sheltered by all our preattentive layers. For we constructed these layers to admit only those things that our conditioning led us to believe were relevant. Sheltered by our biased preselection processes, we mindlessly perpetuate old unfruitful habits and prejudiced attitudes. Moreover, much of this preattentive protection makes it very difficult for perception to fully open up to the true miracle of each event of everyday living. Can Zen training become "sensitivity training?" Can it actually reshape what finally enters our brains?

It can't be an easy matter. We have available only a fixed quantity of resources for visual processing according to most theoretical models of attention. This means that only by shifts in priorities can preattentive mechanisms enable change to occur. On the other hand, inherent within parallel processing rests some of this capacity for change. Why? Because it has three modes of operating: spatial, temporal, and functional.[12] *Spatial* processing will apply the same kind of parallel operation at the same time to all visual items wherever they are placed in space. This mode enables us to generalize and to make such distinctions as "inside" from "outside," "self" from "other." Its partner, *temporal* processing, applies different operations. These address different items which arrive at various times. *Functional* processing also applies different routines, but all at the same time, and to one place in space.

One wonders: suppose a person were suddenly to drop all the old premises which had governed these three ordinary processing modes. What would happen? One result would be a state of consciousness empty of its former preattentive criteria, an experiant who was no longer set up to process—the same way as before—those basic distinctions: "self" from "other," "now" from "then," "here" from "there." This opening and awakening is the insight of kensho.

Meditators also have available other, slower-acting techniques which can enable them to break away from habitual forms of automatic processing. Deikman used the term "deautomatization" to describe these techniques.[13] The age-old meditative practice of "mindfulness" is one step in this direction. Mindfulness, we recall, means paying *bare* attention to ongoing perceptions. In doing so, each such action, and perception itself, gradually becomes invested with much more than the outworn careless amount of inattention. Events are no longer processed automatically. Now, reattended to *individually*, they finally become *de*automatized.[13] *This* breath. *This* step. *This* mouthful.

But to become *this* mindful of the world, the person must first slow down. Only then does one begin to *really look at life, observe it,* and start to *see it afresh* for what it really is. And this is one of the major functions of meditation: to reduce distractions and slow the flow. With time, the person regains that inherently open perspective which deepens to appreciate the whole rich tapestry of living. Slowly then, one can begin to revise that preexisting, biased rush toward judgment through innumerable synapses. Gradually, one starts to establish whole *new* patterns of impulse flow in different association networks.

Openness, revision, and restructuring. Zen's major tasks. None of it is easy.

64

Laboratory Correlates of Awareness, Attention, Novelty, and Surprise

Is it a fact—or have I dreamt it—that by means of electricity, the world of matter has become a great nerve, vibrating thousands of miles in a breathless point of time?
Nathaniel Hawthorne (1804–1864)[1]

Step by step, throughout part III, we have been describing the functional anatomical substrate on which psychophysiology is based. Until recent decades, researchers had no practical ways to define the dynamic functions of these regions in human subjects. Now many tests are available to clarify the kinds of functions of special interest to Zen.

PET Scans

One technique is positron emission tomography. Its acronym is PET. A PET scan is a kind of "metabolic map" of the living brain. The method centers on a simple principle: nerve cells burn glucose for energy. They use more glucose when they fire actively. By using a form of *tagged* glucose, researchers can localize the place where it is burned in the brain. One can tag deoxyglucose, for example, with the element fluorine 18, which emits a positron. After this labeled glucose analog is injected into an arm vein, it goes to the brain. Here its positron "lights up" the most metabolically active regions. These most active sites are then refined into an anatomical image with the aid of computed x-ray tomographic techniques.

In figure 12 and the color plate, the viewer is looking down at a PET scan of both sides of the brain. What it shows are metabolic images projected on a kind of "slab," called a transaxial section. The frontal lobes are at the top. The right side is at the viewer's right. Red equals the regions of highest metabolic activity. Blue represents inactive regions, including the fluid spaces inside the brain.

I was the subject of the deoxyglucose images in this figure. I was lying quietly with eyes masked, and ears plugged lightly with cotton. I was resting, letting go of thoughts, concentrating on the movements of abdominal breathing. Aware. No koan.

Metabolic activity is prominent in two of my basal ganglia nuclei, the caudate and putamen, and in the thalamus. Up in the cortex, activity is prominent over the middle, inferior, triangular, and opercular regions of the frontal lobes, as well as in the transverse and superior temporal gyrus. Still more posteriorly, metabolic activity is also especially high in the innermost depths of the parietal lobe, the precuneus, and in the cuneus, which itself lies farthest forward in the occipital lobe. Some activity is also shown in the hippocampus and in the posterior cingulate gyrus (compare with figures 2 and 3).

The viewer notices more red on the *right side* in each of the cortical regions cited. This right-sided preponderance of cortical activity is evident especially in the deeper regions of the parietal and occipital cortex. There it lies within the retrosplenial region which extends next to the midline behind the corpus callosum.

The subject is strongly right-handed, right-eyed, and from a family of right-handers. The left hemisphere is presumably dominant for language. So, the differences between the data from the two sides reflect, therefore, the conditions of the study: a nonverbal state of mental and physical relaxation, of external visual and auditory blockage, and of awareness simplified—at least to the degree that the field of awareness can be simplified while one is practicing meditation as an experimental subject in a relatively quiet laboratory setting.

Additional PET studies were performed during the same period in this same laboratory on twenty-eight other normal control subjects.[2] The conditions were slightly different. These controls were merely resting, not meditating. Their eyes were closed, but their ears were not plugged. Still, the results showed trends in the opposite direction: higher oxygen metabolism over most *left* cortical regions. And, as noted in chapter 23, it is in their *right* hemisphere that normals tend to *drop* their metabolism the most after both hearing and vision are blocked.

Other PET studies elsewhere have chosen expectant subjects who, again, were *not* meditating. Their goal was to sustain attention on an auditory discrimination task. This meant that they were expecting to be presented with a tone which would arrive through *both* earphones simultaneously. The tone could be at

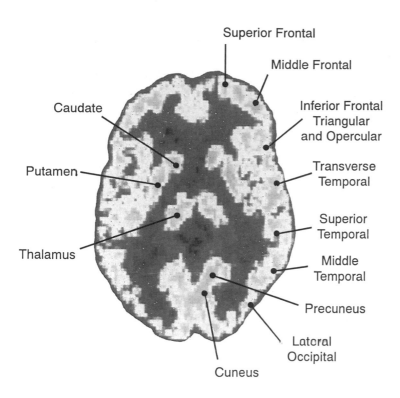

Figure 12 A positron emission tomography (PET) scan during a period of relaxed awareness
Before this scan, 7.2 millicuries of ^{18}F-deoxyglucose were injected intravenously (iv) and equili-
brated during the next hour. Following this, recordings were obtained using a Headtome IV
scanner throughout the subsequent two hours. These studies were performed in 1988 in the
Radiology and Nuclear Medicine Department of the Research Institute for Brain and Blood Vessels, Akita, Japan. I am greatly indebted to Drs. Hidehiro Ida, Iwao Kanno, Fumio Sushido, and
Kazuo Uemura for performing the PET scan, and to Dr. Hideaki Fujita for his assistance in localizing the metabolic activity neuroanatomically. Refined neuroimaging technologies are now available which make it possible to study many meditators quickly, in greater detail, and to draw
statistically significant conclusions.

any one of three intensities, varied at random: loud, louder, loudest. Their task
was to signal only when the faintest tone arrived. Under these conditions, the
right middle frontal region also showed the greatest increase in metabolism, some
5 to 7 percent.[3]

A subsequent PET report was based on eight subjects, studied during yoga
meditation.[4] The general trend was toward reduced metabolism in the posterior
regions of cortex. In this report, neither the control period nor the period of yoga
meditation revealed differences between the right and left hemispheres.

The PET technique, good for general mapping, misses small details. It also
has certain physiological limitations. Suppose metabolic activity does increase in
one location. A PET scan *alone* cannot tell you that the local increase comes from
the activity of nerve cells which serve only excitatory functions. It might represent
cells which are also burning glucose while in the act of serving inhibitory functions. And quantitative measurements are required. Otherwise, one can't be sure
how much of the greater activity on one side is the reflection of lesser activity

on the other side. To arrive at absolute measurements involves drawing blood samples through the wall of an artery, an invasive procedure which causes some pain, apprehension, and is not without complications. Current methods require very long sampling times. Therefore, they miss the more interesting changes taking place in seconds or a few minutes.

A newer technique of imaging is called functional magnetic resonance imaging (functional MRI or fMRI). It offers a faster way to image the activity of the entire brain over the course of several seconds. This technique is based on the principle of following patterns of blood flow as the flow shifts toward the most active parts of the brain.

Brain Potentials

Figure 12 illustrates that a brain does not remain passive at rest. Its screening functions go on, preconsciously, in milliseconds which race too fast for thoughts, and far too fast to be measured by ordinary EEG methods. Fortunately, researchers now have available other sensitive "electrical" techniques. They begin by delivering standardized stimuli such as flashes of light or sounds.[5] Then, as Hawthorne anticipated, the brain vibrates with faint electrical potentials, radiating them throughout its universe. Again, investigators depend on computers to amplify a series of weak signals into measurable physiological waveforms, responses called *evoked potentials.*

The early peaks are high and jagged. They reflect the initial leaps which nerve impulses take across the first several sensory synapses. These early potentials arise in circuits which are basically fixed and "hard-wired." Thus, when a flash of light enters the small brain of a cat, it generates a peak twelve milliseconds later in the visual cortex. Not until thirty milliseconds later does a peak arise in an intralaminar nucleus of the thalamus, and not until forty-five milliseconds later, in the reticular formation.[6]

Attention takes on special interest in Zen. So do sudden, surprising, triggering events. Several refined tests, now available, make it possible to study meditators repeatedly, at deeper meditative levels, and to monitor their brains' electrical correlates of attention, novelty, and surprise. One such test monitors the potential which develops when a person pays *special* attention. Imagine that you are the expectant subject. You are waiting for the arrival of a well-anticipated stimulus. *Which* stimulus are you expecting: a sound, touch, or visual flash? Will it come from one or both sides? It makes a difference. If your brain has been poised to respond to a *visual* flash, the stimulus will shift one of its early visual evoked potentials farther off than usual in the electronegative direction. Normally, this *selective attention potential* begins its shift in the negative direction some sixty milliseconds after the visual stimulus arrives, and it keeps shifting for as long as the next half-second.

Electrodes that record from the right frontal region show the most obvious evidence of this extranegativity during selective attention. But the negative potential clearly has deeper, *subcortical* origins, because the interval is too short between stimulus and response for it to have arisen up in cortex alone. Candidates among the subcortical sites are the lateral geniculate nucleus, the superior colliculus, and the pulvinar.[7] One inference is that these deeper subcortical regions constitute a system of several "gates." Another is that the right frontal lobe will "consult" its own prior sets of attention or intention, before acting in a sense to "nudge" such gates so that they open more widely.

Suppose your next task as a subject is to *listen* with anticipation. You know you will hear a *random sound* stimulus at some time or other. But you don't know which earphone it will come into. Note that this task differs from the one chosen for the last PET study cited above. For now, your task requires you to stay globally alert. A sound could come from *either* direction. Under these circumstances, your *left* prefrontal region then tends to show the greater negative shift. In contrast, when you deploy attention toward tones which you've already been informed will enter only the left ear, it is your *right* prefrontal region which predominates. Patients don't develop these normal anticipatory negative potentials to sound stimuli after they have sustained damage to their prefrontal regions, especially to those on the left side.[5]

The studies cited above raise intriguing questions. Suppose some of our usual "attentive," prefrontal circuitries—on *both* sides together—were to greatly *enhance* their activities. Could researchers measure what would happen? Could such amplified frontal states spill over to increase the efficiency and the scope of their parietal counterparts? If so, then what new experiential dimensions could be generated by such amplified "tuning-in" processes? As we see next, the answers will not come easily. The studies must take into account the fact that many of our frontal lobe contributions are "soft." They hinge on what our prevailing mental set is. They will vary, depending on what next we are expecting the overall setting to yield.

Novelty and Surprise

Consider, for example, what happens when the frontal lobes encounter novel situations. Now they can contribute to a different kind of potential. Why is it known as the P300? Because it is a positive (P) waveform which doesn't arrive until a long 300 milliseconds *after* some outside signal, such as the stimulus of a sound.[8,9] If a stimulus takes this long, 0.3 second, to evoke a potential in the human brain, it has been filtering through layers of synapses. Some of the resulting impulses could have been conferring (or related to) our prior "cognitive sets" or other "soft-wired" associative mechanisms. Indeed, when a potential arrives this late, and is shaped more like a rounded foothill than a jagged peak, it would seem as though the brain had been making quasi-mental, reflexive associations at several different levels.[8,10]

When researchers test for the responses to novelty in the laboratory, they select only a certain kind of sound stimulus. It will be (a) one so exceptional that the person never expects it at all, or (b) one delivered infrequently. Suppose, for example, you are again a naive subject. Much will depend on which mental set you're in. Your prior set determines both the shape and the distribution of your subsequent potentials. If the sound stimulus takes you totally by surprise, your

P300 waveform comes earlier. Furthermore, it is then most prominent over your *frontal* regions. In contrast, if the uncommon sound was one that you had reason to anticipate, your *parietal* regions show the maximum potential.

In each instance, the acoustic aspects of the sound stimulus stay exactly the same. Same sound. *Different mental set.* Your brain responded preconsciously. Each split-second distinction preempted thought, bypassed internal language, and sharply differentiated the novel stimulus from its identical twin, the stimulus you had been expecting.

The differences between the two responses highlight the contrasts between the functions of our frontal and parietal lobes. To oversimplify, one might speculate that a totally new sound stimulus presents an element of shock-surprise. The brain reacts almost with a kind of what-was-that? response. Noteworthy is the frontal distribution of this potential. Perhaps herein lies the hint that subcortical circuits leading up to the frontal lobes are starting to prepare for whatever their next best course of action should be (see chapter 57). It is of interest that patients lose much of this endogenous "surprise"-type response to novel stimuli after having had damage to their prefrontal lobes.

In contrast, the element of surprise is much less when a long anticipated stimulus finally arrives. Then the mental configuration seems more in the direction of, There it finally is! This particular "there" response has a more parietal distribution. Perhaps it reflects the fact that parietal circuits are poised to ask "where" questions, and have cells which participate in a variety of attentive functions (see chapter 55).

Imagine, finally, that you are still a normal subject, different only in that you have been meditating frequently during a long retreat.[11] Now you are not merely calm. You have become deepened, open, and extra aware. Even so, you are still not expecting suddenly to be overwhelmed by any stimulus event from the outside world. Abruptly a novel stimulus strikes. It is a total surprise: a sudden CRACK of the wooden clappers; the CRASH of a cup, the CLACK of a pebble against bamboo. Or a roshi's shout, designed to jar you. Given your prevailing mental set, and in this setting, the depths of your brain might respond with a major frontoparietal response.

So we have come to one of zazen's less appreciated contributions. It creates more detached pauses which last longer and go deeper. Into these gaps, random novel events might sometimes thrust swiftly, deeply, productively. Soon we will go on to explore states of consciousness (see part IV). Later, we return to consider how the impact of such triggering events can precipitate the awakening of kensho (see chapter 105).

Biological Theories: What Causes Mystical Experiences?
How Does Meditation Act?

What is all science then
but pure religion seeking everywhere
the true commandments?

Alfred Noyes (1880–1958)

It helps to know about old theories. They're useful. They remind you that your own theories can be outgrown as soon as more facts become available.

After the studies of Hess, it became customary to think that two functional systems managed our energies in opposite ways.[1] However, these early trophotropic/ergotropic distinctions lacked precision when they were tested, especially in humans and other socialized primates.[2] Soon the ambiguities were compounded, because Gelhorn and Kiely tried to use these same two opposing systems to explain meditation and mystical states of consciousness.[3] They hypothesized that the reduced muscle tone during meditative relaxation led to a loss of the "ergotropic tone of the hypothalamus," a loss soon to be followed by a "dominance of the trophotropic system."

And what was an "emptiness of consciousness?" They regarded it as the psychological concomitant of shifting into the trophotropic mode. Moreover, in their view, when a person made an intensified effort to maintain this "emptiness"—but not to lose consciousness—then this effort would cause an increase of excitation within the ergotropic system. It followed, they believed, that yogic ecstasy represented a further heightening of such ergotropic activity. A grain of truth in each proposition.

Yet, in many instances, the evidence cited by Gelhorn and Kiely was based on destructive lesions too large and electrical stimulations too intense to be appropriate in the light of our present knowledge. Mills and Campbell further contended that the theories had (1) ignored basic differences inside and among the various meditative traditions, (2) failed to consider important findings in yoga meditation, and (3) provided an ambiguous interpretation of the way the opposing systems might affect the orienting reflex.[4] Kiely's rejoinder suggested that ecstatic states corresponded physiologically with REM sleep, in the sense that each had low voltage fast EEG activity plus an increased heart rate, coupled with a lack of increased muscle tension.[5] He also argued that the two states of ecstasy and REM sleep corresponded psychologically. That is, they each blurred the sense of time, place, and personal boundaries.

Fischer went on to develop a cartography that would define mystical rapture as an ecstatic state placed at one extreme end of the ergotropic scale.[6] He then regarded yogic samadhi as the opposite extreme, and placed it at the other end of the trophotropic scale. His map went on to connect the two, rapture and samadhi, with a figure-eight–shaped loop. The loop was intended to represent "the trophotropic rebound, which is observed in response to intense ergotropic hyper-arousal." The rebound, which was proposed to go from ergotropic ecstasy on the one hand to yogic samadhi on the other, was believed to engage that particular form of yogic samadhi which had no thought content. In Fischer's circular version of this map, a subject could travel to inner space and lose the personal I by follow-ing either of two paths: the route of perception-hallucination, or the route of perception-meditation.

Davidson suggested that the techniques of hyperexcitement used by the Sufis and by various revivalist groups represented a hyperactivated ergotropic state.[7] He accepted the idea that shifting back and forth from ergotropic to tropho-tropic states could be conducive to different states of consciousness, as it would be to meditative and mystical experience in general. Still, he emphasized that the total cognitive set and setting would be decisive. These were the elements that would determine both the content of the conscious experiences and the way that the subjects interpreted them, based on their own particular belief systems. Even then, he pointed out, such a model was "unsatisfyingly vague." Why? Because it didn't clarify what had *caused* the person to switch from normal to alternate states of consciousness. A model must specify cause.

In this regard, Mandell developed a theory of "transcendence" heavily weighted toward serotonergic mechanisms as being the causal agents[8] (see chap-ter 42). It drew not only on the pharmacological effects of the amphetamines, on cocaine, and on the hallucinogens, but on several other phenomena as well. The drugs were postulated to induce "an acute loss of serotonergic regulation of tem-poral lobe limbic structures, releasing the affectual and cognitive processes char-acteristic of religious ecstasy and the permanent personality changes associated with religious conversion."[8] He cited two other circumstances as also causing a loss of ST inhibitory tone: (1) previous excessive firing of median raphe cells caused by stress or by hyperactivity. This in turn was postulated to cause a sec-ondary arrest of firing in the same raphe cells mediated by their own ST autore-ceptors; or (2) reduced firing of serotonergic cells as a result of sensory isolation or of meditative quieting.

This more contemporary, biological theory had a number of assets. Included among them was the way it moved beyond the traditional constraints of a seesaw relationship between acetylcholine and norepinephrine (a notion which had be-gun long before, out in the autonomic nervous system) to consider newer data about what might happen when ST nerve cells varied their firing rates. For this theory also went on to affirm that hippocampal firing rates would increase when ST no longer played its usual role in inhibiting hippocampal CA3 cells. It was theorized that this increased firing would lead to hippocampal-septal high volt-age slow-wave activity. The subjective correlate of this was speculated to be "tran-scendent bliss consciousness," an emotional flooding called ecstasy. Basically, the theory envisioned that once the firing of ST cells had been arrested, *other cells* would then show a corresponding, disinhibitory, increase in their firing. Theoreti-cally, this would lead to an "activation of the temporal lobe limbic system" where "either ecstasy or agony waits to emerge, depending on the degree of excitation and/or lateralization" at the time.[9]

Mandell speculated further: releasing the left temporal lobe limbic system would shift the reaction in a negative direction, leading to obsessions, depressions, paranoia, and fear. In contrast, release of the right side would be associated with states of pleasure and hyperactivity. Moreover, hippocampal pyramidal cells would die from overfiring, after having been released from their usual inhibition. Which hippocampal cells would be especially susceptible to death caused by overfiring? The cells we have just seen receiving their usual input from the medial septal nucleus and from the entorhinal cortex. Cell death, it was speculated, would account for the way religious transcendence caused permanent personality changes. The issues raised are basic in neurobiology, and the validity of the above speculations will be commented upon throughout this book.

How does meditation itself cause *its* various changes? So many theories have been invoked that, by 1980, Shapiro could list some eighteen possibilities.[10] He believed that an adequate explanation would require a multidimensional model, because no one possibility was satisfactory. I agree. For this reason many of the currently plausible mechanisms are summarized in part II, in chapter 83, and in the chapters whose titles contain the word *Mondo*.

For the moment, it will prove useful to condense many of the previous theories about meditation and to restate them in three bland oversimplified generalizations: (1) Meditation offers a respite, a welcome relief to those whose lives are otherwise distracted by thought pollution and sensory overload. (2) Meditation might help persons arrive at more integrative states of awareness in everyday living, by mechanisms that change integrative physiological processes deep in the brain. (3) Meditation does involve sensory (and motor) deprivation. And some of its side effects—such as hallucinations and disorganized mentation—do resemble those which occur during conventional forms of sensory (and motor) deprivation.

Later chapters will expand upon each of these issues. And future research could yield valid answers to resolve many of our questions. But research will do so only if the rules of evidence are followed, the scientific method is used rigorously to challenge the data, and critical attention continues to examine the *fervor* to believe.

Where William James had once spoken about our usual "will to believe," Bertrand Russell chose to express the requisite mental posture rather differently. "For my part," said Russell, "I should wish to preach the 'will to doubt' . . . What is wanted is not the will to believe, but the wish to find out, which is the exact opposite."[11]

Yet it is a well-recognized occupational hazard of the academician to become enthralled by the fervor to doubt someone else's project. For example, it would be easy for a skeptic who scans this book to say, What good will come from a project so ambitious that it ventures to pull together the huge neuroscience literature, and then seeks to relate it not only to the mechanisms underlying meditation and Zen experience, but also to the processes underlying everyday consciousness and selected neurological disorders?

The kind of "map" I hold in my hand could help answer this "so what?" question. It is a new *long-term* "weather map." Not so very long ago, the original weather map makers were subjected to similar kinds of skepticism. You may remember what those years were like. It was an era B.C. (Before Computers), when forecasts were barely more accurate than folktales, caterpillar fuzz, and the *Farmer's Almanac*. But today, anyone can obtain this new weather map. It is called the *Climate Outlook*. It is generated by the Climate Analysis Center of the National Weather Service.[12]

This "map" is the distillate of decades of experience and analysis. It goes so far as to predict—over the next *year*—a series of changes in temperature and precipitation that are *likely* to occur in regions throughout the United States. How can it do this? Obviously on statistical grounds only. Because the climate experts have finally correlated the weather we previously had in this country with the still-earlier corresponding data that had been patiently gathered about the behavior of the El Niño and Southern Oscillation patterns. Repeated testing has shown that these earlier weather patterns—where weather "begins" off in the Pacific Ocean—do in fact anticipate, by many months, the trends through which our own climate will evolve.

The third millennium will soon project us into a "brave new world," an era far over the horizon from even Huxleyan imagination. Can the necessary "will to doubt" block our developing the bold new techniques that can study and predict some events of our own "inner weather?" Inner weather was the interesting phrase that Kobori-roshi used to describe the larger climate which governs our thoughts, feelings, and behavior. So, yes, one may doubt, *needs* to doubt. But can one dismiss the likely possibility that the several kinds of functional anatomy correlated in this book—representing many disciplines—carry the potential to help us live better and healthier lives? And that the improvements will also be documented by future "brain-mapping" techniques, whose neuroimaging capabilities will be far beyond what anyone could conceive of today?[13]

We have been emphasizing that, in Zen, the very process of going through a *struggle* can lead up to a positive outcome. And so can it be for the readers of part III. For those of you who have struggled uphill, through what Pavlov called the "groundwork" of neuroscience, will now have emerged ready to take a critical, balanced look at the basis of consciousness, prepared not merely to believe, or to dismiss, but to *find out* about its more extraordinary forms.

Part IV
Exploring States of Consciousness

The fact that there is a religious movement upon which many brilliant minds have worked over a period of many centuries is sufficient reason for at least venturing a serious attempt to bring such processes within the realm of scientific understanding.

Carl Jung (1875–1961)
Psychology and Religion

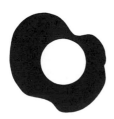

Problems with Words: "Mind"

"When *I* use a word," Humpty Dumpty said . . . "It means just what I choose it to mean—neither more nor less."

"The question is," said Alice, "whether you *can* make words mean so many different things."

"The question is," said Humpty Dumpty, "which is to be master—that's all."

Lewis Carroll (1832–1898)[1]

Anyone who probes states of consciousness soon runs into the word "mind." No such word captures the object it tries to describe. Shakespeare settled this issue for all time when he observed: "What's in a name? That which we call a rose by any other word would smell as sweet."[2] In any century, the rose exists, as *it* is, in *its* own timeless suchness.

"Mind" creates more problems than do many other words. For years, this slippery word has been used to mean many different things. The sole assumption this book makes about mind is that it originates in the brain. Even then, we know we are deceiving ourselves, because any human brain passes down a long hall of mirrors when it tries to solve the puzzle of how human mental processes function.

The several meditative disciplines, including Zen, have added to our semantic confusion. Consider the steps of Zen meditation. First the meditator keeps a minimal soft focus on the rise and fall of the breath. Then, after stimulus and response patterns have dropped out by themselves, the entry occurs into a phase called "no mind." The old Zen term for this was *mushin*. It is frequently translated into English as "no mind." But it really implies *two* things: without mind *and* without heart.[3] Such a "no mind" is not heartless. Nor is it blankness, sleep, unconsciousness, or coma. It implies that a wakeful brain has finally disengaged itself from its personal mythologies, its soap operas, and all other self-referent activities. Now it remains, simultaneously, both highly receptive *and* dispassionate. So the "no mind" of Zen implies a mental posture in which at least two things are going on: (1) bare attention still registers percepts, but (2) *there are no emotional reverberations*. In this manner does the meditator's "no mind" pass beyond simple, alert non-thinking. It enters the depths of that ongoing, perceptual awareness beyond emotional echoes.

Once over this semantic hurdle, the novice meditator, or reader, comes up against another confusing term: mind*ful*ness. Unfortunately, one of our first responses is that it must mean a "full" mind, one full of thoughts. Even though mind*ful* bears only a single *l*, one still leans toward dictionary definitions which imply keeping *something* in the back of your mind. Moreover, lurking in one's memories are such old expressions as: "Mind, you don't fall down the stairs!" These add to the impression that "mind" might even imply something to worry about. Yet, the two terms—"no mind" and bare "mindfulness"—which at first sound diametrically opposed, still point toward similar modes of meditative practice.

Words aside, what matters is how Buddhist meditation applies the method of bare attention to slowly rinse the brain of excess associative content. Then, the process which began on the cushion during zazen continues afterward as an ongoing mode of uncluttered living. Not only is this gradually increasing clarity the setting into which lesser insights can enter. On rare occasions, it will also serve as the foundation for the entry of extraordinarily clear states of consciousness, shaping their form and enhancing their impact.

Many neuroscientists raise other objections to the use of "mind." Too easily do its interpretations spin off into soft topics such as "mind reading," ESP, or into whatever some people imagine when they talk about the "universal mind," the "mind at large," or "fields of pure consciousness." These phrases share many of the same multiple misinterpretations as do words like "collective unconscious." They hint at "things," "forces," or "vibes" vaguely out there in the ether, penetrating the skull, influencing our nerve cells.

The Far East was not the sole source of these grander abstractions. Long before Emerson spoke of the "oversoul," early Middle Eastern and Occidental cultures had already concluded that a higher, theistic "overself" indeed exists. The faithful adhered to the doctrine that God inhabited His Heaven on *high*. The result was inevitable: a high/low dualism. It reduced mankind and earth to lower levels, and made possible the extinction of disbelieving heretics by every imaginable means.

Comparable dualisms still exist. They prompt semantic problems (and can be invoked to excuse ruthless behavior) at all levels: personal, scientific, and philosophical. At the personal level, dualism implies that separate entities exist: *I* am the subject; *it* is the object. Zen steers away from such dualisms and from all other imaginings. In science, the word *dualism* is used in yet another sense. A very few neuroscientists remain outspoken dualists. They contend that a *separate* "self-conscious mind" exists, and that it operates at some level removed from the other activities of our own basic modular, personal "liaison brain."[4] In contrast, most neuroscientists, including myself, are monists. To us, the brain is the organ of our mind. In fact, many monists stand so far inside the biological and humanist frame that they regard this dualistic "mind-brain problem"—which others find so vexing—as something artificial and not worth arguing about.

In the annals of Zen, a precedent for their seemingly casual approach can be dated back to the year 676. A temple banner was flapping in the breeze. Monks were arguing about it. One said, "The banner is moving." "No," the other argued, "the wind is moving." The dispute went on and on. Finally, the Sixth Patriarch said, "Neither the wind nor the banner is moving. What is moving is your own mind."[5]

If monists were forced to consider the issue seriously, perhaps we would lean toward some viewpoint which might be called the "partial promissory materialism theory."[4] Here, the word "partial" acknowledges that we will never completely understand the brain: each research question answered merely spawns others to take its place. The next two words imply that as we gradually discover more about the brain we hope to use rigorous terms to describe how it all works. Words that will have clear structural, numerical, and materialistic counterparts, not soft "mental" terms.

In yet another sense, "partial" will be a key concept in any book entitled *Zen and the Brain*. It will acknowledge that the neuroscience literature is full of words and wiring diagrams that have yet to fully address the possibility of awakening, let alone clarify the process. Moreover, most aspirants, perhaps authors in particular, will remain at best only partially enlightened. In this regard, William James observed how "every science confesses that the subtlety of nature flies beyond it, and that its formulas are but approximations."[6]

Zen itself isn't preoccupied with such gradations and details. It proceeds from the premise, born of experience, that human beings, their bodies and brains, like everything else in the universe, are now already one indivisible whole.

"As soon as you talk about a thing you miss the mark" is an old Zen saying. When Zen cautions about the pitfalls in words, it isn't sticking its head in the sand. It has already seen into them, and then sidestepped them, as it prefers to do with every other proliferating abstraction. In so doing, Zen takes the most open and pragmatic of perspectives, also born of experience: *words and other distractions interfere with the way our ordinary consciousness keenly appreciates this present moment.*

With mind now behind us, what *is* this ordinary conscious awareness?

67

Ordinary Forms of Conscious Awareness

Consciousness will always be one degree above comprehensibility.

Gosta Ehrensvard[1]

Everyone knows what ordinary consciousness feels like. We're *in* it. But like being in love, no words in any dictionary define it satisfactorily, nor has a scientific study. So the problem begins, as Gloor has observed, with the fact that consciousness is "a linguistically formulated concept." The words we're using to describe consciousness "evolved to meet the needs of human social communication, and brain mechanisms do not embody linguistic concepts."[1]

Gloor also went on to say, "Subjectively, consciousness is a unified experience with a measure of continuity in time and with an invariant central reference point, the 'self.'"[2] True, for ordinary circumstances, as Jung had also noted. But soon we will be describing properties of the special, *extraordinary* states. Then such statements will not hold. Realities change during these states. Why? In large part because the experiant no longer starts from the old Ptolemaic premise that the "self" is the central point of reference. What will be the hallmark of the more advanced of these new experiences? *The self drops out. This enables the rest of consciousness to reach a remarkable new perspective of comprehension.* So, for the serious student of consciousness, the "peak experiences" have a crucial fringe benefit. They force us to step back and take a hard look at each new chimerical theory about consciousness. Let us start with ordinary consciousness, and then consider its variations. Do any of their premises seem a little shaky?

To begin with, ordinary consciousness unfolds when two simultaneous processes interpenetrate each other: (1) the brain encodes outside events in *their* setting, generating the sense of "other"; (2) the brain sets *us* up as the central agency which experiences events—both from its own internal sources as well as these external sources. This latter melding creates our sense of "self."

On occasion, after they recover from anaesthesia, patients report that they had retained a core of consciousness even while they were still anesthetized.[3] Part III has prepared us to appreciate that they had remained aware because some regions in their brain were less anesthetized than others. These patients remind us that several major ingredients of consciousness can elude us, by slipping through large gaps in our existing methods of detection. Because no outsider, using secondhand tests, can measure everything we perceive, know, think, feel, and believe. At the instant they enter, the particular *qualities* which make up the content of our consciousness are always personal, and they remain private.

Meditators discover a surprising fact when they finally arrive at moments of "no-thought": *they do not have to think to be conscious.* For consciousness starts with *being aware.* The awareness has a receptive flavor. Its normal landscape is not a level plateau. Instead, it rises and falls as a series of peaks and valleys. What determines the full topography of our awareness? It turns out that at least five aspects of awareness help describe how our consciousness in one state differs from that in another. In brief, as our awareness changes, it varies in terms of its *field, intensity, structure, properties,* and *flow.*[4]

1. The *field* is the major topic. Its subject matter can represent either our interior world or the outside world. Which field will the person attend to? The subtle motoric properties of attention help select whether the focus is internal or external.

2. *Intensity* adjusts the amplitude. It starts with the subliminal, grows to a bare awareness, and culminates in that extraordinary hyperawareness called absorption. Usually, we have some say in how much intensity we will apply and whether we will direct it inward or outward. But note: in major absorptions, both direction and intensity will change *involuntarily.*

3. Existing within our awareness is at least some degree of organization, called *structure.* In its usual foreground is that chaotic play of present scenes, memory images, scenarios of the future, vague fantasies. Yet off in a distant background, is another part of us. It stays vaguely oriented to current time, place, and person. Also residing there, on several other remote planes, is a kind of aerial view of our self observing the present action. It is an "overview self." It paraphrases Descartes down its own long hall of mirrors, murmuring sotto voce, I am aware that I am aware. Therefore, I *am.*

4. Our ordinary awareness has certain *properties.* It can be clear or indistinct, expanded or contracted. It can perceive what is meaningful or meaningless, real or imaginary. Consider one advanced state, the flash of insight-wisdom. During it, which special property becomes so characteristic? The way awareness still takes in that very same field of basic sensory data from the outside world as it had during the instant just before. But in milliseconds a fresh grasp of this scenery has totally reinterpreted it into a new realm of absolute reality. In this instant, what had happened to that former self, the central agency which might otherwise have presumed to claim so rare a moment for its very own? Nothing remains: no background self, overview self, bodily self, or psychic self (see table 11).

5. A final attribute of our usual awareness is the way it *flows*. It is constantly in motion. Ordinarily when we watch TV or movies, the action flows seamlessly from one scene to the next. But sometimes the projection equipment stops. Recall what happens. The scene is frozen in midaction. Especially during internal absorption does this arrest of flow invoke a strong sense of stasis, of being placed on hold.

In *Ulysses,* James Joyce was merely presenting his readers with what they already knew: they were possessed by a "stream of consciousness," swirling and bubbling with thoughts. No one appreciates this fact more than the mindful meditator. Indeed, special research techniques now confirm that it is typical of a normal brain to be in so dynamic a state of flux that it undergoes distinctive electrical changes many times each second.[5] Even the brain waves of the old-fashioned EEG can be seen to pass, at random, through a large series of different configurations. Among these, an average segment might last one-fifth of a second (200 milliseconds). But some intervals are as short as 50 milliseconds, and others last as long as 500 milliseconds or so. When scientists try to correlate the data from the different levels of analysis, they are still uncertain which of our neurophysiological microstates are being reflected in such brief EEG landscapes, and how either of these episodes relates to the Joycean stream of topics which swirls around in our subjective mental field.

But suppose we consider the longer EEG segments noted above. Lasting one half of a second or so, they are getting close to how long a subliminal stimulus must last before it develops enough substance to penetrate conscious experience.[6] Moreover, the ordinary range of human activities has also been monitored using standard polygraphic techniques. And a few such studies employed much longer sampling windows. These measured intervals lasting as long as thirty *seconds.*

Even from such limited studies it has been shown that we pass through at least *six* distinct physiological stages during our everyday waking lives. These stages can each be identified by obvious differences in our EEG, eye movements, and muscle movements.[7] One aspect of the study cited is of special note: the moments of *attention* are one of these six stages. And *distinctive of attention is the way all eye movements stop.* Perhaps it is not surprising, then, for a subject to sense that gaze functions no longer pursue their usual to-and-fro scanning mode during the advanced states of *hyper*attentive absorption. Indeed, only as a fact of experience does the meditator discover a special distinctive attribute of such a moment: awareness itself conveys the unique, almost palpable, sensation that it is being placed on hold (see chapter 84).

Aside from the phenomenon of this arrest of awareness, the discussion so far will have emphasized two other aspects of consciousness. First, that its dynamic properties do not allow it to hold still long enough to be easily characterized. Second, that the full content of consciousness remains private, internal, and brain-bound. If so, then each person's private consciousness would not seem—in and of itself—to bear any *direct* cause-and-effect relationship with other events elsewhere in the universe. A great many people think otherwise. It is instructive for an open-minded reader to be presented with a small sample of the words of the counterargument. For example, one proponent would start from the premise that consciousness is a *non*physical entity. In his view, consciousness is connected with physical reality by means of one fundamental quantity. This quantity, he believes, is a "state vector" for a quantum mechanical process which links many synapses of the brain.[8] A state vector is considered to be a collection of all the states representing solutions to one basic equation which expresses the same complete set of boundary conditions.

In the type of quantum theory which is being proposed above, the meditative state itself would correspond to 10^8 bits. For a person to proceed thereafter into what was called the experience of "revelation" would correspond with the raising of "consciousness interconnectedness" from its initial, nominal 10^8 power bits per second up to some 10^{12} bits per second. So, at least according to such calculations from quantum mechanics, when we have finally arrived at our most refined analytic perception of "objective consciousness" it will represent "a direct channel to an extensive nonphysical reality." According to this thesis, enlightenment is really real, and not merely a vast illusion. Old Master Huang-po would have nodded in agreement.

Brain-bound neurologists, including myself, may be dizzied by such heights of abstraction. And even theorists of long experience in the stratosphere of this field acknowledge that "quantum mechanics . . . does not explain the large-scale world."[9] Yet, meanwhile, whatever "Buddha mind" is, or implies to various persons, every novice struggles to enter its vast, cosmic expanse. A further difficulty, for neurologists in particular, is that we tend to be cast in an unfamiliar role whenever we run up against the extraordinary *heights* of consciousness, awareness, and performance. Our training has inclined us to search for the *reduced* functions, those that localize which circuit is damaged. Our "bag" is trouble. And even when our patients do develop "positive" signs and "overfunctions," they are usually only caricatures of normal movements or behaviors.

We might benefit from some fresh perspectives, as long as we still keep our feet on the ground.

68

Variations on the Theme of Consciousness

> The roots of humanity's troubles run very deep. There are no simple prescriptions to overcome them. . . . What is needed are changes in consciousness, in relations between people, between nations and in their attitudes toward nature.
>
> Mikhail Gorbachev[1]

> Wisdom is the principal thing; therefore get wisdom: And with all thy getting get understanding.
>
> Proverbs 4:7

Glasnost. Perestroika. If these words are taken as loose metaphors, they suggest potential remedies which might be prescribed to treat a few of humanity's troubles. If so, could we somehow open up and restructure our present states of consciousness? Change our own attitudes, steer clear of future troubles? But before embarking on any ambitious changes, perhaps it would be wise to begin by understanding something else: how we structured consciousness in the first place.

William James looked into this matter by breathing nitrous oxide (see chapter 98). In doing so, he discovered that he had layers of consciousness. He found them really rather filmy. It was in the context of these experiments on himself, using N_2O, that he would call our attention to two aspects of consciousness. First, to how many kinds there were. Second, to how totally different they were from our "normal waking consciousness." A student of consciousness soon becomes lost among so many different filmy layers. One feels the need for support from some kind of intellectual scaffolding. Bearing this in mind, Krippner identified twenty states of consciousness, but he also noted how much they overlap.[2] "Lumpers" could develop fewer categories; "dividers" create lists ad infinitum.

In these pages, it is expedient to adopt a middle way—a system which both groups and separates. The next three tables are intended solely to provide a springboard for the discussion throughout this book.

Table 9 presents a simplified summary. It begins with the states that we slide into and out of during a ordinary day: waking (I), sleeping (II), and dreaming (III).[3] It continues, in the interests of simplicity (not accuracy) by lumping together the various levels of meditation into a provisional "fourth state."

After trainees undergo intensive meditative experience, it becomes more likely that they will access extraordinary alternate states of consciousness. Table 10 summarizes three of the preliminary forms.

Table 11 presents two advanced forms of extraordinary alternate states, and a later stage entitled "ongoing enlightened traits." We further develop each of these categories in the discussion that follows, and will continue to describe them in subsequent chapters.

Now, it is clearly arbitrary to represent the full spectrum of consciousness in a mere ten provisional working categories. But ten will provide a conceptual framework for dialogue, even though they do not represent a hierarchical outline of successive physiological levels. There is no reason to believe that these ten categories can be carved in stone, any more than were other attempts presented elsewhere.[4,5] The reasons are several: (1) physiologically, the categories are not equidistant each from the other; (2) experientially, categories each shade off into a continuum; (3) they can be further subdivided; (4) even when subdivided, most categories remain mixtures—apples and oranges. For instance, the first three of the last four are decidedly otherworldly. Moreover, the tenth and last category represents an ongoing *stage*. Think of it as a prolonged change in *trait*, not a brief change in state.

To return now, in table 9, at right, to the meditative states. Here, subsumed under the large category IV, one can lump meditation (with obvious reservations) into its shallower and deeper levels. If the meditator focuses attention narrowly, the type of meditative mode can be described as "concentrative." If the focus is open and widely deployed, it can be termed "receptive." At deeper levels, some trainees might probe a *koan* in the setting of their relaxed, clear awareness.

Then, after trainees undergo months of intensive meditative practice, many will access *extraordinary* moments of consciousness. Table 10 summarizes three

Table 9
Ordinary and Meditative States of Consciousness

	I Ordinary Waking States	II Slow-Wave (S) Sleep	III Desynchronized (D) Sleep	IV Levels Reached During Concentration and Receptive Meditative Modes	
				Shallower	Deeper
Type of awareness	External and internal	External and internal	Internalized	External and internal	External or internal
Awareness of	A flow of perceptions, thoughts, feelings, and images	Usually no content	Vivid, imaginative dream material during REM episodes	Recurrent thoughts, sensations	Transient thoughts, sensations; later, no thoughts
Intensity of awareness	Usually 2–3	0–1	1–2	1–2	1–2
Usual, experiencing, bounded self	4–5	0	0–1	2–3	1–2 transient
Sense of time and place	4–5	0	1	2–3	1–2 transient
Sensate perceptions registered	4–5	0–1	0–1	2–3	1–2 transient

Positive affect	Variable	0	Variable	Variable	2
Duration	Minutes to hours	Minutes to hours	Minutes to hours	Minutes	Seconds to minutes
Detachment from cravings/aversions	0	2–3	1	1–2	2–3
Events that follow	Provide the basic foundation for ordinary consciousness	S-sleep is preceded by drowsiness and followed in the A.M. by reverie; subsequently, it is generally replenishing	Cumulatively refreshing	Tranquilizing	More tranquilizing, clarifying, refreshing; rarely proceeds to States V and VI
Comment	May be interrupted by daydreams and by other periods during which there is a variable access to the usual self	A few normals may have vivid hallucinations during transitional phases when going in or out of sleep	Rarely, dream material yields a comprehensive, resolving insight	More reproducible; with regular practice, a feeling of relief may occur	Approaching shallower levels of absorption, there occurs a feeling of becoming continually one-pointed with enhanced perceptions

0 = none; 5 = maximal

Table 10
Extraordinary Alternate States of Consciousness

	V Heightened, Emotionalized Awareness without Sensate Loss	VI-A Absorption without Sensate Loss: External Absorption	VI-B Absorption with Sensate Loss: Internal Absorption
Type of awareness	External and internal	Focused on some external source, or on personal action	Internal Focal and contracted Diffuse and expanded Ambient
Awareness of	Sensate impressions, peace and joy	Ongoing events	Awareness itself, permeated with black, silent space
Intensity of awareness	3	3–4	4–5 Absorption is held
Usual, experiencing, bounded self	1–2	1–2	0
Sense of time and place	1–2	1–2	0
Sensate perceptions registered	3	3 Quickly, automatically, efficiently	0
Positive affect	2–3 Joyful, loving, happy, peaceful	Calm	Enchantment, bliss, rapture, ecstasy; awe and some sacramental quality on emerging
Duration	Seconds to many minutes	Seconds to minutes	Seconds to minutes
Detachment from cravings/aversions	1 Temporary	3 Temporary	4 Temporary
Events that follow	Memorable, not transforming	Memorable, not transforming	Alerting, quickening, feelings of lightness; memorable and temporarily transforming
Comment	A heightened plane or "plateau" experience (Maslow); epiphany*	Variable in degree; heightened awareness is not emotionalized†	More common after concentrative meditation approaches; sensate loss is distinctive; variable in depth, duration, quality‡

0 = none; 5 = maximal.
*"Adamic" episodes (Laski) of "profound peace" (Greeley).
†"Positive samadhi" (Sekida); play absorption.
‡"Absolute samadhi" (Sekida).

Table 11
Advanced Extraordinary Alternate States of Consciousness

	VII Insight-Wisdom Kensho, Satori	VIII Ultimate Being, beyond Expression	IX The Stage of Ongoing Enlightened Traits
Type of awareness	External; eternal	Ultimate source	Unbounded external and internal
Awareness of	Suchness One-ness	Primordial emptiness, a groundless void beyond oneness	The suchness of all things
Intensity of awareness	4	5	3
Usual, experiencing, bounded self	0	0	Free access without bounds
Sense of time and place	0	0	Free access without limitations
Sensate perceptions registered	5	0	4
Positive affect	Perfection in all things just as they are; no fear	Inexpressible	Selfless compassion
Duration	Seconds	Seconds to minutes	Ongoing
Detachment from cravings/aversions	5	5	5 Permanent
Events that follow	Memorable; more permanent transformations of attitude and behavior	Memorable, but ultimately "nothing special"; markedly transforming	Not readily traceable back to the person
Comment	Enlightenment, awakening, seeing into your true nature, seeing your original face; at least four levels progressing toward increasing oneness	Rare experiences, beyond seeing and knowing (Johnson); nirvana*	So in the flow of events that positive things happen with a light touch†

0 = none; 5 = maximal.
*"The peace of the summits" (Underhill); "pure being, beyond subject and object" (Merrell-Wolff).
†Stages 9 and 10 in the oxherding drawings; "self-fulfilling" activity (Dogen).

preliminary forms of these alternate states. I invite the reader's particular attention to the list of criteria in its left-hand column. There are eleven criteria. And this *same* list proved useful in describing the various *ordinary* states in the preceding table. Consider, for example, that relatively common event when a person experiences a heightened, emotionalized peaceful awareness. During this state V, most of the usual bounded self still remains. On the other hand, during state VI-B, the sensate physical self drops out. Therefore, this criterion—*the presence of self*—is helpful to distinguish state V from the most advanced state of absorption.

The "epiphanies" of state V often occur in natural outdoor settings, and at times other than those devoted to formal sitting meditation. Awareness now becomes amplified and directed externally. The world of outside sensory stimuli takes over. Consciousness is then witness to a field of enhanced sensate impressions suffused with a positive affect. Maslow calls this a "plateau" experience. Laski refers to it as an "Adamic" experience. During such episodes, the observer's sense of time, place, and person can fade momentarily, but none of their deep roots disappear.

State VI represents a much greater change in consciousness. The outcome is called *absorption*. As noted earlier, it is an extraordinarily clear, intense, involuntary awareness. Captured in the foreground field is either world, the exterior or the interior. For example, the process turns inward during absorption's more advanced *internal* form, state VI-B. In doing so, it preempts or otherwise sweeps past the ordinary checkpoints of personal overview. Brief hallucinations may occur at moments when excitation reaches such positive heights. But the brain quickly snuffs them out, summoning powerful reactive inhibitions. What happens within consciousness as a result of these latter, negating, inhibitory properties? Now, vision, hearing, and body sensations come to a definite halt. And bypassed, at the same time, are the person's next adjacent filmy layers: the notions about time, place, and the bodily self.

What is then witnessed is a vast void of silent space, a new visual overview remarkable in scope. A term, *absolute samadhi*, is sometimes used to describe this state. Some of these moments of internal absorption will present themselves during deeper levels of meditation. When they do so, their prelude may consist of a plunge into a vacant, blank interval of no consciousness. This gap in consciousness may seem, in retrospect, to have been a "dropping off of body and mind."

Table 11 goes on to summarize the three most advanced categories of alternate conscious experience. Again, the same criteria are used in the left-hand column. The three form a distinctive group. The first, state VII, is the state of awakening, of sudden enlightenment. In Zen, the technical term is *kensho* or *satori*. In one flash of deep, objective insight-wisdom this state cuts off every self-referent bodily *and psychic* tie. The experience sets in motion a series of other, subsequent events. Positive attitudes infuse awareness. Afterward, the person's behavior changes in everyday life. Episodes of *kensho* can recur. Traits of character are then more likely to be transformed. When, in point of sequence, do such brief awakenings to profound understanding occur? They tend to enter after the first of the absorptions.

The next rare state is VIII, Ultimate Being. Capital letters are often used in association with the phrase. They do little more than hint at its inexpressible properties. This state of grace is reserved for the very few. They are persons who are far advanced in their practice of the spiritual path, and who have previously undergone several awakenings.

Finally, one comes to the rarest subjects of all, those who go on to reside totally, and continually, within what lies next beyond. For level IX is the exceptional ongoing *stage* briefly referred to above. It implies that *two* things have truly changed: *consciousness and traits of behavior*. First, because consciousness, in this stage, will finally have evolved in the direction of true equanimity, simplicity, and stability. Moreover, genuine compassion will finally have transformed the person's behavior.

Gradations

In order to distinguish among these several categories of states of consciousness, it has proved useful to *grade* certain of their attributes. The rating scale used in each table is derived from the one used in clinical neurology. Zero (0) means absent; 0–1 implies a trace; 1 means definite; and 2 represents about twice that much, namely the level that might be expected in the average person under "normal" conditions. Using this numerical system has advantages. It paves the way for going on to rate several properties of awareness and consciousness, even when they rise to levels either much higher (5) than normal or descend to those much lower (0).

As the person passes in sequence through the last four categories, from VI through IX, two aspects of consciousness become quite extraordinary. Now the reader may begin to appreciate why previous chapters have so emphasized these two topics. One is the content, scope, intensity, and clarity of the field within awareness. The other aspect is the subject's progressive loss of the *I-Me-Mine*. Therefore, two striking facts stand out in the final stage: (1) the fully enlightened person has now become totally detached both from cravings and aversions; yet even so (2) has remained fully aware and responsive.

This combination alerts us. It tells us that enlightenment of this degree is a true transformation of the brain. It would be an error to regard this as merely a superficial change of habits of thought.

69

Alternate States of Consciousness: Avenues of Entry

> Our main research task of the future is accurate delineation and specification of individual differences in various discrete states of consciousness. We need detailed mapping of the experiential spaces of individuals before making generalizations across individuals.
>
> Charles Tart[1]

How does any brain manage to bring together and blend the ingredients of its various states of consciousness? Tart offers some psychological viewpoints which begin to organize the way we think about the whole process.[1-4]

Start with you. You know you are the person reading these lines. You have a discrete and stable sense of who, what, and where you are at this very moment. Yes, your present state of consciousness does seem to be a seamless, unitary phenomenon. In fact, it is a conglomerate of subsystems, functioning in many separate, but interacting, dynamic configurations.[1]

Tart's theories propose that such subsystems of consciousness are primarily "psychological." (One can interpret this to mean that all their physiological origins remain to be clarified.) Each subsystem might be operating at a high, normal, or low level. And each might also be invested with attention to a greater or lesser degree. Given all these permutations, any single one of our many discrete states of consciousness would seem to be a mere temporary aggregation of substates, a "temporal clustering of the content and organization of consciousness."

But what kind of glue could hold all this together? And why are our ordinary discrete states of consciousness so relatively stable and pervasive, despite all this diversity? Tart points to several mechanisms which usually stabilize them.[1] For example, most of us soon become trapped in the web of our routine day-to-day activities. Or we get tangled up in imagining scenarios which might help us plan for them. So when friends ask, "Keeping busy?," to answer "yes" is almost a matter of pride. How often do we chose to take up the meditative path and to enter its moments of calm, mindful awareness?

Yet there are no fixed boundaries along our major ordinary conscious states. Only edges, in constant states of change. For our waking hours finally give way to sleep; sleep shifts into dreaming. The dreamer may awaken, or slide back into ordinary sleep. In short, our consciousness has many *alternative options.*

It is for this reason that Zinberg suggested using the word *alternate,* not "altered," to describe them.[5] In full agreement with this view, I have chosen to use the term *alternate states* of consciousness throughout. As a term, *alternate* carries no pejorative connotations. It states the obvious: many optional states occur. And they differ substantially. Suppose, for example, you have etched an especially vivid daytime incident into memory. There it will lodge in a special way that seems different from an ordinary dream. Each episode has become a separate constellation of psychophysiological events, a distinctive microstate, a *discrete* state of consciousness.

In Tart's theoretical framework, each discrete state of consciousness starts out as a private configuration. It is *unique for a given individual.* Each person recognizes that *this particular pattern* of conscious experience is distinct from some other discrete state of consciousness and not merely an extension of it. Each person then concludes, "This condition of my mind feels *radically different* from some other condition."[3] But note that the person must be able to hold such a discrete state in the forefront of awareness for a sufficiently long period of time. Otherwise, it won't stand out and be recognized as a definite entity.

So we have now cited at least two general categories of phenomena which people commonly experience: (1) ordinary consciousness, and (2) ordinary discrete alternate states of consciousness. It is true that transition periods—such as drowsiness or ordinary daydreaming—are a third category set in between such discrete states. But it is hard to characterize the dynamic mental field of these ordinary transition periods because it changes constantly.

Moving beyond these ordinary states and their transitions, leads one to a borderland even less well-defined. For, during our waking hours, we do not always maintain the same, stable grasp on reality. Reality isn't always here and now. When we slip into and out of states, we sometimes slide off for very long distances. For example, surveys of college students showed that between 39 and 46 percent of them had curious "borderland" experiences.[6] During these episodes, the subjects might lose the experience of their own bodies, or might seem to be detached observers of a distant scene. Even long-familiar experiences in the outside world might either seem unfamiliar or frankly unreal. In the student population surveyed, drug use was not an explanation for the high incidence of these phenomena. Rather it reflected the greater freedom that the younger generation had during the 1960s in being able to talk openly about such experiences. In any decade, how can we, as outside observers, interpret such depersonalizations and derealizations? Many of our own problems of definition will still hinge on the subjects' own *private* opinion. Did *they* believe the borderland event was something "ordinary?" Was it *extra*ordinary but forgettable? Or was it both extraordinary *and* unforgettable?

Yet now the caveats mount, for the next step will lead us to consider distinctly *unusual* states of consciousness. Tart forewarns us of the impending "paradigm clash" whenever we move on past the "ordinary" borderlands. For "paradigm" implies much more than those assumptions and frames of reference we all share about what constitutes reality. It also includes what kinds of questions society has decided are appropriate for us to ask when certain topics venture off at the fringes of this reality.

Reflect on how uneasy we feel about our *own* subconscious processes. It is hard to deal with the notion that *we* have "hidden, unconscious compartments." Somebody else, yes. But not *me*. Our slips still embarrass us. Decades after Freud we still don't totally accept the fundamental fact: many mental activities go on unconsciously, especially those over which we feel we "should," or "must" exert some control.

Science reflects society. Scientists partake of the paradigm clash, and scientists share the same unease. Especially do they tend to reject outright or to misperceive data when they are called upon to judge states that are alien to their own experience. Many scientists share another prevailing tendency: that of dismissing *all* phenomena of such alien states merely by the act of labeling them "subjective" or "ephemeral." Alter*ed* states of consciousness do seem subversive enough to threaten many people's prejudices. Indeed, the few scientists who work in this general area tend to be defensive about their research, because much of it still has to gain full scientific respectability.[5]

So after this preamble about the ordinary, transitional, and borderland states, we are now prepared to take up the *extraordinary discrete alternate states of consciousness*. By definition, these are rare, highly valued, distinct states which represent *a sharp break from other states of perception or intuition*. We would concur with Tart that up until now, the status held by each such extraordinary state has seemed to have been that of a "psychological experiential construct." This book is different. It will venture far beyond the usual psychological constructs. The aim of this book is to propose very specific psychophysiological correlates for each state. These proposals are based on the functional anatomy reviewed in part III, and they can be proved or disproved by research methods, especially by the latest, ultrafast, neuroimaging techniques.

However, at this point, it may help to consider a simplified global analogy. For geologists have also been busy. They now have remarkable evidence about Earth's active early history. Our planet's crust sinks, thrusts up, breaks apart, drifts, and reassembles in new configurations. Subterranean forces are still causing our continents to move. Even viewed in slow motion, these dynamic geologic changes are a useful metaphor for the active processes that create the astonishing mental landscapes and deep, V-shaped ocean trenches of our extraordinary alternate states. And it is also true that the experiant, like a wide-eyed Marco Polo, will be witness to novel *continents* of experience, worlds that could never have been imagined.

For millennia, humans have resorted to all kinds of physical and mental measures, trying to evoke these extraordinary states. Tart reduces the many techniques to two basic operations. The first *disrupts* consciousness. The second *repatterns* it. To be effective, several disrupting influences must combine, be extra strong, and prolonged. Sometimes, too, they may need to converge into an especially vulnerable physiological crevice, to thrust deeply into it, and to do so at precisely the right time. For until a series of events does come together, no brain can plunge readily into an alternate state, especially if the subject's previous personality structure has been well organized. Why this resistance? A major reason is the way the brain holds on tenaciously to its conventional states of consciousness. Their basic routines have been "overlearned" and well balanced for many years.

Destabilizing Influences

But suppose you upset this relatively stable physiological equilibrium. Things become unsteady when you bring to bear the following types of destabilizing influences.[1,7]

1. "Overloading" implies an excessive burden of stimuli. A barrage of stimuli can come in from the outside. Or the subject can be overcome by the kinds of heightened arousal associated with excessive motor activity and overflowing emotion.

2. Sensorimotor deprivation.

3. Unusual stimuli, "triggers."

4. Increasing alertness or mental involvement, as occurs in the course of highly focused concentrative meditative techniques.

5. Decreasing alertness, to the point at which the subjects relax their critical faculties and develop a detached, passive state of mind.

6. Disruptions of the usual sleep-waking cycles.

7. Pharmacologic agents: anesthetics, psychedelic and other drugs.

In subsequent chapters we focus on the last six destabilizing influences. Here, it suffices merely to expand on the first. Overloading is a prelude to the kinds of trance states which subjects undergo at tribal dances and at revivalist meetings. Indeed, hypnotic trance states can also be produced experimentally. First, one induces a hyperalert period of high arousal and increasing tension. During this pressured interval, thoughts and sensations race at such high intensity that they preempt any narrowly focused, concentrated attention. After five to twenty-five minutes, the trance starts.[8]

What happens when two or more of these seven destabilizing forces converge? First they shatter the physiological links which had previously held together the preceding state of consciousness. This disrupts and depatterns. Next comes a critical moment of flux. This brief interim moment is not to be confused with a *state*. For a state, in the traditional sense, lasts longer and is much more stable.[1] Rather is this another kind of short transition period, an interval so dynamic that the subject's ordinary consciousness becomes suspended or highly disorganized.

The experiential correlate of such a transitional interval might appear to be a blank period, a moment when no mentation takes place. Afterward, the person may think, I must have fallen asleep (see chapter 112). However, even during this brief interim phase, *repatterning* forces are already gathering momentum. Soon they will help influence the content of the experience yet to come.

The next moment is also a fragile one. Now, the new discrete alternate state is coalescing. An *extraordinary* state, not your ordinary variety. As this new state enters consciousness, it is relatively unstable. But supposing there had been a long prior period of meditative practice? Could this have influenced its form and content? For if it had, then one can envision that the elements of the new state will enter a matrix of consciousness that had been progressively shorn of the trappings of self. Free from the sticky distractions and old distortions of that person's subjective ties, these novel functional components may stay joined longer.

Finally, years later, and after several such awakenings in the interim, the reconfigurations may go on to remain together permanently, seamlessly. What could explain their subsequent staying power? Ultimately, it could reflect the stability of a whole new simplified neurophysiological baseline. What is this extended condition we are now attempting to capture in words? It is that same remarkable transformation which is the basis for the exceptional ongoing *stage* of enlightened traits (category IX in table 11).

Some Properties of Alternate States

Suppose we continue to employ psychological terms. Which are the best terms to use to characterize the attributes of extraordinary alternate states of consciousness? It is instructive to review the historical background which led up to two separate lists of such words. The first list, presented just below, was drawn up during the 1960s.[7] At that time, it was thought to be the *general* characteristics of alt*ered* states of consciousness. The ending on the word, *-ed*, serves as its own commentary. It reflected an orientation to the drug scene. It arose during that particular era when psychedelic drugs seemed an easy way to *alter* your consciousness.

1. Alterations in thinking
2. Disturbances in the sense of time
3. Loss of control
4. Sudden, unexpected expressions of primitive and intense emotions
5. Detachment
6. Changes in body image, including a dissolution of boundaries
7. Perceptual distortions
8. Profound, insightful changes in meaning or significance
9. The sense of the ineffable; the experience cannot be communicated
10. Feelings of rejuvenation; a new sense of hope, rebirth
11. Hypersuggestability; an increased tendency to believe

The second list evolved much later, in 1975. And it would represent, in that year, the efforts of a conference committee set up to address the same topic. But now the states were being described as "alter*nate*," not "altered."[5] In 1975, what would a committee consider to be *general* properties of alternate states of consciousness? The members spent one morning discussing this very issue. They concluded that certain properties were easy to rate. For example, if they set up a numerical scale which ascended from 1 to 9, it seemed simple to quantitate each of the four psychological attributes listed below. Because, with the aid of this scale, an alternate state could be inferred whenever there occurred a *marked* departure from the norm of the following four standard properties:

1. Vividness
2. Absolute conviction that one was either in the usual state of consciousness, or in the *un*usual alternate state
3. Connectedness to ordinary feelings
4. Generalized affective reactions

But something was missing. The committee had only a partial answer. It was as though the members had blindfolds on, and had only been feeling the four legs of the proverbial elephant. Now they needed to grapple with the tough, axial issues of self. And that particular numerical rating system—because it ascended from 1 to 9—just didn't work well in the context of self. Why not? Why did they need a different system? Because it would have to do two things: (1) it would need to express the *normal* levels of a person's self-related properties; (2) it would also need to leave plenty of room *below these levels*. Otherwise, no researcher could rate those properties of a self which could later drop out.

Their solution? They went on to specify certain psychological properties that were clearly related to the sense of self. Then they assigned to "normal" not the number 1, but the higher number, 5. A minor adjustment, you might think. A trivial step. Yet, consider how much the new gradations implied. These were committee members who had grown up thinking about the "self" in Western terms. Now they had an intellectual grip on the puzzling, but age-old Eastern concept: *this egocentric self could be downgraded, as it were, toward zero.* Previously, such a notion had either seemed counterintuitive or inconceivable.

The lists themselves were drawn up almost a decade apart, and the second one is now over twenty years old. Yet the contrasts between the two still provide useful lessons. No surprises reside in the message that different professionals can reach different opinions about the psyche. But it is encouraging to find that a committee can develop a fresh orientation, and can introduce a new set of psychological criteria into its later list.

Which criteria did the committee members select, in 1975, as properties related to the concept of *self?* They had finally come to focus on such issues as

1. A person's awareness of self.
2. The sense of exerting active "self control" over events, as opposed to merely passively observing events as they passed by.
3. The way the person differentiates self from other, along that self/other boundary which separates our inner self from the outside world.

So the students of consciousness in the West seem to have been evolving. The trend in recent decades is to shed the earlier preoccupation with psychedelic drugs and their epiphenomena, to become more aware of the pivotal construct of self, and to appreciate the time-honored meditative approach to the dissolution of this self. Zen Master Dogen would have nodded in approval.

In closing, let us continue to heed the caveat in Tart's quotation which opened the present chapter. For yes, it will always be vital to have *individual subjects* looking, highly critically, at their own experiences. They alone can map what their experiences were, from the inside. And by way of a preview, this will indeed be the plan of this book as we go on later, in parts V, VI, and VII, to examine one person's experiences. I make one obvious disclaimer: there are many more permutations of mystical experience than happened to me. For this reason, other persons' experiences and even psychedelic reports are included when it seems appropriate.

70

The Architecture of Sleep

> Sleep is really the outward manifestation of a number of processes that are going on independently, simultaneously, in combination, at different times, with different relationships.
>
> W. Dement and M. Mitler[1]

Like waking, sleep is a dynamic product, a fluid continuum of substates. These are usually linked together, but they can be dissociated. We have much to learn about sleep states, substates, and the transition periods between them. Few topics can teach us so much about Zen and the brain. Why? Because some sleep mechanisms become relevant to internal absorption. Still others help clarify how clusters of physiological functions break apart—and then fall together—during "quickenings," and even during extraordinary states. For these reasons, the next four chapters emphasize the normal brain mechanisms which shift us up and down, back and forth, between several hypo- and hyperactivated states.

Again, the definition of a *state:* it is a set of recurring physiological changes which tend to cluster and to last for a finite period of time.[2] In our daily sleep-waking cycle, our *wakeful* state (W) descends into *slow-wave* sleep (S). This in turn gives way to brief episodes of *desynchronized* sleep (D). *We may or may not dream* during D-sleep. But as a memory device, some find it helpful to recall that they are *sound asleep when in slow-wave, synchronized S sleep. Whereas *dreaming sleep is most likely to be D-sleep.

Our three basic states, W, S, and D, can usually be distinguished by asking three questions: (1) Does the EEG show low voltage fast-wave (desynchronized) activity? (2) Are rapid eye movements (REMs) present? (3) Are the midline, antigravity muscles actively contracting?[2] In the animal research laboratory, the three states separate further when subjected to three other criteria. These are based on how fast certain nerve cells fire in different parts of the brain stem.

During the waking state, cells discharge at relatively high rates in the midbrain reticular formation, the locus ceruleus, and in the raphe nuclei. In contrast, during D-sleep, firing rates *slow* markedly in these same norepinephrine and serotonin nuclei. And, again during D-sleep, acetylcholine cells *increase* their firing rates in selected regions of the medulla and pons, especially in nuclei that help generate rapid eye movements (REM).

These clusters of rapid eye movements are hidden under closed lids. They had always escaped notice. So there was great excitement when they finally caught the attention of Aserinsky and Kleitman in 1953. Shortly thereafter, the presence of rapid eye movements led to the whole length of desynchronized sleep also being known as REM sleep. Then other findings presented a paradox. In D-sleep, why were the chin, neck, and other axial muscles so paralyzed, when other muscles were still contracting? Soon this curious state, described as "an active brain in a paralyzed body," also became known as "paradoxical sleep."[3]

Sleep then turned out to have an almost architectural profile. Something like an ancient pyramidal temple, it seemed to have different levels connected by steep staircases going up and down (the left portion of figure 14 illustrates something of the general effect). Each night, over a seven- or eight-hour period, we run through four or more sleep cycles.[4] The first cycle takes us from wakefulness (W) quickly down through sleep stages 1 and 2. The descent continues, more slowly, with a plunge into the depths of stage 3 or stage 4 sleep lasting one or more hours.

The alpha EEG rhythms of waking evolve, during ordinary stage 1, into slower theta activity at 4 to 7 cps. Further slowing occurs as sleep descends to its deepest levels. Then, on the way back up, we rapidly *ascend* back through stage 2 to reach the first brief interval of D-sleep. Typically it unfolds some 90 to 100 minutes after we first drop off to sleep. It lasts ten minutes or so. Part of the time there will be some rapid eye movements.

Next, the second cycle of sleep unfolds. Again it descends to stage 3 or 4, then climbs back up to stages 2 and 1 to enter the second REM period. It lasts longer, perhaps twenty minutes. Through the night, several other similar cycles then develop. On each occasion, segments of D-sleep occupy progressively more of each cycle, bringing longer episodes of rapid eye movements. And those periods of deeper S-sleep also occupy less of the cycle.[4]

People differ physiologically. Some are light sleepers, others deep sleepers. Why? Suppose you awaken subjects from those segments of D-sleep during which they are having REM episodes. Then, both light and deep sleepers report generally similar kinds of dream mentation.[5] But if you awaken the light sleepers out of S-sleep, they report two and a half times more dreaming episodes than do deep sleepers. Moreover, they also show faster heart and breathing rates, higher body temperatures, more awakenings, and more gross body movements.

The evidence above suggests four important points: (1) people who are light sleepers seem to stay up at a lighter, *relatively more aroused,* level during their S-sleep; (2) dream mentation reflects what a person's general level of arousal is at the time; (3) reports of dream mentation also hinge on one's becoming awake enough to remember the latest dream well enough to report it afterward; (4) dream mentation can occur both in REM episodes *and during S-sleep.*

Some subjects give "dream" reports even though their EEG still shows an alpha rhythm.[4] When their alpha activity coincides with rapid or with slow eye movements, the subjects commonly report that emotion invests their visual images. In contrast, *affect drops out when subjects move down from stage 1 to 2.* This means that by the time stage 2 occurs, the dreamlike content tends to be *emotionally flat.* Still, during their earlier sleep stages, most subjects remain active participants in their dreamlike mentation, not simply passive observers.

Drowsiness and "Active" Sleep

Drowsiness is not prosaic. It is a dynamic interface full of potentials, when events are in transition. Drowsiness is so complex that a whole book has been devoted to its experiential and physiological aspects.[6] Remember how frequently meditators slide in and out of drowsiness? In the process they will open up to many variations—and some mutations—on the themes of ordinary consciousness.

During drowsiness, the brain is switching its pacemakers. Even a few normal persons show brief paroxysmal EEG discharges resembling those in epilepsy. Sometimes these sharp bursting patterns are widespread. At other times the bursts project more over the frontal and central regions. Diffuse theta activity also occurs. Drowsiness itself varies, even in the same person. Indeed, quite different EEG patterns may show up even though the same person is traversing successive cycles of drowsiness. As we first drift down toward stage 1 sleep, an early period of reverie may last from four to ten minutes. Then, when we descend into stage 1 sleep, we lose much of our contact with the outside world. This is a suggestible period. If verbal suggestions are made, they tend to be accepted uncritically, a point of interest to students of hypnosis.[7]

Drowsy transitional states have been studied in animals with the aid of deep electrode recordings. The particular transitional intervals which descend from waking to sleep, represented as W → S, reveal especially dynamic changes. For instance, spindle-shaped waves invade the EEG. They are, in fact, rhythmic spike clusters. And in their waxing and waning they indicate that the deep thalamic relay nuclei are being *prevented* from firing, not that they fire more.[8] Indeed, sensory transmission through these relay nuclei drops off markedly during this drowsy transition period. This drop occurs long before the animal nods off or otherwise appears sleepy. In effect, *barely starting to fall asleep results in a markedly deafferented brain.*

The descent continues. From waking, next through this dynamic W → S transition period, the brain finally enters the state of synchronized, slow-wave S-sleep. At this time, tall EEG spindles cover the frontal and other association cortex. They cycle eleven to sixteen times per second. Some "sleep spindles" also occur as far down as the midbrain reticular formation. Even so, other parts of the brain still remain "awake." Yes—later on—these regions will finally fall into "sleep." But it will be only in their own particular ways, and on their own time-tables. For example, low voltage faster-wave activity may still prevail in some specific sensory thalamic nuclei, in the pulvinar, and in the lower brain stem.[9,10]

So what? By virtue of their *still staying* awake, *these regions remain available to be swept up by sudden surges of activity, even though the rest of a meditator's brain has slipped into an otherwise drowsy or sleeping condition* (see chapter 112). Once slow-wave S-sleep is sustained, however, brain metabolism plummets. This drop will dampen the functions of two sensory systems in particular. One of these had been mediating hearing, employing the medial geniculate body and the auditory cortex. The other system had been involved in visual functions, using the superior colliculus and the pulvinar.[11] So, after a person stays in deep S-sleep for many minutes, some hearing and visual functions are likely to be relatively inactive.

Drowsy meditators, and students who nod off in classrooms, could begin to draw some comfort and understanding from the way Pavlov's trained dogs sometimes fell asleep. Suppose the dogs had been placed in a new test situation, one in which their task was to *withhold* a response they had previously learned. Soon, these canine trainees nodded off. Pavlov might have stopped there, lured by an easy conclusion: his dogs had simply become bored. Instead, he arrived at a startling deduction: his dogs' sleep expressed a relatively high-level function. Their sleep was an *active* "internal inhibition," not a passive phenomenon.

Hess preferred to study cats. Cats, he observed, could be sent drifting off into a natural sleep as soon as he actively stimulated their lower thalamus and anterior hypothalamus at *low* frequency rates. This finding mobilized his thinking. Now he could conceive that these sites were active regions which could save or restore energy.[12,13] At two other sites, *low* frequency stimulation also produces synchronized EEG patterns. These are the intralaminar nuclei of the thalamus and the nucleus of the solitary tract in the brain stem.[14,15]

So S-sleep, as Pavlov suspected, is more than the mere absence of waking. We can now summarize four brain mechanisms which *actively* promote falling asleep. They reside in (1) the anterior hypothalamus and preoptic regions;[12]

(2) the basal forebrain region;[16,17] (3) the central projections of the ninth and tenth cranial nerves;[14] and (4) the actions of several hormones and sleep-promoting substances.[18–20]

During the earlier epidemics of sleeping sickness, a few patients, paradoxically, stayed wide-awake. It turned out that, in these insomniac patients, the encephalitis virus had damaged the *anterior* parts of their hypothalamus. This raised the question, Did the same region help normal persons sleep? If this were true, then sleep might also occur when animals were stimulated *chemically* in this same general region. And, indeed, animals also went to sleep when acetylcholine agonists were used to stimulate this anterior region.[21] Stimulating the nearby basal forebrain area, by locally warming it, also induced the phenomena of sleep.[16,17]

This anterior hypothalamic, preoptic "sleep" region appears normally to be held in check by signals relayed up from the midbrain reticular formation.[22] And it is also very sensitive to light falling upon the retina. Even the faintest rays of light can be sufficient to stop its sleep-promoting functions. In Zen meditation, the age-old directions to keep the eyes partly open appear well-founded.

Under certain circumstances, transition periods can be short, and steep on each of their two sides. Later, the meditator may be unsure: did I plunge into sleep, and if so, which kind of sleep was it? Chapter 112 illustrates this point. But in the sleep research laboratory, this pivotal "moment of sleep" can be reliably defined.[1] Perception stops. At the same time, visual fixation breaks off. Now *slow eye movements* begin. Changes deep in the brain determine these three events, changes starting seconds before the scalp EEG itself develops its sleep spindles and its slow waves. When humans lose sleep and build up a "sleep debt," they sink easily into the little microsleep episodes. These catnaps last up to a minute or so. Naps are brief downward thrusts, produced when the pressure of sleep indents the downsloping W → S transition line.

But what about *upward* thrusts? Because transitional states do not occur only as we descend into deep sleep. Indeed they also develop each time S-sleep *ascends* to D-sleep. In cats and rats, the brain needs only one to five seconds to ascend from S to D. Again, during this ascending transition period, studies show that *sensate messages are blocked from rising through the thalamus.* How effective is this *physiological* process at cutting off the sensory supply to higher cerebral structures? The researcher compares its afferent blockade with that of a *surgical* slice through the brain stem at the high midbrain level.[23]

Our short transition periods—down into S-sleep and up from it—are not like the smooth ascents and descents of an airplane flight. Nor are the brief "downdrafts and updrafts" during sleep comparable with the way our senses get buffeted in an airplane seat at times. Because certain sleep transitions carry the potential for a strong sensate blockade. And each time the sensory input is cut off from consciousness the meditator confronts a recurrent challenge: *How do I hold on to awareness and attentiveness, even though (without my knowing it) my physical self is being subjected to deafferentation?*

Back in part III, we considered how such attentive skills originate in successive physiological layers (see chapters 37 and 62). And the reader may also recall an earlier series of chapters. These emphasized how Zen has always focused on the training of attention (see chapters 15, 16, 18, and 21). So one begins to wonder: could such training be, in a sense, a kind of "exercising" of one's attentional networks, and at levels higher than before? An involvement of more rostral circuits which perhaps, if they spread, might engage "insightful" loops in the frontal regions of one's brain? (see chapter 141).

Meanwhile, the brain is undergoing other striking changes whenever it draws near D-sleep. For now, more obvious activating phenomena are taking over. The next three chapters present one paradox after another.

71

Desynchronized Sleep

Don't tell me what you dreamed last night, for I've been reading Freud.
Franklin P. Adams (1881–1960)[1]

Dreams are mere productions of the brain, and fools consult interpreters in vain.
Jonathan Swift (1667–1745)

This chapter emphasizes not the content of dreams, but what our capacity to dream implies. Dreaming means that, while still sleeping, we reactivate many of the mechanisms of awakening.

In overview, desynchronized sleep, D-sleep, enables our brain (a) to reactivate itself during its otherwise drugged stupor of slow-wave sleep, but (b) to accomplish this so gently that we're not sent all the way up to the waking state.[2] During our waking hours, stimuli from the outside shape consciousness. But during D-sleep the field of awareness can turn inward. Now it can pursue directions other than those dictated by new sensory stimuli entering from the outside. In many other respects, D-sleep and wakefulness seem to be "fundamentally equivalent brain states."[3]

Two aspects of normal D-sleep are most relevant to Zen. One is the evidence that D-sleep activates most of the brain. The other is the evidence that normal subjects can dissociate the substates of D-sleep and displace them. These two phenomena are of greater present interest than are either the florid dream imagery or those fast movements of the eyes which first gave rise to the acronym REM. For these reasons it has seemed preferable to use the more inclusive, generic term, *D-sleep*, to refer to a state which is of much greater general importance than are its rapid eye movements per se.

D-Sleep, an Active State

The brief phasic, and longer-lasting tonic events in D-sleep tap many sources within the brain stem.[2-6] Here, acetylcholine mechanisms do interact with those of norepinephrine and serotonin. Yet several striking examples illustrate how important ACH itself is. *Direct* cholinergic stimulation of pontine reticular cells can trigger REM episodes.[7] And by giving physostigmine, researchers can increase the synaptic levels of ACH. This drug precipitates human subjects into D-sleep when it is injected intravenously during stage 2 of sleep.[8] In marked contrast, the firing rate of ST and of NE nerve cells drops off sharply at the start of D-sleep.

Item: LSD also causes a sharp drop in the firing of ST nerve cells. This drop has long suggested that when a person's ST firing tone is reduced, this pause might help to generate D-sleep in general and be responsible for many of the mental effects of LSD in particular (see figure 14). But one cannot immediately assume that the slowing of raphe cells alone is the primary causal agent. For raphe firing rates also slow, secondarily, during any general reduction in motor activity. Why? Because when motor systems "rest," the quiet state itself deprives many nerve cells of the usual sensory stimulation they would otherwise have received as the result of active movements.[9]

Early studies suggested that D-sleep itself depresses muscle reflexes,[10] and that it also periodically blocks sensory impulses from entering their usual pathways at multiple levels.[11] This sensory blockade frees the sleeper to engage in dream imagery and other *internal* quasi-sensory activities.[12] Indeed, measurements show that such higher-level sensory systems do become more active. Take, for instance, the nerve cells which send their long axons out from the sensory association cortex. During waking hours, these larger parietal lobe cells fire only eleven times a second. During S-sleep they discharge only nine times per second. But they fire seventeen times a second during ordinary D-sleep, and twenty-two times a second when REMs intrude into D-sleep.[13]

Elsewhere in the brain, many other nerve cells are also firing much more in D-sleep than during S-sleep. This increases their local metabolic rate.[14] To illustrate: when a cat is in D-sleep, its activated groups of nuclei include the cingulate gyrus, nucleus accumbens, and nearby basal forebrain, as well as the ventral anterior nucleus of the thalamus.[15]

During D-sleep, the reticular formation shows a relatively greater increase in its metabolic activity than it does during wakefulness, when viewed in relation to the metabolism of the rest of the brain. And sensory relay nuclei in the back of the thalamus also become more metabolically active than they are in S-sleep. *Except for the* pulvinar, a noteworthy omission. So, when we ask how the large pulvinar can contribute to specific alternate states, we will need to remember that its usual functions are chiefly associated with an actively awake brain.[14]

Over a century ago, a physician, Dr. E. Clarke, happened to be looking at his patient's brain. He was surprised to see it becoming so engorged with blood that it protruded through the opened skull case.[16] The patient was dreaming. We now have the explanation: when nerve cells increase their firing rates, the increased metabolism quickly translates into more blood flowing into the brain. Refined studies now show that we increase our blood flow during REM sleep as much as 47 percent in the brain stem and cerebellum, and 41 percent over the cerebral hemispheres.

Some evidence hints that our two hemispheres dream asymmetrically. Thus, blood flow may double in the *right* parieto-occipital and posterior temporal regions at the particular moments when patients are having vivid visual and auditory dreams.[17]

Yet it is also true that prolonged D-sleep *quiets* certain other functions. Of note are the preoptic and anterior hypothalamic regions. Here D-sleep slows the firing of the special nerve cells sensitive to temperature. And when these "thermostat" cells slow, the brain suspends the vital functions which had been regulating body temperature.

How was this discovered? By observing a rabbit's ears. Normally, a sleeping rabbit's ears become cool if the outside temperature drops. This occurs because animals shut down the circulation in the skin of their ears in the process of conserving heat. But suppose S-sleep has shifted up to D-sleep. Now the blood vessels dilate. The rabbit's ears become warmer and pinker. So the otherwise stable and dependable hypothalamus develops an unusual *in*stability during D-sleep. It now becomes "free to drift out of the normal range of homeostatic regulation."[18]

Rabbit's ears? How important is this evidence that even the hypothalamus can become unstable? The finding is relevant when we search for the underlying cause of many other physiological instabilities that develop during a prolonged meditative retreat. Indeed, in order fully to understand Zen and the brain we will need to carefully study meditators during their formal *nighttime* sleeping hours, not merely during the day. One question to be tested in these future studies can be stated as follows: Do intensive meditative retreats—by increasing the *range* of the physiological drifts—set the stage for the brain's subsequent shifts into fragmented desynchronized states and substates? (see part V).

D-sleep activates the brain through a series of steps. Put simply, it turns out that when the brain stem activates the thalamus, the thalamus then activates the cortex[4] (see chapter 37). Again, we observe that throughout these operations the brain functions economically. *For it employs similar basic mechanisms whether it is in the course of activating itself naturally during D-sleep, or during waking behavior, or has become activated artificially as a result of direct electrical stimulation to the midbrain reticular formation.*

One may ask, what is so special about an "activated" nerve cell during either of these three conditions? *It stays ready to respond.* It remains on the alert, a term which originally described the sentry on his lookout high in a watchtower. First, the nerve cell membrane tends to lose its opposing charges. It then *de*polarizes. Not much. Just enough so that the next stimulus will send it leaping instantly past its threshold and cause it to discharge. Yes, this cell does pause briefly after each firing. But it remains poised instantly to respond to the next incoming message.

Midbrain reticular nerve cells are sentinels. They are vital to the process of awakening the rest of our brain and body. In animals, these small sentry cells begin firing faster some eighteen to twenty-two seconds *before* the scalp EEG suggests that arousal has begun.[4] Moreover, midbrain reticular cells are already wide-awake and firing *tonically* fifteen seconds before the EEG itself finally shifts into its low voltage fast activities and the rest of the animal begins to stir into frank behavioral awakening.

Now, this same sequence outlined above is put into use multiple times. It also operates during that particular transition period when, after S-sleep, the next destination is *D-sleep*, not waking. Not only do midbrain cells fire earlier but now the hippocampus desynchronizes. And cells up in the intralaminar nuclei of the thalamus also become more excitable. They start to discharge as long as six to twelve seconds before the surface EEG desynchronizes.[19] And the brain runs through this repertoire whether S-sleep switches all the way up to full waking, or stops short to enter D-sleep.[20]

But suppose you remove these midbrain reticular sentinels. To do so, you employ the local excitotoxic properties of kainic acid. Even then, the animal can still ascend into D-sleep from S-sleep. At first, this was puzzling. Could the brain draw on resources *outside* the midbrain in order to prompt its desynchronizations? If so, where are they?

Some come from the medulla. It was down in the medulla, during waking, that we first met the extra-large ACH reticular nerve cells (see figure 5). The more important of these is the *magnocellular group*. They fire in long tonic runs. The other, *giganto*cellular, set of nerve cells also project up to the intralaminar thalamic nuclei. They discharge more phasically.[4]

Large cells can fire rapidly, speeding messages along large axons to their targets. The magnocellular cells send their impulses up to the thalamus by e-mail—twice as fast as do their smaller counterparts in the midbrain reticular formation. Moreover, they can influence the thalamus selectively, and the cortex widely. Once their messages enter the ventromedial nucleus of the thalamus, their influence can then relay up to *the whole anterior neocortex*, there to bias its foremost layer of excitabilities.[21,22] But these two sets of large ACH cells in the medulla can accomplish only so much. Although they can still influence vision and hearing indirectly, neither has a *direct* route into either the lateral pulvinar or the geniculate nuclei.[4]

Day or night, the brain can operate only through its systems of checks and balances. Down in the medulla and pons reside covert inhibitory circuits. They are easy to overlook. But *sleep uncovers them*. Sleep reveals how they normally hold desynchronized states in check. This finding becomes especially relevant to the set of experiences which meditators have after they doze off and drift into blank moments (see chapter 112).

Recall the barbiturate experiments in which a weak dose of barbiturate was infused into the arteries nourishing the medulla and lower pons. In a waking cat, nothing happens. Its EEG does not change; neither does its behavior. But suppose the cat is already sound asleep, and in S-sleep. Now inject the same dose of this depressant drug into the same region. Does this "sleeping pill" drug make the cat sleep more soundly? No. Instead, the cat shifts up out of its slow-wave sleep, ascends into its natural D-sleep, and shows rapid eye movements! If you then add a slight sensory stimulus, the cat wakes up.[23]

Why such unexpected results? Barbiturates enhance GABA functions. Local GABA mechanisms are important in the covert inhibitory circuits cited above. So the findings in the barbiturate injection experiments point to delicate balances. Here, in the lower brain stem, the circuitries are highly leveraged. When their set-points change, they can tip the rest of the brain into either of our two natural, activated states—D-sleep or waking. One begins to wonder: could a series of events starting this low down in our brain stem underlie some of those thin, filmy veils of consciousness that William James had once referred to?

Paradoxes in D-Sleep

The early researchers called it "paradoxical sleep" for good reasons. One surprise was the way a few REM episodes slipped in only a few minutes after sleep began. These early episodes are called *sleep-onset REM*. It turns out that many conditions can displace REM episodes forward in this manner, *into the early minutes* of each sleep cycle. Normal newborn babies show them,[24] as do depressed patients,[25] patients with narcolepsy,[26] normals who are isolated from all time cues,[27] and normals who receive doses of L-tryptophan, the serotonin precursor.[28]

Sleep-onset REM episodes are also prone to occur among those normal subjects whose core body temperatures remain stable. REM episodes also arrive early whenever there occurs a general flattening in amplitude of the otherwise large tidal up-and-down swings between the sleep cycle and the arousal cycle.[29] It is possible that the person who continues to meditate on a regular basis during the daytime could dampen such swings in a manner that might contribute to this overall process of flattening.[30]

Another paradox. Consider what happens when normal people respond to stressful circumstances. Soon they develop "ambiguous" periods. *These intervals combine elements both of D-sleep and of S-sleep.*[31] True, their EEG does become desynchronized, as in typical D-sleep. However, these subjects still keep up their *waking* muscle tone, and they do not go on into rapid eye movements. Even *unstressed* normal people also enter ambiguous periods, positioned between D-sleep and S-sleep. These episodes take up as much as 1 to 7 percent of their total sleep time.

Normals also undergo brief, "micro-REM" episodes lasting from one to fifteen seconds. And they sandwich these micro-REM episodes *into wakefulness*, not only into S-sleep.[32] There is nothing ambiguous about the implications of these findings. Consciousness is a mixed bag. *We are more often on the brink of falling into D-sleep than we realize.*

But sleep is most obviously destructured in one disease condition, called *narcolepsy.* Patients with narcolepsy have many sleep-onset REM periods and REM-like, ambiguous periods. They also become excessively sleepy and undergo sudden losses of tone (cataplexy) during the day. Moreover, they hallucinate and develop episodes of sleep paralysis as they enter and leave sleep.[33] Like meditators, many narcolepsy patients are not aware how frequently they "drop off." Looking back, they may realize that there was a gap, caused by a short "sleep attack." Even in a research laboratory, they fall sound asleep within three and a half minutes. There, slow rolling eye movements and abrupt microsleeps betray their strong tendencies to drowse off.

Short naps can cause episodes of sleep-onset REM not only in patients with narcolepsy[26] but also in normal subjects.[34] During morning naps, for example, normals may slip into REM just after they enter stage 1 sleep. This finding again illustrates how easily any meditator might slip into D-sleep, unexpectedly, while dozing off during zazen. Not enough attention has been paid to all the ways this might affect the meditator (see part VI).

A critical look at our usual dream mentation shows much of it to be disorganized and illogical. On the other hand, it can be reassuring to know that D-sleep does enhance many brain functions in a more coherent manner. When normal subjects are awakened directly out of D-sleep they are not confused. Indeed, they react almost as fast as they do during the waking state. When given various tasks, they perform relatively better on the visuospatial tasks associated with *right* hemisphere functioning.[35] In contrast, if the subjects had been awakened from the two deeper levels of S-sleep, they remain confused and show slow reaction times for several minutes.[36] Moreover, at this time, the tasks on which the S-sleepers perform relatively better are those considered to reflect *left* hemispheric performance.[35]

Could our mentation become incoherent during D-sleep because it changes the ways the two hemispheres usually interact? When cats are in D-sleep, measurements show relatively little neuronal activity passing along those nerve fibers of the corpus callosum. These fibers normally transmit messages back and forth between the two cerebral hemispheres.[36] We don't yet know if humans have similar evidence suggesting that D-sleep reduces the cross-transfer of information between the two sides of the brain. But if they do, then during D-sleep and related states it could be difficult for subjects say, to access the language attributes of their left hemisphere in order to clarify events that had first entered into experience within compartments of the nonverbal right hemisphere.

How does prior sleep restore the brain? We still don't know. Some speculate that the processes of REM sleep cause us to "unlearn" false associations.[37] Others counter with an argument in reverse: it turns out that more D-sleep and REM episodes occur *after* some learning has already taken place earlier. In fact, animals cannot retain what they had learned earlier *if* you eliminate their D-sleep in the follow-up period.[38] Moreover, only certain rats become the "fast learners" of new tasks. Which ones? The "dreamers," the rats whose innate capacities already allowed them to enter into more D-sleep initially than did their slow-learning controls.[39] Meanwhile, human animals need not subscribe to any set theory about dreams. We can still go on appreciating what a good night's sleep contributes, enjoying the way it restores fresh attitudes. And we remain free to marvel at that rare dream which either resolves our deep irreconcilables or clarifies them in some curiously satisfactory way.

If you deprive the brain of REM sleep on one night, it rebounds the next night. This phenomenon makes up for what was lost. And if you give animals the opportunity to do so, they will learn to keep pressing a lever switch which keeps delivering stimulating pulses of electricity to their own medial forebrain bundle. Suppose you then deprive these trained "self-stimulating" animals of *their* REM sleep. What happens? They stimulate themselves even more, and they respond more sensitively to it.[40] How much more of the extra artificial self-stimulation do they then add? It turns out to be *just enough* to cut back on that extra amount of "REM rebound" which they would otherwise have developed naturally. These studies are intriguing. They suggest that the two states—the one of self-stimulation, and the other of D-sleep with REM—do resemble each other. True, they differ in obvious ways. But each appears to yield, in a sense, an "equivalence of activation." It seems almost as though an animal will seek out more brain stimulation (even though it is artificial) to make up for the amount of prior activation it had lost in the way of authentic D-sleep.

At this writing, humans have yet to be tested along these same lines. But it is clear that many persons are prone to abuse stimulants. And it is also evident that many are also engaging in other stimulus-seeking behaviors inappropriate in kind or degree. Could we be driven, unknowingly, into some of our subtler appetitive behaviors as part of an attempt to satiate deep, unmet physiological needs for stimulation? Could we reverse this situation by getting equivalent amounts of D-sleep? Moreover, in the process, would we be able to rechannel our drives toward more fruitful kinds of equivalent activities during our waking hours, kinds which don't entrap us in disadvantageous forms of appetitive stimulation? Such questions would seem to merit further study. Meanwhile, there may be unexplored benefits to meditative approaches that sharpen the senses and enhance mindful awareness during the day. In ways now hidden, heightened attention might be contributing subtle degrees and kinds of positive stimulation that could prove beneficial.

D-sleep itself may keep open, at least partway, certain narrow windows of awareness which still allow especially meaningful outside stimuli to penetrate the brain. It is when the sleeping mother is in D-sleep that she responds most readily to her baby's faint cry.[41] One recalls here the ideal embodied in the image of the Bodhisattva of Compassion. This Bodhisattva, a model for all Buddhists, hears objectively and attends with penultimate detachment to the cries of the whole suffering universe.[42]

Decades of complicated research are summarized in this chapter. The evidence has opened up a Pandora's box. Sleep, that once seemingly quiet period, has now had the covers thrown off. Revealed instead is a dynamic turmoil, full of shifting checks and balances. The modules and functional systems which usually generate our sleep and wakefulness each tend to cling together physiologically. They rise and fall together during alternate cycles of rest and of activity. But sometimes this regular, organized pattern becomes unstable. It may then overshoot in either direction. Then, substates may split off. These give us novel perspectives on the relationships between Zen and the brain.

72

Other Perspectives in Dreams

> Our dream images are like pictures sent back to earth from a camera located on a satellite in space. The broader scene emerges.
>
> M. Ullman and N. Zimmerman[1]

Some still believe, as did Freud, that dreams are the "royal road" which leads to our understanding the unconscious. Others have taken the plebeian view that to engage in formal dream analysis is like trying to find a meaningful poem in a bowl of alphabet soup. Truth may reside in-between these extremes. A few dreams are useful because they enable us to step back, and "to view the system we are examining from a point outside the system."[1] In this sense, the dreams do let us see, objectively, into our mental processes. Rarely, such dreams give us very direct *insights*, *intuitions*. Otherwise, in most dreams, the forebrain seems to be scrambling, improvising scenarios which might seem to provide the best fit for an otherwise inchoate turmoil of nerve cell firing.[2]

Piaget found that children first realize about the age of five years that *they* create their own dreams, not some outside influence. Meditation is like that. It also helps meditators discover how much of their own discomfort arises from within. Gradually, suffering is seen to be self-inflicted, the product of a self which had constructed its own daydreaming world of illusion and delusion.[3]

Dream awareness focuses inward. That is, it orients not toward the details of our bedroom but toward those interior images that establish the dream's structural foreground. And we usually maintain that sense of self which relates our dreams to our waking situations.[4] The usual dreams include hallucinatory-like material, but frank hallucinations are uncommon, found in less than 8 percent of dreams.[5] Still, they are impressive, because they transport the person into a distinctly different setting which seems especially "real." These same two attributes of "otherworldliness" and "hyperreality" are amplified in alternate states of consciousness. Two more reasons to emphasize desynchronized sleep in the context of Zen.

Some studies suggest that our left posterior hemisphere is dominant for dreaming. True, damage to this back part of the brain does interfere with *recalling* dreams.[6] But the right side also seems to make another major contribution. The blend from each side makes for a dream content fully as complex as is the turbulent flow of Joycean thought streams during our waking hours. Moreover, recent studies reveal a surprising fact: dreamers *reduce* the blood flow to their inferior frontal regions by 9 percent. We have noted that the more *medial* aspects of this part of the frontal lobe are normally associated with drive and motivation (see chapter 57). Perhaps some reductions of these drive functions might contribute to the passivity, acceptance, and loss of ordinary time sequences which are so familiar to us as features of dream experience.[7] Moreover, any reductions of those normal impulse-control functions of the adjacent *orbital* frontal regions could release the dreamer into more primitive kinds of mentation.

We usually think that our dreams take only a visual form. Closer inspection reveals that dreams embody a kind of "story." The yarn unfolds in *narrative* form. Recent evidence suggests that we don't process these storybook qualities of our REM dreams the same way that we process their visual counterparts. For example, one intelligent patient was studied after having had major damage to the *right* temporo-parietal region. This patient's dreams during REM sleep lacked their previous *visual* imagery. "It was almost like I had a complicated story going on rather than a complicated movie going on."[8,9]

Such evidence makes it clear that during D-sleep *we also construct a story line using nonvisual kinds of information.* Moreover, while doing so, we can transmit certain forms of knowledge in a relatively coherent, organized form *without a word being spoken.* The following point is worth emphasizing: while awake, and during the usual process termed *insight,* we infuse some of these same narrative qualities with *understanding.*

Yet one other aspect of dreaming is less clear. Why, only rarely, does a dream state access that major class of insight-wisdom which seems to be an equivalent of kensho? The classic example was provided by Master Hakuin, who recounted a dream he had when he was thirty-three. His dream narrative was illustrated, and in this instance it led up to an impressive closure. His mother was handing him a violet robe. In each of its two sleeves was a heavy mirror. The right-sided mirror penetrated deep into his heart, at which point the whole earth and his mind became transparently clear. Then the left mirror flashed out a broader beam, a million times brighter. At this memorable stage in his dream, Hakuin finally experienced oneness with the whole extent of the Buddha nature.[10]

In the previous chapter, we noted how both D-sleep and waking activate the brain. The similarities have prepared us to conclude by acknowledging a subtle but important point: those mechanisms that will shift a person into a kensho-like closure are not always confined to the waking hours.

73

Lucid Dreaming

[On lucid dreams] The union of separate elements, dreaming and consciousness.

S. LaBerge[1]

Sometimes, while dreaming, we realize it is "only" a dream. And when the term "lucid" is applied to dreaming, it refers to just these moments. *Lucid*, then, simply means that the dreamer has become conscious of dreaming. A few persons become skilled lucid dreamers, so adept that they attain much of the same clarity and coherence as they did during the waking state. Moreover, strange as it may seem, these exceptional subjects—while still dreaming—can reason, remember, and act volitionally.[1]

Lucid dreams are not mere tricks to be studied in a laboratory bedroom. They emphasize two fundamental points. First, if you dissociate brain states during transitional intervals, their substates can reassemble in the form of some very curious hybrids. Second, we rarely engage in lucid *waking*. Consider how seldom we truly grasp our immediate situation, and realize that we are now fully alive and awake!

At night, in bed, we usually lack that full, keen understanding that *we* are individuals who are actually in bed, dreaming the dreams. But suppose we then let awareness enter a dream, so much so that it now takes in the *total* situation. At this point—once we conclude that "this is a dream"—then we perceive something singular: this particular moment is also marked by genuine mental clarity *in general.*

A person can cultivate this tendency for a lucid quality to enter dreams. One technique is to break frequently into daytime consciousness, asking the question, Am I dreaming? Another technique is to keep mentally awake while becoming physically relaxed, by repeatedly focusing attention on some ongoing mental action.[1] Obviously, these procedures resemble some standard techniques used in meditation. Both approaches cultivate an attentive, mindful awareness of the present moment, the Now. Well-motivated subjects have more lucid dreams if they remind themselves, before going to sleep, to become lucid during the next dream.[2]

On two occasions, while still sleeping, we are rather close to being awake. One occurs just as we first drop off to sleep; the other is later on, just before we rouse. And most lucid dreams also occur when the subject is at or near these same, more *wakeful*, ends of S-sleep. Of LaBerge's own nearly 900 lucid dreams, 8 percent began when he maintained a "continuous reflective consciousness while falling asleep." What techniques does he use to cultivate this kind of lucid dream? They proceed in the following manner. When he first awakens from a dream in the morning or in the afternoon, he tries to maintain reflective consciousness. He then drifts into a period of imagery (of the kind that one usually has at the *onset* of ordinary sleep). Following this imagery, he slides into a lucid dream scene. His lucid dreams during the daytime hours are basically the same as those which emerge after longer periods of nighttime S-sleep.

It is noteworthy that after LaBerge generates hallucinatory (hypnopompic) imagery, on the way up from sleep to waking,[3] he may then suddenly find himself already "fully in the dream scene, and lucid." In his case, this particular sequence of events typically falls into the following order: (1) starting to awaken; (2) hallucinatory imagery; and (3) the abrupt onset of lucid dream mentation *with no interim period of ordinary dreaming*. It will help the reader to keep this sequence in mind. It bears a remarkable resemblance to the series of events at the start of the present author's episode of internal absorption (see chapter 108).

But there are also major differences. Table 12 compares lucid dreams with other states relevant to meditative experience.

Lucid dreamers still "own" their dreams. They remain clear about the fact that the dreams are their very own, ongoing productions. They still sit in the director's chair, willfully creating their own actions and fantasies. And when LaBerge does so, he is almost always a *participating actor as well, not only an observer.*[1]

When lucidity arrives, it can usher into the dream a host of other new and interesting qualities. For instance, even LaBerge's most prosaic lucid dreams tend to begin with "an unmistakable sense of excitement and delight." Space expands as this positive affective tone blends into enhanced perceptions. The intensity of light also increases, and the dream scene takes on a richly beautiful luster. *Lucidity, therefore, can be accompanied by unusual perceptual clarity, visual enrichment, and delight.* Still, it is the instability of a lucid dream—not its vivid quality—which serves as the best criterion for distinguishing this dream from ordinary waking reality. For a lucid dream is a delicate moment. It is easily disrupted until the dreamer has learned how to let go. This allows the dream experience to then flow by itself, without entangling the dreamer in it emotionally.

Out-of-body experiences are not a regular part of lucid dreaming.[1] LaBerge's rare out-of-body experiences occurred only at times when he felt that he was already having some unusual problem thinking critically or remembering. However, having first noted that *fully* lucid dreamers *might* go on to surrender their

Table 12
Some Differences between Samadhi-absorption, Dreams, and Certain Other Relevant States

Aspect	Usual Waking Consciousness	Usual Dreams	Lucid Dreams	"Out-Of-Body" Experiences[†]	Samadhi with Internal Absorption[*]	Comment
Loss of the usual, bounded self, sense of unreality	0–1	0	0–1	0–2	4	*None of the perjorative connotations of depersonalization or derealization
Impersonal detachment	0–1	1	0–1	2–3	4	
Complete, ongoing appreciation that one is really awake, or dreaming	3–4	0	2–3	1–2	4	*Awareness witnesses; awareness in the absence of self
Hyperlucidity and hyperawareness	0	0–1	1–2	2–3	4	*Awareness witnesses; awareness in the absence of self
Valued in retrospect	0–1	0–2	1–2	1–3	3–4	†More valued in the near-death context
Accurate time sense preserved	3–4	2	2	0–1	0	*Notions of the sequences within the experiences persist

0 = none; 5 = maximal. The numbers suggest only relationships, and are not absolute.
†Note that, at the moment of, and in a near-death experience, many subjects feel that their *essential* personal self still continues, and that their vivid, ongoing awareness views their physical self as detached and distant.

own self-image, he goes on to conclude that "Fully lucid dreams are transcendental experiences."[1]

The skeptic may well ask, What's the proof that the subject is both dreaming and also awake? Lucid dreamers lose the usual EMG evidence of muscle contractions in the chin and in other muscles along the long axis of the body. This same silent EMG is also typical of the usual form of D-sleep. Nonetheless, lucid dreamers can still make complex volitional movements, planned in advance, using their fingers and other distal muscles in their extremities. They can also perform willed tracking movements with their eyes.[4] They can also send out other signals such as a series of extreme eye movements having a predetermined sequence, or a series of squeezings of the fist in Morse code. And all the while these willed movements are going on, the dreamers still show the other classic evidence of D-sleep. This not only persists in their EEG and EMG recordings but continues for the next minute or so.[5]

It is evident from careful polygraphic monitoring of lucid dreamers in the sleep laboratory that they have indeed entered an unusual state. It displays a conglomerate of features compatible *both* with dreaming *and* with being awake.

But the timing of this state is also a most important feature. *Most lucid dreams occur when the general tidal level of waking consciousness is on the rise.* At such vulnerable transition periods, the sharp clarity of the waking state briefly penetrates the previous state of dreaming, and the two overlap.

Not surprisingly, the *surface* EEGs during lucid dreams show variable results. They differ from subject to subject and from laboratory to laboratory. Some reports describe a relatively low voltage, mixed frequency EEG,[5] even a theta wave–dominant EEG.[4] Others suggest that lucid dreams occur when alpha activity rises to a peak during an ongoing state of D-sleep which had been in its phase of rapid eye movements.[6] Still others find that lucid dreams start during an alpha rhythm, of relatively high amplitude in D-sleep, when it falls to a moderately low amplitude just before the subject rouses.[7] However, ordinary people can display higher amplitude alpha waves during D-sleep without being in a lucid dream.[7] And some persons can export motor signals out of their lucid dreams without being in such alpha rhythms at the time.[5]

To conclude: lucid dreams provide an excellent example of those same basic principles of sleep physiology reviewed in the previous two chapters. They illustrate, in ways that strain credulity, one more paradox of paradoxical sleep: that a wave of conscious awareness can pierce a dreamlike state, riding on the crest of its own independent biological cycle of wakefulness.

74

Conditioning: Learning and Unlearning

> If we could look through the skull into the brain of a consciously thinking person, and if the place of optimal excitability were luminous, then we should see playing over the cerebral surface a bright spot with fantastic waving borders, constantly fluctuating in size and form, and surrounded by a darkness, more or less deep, covering the rest of the hemispheres.
>
> Ivan Pavlov (1849–1936)[1]

> In the pursuit of knowledge, everyday something is added. In the practice of the Tao, everyday something is dropped.
>
> *Tao Te Ching*[2]

Those outside Zen think it is an esoteric oriental philosophy or religion, something they can "add" to their store of information. Those inside Zen know it involves a subtraction, a dropping off, an unlearning. Kobori-roshi emphasized how much prior conditioning we had all undergone. And yet he also stressed that vibrant central core which remains when it drops off: our "unconditioned self." What does "unconditioning" mean? One can better understand by asking, how did we all become conditioned in the first place?

In Pavlov's metaphor, each consciously thinking brain was a shifting play of excited highlights. In the surround were dark inhibitions. His key studies of higher reflex functions were the product of his later years. His Nobel Prize had come for his earlier pioneering studies of the physiology of digestion. But in the course of watching his dogs salivate, Pavlov became fascinated. He realized how crucial a function was actually going on: they were attaching *meaning* to substitutes for their food! Central to Zen is every process which attaches meaning to our basic unconditioned brain.

At first, Pavlov's dogs ignored the sound of a bell ringing, in and of itself. After all, to a naive dog, the ring means nothing, only another sound, nothing to salivate about. But then Pavlov rang the bell a few times just before feeding. Now the dog caught on, made a connection. It *associated* each ring with the pending arrival of food. Now the ring had become that of a *dinner* bell. Gradually the dog became *conditioned*. Finally, it salivated to the ring of the bell alone.

In these experiments, the food starts as the dog's basic natural, *unconditioned* stimulus. Next, the dog brain learns to link the two stimuli together. Finally, the bell itself comes to predict food. Bell means food. Its sound has been transformed into the *conditioned* stimulus. To us, it would be a dinner bell. It certainly is for the dog. The sequence evolves:

$$\text{Food} \rightarrow \text{saliva}$$
$$\text{Bell} \rightarrow \text{food} \rightarrow \text{saliva}$$
$$\text{Dinner bell} \rightarrow \text{saliva}$$

But the bell is still a mere sound. What happens in the brain? How do its circuits change over the properties of the very same bell signal so that a once-neutral stimulus becomes a conditioned stimulus? And salivation—at first the drooling was the dog's natural unconditioned response. What changes *it* into a conditioned response? Which synapses in the brain are the agencies of change? Theories have multiplied.[3]

Sensory and Motor Limbs of Conditioning

In his day, Pavlov thought his dogs would need a cerebral cortex to be conditioned. More recent experiments show that a cortex is not needed, neither to acquire conditioning nor to retain it. It turns out that learning goes on all over the nervous system. Various isolated segments, at levels high and low, can "learn" certain well-defined tasks.[4]

Suppose you begin by lightly touching the cornea or lid of a rabbit's eye. Its thin nictitating membrane quickly contracts to protect the eye. The basic circuitry of this blink reflex originates in the brain stem. It then loops up to enlist the cerebellum.[5–7] After the rabbit is conditioned, its eye-blink membrane will contract in response to a sound, rather than just to a touch.

Do different neuromessengers make different contributions? Yes. Animals acquire this conditioned blink reflex more easily if you have given them drugs which mimic or enhance the actions of dopamine, norepinephrine, and serotonin. Included among such drugs are LSD and the amphetamines. If you release NE locally in the hippocampus, it makes it easier for hippocampal cells then to respond to the kinds of conditioned stimuli that will become important behaviorally.[8] But certain other drugs make it *more difficult* to become conditioned. These drugs block the effects of acetylcholine and DA. Included among them are scopolamine, haloperidol, and morphine.

Each of these drugs can act at several levels. To begin with, it can act on the much earlier *sensory* limb of the blink reflex, the first part, which delivers the "raw" sound signal. A drug that acts on sensation will change the incoming messages relayed from the stimulus itself (much as we had observed occurring in *Aplysia*) (see chapter 49). So now the sound stimulus could become either a more effective or less effective substitute for the original threat posed by being touched near the eye.

LSD serves as an example of this early, "sensory limb" principle. For LSD helps a rabbit learn the conditioned reflex to sound. How? By enhancing the excitatory properties of the sound stimulus itself. In contrast, the blocking drugs (scopolamine, haloperidol, and morphine) mute a sound's excitatory conditioning properties. Opioids act on their mu receptors to slow classical conditioning,[5] and endorphins also dampen the impact of that initial noxious stimulus on which hinges the process of aversive conditioning.[9]

Suppose you want to interfere with the *development* of conditioned learning. These studies suggest how to do so. You can either cut down on the tone of the biogenic amine and ACH systems or you can increase opioid tone. Then what about all those "things" that Lao-tzu had said would drop out "in the practice of the Tao?" What about the *un*learning, and *de*conditioning of established habits? Could even more drastic measures actually *reverse* the brain's conditioned responses *after* they had once been well-established? It was purely by chance, during the major Leningrad flood of 1924, that Pavlov discovered answers to these questions.[1] When flood waters surged high into Pavlov's kennels, his terrified dogs, still in their cages, had to paddle for their lives, nostrils held barely above high water level. Many of the survivors, rescued in the nick of time from this major stressful circumstance, then broke down, following a pattern resembling the state of shock shown by many human survivors.

Before the flood, Pavlov had already trained one group of his dogs to show certain positively conditioned behavior patterns. After the flood, he retested his dogs. To his surprise, he found that the particular dogs who had broken down had *un*learned their new tricks. Something had caused them to "forget." Something about their profound excitement and state of shock seemed to have washed away those conditioned responses that he had previously worked so hard to implant.

Pavlov had discovered a way to make old dogs *un*learn new tricks. His pioneer work ushered in a complex field, one to which the term "brainwashing" would later be loosely applied. In psychology, a general technical term for this process is *extinction*. And the reader, recalling that nirvana also implies an "extinction," may now begin to wonder: could there be any connection between these two words? Several lines of research hint that, in one sense, there might be.

Extinctions and Behavioral Inhibition

You can study *un*learning in a rat. First, it has to learn. So you train the rat to perform in a certain way that will finally give it the reward of food or drink. Then you change the rules of the game. You omit the reward. The rat is in a quandary. It must now forget your previous appetitive rules and learn something different. Extinction is equivalent to forgetting those old rules. It implies that an earlier behavior, previously learned and rewarded, is later extinguished.[10]

Now you can continue toward your original goal, that of studying *un*-learning. One technique is to increase some of the rat's cholinergic functions. A number of animal studies suggest that the normal brain uses ACH—acting on ACH muscarinic receptors in certain circuits—to withhold, or suppress, particular kinds of behavior. Moreover, *two* messengers—ACH and NE—can work cooperatively in the direction of this unlearning, because increasing NE activity can also enhance extinction in some instances.[11] Perhaps, on the other hand, you and your rat are comfortable with the status quo, and would prefer to thwart extinction. It isn't easy. Even after the blockade of *both* their NE beta-receptors and their ACH muscarinic receptors, rats still manage to "forget" practical lessons, learned earlier, which had helped them avoid aversive foot shock.[12]

Yet, imagine what severe stress responses the Leningrad dogs must have undergone in their flooded cages! Major changes in ACH and NE turnover could have helped them extinguish their *old* conditionings, and major increases in the turnover of DA, NE, and ST could have favored the emergence of *newer* ones. And this is not yet to mention the effects which the canine variety of near-death experiences would have had on other transmitters and messengers (see chapter 104).

Four chapters earlier, we referred to Pavlov's other studies on dogs, the ones that had dozed off in class. Observing these dognaps, Pavlov had postulated that their brains were then using an *active inhibitory process*. This "internal inhibition," he thought, was the kind of process which could turn off a response whenever it was not later reinforced.[13] There is a classic way to find out if such "internal inhibition" is present. It is to observe how any goal-directed subject behaves in a simple maze.

Now a simple maze has two arms, but no reward will be hidden at the end of either arm. What happens when a sensible hungry person, or rat, finds no reward in the right side? They will turn into the left arm 85 percent of the time on their next trial. Conclusion: "inhibition" has stopped the subject from returning to that vacant first arm. Young rats prove highly competent at this kind of a maze. By only four weeks of age, they have matured into their adult level of performance, scoring at the 85 percent level. And human children? We need four years before we can progress beyond our original, chance alternation rate of only 50 percent and attain adult levels of performance.

Maze learning skills depend on the interactions of several small units of the brain. After hippocampal lesions, if the animals are no longer reinforced, they can't use those particular spatial cues—the ones which they had learned, earlier, *would* work—as landmarks in order to gain their reward.[13] And after lesions of the basal-lateral amygdala and ventral striatum, they lose other relevant skills. These are the techniques which could have previously moved them to *seek out* the best location by virtue of infusing their behavior with "quasi-affective" or "motivational" elements.[14]

Drugs which block ACH (such as atropine or scopolamine) also interfere with correct maze behavior. In contrast, maze performance improves when low doses of prostigmine are used to increase the effects of intrinsic ACH. Once again, the results illustrate how many contributions are made by ACH. For the particular drugs which enhance ACH functions encourage more adaptable responses in general, and these ACH-like drugs also help animals drop off certain of their older behavior patterns which are no longer reinforced. ACH is a transmitter to remember (see chapter 38).

As tested by simple maze behavior, Pavlov's internal inhibition appears to be almost a kind of "common sense" which would stop any subject from doing the "dumb" thing. In its wider general applications, what kinds of normal mechanisms enter into such behavioral inhibition? They are of two kinds. Again, we can view them broadly as "sensory" and "motor." A sensory line of explanations runs as follows. Suppose you stop sensate rewards from coming in. This shuts off the reinforcements of added food and drink. Theory would predict that a number of networks would then "learn" to shut down once this appetitive sensory data no longer resonated, as before, throughout the hippocampus, the reticular formation, and their extensions.[13] Before too long, any *un*rewarded stimulus will then be left dangling, as it were, incapable of enlisting a full motor response.

Other disconnections along the "motor limb" of behavior could further dampen that stream of messages which usually flows out initially through the amygdala, ventral striatum, and hypothalamus. Disconnections along these sensory and motor limbs—and at their interfaces with motivation—could also help explain some of the nonattachment associated with Zen. For such an hypothesis would propose that disconnections in these specified locations would do two things: (1) cut down on the resonances of the sensate input which had been driving certain affective responses (2) prevent these messages from passing out into behavior.

Still another kind of conditioning is called *operant conditioning*. This means that the investigator is encouraging certain of the animal's natural responses. In studies of operant behavior, food or drink is the typical bribe, although research papers still refer to the process as *reinforcement*. Having been reinforced repeatedly, the desired response occurs not only more frequently but it also recurs in an unconscious, automatic fashion. Again, operant conditioning techniques do not require the cerebral cortex, even in higher mammals like rats and rabbits.[3]

Human Learning and Unlearning

Back in their own homes, with their pets, it dawned on obedient researchers that their own dogs and cats had been conditioning *them* to give out food. At this point it appeared reasonable to assume that the principles discovered during operant research in lower animals might readily transfer to humans in general. Not only in jest were such phrases used as, "I have not been programmed to respond positively to this." Perhaps to pet-owning behavioralists in particular, it might have begun to seem that each input would automatically lead to output, every stimulus to a response.

A long article challenged such views. Its title asserted: "There Is No Convincing Evidence for Operant Classical Conditioning in Adult Humans."[15] Brewer contended that *humans* are different. Rarely do we use simple automatisms. Moreover, our responses are *not unconscious, nor are they automatic,* when we are the subjects in standard operant conditioning experiments. After all, we do have large frontal lobes. We develop *expectations* about what *may* happen. We anticipate, project, plan. And all these cognitive variables contribute in a major way to human conditioning.

In fact, how do humans and other primates cope with their social intricacies? Only by having built up a huge repertoire of optional responses. Each of these is much more sophisticated than is blink reflex. We insert a host of higher associations into every millisecond of that magical interval which separates stimulus from response. Countless examples illustrate such associations. Consider one: ACH nerve cells up in the basal forebrain fire more when the monkey learns the *meaning* of a certain outside stimulus, by connecting this signal with the fact that an apple will soon arrive as a reinforcing reward.[16]

Pavlov's original experiments were simple. They focused on how a single stimulus caused a response. Diagrammatically, one can represent this basic sequence as $S \longrightarrow R$. But human social interactions require many complex associations, and they also yield many varied responses. So, let n stand for any large numbers of either of these. We can then extend the point of the arrow on the $S \longrightarrow R$ line. This allows us to represent most human situations as: $S \xrightarrow{associations_n} R_{(n)}$. True, this leaves us better off, at least in the sense that we can represent why dog owners have far more behavioral options than do their dogs. But ours is a mixed blessing. Because many human responses can likewise go astray, chasing associations and running off in directions which prove highly counterproductive.

As lowly *Aplysia* withdrew, it could be taught to habituate, or to be sensitized. None of this simple learning at the mollusc level hinged on *time* sequences. But higher forms of life depend on *associative learning*. So, too, do the more advanced techniques of classical or operant conditioning. And all this associative learning *hinges on time-linked sequences.*[17] What is so special about time-linked sequences? They set up cause-and-effect relationships: *this* means *that.* Fire-hot-burn-*hurt.* In fact, we travel along this same "one-way" avenue when we build up our private concepts of "time" itself. For the sense of time also builds on such sequences and their consequences. It becomes an emergent function of all those many kinds of hyphenated connections which link a given earlier event with the specific consequences that follow it (see chapters 134 and 135).

A brain begins to learn these lessons early in life. And the lessons make an actual histological impact. One can appreciate this by returning, briefly, to the topic of those young but maze-competent rats. Between 16 and 23 days of age, the brain of a young rat will be going through a growth spurt. Suppose, during this critical growth period, we condition the young rat. We teach it, by operant techniques, that when it presses a lever it will obtain food. This whole procedure makes an impression on the developing brain, deep enough to change its very structure. For example, more branches and twigs now grow out from the dendrites of its pivotal CA3 pyramidal cells.[18] Why are some of our own behavioral traits so hard to unlearn? Perhaps because they had also been reinforced at critical early stages, and had been woven intimately into the very architecture of our nerve cells.

True, at birth, we were still essentially *unconditioned*. But gradually, life's events conditioned us. Limbic and brainstem circuitry soon learned to make us blush with shame, flush with anger, glow with pride, blanch with fear, and clutch with desire. Are these the conditionings which Zen would have us shed? Yes, indeed. This is what is implied in getting back to our unconditioned self.

The word may sound scary, but "unconditioned" remains an excellent term. On the other hand, misunderstandings do arise about another term. When Master Bankei referred to the "unborn," he was speaking metaphorically. It bears reemphasis that enlightenment does not return a person's brain literally to the primitive physiological status of an unborn fetus. Rather does the word point to the ways in which a *mature* brain enters into the direct, comprehensive experience of the world as it now is. Now, rinsed free of *inappropriate* conditioning, the mature brain responds creatively, drawing on its adult resources. The keyword is *in*appropriate. For it will be out of this ripened state that fresh responses again flow in an unqualified fashion.

Why do newly enlightened persons behave so energetically, react so spontaneously? Why not? Now they don't have to leaf back serially through every cause-and-effect relationship they had learned. Finally, they are rinsed free from all those (*n*)-numbers of old ambivalent and counterproductive associations (see chapter 155). They are *de*conditioned of the old mental baggage of nit-picking thoughts the cumulative weight of which had once so burdened the brain.

Meanwhile, have you ever trained your own puppy or kitten to stop doing something really "bad"? If so, how? Many owners condition their pets by linking the undesired act with the threat of an unpleasant stimulus. Circuits passing through the amygdala help *initiate* this kind of avoidance behavior. Subsequently, however, different circuits then perpetuate the late phases of conditioned avoidance behavior. And one pathway which then *maintains* this conditioned avoidance behavior is the mammillothalamic tract.[19] (As medical students, we were attracted by its more exotic name: the bundle of Vicq d'Azyr.) Along this major tract, messages speed from the hypothalamus up to the anterior thalamic nucleus (see figure 6). Perhaps there, a lower-order tier of limbic valences can be refined so that on their next relay they might further influence the cingulate cortex.

In this book, little will be said in favor of the extra-harsh extremes of *aversive* conditioning which were once used to force-train wild animals in the past. In humans, such methods too can produce results, but only by setting up painful or unpleasant associations. Yet, as Schloegl observes, the old harsh taming methods do not apply to contemporary Zen, or to the ways it conducts its behavioral unlearning and retraining. Zen will diminish the I, but it does not intend to break the spirit or to leave behind some neutral, lifeless, unresponsive product. No, the Zen approach does not try to quench the fires under the old misdirected energies. Instead, it will stir them up and jar them into kensho, from which they will be rechanneled. In the Western setting at least, most Zen procedures resemble more the very gradual and sophisticated "gentling" of a horse.[20]

Nor does authentic Zen deconditioning lead to license. In genuine emancipation, the moral compass remains. It still points to true north, and each year it wobbles less on the way. Can prolonged conditioning enable a person to express humane values with emerging compassion? Does this involve some kind of moral and ethical alchemy? The skeptic may find a contemporary answer in Tenzin Gyatso, the son of a Tibetan farmer. Raised from infancy as the Dali Lama, immersed in Buddhist traditions, struggling against oppression on a massive scale, he endured to become an inspired leader. And he would be later recognized, by the Nobel Peace Prize Committee, for his efforts as an exemplar of the world movement toward nonviolence.

75

Other Ways to Change Behavior

> When one of these monkeys is approached by an investigator and its face is lightly stroked with a glove, instead of reacting as usual by opening the mouth, showing the teeth, and attempting to bite, the animal simply turned its face away without signs of distress or hostility.
>
> J. Delgado[1]

Conditioning can establish behavior, and deconditioning can extinguish it. How else could Zen bring about lasting changes in the brain? This chapter summarizes reports which describe the results of stimulating the brain, of making small lesions in parts of the brain, and of adding certain drugs and hormones which act on brain receptors.

A rat learns quickly to stimulate certain parts of its own brain. It will press a lever repeatedly to deliver the electrical stimuli through implanted wires. Are human beings above this kind of artificial self-indulgence? No. We, can learn to engage in electrical self-stimulating behavior.[2] In animals, one especially potent stimulation site is the median forebrain bundle. It contains fibers running in both directions, to and through the hypothalamus.[3] When stimuli enter this bundle they exert a profound change on behavior. The starving rat, given a choice, prefers to stimulate its own brain rather than eating the food placed nearby!

When researchers discovered this powerful tool, they first referred to it as "brain stimulation reward." The phrase carried an implication: their animals were "feeling something good" at some vague sensory or emotional level. Therefore, they kept pressing the lever simply to get more of it. Then it was found that drugs changed the behavior. Drugs that increased the effects of dopamine and norepinephrine would enhance self-stimulation behavior, whereas small doses of opioid drugs reduced it. The most recent interpretations suggest that DA acts on the *motor* limb to energize behavior and does so *non*specifically. These concepts of DA function are tilted toward the "output" side of the equation. They downplay the previous notion that the rat must be feeling something "rewarding" in any pleasurable sensory or emotional sense.[4] They imply that when brain stimulation does increase DA turnover, this extra DA merely increases the "motoric" *probability* that the rat will then press the lever more often.[5]

Even though you stimulate certain key sites locally, *distant* regions become activated. Consider what happens when a rat self-stimulates its own ventral tegmental area. Metabolic activity increases, especially in many of its limbic regions, including the amygdala and the hippocampus. In contrast, self-stimulation of the substantia nigra goes on to increase metabolism more in the anterior cingulate gyrus and caudate nuclei.[6] And several stimulant-type drugs enhance the functions of the nucleus accumbens, making animals generally hyperactive.

It is relatively easy to provoke lower animals into aggressive behaviors by delivering electrical stimulation to various other sites in the brain. In contrast, primates such as rhesus monkeys do *not* develop directed forms of aggression even though researchers stimulate them in many of these very same aversive sites. In fact, monkeys only develop aggressive behavior when they are stimulated in a mere 14 out of 174 potential "aggressive" or "noxious" sites. What monkeys usually do, instead, is try to escape. Or they display submissive gestures.

Why do monkeys express so many varied, individual differences between aggressive and submissive responses? *It depends on where that particular monkey fits into the social hierarchy.*[1] These primate studies carry a message: our own behavior hinges on how many options we hold in reserve. Our brain has a wide variety of socially conditioned subsystems. Each one is capable of conveying one fragment of our varied behavioral repertoire.

Gross lesions of the nervous system do not allow us to draw firm conclusions about behavior. An apocryphal story illustrates why. The tale is about the child who suddenly sees a snake appear on the television screen. Afraid of snakes, the child strikes the side of the TV set with a baseball bat, and the snake image promptly disappears. No adult viewer would conclude that the blow had wiped out some special snake center in the television set. Nor do the brain's intricate circuitboards allow one to draw any similar conclusions. However, researchers can create a discrete "pharmacologic" lesion at a small site in the brain. This approach can overcome some of these limitations.[7]

Take the monkeys who had been the subjects of the opening quotation of this chapter. They had been injected with a local anesthetic in the region of the hippocampus. This created a pharmacologic lesion. The "numbness" briefly suppressed the local electrical activity. The monkey turned its face away. You might even consider making a literal interpretation, for the monkey did seem to be "turning the other cheek." Yet no evidence indicates that the hippocampus, or especially the amygdala nearby, is *the sole* site responsible for briefly "taming" the monkey, let alone for the long-range kinds of effective "gentling" which will still leave *all* other functions intact.

Suppose, for example, that a monkey has a larger structural lesion localized to the frontal lobe on one side. As you watch it behave, your first impression might be that this animal had been tamed. For this lesion does cause the monkey to neglect cues coming from the opposite side of the environment. Indeed, the monkey no longer becomes startled or orients to stimuli coming from this particular neglected side.[8] But watch out! Don't reach over to grasp this monkey or to stimulate it on its *intact* side. For now the monkey behaves in its usual manner—avoidance or aggression. Removing the cingulate gyrus on both sides also makes monkeys docile and appear less fearful.

So behaviors build upon those basic foundations already set into place by our arousal and activating systems. But thereafter they go on to be shaped by functions and events throughout many regions of the brain. If Zen is behavior modification, what is its laboratory? The usual events of each day. The trainee focuses attention on them. The process is called daily life practice. Nothing mysterious. It begins by just paying mindful attention to whatever is going on—noticing, enduring and introspecting.

Many behaviors are latent. They can't express themselves until other behaviors are first turned off. As children, we observed how female cats or dogs behaved. The female would either aggressively strike out at, or run away from, the advancing male if she were not in heat at the time. In sharp contrast, during estrus, we saw an affectionate female turning receptive and assuming a mating posture: her back becoming low and straight, or curving into the posture of lordosis, while her head was then elevated. This innate posture is permissive for mounting. It serves admirably the need to perpetuate the species.

Which nerve cells subserve these "in season" episodes of mating behavior? In the cat, they begin back in the posterior mammillary region of the hypothalamus and run forward to the anterior preoptic region.[9] The cells are highly sensitive to estrogens. After one pulse of estrogen is given intravenously, the brain promptly concentrates this hormone both in the medial hypothalamus and in the lateral septum. Still, it will take *three more days* before these nerve cells change. And only after this three-day delay does the brain turn off its old hostile and evasive behavior. Now the "new" behavior can come forth. Why does it take so long before the female cat finally behaves in an affectionate and receptive manner? Some of the delay reflects how long it takes to restructure nerve cells. For during these three days, the initial hormonal signal must wait for the leisurely metabolic responses of second and third messenger systems to catch up (see chapter 48).

Are changes high up in the cortex the explanation for the major adaptive behavioral transformations implicit in Zen? (see chapters 148 and 155). The foregoing lines of evidence suggest that they are not. For deep structures will first need to change: such as the hypothalamus, the lateral septal region, the central gray substance, and the amygdala. Only then can human behavior itself begin to make any major, *enduring* shift in the direction of receptive submission or surrender (see chapter 152). Indeed, the hypothalamic region remains a key integrator for these basic brain mechanisms, as it does for many other behaviors that preserve our species. And, as a further illustration of the behavioral potentials of the hypothalamus, we turn next to the way it plays a dramatic role in promoting another process of awakening, that from hibernation.

The Awakening from Hibernation

Toward the anterior part of the aqueduct of Sylvius and the side of the floor of the third ventricle, there exist . . . centers of slowing and acceleration on which hypothermia and re-heating, torpor and wakefulness, depend equally.

R. DuBois[1]

Woodchucks, marmots, and ground squirrels hibernate during the cold winter months.[2] And some Russian researchers also hole up in Siberia during its long winter to study these animals intensively.[3] But are ground squirrels relevant to those of us who live in more temperate zones, and are interested in Zen? If so, how?

Because they help clarify how we drop off into sleep and awaken naturally. We now understand that we wake up each morning not simply because we have been globally released from the inhibitions of sleep. Rather, what arouses us is an intricate blend of selective excitations and inhibitions.[4] And one reason we study hibernating animals is because each time they descend into their dramatic hibernating state, and rouse from it, the processes responsible can be studied in slow motion.

Say that winter is approaching in Siberia. Imagine what it would be like to be a ground squirrel. As you were descending into hibernation from sleep, you'd drop your body temperature from 38°C to *near zero*. Gliding into hibernation over a six- to fifteen-hour period, your heart rate would fall from 200 down to only 10 beats a minute, and your metabolic rate would plummet 100-fold. Then, after having bedded down for two weeks in deep hibernation, you'd rouse briefly to relieve yourself. Following that, you'd reenter hibernation, and would not emerge until spring beckoned.

Why do mammals hibernate? In a harsh climate, it helps them survive by conserving energy when there is little food. Because hibernation conserves energy much more efficiently than does sleep, Dubois wondered, which parts of the brain turned things off, and what started them up again?

A century ago, it was no easy task to answer these questions. Undaunted, he proceeded by removing different parts of marmot brains. Finally, in 1896 he reported that regions in and around the hypothalamus were vital for coordinating hibernation. Since then, it has become clear that several discrete mechanisms are involved. If there is damage to the posterior hypothalamus, hamsters cannot descend into hibernation. If one makes a lesion in the anterior hypothalamus, ground squirrels will enter it, but not arouse from it.[1]

But hibernation is not coma. If you stimulate the animals, they will still move around in their nests. Surprisingly, they move even though their brain temperatures have fallen to as low as 6°C. And they still continue to show low amplitude EEG activity in such vital regions as the midbrain, hippocampus, septal area, and hypothalamus.[5] Which two of these sites will take the lead when the animals finally awaken? The hippocampus and hypothalamus.[6,7] Researchers can trigger hibernating ground squirrels into arousal by injecting either acetylcholine, norepinephrine, or serotonin into their preoptic or anterior hypothalamic region. But of these three, only ACH also triggers their arousal when it is injected into their midbrain reticular formation.

Another especially potent arousing agent is a tripeptide. It is called thyrotropin-releasing hormone, or TRH.[8] Even when TRH is microinjected into the hippocampus during the descending phase, it soon triggers an awakening which seems as natural as a spontaneous arousal. Twenty-five minutes after the injection of only 100 nanograms of TRH, body temperatures start to rise from 5° up to 35°C. How potent is this peptide? TRH can awaken monkeys right out of a sleep induced by barbiturates. In this experiment, the TRH is microinjected either into the septal region or into the medial anterior hypothalamus.[9] Microinjections of TRH into the nucleus accumbens appear to activate the animal by increasing the local release of dopamine.[10] In the human brain, there are three potential sites at which TRH might awaken us: we concentrate TRH receptors in our amygdala, hippocampus, and superior colliculus.[11]

Researchers are still discovering how the descent into and ascent from hibernation is shaped by opioids, by other messenger molecules, and by their receptors.[12,13] Meanwhile, the hibernation models do more than highlight some of the steps through which we enter and emerge from a natural sleep. They also provide study time *in slow motion*. This has enabled researchers to appreciate how the discrete release of ACH, or of tiny amounts of peptides, can trigger striking physiological changes. The sensitive sites reside both in the dormant hypothalamus and in the three other deep midline regions lying successively in front of it. These are the preoptic area, septum, and nucleus accumbens.

It is a noteworthy fact that the arousing brain also undergoes structural changes. As animals ascend and awaken from hibernation, they again establish synaptic contacts between their mossy fibers and their CA3 cells in the hippocampus. These synaptic connections had dwindled and been lost during their earlier phase of wintry torpor[14] (see figure 6).

77

Tidal Rhythms and Biological Clocks

> Everything passes
> Everything ends;
> After every December
> There's always a May.

German popular song, 1945

Once every eleven years in the solar cycle, sunspots reach their peak. When their high-energy particles finally reach our atmosphere, we witness the luminous bands of the aurora borealis, or northern lights. Living things also undergo cycles of illuminating activity. These cycles are as regular as clockwork, as dramatic as hibernation. A century and a half ago, Linnaeus found that certain flowers open, and close, at distinctive times of day. On his nature walks he observed the water lily unfolding between six and seven o'clock in the morning, but the scarlet pimpernel did not open until 8 to 9 A.M. Based on this kind of factual knowledge, Linnaeus could tell what time it was. The records of this Swedish botanist do not inform us at what hour the Asian lotus opens.

Botanical clocks have their counterparts in neurobiology. The brain parses its rhythms even at the level of a single nerve cell. Here, after each sharp spike of synaptic excitation, one can observe the neuron issuing waves of inhibitory postsynaptic potentials. Their shoulders restrain the peak of excitation in each nerve cell, sculpturing its response both in space and time.[1]

The brain also has much longer cycles. One of them dramatically changes our whole state of consciousness. About every twenty-four hours, it alternates us between waking and sleeping. This is *circadian rhythm,* so called because it recurs at intervals around (*circa*) one day apart. Our sleep-waking cycle reflects major tidal rhythms going on deep in our brain.

The term *cycle* comes from the Greek. It implies that a circle—a round of related phenomena—returns to the same starting point. It is a simple matter to design a larger clock face that also places *one entire day on the whole circle,* not our half-day, as is usual. Then, when the hour hand completes the full circle, it will have touched each one of the twenty-four hours on this clock face. There are advantages in this arrangement. Now one can appreciate that some functions do not represent themselves uniformly on our biological clock in a perfectly round fashion (figure 13). In fact, our personal level of wakefulness expresses itself in an irregular manner, as shown by the large blob on the left side of the figure. At times, we are very wide-awake. At other times, only covertly so.

When are we most awake? Not when you might think. Researchers found this out when they defined the peak of alertness as that period when we are *least* likely to fall asleep. Looked at this way, we are most alert between 6 and 11 P.M.! Indeed, not until the evening hours do we perceive most acutely, reach a higher body temperature, and achieve the best results on many of our tests of performance.[2] Why then? Perhaps being more alert later in the evening was an advantage for our hominid ancestors. After the sun went down, it would be a very good thing to stay alert long enough to find a safe spot to bed down in, using the extra hours to secure food and shelter against a long, cold night ahead.

In contrast, many memory functions don't reach their peak until after our body temperature reaches a lower level, as it does in the morning. Note the bulge in figure 13 starting at about 7 A.M. Here, the area representing the amount of our wakefulness again extends itself for the second time. Moreover, every hour and a half or so, little semiwakeful activations also insert themselves into sleep. These are the same normal, brief radial projections of desynchronized sleep with REM episodes that were discussed in chapter 71.

What significance do these rhythmic aspects of natural awakening have for the Zen meditator? In fact, they are predictive. *They suggest moments when the meditator might be most likely to enter periods of enhanced awareness.* Take, for example, that major wave of awareness which rises to its extraordinary peak during internal absorption (see part VI). When might it reach its greatest heights? Perhaps if it came in during the evening. Note again that higher tide of peak awareness at around 9 P.M. And suppose it did happen to occur at that time. It might then be more likely to sweep in on its surface a flotsam of adjacent phenomena. For standing nearby is either a transitional period or sleep-onset REM. If any loose fragments were dislodged from either of these substates, they could quite readily be displaced into the surge of the wakefulness cycle during the evening's "high tide."

The brain's usual activating mechanisms go through their rhythms as naturally as does the opening of a lotus. Each day, essentially similar mechanisms are doing more than cycling through our usual rhythms of awareness and attention. For many of them are also being channeled into our episodes of desynchronized sleep. The thesis proposed above can be extended to absorptions as well. The implication is that absorptions, too, will first build upon the foundation of these mechanisms natural to the human brain, and then *amplify* their functions. Such a theory remains open to three possibilities: (1) that an episode of absorption could either be induced by meditation, or (2) by certain drugs, or (3) might seem to have occurred spontaneously. Pharmacologists have learned that the same drugs may have different effects at different times. Much depends on exactly *when* the drug arrives in relation to that person's daily cycles. Meditation, too, could have

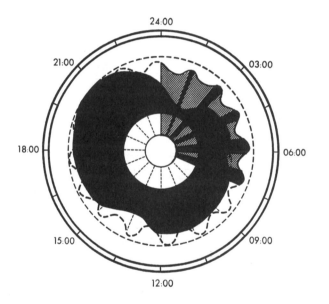

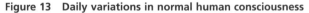

Figure 13 Daily variations in normal human consciousness
This is a composite *24*-hour clock. Therefore, it summarizes, on *one* circle, the endogenous rhythms, both circadian and ultradian, during a whole day. Midnight is at the top, and noon is twelve hours away, at bottom. Note the expansions of the large, somewhat doughnut-shaped, black structure. They emphasize the times when we reach our maximum levels of waking consciousness and performance. The peak occurs from about 19:00 to 21:00 hours, that is from 7 P.M. to 9 P.M.

Diagonal lines placed close together indicate the nighttime hours of S-sleep. Five maximum peaks of D-sleep activity are shown as blunt black ribs, superimposed. They radiate out in the fanlike arrangement in the right upper quadrant. Wavy, interrupted lines, peaking every 90 minutes, suggest tendencies to other periodic fluctuations during the day. (This composite figure is adapted from figures 2 and 3 of R. Broughton. Biorhythmic variations in consciousness and Psychological functions. *Canadian Psychological Review* 1975;16:217–239. Copyright 1975. Canadian Psychological Association, With permission.)

different effects at different times. The hypotheses developed in this chapter are testable and invite experimental challenge.

25+ Hour Days

Society imposes many customs. Every day we live within the rigid boundary of a 24-hour clock time. But suppose we are left to our own devices. No clocks. No changes in illumination. Isolation from all other time cues. Then each person's brain reasserts itself. Now it can express its personal cycles of rest and activity. Most "days" then drift out to become *twenty-five* hours long. A few days might even stretch out for thirty to fifty hours.[3] Under such free-running conditions, when do the sleep-onset REM periods slip in? Less than ten minutes after sleep begins, even though the *total* percentage of time spent in REM periods does not change. Clearly, *REM segments are free to shift around within the total sleep process.*

This instability of REM episodes is noteworthy. It suggests that they are thrust up under the influence of some deep biological rhythm oscillator(s). Hormonal data support this interpretation. Already—a few minutes before these sleep-onset REM episodes begin—the plasma levels of adrenal cortisol have jumped to readings almost twice normal. This means that the hypothalamus (via its pituitary-adrenal connection) has already anticipated these early REM episodes.

Sleep-onset REM episodes can occur in normal healthy persons who disturb their sleep-waking cycle in several ways other than those which we have cited earlier. Indeed, REM episodes occur early when subjects shift time zones rapidly, or if they extend a "day" so that it now becomes forty-eight hours long.[4] And by depriving subjects of their usual REM later in the night (selective REM deprivation), they will later go on to develop premature REM periods at the start of sleep.[5]

The hour at which we wake in the morning is of critical importance. It entrains our natural twenty-five-hour sleep-waking cycle, and helps squeeze it to fit into our twenty-four hours of clock time. We get inklings of this twenty-five-hour biological cycle on laid-back weekends. If we are free to get up without an alarm clock on Saturday, we may rise as much as an hour later that day. On Sunday morning we might add one more hour of late arising. No wonder, when the alarm clock goes off on Monday morning at its usual time, it now seems two hours too early! When our personal time differs this much from alarm clock time, it contributes to the sluggish Monday morning blues.

Sometimes, prolonged intensive meditative sessions also generate a much longer period of true depression, a "dark night." And severely depressed patients do show profoundly disturbed sleep cycles. Recently, a technique of sleep deprivation has been found to relieve some patients of their depression. The approach used is sleep deprivation during the *second* half of the night.[6] We now know that this is when most D-sleep occurs (see figure 14). As a therapeutic technique, this selective, partial, sleep deprivation provides only temporary benefits. But as a research tool it focuses our attention on two large issues of critical importance: (1) how biological clocks might interact initially to precipitate depression; (2) how waking up very early might later enable the brain to shift into temporary activated states.

In general, the prime time for D-sleep is that hour or two just before we wake up in the morning. Then, D-sleep has more momentum, and it lasts longer. Then, too, are we also near the bottom of our daily temperature rhythm.[3,7] Later, throughout the day, and during the night, the brain couples its arousal cycles more closely with our daily body temperature cycle. Our core body temperature warms up during the *second* half of the day. So it will be then that our arousal cycles recur more frequently. Among depressed patients, it is those persons who maintain lower average body temperatures who will tend to be improved by techniques that temporarily deprive them of D-sleep.

Resetting Biological Clocks

Let us suppose that we have suffered jet lag after a very long flight. A meditative retreat or working a night shift could cause similar dislocations of the sleep-wake cycle. Any disruption of sleep habits causes major consequences. Now we may fall asleep when our body temperature is *lowest*, whereas previously we didn't drop off into sleep until some hours *after* we had reached our *highest* body temperature. Our sleep-wake cycle has now become dissociated. Some of its D-sleep phenomena—now uncoupled—enter during sleep-onset REM episodes. In fact, a subgroup of patients who suffer from endogenous depression do seem to have displaced their circadian rhythm in this very same manner. As a result, they enter D-sleep prematurely.[8]

We think we stay awake all day, forgetting how many daydream fantasies we indulge in. Their cycles recur every 90 to 100 or every 180 to 200 minutes.[9,10] To these, the name *ultradian* is applied. It means cycles which recur at intervals of *less* than twenty-four hours. Of course, the most thoroughly studied ultradian rhythm is none other than desynchronized, REM sleep, which recurs every 90 to 110 minutes or so during the night.[11] What is sorely needed are equally careful studies of the rhythms of our *intuitive* functions, starting with those which enter during morning periods of reverie.

Sleep specialists now favor the view that our basic, central arousal mechanism has *alternate* ways of expressing itself: (a) as periods of D-sleep and of rapid eye movement during our sleeping hours; and (b) as active wakefulness during our waking hours. Are these really equivalent? The answer becomes highly relevant to Zen.

For meditators may rise as early as 2 or 3 A.M. during some rigorous Rohatsu sesshin. What happens when you first shorten sleep and get up this early? It markedly destabilizes the basic rest-activity cycle, and it disrupts other cycles as well. It means D-sleep deprivation, S-sleep deprivation, and a phase advance of arousal. The consequences are foreseeable: (1) wide-awake hyperarousals recurring at unusual times; (2) waves of sleepiness; (3) REM-like dreaming activity. The dreaming episodes plunge in after brief moments of drowsiness or no-mindedness, and persist for seconds or more. Every aspirant at a Zen sesshin is familiar with each of the above. Unfortunately, none of these episodes of activated arousal phenomena have yet been studied in full detail. The results of future experiments could shed light on why major swings in mood, awareness, and attentiveness recur during intensive meditative retreats.

You can change your mood. How? By resetting your biological clock, and making major changes in your sleep-waking cycle. But note: the changes in mood are *delayed*. For example, after normal subjects have been kept awake under laboratory conditions for thirty-six to seventy-two hours, they soon fall into a long recovery sleep. Only later, the *following* morning, do many of the subjects become animated, extra-talkative, almost euphoric. Their positive mood can persist for a day or so. A skeptic might say that they feel better only because, having gone through an ordeal, they can now think of themselves as "liberated." But this is not a matter of mere thoughts, nor a simple feeling of relief. For it is very stressful to stay awake for a long period. In response, the hypothalamus releases a number of peptides directly into the brain, as described earlier. These include such excitatory peptides as thyrotropic-releasing hormone (TRH) and ACTH, as well as beta-endorphin. Staying awake also increases the levels in the blood of the thyroid metabolic hormones T_3 and T_4 for the next four to five days.[12]

Deeper levels of zazen unleash destabilizing forces which have physiological consequences. What happens when you vary the timing, depth, duration, and content of deep meditation? *It could displace both the moment of entry and the momentum of whatever underlying cycle is then being impinged upon.* Zazen performed several times during the day would obviously have an influence on the underlying ninety-minute ultradian cycle. Zazen performed later at night (when it had been the meditator's usual habit to be asleep) could displace the phase entry time of the circadian cycle and change its momentum. Moreover, the person who meditates later at night might then drop into S-sleep faster, and proceed to experience the several phenomena of D-sleep much earlier than usual.

Each day, the tidal mechanisms that drive our wakefulness press against the strong currents of those that promote sleep. Suppose we decide to stay up and watch the late TV show. Now, our stronger wakefulness cycle overrides our sleep cycle. But the next day, even though seeming to be "awake," we can doze off into catnaps at any time between 7 A.M. and 5 P.M.[9]

Up to now, we have been considering the usual mechanisms of both sleep and awakening. In Zen, however, a special meaning attaches to the word "awakening." When Zen uses the term, it does not refer to these lesser variations on the theme of simple arousal. The word implies extraordinary enlightenment experiences. These reach the peak of an insight-wisdom that awakens one to the miracle of otherwise prosaic events. Even so, lesser "quickenings" also occur (see part V). And some of these do resemble our smaller, everyday awakenings. That is, they are basically (a) moments of intensified awareness or (b) intervals when emotions and mentations are amplified to somewhat less than peak levels.

Matters of Timing

As a preamble to part V, it will help to specify here the *timing* of some pivotal mechanisms which usually serve to awaken us in one way or another.

When do we waken? If we happen to wake up during the night, we tend to do so when we are already in a period of D-sleep. Cues from our internal clock prompt these spontaneous rousings from D-sleep.

What is the best *way* to awaken? It depends on what needs to be done. Subjects who awake from desynchronized sleep perform best on tasks which involve certain kinds of orientation in space. These particular tasks are associated more with *right* hemispheric functions. And some studies even report that awakenings from D-sleep yield *above-normal* capabilities of the kind associated with right parietal lobe function.[13] But slow wave sleep is different. Subjects who awake when their S-sleep reaches its maximum—between 1 and 3 A.M.—do relatively better on tasks related primarily to *left* hemispheric functions.

By referring back to the simple principles of sleep physiology, and also to issues of *timing*, one can further understand the basis for those techniques researchers use to cultivate lucid dreams (see chapter 73). First, they waken their subjects and get them up in the middle of the night. Most of the sleep lost will be the major episodes of D-sleep. Second, their subjects return to bed in the later morning hours. (Note: At this time, their usual tidal level of morning conscious awareness is starting to rise.)

What do these events imply? First, that the subjects will now have an opportunity to rebound into their lost D-sleep. Second, that *these rebound phenomena will be superimposed on that morning's increasingly higher covert background level of conscious awareness.* So it will be at this particular time—still dreaming—that the subjects are now able to accomplish all their remarkable *willed* movements. Put simply, lucid dream phenomena imply that the brain is displacing functions from one of its major cycles (D-sleep) and transposing them into another cycle (waking).

The same principles apply to slow-wave sleep. Segments of S-sleep can also be shifted around. One technique used to uncover the underlying rhythm of S-sleep is perceptual deprivation. It releases episodes of S-sleep with great force and regularity.[14] Now we can understand another reason why there is an advantage in performing zazen with the eyes open. It yields lesser degrees of sensory deprivation, and reduces one's tendencies to slip off into those intrusive naps of slow-wave sleep.

Noting how readily our sleep segments can be manipulated, it would seem that what we call the "biological clock" is something of a misnomer. It is a large number of clocks, engaging a vast series of gears. *Each physiological component usually turns at its own rate.* But while each gear does turn over on a cycle of its own, it also tends to synchronize with the others in *relatively stable* phase relationships.

What happens when you destabilize the brain, uncouple its waking and sleeping physiologies? A very long list of alternative combinations now emerges. In the course of such readjustments, our endocrine cycles do not remain passive. In fact, these hormonal functions shape our other activity cycles, not merely react to them. In one unique personal study, Hamburger followed his own adrenolcortical stress hormones for over fifteen years.[15] He monitored ketosteroid levels in the urine. (These were the metabolic byproducts of the adrenal glucocorticoids in his blood.) His adrenal stress hormones showed *three* rhythm peaks. One recurred about once a week. A second cycled once every thirty days; the third recurred at yearly intervals.

His weekly rhythm peaked every Wednesday and Thursday. These were the busiest days in his professional workweek. His adrenal steroids were helping him cope with this hectic pace of events. Each year, his ketosteroids peaked in the month of November. Why November? It exemplifies that critical interface between fall and winter. Now the rate of change accelerates in many biological rhythms. Before then, around the time of the fall equinox in late September, we had woken early and gone to sleep early. Afterward, by the time the winter solstice has arrived in late December, we are waking up later and tending to go to sleep later.[16] No person stays the same throughout the year, physiologically or metabolically.

It is easiest to observe the behavior cycles of someone else. But subjects can also keep track of their own ups and downs. In one study, over a fourteen-month period, sixty-four subjects wrote down how many hours they slept. To these sleep data, they added comments about their own general levels of energy, anxiety, and mood. Normal subjects were studied in addition to those who underwent mood changes in association with their affective disorder.[17] Most subjects showed "psychic" cycles. These had a periodicity longer than one day. Indeed, about 35 percent of these cycles peaked with the *seasons*, every 85 days. Another 15 percent followed more of a monthly cycle. This ranged between twenty-six and thirty-seven days. A final 14 percent recurred at weekly intervals or less. What features distinguished the patients who had affective disorders? Their mood cycles came more frequently, and their mood swings were much greater in amplitude.

Some persons become keenly aware that they cycle with the seasons. The greater the ambient light, the more they increase their output. They feel full of energy during the brighter, warmer months. Indeed, between March and August they become more emotional, and their thoughts tend to race more. Later, during the darker months from September to February, they feel drained of energy and become moody.[18]

Light does have powerful effects. Light causes an increase in the number of NE alpha-receptors in the animal forebrain.[19] In the human brain, serotonin and norepinephrine levels also change substantially during the year.[20] A critical period for ST is that particular interface when late fall is changing to early winter. Autopsy studies show that ST reaches its peak levels in the hypothalamus in the late fall. Indeed, when ST rises to these peak levels—in October and November—they are then over twice as high as are the ST levels during winter's depths, a mere two months later in December and January.

Moreover, ST levels also vary markedly throughout a twenty-four-hour day. High levels occur around 5 A.M. This ST peak is twice that of the two trough levels. Two subsequent peaks occur. The first is two hours later, at around 7 A.M. The second occurs at 2 P.M. Serotonin also increases its turnover in the brain during these peaks. As an index of this, its breakdown products follow a parallel course. This implies that ST is not being "unused" because it has been dammed up in some compartment at the time. Instead, ST is actively being used in synapses over and over again.[21]

Norepinephrine is different. Human NE levels do vary during a day, but they do not vary in obvious ways with the seasons. NE levels rise to a peak in the hypothalamus around 1 to 2 A.M. Later, by around 7 A.M., NE falls to levels only half that. NE drops to low levels in the medulla during the morning hours, between 6 A.M. and noon. Clearly, our brain ST and NE levels are engaged in several crosscurrents. This is especially true during that dynamic period of awakening from around 5 to 7 A.M.

Syzygy and the Meditative Way

Early in January 1987, newspapers carried stories of extraordinarily high tides on both coasts of the United States. Massive waves were swept still higher by winds. Washed away were high sea walls and beach properties. Why such huge tides? We began to hear about a new word.

Syzygy is a normal phenomenon that recurs twice a month. Nothing exotic. At these times, the orbits of the moon and the sun place them *in line*, both off on the same side of the earth. Now, in conjunction, they exert a big gravitational pull. But also in January 1987, two more cyclic factors came into play. As they converged, they exerted an extra-strong pull on our planet: (1) the moon in its monthly cycle had come closest to the earth; (2) the earth in its yearly orbit had come closest to the sun. This fourfold confluence of events was rare, the National Weather Service told us reassuringly. A mere three had occurred since 1912. Parenthetically, nothing in this convergence of natural physical forces is to be equated with vague metaphysical notions about astrology or other "harmonic convergences."

Our early ancestors also needed to explain why the tides rose and fell. Imagine the mythologies they had to invent! Mankind now knows better. We have come up with sound, interdisciplinary associations. We have learned to take the basic principles of gravity from physics, and to correlate them with facts from astronomy and meteorology. Now we can predict when cycles will align and crest together to have rare, but earth-crunching effects. Neuroscience has the potential to integrate corresponding degrees of knowledge. On the one hand, it can use the experiential reports of "inner weather," plus the subjects' observed behaviors. On the other hand, it will have data from the physiological cycles, plus those up-and-down rhythms in human neurotransmitters, hormones, and other chemical messengers. Finally, once we have understood our own internal rhythms in an equally comprehensive and integrated way, humankind will be able to correlate the two sets of data. Then, we will be able to forecast—and encourage—those rare conjunctions when biological systems, joining forces, go on to transform our bodies and brains (see chapter 65).

Meanwhile, how do we get started? What will we need to clarify *how* meditation acts to cultivate absorptions and enlightenment? A new paradigm. And this means multidisciplinary studies several orders of magnitude more complex than any reported thus far. Why? Because the periods spent in meditation must be studied not as isolated events, as they are now. Meditation must be examined in the context of the remarkable cycles already going on in that same person's body and brain. *So once research has first defined the meditator and the kind of meditation, it must also specify exactly when and how this meditation is affecting the person's biorhythms going on at that time.*

Does it help to understand that our rhythmic brain functions can be scrambled and reassembled in many different combinations? Yes. It enables us to appreciate the basis for one other finding, a key fact otherwise inexplicable: rarely does a particular person's mystical-religious peak experience ever repeat itself in exactly the same manner. And the more variables there are, the less likely they will all be to align themselves together again in the very same manner.

78

The Roots of Our Emotions

Any physiologically based formulation of emotion must specify the fashion in which physiological processes interact with stimulus, cognitive, or situational factors.

S. Schachter[1]

We see a watercolor painting. Its white areas sparkle, and speak to us in some subtle, telling way . . . we *like* it. What caused the connection? How did we link our interior aesthetic sensibilities with the painting's purely optical aspects?

The emotional life has complex roots. One early theory attributed an emotion, such as fear, to the sensory feedback we received when our heart beat faster and our muscles became tense. This James-Lange theory never caught on. Why has it recently undergone a modest revival?[2,3] Because facial muscles do more than outwardly express the emotions generated by our subjective internal states. It turns out that subjects who voluntarily create happy or sad faces tend also to shift their emotions in the corresponding direction.[4]

The later Cannon-Bard theory held that our emotions stem from *central* sources, primarily in the brain. It proposed that these same regions also went on, secondarily, to cause our heart to beat faster and our muscles to tense in the rest of the body. The Papez theory went further. It specified that limbic circuits were the source of our emotions. How does the limbic system get its information?

The first route in is short and quick.[5] Its sensate input speeds through the relay nuclei of the thalamus and funnels chiefly into the central and lateral nuclei of the amygdala. This fast pathway provides subliminal value judgments.[6] Because these affective reactions are deeply rooted in our very core, they seem effortless, "visceral," difficult to put into words and hard to override. Other pathways are slower, because their sensory input will be processed in relays through the pulvinar and parahippocampal gyrus.

Big bears roam the dark woods ahead. A large pine cone crashes down. *Instantly* you jump, then know fear. We have just seen that the fearful amygdala helps trigger *conditioned* emotional responses. It makes a key contribution to such split-second reactions, as has been made clear by experiments in which rats were first classically conditioned to fear a certain sound. Later, a small lesion was made. It was so small that it cut only the fast input on its short pathway *before* it could enter the amygdala.[7] What does this particular quick, hearing → fear connection do normally? It links the medial geniculate nucleus (where some "early hearing" occurs) with its next target field, the amygdala (which contributes to primal fear). Note that *these rats are still able to hear.* But something has dropped out of their behavior. This particular something is crucial to our understanding of Zen. For the rats lose *only* a certain kind of fearful behavior: only that particular kind which they had learned (from their earlier conditioning) would be associated with that specific fearsome sound.

As children, we heard Grimm tales about dire events lurking in the forest outside. And maybe that night the moaning noises of the wind made our hearts beat faster. But with maturity, we *weigh* such decisions. Our slower, *cortical*-limbic pathways superimpose more thoughtful discriminations. Still, primed as the above geniculate-limbic circuits are to respond quickly, no wonder we remain suggestible and jump to conclusions! These fast circuits—with their sensitivities tuned to every primitive stimulus feature of darkness—still raise the gut-level issues of survival, whispering a "be careful" bias about things that lurk outside. And if arousal has first stirred up our emotions, nonspecifically, we very quickly label the next event with an emotional valence. Will it be labeled positive or negative? This depends on which kinds of meaning and context are close at hand.

In a clinical study, Schachter found that it was relatively easy—once his subjects had become aroused—to tilt them toward different emotional states. Which particular state emerged: euphoria, or amusement, or anger? It hinged on how they had sized up their external circumstances at the time.[8] First, in order to arouse his experimental subjects, Schachter gave them epinephrine subcutaneously. He then placed a stooge in the same room with the unsuspecting subjects. The stooge's task was to manipulate the situation by behaving in a manner that was either humorous or angry.

Suppose his subjects had not been told in advance that epinephrine was the primary cause of their symptoms of arousal. In this case, they tended to label their new amusement or anger in keeping with whatever situation they believed was then going on. In contrast, if they had been told exactly what symptoms to expect from the epinephrine, they remained relatively immune to the stooge's manipulations. It is of interest that even this thin veneer of insight was helping them avoid getting carried away by their emotions.

In other experiments, subjects were also injected either with epinephrine or a placebo. They were then shown a comedy film. The epinephrine subjects became openly amused and laughed heartily. The placebo subjects tended to be only quietly amused. Such evidence suggests that when the human brain puts a "label" on emotional states, it pulls together a variety of refined perceptual, cognitive, and situational factors, and integrates them with its resonances of raw physiological arousal.

Schachter warned us that we would feel uncomfortable using these psychological constructs to understand his data. Why? Because we could not reduce them to physiological terms. Yet, he continued, "if we don't use such vague concepts as 'perception' and 'cognition,' my guess is that we will be just about as successful in deriving predictions about emotion or any other complex behavior from a knowledge of biochemical and physiological conditions as we would be at predicting the destination of a moving automobile from an exquisite knowledge of the workings of the internal combustion engine and of petroleum chemistry."[8]

And so it is, throughout this book, that we will also be obliged to use over-simplified words even more vague than "perception" and "cognition," to resort to shorthand words derived both from Zen and the brain, in order to discuss the many ramifications of the emotions. But if we would understand their *basic* mechanisms then we must still open up our mechanic's manual (as in part III), to look under the hood, and to examine the engine.

Many patients have epileptic seizures. But only rarely, in less than 1 percent of epileptic patients, do seizures *begin* with emotions of pleasure or unpleasure, feelings which are a primary, integral part of their symptoms.[9] Fear can arise when a focal discharge into the anterior temporal lobe gains access to the amygdala. Feelings associated with pleasure or unpleasure are different. They tend to correlate with focal discharges into the *posterior* temporal region.

One woman had an exhilaratingly pleasant feeling in association with her posterior temporal seizure focus. Along with this feeling was the sense that "I must get to the bottom of it," together with an hallucination and with depersonalization. Another patient had a compulsion to look off to the left side, accompanied by a mood of pleasure and a feeling that *space seemed to open up.* A third patient had the sudden feeling of being lifted up, of emotional elation, plus the feeling, "I am just about to find out knowledge no one else shares—something to do with the line between life and death."[10]

These are anecdotal reports. Still, their form and content suggest that functions related to the posterior temporal region can be especially relevant both to absorptions and to kensho. For here the brain seems capable of mobilizing several ingredients: elements of hallucination, depersonalization, pleasure, and the opening up of space, *along with* profound complex interpretations. Yet in most cases of seizures the feeling tone ranges merely from pleasantness to elation. It seems to fall short of those extra degrees of deep blissful rapture which we will consider in part V.

Over a century ago, Hughlings Jackson focused on the few of his epileptic patients who did have an emotion at the onset. When this earliest phase, the aura, was emotional in nature—such as a "dreamy" reminiscence or a fear—it was most likely to herald *a seizure which began on the right side of the brain.*[11] Today, several lines of evidence support his prescient clinical suggestion that the right hemisphere is the more "emotional." Suppose, for example, that emotion-laden films are channeled into one hemisphere or the other. The right hemisphere subjects secrete higher levels of adrenal stress hormones like cortisol, and their blood pressures reach higher levels.[12] Other observations have been made of patients after a barbiturate had been injected into the arterial supply of their right hemisphere. As the first effects of the drug are wearing off, the subjects tend to laugh more, and their mood becomes elevated. In contrast, left-sided injections tend to be associated with crying.[13] Our right temporal lobe also plays the major role in decoding the particular emotion we see expressed on another person's face.[14]

To Charles Darwin, disgust was a basic emotion. To be disgusted was to be repulsed by the very notion that an offensive object might be taken in by mouth.[15] By the time children reach the age of eight years, their disgusts are firmly established. Disgusts can be weakened, but what do such unpalatable notions imply? Strong physiological prejudices that are very difficult to unlearn (see chapter 50).

Emotions are not "bad." At the *roots* of our emotions are primal energies which can be put to fruitful use. Indeed, there is an old Mahayana Buddhist saying, which in its Japanese equivalent becomes the phrase: *Bonno-soku-bodai.*[16] One of its implications is that the *energy* of enlightenment arises from the very same natural origins as those which give rise to our everyday passions and emotions. In this context, Schloegl points out that, because the egocentric self has become so deeply entrenched, only the strongest countervailing forces—emotional energies, in the broadest sense—will be capable of pulling it all out.[17] Freud's view that a person's energies were contained within the *id* would seem to leave room for related psychological interpretations.

Thus far, we have seen how the limbic system sends its resonances reverberating throughout still higher levels of associations. These "vibes" strongly bias our more conscious decisions about good and bad, right or wrong. So, at this point, several issues will be coming to the fore. Leading to questions such as, How might we dampen our big, unwanted emotional overloads? More narrowly, How could Zen training be *selective?* How could it, on the one hand, reduce our cravings, our hungry *reaching out* to grab things, while at the same time stopping the opposite reaction: our *recoiling* with disgusts and aversions? And suppose Zen training does dampen emotions such as fear and hate. By what means could it also enhance the reciprocal ones of compassion?

Some answers will hinge on what one can learn, secondhand, from the kinds of research highlighted in part III. Other answers will come only to an experiant. And then, only when that anonymous subject undergoes the kinds of firsthand comprehension and acts of *un*learning which we will be taking up in parts VII and VIII.

79

The Spread of Positive Feeling States

> When you entertain evil thoughts like hostility and hatred, there is no joy in your heart and you are a nuisance to others. On the other hand, if you develop kindness, patience and understanding, then the whole atmosphere changes.
>
> The Dalai Lama[1]

> True illumination, like all real and vital experience, consists rather in the breathing of a certain atmosphere, the living at certain levels of consciousness, than in the acquirement of specific information.
>
> Evelyn Underhill[2]

You don't need to have been nurtured in a Buddhist atmosphere as a child in Tibet to get a lift from a benevolent culture. Indeed, at particular times when your mood becomes elevated, you will engage in positive brotherly and sisterly acts toward other persons. These common courtesies have now been documented.

Changes of "atmosphere" may sound rather soft. So let us consider four specific situations showing how humans can indeed "accentuate the positive." The subjects were responding spontaneously, not aware that they were being studied under controlled experimental circumstances. First, some "nice things happened." A simple matter of "finding" a dime in a phone booth.[3] Or the pleasant surprise of receiving a "gift" of cookies while studying in the library. Suppose you were the "lucky" person who had found the (planted) dime. Several minutes later, when someone else dropped their papers, it would turn out that you would bend over to pick them up. Or, if you had received the cookies, you would then volunteer more readily to help another student. Moreover, if you were the cookie receiver, you would do more than become helpful in positive ways. For in a sense, you would then be "delivered from evil": you would reject any nasty suggestions to annoy other students.

In a separate experiment, certain subjects received a free gift, such as a note pad or nail clipper.[4] Afterward, they were asked to evaluate a most sensitive matter: how did their own cars *really* perform? If you had been the gift recipient, your mood would have become positive to such a degree that you would later give more optimistic reports about your automobile's performance. But the nonrecipient control subjects remained in the usual, more circumspect mood of the average car owner.

The third study focused on "victorious" subjects. They had just "won" at a computer game, and had been pumped up into an elevated mood state.[5] Earlier, this group of subjects had listened to a list of words played on a tape. Some of these thirty-six words had positive connotations; others carried a negative emotional valence. If you had been declared a "winner," you would later be able readily to recall from memory the positive words on this earlier list. What about the nonpositive words? Your high spirits didn't make *them* more accessible.

In a final study, one group of students performed a perceptual-motor test. The researchers then induced a positive affect by telling these subjects that they had just scored a high 97 percent![6] The control group merely evaluated these same tests. Both groups then went on to a separate project. This second task involved sifting through fifty-four items of data. Their goal: to select the best automobile from a list of nine candidates. If you had been in the "high-scoring" group, you would screen the items more rapidly and reach decisions sooner. You would focus on the key issues of high priority and discard irrelevant information.

Cookies, the plaudits of the crowd, and automobile game-playing? You might think that they have nothing to do with Zen. But the studies are not as banal as they might seem. Indeed, one message seems clear: people change when they feel happy and confident about themselves, and comfortable in the world at large. Their positive feeling states spread out and become linked to

1. Being helpful
2. Avoiding being unhelpful
3. A more ready access to positive material in memory
4. Rapid screening and efficient decision making

Now, drugs which activate opioid receptors or serotonin receptors also help elevate mood. The person "feels good," at least for several hours. But Zen is concerned with *major enduring attitudinal change*. How can positive affective states go on to influence behavior in a more *lasting* way? In part III, we noted how several pathways from the limbic system can infuse their positive or negative limbic valences into frontal lobe functions. And, in the present context, it is appropriate to cite another limbic avenue which could affect mood: input from the cingulate gyrus. For when the cingulate gyrus itself is stimulated, it can excite the prefrontal cortex. Indeed, frontal excitation occurs if one stimulates the cingulate gyrus at frequencies ranging from one to twenty times a second.[7]

Later (in chapter 150), we will go on to consider how more enduring behaviors, somewhat similar to the four listed above, could create the kind of positive "atmosphere" the Dalai Lama is talking about, the kind that exerts a lasting salutary influence, both on the person and on society at large.

80

Pain and the Relief of Pain

Bite your tongue. Get a cinder in your eye. When you feel good, you feel nothing.
Buckminster Fuller (1895–1983)[1]

No strain, no pain.
No pain, no gain.

Old saying

Once again, you grabbed a rough piece of wood in a hurry. As the sliver of wood pierced your hand, the reflex arc in your spinal cord jerked your hand away. You had no time to think. Signals leaping up to your brain stem and thalamus localized the stab to a finger, and pain gathered another strongly aversive valence in the lower parietal cortex.[2] The sliver went deep, and already you're feeling a bit anxious. Two forward-looking frontal lobes begin to worry about infections that follow deep puncture wounds. And, for as long as the nagging, two-way dialogue continues between these regions and the limbic system, you will keep painfully attending to that wretched sliver.

How much pain can a person endure? Your sensitivity to pain per se is but one of many influential factors. If you should wish to raise the pain threshold, a frontal lobotomy is not the solution. Yet it does increase a person's ability to *tolerate* a given level of pain. Other factors which help subjects cope include analgesics such as aspirin, alcohol by mouth, white noise, or an episode of schizophrenia. And, as Bucky Fuller noted, the more elevated your mood, the less bothersome even a cinder in the eye becomes.

The sliver of wood set off pain of two major types.[3] The first stab was "fast pain." Most everyone has about the same threshold for fast pain. As its signal ascends, it becomes increasingly localized. "Slow pain" takes on diffuse aching to agonizing qualities. Its unpleasant properties are poorly localized. When they dominate the foreground of consciousness, we feel distressed. Some of these ill-defined aversive resonances become the neural basis for suffering.

Opioids block slow pain much more than fast pain. This was an old clinical observation. Recent evidence suggests why: a blanket of opioid receptors envelops the slow pain pathways from the spinal cord on up (see chapter 47). Indeed, evolution went so far as to provide two general endogenous systems for *relieving* pain. One kind is opioid. The other is nonopioid.[4] Rats, being highly competent animals, use both kinds. Brief noxious electric shocks to a rat's paws produce analgesia, because they activate each of these two pain control systems. But after the *front* paw is stimulated, the opioid system is the more effective in relieving pain.[5] In contrast, shocks to a rat's *hind* paw tend more to activate the separate, *non*opioid, pathways for analgesia. One of these lies within the spinal cord; the other descends through it.[6] It seems that the nervous system has ways to treat leg pain somewhat differently from finger pain.

> Once, during the deep leg pains of a difficult sesshin, I just kept on going. Finally, meditative awareness entered some nether, detached region. A place where even agonizing leg pains dropped away. This relief of pain hinged on an ever-so-subtle shift of focusing. Awareness was steering itself toward a vague layer beyond thought. *Here, pain alone could be turned off, pain in and of itself.* Something resembling a residual *I* was still around, for I could still feel and envision my leg. I had not become completely indifferent to pain. Instead, there was the sense of employing a soft-edged mental focus to plumb some deep centering point. Once "there," a gentle nudge from somewhere promptly shifted *all* the pain away. Later, when the pain slid back in again, returning back "there" soon dropped it out again and again. None of this pain relief was associated with any obvious mental "high." So it is possible that the pain may have been relieved either by some of the nonopioid mechanisms referred to above, or by the opioid systems lower down. Exactly where and how such a remarkable process takes place in humans is not yet evident, nor can I bracket it with any other positive or negative attributes. The most to be said is that one sinks into its depths using, as rudder, a soft concentrative focus.

Experience, not words, helps one navigate such inner depths. Yogis who have many years of interior experience have refined similar abilities. They can use them to steer wordlessly either toward relieving that pain which comes from lying on a bed of nails, or into other alternate states of consciousness. Recently, studies were conducted on this ability of a yogi to tolerate lying on a bed of nails. (The investigator, who tested the bed himself, could not tolerate it even though its nails did not have sharp points.) Taking naloxone did *not* make the procedure more *in*tolerable. This particular observation suggested that nonopioid mechanisms were involved.[7] Nor does naloxone reverse the analgesia associated with hypnosis. This latter observation suggests that most of the pain relief which hypnosis confers may also originate in some nonopioid mechanisms.[4]

In humans, chronic pain can improve for several weeks after the central gray substance is stimulated high up near the posterior commissure just behind the third ventricle. It is clear that opioids contribute to this analgesia. The facts are that naloxone blocks the pain relief, and that the stimulation releases beta-endorphin.[8] Serotonin nerve cells also appear to be involved in this pain relief mechanism, because stimulation to the central gray relieves pain more effectively after the patients are given tryptophan, the ST precursor.[5]

Continue to sit in zazen for many hours, and the side effects will soon enlist your sympathies for any rat studied in pain experiments. Back, shoulder, and leg aches penetrate your deepest instincts for self-preservation. Your body and instincts may be different from mine. It turns out, physiologically, that we are not all created equal. Some persons tend to be more "sensitive" in every meaning of the term. Others are on the opposite end of the bell-shaped curve. They reduce the bare stimuli they register.[9]

Reducers and Augmenters

Researchers blindfold their subjects when they test for these opposing tendencies. First, each subject estimates how wide a block is, focusing on the width of the gap between thumb and forefinger of the *right* hand. Then, with the *left* thumb and forefinger, the subject next feels along a long, *tapered* measuring bar. The question: Where on this separate measuring bar lies that very same width which had been perceived earlier with the fingers of the right hand?

Thereafter, the right thumb and finger proceed to rub a much wider block, and for a longer period, lasting one to two minutes. It turns out that this second procedure alters the perception of size. And the person who is an extreme "augmenter" will now go on to perceive the same measuring bar as having increased some 50 percent over its actual size. In contrast, the extreme "reducer" perceives this original bar as having decreased 50 percent. These two groups of subjects represent the opposite ends of the human continuum in the way they process data from their sensory environment.

So what? The observations take on interesting behavioral affiliations (table 13). As might be anticipated, the augmenters do not tolerate painful stimuli. It does not seem to matter whether the stimulus evokes fast pain (from local heat applied to the skin of the forehead) or slow pain (from strong pressure applied to the bone in front of the lower leg, the kind of slow leg pain that meditators are very familiar with.) Speculation: Could augmenters have developed, on the basis of their having undergone more pain themselves, a better understanding of the way pain feels? And would this help them to develop greater empathy and compassion for pain in others?

Moreover, augmenters seem also to begin with a high tolerance for isolation, for measures which restrict their activities, and for sensorimotor deprivation in general. Speculation: Is this because they still go on perceiving relatively "more" stimuli, even after these three circumstances curtail most cues that had entered from their sensory environment?

Then what about the reducers, those at the other end of the spectrum? These persons tend to reduce sensory stimuli from their environment, and they tolerate pain better. However, they tend not to tolerate sensorimotor deprivation, perhaps because they already begin with a kind of relative "sensory scarcity."[9] The above hypotheses remain to be tested critically. The results could help us understand why some meditators are sufficiently stoic to endure a rigorous sesshin, whereas others are not.

Table 13
Differences between Augmenters and Reducers*

Aspect	Augmenters	Reducers
Response to the sensory environment	Tend subjectively to enhance the perceived intensity of stimuli; sensory gates open	Tend subjectively to reduce the perceived intensity of stimuli; sensory gates closed
Pain	Less tolerant	More tolerant
Sensory deprivation	More tolerant (still receiving stimuli)	Less tolerant (are below their comfort level)
Empathy for pain in others	May better understand from own experience	May not understand as well from own experience
Compassion	May develop greater concern	May develop less concern
Need for exercise	Lesser	Greater
Need to be alone	Greater	Lesser
Degree of extroversion	Lesser	Greater
Degree of neuroticism	No correlation	No correlation
Correlation with psychotic states	More with manic-depressive psychosis	More with schizophrenia

*After Petrie[5]

In summary: Fast splinter pain and slow bone pain arise at many levels throughout the nervous system. But two systems, opioid and nonopioid, help us relieve these pains.

81

Suffering and the Relief of Suffering

Abominating Hell
longing for Heaven
you make yourself suffer
in a joyful world.

Master Bankei (1622–1693)[1]

The spiritual path involves suffering. Suffering takes many physical and mental forms. Legends say that even when Siddhartha was a child, he was distressed when he found how living things consumed one another in the food chain. Still later, outside the walls of his privileged enclosure, he was deeply moved when he first confronted old age, sickness, and death. Brooding about these existential questions, he left his princely life and family to set out on a serious quest. In those days it meant the long, hard road of an ascetic pilgrim.

His wanderings in Nepal and northern India over the next six years were difficult ones at best. They brought him no lasting relief. But then enlightenment struck. Its basic wisdom was implicit: now he clearly understood what caused suffering and what relieved it. He then went on to sum up the essence of his teachings as follows: "Suffering I teach, and the Way out of suffering."[2] The central issue, he believed, was to know all about suffering. Of much less significance were the abstract questions such as the relationships between body and soul, mortality and immortality, or whether the world was finite or infinite in nature.[3]

His followers transmitted the Buddha's basic message. A person couldn't avoid some sufferings. They were predetermined by past events and other people. But the rest were self-inflicted, more or less, and these could not truly be laid at someone else's doorstep. They stemmed from one's own ignorance, from one's own cravings and hostilities. Suffering fades away when such emotions and attitudes fade away as a result of the person's long-sustained, appropriate daily life practice and insights.

True, early on, it is certainly pleasant to fulfill our desires. And it is also true that many desires are essential and useful, because they harness the energies which help individual persons and their societies survive. Indeed, one useful desire is to embark on the Buddhist Way or on any similar path of transformation. But tradeoffs occur. Sooner or later, sufferings of some kind can be observed to complicate the harvest of wishes fulfilled. So what each person needs especially to address are the *nonessential* desires and aversions, the substance of our distractions and delusions. For these, when coupled with ignorance, often make for the most suffering.[4]

But it is profoundly disturbing, and highly unpleasant, to be asked to change one's firm opinions. Adults don't like to change sets. No one likes to surrender his or her most cherished fantasies, or any other rigidly fixed, well-guarded "mental" domains. We rebel like a one-and-a-half-year-old child. There are messages here. What could they be telling us? Do we need to gentle our *I-Me-Mine?* Would it help us to sever some of those links that allowed it to spread *negative* feeling states throughout our affective defense and pain-linked circuitries?

Most human beings exist in a state of chronic dis-ease. The Buddha prescribed a way out. His eightfold path out of suffering combined the following positive steps: proper views, aspirations, speech, conduct, livelihood, effort, mindfulness, and meditative concentration. *Acting together,* synchronized, each element could reinforce the others. To follow this eightfold path is to pursue a *moderate course.* It leads to the cessation of cravings, *and* it thereafter relieves the suffering linked to these cravings. This *Middle Way* steers flexibly between two radical extremes: the one of self-indulgence with no restraints; the other marked by painful forms of self-mortification.

Suffering is a heavy topic. Yet no great teacher could have reached the Buddha's stature without also having emphasized the joy of living fully in the everyday world. Like other enlightened persons who had come before and who would follow him, he put into his teachings the practical, simple wisdoms he had learned growing up. They're still needed. Today, some studies estimate that the average American is afflicted by *high-level* suffering, severe enough to interfere with daily living, for as many as sixty days each year.[5] Moreover, it is hard to overlook the sobering truth of the heavy opening line of the recent *Declaration of a Global Ethic:* "The world is in agony." So suffering is a fact of life. It is a reality declared by the latest Parliament of the Worlds' Religions in 1993, not some topic overemphasized by the early Indian Buddhists.

Master Bankei was a popular Japanese teacher who came two millennia after Buddha. Why do we suffer? He said it was because we long for heaven and abominate hell. In all the centuries before and since, people have discovered that "life is no bed of roses." But life's thorns are merely painful. The really troublesome aspects of life are the agonizings: guilt over the past, hassles in the present, worries about the future.

Anguish has obvious motor counterparts. The furrowed brow and sagging posture tell us when someone else is suffering and depressed. We can also appreciate why tones of distress enter into our family dog's bark. He sees a rival dog threatening to violate *his* space! Yet, it still takes us a long time to appreciate a subtle aspect of mental suffering: it has a deep internal *sensory counterpart*. When people sink into the trough of their "down" cycles, they suffuse ill-defined discomforts into their other levels of conscious experience. And D. T. Suzuki knew that such agonizing would not stop simply because the person took up religion. Indeed, he concluded, "The spiritual life is pain raised above the level of mere sensation."[6]

One striking feature about morphine and the other opioids is the way they do more than relieve physical pain. Why do the patient's pains then become less immediate? Because opioids relieve suffering, the "psychological" response to pain. Not only do the patients' original pains improve but those that remain seem to *bother them much less*. The patients have become "emotionally detached" from their pain. A gap seems to have opened up between the perceptive and the responsive. This "distancing" is a noteworthy phenomenon. Zen, too, illustrates this kind of nonattachment, at several levels. And not only with regard to pain but also with regard to emotional responses that can extend in positive or negative directions.

From his experiences with wounded soldiers, Beecher concluded that "the intensity of suffering is largely determined by what the pain means to the patient."[7,8] If you immerse your arm in ice-cold water you will experience intense pain. But extensive meditative training can help reduce the distress associated with such pain. In one study, TM meditators (who had practiced for an average of nine years) were significantly less distressed by the cold water than were controls. The TM group did not differ otherwise in their pain threshold level, nor in how much their heart rate increased, nor in how much their skin resistance decreased.[9] Certain brain operations such as prefrontal lobotomy and cingulumotomy can increase patients' abilities to *tolerate* pain, without raising the threshold at which they originally perceive the sensation of pain.

Some subjects have reported that, under the influence of LSD, they can have pain which "does not hurt."[10] The greatest aid to experiencing such nonhurtful pain is to have an exemplar who has been "there" once before and who is not afraid. In Weil's view, the fear of pain is itself the greatest obstacle. He believes that a subject can experience nonhurtful pain, without LSD, when both the mental set and the setting are appropriate. In the presence of pain, the technique involves first deepening one's concentration, then turning attention away from verbalized thoughts and directing it toward the feeling itself. In the previous chapter, I described a personal episode, during meditation, of becoming aware of a related phenomenon. It differed, however, in that *all* pain disappeared.

Psychologists usually emphasize that our life crises create negative influences. These then go on to *cause* behavioral disorders. Yet, in the long run, some clouds have a silver lining, and some cloudbursts expose a vein of gold. Recent studies suggest that many healthy young people place a *positive* interpretation on their most painful life crises. In fact, of the 42 percent of them who do, the vast majority (88 percent) report that the crisis enhanced their sense that life has meaning.[11] Moreover, at least as far back as the sixth century, in the traditions associated with Bodhidharma and his followers, it has been appreciated that suffering—and adapting to it—has the potential to infuse something positive into Zen practice.[12] This same principle has a contemporary acknowledgement: "those who have suffered and lived in pain can attain enlightenment more quickly than those who approach enlightenment only by abstract meditation, especially if the suffering and pain are really serious."[13]

So a variety of unforseen benefits accrue to those who keep going through pain and then beyond it. Among them is a change in their attitudes about pain. After a sesshin, one young Zen monk spoke to us about it in the following way: "I am grateful for all the aching in my legs and for my stiff and tortured back. Through these I came to know that all such pains can become insubstantial and have no meaning. I don't know how to express in words the depths of this realization."

82

Bridging the Two Hemispheres

Subcortical structures do not serve simply as pathways linking the two hemispheres but play an essential coordinating role in the integration of hemispheric activity.

J. Sergent[1]

Since the conscious properties of the left hemisphere are obvious through a subject's verbal behavior, our main concern has been with the silent inhabitant of the right side of the cranium.

J. LeDoux, D. Wilson, and M. Gazzaniga[2]

Silent, but influential. How much the right hemisphere contributes became clear only after neurosurgeons began to split the corpus callosum. This is the broad uppermost bridge which joins the right and left hemispheres (see figure 3). The surgeons cut it along its midline in an effort to stop the spread of severe generalized seizures. When Roger Sperry first studied such patients, he used a technique which channeled visual stimuli from one side of space into the corresponding hemisphere on the opposite side of the brain. For this pioneering research in humans and monkeys, Sperry received the Nobel prize in physiology or medicine in 1981.

Our vocalizing left hemisphere had more obvious functions. Its specialty was language and the analysis of those kinds of items which language can categorize. Moreover, for many years it has both directed our own speech and listened to what it sounded like. By now, it must retain a host of subtle memory traces convincing us that our "verbal self" does exist.

But our right hemisphere takes a different tack to "thinking." Its version uses visual strategies, is nonverbal, works best in gestalt, and tends to draw global conclusions based on the whole visual picture. It is more proficient in grasping personal and spatial interrelationships. And in order to do so, it needs to deploy attention into certain higher-order constructs. Why are these constructs so relevant to Zen? Because they represent our personal self as it interfaces with the outside world on both sides of the midline.

Wedded by the broad band of the corpus callosum, our two hemispheres normally yield a single, unified system of attention. But what happens, then, in the so-called split-brain patients? At first glance, rather little. Under most circumstances, split-brain patients seem normal. They behave, without hesitation, as unified persons in an integrated, reasonably coherent manner.[1] But suppose you test the patients under certain artificial experimental situations. Now the split becomes evident: they are not so much married as separated and living together. They turn out to have two separate attention and action systems. Yet, sometimes, this helps them achieve the impossible. For example, a patient's right hand can busily sort out one simple object from a mixture containing beads or small cylinders. Simultaneously, the left hand is successfully sorting out two *other* kinds of objects! The rest of us find this a daunting task.[3]

Still, with practice, even normal subjects can learn to automate the techniques for sorting different objects. How? By learning—as a trained juggler does—to free the task from *too much egocentric intrusion*. It is not easy. Soon we slip back into our old habits, worry about what we are doing, and then fumble around again. Like learning to meditate.

Normals go through a three-step process to learn these two-handed sorting tasks. First is the basic training to become competent. Following this comes increasing confidence in one's abilities. Finally, it is necessary to "let go." All three are the essence of Zen, especially this last step. *For it means trusting one's brain to do the correct thing.* The brain has a highly competent automatic pilot. It will enhance performance only to the extent that one's *I-Me-Mine* learns to stop wrestling for control of the stick.

But is it true that we lateralize certain brain functions to only one hemisphere? Claims and counterclaims have grown apace.[4] In the process, a topic of Nobel caliber has been reduced to an either/or, right/left issue, and has fallen into caricature in the tabloids and comic strips. If a given function were indeed a lateralized one, then any researcher who says it must exit on one side would already have a 50 percent chance of being correct. Many earlier claims that the two hemispheres show major differences have not withstood the test of time.[5,6]

What now seems clear is that our right and left hemispheres are allies in an uneven alliance. Though usually linked in tandem, the right may take the lead in some respects, the left in others. This chapter emphasizes new evidence about what kind of silent dialogue passes *between* the hemispheres. And this book emphasizes what these two allies accomplish when they join certain of their forces—while dropping out other functions—in very special ways.

The separated right hemisphere only *seems* silent and nonverbal. In fact, it recognizes, and acts. Consider how much the right side already *knows* about apples. Place in front of the patient a multiple choice situation: a selection of fruits and other objects. Then flash the picture of an apple solely into the domain of this right hemisphere, namely, into the patient's *left* visual field. True, this right brain may not, by itself, then be able to *speak* the word "apple." But it does know what to look for. Immediately it directs the sensorimotor functions of its left hand to search for *just* the apple.

The refined techniques now available can be used *in normal persons* to channel visual stimuli to only one hemisphere. And these studies (the corpus callosum being intact) confirm that the normal right hemisphere does take in the big picture by using its global, visuospatial processing strategies. Show this right hemisphere some random items in a disorganized scene, and it will quickly discern that box, tire, axe, and spool share no common overall theme.[7] In contrast, the normal left hemisphere is better at picking out more detailed incongruities. It spots the Eskimo and igloo, given a scene which also includes pictures of a farmer, a horse, and a barn. And this left hemisphere is also better at synthesizing the kinds of imaginative interpretations which carry a story line. It can infer boiling water, given the presence of a pan plus some water.[8] The story line is important because it gives a sense of meaning (see chapter 72).

Instantly, we know whether another person wears an expression of greeting, grief, or disgust. On balance, the right hemisphere is the more facile at discerning these emotions. Some normal persons become especially skillful at expressing their basic, Darwinian countenances. Most of these nuances come from contracting the muscles of the lower left side of the face. In such instances, the right hemisphere may be contributing the greater emotional input. Even so, it will be the deeper brain regions on *both* sides which yield most of the components of our spontaneous expressions.[9]

The right hemisphere has other subtleties. These go beyond recognizing emotions and generating different kinds of affect. For when Penfield stimulated the right side, the patients reported almost three times as many experiential flashbacks, especially when stimuli were delivered to the cortex of the right temporal lobe.[10]

But much confusion arises if it is tacitly assumed that everyone's hemispheres are "wired" the same way. In fact, human brains are a genetic mishmash, hybrids emerging from a vast DNA pool. We differ in the ways we process information and express it.[11] True, some patients, and some normals, do appear to lateralize their emotions more so than do others. However, when large populations are studied, the results are less clear. The simplest interpretation is that everyone does not generate positive and negative emotional valences *consistently and to the same degree* from the domain of either hemisphere.[8,12]

And language skills, likewise, can sometimes arise in both hemispheres, not only in the left. In one such instance the person underwent a split-brain operation.[2] Now it became possible for researchers to carry on a *symmetrical dialogue with each hemisphere's mental functions, individually.* Words were then displayed, to each hemisphere. Each side could rank the words along its own scale of good to bad. What was the functional mood of the right hemisphere? Well, this side tended to be in a "bad mood." That is, it usually ranked the test words more negatively than did the left. Indeed there were days when the two hemispheres were very far apart in the way they evaluated the same word. And on these discordant days, the patient was also more anxious, and behaved poorly.

But then, too, there were other days. Now the two hemispheres "agreed," evaluating the outside world in the same way. And at these times, the patient was calm and socially appealing. Such observations are intriguing. (To some, they might seem to prove that being mentally "unified" goes on to have positive social benefits. But we will need more than the concords—or discords—among words in a single patient to generalize about the rest of human social behavior.)

One other unusual split-brain patient spoke with his left hemisphere after information had first been presented to his right hemisphere. Where had this patient's speaking hemisphere (his left) gotten this information? *It had no idea.* It was not *consciously* aware that it had indeed received any covert messages from his right (receiving) hemisphere. Perhaps, Gazzaniga suggested, the particular kind of information transmitted from right to left was *non*cognitive in nature.[13] If so, it was speculated that when these signal messages from the right side did cross over to the left, they engaged there a kind of "response readiness." On this left side, potential speech responses would be already well rehearsed, and ready to be uttered.

Zen and the Subcortical Bridge

Why do the split-brain patients still *behave in a unified manner* during their everyday activities? How can they be unified after their main *transcortical* bridge has been cut? To Sperry, this behavior suggested that our system of consciousness is shaped like a Y. True, the system is bifurcated above, up there in the hemispheres. But it remains undivided below.[14] Unified behavior strongly implies that the patients are using other major avenues to exchange messages between the two sides of the brain.

In the present context, we shall refer to all these lower avenues collectively as the *subcortical bridge*. One major portion of this bridge conveys neuronal traffic back and forth across the diencephalon∗ and upper brain stem (see figure 3). This region is represented at the site where the three lines of the Y come together. Does this mean that some of our higher-level messages must go down as far as the diencephalon and brain stem, then cross over, and climb back up again? Yes, it does. We have seen similar circuitous steps in operation before, as in chapter 37. So, even though all the spans and abutments of the subcortical bridge are hidden deep and out of sight, they are hardly out of mind. For they still enable two-way traffic to join the two hemispheres, simply to link them at a level much lower than does the corpus callosum. Two lesser footbridges also remain: the anterior

---

∗ The diencephalon includes both halves of the thalamus, the subthalamus, and the hypothalamus

and posterior commissures. It is not clear what sorts of affective messages might traverse the small anterior commissure.

The newer techniques of visual projection allow researchers to test which kinds of messages pass across the subcortical bridge. Suppose, for example, that the investigator projects the picture of an apple off into the left side of space. A stimulus from out there will register on the right half of the retina in each eye, and its image will take shape directly in relays only in the right hemisphere. This right side then spins off its many abstruse associations to the apple. These are coded messages containing loose inferences. They relate to the *context* of the apple, rather than to its purely optical properties. The right side then relays these encoded messages via the subcortical bridge—down, across the intersection of the Y, over and up—to the left side of the brain. En route, neighboring nerve cells along the bridge have an opportunity to elaborate upon the messages.

Let us first seem so contrary as to ask, What kinds of messages *do not* exchange readily across the subcortical bridge? Language-based information doesn't move freely. Nor does complex geometric information. Things like apple pie, or the roundness of an object, don't pass. These are the more concrete associations we might make when we see the apple's literal visual image or think about its word image.

Then what sorts of messages *are* readily transferred? In general, information which conveys nuances of feeling about the subject, useful hints about which giant category it belongs to, or abstract concepts that are even higher and softer.[15] Which of these kinds of messages cross best? Those that are *nonverbal,* as well as highly abstracted. Even so, their codes still convey useful information. And this information can then enter into unified behavior. To illustrate: the nonverbal messages include such data as hints about gender, race, and occupation; whether numbers are higher or lower in value; whether a number is odd or even; and so forth.[1] Put simply, *what crosses best are unconscious or preconscious codes, nuances we can never attach a name to.*

So we have come into the presence of *precognitive murmurings.* Overtones tinged neither by language nor by spatial geometry. Qualities so intuitive that they escape easy definitions. These are the soft messages which travel best across the spans of the subcortical bridge. Zen would seem to be on familiar ground in this deep, ineffable domain. For intuitions, too, contain inexpressible messages. Their codes elude the metaphors of poets and philosophers alike. In these recent research findings are implications which help us understand certain alternate states and behaviors, if only by analogy. For when sudden major insights are indescribable by ordinary language, we need to keep asking, Why? Indeed, when a person's experience is ineffable, could it signify that the coded functions of some of these subcortical mechanisms have been amplified?

Directional Preferences

To begin to answer, it may help to ask, Do any of these coded messages pass more easily *in one direction* across the subcortical bridge? Yes, some do.[15] Some messages move more readily from *right to left.* These are hotline messages, alarms. These emotionally linked messages convey impressions of danger, sudden movements, and potential violence.

But certain other concepts do *not* pass easily from right to left. Their associative codes rank low on the scale of emotionality. What do these cooler messages have to do with Zen? They could be presenting us with something more than a remarkable coincidence. For they express concepts of *time,* of *lack,* and of *silence.*[15] Later, we will find the first two of these same *un*sentimental qualities emerging from the arctic moonlight of kensho. At that point, the descriptive words used to discuss the properties of time and of lack will include eternity and emptiness (see chapters 135, 137, and 138). Later still, we will take up the issue of an ultimate silence (see chapter 146).

So there seem to be "one-way traffic" signs, as it were, on some sections of the subcortical bridge. What could be the result of these intrinsic signs? They could shape the way the person experiences an alternate state, and then tries vainly to describe it thereafter. Because it is never any simple matter to construct abstract concepts of issues as vital as time, lack, and silence. And some portions of these interactive processes could be arising—and entering into consciousness—more on the right side. If so, then they might tend to stay put, as it were. Being relatively isolated, they could prove difficult for the left hemisphere to access. So the inherent limitations of one-way traffic could render such cool messages—when they arose on the right side—difficult to put into words, ineffable.

But this is not to ignore the evidence that, in their usual state, split-brain patients go on behaving in a unified manner. Implicit in this observation is the fact that the two-way traffic which does pass readily across the bridge is very good at integrating complex nonverbal behaviors. Indeed, codes of this kind might be serving as the basis for the nuances of *body language* we call pantomime. And similar bridging functions will later become one part of the explanation for why fast, efficient behavior is so typically associated with Zen training (see chapter 155).

The evidence just cited leads one to a rather different perspective on the earlier split-brain studies. The issue is not whether the cortex of one hemisphere is "smarter" than the other, or more capable. What matters in the Zen context is how facile—and yet how selective—our many subcortical *bridging* systems have increasingly been revealed to be. Here, in the core of the brain, a highly competent automatic pilot has available for its use many sophisticated precognitive operations. What does precognitive mean? Precognitive functions are the kinds which allow the jazz musician to take off from his familiar terrain of melody, and wing it on impossible flights of improvisation. No pilot's license is required, certainly not one written in ordinary language or notation.

Lateralizable Functions and the EEG

When we are in our usual resting state, the EEG amplitudes on the two sides of the brain resemble each other. But when one hemisphere becomes more activated, it adds more low voltage fast-wave frequencies. Now, its average EEG amplitude is reduced. And at that same moment, the EEG amplitude on the opposite side also decreases some 70 percent of the time. However, if you deprive human subjects of sensory input for only twenty to thirty minutes, the brain waves of their two hemispheres become more independent. At this point, you can no longer predict what the EEG amplitude of one side will be, based on the height of the waves on the other side.[16] What happens during those particular kinds of meditation which also have the effect of reducing the input of patterned sensate stimuli? Could this reduction make it more likely that the two hemispheres would express themselves in more dissociated, *independent* feelings and behaviors? And if the two sides were less inclined to function in synchrony, would this be a "good" thing? These questions remain to be critically tested.

Mystical absorptions resonate in metaphoric ways, and sometimes these transports seem to overlap with feelings of sexual love. It is in this context that several other case reports are of interest.[16] None of them, it should be noted, are based on split-brain patients. In one instance, a nineteen-year-old schizophrenic woman showed a right temporal lobe preponderance of EEG activity when she experienced "feelings of love" for her boyfriend. In another, an eighteen-year-old schizophrenic youth shifted to a predominately right temporal EEG activation when he first felt a "deep religious ecstasy." So some feelings termed "ecstasy" or "love" may appear to correlate with right brain activations, at least in some patients. However, they do not correlate with the EEG findings recorded from other patients when they reach sexual climax. In fact, during orgasm itself, the left cerebral hemisphere tends to show the more activated EEG.[17] Few would contend that left brain phenomena would afford an adequate explanation for all the sensate, motoric, and affective aspects of orgasm.[18]

A third extraordinary case report describes a woman who had learned to select, *at will*, one of two mental states. One of these states reflected predominant activity in her right hemisphere, the other in the left.[19] When she was a young child, her two mental states switched by themselves. But by the age of sixteen she had learned the art of control. Now she could shift *voluntarily* from one state to the other. How? She began either by closing her eyes, or by looking off at the horizon. Then she simply allowed her conscious decision to take effect.

We have been searching, of course, for the origins of the *I*. Therefore, it is of some interest to note the word she used to describe her *left*-sided state. It was "I." And, whenever she was in this state, the investigators concluded that her usual cognitive modes were more "left hemispheric" in type. Moreover, her left-sided EEG leads also showed the correspondingly greater activation. In contrast, she referred to her other state as "it." "It" showed more *right* hemispheric EEG activation. "It" was also the more spatially adroit. So far, everything seems to fit the conventional notions outlined at the start of this chapter.

When she was in her right hemispheric active state, her behavior appeared more open, enthusiastic, and forthright. But (and here any wistful, simplistic analogies start to break down), she was also more impulsive, emotional, and had more definite likes and dislikes. In contrast, her left hemispheric active state was the more defensive one. She was guarded, cautious, and restricted, yet also more *indifferent* to matters of picking and choosing. (How could what we have already learned about Zen represent functions that must arise from *only* one of her two hemispheres?)

Even so, other EEG studies support the view that the right hemisphere does take the lead at the active interface between our attention and intention.[20] The findings suggest that we activate primarily the right parietal lobe when we attend to either or to both sides of the outside world. Moreover, subjects have been studied at the moment when they shift into three-dimensional modes. Their visual task is to view simple figures which have been drawn so that their planes shift in and out like Necker cubes. Again, the evidence indicates that the *right* temporal and parietal regions are involved to the greater degree.[21]

Still, the right hemisphere is not the sole generator of visual imagery, including that during dreams. The same *number* of dreams occurs during sleep whether the EEG of the right or the left hemisphere was the more activated at the time. Moreover, if EEG asymmetries do occur during desynchronized REM sleep, they lateralize to the same side as they did when the same subjects were in synchronized, *non*-REM sleep.[22]

On the other hand, when subjects respond to affective test situations their EEG correlates are more predictable. This correlation begins early in life. Even at ten months of age, the particular female infants who already show a greater right frontal EEG activation will be the ones temperamentally disposed later to cry more when their mothers leave the room.[23] In adult women, the EEG becomes relatively activated in the right frontal regions during negative emotions, whereas a left frontal activation predominates in association with positive emotions.[24] And pharmacologic evidence supports the view that our left hemisphere is the more specialized to release positive, euphoric emotions, whereas the right tends to release negative, depressive emotional expressions.[25] Overstated simply, and far too loosely: the left side tends normally to be the "upper"; the right side is normally the "downer."

Left/Right Aspects of Meditation and Alternate States

Thoughts drop out during meditation. Moreover, some quickenings occur which are difficult to put in words. Given these observations, it is easy to understand why meditation has been believed to reduce the verbal-analytic activities of the left hemisphere, and to enhance the nonverbal functions of the more "holistic" right hemisphere.[26,27] However, a person's meditative mode shifts both during a single sitting and from one day to the next. So let us look critically at the notions that meditation enhances, indiscriminately, the functions of the *whole* right hemisphere. Would this really be a good thing? Especially if the right side is normally a downer? Where do such all-inclusive theories lead?

The evidence just cited (in references 19, 23, 24, and 25) suggest that negative emotions might rise to the fore under these circumstances. Does such a view support the wholly beneficent flavor of meditation, at least as it is described by some of its proponents? Then, too, some investigators believe that the right hemisphere plays the greater role in generating our sense of *personal* familiarity. You might think of this as the egocentric tug which mutters, convincingly, "these are *my* car keys."[28] Again, let us stay within the Zen context of alternate states. It has been teaching that it is desirable to *dissolve* the self. As long as we retain this perspective, the proposals that a meditator becomes *wholly* "right-brained" cannot be supported. For a valid theory needs to clarify how meditation proceeds to *dissolve* this particular function of personal relevance, not to enhance it.

When our left hemisphere recognizes things, it seems to use more tightly organized templates than does its partner. Recent studies of normal persons illustrate these two different approaches to data processing. Start with one of those pictures containing several items. Next, use that same kind of visual device which channels this scene first into one hemisphere and then the other. In normals, the more critical left side quickly detects the incongruity: a giraffe does not fit in next to that Eskimo and his igloo.[7]

Can one turn around the implications of such findings? Would they mean that our most critical functions—those led by the left side—*leave* during those rare moments when all distinctions drop out? For it is true that discriminations drop out during the unity of kensho's vision. Does this suggest that kensho briefly suspends the usual, more left-sided discriminative functions—those which had quickly enabled the person to pick out incongruous details? Such questions may be too simplistic. At least under usual circumstances, both of our hemispheres act together to process novel scenes. And when they do address the unexpected, it is with a blend of their two different strategies, not with one alone.[7]

On balance, the evidence reviewed throughout this book suggests that the brain undergoes no complete right/left split in its functions. Not during meditative states, not during absorptions, not during insights. Instead, the data suggest that far more complex (and interactive) neurophysiological principles are involved. They are not the simple ones which stress dichotomies. They won't suggest that the brain's functions can be divided, as by a surgeon's knife, into two disparate halves. Indeed, studies pursuing the view that meditation must be solely a right hemispheric phenomenon have so far yielded very mixed results.[27,29,30]

Which wing, the right or left, is more important? Would one pose such a question to a hummingbird? Or to a Lindbergh straining to reach the other shore on a transatlantic solo flight? The central truth is different: *each hemisphere is specialized in ways that are complementary to the other.* This conclusion will not ignore all the recent research that would divide brain functions into categories that are mostly right- or left-sided. Rather it allows one to say that such tidy categories as holistic/analytic, nonverbal/verbal, simultaneous/sequential, and so on, have not prepared us to understand *all* the extraordinary features of alternate states.

A View, from the Bridge, toward Awakening

Consider kensho, for instance: the prime example of a brain uncovering its latent, insightful qualities and heightening them. Where do these qualities come from? An earlier paragraph in this chapter raised the possibility that some of the more subtle properties of insight come from events at specified subcortical levels. And that thereafter, when these ingredients entered conscious awareness, they could still be in the form of abstract coded messages which research has only barely begun to understand.

Yet what else happens in kensho? Its awakening *suspends* many of the brain's other functions. It does *not* enhance them. So when we go on to consider *both sets* of findings further, we soon discover that the resulting state is a very mixed bag. Even when the properties of awakening are oversimplified, they still resemble a huge checkerboard pattern, a design so vast that it leaves wishful thinking and simple notions far behind (see chapter 142). Could kensho then be the expression of only two contrasting sets of functions, each unique to its own hemisphere, one half of each set suddenly illuminated, the other blacked out? No. Our perspective here is that *awakening has selective properties*. They have a distinctive pattern. The way this pattern transcends any simple right/left differences has yet to receive sufficient attention. Indeed, in a sense, there is an almost "savant" aspect of insight-wisdom.[31] For yes, kensho enhances only certain rare faculties, and does so at great speed. But equally striking is the way it loses all concepts of self, of time, and dissolves the old sharp-edged affective distinctions.

In parts I and III we slowly became familiar with the *I-Me-Mine.* We observed how its fears and desires arise from the networking of multiple modules, at levels high and low along the neuraxis, and on both sides. How could kensho, at one stroke, bypass or destructure such constructs, while still sparing the patchwork quilt of one's other functions? It is by focusing on the *total pattern of functions*—some being heightened, others dropping out—that we will arrive at a better understanding of Zen and of its phenomena.

The general approach we must now follow will continue to elaborate on a series of experiential distinctions. We will continue to distinguish between meditation and quickening, between absorption and insight-wisdom. But our explanations will now increasingly rely on the different physiological systems that we have seen *in interaction within the brain as a whole* (see part III). And our theories will further acknowledge two facts: first, that our two hemispheres have complementary functions; second, that they engage in subtle dialogues across the subcortical bridge.

83

The Pregnant Meditative Pause

> How can you even hope to approach the truth through words? . . . full understanding can come to you only through an inexpressible mystery. The approach to it is called the Gateway of the Stillness beyond all Activity. If you wish to understand, know that a sudden comprehension comes when the mind has been purged of all the clutter of conceptual and discriminatory thought-activity. Those who seek the truth by means of intellect and learning only get further and further away from it. Not 'til you abandon all thoughts of seeking for something, not 'til your mind is motionless as wood or stone, will you be on the right road to the Gate.
>
> Master Huang-po (died 850)[1]

It is a long road to the Gate. If you conceive of it as two goalposts, they will keep moving farther away. To Huang-po, a still, motionless mind was the prelude to sudden comprehension. Nature builds in quiet pauses everywhere. In the heart, diastole is prelude to each resurgent systole. In the nervous system, pauses occur at each organizational level, from single nerve cells up to the behavior of the whole organism.

On a printed page, words leap out because they have spaces around them. Commas and periods are also pauses, strategically placed. When a single neuron fires its tiny spike, it will be those intervals on either side which make its signal stand out high above all the other background noise. In neurobiology, the same general phenomenon takes on another dimension. It has evolved into a notion called the "rest" principle. This theory suggests that an actively used connection will become "stronger" if it is allowed to rest briefly.[2]

A single nerve cell has several ways to "rest" itself. For example, some cells send out small axons which branch off from its main fiber. Then, after these side branches curve back to the main cell, their impulses give this cell the negative feedback which will its slow firing rate. Farther down still, already past the synapse, the next neurons can enlist the help of adjacent smaller GABA interneurons. Here, GABA fibers also curl back to provide negative, inhibitory feedback in local circuits (see figure 4). Lacking such restraints, a prodigal nerve cell can quickly burn itself out in runaway overfiring.

What happens to an assembly of larger nerve cells when all incoming excitation slackens off? While this quieted system is undergoing its long-drawn-out pause, one may speculate that it does not "need" as much restraint from its customary GABA inhibition. Then when GABA inhibitory mechanisms themselves become quieted way down, they will use up fewer GABA molecules and won't be receiving the usual stimulation they require to synthesize new ones. Lulled by long hours and days of such relative quiet, GABA systems may then be operating at less than peak efficiency. At this point, with their guard down, so to speak, GABA systems might then be overrun by the next brisk surge in activity of the larger cells. In this manner, when a long-delayed excitatory surge finally does enter a quiet interval, its impact will be greater, its effect longer-lasting.

An experimental model already exists that shows what does happen after synthesis slows. First, the researchers give a drug which stops the brain from making new dopamine molecules. Within two hours, the treated rats will have used up their previous supply of DA. Now their brain levels of DA fall. No longer stimulated by any fresh DA, their DA receptors become relatively quiescent. At this point, even a weak dose of a DA agonist greatly energizes the rats' behavior.[2] Why? Because after the existing DA receptors on postsynaptic cells have "rested" briefly, they become *extra*-sensitive to the next pulse of the DA agonist. In separate experiments, the rats' DA receptors can be blocked by the DA antagonist haloperidol. Again, these rested receptors later become extra-sensitive to DA. And in this instance, some of the rats' exaggerated behaviors now reflect the fact that they have increased temporarily the *numbers* of their DA receptors.

Similar feedback mechanisms regulate the "strengths" of the connections within norepinephrine systems. Many NE terminals are encrusted with presynaptic alpha-receptors. Once these receptors are activated, the result is like shutting down the nozzle on a garden hose: less NE is released into the synapse. The postsynaptic cell compensates for having had too little NE released on it. Later, it generates an *extra* surge of its second messenger when it receives a pulse of NE (see chapter 48).

The dominant effect of biogenic amines like DA and NE is to *hyper*polarize the next cell. Then why does this next cell pause? Because, at this point, no average-sized excitatory stimulus can easily *de*polarize it. But next, let a critical mass of excitatory impulses arrive. Now, when the once-rested, hyperpolarized cell finally does topple into its firing mode, it will discharge in very long bursts.

In neuronal terms, this process is reminiscent of the French phrase *reculer pour mieux sauter*. Kids learn the technique early. It is that stepping far back from the bank of the creek, the better to run and to clear it on the next leap forward. In nerve cells, the delayed burst firing is itself followed by still another long pause. So, in the brain, say at times when the other nerve cell systems have been droning on at one of their regular discharge rates, fresh pulses of dopamine, norepinephrine, and serotonin can surge in to break the monotony. For now there occurs a *triphasic* firing sequence: slowing, burst firing . . . long pause. Each trough of local inhibition has become the springboard from which the next incoming signal can take off. In such indirect ways can relatively few biogenic amine nerve cells make tall waves on an otherwise flat seascape.

How do such observations translate into the functions of our large assemblies of nerve cells, in ways that are relevant to Zen? By way of an example, consider what kind of vision we need when we are first starting to awaken. We certainly need to see the world *clearly*. And to help accomplish this, geniculate nerve cells can be tuned to fire in *single* spikes, not in bursts of spikes.[3]

Waking up is one of those moments in the nervous system when less is more. (And much the same could be said for the awakening of kensho.) Suppose, for example, that one's arousing retina had sent many fresh volleys of visual impulses on back to the lateral geniculate nucleus. And suppose, at this very same time, that the geniculate was already preoccupied—it was having too many of *its own* internal long burst discharges. In this case, the geniculate (which should relay visual signals accurately) might garble these incoming retinal messages. Waking up is not a good time to have any kind of information jumbled in transit. The less confusion, the better.

So the optimal solution, which in fact *does* occur during actual arousal, is to constrain the lateral geniculate nucleus. To bias it, so that it responds with *single*-spike activity. Now it can relay its incoming visual messages with great fidelity. No clutter of extra background noise en route. The result is a clear *visual signal* sent on to the visual cortex.

Now, NE makes two contributions to this single-spike firing mode during arousal. First, NE acts directly on the visual relay cells in the lateral geniculate. Here, it constrains them to fire *one* spike, and then to pause. No long spike bursts. Second, NE also acts on the reticular nucleus. Here, it shapes both the kinds and numbers of sensate messages that this nucleus will allow to pass through the thalamus. When humans experience brief moments of visual or even mental clarity, similar processes may be operating on a larger scale. Then NE could be contributing both to the amplitude *and to the clarity* of the moment.

But what about all those diastolic pauses in mentation and behavior, the ones that we undergo in the course of an ordinary day? Sometimes, acknowledging such gaps, we say: "I must have drifted off," or "I guess my mind was somewhere else." Researchers have been studying these phenomena of pause.[4] It turns out that we insert *many* blank pauses into an average day. In fact, we spend about 5 percent of our time staring or standing, *not thinking, not doing anything*. Not even daydreams intrude into these blank periods. Ostensibly awake when we enter them, we may even continue to wash and dry our face, comb our hair, walk, drive, and so forth. Moments later, we pick up where we left off. Once again we become aware of what we are thinking, knowing, and doing. Of course, meanwhile, some of these "no-mind" moments will have effaced many of our usual *I-Me-Mine* boundaries.

Now, suppose a set-point shifts. A thin wedge thrusts up from a major energized brain state. Suppose that it impaled one of these major blank moments, and did so during an especially vacant interval when we had drifted far away from our usual *I-Me-Mine* mode. Such an experience would then consist of the basic triad: (1) a blank moment, (2) no self around, (3) this blank, no-self moment penetrated by the clarity of enhanced awareness.

Five percent of one's time isn't very much to spend in blank periods. Perhaps if Huang-po were right, meditation would help us to cultivate a few more of these fertile triads. One could then envision a basic function of meditation as sponsoring the following confluence of events: (1) the occurrence of more frequent, deeper, longer blank periods; (2) some loosening up along the boundaries of our usual rigid cycles of rest and activity; (3) a partial dissolution of our *I-Me-Mine* connections; (4) their being completely cut off during the well-timed entry of a major activating surge.

Zen mediative training does facilitate each of these four requirements. Of course, the sequences of training evolve over a period of months and years, unlike the brief series of events which a single cell runs through in the course of its daily rhythms. Still, the initial event is a pause, a meditative quiescence. Gradually, meditative training goes on to cultivate a repertoire of pauses. These could affect the usual transition zones between the states of waking, sleeping, and dreaming. In this manner it could set the stage for rare surges into absorptions, for example (see part VI).

In a larger sense, meditation is itself a pause, something like the sabbath. It opens up our simpler sensibilities. Refreshed, they perceive deeply the sacramental beauty of the world in which we live. And before long, other kinds of pregnant pauses begin to occur. These become the brief plateau experiences of "really seeing," as opposed to ordinary looking. Of "really hearing," as opposed to ordinary listening. Of deep *understanding,* instead of merely knowing more facts. During such openly receptive moments, we get intimations of the elegant simplicity of *being,* uncluttered by legions of proliferating thoughts.

The pause is prelude. Its sequelae afford a plausible glimpse of how the Zen meditative path might lead toward that gateway of which old Huang-po spoke. And in every era, those who pause to meditate have increased the frequency, depth, and duration of the quickenings that next ensue.

PART V

Quickening

The flowering of man's spiritual nature is as natural and as strict a process of evolution as the opening of a rose or a morning glory. But there is this difference: While the plant must have a congenial environment . . . the human flowering often takes place amid the most adverse surroundings . . .

John Burroughs (1837–1921)

Side Effects of Meditation: Makyo

Was it a vision, or a waking dream? Fled is that music:—Do I wake or sleep?
                                                    John Keats (1795–1821)[1]

Meditators experience unusual body sensations and perceptions. They see a play of colors, hear noises, experience feelings of heaviness, lightness, or tilting. Zen downgrades all such hallucinations, either during meditation or at any other time. Soyen Shaku, for example, clearly excluded many of the visionary phenomena and related "psychical aberrations" from contributing to the true Zen "realization of the religious life," even though, in the meditative traditions of India, they might have been included among the states called samadhi.[2]

Now that we have just observed the centennial anniversary of this first trip by a Zen master to the United States, it is worth noting which epiphenomena he specifically *excluded:* (1) the sensation of being lifted up in the air like a cloud; (2) the feeling of the presence of some indescribable luminosity; (3) the experience of supernatural joy; (4) the clarification and transparency of mind such that it appears to reflect all the world like a very brilliant mirror; (5) the feeling as though the soul had escaped bodily confinement and had expanded itself out into the immensity of space; (6) a return toward that definite state of conscious awareness in which all mental functions are present, and the past, present, and future reveal themselves; (7) a feeling of nothingness in which no mentation is present; (8) a state neither of loss of consciousness nor of consciousness of anything in particular, considered by some to be the highest stage of samadhi.

What purpose did his exclusions serve? They gave early notice to East and West: *Traditional Japanese Zen would concentrate on the high ground of insight-wisdom.* It would deemphasize the hallucinatory and sensate phenomena of the "vision quest." The conservative core of the Christian mystical tradition adopts a similar position.

If Zen downgrades all these side effects as epiphenomena, then why waste time discussing them? Because they are excellent examples of how meditation influences brain functions. They illustrate, in particular, what can happen when the brain opens up some barriers which would otherwise separate its states of waking, sleeping, and dreaming (see table 9). One's early months of training yield obvious physiological swings. Indeed, volunteer subjects can experience distortions of perception, affect, and of their sense of time within ten minutes of relaxing into a passive attitude in a psychology laboratory. Moreover, these side effects become more prominent when the subjects focus attention on them.[3] A technical term for this is *introspective sensitization.*

The side effects of meditation tend to stop when each meditative period is shortened, and will fade when meditation is practiced regularly over a period of months to years. Their basic cause stems from no specific psychodynamic correlates. Recalling that even the Buddha took over six years of practice to become fully enlightened, one comes to appreciate the long-range Zen view: these early "by-products," termed *makyo* in Japanese, are of no consequence. One observes them, accepts them, and finds that they drop off by themselves.

Among the Americans in Andrew Greeley's survey who did have a mystical experience, 14 percent acknowledged "a sense that I was being bathed in light."[4] Greeley emphasized that the colors were a pale "diffused blue or rose." I regularly experience a *central* haze of blue-pink when engaging in open-eyed meditation in subdued light. This phenomenon occurs when I am sliding into that early stage associated with peaceful relaxation and with thoughts dropping off. Later, the dark lines of a pattern on the wall or floor may become more blue, while rose colors develop in the larger intervening spaces. Later still, yellow-green and contrasting blue-purple colors may enter as highlights which further enhance the texture of a surface. These phenomena serve only to remind one that, during successive meditative levels, many pathways in the large visual brain are interacting with retinal signals in ways that reorganize the usual flow of impulses.

Olfactory hallucinations are as rare as visual ones are common. Dogen's Chinese teacher told him that if he had practiced zazen long and continuously, he would finally "perceive a sweet, exquisite fragrance which has no equal in the ordinary world."[5] However, monks were exposed to very intense and stressful training methods in those early days. One notes that this same master had also advised Dogen to practice zazen as zealously as though you were "putting out a fire on the top of your head."

Intensive meditative concentration for weeks or months invariably yields visual or auditory aberrations, hallucinations, or unusual somatic experiences. Again, in the Theravada Buddhist tradition, these are regarded not as signs of a serious psychic disorder, but as the "normal perceptual changes happening in predominantly healthy individuals" who embark on the rigorous training of mindfulness.[6]

In the study cited above, involuntary jerks or pulling forces were most commonly observed. Sensations could drop off from the hands or from the body. Visual perceptions were often enhanced with the eyes open, and this sometimes coincided with episodes of heightened concentration or with states of rapture. If the eyes were *closed*, there might occur flashes of light, or very bright lights. Many meditators reported dramatic swings in mood between intense emotions of anger, fear, sadness, and joy. A blissful experience of some kind occurred in 40 percent of those meditators who had meditated for only two weeks, and in almost all subjects who underwent three months of training. These blissful moments were associated with mental concentration, with periods of no pain or of reduced body pain, with lightness of the body and unconstricted breathing.

During the three-month meditative retreat, the hours spent sleeping dropped some 25 percent, and food consumption fell by one third. The meditators' sense of general awareness increased both before, during, and immediately after sleep. They commonly experienced vivid dreams and even nightmares.[6]

What causes nightmares? During childhood, these distressing sleep terrors occur during the early phase of *synchronized* sleep. Both the basolateral amygdala and the ventromedial hypothalamus convey strong emotional potentials. So it is noteworthy that cells in these two sites are among the exceptional few which do fire faster in S-sleep.[7] On the other hand, D-sleep is the time when we adults have our ordinary "bad dreams." At this particular time, the hippocampal part of the limbic system is metabolically more active.[8]

John Burroughs would characterize many contemporary retreats as "adverse" situations. Meditators trained in psychology have described their own retreat experiences in ways that convey their emotional flavor.[9–11] Reputable organizations screen their candidates both medically and psychologically, for good reason. Even so, a few meditators who pursue ill-advised practices then go on to develop substantial psychiatric complications. These include anxiety, depression, suicidal attempts, schizophrenic reactions, and other psychotic episodes.[12] How often do these problems arise?

In one survey of over 890 persons on the transcendental meditation mailing list, most respondents (52–64 percent) reported no major complications. However, TM teacher-trainees who had practiced for almost four years reported more problems: antisocial behavior (14 percent), frustration (10 percent), and restlessness (10 percent), as well as anxiety, confusion, depression, and procrastination (all 9 percent). Otis concluded that TM was not innocuous, and that patients experienced more adverse effects if they already had psychiatric disorders.[13] Deikman adds that the mystical path is no substitute for psychotherapy, or vice versa.[14]

Most meditators confront other, more specific, difficulties. They need to work through such problems as: "submergence," distraction, excitement, dullness, and "sinking." "Submergence" is a shallow, temporary, untroubled emptiness. It comes from getting too wrapped up in meditative states. It includes some degrees of happiness, clarity, and energy, but it is not to be confused with awakening.[15] "Sinking" involves difficulty grasping and remembering the object of meditation.[16] Meditators are also bothered by their glacially slow rate of progress and by their fixation on inner thoughts, feelings, and sensations. They develop strong transference reactions to their teachers, complicated by childhood difficulties in developing appropriate relationships with other key interpersonal figures.[17] Those meditators whose sense of self is already the least cohesive and integrated may find it difficult to detach from what self they already have.

Positive spiritual experiences do not always occur. Indeed, for some meditators, the long-delayed "awakening" is a profound "bleak experience." Reports of such negative, dysphoric states seem more common if their meditation has not taken place within an authentic, supportive context. An additional set of fears can arise at still deeper levels of practice. These fears seem to be prompted by a loss of sleep, and they coincide with concerns about the loss of the egocentric self.

Meditators do not make linear "progress" on their path. Those naive beginners who cling to unrealistic expectations are prone to become disillusioned. No student realizes how many hours must be devoted to meditative practices each day, how many years it will take to effect long-range spiritual growth, and what kinds of unusual sensate, emotional, and other psychological experiences must be worked through in the interim. Our plan in part V is to provide instructive examples of such unusual events, many of which are drawn from personal experience.[18]

It is no accident that these episodes, next to be described, will also serve to illustrate various aspects of the same kinds of functional anatomy which have just been discussed in parts III and IV. Then why call them "quickenings"? Not merely for lack of a better term. For in women of childbearing age, quickening signals the presence of a moving fetus, of a biological process which may, or may not, go on to the birth of a viable, full-term infant. Makyo events are also preliminary signals. Yes, at first glance, they might seem to be trivial stirrings. But we are not going to disregard them. For us, their overall message is also pregnant with physiological significance. Because vital and interesting processes are going on. And by using their clues as probes, the mechanisms underlying makyo are going to help us understand both Zen and the brain.

85

The Light

> The light shined in darkness; and the darkness comprehended it not.
>
> John 1:5

> Bright light bathes me on all sides, intense as the midday sun. Its dazzling brightness extends far behind my head and upper back. Instantly I am wide awake. Lying quietly, with eyelids still closed, I quickly run through the possibilities.
>
> Much too bright for the bedroom light, or for a flashlight. Not a white beach in the sunshine in a dream. I'm wide awake, very clear about the time and place. Clear about the fact that something is happening to me. This feels like the middle of the night, and I know that I have just been sleeping soundly in bed, and am lying on my right side.
>
> Only this all-pervading light. Nothing else accompanies it. No other sensate elements or loving affect. No extra quietness in the background. The light lasts perhaps only three or four seconds, then subsides over another two seconds or so. I remain wide-awake, without fear, wondering: What is going on?

I am still wondering. We do know that prior darkness causes a huge increase in the sensitivity of the visual system. When the retina adapts to the dark, for example, it increases its sensitivity to light up to ten thousand times. But this was no process limited to the retina. For the light enveloped a wide volume *behind me.* This fact suggests that the enveloping light arose farther on in the interior of the brain. Here it could soon engage some of the same visual coordinates which represent my basic matrix of three-dimensional space. Chapters 114, 115, and 116 of part VI will be explaining the nature of this process in greater detail.

My awakening was smooth in onset, without startle, and it was not provoked by any obvious trace of a remembered dream. During normal slow-wave sleep, the relay cells in the lateral geniculate nucleus slow their firing rate. Then, later, S-sleep begins to lighten. At this particular moment—just as it starts to ascend toward D-sleep—the lateral geniculate cells discharge, stimulated by acetylcholine cells down in the brain stem. So a plausible explanation for the light is a sudden surge in firing. First, it causes an excessive degree of visual transmission. Then, as it spreads farther, it generates a sense of "envelopment."

Moreover, the bright light was diffuse. It contained no individual lights, nor did it go on to develop any formed hallucinations. These observations also suggest that some of the impulses may have originated in the lateral geniculate nucleus, or near it, and then gained access to their usual visual relays farther back in the superior colliculus and beyond (see chapter 54).

86

Bright Lights and Blank Vision

Wisdom excels folly, as far as light excels darkness.

Ecclesiastes 2:13

Many persons have had similar, striking experiences of being enveloped by a blinding light. Brighter than sunshine, it comes from all sides. Sometimes it emanates from a diffuse source directly in front. It is less well appreciated that such a light may occur as an isolated, entirely independent phenomenon, and take the form of a fragment as in the event just described. If asleep, the person wakes with the impression that an intense light has just been turned on in the darkened room.

Of course, this same "seeing the light" can also be included—as an early sensory event— in a sequence with several others, in a much more complex mystical experience. In such an instance the light remains a literal *sensate* fact in itself. It is not a loose metaphor. It does not allude to the way the person is "illuminated" *mentally* by a new insight which may have flashed in shortly thereafter.

Once impulses have passed back beyond the retina, many central factors decide what we then "see" when these messages enter into the rest of our visual experience. Even sites as low as the brain stem can contribute to what we perceive visually. This was discovered during operations on the human brain. At these times the outer surface of the brain stem was stimulated at locations extending from the superior colliculus as high up as the pulvinar (see figures 3 and 11). On a *few* occasions, these stimuli yielded a "positive" sensation of "light." The patient perceived this light on the side opposite the stimulus, or saw it in the fields of vision on both sides.[1]

Our visual brain covers a very large territory. When, and how, do impulses which gain access to its diverse parts give rise to seeing a bright light? The basic fact, of course, is that many more visual impulses relay through the lateral geniculate nucleus *when the brain is in transition to its desynchronized states* (see chapter 71). And this happens whether these activated states surge up as part of waking itself, or as interruptions inserted during sleep or moments of drowsiness.[23] Moreover, these brief moments of drowsiness are especially prone to enhance visual transmission if, at the same time, the midbrain reticular formation is then stimulated.[4]

What could initiate such a light? The stimulus path arising from inside the parabrachial nucleus is direct, and it quickly excites both the lateral geniculate, the pulvinar, and other thalamic nuclei.[5] Moreover, this direct acetylcholine pathway instantly activates nicotinic ACH receptors. Next comes the second wave of ACH effects. Now, ACH is acting on its nearby muscarinic receptors.[6] Their actions prolong a positive visual excitatory response, perhaps for as long as 21 seconds[7] (see chapter 38). Still other mechanisms will enhance the flow of visual impulses by acting *in*directly. For example, those which inhibit the reticular nucleus of the thalamus.

Suppose you stimulate two other sites at the same time: the posterior hypothalamus *and* the lateral geniculate nucleus. Now the visual cortex itself becomes much more responsive.[8] It seems likely that a person could further amplify the experience of seeing positive visual phenomena by enlisting parts of the hypothalamus into higher levels of arousal.

On the other hand, patients *usually* experience "negative" phenomena when the outside of their brain stem is being stimulated.[1] This means that they can't see *anything* on the side opposite the stimulus.[1] And even normal experimental subjects are surprised to discover that their vision can blank out briefly. In this instance, the technique used bears a resemblance to open-eyed meditation. It involves looking continuously at a homogeneous visual field, and adapting to it during low illumination (the *ganzfeld*).[9] But these normal subjects draw a distinction between this blank vision and *black* vision. True, their *sense of vision* may have disappeared. But in fact, they do not go on to experience a dark *black* field. Instead, they say: "I feel blind. I'm not even seeing blackness. This differs from the black when lights are out."[9]

By way of beginning to explain such a symptom, one inhibitory loop does descend from the occipital cortex which inhibits lateral geniculate nerve cells.[10] And the subjects who look at something for a very long time might tap into inhibitory circuits of this general kind. It is of incidental interest that alpha EEG activity briefly increases both when a person stabilizes an image on the retina and when vision "blanks out" while looking into the ganzfeld.[11]

On all other normal occasions, we assume that when we "look" at something we're actually going to "see" it. However, certain patients "look," but can't "see." Suddenly, the scene vanishes in front of them, even while they are normally fixing their gaze on its contents. What kind of process could uncouple their motor act of fixation from their conscious visual awareness? This peculiar "negative" symptom is caused by dysfunction of the upper part of the visual association cortex on both sides[12] (see figure 2).

When we close our eyes in the dark, it is not absolute blackness that we see. Rather, it is what William James aptly called "a dark visual field in which a curdling play of obscurest luminosity is always going on."[13] Why? Even when no light enters our eye, our retinal nerve cells still stay "awake."[14] Many retinal cells keep firing actively and spontaneously. And some will discharge more, even in total darkness.[15]

Meditation sponsors many kinds of positive, negative, and complementary visual phenomena. The following two simple examples illustrate the point.

> I am sitting in zazen. A small oval hazel-gray area appears. It is no bigger than the eraser on a pencil held out at arm's length. It occupies a light spot in the right lower quadrant of the visual field of my right eye only.[16] Indeed, at first, it is *lighter* than the wall in the background. But several seconds later, it transforms itself. Now it becomes even *darker* than the background in the dim room. It stays the same size and shape. After perhaps five seconds, this dark black oval itself fades away.

Perhaps what produced the initial lighter, "positive" visual image was a small zone of excitation in the retina of the right eye. Then, a few seconds later, this same region was suppressed, inhibited, blacked out. This sequence, local excitation → inhibition, occupies but a few seconds. It is a noteworthy phenomenon, typical of the many other circuitries we have described throughout the rest of our visual system. For such circutries are poised to surround and to invade with their dark zone of inhibition whichever item may have become overemphasized in the perceptual center.

> I am meditating in a relaxed but alert manner, with eyes open in dim light. After ten to fifteen minutes or so, the usual prelude of central bluish-pink colors yields to a play of their *complementary* colors: green, yellow, orange. Clearly, meditation must be influencing color vision as well. How? Where?

Goethe, who painted as a hobby, once pointed out that a colored object soon elicits its complementary color. Blue calls forth orange, purple reaches for yellow, green follows red, and vice versa. And Newton, watching his prism, observed how it split ordinary white light into several components: separate wavelengths which yielded red, green, and blue. Even when the meditator is in a dimly lighted room, these same faint light waves will still be stimulating the retina. And then, as the meditator adapts to darkness during the first fifteen minutes, which color-coded cones will become the most sensitive? Those cones sensitive to *red* wavelengths. Moreover, even the light-sensitive rods become more sensitive to *blue* during the first thirty-five minutes that they are exposed to darkness.[17] So, as the signals from these cones and rods start out from the retina on their long journey of transformation in the brain, the meditator's shades of red and blue may someday begin to yield some simpler explanations of colors to physiologists who specialize in color perception.[18] This hypothesis is testable.

87

Faces in the Fire: Illusions and Hallucinations

> The electrical stimulation can call back a sequence of past experience . . . a previous experience—its sights and sounds and thoughts—seems to pass through the mind of the patient on the operating table . . . he re-experiences some period from his past while still retaining his hold on the present . . . The re-experience seems to be more real, the voices heard are more acute, and the objects or people seen are more vivid than when the event actually happened.
>
> L. Roberts[1]

Hughlings Jackson believed one image was as valid as any other. They were "real," whether we "saw" the image in our normal perceptions, in a dream, in an illusion, or in a hallucination. He added that we all share a common visual illusion: we see "faces in the fire." When we look at burning embers, he said, we find that they do more than generate exact images of themselves. Soon, the flames "produce faces in us."[2] Jackson believed such imageries were the expressions of release phenomena. Back in 1879 he stated, "I believe all *elaborate* positive states occur from, or arise during, an increased energizing of centres permitted by removal of control of higher centres."[3]

Like a Zen master, Jackson was well aware of the subject/object distinction. He knew that the moment we set up this self/other boundary we created two categories of consciousness. So he applied the capitalized term, "Subject Consciousness," to those occasions when we were aware of *our self* throughout all of its extensions. And his "Object Consciousness" referred to that awareness which perceived *other things*, those in our outside environment.

He provided the following sentence as an example: "I see a brick." In this instance, subject consciousness was in every aspect concerned with the "I." Object consciousness was symbolized by the "brick" *alone*. Jackson concluded that seeing faces in the fire meant that we had relaxed our usual level of outer-directed, objective consciousness and had shifted into our own subjectivities. Jackson's intuitions are a useful starting point. They make it possible to place into one neat subjective category all of our self-generated daydreaming imageries, as well as the phantasies driven by our fired-up imagination. After this distinction is established, there remains the other *selfless* category—that of *Object Consciousness*. Later we will find that its objective vision turns out to be the essence of *insight-wisdom* (see chapter 138).

The face we see in the fire is a visual *illusion*. An illusion is a misperception which begins with some natural stimulus. We not only inhabit a world of sensory illusions. We actively create it. There is no denying the fact that, after the train comes to a stop, those trees outside still convey the illusion of movement. The illusion is just as compelling even when we neurologize it and attribute it to some vestibular connections which keep our eyes moving. The moving trees are convincing evidence that mechanisms rising from the brain stem can influence what we perceive.

Sensory illusions can harden into mental sets. Suppose, for example, you had lived all your early life simply taking one fairly obvious perception at face value: every glass rod bends at an angle just as it passes beneath the surface of water. If so, you now might harbor a very strange notion: water bends glass. Or you might even think that all glass rods are bent. Each is a false belief, a *delusion*. But they are testable.

One can quickly dispel each delusion by a simple direct experiment. Withdraw the rod from the interface between its dual environments, air and water. Now one sees the way things really are: a simple glass rod in all its clear straightness. The rod distorts only when its world is divided into two phases.

Of course, differences in the refraction of light are the physical basis for this illusion. But could we ourselves inhabit similar dual worlds? Don't they start as soon as we create our own self/other opposites? For, unsuspectingly, we have gone on to construct whole lifetimes filled with other distortions. Yet these, too, can finally vanish. As soon as that *one-phase world* of enlightenment opens up, a totally objective consciousness prevails.

Our ordinary visual illusions have an either/or aspect. Consider the familiar illustrations. One is the picture which shows a standard figure-ground illusion. Looking at it, we'll see either the two curves of the white vase in the center, or the two dark facial profiles facing inward. Another illusion arises from the Necker cube, where the lines of the cube are so drawn that it seems to have edges in three dimensions. The cube flips, first one way, then the other. Each mental set is separate, irreconcilable. The pictures themselves remain the same. It is *we* who can't transcend sets. We're the ones who can't see *both* possibilities at the same time.

Hallucinations

Hallucinations are something else: strange sensate perceptions that occur even though no appropriate external stimulus is present. The origins of the word "hallucination" imply a wandering in the mind.[4] After you recover from an hallucination, it is hard to shake the notion that your mind must have indeed wandered very far off in the wrong direction. Accordingly, many investigators chose to describe such events using benign terms. The terms are "visual imagery,"[5] "visions,"[6] "aesthetic images," or "eidetic images."[7]

Here, we use the term *hallucination* to describe any unusual sensate experience that develops outside dreams and which is unexplained by any natural peripheral stimulus. This means we regard as hallucinations one class of vivid, internally generated imagery which arises at certain special times in the sleep cycle. One of its varieties rides on the leading edge of sleep. It occurs during a person's first *descent* from the waking state toward the sleeping state. These hallucinations are called *hypnagogic*.[8] They are usually positioned between the first drowsy period and the first transition period of the night.

Hypnagogic hallucinations, both visual and auditory, are not abnormal. They are highly instructive. Indeed, they help us understand the mechanisms of internal absorptions (see chapter 113). Nor are they rare. In one survey based on young Finnish military recruits, 14 percent (of 2537 subjects) reported having had them.[9]

Hypnagogic visual hallucinations are *not* dreams. They occur *before* the first dreams. We begin to insert dreams somewhere between our initial transitional period and light sleep itself.[10,11] Moreover, these early hallucinatory events start quickly, and tend to remain stationary. What makes them more vivid than dreams? First, they are *highly colored and etched with enhanced textural details*. Second, these hallucinations arrive at a particular time. They occur when there is "a relatively large degree of awareness."[12] Finally, they also invite a strong aesthetic response (table 14).[12,13]

Hypnagogic visual hallucinations have other features of note. They elicit detached observation, not active participation. The images usually enter when the eyes are closed, but may be experienced with the eyes open. Some kind of separate thought stream tends to continue, and ordinary perceptions may still go on. These several lines of evidence convince the subjects that they are very wide awake during the hallucination.

The hallucinated images arrive full-blown at onset. No gap intervenes between their arrival and their being broadly characterized and identified. As Sartre noted, "suddenly knowledge appears, as vivid as a sensory manifestation: one becomes aware of *being in the act* of seeing a face."[14] Yet if a whole face is seen, it is *not usually recognizable* as a specific person at that particular moment. This suggests

Table 14
Hallucinations and Dream Imagery during Sleep Transition States

Aspect	Hallucinations during Drowsy Periods (Hypnagogic/Hypnopompic)	Imagery during S-Sleep	Imagery during D-Sleep
Usually vivid	5	1	1–2
Image moves	0–1	3	4
Intense colors	5	1	3
Enhanced textures, contours, details	5	0	1–2
Involuntary; not subject to control	5	4	3
Quick onset and offset	5	2	2
Strong aesthetic response	5	0	1
Invite interested observation, not participation	5	1	0–1
Smooth, organized narrative flow	0	2	4
Strong affective response	0–1	1	2
Quick "snapshot" quality	5	1	1

0 = none; 5 = maximal

that the subject is also experiencing some difficulty in recognition memory (as is described in chapter 109). Yet at other times, the subject can easily sense that the source of the hypnagogic hallucination is some specific visual incident in past experience. But many hallucinations still remain impersonal, and are difficult to account for. Some are interestingly foreign, others alarmingly so.[13] The more detached the observer, the more evident it becomes that the images are "not real" but hallucinatory in nature.

Some of the initial hypnagogic events skip along at a much faster pace than do the moments they appear to represent. How do the events condense time? One way is by omitting visual continuity. This speeds up the visual imagery. So much so that it then becomes "something more like a succession of snapshots than like a movie" (see chapter 90). In contrast, during an ordinary REM dream the action unfolds at about the same pace as it actually does during waking hours. Moreover the visual content of the earlier hypnagogic periods seems more like a brief "dreamlet."[15] It lacks the well-developed plot that occurs during longer REM periods.

Normal persons have been studied who were having hypnagogic visual hallucinations during their first drowsy period before sleep. Their EEGs tended to show a reduced amplitude of alpha waves or slower frequencies, or both, nearing the theta range. When the hallucinations began, the subjects were relatively less aware of their surroundings, even though their EEG might have changed very little.[14,16] The fast roving eye movements (so typical of REM dreams) did not occur, and EMG activity was reduced only slightly in the forehead muscles.

Mechanisms of Hallucinations

It is essential to appreciate that meditators experience several kinds of visual hallucinations, and for different reasons (see table 14). Many images are fully consistent with hypnagogic hallucinations. During long periods of zazen, meditators slide in and out of that drowsy—but dynamic—transitional zone. Now one understands the basis for the old Zen caveat: stay erect and keep your eyes open. Accordingly, those meditators who can hold an erect posture and keep their eyes open do find it easier to maintain a higher level of arousal and to avoid nodding off into sleep. The Zen caveat is confirmed in studies of narcoleptic patients whose task is to sit on a stool. Despite their heavy sleep pressure, this precarious position stops the patients' strong tendency to drop into sleep-onset REM periods.[17] But even while sitting on a stool, some narcoleptic patients still enter brief, "micro-REM" episodes or show lapses in body tone when they become drowsy.

No study both accurately describes in graphic detail the full content of hypnagogic hallucinations while also correlating them with contemporary polygraphic measurements.[12] When meditators are doubly monitored in this manner in the future, it will then be possible to specify which hallucination occurred during that interval when they were "descending" from waking (hypnagogic), and which arose during that other interval when they were "ascending" from sleep toward waking consciousness. Following convention, this latter *ascending* variety has been given another term, *hypnopompic*.[18]

Now, it is not difficult to assign the term *hypnagogic* to an hallucination which occurs on the leading edge of sleep when the person is *first* dropping off into a long sleep at night. Nor is it difficult to reserve the word *hypnopompic* for those episodes that enter many hours later when the person is finally starting to wake up the next morning. But what about similar hallucinations that occur *on either edge* of a brief nap? Short naps can blur the distinction between the leading edge and the trailing edge, posing semantic problems. Does it matter?

Yes, because more than wordplay is involved. Suppose that an extraordinary degree of awareness were to thrust up at a time when most functions of the sleep cycle were already starting their descending phase; that this surge entered at a time during the *first* part of the night when you might assume that only a "descending" (hypnagogic) hallucination would occur; and that at this point, much of the brain then reversed course and the person became especially wide-awake. Chapter 108 provides a personal example of such a "nocturnal" hallucination. And at first you might be led to think—from its "bedtime" position alone—that it had entered on the way "down" near the first period of sleep. But the other details of the experience are critical. They suggest that this subject was actually on his way "up," and starting into an extraordinary episode of wakeful hyperawareness (see figure 17).

Human beings pursue alluring visions. The vision quest is an age-old phenomenon. Contemporary religions are more skeptical. Conservative mysticism shuns spectaculars, including hallucinated apparitions. Indeed, the Christian mystical tradition holds that if you have seen God clearly you have not really seen God.[19] Buddhist injunctions against seeing Buddha are even more emphatic.

Herein, hallucinations, locutions, and ecstasies will be viewed as phenomena suggesting only that parts of the brain are in an excitable, quickened state.

Which parts? Where do hallucinations come from? Stimulating the temporal lobe electrically can evoke visual hallucinations.[1] It may be that some patients are more vulnerable to hallucinations if their brains have already been affected for years by epileptic seizures or chronic schizophrenic disorders.[20–24] In Penfield's pioneering studies, stimuli delivered to cortical sites over the *right* temporal lobe had a visual bias. They tended to evoke mostly *visual* hallucinations or visual-experiential phenomena.[21] In contrast, the patients showed no tendency to lateralize other flashbacks of prior experience which contained visual imagery, *or* auditory imagery, or combinations of the two. Their temporal cortex on *both* sides gave rise, about equally, to these flashback mixtures. Penfield concluded that "The evoked experiential response is a random reproduction of whatever composed the stream of consciousness during some interval of the patient's past waking life."

Even then, his patients reported rather few experiential flashbacks: only forty were reported in his series of 1132 patients. In one other series, less than 1 percent of the brain stimulations evoked either a visual hallucination or a vivid visual thought image.[23] When stimulation does evoke a patient's visual hallucination, the image takes on a definite, formed shape. Only occasionally is this hallucination projected out into the space of the actual external world.[22] Precisely when are these evoked images projected into awareness? Usually *after* the initial electrical stimulus to the cortex itself has stopped. At this particular moment an ongoing deeper afterdischarge is actively going on in the posterior hippocampus or amygdala. By the time another three or four minutes have elapsed, the patients have forgotten many details of their recent complex evoked hallucination.[22] (This is in keeping with the kinds of disruption that a very artificial stimulus causes when its impulses spread to disorganize deeper sites.)

An evoked hallucination is indeed a "random reproduction." Many never repeat themselves, despite the fact that a second stimulus through the same electrode has later excited the very same spot. Moreover, a given experience can first be evoked electrically, and then recur later as a spontaneous hallucination, *even after the stimulation site which had first yielded it from the medial temporal lobe had already been surgically removed.*[24] This observation tells us that an "experience" is widely distributed. How, then, does the stimulation act? It seems to evoke the experience by tapping into its large network at one of several potential sites, and by doing so *at one particularly responsive moment.* Even then, each experience has been undergoing a substantial editing. Consider this singular fact: *only one previous experience has been selected to take place at any one moment,* whereas the electrical stimulus must have been passing across the links of many other potential memory circuits.[21]

Where do the subjects perceive their visual hallucinations? In the *opposite* half-field of vision. That is, if the local electrical stimulus prompts one region to discharge on the right side of the brain, the patient's hallucination appears off to the left. Only the simpler, *un*formed hallucinations arise when the brain is stimulated back in the primary visual (occipital) regions. These unformed images consist of abstract, elementary shapes. In contrast, *formed* hallucinations look like real things, like actual birds or inanimate pebbles. Formed hallucinations of this kind arise from sites farther forward, say in the temporo-occipital or other association cortex. Again, they begin more often in the right side of the brain.[25]

Schizophrenic patients show a different tendency. They lateralize their visual hallucinations more in the *right* visual half-field (*if* it happens that their hallucinations are lateralized).[26] And brain mapping techniques confirm this tendency toward a left-sided arousal. They show fast electrical activity at frequencies between 28 and 32 cps, most obviously occurring over the *left* posterior cortex.[27]

Certain other neurological conditions help us understand what causes hallucinations. A few patients develop elaborately detailed, colored, formed visual hallucinations *after* they suffer damage to their primary visual cortex or to the earlier visual pathways.[28] Some items in this hallucinated material are obviously derived from the patients' own past visual experience. The topics include cats, the queen of England, a tree branch, etc.

Following the early lead of Hughlings Jackson, one assumes that such hallucinations represent the release of latent images, generated internally. This interpretation implies that the patients had first registered the original raw visual data back in their primary visual cortex at some earlier time. Then, to account for their complexity, these earlier images would need to have been resynthesized into representations laid down in other circuits many synapses farther on (see chapters 54, 55, and 56). So it is important to note *where* these particular patients later go on to project their long-delayed, *internally* generated hallucinations. They project them into the "blind" visual field. The image—cat or queen—appears in that very same area within which the patients are blind to other visual stimuli entering from the real *outside* world.

How is this possible? How can a brain see "internal" things within a visual field that is blind? The explanation brings us back to the inhibitory processes which normally enable our large visual brain to function (see chapter 54). Think of how distracting it would be if cats, royalty, and tree branches were spinning up, at random, into our ordinary ongoing vision! To avoid this, the brain depends on its array of inhibiting mechanisms (see chapter 86). These normally hold in check those of its more excitable internal memory circuits. Unsuppressed, they would otherwise sponsor images at the slightest encouragement. Especially do these processes of suppression operate when we keep our eyes open and engage our earlier visual pathways. The symptoms of the patients just cited above allow one to arrive at a plausible explanation. For, more than likely, these localized lesions destroyed the patients' normal *inhibitory* functions, not only their "positive" seeing functions. And this deficit of inhibition then released hallucinations which previously had been held in check.

Many persons have been impressed by the vivid quality of their "ether dreams." Why are they so vivid? Again, it is reasonable to postulate that several mechanisms are converging. Some are inhibitory, some *dis*inhibitory, others directly excitatory. Where do *general* anesthetic agents insert the "blockades" that cause anesthesia? One of the target sites for the anaesthetic blockade is the system of widespread wakeful excitations created by glutamate which normally help keep us awake. Much later, as the level of anesthesia begins to lighten, resurgent swings of glutamate transmission then occur. These surging glutamate (and other) excitations are candidates for some of the dramatic alternate state phenomena which anesthetized patients undergo.[29]

Some psychiatric patients are caught in the grip of a major obsessional neurosis. It becomes so unrelenting that they elect to have their anterior cingulate gyrus operated on bilaterally. During the first three days of their postoperative period, while still quite alert, they experience a temporary flood of vivid, clear thoughts and dreamlike mentation. This imagery becomes so vivid that the patients cannot separate fantasy from reality. Each time they close their eyes, their visual and auditory hallucinations intensify.[30] How do the patients escape from being disturbed by their fantasies? The old Zen way. They learn to keep their eyes open. Bodhidharma would have approved (see table 19).

88

Stimulating Human Brains

> There is no convincing evidence that stimulation of any brain region specifically activates or inhibits one and only one motivational system.
>
> E. Valenstein[1]

When a patient's brain is stimulated, the results are less straightforward than might at first appear. True, Penfield's patients developed what he called "experiential" phenomena when he stimulated the outer layers of their temporal lobe cortex. But most of his patients were epileptic. Normal brain is not as responsive. When relatively *normal* brain tissue is stimulated, either rather little happens, or it happens inconsistently.[1] In one large study of 1500 electrical stimulations, euphoria and pleasant feelings occurred only once. These emotions were prompted by stimulating a site deep in the anterior cingulate gyrus.[2]

More recent studies emphasize a point which assumes great importance in Zen. Not what makes a vision vivid, but *what makes a percept "ring?"* What causes it to develop a sense of compelling experiential immediacy? This happens only when the *deep* limbic structures are stimulated directly, or when they are involved in the spread of a seizure discharge.[3] Indeed, many of those direct, immediate qualities we associate with "higher" states of consciousness are probably attributable to physiological events arising well below our neocortex.

In most instances (92%), stimulating *medial* temporal lobe sites produces no gross overt subjective or objective change.[4] A few sites do seem to produce mental phenomena *after* the electrical stimulus itself stops, but only *if* the stimulus has gone on to generate repetitive afterdischarges. In these instances, the experiences are distinctive for *that particular person*. They are not specific for one particular, constant anatomical location. Moreover, the evoked experience hinges on how that person *feels* at *that very moment*.

Suppose the stimulus happens to generate an olfactory hallucination. Will this patient decide that it is a nice smell or a foul smell? Will it seem good or bad? *This judgment call can be shaped in either direction.* What causes it to shift from pleasant to unpleasant and back again? The pivotal issue is the underlying emotional tone of the discussion going on between doctor and patient at that moment. *These emotions are swaying perception.*[4]

Suppose the undersurface of the frontal lobe is stimulated. Here, a few sites do yield relaxing and pleasurable responses. These sites tend to be located deeper and nearer the midline than are those other spots which sponsor negative feelings of anxiety and irritation. Deep stimulations around the hypothalamus cause the most vigorous responses, in either positive or negative directions. And a few stimulations around the midbrain have yielded euphoria. The patients laugh aloud and seem actively to enjoy themselves.[5]

Let us not be confused by all these stimulation studies. Their diverse results help us understand why alternate states of consciousness are so variable. True, as noted earlier, several categories of alternate states do contain reasonably uniform features. However, as William James observed, religious experience occurs in many "varieties" which differ from person to person in many other fine details. Moreover, when one person undergoes several "experiences," either of absorption or kensho, each will differ substantially from the others even in the same general category. Why? To begin with, some of these varieties of religious and mystical experience surely reflect the ways that nature and nurture had combined to give each of us distinctly different brains, which express themselves in our unique personalities. But from then on, we must develop a coherent set of explanations to account for the range of the differences. Some have already been presented (see chapter 77). Others follow shortly (see chapter 105). Put simply, the Jamesian varieties also reflect the *varying circumstances of the seasons and of the moment.*

When the temporal lobe is stimulated briefly, physiological studies reveal that neuronal activity is *depressed* locally, and for the next several *minutes,* as part of the secondary response to this localized excitation. And during these minutes, the patient often shows confusion and impaired thinking. None of these observations support the possibility that a "seizure" of similar kind could be the cause of internal absorption or of kensho. For if seizures were the explanation, then one might expect that *ongoing* memory would also have dropped out at the same time (see chapter 42). And, even if one were to focus solely on the issue of memory alone, then both internal absorption and kensho would still provide us the sharpest possible contrast with the amnesia of a seizure. For during each of these two alternate states, and after them, the experiant's *ongoing* memory processes are hyperacute, and the positive qualities of the experience remain indelibly in memory.

The Ins and Outs of Imagery

That idea of red, which we form in the dark, and that impression which strikes our eyes in sunshine, differ only in degree, not in nature.

David Hume (1711–1776)[1]

Does a cat's tail curve forward or backward? Which is larger, a mouse or a ground squirrel? To answer such questions, we resort to visual imagery. We envision. It *is* internal seeing. Images evolve in our dreams, enrich the matrix of our creative imagination, sometimes enter as hallucinations.[2]

How do we accomplish this remarkable feat? Our answers sound vague. It seems as though a deep projection screen were located inside one's forehead. Researchers venture more formal explanations. They define imagery as a "quasi-pictorial" representation, one which our brain first extracts from its memories and then reconstructs.[1] But exactly how does our "mind's eye" do all this? How does it select what to tune *out* as well as in? These matters are still elusive.

Ordinarily, when we are awake, the images we envision are not stable. Nor are they nearly as vivid as their original counterparts. However, people who show fewer and slower eye movements tend to generate the most vivid images.[13] These findings suggest that *the physiological act of fixing eye movements on a target* while one is concentrating is one other way to enhance the processes that create vivid images (see chapters 87 and 109).

Our right hemisphere seems to be the more "visual." During imagery, blood flow increases, especially in the lower (basal) regions of the temporal lobes, where the flow also tends to shift to the right side.[4] Still, the usual forms of visual imagery do not spring solely from right hemispheric functions.[3] Indeed, our left hemisphere appears to play a more obvious role when special visual discriminations enter into the task of generating images.[5] So once again it seems that both hemispheres are involved in generating simple mental images and in using them. The right side helps to arrange the images in terms of their spatial relationships, while the left adjusts their parts in terms of categories.[6]

Suppose you ask subjects to imagine a cube. Then to position it in space. And finally to rotate it *in relation to space*.[7] Special EEG mapping techniques show that men handle this imaging task in a different way than women do. Men develop more theta and beta activities in their right parietal region. Women develop more theta and faster beta waves in their left hemisphere, yet both hemispheres participate in the task.

"Overlooking" the Obvious

Many campuses have an apocryphal tale about some absent-minded professor. If it is a math professor, he will have become totally absorbed in visually imagining an equation. As a result, he will have walked far past the door of his own mathematics building, and will finally have come to, say, in front of the gym. The easy assumption: the don was simply "distracted." He hadn't paid sufficient attention to all those visual clues that were obviously out in plain sight, if not right under his very nose. Another possibility exists.

Back in 1910, Perky asked his human subjects to generate the image of a banana. While they were describing it, he then placed a facsimile of a banana directly in front of their gaze. The dangling artificial banana was clearly in plain sight. Surprisingly, while Perky's subjects were imaging, they didn't register this facsimile, nor did they identify it. How could anyone overlook a banana?

The "Perky effect" is more than a curious bit of trivia. The effect has since been confirmed and extended far beyond bananas.[8] Indeed, subjects still neglect the external object in front of their line of sight. It doesn't have to be the same item as the one which they are actively imaging. This fact can be demonstrated by asking normal people to revisualize some common item out of memory—a leaf, a glass of orange juice, etc. Now, at this same moment, other actual objects simply *drop out from the scene* in front of them, as do even simple, colored, obvious geometric forms. Clearly, we share, with the professor, an ability to blot out other visual functions while in the act of pulling up images into the mental foreground. This is *an active process of suppression*, not one that merely overlooks an object that has received a slightly lower priority. Imaging *in*, blots *out*.

In separate experiments, a third of normal subjects were able, voluntarily, to alter the visual potentials which strong visual stimuli were evoking in their brains (see chapter 64). How did they accomplish this? By "mentally tuning out" the visual stimulus pattern. They tuned it out either by using some meditative technique or by shifting their concentration elsewhere.[9] Beyond this, a few people are gifted with an incandescent imagination. Schatzman studied one such woman who could hallucinate apparitions at will. Her technique was first to *stop* paying attention to everything around her. She then concentrated her mental processes solely on creating the image of the person she wanted to hallucinate.[10] As might be expected, this act of generating images in the interior of her brain caused no change in the way her retina functioned. That is, her electroretinogram still went on responding normally to each standard visual stimulus—a flashing light coming in to her eye from the *outside*.

But then she concentrated, totally, on trying to project her apparition. (This willful act of intense concentration, itself, is the most critical aspect of the phenomenon.) Again, the same standard visual stimuli from the external light source flashed in through the retinas of her eyes. But, now, at this point, these flashes no longer gave rise to the expected evoked potentials in the *back of her brain*. Why not? Was something occult going on?

No. No bizarre hypotheses. The findings suggest that an active inhibitory process had taken place within her first visual system (see chapter 54; table 5). By now, the reader will have guessed that her intense concentration would have imposed a physiological block somewhere in or behind her lateral geniculate nucleus. And, during such a period of extra-heightened concentration, such an inhibitory barrier could stop the transmission of her light impulses. Now they could not be relayed on to her visual cortex where they would otherwise have shown up as visual evoked potentials. But that wasn't all.

By highly focusing her concentration, she could also stop the transmission of *sound* impulses through her auditory pathway and block the development of her auditory evoked potentials.[11] So this woman's particular talent provides another example of how much can drop out when the reticular nucleus of the thalamus stops impulses from passing into the rest of the human brain, a topic cited in many parts of this book. In her instance, one might speculate that the talent of deliberate *willful* concentration, perhaps by engaging the frontal cortex and basal forebrain, was a major access route which helped close the thalamic sensory gate (see chapter 60). This hypothesis is testable.

At the other extreme are those few persons who are not nearly so talented. These subjects cannot regenerate visual images at will.[12] For example, they are unable to *re*visualize the curves of the numeral six. They are "*re*visually challenged." But their difficulty does not prevent them from visualizing a real 6 when they see it placed before them in the outside world. Or stop them from remembering it for a few seconds.[13] A few chapters farther on, it will become of interest to recall that these same persons, although they *cannot* regenerate visual imagery, do have one advantage over normal subjects: when they take LSD, their visual perceptions remain relatively undisturbed[14] (see chapter 100).

It is one thing for the normal human brain to summon up the image of a specific object and to project it into the mental foreground, whether the image be a red leaf, a banana, or the shops along the plaza in Milan. But how could one's brain develop an internal image comprising vast, empty space? This is quite another matter. And yet some kind of *space* is the implicit setting within which an imagining takes place. We cannot afford to overlook this background of space. And we won't. For the plan is only to defer, until chapter 114, the discussion of its vital properties.

90

The Tachistoscope

Write the things which thou hast seen, and the things which are, and the things which shall be hereafter.

Revelation 1:19

It happens during the final evening sitting in the zendo, around 9 P.M. Very calm, quiet, relaxed; eyes half-open. Abruptly, a run of images starts just below the center of gaze in front of me. Each is a snapshot, seen as if one were flipping through an album of old, faded color prints. It snaps in with a faint, almost physical impact, stays in view for the same fraction of a second as the one before, then vanishes softly. Each frame is a fragment of some actual scene out of the past, clear but not vivid. I am aware that these are actual people and places. Selected at random from separate decades, they fall into no obvious temporal sequence and are linked by no obvious unifying theme. Each snapshot carries instant recognition, but none captures a memorable event. After perhaps ten to fifteen seconds, the slide show stops. There is no other associated change.

What was going on? Normally, our visual system takes a chaotic stream of stimuli and processes it into a series of chunks.[1] Each of its "time windows" lasts a mere 120 milliseconds, or one eighth of a second. Sometimes, drowsiness provides the requisite setting, at which time these memory frames are released and rush into a dynamic transition phase. Then their images flip by as quickly as do those of a tachistoscope.[2] Electrical stimulation of the human temporal lobe cortex also occasionally yields runs of similar images. Moreover, when Albert Heim described his near-death experience of falling off a cliff, he too would compare his images with those "from a film sprung loose in a projector or to the rapid sequence of dream images"[3] (see chapter 104).

No snapshot I projected that evening would pass a test for relevance. No circuits designed for salience would have lingered over such scenes. Each was a most ordinary slice of life. Long-forgotten image chunks had suddenly fallen out, quick-thawed and sliced by some obscure rhythm in the brain, as if from some mammoth, frozen unaccountably in a glacial age past.

No matter. As each frame sprang up, it was already tagged with recognition. Each snapshot was instantly self-explanatory, self-contained, infused with its own intimate déjà vu–like quality. So this tachistoscope had not been totally objective and free of self. Nor, on the other hand, had it arranged its scenes in any obvious sequence. And yet these private snapshots sponsored no other affective response. For, aside from the bare fact of personal recognition, they were witnessed at a mental distance once removed.

Physiological phenomena of great complexity had thrust up into the active interface between wakefulness and sleep. Based on the studies already reviewed (in parts III, IV, and chapter 87), one may speculate about their mechanisms. Suppose first in sequence, many years ago, that visual transmission happened to have been interrupted though the lateral geniculate nucleus. Say that vision was inhibited only for a relatively short period of a half-second or so. Maybe then, the *next chunk* of information would have been transmitted and processed during the secondary *heightened* rebound burst of firing which followed. This might have caused a brief episode to stand out with a high profile in its memory storage site, as might any scene frozen at random by the flash of a stroboscopic light on the stage of an otherwise dark theatre.

In my case, that evening in the zendo, the responsible agency seemed to have been a deeper level of meditation, with a core of awareness still preserved (see chapter 83). No tachistoscopic episode had ever occurred before or since. Moreover, the observations suggest that these hallucinogenic phenomena may represent the kind of release from prior inhibition that Hughlings Jackson had often invoked (see chapter 87). In this particular instance, one can specifically postulate the release of visual memory mechanisms accessed through the temporal lobe (see chapter 42). For each image constituted a facile process of memory recall. It was a process which could silently flip through decades of memories in its card index, and extract a string of random moments that were each instantly interpretable. Similar processes appear to be activated when the temporal lobe is stimulated directly. Clearly, when we understand these film projector–like mechanisms, we will have a better idea of what caused the early visual events in Heim's near-death experience.

The Descent of Charles Darwin: Computer Parallels

> I had, as a very young boy, a strong taste for long solitary walks; but what I thought about I know not. I often became quite absorbed, and once, whilst returning to school on the summit of the old fortifications . . . I walked off and fell to the ground . . . the height was only seven or eight feet. Nevertheless, the number of thoughts which passed through my mind during this very short, but sudden and wholly unexpected fall, was astonishing, and seemed hardly compatible with what physiologists have, I believe, proved about each thought requiring quite an appreciable amount of time.
>
> Charles Darwin (1809–1882)[1]

In these words did Charles Darwin later recall his boyhood fall. Since then, many other persons who survived much longer falls have also described extra-fast mental processing. The mental flood takes place in the first second or two. This is long before the body's adrenal glands could release amines which might secondarily speed up the brain. Moreover, some situations happen so quickly that they preempt fear. "I didn't have time to be afraid" is a common afterthought.

But each passing second further stimulates the intrinsic stress responses of the survivor's brain. Then, sometimes—and only after an ensuing delay of many seconds—do alternate state experiences occur. Several of these later phenomena carry the stamp of a profound personal and universal portent, and we will shortly be considering them under the heading of "near-death" experiences. Here, we begin by focusing on what happens when the brain *first* senses a yawning abyss. At this early instant, the person's experience still retains its clear "near-*life*" quality, not some near-death one. In these early milliseconds, the brain markedly sharpens and speeds up its perceptions and recall. The fact that mentation shifts into high gear during this first second or so has an important implication. It suggests that fast-acting neurotransmitters intrinsic to the brain are starting to flood their receptors.

Some patients with chronic neurological diseases may show the opposite trend. For example, a few patients who have Parkinson's disease continually think slowly. In these instances, the name *bradyphrenia* is given to their chronically slow rate of cognitive processing.[2] To describe Darwin's acute burst of extra-fast mentation the term *tachyphrenia* suggests itself.

Darwin, born in 1809, lived until 1882. So his boyhood fall could have taken place in the second decade of the last century. His autobiography was not written until much later, and was signed in 1876. His quoted remarks reflected the fact that in those early years pioneer physiologists had few hard facts about how fast thoughts could arise. But anyone in any century could share Darwin's astonishment. How *could* so many thoughts take place so quickly? When human brains become too amazed by their awesome processing capabilities, they may drift toward supernatural explanations. Our task here is to develop only conventional explanations for the scope of such fast processing.

One can agree with Darwin that vast amounts of information do flow during such remarkable states. So let us begin by considering a mildly preposterous analogy. We turn first to the events which proceed at their usual pace through the brain's synapses during our ordinary relatively slow thinking. We then propose to regard them as akin to the usual streams of traffic in downtown Manhattan. Both are stop and go, more linear than one would like. Despite attempts to synchronize traffic signals, the flow of traffic is still sluggish and disorderly. Jams occur, especially at rush hour.

But now envision that a switch has been thrown. An overall master plan has come into operation. Feedback comes in from sensors on every street. They monitor and help synchronize the timing of every light in relation to each car, bike, and pedestrian. Traffic flow is now liberated, reaching peak efficiency in all directions. The air becomes transparent, clear of smog, free from the angry honks of frustrated drivers. After years of being harassed by gridlock conditions, cynical taxi drivers will scoff. How could such utopia occur in New York City?

In fact, a European consortium has already pulled together most of the requisite technical details. The result is a huge seven-year project, appropriately named Prometheus.[3] If a similar program were to be assembled in our largest cities, and *working*, we could surely breathe a prayer of thanks. But could we insist that some divine intervention had been the miraculous agency which alone could have loosened our bonds?

Parallel Operations in Brains and Computers

Only a few years ago, ordinary computers also crept along slowly. Constrained by the limitations of only a single central processing unit, they were obliged to solve problems in serial fashion, one step at a time. But soon, our daily papers described a "fast" computer. What made it special? It deployed many processors in *parallel*. By coordinating them, it could solve, simultaneously, the many smaller parts of a large problem. This gave it a one "megaflop" capability: 1 *million* basic operations per second. Next came a "superfast" computer. Only slightly larger than a breadbox, its 64,000 individual processors conferred a "gigaflop" capability: 1 *billion* basic operations per second. "Teraflop" capabilities will yield 1 *trillion* calculations per second.[4] That's fast!

Is computerized "artificial intelligence" a new development? Yes and no. It turns out that these recent advances occurred only when the experts designed computers which mimic the way, eons ago, ancestral brains had evolved. An essential step, in each instance, was to incorporate processes which made possible a "random access" into larger parallel circuits. At the very instant that young Darwin's brain descended, it may well have tapped into some of these primal ultra-fast, high-capacity circuitries. Nowadays, to describe the way that the brain integrates its many functions, the term "massively parallel distributed processing" has come into vogue.

Indeed, well over a century ago, young Charles Darwin's brain was already a prime example of "biological intelligence." And its remarkable capabilities were so distributed, from top to bottom, that it would never need to feel intimidated by a computer, even if Darwin's thought had somehow been privy to our most recent flip-floppings of artificial intelligence. Darwin might have been intrigued by how many nerve cells one human central nervous system contains. Perhaps it holds as many as 1 trillion neurons, more or less, if one were to round off the more generous estimates.[5] In an era when we count our national debt in the trillions, a trillion nerve cells might seem to be a relatively small number. But it's their *interconnections* that count.

The majority of the nerve cells reside up in our convoluted neocortex. We devote some 85 percent of these cortical cells to our higher *associative functions*. They are cells which have been relieved from the burdensome obligations of having to receive every sensate message *directly* from our eyes, skin, joints, auditory, or vestibular apparatus. Instead, this highest cortex relies on other facile subsystems deeper in the brain to scan this vast information, decode it, repackage bits of it, and send the results up for review. And one can hardly minimize the brain's extensive *subcortical* processing and bridging functions. For these deeper operations, linking both sides of the brain with its central core, assume major importance. Indeed, if the neocortex alone were to contain perhaps 70 percent of all the nerve cells in the entire brain, this would still leave another 300 million other cells at lower levels to sponsor its other vital networking functions.

High up in our cortex, nerve cells are not scattered at random, windblown, as it were. Instead, they band together in tall, vertically organized columns. These plunge down perpendicular to the outer cortical surface. Each columnar unit begins as a slender minicell column, not much wider than a few red blood cells. Yet this unit contains some one hundred to three hundred nerve cells, each carrying on an active conversation in both directions.

At the next level of organization, these individual minicolumns merge into larger processing units, called modular columns. A single large modular column, say one in the visual cortex, could bundle together two hundred or so minicolumns. This modular column, in turn, enters into much larger circuitries, strung together into long loops. We distribute these loops widely throughout our brain, interconnecting many of its cortical and subcortical modules.[6] What good is one individual nerve cell? Its power comes from the ways it is *interconnected* into minicolumns, modular columns, and larger circuitries, looping high and low, right and left.

It follows, then, that there is no "simple" way to account for even our elementary perceptions and memories, or our most routine behaviors. They are the result of many smaller functions drawn together into very large constellations. They cannot be localized to any one lobe. Nor to any single part of the cortex, nor to any other particular spot in the brain. Instead, each represents a dynamic emergent function, expressing the integration of these many widely distributed columnar systems. All our acts are interactions.

Studying these interactions, neuroscientists are increasingly awed by the brain's complex table of organization. Some might be tempted to draw lines connecting a few of the "boxes" which represent its many nuclei. But they will soon run out of "arrows." However, even a glance at our present wiring diagrams does show ample numbers of *parallel connections* to account for Darwin's high rate of processing. Indeed, when one surveys the architecture of the brain's "early warning" functions, one can envision how—in the first milliseconds of compelling urgency—they could shift the brain instantly into brand new configurations.

Parallel distributed processing throughout vast neuronal systems—this is how the human brain evolved its lightning speed, scope, and creative flexibility.[7] What makes this relevant to Zen Buddhism? The sudden enlightenment called *kensho* or *satori* also strikes like a flash of lightning (see chapter 131). Why can't we "think" our way into it? Well, even during our more routine moments—at times when we're processing and translating conventional information at reasonably fast speeds—things are already rushing by so quickly that the rest of our conscious brain can't easily reach in and modify them.[7] So, in a very real sense, when the peak moments of insight-wisdom flash by, they have become totally inaccessible to any of that person's previous patterns of conventional thoughts. These moments are now so far beyond reach as to be "cognitively impenetrable."[7] This very fact contributes to their otherworldly quality.

In the following chapters we begin to clarify several other mechanisms that converge into this unusual kind of processing.

92

Bytes of Memory

> From the beginning, all beings are Buddha.
>
> Master Hakuin, in the *Zazen Wasan*

The *Zazen Wasan* is Hakuin's oft-recited chant in praise of zazen, treasured in the Rinzai tradition. After one has chanted it many times, the verses flow automatically like those of an old familiar Christmas carol. Its first line, quoted above, is a masterful distillation of Zen. It serves to cue the subsequent line, and so on, until the momentum of recall carries you through the closing line of the chant without pausing for thought.

The chant lasts a long minute and a half. It has twenty sentences or so in its English versions, and contains some three hundred words. So, once you have started the first sentence, you might sense a distant glimmering of the one or two lines that will come next in sequence. But ordinarily it is impossible to grasp large, intact portions of the chant. You can't hold these either in thought or in your mind's eye at any one moment.

> Tonight is the weekly formal evening sitting in the zendo, and it is around 9 P.M. After three deep sessions of zazen, I begin Hakuin's chant, totally relaxed, and awake, with eyelids unaccustomably closed. Suddenly, *all verses* in the whole first quarter or so of the chant are THERE, simultaneously. They are in their normal sequence, but not in vision. They are *known* and *heard*. These known-heard verses are in my own voice. It is projected out vaguely in front of me in the form of clearly heard thought-knowledge. I continue to chant and hear myself doing so, line after line at my usual pace. Yet at the same time these other familiar heard-thoughts race far ahead. Effortlessly scanning the later verses, they engulf in one big byte each quartile or so of the remainder of the chant.[1]

All verses are explicit in each of these large bytes. The words are as clear at the end of the byte as when they issue from its beginning. This fast-forward scanning mode skips along quietly. It operates at a mental distance once removed from my actual chanting. Off there, it does not distract from the particular line I happen to be reciting aloud at that same moment.

Something of an *I-Me-Mine* remains. Enough to make two other observations. One is that this recall process operates equally well in fast-forward and fast-reverse modes. Indeed, it is so agile that the faintest mental steering sends it skipping *back and forth*, in either direction. The second is that I register a sense of my own ongoing amazement at this enormous, new flexible expansion of a brain's processing abilities. This facilitated state extends throughout the rest of my chanting. Then it phases off smoothly within the next several seconds.

What was happening? Once again, the quickening occurred shortly after the end of formal sitting meditation, in the evening, around 9 P.M. This time, it highlighted a different category of mental functions. A nimble, superordinate, mode of thought had grasped huge chunks of relevant material. Not visual snapshots this time, but heard-thoughts which issued directly in front of me. How fast was I retrieving auditory memories into that frontal space? I estimated the speed just afterward to have been perhaps five to ten times faster than usual. Moreover, during the episode I also had the impression that my vocal fluency had potentially increased. Had I wished, it felt as though I could have chanted, in my regular spoken voice, perhaps three times faster than usual.[1]

Experientially, the episode was like going along in the old routine act of typing out some well-known text on my old, slow personal computer. And then suddenly becoming aware that a new window had appeared in the middle of the screen. This "thought-window" had opened up into some of the word-processing capacities of a supercomputer. Yet my whole field of consciousness didn't really feel "split." It still seemed normally unified. Instead, two functions, actual chanting and byte processing, were each going on in one awareness. They were proceeding, naturally and independently, in much the same way that a person doodles with pen on paper while still talking and listening on the telephone.

The phenomena invite speculation. It is reasonable to postulate that the subject who is vocalizing a familiar, overlearned chant is using multiple networks, some of them looping deeply. The bytes of memory I recalled were very large and clear. Yet they moved with great agility to and fro. These facts suggest that the prior meditation had uncovered some unusual executive speech functions, and had integrated and amplified them by fast parallel processing.

Sometimes, frontal lobe seizures also begin with a stream of thoughts. The patients describe their new thought stream as "crowding into the mind." This phenomenon is called forced thinking.[2] Could some of my heard-thoughts have been issuing from frontal and subfrontal origins?

The question leads us toward a language disorder recently described. It resembles the *converse* of my experience.[3] The patient had suffered a mild disorder of expressive speech. It was the result of a stroke which involved the dorsolateral aspect of the left frontal lobe. But this mild Broca's aphasia was not the patient's chief problem. His major deficit related to the *sound of words.* He could not scan his verbal memory to find the correct *sound* of a word. It is plausible to consider that my brief experience, similar to the reverse of his, might have been the result of a hyperfluent functioning within similar frontal networks.

If so, their loops were not only retrieving and projecting extra-large chunks of word-thoughts into my field of consciousness. They were also creating the added impression that batches of verse were already poised on the tip of my tongue, ready to be spoken. The average person who speaks in the English language will utter meaningful correct sentences at rates of 140 to 180 words a minute, and will spend as little as 126 milliseconds on each syllable.[4] I speak slowly, but even so the impression remained that this new potential motor capacity could have allowed me to vocalize the entire chant in only thirty seconds or less.

Following this episode, Hakuin's chant became more deeply etched in memory. Ever since, I seem to have moved more easily through it without stumbling or getting lost. And I have never lost something else: my astonishment at having been able to speed through huge bytes of it. To this neurologist, it was a startling illustration of how the brain sometimes amplifies its capacities when one emerges out of meditation.

It's becoming interesting to observe that this kind of extra surge seems more likely to occur around 9 P M The issue of timing, first discussed in chapter 77, is going to come up again in chapter 121.

93

Where Is the Phantom Limb?

> The man whose arm has been amputated, has not merely the perception of pain being seated in that arm, but he has likewise a sense of its position.
>
> Charles Bell (1774–1842)[1]

You and your arm occupy a position in space. You're certain that you both exist there. Why? Because you've laid down a convincing and (almost) indelible sense of your body image. Even after you close your eyes, you still know that your own left arm exists. And you can still go on "feeling" this arm even after all the sensation from it has been blocked by local anesthetic injections, made around the shoulder. Similarly, patients can still "feel" their legs even after their lower spinal cord functions have been blocked by spinal anesthesia.[2]

These observations imply that the spinal cord and higher levels of one's central nervous system have a kind of "memory." They remember the version of one's body with which they have long been familiar. Their creations are called phantoms. Note that phantoms do not depend on sensory impulses continuing to arrive, as usual, from the arm or leg. Therefore, in this respect, they seem almost like a *sustained* somatosensory counterpart of those other brief processes in the visual sphere which might cause a queen or a tree branch to quickly pop into a patient's blind visual field (see chapter 87).

When one arm or one leg is blocked with local anesthesia, as part of a research study, the person's vision is also masked. So these normal subjects can't see where their anesthetized limb really is.[2] Nonetheless, they develop a vivid impression of where it *seems* to be: their phantom limb feels *half-bent*. This semi-flexed posture of the acute phantom limb is that of alert readiness. It is the opening stance of a skier or of a sumo wrestler.[2]

Why do these subjects feel that their phantom limb image is *flexed?* Perhaps the flexed position represents no more than a statistical average of all the previous positions the arm or the leg had been in before. If so, then the semiflexed feeling might be some kind of quick distillate of countless, softwired, older autobiographical memories.

But perhaps the phantom's flexed position dates back to much more ancient times. Perhaps it discloses the presence of an underlying, widely distributed inborn "matrix." An "inherited neural memory." A basic internal standard of reference that was part anatomical, part physiological, and was also capable of being modified by later experience.[3] After all, half-flexion is the optimal position. From half-flexion, you can move quickly into either full flexion or full extension. Perhaps, therefore, half-flexion reflects the ancient postural patterns which natural selection had shaped into our basic hardwired attitude of readiness, almost a kind of "physiological fossil image."[2]

As Bell noted back in 1830, his patients most frequently suffered phantom limb phenomena if they had completely lost an arm or leg. And the amputee's vivid, ongoing illusion—that *this missing limb is still attached*—is so convincing that it can set the stage for delusions. Admiral Horatio Nelson, whose right arm had been amputated after the battle of Tenerife, became so attached to the illusion that he took his persistent phantom arm as compelling evidence that his soul, too, would be eternal in nature.[4] Zen has long emphasized that our delusions also build on illusions. The net result is that vivid complex of notions which compel us to see ourselves in isolation, not as part of the whole.

Certain other neurological patients afford a sharp contrast: they *lose* the normal topography of their physical self, the sense of their bodily I. Of course, to dissolve the physical I on both sides of the body takes a relatively large lesion. It is usually centered around the superior parietal lobule (see figure 2). Damage to this degree disrupts consciousness in too many other major ways to be relevant to our discussion here.

However, still other patients have selective damage, localized to the *right* parietal lobe. This can cause a loss of awareness of the opposite half of their body. In this instance, the disorder of self-topography is called *autotopagnosia*. Moreover, some of these patients go on to vigorously deny that the paralyzed left arm and leg which occupy their bed are their very own, even after they see and touch these deadened limbs.[5]

Their "denial," so called, is not to be understood as merely a kind of superficial negativism. One must realize that underneath it there exists a profound physiological deficit. For these patients have lost their higher-level elaborations upon perception. These lost refinements are in a far category from those other elementary sensations of touch which we would lose if some of our peripheral nerves were simply blocked at a low level by local anesthesia. For, as a result of their right parietal damage, these patients have lost their capacity to image, to reimage, and to imagine one other crucial matter. A subtle skill, which we normals take for granted. Namely, how our own limbs are articulated, and how they act on our behalf, within our personal envelope of left-sided space (see chapter 55).

94

The Feel of Two Hands

How wondrous this, how mysterious!
I carry fuel, I draw water.

Layman P'ang Chu-Shih (740–811)[1]

Let us now expand on this topic of how our elementary sensations are elaborated upon at higher levels in the brain. Take, for instance, the human hand. Its skin is a glove rendered sensitive by some 17,000 touch receptors. Our ordinary consciousness tunes out this vast tactile world. But anyone can coax his or her signals back into awareness. Try running the fingertips of one hand very lightly down along the fingers and palm of your opposite hand. You'll discover a hand you had forgotten was there.

On one occasion, I felt this latent tactile world leap out by itself. It did so, unannounced, in the following manner.

> On an average morning, after 25 minutes of zazen, I will shave and casually rinse my face. Then, eyes closed, rubbing rhythmically with both hands, I'll dry it off with a towel. It's an old routine, overlearned for decades. I am not thinking at the time, nor will I be paying any special attention to the way messages from either hand enter my sensate consciousness.
>
> So at first, nothing about this particular Saturday morning seems different from any other.[2] Around 7:30 A.M., five minutes after zazen ends, I shave, rinse my face in my hands with cold water, pick up a towel, and then start to dry my face as usual. Suddenly, for the first time ever, I *really feel* both hands. Abruptly, during toweling, my tactile sensations are enormously enhanced. Perception increases dramatically on the right hand and shades off around the elbow. On the left, it increases perhaps one-third that much and extends above the wrist. Only the sense of *touch* is enhanced, as it is elicited by the towel in my *hands*. The way the towel feels on contact with my face is the same as usual. I still retain all the usual distinctions between myself as subject and the towel as object. Vision, hearing, and other sensate experiences are unchanged. My hands are as strong as before. No fingers are jerking (as they might if this were some kind of a seizure.)
>
> Astonishing, delicious perception! How much richer this tactile experience is than ordinary feeling! The episode lasts perhaps five to ten seconds, then gradually fades over a second or two.

Never before, or since, has my tactile sense so vastly expanded. For five or ten seconds, I was witness to acute touch perceptions which sober estimation placed as being amplified perhaps fifteen times more than usual. These were perceptions that one usually tunes out. What had released them?

Looking back, the only distinctively unusual event was getting up an hour earlier. I had done so in order to make a train trip to Cambridge later that same morning. The taste of kensho had already occurred in London a long four months earlier. The only other vaguely immediate prelude I could identify was a subtle interval of no-thought while toweling, although this was not unusual. Obviously, the episode of extra feeling in my two hands was intimately related to all the extra tactile input that was already coming in from the rubbing. But how could ordinary rubbing amplify sensate experience so profoundly?

Explanations start with those thousands of tiny specialized touch corpuscles embedded in the skin, each performing its silent, minor miracle. Collectively, they transform—that is, transduce—touch stimuli into nerve impulses. After these impulses from each hand funnel up through the opposite thalamus, they finally reach the opposite somatosensory cortex. This occupies the front part of the parietal lobe (see figure 2).

In case you had ever wondered how neurophysiologists spend their time, it turns out that some researchers study precisely how these incoming sensory impulses change the firing rates of parietal nerve cells. In fact, a few of them remain very down-to-earth about which behaviors they select to study. They have chosen to perform model experiments at the particular times when animals were washing and grooming themselves with their forepaws! Now, these natural washing and grooming movements create a major *excess* of sensate input. And, as one might expect, the normal brain is designed to adjust to this brief sensory overload from the forepaws. Indeed, while the animal grooms, the brain now suppresses its momentary excess of sensory input, and inhibits the sensory cortex some 40 percent.[3]

These same physiologists didn't stop there. They now know, in surprising detail, what happens when the parietal cortex undergoes an increase or a decrease in its excitability. Again, as in the thalamus, the process is called "gating," because it resembles the opening and closing of a sensate gate.[4] And the gate not only closes early, it anticipates events. In fact, we humans have already started to inhibit the parietal sensory cortex which serves our hand region 100 milliseconds *before* we normally move the muscles in our hand. This kind of preparation is only the beginning.

Next, this primary sensory cortex sends major volleys of impulses back into our parietal *association* cortex. Here, in the superior parietal lobule, lie those same neighboring nerve cells described in the last chapter. They will synthesize and elaborate our much higher orders of sensory processing.[5] These neurons also help us perceive both a towel's rough texture and the position of its folds in three-dimensional space. At the same time, our deeper kinesthetic sense is also informing us what positions our own fingers are in as they hold the towel, and how these fingers are moving along with the rest of our arms.

Now it becomes important to note, in this regard, that certain cortical nerve cells here are responding each time these several joints move. Others fire only when the skin is touched. Still other cells have a curious dual property. They are called "joint *and* skin neurons." *They fire only if the elbow is flexed, while at the same time the touch receptors of both the skin of the palm and the forearm are being rubbed.*

Imagine you are at the washbasin. Reflect back on what you do when you wash, rinse, and dry off your face with your hands. Your normal movements duplicate precisely those "special" mundane conditions in the laboratory, the procedures which we now know fire *these particular nerve cells* up in the parietal association cortex.

It might seem a trivial matter to demonstrate that specific paw movements excite certain cells. But this whole line of parietal research has provided us with a highly useful experimental tool. And the results are also going to help us understand quickenings. How? To begin with, a set of further studies of the paw model have amplified our previous working generalization: *the brain excites nerve cells quickly using acetylcholine and glutamate, while also relying on GABA to inhibit them* (see chapters 38 and 45).

Indeed the physiologists observe that when ACH is released in sensory cortex, it speeds up the firing rate of local cells for up to a minute.[6] At first, the added ACH excites both parietal sensory cells *and* their GABA interneurons nearby. This GABA workhorse function tugs on the reins. It gentles excitation, and prevents the sensory receptive field from spreading excessively.[7,8] But once ACH's muscarinic response does gather momentum, its excitation overrides the GABA inhibition. Now what happens to the parietal sensory cells? Each time the paw is touched, they respond *three times* more than before.

Now suppose that all the GABA inhibition had first been removed. This leaves ACH unopposed. At this point, sensate responses become strikingly enhanced. And the enhancement lasts for a very long time—from eight minutes up to an hour.[9] Moreover, the results of adding glutamate are confirmatory. When glutamate is released locally, it also excites quickly. Within seconds it stimulates the sensory cortex into a similar increase in its responsivity. At higher concentrations, glutamate can even take over and drive the cortical firing response.

Usually, we depend on at least two aspects of the forces of excitation and inhibition. We need them to both mesh smoothly and to counterbalance each other. The toweling incident that morning is a model of an exception to the usual rule. It shows how a person undergoes a major perceptual change when these relationships become unstable. A surge of excitation seemed to have bolted through one part of the perceptual field. Inhibition appeared to have slipped out of phase, its reins dragging behind.

The feel of two hands seemed to be more than a mere increase in the quantity of raw touch. My *discriminative* abilities had also increased, especially those in the right hand. The physiologists' findings support this clinical observation. They lead one to expect that toweling movements could amplify those special, topographical discriminative functions farther back in the parietal association cortex. In the next chapter, we describe other mechanisms in the thalamus which could also be contributing to enhanced perception.[10] Moreover, a minor extra pulse of norepinephrine could have participated in the episode (see chapter 44). For when the locus ceruleus is stimulated, its release of NE further enhances the response of the sensory cortex to each touch stimulus delivered to the forepaw.[11]

What I experienced, in both hands, was an awesome sensory overload. It was a degree and kind of feeling almost too much to bear had it *stayed* at this same perceptual level, five to fifteen times higher than usual. But suppose a person's senses were attuned to remain keenly aware of simply living each wondrous moment. Suppose one were continually to live within that same level of awareness as did layman P'ang Chu-Shih. To live at a sage level, to see all life impregnated with salient meaning. Would not this be another matter?

And so this simple clinical and experimental model leads one to wonder: If a person's parietal cortex can overrespond to this degree in the sensate realm, then what happens during a similar brief physiological imbalance—between ACH, glutamate, and GABA—when *other* regions are uncovered?

Earlier chapters have emphasized that, in regions like the frontal and temporal lobes, our repertoire of major insightful and interpretive functions is much wider and richer. When the meditator releases these higher elaborations, what would they contribute to the form and content of the other, extraordinary, experiences on the spiritual path?

95

The Attentive Cat

> Believe in the simple magic of life, in service in the universe, and the meaning of that waiting, that alertness, that "craning of the neck" in creatures, will dawn upon you.
>
> Martin Buber (1878–1965)[1]

The cat lies in wait, alert, by the mouse hole.[2] She *is* Buddha nature, and her nervous system is totally "in service in the universe." More so than she knows, for she is also being studied in the laboratory. There, alert human beings are craning their own necks to watch her. They are researchers. The service they perform for the rest of us is to find out what causes her behavior. In doing so, they can't help but be awed by its inherent magic.

For they are focusing on some localized fourteen-per-second rhythms in her electrocorticogram. These discrete rhythms occur in only two small sites. They are the areas of cortex on each side that refine the primary sensation of her right and left forepaws. Far below, in the thalamus, is the corresponding set of pacemaker cells which drives these two cortical paw regions. This set is also highly localized, being limited in this particular case to the paw region of each ventroposterior nucleus (see figure 11). Here, in the thalamus, the cat has ways to shift either rhythm independently. This means she can enhance the cortical sensory functions of her right paw on one occasion. Or she can shift over to her left paw on another occasion. And here too, she would be able to enhance the *feel of two paws* at the same time. This may begin to sound familiar . . .

Suddenly, a live mouse appears in the hole. The mouse will suffer no harm, because it is enclosed in a transparent shell of clear, hard plastic. As the cat snaps instantly to attention, two more cortical regions now develop a fast rhythm. One of these areas is back in each parietal association cortex.[3] The other lies forward in each motor cortex. It would be easy to overlook the new 36-cps fast wave activity in these latest two sets of excitable cortical regions. Both are very small.

Indeed their surface area, a mere three to ten millimeters square, is comparable with one of those single macrocolumns of cortical cells described four chapters earlier.

Now, the set of thalamic pacemakers which drive the right and left fast rhythms up in the parietal *association* cortex are different from the previous pair. This latest set arises from other cells down in each posterior nuclear group of the thalamus. So they are not the usual sensory relay cells of the thalamus, the ones that will respond directly to an actual light touch on the cat's paw. Instead, they probably export "semisensory" signals from thalamus to cortex. These associational messages might be anticipatory in nature.

Having confessed to neurologizing, let us at least hazard a notion about what kinds of thalamocortical messages the attentive cat is now processing. If *we* were in the same role as that cat when it first began its vigil outside an empty mouse hole, what would we need? We would need to have the capacity to develop extra feeling coming from our two paws. For example, one of our next moves might be to probe for a potential mouse with either paw inside the hole. This would require heightening the cortically refined sense of touch.

Next, if *we* then became as transfixed as was that cat when a real live mouse appeared, it would also be useful to have close at hand, as it were, the *full* behavioral repertoire of our own two paws for their imminent pounce and final clutch.

Note that any "pure" motor programming, by itself, is not going to catch this mouse. Motor functions must be integrated. They must be informed by the total kinesthetic sense of *where—in the envelope of adjacent space—*one's own limbs, trunk, and head are placed in relation to one's target. So to us, Buber's waiting animal serves to demonstrate more than a philosophical issue. This is how the thalamus interacts with the frontoparietal regions when a brain refines its attentive functions[4] (see chapter 62).

Then, once the mouse appears, what makes the cat especially attentive and further increases the fast activity in its cortex? Any measure that enhances the release of dopamine or of acetylcholine up in its cortex.[5,6] In brief, when the brain snaps into a state of intensely focused attention, it will be a complex act paced by the thalamus, further enhanced by DA and ACH, and associated with localized fast cortical EEG rhythms.[7]

Immobility can be deceptive. Hunting dogs go on point, and rabbits freeze, yet their brains remain dynamically active. One can induce an "immobility response" in a rabbit by gently turning it upside down and keeping its limbs motionless for a few seconds. What happens next is *not* a passive state. Yes, this rabbit's muscle tone does soften. However, its eyes become open and fixed, and low voltage fast EEG activity develops in its cortex. Several minutes later, a second phase begins. Now, muscle tone decreases further, the heart rate and breathing rate slow, and the EEG shows high voltage *slow* activity with cortical spindles. Sometimes, this very high amplitude synchronous EEG activity resembles seizure activity, yet no overt clinical seizures occur.[8]

When a rat freezes into its version of this dynamic immobility response, it dampens the *spontaneous* firing of cells up in its sensory cortex. However, these same sensory cells respond much more than before to fresh incoming sensory impulses.[9] This evidence speaks for an enhanced signal- to-noise ratio. The point becomes of interest, because it suggests the possibility (as yet untested) that norepinephrine may be responsible for some of their enhanced response (see chapter 44).

The immobility response of animals resembles—at least superficially— some aspects of the several immobile trance states observed in humans. However, all animal experiments lack a crucial dimension. The question remains, what do we humans *experience* when we enter our extra-emotional or extra-attentive states? True, our quickened moments are qualified; they have an inherently subjective component. But our introspective accounts do yield the vital, and otherwise missing, "facts of personal experience." These data, William James knew, would always be essential.

96

Emotionalized Awareness without Sensate Loss

Seeing is believing, but feeling's the naked truth.

John Ray[1]

It is the seventh and final day of the early winter Rohatsu sesshin.[2] It is 11:30 A.M., and I am standing quietly outdoors, basking in the warm sunshine, waiting in the lunch line, bowl in hand. Abruptly, the sacred quality of all life overcomes me. Tears of gratitude and pure joy well up into my eyes, and my breathing becomes all choked up. Tears flow repeatedly over the next ten minutes, associated with the feeling that all tensions have dissolved. I haven't cried this way since I was a child.

This singular kind of profound knowing is touching sacramental depths. Yet, at the same time, it still has not cut off the physical or psychic core of the personal past. Diminished, but not lost, is my observing self. Even so, I slowly comprehend something during the first minute: this lesser self is an integral part of all the special intrinsic beauty of the whole world.

The experience had three distinctive features. The first two occupied the foreground. First, its sudden onset. Second, the immense power and elemental raw force behind its emotional surge. Third, the softer qualities of its background theme. For at whatever level of amplification it may enter, this theme of a joyous and tearful unification is a memorable event. By itself, it leaves the traveler feeling rinsed and refreshed for the long path ahead. While this level of understanding plumbed depths deeper than those of a mere intellectual idea, it somehow lacked the essential penetrating quality and the otherworldly "feel" of being potentially transforming. That earlier experience of dry-eyed kensho had enabled the subject to appreciate the difference.[3]

Seizures, Religious Experience, and Patterns of Behavior

If any man among you seem to be religious, and bridleth not his tongue, but deceiveth his own heart, this man's religion is in vain.

James 1:26

Some patients can later remember what happened when it started. To them, the aura was the earliest part of their epileptic seizure. They felt this happen just before they lost consciousness.[1] To the physician, the aura is the heralding symptom, the "focal signature." It pinpoints that spot in the brain where the focal discharge begins.

Over a million Americans have recurrent seizures which are caused by a primary source in their brains. Yet it is exceptionally rare for a seizure to *begin* with an aura of profound bliss or ecstasy, a moment which patients might interpret as being of religious significance. Indeed, Gastaut commented that during his lifetime spent studying seizures, he had encountered only "several rare cases of positive auras," and had never yet observed a patient whose aura was ecstasy.[2]

Even so, for many years, it was widely believed that some of Dostoevsky's seizures had begun with an ecstatic aura. These would have arisen, it was inferred, in the temporal lobe. Current opinion now holds that Dostoevsky had primary *generalized* epilepsy.[2] This means that he did *not* have focal seizures starting in one temporal lobe.

The vast medical literature contains few reports of ecstatic seizures, and they are usually incompletely documented. One recent case report in point describes a thirty-year-old man whose seizures began at age thirteen.[3] In these brief episodes he stopped, his consciousness lapsed, and he became inattentive to his external surroundings. Yet during them, his whole being was pervaded by an ineffable sensation of joy. His bliss was so intense and pleasurable that it was like nothing else in reality. His episodes usually struck when he was relaxed or drowsy. The EEG, performed during sleep, showed that his abnormal focal spike activity arose in the right temporal region.

One thirty-two-year-old woman experienced an especially meaningful moment after she had been meditating for nineteen minutes. Now, she felt very close to "the cosmic whole."[4] And at this same time she developed—in her temporal EEG leads only—an unusual kind of slow EEG activity which had an aberrant spike and slow-wave profile. This lasted for fifteen to twenty seconds. It was not possible, for technical reasons, to assign her EEG abnormality to the right, left, or both temporal lobes.

Researchers can record their subjects' EEGs, day and night, using scalp electrodes or deeper leads. These twenty-four-hour–monitored EEGs commonly reveal that seizure patients have lesser, "microseizures." But such "electrical" seizures finish so quickly and remain so localized that most patients never know they are having them. Do these subclinical discharges go on subtly to affect nearby brain regions, or to influence the physiology of more distant circuits? This possibility has raised controversy. The disagreement focuses especially on patients whose clinical seizures have already been shown to arise in the temporal lobe. Normally, it is in our temporal lobe circuitry that we weave the most subtle fabric of interpretations out of the strands of sensory perceptions, affective tone, cognitive activity, and past experience[5] (see chapter 56).

Neither epilepsy nor schizophrenia nor behavior nor religious experiences are simple topics. Any interface between them is sure to generate controversy.[6] Indeed, a heated debate has been going on for the last two decades over a straightforward question: *In between* their overt seizures, do otherwise alert patients with temporal lobe seizure foci show *distinctive* behavioral abnormalities? The issue gathered momentum when Dewhurst and Beard reported that several diverse experiences of a "religious conversion type" had occurred among sixty-nine patients who also had a schizophrenic-like psychosis and epilepsy.[6] Now, schizophrenia by itself can prove difficult to evaluate (see chapter 6). Moreover, careful reading of this report shows that no discrete religious conversion was consistently traceable to *one single seizure*. The authors did believe that *if* schizophrenics superimposed a religious conversion experience, this event tended to occur while their mood was shifting *up*, from depression to exaltation (see chapter 140). Few religious preoccupations occurred in patients who were stuck in periods of depression alone.

A minority view holds that, in between their overt seizures, patients with temporal lobe epilepsy show a distinctive psychological profile. Among its features, this profile is said to include a deepened affect, strong religious and philosophical interests, a preference for circumstantial details, a desire for social affiliation, and so forth.[7] Other investigators, in contrast, find that these same traits occur as frequently in patients who have various types of seizures other than temporal lobe seizures.[8,9] Currently, no compelling evidence establishes that, as a group, the patients who have temporal lobe seizures are also subject to some consistent, predictable, *specific* personality disorder. Nor do the data show that, whatever disorder of personality a given patient may sometimes have, it differs depending on whether the right or the left temporal lobe is the site of the seizure focus.[10,11] Put simply, temporal lobe seizures may coexist with hyperreligiosity in a few patients, but the association does not appear to be one of direct cause and effect.[12]

Yet the temporal lobe of some patients, in between their seizures, does display several other ongoing abnormalities. Mu opioid receptors are slightly increased, averaging some 9 to 15 percent, in the temporal cortex on the same side as the seizure focus.[13] And the metabolic activity of the affected lobe also tends to be *lower* when studied by positron-emission tomography (PET) scans.

Auras of a psychic nature do usher in more frequently those seizure episodes that begin in the right temporal lobe. In such patients, the term "psychic" is qualified. It implies only that the symptoms could be chiefly affective, or déjà vu, or cognitive in type (see chapter 78). And perceptual changes, such as structured hallucinations or illusions, may also occur.[1] Some patients, whose seizure focus is in the right temporo-occipital lobe, have longer episodes of REM sleep than do their controls.[14]

Two aspects of sexual behavior tend to be different in subjects who have seizure disorders. First, patients with temporal lobe epilepsy show a global tendency toward reduced sexuality.[15] Second, in those rare patients whose seizures are accompanied by orgasm, the EEG focus is usually in the right hemisphere.[16]

Tendencies do not mean always. Nor is everyone who shakes, quakes, or trembles having a genuine epileptic seizure. Human beings are suggestible. Pseudoseizures are common. Another group of aspirants who pursue the concentrative meditation techniques with too much zeal will develop makyo and other misadventures in their quest for spiritual advancement. So, in conclusion, the evidence indicates that seizures remain fundamentally different from peak experiences, and there are no real grounds for confusing them with the extraordinary alternate states of absorption and insight-wisdom.[17]

98

The Fleeting "Truths" of Nitrous Oxide

With me, as with every other person of whom I have heard, the keynote of the experience is the tremendously exciting sense of an intense metaphysical illumination. Truth lies open to the view in depth beneath depth of almost blinding evidence. The mind sees all the logical relations of being with an apparent subtlety and instantaneity to which its normal consciousness offers no parallel.

William James, 1882[1]

Truth revealed! All logical relations of being, instantly illuminated! This sounds like enlightenment. What was William James referring to? He was describing the way he felt when breathing nitrous oxide. It was these N_2O experiences which would force upon him that one unshakable conclusion, much quoted since: "It is that our normal waking consciousness, rational consciousness, as we call it, is but one special type of consciousness, whilst all about it, parted from it by the filmiest of screens, there lie potential forms of consciousness entirely different."[2]

Many others had experimented with nitrous oxide a century before. Joseph Priestley, who also discovered oxygen, described nitrous oxide back in 1772.[3] Thereafter, N_2O would soon become known as "laughing gas." Among the many users of this recreational intoxicant was Peter Roget, to whom we are indebted for his *Thesaurus*. But even he admitted that nitrous oxide's effects were difficult to put into words. The problem, he said, was that "the nature of the sensations themselves . . . bore greater resemblance to a half delirious stream than to any distinct state of mind capable of being accurately remembered." A "half delirious stream . . ."

Roget soon teamed up with Humphrey Davy (who discovered potassium) to study gases in Thomas Beddoes' newly opened "Pneumatic Institution" in Bristol, England. Beddoes' circle of notables soon grew. It included the influential poets Samuel Coleridge and Robert Southey, together with the inventor James Watt and numerous other creative spirits. By the turn of that century (1799–1800), Davy had parted the filmy screens often enough to write a very large book on his experiments with N_2O. He credited a patient with having described the effects of N_2O in that memorable phrase: "I felt like the sound of a harp."

We also have Davy's own words. They describe how, in its "highly pleasurable thrilling . . . objects around me became dazzling and my hearing more acute . . . at last an irresistible propensity to action was indulged in . . . sometimes I manifested my pleasure by stamping or laughing only; at other times by dancing round the room and vociferating." Moreover, there were also residual effects. Indeed, many hours after Davy had first breathed N_2O, recovered from it, and then slept, he still noted that he might awaken having "the feeling of restless energy, or that desire of action connected with no definite object."[3]

So people already appreciated, two centuries ago, that N_2O had mental effects, activated motoric systems, and energized impulsive behaviors. But most impressive were the "metaphysical illuminations," the events William James would later emphasize. Among them, James recalled that, while breathing N_2O, one authenticated truth had made a lasting impression. It was that "every opposition, among whatsoever things, vanishes in a higher unity in which it is based; that all contradictions, so-called, are of a common kind; that unbroken continuity is of the essence of being; and that we are literally in the midst of an infinity, to perceive the existence of which is the utmost we can attain."[3] One recognizes many ancient truths of Zen in this statement. Had Priestley's advance in chemical technology gone on to teach old dogmas new tricks?

But N_2O soon disappointed even its proponents. As Roget noted, its half-delirious rush of highly compressed insights halted as soon as the gas was turned off. James also concluded, regretfully, that "As sobriety returns, the feeling of insight fades, and one is left staring vacantly at a few disjointed words and phrases, as one stares at a cadaverous-looking snow peak from which the sunset glow has just fled, or at the black cinder left by an extinguished brand."[3] Still, James wrote furiously during his intoxications, sheet after sheet of phrases "which to the sober reader seem meaningless drivel, but which at the moment of transcribing were fused in the fire of infinite rationality." Consider the two following examples of James's sentences: "That sounds like nonsense, but it is pure onsense!" "There are no differences but differences of degree between different degrees of difference and no difference."[3]

So nonsense was embedded in those same "truths" which James had labeled as authentic only moments before. Despite this, James would add, "Nevertheless, the sense of the profound meaning having been there persists; and I know more than one person who is persuaded that in the nitrous oxide trance we have a genuine metaphysical revelation."[4] But many others would be less impressed. Given how ephemeral and subjective was the quality of such infusions of profound meaning, how could any such drug deliver a genuine, *lasting* truth that was objectively verifiable? And even if it did, which parts of the brain was it acting on?

Because nitrous oxide displaces oxygen, breathing 100 percent N_2O produces anoxia. Even in the present century, patients recovering from N_2O anesthesia have still shown mild degrees of anoxia lasting nine minutes or so *if* they were first switched to breathing only room air.[5] So, brain anoxia may have contributed to the earlier experimenter's many symptoms. However, when enough oxygen is added to prevent anoxia, even N_2O concentrations as low as 40 to 60 percent will still produce the classic N_2O mental effects described above. And after sufficient oxygen is added, N_2O does not depress vital brain stem reflexes, or cause major changes in the size of the pupils or in the intracranial pressure.[6] In fact, when humans breathe N_2O in concentrations higher than 50 percent, it causes fast beta EEG activity over the frontal regions.[7] So one source of the highly pressured *associative* stream of the delirious state might come from the way N_2O is activating associative functions of the frontal lobes.[8]

Some recent metabolic studies in rats confirm the old impression that N_2O is indeed a relatively "physiological" anesthetic, one that slows overall cerebral metabolism only slightly. Metabolism does drop more in rat neocortex (-35 percent) than elsewhere (-15 to -20 percent).[9] But still other experiments show that *certain* parts of the brain do *increase* their metabolic activity when rats breathe 70 percent N_2O. Given the way humans report a delirious rush of auditory and visual images, it is of note that the regions showing this increased activity include the lower-level pathways which help us see and hear: the two geniculate nuclei which are poised at the gateway of the thalamus; and the superior colliculus in the upper brain stem. Metabolism also increases nearby in the red nucleus in the midbrain. This finding becomes of further interest in view of Davy's vigorous impulse to dance and shout. In contrast, N_2O reduces metabolic activity at such higher motoric levels as the nucleus accumbens and the sensorimotor cortex.[10]

In its heyday, Beddoes' Pneumatic Institution must have generated more than a full share of hilarity. But two centuries ago, it fell gradually into disrepute. Davy, however, had already made a shrewd observation: a few breaths of N_2O reduced pain from the gums. Later, this pain-relieving property of N_2O would be embraced by dentists and physicians. They now had a useful agent for producing analgesia and mild anesthesia! Subsequent research went on to show that humans who breathe 80 percent N_2O do lose most (88 percent) of their sense of pain. Yet only recently have we started to appreciate the opioid implications of this N_2O analgesia.

Suppose we reconsider the painful sliver that got stuck in your finger. If you were to breathe N_2O, it would still allow most of these pain signals to register as impulses higher up in the spinal cord. However, the pain message would then dwindle as it continues to ascend.[11] This suggests that N_2O dampens pain messages in those higher pathways which lie somewhere between the spinal cord and the cortex. Could opioids be acting at these levels? (see chapter 80). Indeed, both mu and kappa opioid receptors appear to be involved in mediating the analgesic effect of N_2O.[12]

And there are further reasons to implicate endogenous opioid mechanisms: the N_2O analgesia is partially reversed by the opioid *antagonist*, naloxone[13] (see chapter 47). Additional evidence suggests that *N_2O directly stimulates endorphin nerve cells* up in the arcuate nucleus of the hypothalamus.[14] When stimulated, these endorphin cells can release enough beta-endorphin to block pain impulses down in the central gray substance. Indeed, 60 percent N_2O does double the beta-endorphin content in the rat hypothalamus, and it also increases endorphin levels in the diencephalon and central gray.[15] The central gray is clearly an important site in N_2O analgesia, because the analgesia does not occur after prior lesions have damaged its key ventral lateral portion[16] (see chapter 52). Some of nitrous oxide's effects might also reflect the release of one other opioid, dynorphin.[17]

Recent research also confirms Peter Roget's old observation. Nitrous oxide does create a rush of associations, causing them to rush in *and to rush out* faster than they can be assimilated. Even low concentrations of N_2O, say between 15 and 35 percent, still slow the way the human brain reacts to names. Moreover, evoked potential studies reveal that N_2O also delays the P-300 waveform. This finding suggests that N_2O reduces the brain's capacity to evaluate outside stimuli[18] (see chapter 64).

The Sounds of the Harpstrings

Nitrous oxide's fleeting euphoriant and insightful experiences represent a mixture of phenomena. These include the quieting of many higher inhibitory circuits and the enhancing of other circuits, coupled with the release (and rapid turnover) of endogenous opioids in the core of the brain. And, because it is relatively easy to breathe the gas, N_2O continues to have the potential for abuse. A century ago, William James considered that N_2O inhalation was "short and harmless enough." He concluded, "I strongly urge others to repeat the experiment . . . The effects will, of course, vary with the individual, just as they vary in the same individual from time to time."[3] Today, we appreciate that this seemingly simple gas has complex chemical and physiological actions.[19] The serious damage that nitrous oxide abuse causes to the spinal cord and peripheral nerves has been attributed to its interfering with vitamin B_{12} metabolism.[20,21]

Nitrous oxide, like many other drugs, produces an overabundance of phenomena. And their half-delirious stream no sooner reveals than it obscures. When subjects are actually breathing N_2O, some of their outbursts of laughter reflect their general tendency toward motor activation. But the happy laughter fades, as do the fleeting moments of conviction, once they stop inhaling the gas. In contrast, the insight-wisdom of kensho goes on resonating for hours.

As we step back and look at alternate states in general, what do laughter, crying, or other emotional outbursts imply? They simply confirm that the person has undergone an experience *of some kind*. And they indicate that this episode has been associated with some kind of a motor and psychic release. But in no absolute sense do these outbursts necessarily validate the rest of the content of the experience itself (chapter 96 affords a relevant example). This caveat is especially applicable when collateral evidence suggests that the subject's arousal mechanisms have been driven up to high intensity and further activated by artificial means.

It would help if we could slow down the kaleidoscopic rush of the N_2O experience. Suppose we could allow it to emerge in slow motion. Then we could study individual segments of its sequences somewhat more leisurely, as they were in the hibernation experiments (see chapter 76). Perhaps in this manner one could better isolate the steps leading up to each fleeting moment of "truth." Such studies could help clarify which neurophysiological and biochemical events actually fuse to create our more impressive intuitions, rather than merely accompany them. Meanwhile, we need many more integrated studies of animals, and of humans, performed during selected stages of N_2O analgesia, anesthesia, and recovery. We could then begin by studying opiate antagonists, highly selective for each receptor type. This could allow us to test the hypothesis that selective antagonists—for opioids and other messengers—would eliminate certain features of the N_2O experience in human subjects.

In the interim, we can only be sobered by the fleeting nature of those depths of meaning which briefly permeate consciousness when subjects are breathing N_2O or ether. These brief artificial states contrast strikingly with the enduring transformations which are the residues of kensho and satori. Why does the insight-wisdom of prajna remain subsequently more readily accessible? Why does it resonate at depths which allows it later to be appropriately validated and channeled?

In the meditator, insights strike from the background of long meditative practice. Insights enter in clear, unclouded consciousness. One may speculate that a meditator who has already learned to hold attention as a result of prior mindful training could then fix these insights in clear consciousness for a longer period of open, uncluttered time. In this way, perhaps for a given moment of equal impact, the whole kensho experience could penetrate deeply, without distractions, into long-term memory storage sites. There it could take the form of enduring traces. These traces would not rush away so quickly.

In this chapter we have drawn one step closer to those sources in the brain which could generate the sense of authenticity. Is authenticity important? Yes indeed! *When this stamp of certainty reinforces a thought, idea, or symbol, it helps empower our rarest and most meaningful life experiences.* Yes, we are hypothesizing that *one* part of this authoritative feeling is associated with a pulse of endogenous opioids. To some, this would be reductionism; to others, heresy. But however it may be challenged, this working hypothesis—that opioids are ink on our imprimatur of certainty—will have heuristic value. There are two reasons.

First, it is a testable hypothesis. It will stimulate researchers to go further. We need to find out how a person's belief system gets ensnared by its strongest motivating impulses. Every century bears witness to the fact that humans do become enthralled by the addictive roots of dogma. And this is quite apart from the separate issue of whether the *content* of a particular belief is true or false in the abstract. Second, the proposal can stimulate us to be renewed on an age-old search. For this troubled humanity does sense that it has been set adrift. Even as its members wallow between monotony and angst, they already realize how to remedy their situations. They must find new ways to infuse a fresh sense—of appreciation and of meaning—into the simplest experiences of their everyday lives. This is an internal, endogenous issue. It will not be solved by adding drugs from the outside.

So what does the topic of nitrous oxide contribute to the quest? It focuses attention on a gap so wide that it might seem unbridgeable. It is the same gap which Zen exemplifies. For Zen, too, brings each person into that same confrontation between sheer nonsense on the one hand and the essence of being on the other (see chapter 26). We may well suppose that both Davy and James, in their day, had also been intrigued by the outrageous notion that an artificial "laughing gas" could help understand the mechanisms that might bridge this gap. They would have been incredulous at the recent finding that *the brain itself can make, and use*, another gas. A gas with a similar name that has even more striking properties.

Nitric Oxide

Two centuries after nit*rous* oxide arrived, this different gas, abbreviated NO˙, has become the latest research fad. It is easy to see why. Even the short list of its properties, as outlined below, helps one appreciate why nit*ric* oxide plays unique roles in normal brain function, and carries the potential to participate both in alternate states and in their residua.

1. NO˙ is made in many neurons. Not only in the short nerve cells that influence local circuits but also in the long acetylcholine nerve cells rising up from the key parabrachial region (see chapter 38).[22] In the amygdala, most of the nerve cells that can release NO˙ are located in the basolateral group of nuclei.[23]

2. Once made, NO˙ diffuses readily. So it quickly exerts a local sphere of influence. Unlike standard messengers, it is not stored in small vesicles at synapses. Nor must it pause to activate receptors on the *outside* of the next nerve cell.

3. Instead, when released, NO˙ speeds quickly to its major metabolic target. This target lies *inside* adjacent cells. It is the soluble enzyme which makes cyclic guanosine monophosphate (cGMP).[24] The result is an increase in cGMP. This second messenger then sets off a cascade of effects which have long-range implications for transforming the brain (see chapter 48).

4. NO˙ increases long-term potentiation in the hippocampus.[25,26] Moreover, it can nudge the oscillatory bursts of thalamic relay cells in directions that seem "conducive to wakefulness."[27]

5. More NO˙ is formed after glutamate and aspartate receptors are activated. Moreover, some of the actions of NO˙ further enhance the toxicity of these two excitatory amino acids.[28] These are impressive interactions (see chapter 152).

6. The small round dot in NO˙ indicates that it is a free radical, unstable and highly reactive. It reacts further with oxygen to form toxic peroxynitrite byproducts. These can further change a nerve cell by damaging its DNA.[29,30]

Having said this, it is no simple matter to be certain exactly where and how a given NO˙ molecule *acts* once it is formed inside a particular nerve cell. Note that the gas molecule can then diffuse back from this first cell's dendrites, or out from its cell body, to influence adjacent nerve cells upstream. To a lesser degree, a few gas molecules might even be emitted father downstream from this first cell's distant axon terminal. Thereafter, while NO˙ may influence excitability directly, its delayed metabolic effects hinge on the answer to one simple question. Does its nearby target cell already have that cyclase enzyme system which can make cGMP?[31]

Is the brain really resorting to passing gas messages? And not only from nitric oxide but from its recently discovered sources of carbon monoxide? Perhaps ideas this ludicrous will have begun to seem out of place in any quasi-religious context. If so, then this chapter on gases will already have served to introduce the next topic, the particular comic spirit so characteristic of Zen.

99

The Roots of Laughter

> The brain of our species is, as we know, made up largely of potassium, phosphorus, propaganda and politics, with the result that how not to understand what should be clearer is becoming easier and easier for all of us.
>
> James Thurber (1894–1961)[1]

Smiles begin very early, a prelude to laughter. A special beatific smile transfigures a baby's face. It is called a "smile to the angels." It flashes in for the first time when the infant is in D-sleep. Only much later will the enchanted mother and father be privileged to see it happen during the waking hours.[2] This first smile is a hardwired phenomenon. Even an infant born prematurely expresses it.

The beatific smile is intriguing when it is correlated with the other events which take place in the brain stem during D-sleep. Here in the pons, for example, are the motor nerve cells directly responsible for tightening the facial muscles. The muscles contract into a smile only when a certain pattern of impulses converges on them. During an infant's first twelve months, the beta-endorphin levels in this facial motor nucleus are among the highest in the brain stem.[3] Alas, as our brain matures and proceeds to remodel its original architecture, it reshapes our original smiles as well. Rarely do our adult smiles regain their original, spontaneous, luminous quality.

But there are two exceptions. In Zen circles, the illuminated face has long been known. According to Kobori-roshi, the countenance of a well-trained monk both regains and *keeps* some of this beatific quality after the monk becomes fully enlightened. My friend Dr. Kiyonobu Katou once accurately described Kobori-roshi himself using these words. "His smile is wider than his face." The illuminated face is a phenomenon which should prove of interest to several groups of investigators, including those who have reported that our external facial expression sends back signals which help us *feel* the corresponding emotion.[4]

Other anecdotes testify to a second occasion when the face can light up. This may occur, briefly, during the inspired terminal moments of a dying patient. Neuroscientists could discover something worthwhile if they went to the source of each of these two "1000-watt smiles." For their studies might someday cast new light on that old Zen term, "original face," and open it up to still other physiological levels of interpretation (see chapter 129).

> Children laugh a lot, but I remember one personal laughing fit in particular. I was six at the time, and we had just switched over from the old, clear-glass milk bottles to the new, opaque waxed cardboard cartons. Although these one-quart cartons didn't shatter, you couldn't see how much milk they contained. It was a summer lunch, and we were all thirsty. The first time my arm lifted up the full milk carton to pour a glass,

its proprioceptors registered how heavy the carton was. Unconsciously, I gauged how much strength I would require the next time I needed to lift the weight of this carton off the table.

Minutes later, I hurriedly reached over and lifted the carton again. But something had escaped my attention. By then, the others at the table had almost emptied it. Now, as I grabbed the opaque carton, not knowing that it was nearly empty, my hand and arm soared high off the table. Surprise! This lightweight carton shattered a heavy expectation. And with this abrupt proprioceptive surprise, a mental set gave way. I dissolved in irresistible gales of laughter, laughing so long and hard that tears flowed and my sides hurt.

The milk carton incident serves as shallow preview of what sometimes happens when a much deeper awakening experience overturns a person's preconceived sets. Trivial as the childhood example might seem, it introduces us to the comic spirit, to the laughter and the tears, which can flow when the innocent truth of Zen is revealed.

Overly religious orthodoxies might view the comic as an affront to the sacred. Not Zen. The comic perspective plays an integral role in Zen, perhaps second only to the cosmic. Zen's childlike, foolish, playful side is embodied in the spirit of Han-shan, that carefree eccentric poet who lived during the Tang dynasty.[5] Does his lighthearted Zen pose a real threat to the sober-sided meditative Zen of Bodhidharma? No, it rounds it out, as does yin to yang. As does the act of that destitute man in the charming fable of the Juggler of Notre Dame. The only thing of worth he could possibly offer Our Lady—and the one she would value the most—was simply that gift of juggling his very best in front of her altar.

Meditation is the foundation of Zen practice. All the more reason for Zen to poke fun at it. The act, so typical, was never performed so humorously as by Master Sengai. His brush (surpassing even Thurber's) once sketched the bare outlines of a frog in his usual seated posture. To the left of this wonderful meditating creature, Sengai began the caption: "If a person becomes a Buddha by practicing zazen . . . " After which, the struggling meditator will have no problem supplying the gist of the remaining caption ". . . then, even though I'm a frog, I should have become a Buddha long ago."[6]

The light touch of this comic spirit is no sacrilege. It confers resiliency, impregnability. The person who has truly realized this spirit in Zen is well on the Way. He has arrived at the same kind of "invincibility that has often been noticed in the person of the clown or fool. He cannot finally be conquered, defeated, or killed; for the Achilles' heel of Ego, attachment and desire is not there."[7]

A good joke requires no explanation. A joke doesn't "work" unless there occurs that intuitive flash which grasps the essentials and senses their incongruities. In this respect, a potentially humorous joke resembles a koan. Both must be "seen into," intuited, realized immediately. This kind of insightful function lies at the core of Zen.

Laughter translates well in any tongue. While many observers keep speculating about what precipitates laughter,[8] here we will consider only four theories pertinent to the issue of awakening. These hypotheses fall into the categories of (1) playfulness, (2) surprise, (3) energized levels of activity, and (4) novelty attached to the collapse of old barriers. What barriers? The ones we had previously set up between categories, that is, between sense and nonsense, victory and defeat.

Although babies do smile in their early weeks, they don't really *laugh* until they are three or four months old.[8] Then they'll laugh during playful situations, like peekaboo. A common element here is a surplus of energy. This energy is more readily discharged when one is aroused and one's spirits are high. Charles Darwin emphasized that people also broke out laughing when some jarring note took them by surprise at a time when they were already in a happy frame of mind. This jarring note could be an event that was either incongruous or unaccountable.

As an example, consider one consequence of our having been conditioned to respect other persons. Suppose we have almost elevated them to a pedestal. Then this high regard will be incongruous with any later image of their also slipping on a banana peel. Our normal cultural tensions compress two such divergent concepts into separate compartments. Laughter erupts when these tensions are released.

Novel things also prompt laughter, things so odd as to be nonsensical. "Something about it struck my funny bone" is one descriptive phrase. Laughter also springs from situations that create an unexpected, new relationship between victory and defeat. Now those old roles are reversed which had once separated the victor from the vanquished.[8]

When we plumb all these roots of laughter, again we discover Zen. For variations of each of the above situations occur whenever the insights of kensho overturn the old *I-Me-Mine*. The new domain is unexpected. It has inconceivable dimensions. So when laughter bubbles out of a pervasive, ongoing, comic spirit, it signifies something akin to that abrupt giving way of boundaries, that melting undifferentiation of barriers, that release of all tensions which *is* Zen awakening.

Novelty, abrupt responses, unpredictability. Zen exemplifies the same attributes in other ways. For, as Muso Kokushi (1275–1351) noted, these are also the standard, stock-in-trade ingredients of the old-style Zen master.[9] And this kind of creative vitality certainly keeps disciples on their toes. Muso Kokushi himself was so lively, so unfettered and unpredictable, that no monk ever knew what he would do next. Nor did he.

Many of the early Zen masters freely displayed eccentricities which might seem "crazy" in the culture of today. Let us give their "unfettered vitality" a provisional charitable interpretation. It was the manifestation of an open, emancipated spirit. Nothing was sacred or forbidden. Nothing either too zany or too serious.

When Master Ma-tsu's kick knocked him down, Shui-lao abruptly realized satori. He rose up and laughed heartily as though the most welcome and unexpected event had occurred. Later on, whenever he was asked about his understanding of Zen, he simply replied, "Ever since master Ma-tsu's hearty kick, I haven't been able to stop laughing."[10]

For in satori lies the great surprise, the ultimate kicker. An unparalleled state of grace suddenly simplifies all prior complexities, within and without. As it evolves, uncontrolled laughter sometimes bursts forth.[11] The laughter can alternate with uncontrolled sobbing, but the tears are those of joyous relief.

Tap goes the doctor's reflex hammer against the tendon at the knee. Patients still tend to be startled by what happens next. A reflex *beyond their control* jerks their leg out! And they hadn't consciously granted it permission to do so! Many subjects laugh when they first feel their own leg suddenly jerking out. Overcontrolled young doctors and nurses are among those prone to laughter.

Darwin noted that the person's facial expression during paroxysms of laughter is not too dissimilar from that during howls of grief. Our everyday language makes the same point. In the process of unleashing one expression we may also lose our grip on the other: "I laughed until I cried," or "I nearly died laughing." It is a fact, learned by experience, that a good cry also rinses away tensions, opens up new depths of compassionate understanding. It is time for a major, in-depth study of the basic psychophysiology of laughter and crying.

Who can resist certain comic strips? They relieve us of the newspaper's daily litany of woe. Leavened by its superb cartoons and those tweaks of newspaper mistakes at the bottom of a page, even the staid old *New Yorker* magazine of yesteryear became more approachable. If there is no access to humor, problems arise from being overearnest, and from endowing one's person, cause, or situation with unqualified seriousness. Overly solemn persons can become especially vulnerable to the heavy burden of their religious preoccupations.[6] Recognizing this syndrome, the old masters and monks spoke of those overearnest persons who had gotten so involved that they "stink of Zen." The antidote for this solemn situation is the light touch, the simple-minded comic spirit. D. T. Suzuki observed that "something in Zen itself makes Zen people laugh at one another, and each singly within himself."[12] And, let it be added, *at* oneself as well.

Perhaps there is a solemn streak in Kaufmann which enables him to contend that most philosophers can't really laugh.[13] He suggests that the old fable about the emperor's clothes affords one explanation for this conclusion. For the tale does illustrate that persons who *pretend* to see something which they don't really see are never in a position to laugh. Let us follow this line of reasoning, but then turn it around. For this modification will enable us to state the emperor's clothes hypothesis in reverse: *a person might be most ready to laugh when every pretense about reality finally vanishes.*

Our genuine laughter gushes out unrestrained. No pretense remains. Watching normal people laugh spontaneously, the pioneer neurologist, William Gowers, observed: "The will is needed, not to effect it, but to restrain it."[14] But neurologists (who have their own sober side, as well) usually find many widely scattered brain lesions in individual patients who have been laughing all the time. Our short explanation stems from Hughlings Jackson's original proposition: having many lesions on both sides releases the "lower levels" from being inhibited by the "higher levels." However, these *dis*inhibitions are only one part of a more complicated story. In fact, "higher" physiological levels enter into both inhibitory and excitory interactions *among themselves* as well as with "lower levels." What does exaggerated laughter imply? Put simply, it means that a *series* of inhibitory and excitatory mechanisms are probably summating at several levels, high and low.

At the higher levels, certain *focal* lesions release laughter. For example, laughter can occur after damage to parts of the prefrontal, temporal, and limbic regions near the midline. Stimulations in the depths of the frontal lobe or thalamus can also bring about smiling or loud laughing.[15] Within the thalamus is one clue about why some of our laughter goes on to tears. For in the intermediate part of its intralaminar nuclei, or in its central lateral nucleus, stimulating at only 25 cps prompts laughter. But crying occurs when stimulating at frequencies twice that.[16] Occasionally, epileptic seizures that activate either hemisphere can also be associated with brief, exaggerated laughter.[17]

Some lesions that damage and deactivate the right hemisphere leave patients with a tendency to laugh more. And this laughter occurs even though the patients neither recognize in others nor express in themselves the full ranges of emotion. In contrast, damage to the left cerebral hemisphere tends to leave some patients depressed and prone to develop abrupt emotional reactions.[18]

Rarely, small tumors or other lesions around the hypothalamic region produce excited or exalted states of consciousness.[14] During brain surgery, merely touching a small part of a patient's hypothalamus (the infundibulum) can prompt such an excited state, leading to whistling or singing. From here, the roots of laughter extend still farther down to their final, common pathways inside the brain stem.

Drugs other than laughing gas enhance laughter. Some subjects are overwhelmed with laughter during the first minutes of their response to mescaline. Parts of this particular laughter may be a secondary reaction to—or coincide with—the subjects' feeling that they have left behind their greatest self-conscious fears. Still later, one subject also felt driven by a different kind of impulse. It was "an intense, almost uncontrollable need to laugh—as intense and organic in quality as a distended bowel or bladder."[19] This is also an accurate description of the raw surge of emotional power which drove *my* tears of joy, as just described in chapter 96.

Another broad category of "overflow" laughter occurs during an ongoing, energized excitement and euphoria. After human subjects are injected with epinephrine in an arm vein, they tend to laugh more vigorously at a slapstick movie.[20] And the more aroused they are, the deeper their emotion becomes. Chlorpromazine stops this enhanced laughter. Why is this point noteworthy? Because chlorpromazine blocks the receptors sensitive to dopamine, norepinephrine, and epinephrine, both in the central and peripheral nervous systems.

From the foregoing accounts, one can appreciate from how many levels smiles, laughter, and the general comic spirit flow from the human brain when restraints drop off. From such spontaneity, it is but a very short trip before we find them entering into the traditions of Zen. A recent arrival is the Zen cartoon book, with that superb title, *The Upside Down Circle*.[21]

But far back, Zen has epitomized something more subtle. From its very first historical beginnings, there has been a Zen version of the tantalizing Mona Lisa smile. On this refined plane, no loud laughter, big gestures, or grand words will ever be necessary. For one of the oldest-rooted of Zen legends relates to that special occasion when Buddha had been asked to deliver a sermon. And when, instead of speaking in words, he simply held up a sandalwood flower. Upon seeing into this gesture, his disciple Mahakasyapa responded with a sublimely wordless smile.

It is with such a wordless smile that authentic Zen, in every age, will go on to elude all self-conscious actions. Not for Zen is that artificial, "say cheese"–type of smiling we are invited to display when being photographed. When will you rediscover your *original* smile? When will it come out of hiding? Sometime when you are observing children or kittens or puppies joyously at play. Then you'll find it already on your face: the enchanted smile of natural delight.

100

How Do Psychedelic and Certain Other Drugs Affect the Brain?

> In its imagery, emotional tone and vagaries of thought and self-awareness, the drug trip, especially with eyes closed, resembles no other state so much as a dream.
>
> L. Grinspoon[1]

A drug like LSD triggers an acute hallucinogenic sequence as soon as it exceeds a threshold level. In humans, the threshold dose of LSD to enter this first, hallucinogenic phase is only twenty-five to fifty *micro*grams, taken either by mouth or intravenously.[2] The result is a mental quickening: a "TV show in the head." During the next four hours, the flow of imagery is a mere "curiosity of the drug-state."[3] A few undercurrents of meaningfulness might arise, but they do not have true religious or mystical import.

During the second phase, these visual hallucinations are no longer compelling, but various ideas of reference can develop.[2] Because the paranoid tone of such reactions may reach psychotic proportions, LSD is also called a *psychotomimetic* drug, one that mimics psychosis. During these two phases, the pupils dilate as a reflection of LSD's *sympathomimetic* actions. The pupils remain abnormally large for as long as ten hours after a dose of 100 to 200 micrograms by mouth.

If LSD is injected intravenously in one quick pulse, it can soon prompt intense visual illusions and semihallucinatory experiences. Some of these resemble individual film clips taken out of a movie strip, a point that will interest those who have had similar tachistoscope experiences (see chapter 90). These snapshot images flick by for several minutes before their pace slows.[2]

When LSD is injected more slowly, over one or two minutes, a *delayed* shift in awareness occurs abruptly, twenty minutes later. Now, objects out at the periphery of the visual field become as salient as do those straight ahead. In addition, minute details are enhanced: the subject now appreciates the fine grain of the wood, not the whole door itself. These just-cited descriptions emphasize the most distinctive features of the *early* LSD experience: the way it shifts attentiveness, heightens arousal, and disorganizes those normal mechanisms which would otherwise suppress or smooth out the flow among the person's different perceptions.[2]

And these *early* perceptual symptoms offer tantalizing hints about where psychedelics *first* act on amine circuits in the human brain (see chapter 103). But it is a different task to localize the sources of those long-delayed mystical, religious, or other experiences. Why? Because they do not develop until many *hours* later (see chapters 101 and 102). One cannot expect to find simple explanations for the experiential flavor of these rare *later* events. At least not in the known *primary* effects of the psychedelic drugs.

Moreover, a drug "trip" is subject to many variables. The variability begins with what the person had been led to expect. Later, as Alan Watts pointed out, it may depend on the way each journey itself unfolds. He believed that during the later stages of an individual LSD trip, it helped him to "go along with the flow." When he became passive, things then became more harmonious, and he seemed about to begin to apprehend consciousness itself.[4] But it is risky to use a drug to "go with the flow." The subject can be swept either into an episode viewed as an isolated curiosity, or into a dramatic mystical event, or into that rarer condition in which disturbing flashbacks recur.

LSD reactions also vary in intensity as well as form and content. Subtle differences change the triggering threshold. They also modify how fully the response manifests itself. It will prove useful to review some of the variables which can influence the degree of the LSD response. For example, subjects respond more

1. After sleep deprivation.[5]
2. If they have hysterical personalities.[6]

Whereas the following conditions decrease the reactions to LSD:

1. "Sensory" deprivation[7]
2. Tightly structured, obsessive-compulsive personalities[6]
3. Overcontrolled patients who cannot relax and let go.[6]
4. Patients who lack confidence in their therapist.[6]
5. Doses repeated after too short an interval.[2]
6. Anterior temporal lobe removal (which decreases the perceptual changes).[8]
7. Chronic medication with a drug that reduces the breakdown of serotonin and other amines.[6]
8. Phenothiazine drugs, such as chlorpromazine.[9]

A few comments are in order about the list above. Ram Dass cites an anecdotal report about his Indian guru. Allegedly, this guru did not respond to LSD on two occasions, even though he had taken very high oral doses of 900 and 1500 micrograms.[10] This account was not documented scientifically, but it has led to the uncritical notion that perhaps there might be an "acid test" for a genuine guru: he will fail to respond to LSD because he is already "there." When one reviews the above long list of *other* conditions which reduce the LSD reaction, it seems obvious that a rigorous formal test of such a hypothesis would be indicated. Moreover, if such a notion were to be validated, one would need to go on carefully from there to define the precise mechanisms responsible. In part VIII, we consider in greater detail what is actually entailed in the psychophysiology of "being there."

The temporal lobes are vital to the perceptual aspects of the LSD response. If normal chimps receive a large oral dose of LSD, they develop "perceptual aberrations and panic."[11] In contrast, they do not react this way if their temporal lobe cortex has first been removed, on both sides, along with its underlying white matter. The temporal lobes' contribution became further evident when LSD was given to patients who had severe chronic, epileptic seizures.[8] LSD caused twice as many perceptual responses when given to patients whose seizures had begun in their *right* temporal lobe, as opposed to those whose seizures had begun in the *left* temporal lobe.

To control these severe focal seizures, the tip of the temporal lobe on the affected side was then removed. The regions removed included the temporal cortex, amygdala, and hippocampus. After the surgery, LSD was given again. Now most patients had far fewer perceptual responses. However, LSD still produced more perceptual responses in that group of patients whose *previous* seizures had started on the right side. In contrast, removing a chronic frontal lobe seizure focus did not change the response to LSD.

The drug nialamide is a monoamine oxidase inhibitor and stimulant. Patients who take this medication on a long-term basis become highly resistant to LSD's effects.[6] The reasons are complex. Nialamide slows the metabolic breakdown of biogenic amines, and it profoundly reduces REM sleep, among its several other side effects.

Phenothiazine drugs such as chlorpromazine are used to stop the severe behavioral reactions to LSD.[9] These drugs appear to reduce the LSD response chiefly by blocking dopamine receptors.

Our plan, throughout part V, is to consider—without prejudice—what causes quickenings of different kinds. In this and the next chapters dealing with drugs, a big question will be sneaking up from behind, as it were. Let us now, both reader and writer, openly confront this issue. Stated simply, do meditative training procedures have "psychedelic" properties? If so, in what sense would one be using this word? Now, with regard to meditation, one could only use "psychedelic" in its most general sense, and not in a manner that might cause the reader undue concern. Indeed, when Osmond, a psychiatrist, first coined this term, it included two concepts: "enriching the mind and enlarging the vision." Psychedelic, then, simply meant "mind-manifesting."[12]

Clearly, some of the quickening effects of meditation resemble some of the quickening effects of drugs. Why? Could they both be sharing certain mechanisms, at levels either shallow or deep, that are worth making a serious effort to understand? If so, then do either one of these two agencies—psychedelic drugs or meditative training—have *specific* effects? The literature clarifies these issues.

The Implications of Carbon Dioxide as an Adjunct

We have just seen how a gas like nitrous oxide can activate mental processes (see chapter 98). Another gas, when inhaled, also releases experiences that in some ways resemble those prompted by LSD. This gas, carbon dioxide, is normally found in low concentrations in our bodies and brains. As an example, Grof found that the kind of reaction he could stimulate by giving his patients arousing concentrations of CO_2 would *predict* which kind of response to LSD they would later develop.[13] Moreover, the next point is especially noteworthy. *Each person's response to CO_2 also evolved—over days, weeks and months—as did that to LSD.*

Suppose the subjects breathe the CO_2 at times in between their *early* LSD sessions. (The gas is administered as 70 percent O_2–30 percent CO_2.) Then it evokes only visions and the reliving of their childhood memories. But suppose you also give the same gas mixture several weeks later on. Now it elicits different *kinds* of experiences. Grof interprets these as resembling the kinds that will occur later in the more advanced phases of an LSD-induced "death-rebirth struggle." And suppose, subsequently, that you allow these same subjects to inhale O_2-CO_2 at times in between their much later, more "transpersonal," types of LSD sessions. Now this same gas mixture will be able to induce still other transpersonal phenomena. These later experiences, driven by CO_2, include both mystical and religious states.[13] Over time, has the person's brain been evolving, psychophysiologically and biochemically? If so, how?

Now, if one were to step back and regard this gas mixture in isolation, out of the LSD context of the present discussion, one's first thought would not be that O_2-CO_2 is "psychedelic." But this high concentration of CO_2 is an *adjunct*. It plays a nonspecific role in driving up and ventilating whatever material has already started to come closer to the surface.[14] Nor, at first, would one be likely to label as "mind-manifesting" those physiological quickenings which surge in as the result of meditative practices. Yet both drugs and meditation sponsor mind-manifesting effects.

What general conclusions can one draw from the above observations? First, that the brain's responses do *evolve*. A prosaic point, yet one so vital to our understanding of Zen that the next chapter will be developing it further. Here, let it serve as a reminder that the brain's second messengers give it a remarkable capacity to transform itself (see chapter 48). Second, that when the brain is already primed and on the brink, a strongly arousing event may tip it over into different kinds of quickenings and awakenings. In chapter 105 we will be considering how "triggers" act in this process.

Physiological Changes after LSD

During everyday physiological circumstances, a normal brain releases only minute quantities of its own fast chemical messengers. It delivers them discretely. Their targets are specific receptors on defined groups of nerve cells. The sequences of delivery and of reuptake are exquisitely timed and well orchestrated.

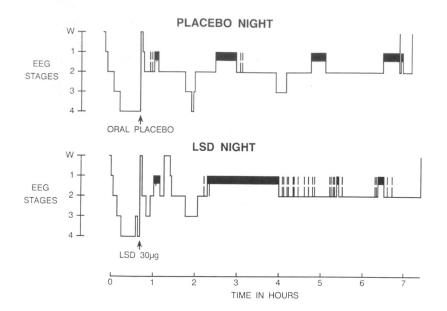

Figure 14   Sleep cycles on two successive nights, before and after LSD

In the top graph, the subject descends, in "staircase" fashion, through the four stages of normal sleep. She is then awakened (vertical line) in the act of receiving an inactive placebo (small upward arrow). On the next night, at bottom, she is again awakened out of stage 4 sleep to receive 30 micrograms of LSD. At this point, she begins the LSD study, again in the waking state (W), at time zero.

The thick black horizontal bars indicate when each subsequent episode of rapid eye movement (REM) sleep began and how long it lasted. Note that most REM episodes enter at times when she is considered to be in stage 1 (REM) sleep as judged by electroencephalographic (EEG) criteria (vertical axis). The other thin lines, plotted in stepwise fashion, reflect the stages, from 1 to 4, through which the EEG evolves as she descends from shallower (1) into deeper (4) levels of slow-wave S-sleep.

This subject's total sleep time averaged just over seven hours on each night. However, after LSD she spent more time in REM episodes. After LSD, REM periods took up 31 percent of her total sleep time, but only 19 percent of the time during the first, placebo control night. Note, too, that after LSD the long black bar of her second REM episode is (a) displaced earlier; (b) almost three and one-half times as long as the corresponding REM bar after the placebo. Moreover, many micro-REM episodes burst into sleep for several hours after LSD takes effect, especially after the fourth hour. (Redrawn and modified with reference to figure 5 of J. Muzio, H. Roffwarg, and E. Kaufman: Alterations in the nocturnal sleep cycle resulting from LSD. *Electroencephalography and Clinical Neurophysiology* 1966;21:320.) with permission from Elsevier Science Ireland Ltd, Bay 15 K, Shannon Industrial Estate, Co. Clare, Ireland.

None of these four statements describes the crude ways in which many drugs affect the brain.

We are still learning about all the places that LSD acts on, and the ways it *inter*acts there.[15] Human and animal studies provide four intriguing leads. *First* is the way LSD enhances early REM sleep. LSD prolongs either the first or the second episode of REM. The effect is substantial: LSD can increase the length of the first REM period some 160 percent. But it does so only *if* it is given either just before sleep, or one hour after sleep begins (figure 14).[16] And the dose of LSD is also critical. Too high a dose will produce frank awakening just as the REM period is about to begin. In one sense, LSD subjects resemble those light sleepers who tread that fine line between waking up all the way or continuing to dream (see chapter 70).

LSD also injects "micro-REM" segments into the next episodes of slow-wave sleep. They last a mere two to twelve seconds. The above human studies are noteworthy, because relatively *low* LSD doses (30 micrograms) were used to enhance REM episodes. Doses this low help to define two vulnerable transition periods which are highly sensitive to LSD: (1) the moment when S-sleep gives way to desynchronized D-sleep; (2) the moment when this same D-sleep ascends into awakening (see chapter 112).

A *second* key observation is that LSD changes the usual rapid eye movements themselves. It reduces both their number and their speed. Moreover, in slightly greater doses (75 micrograms), LSD also markedly reduces the other fine jiggling movements which a normal person's eyes usually make even when they are at rest.[17] What happens as a result of LSD? Now the subject's gaze becomes concentrated. At this point, these other small jerky (saccadic) eye movements are aligned *into one small portion of the visual field*. It is plausible to think that these two features help to create the subject's feeling that visual experience is being focused narrowly and intensely (see chapter 89).

A *third* important finding is the way LSD *excites both cortical and deep limbic regions*. In humans, LSD increases the fast activity in cortical EEG leads.[9] Schizophrenic patients who receive LSD, in doses varying from 50 to 200 micrograms, also develop lower voltage fast-wave frequencies in deeper subcortical structures (including the caudate, amygdala, hippocampal, and septal regions). Some limbic sites then go on to shift their background activities toward slower frequencies, giving rise to localized paroxysmal bursts lasting for one to ten seconds. In monkeys, relatively low LSD doses also cause partial alerting of cortical activity, plus additional bursts of rhythmic 7 to 8 cps theta rhythms.[18]

A *fourth* lead is based on animal studies. After an animal has already become highly aroused by electrical stimuli delivered to its midbrain reticular formation, LSD cannot further arouse it. This original finding, plus the results of related studies in lower animals, led to an early theory about LSD. Called the "sensory system hypothesis,"[19] it proposed (a) that LSD directly increased the way the reticular formation responded when sensate impulses first came into it but (b) that the drug did *not* directly increase the way these reticular cells then relayed their activations farther on up to the cerebral cortex.[20]

One can summarize much of the above physiological research on LSD with a general observation: the two most sensitive targets are those regions which normally promote behavioral and EEG alerting, and those deep subcortical structures which tend to yield paroxysmal bursts, such as the hippocampus.

Responses to Other Drugs

Other drugs also offer instructive parallels. The early symptoms of amphetamine include heightened awareness, "crystal clear thinking," and an acute sense of novelty. Entering at more advanced stages are preoccupations with "beginnings, meanings and essence," plus insights of various sizes (including a few revelations).[21] Amphetamine causes an increased release and turnover of dopamine and norepinephrine, and repeated abuse of the drug can lead to psychosis.

MDMA ("ecstasy") is a derivative of methamphetamine. It promotes a sense of being closely affiliated with other persons. Its initial effect in animals is to release serotonin from serotonin terminals. Later, however, the brain levels of ST fall. Why? Because, unfortunately, MDMA is selectively toxic to the fine ST terminals issued by the dorsal raphe nucleus. And these ST terminals can remain degenerated for as long as a year.[22]

Cocaine is still the street drug of current notoriety. By some estimates, cocaine is the major offender in the hundreds of *billions* of dollars spent yearly on illicit drugs.[23] Under laboratory conditions, when *low* doses of cocaine are slowly infused intravenously, the subjects first feel a sense of calm well-being.[24] Next, in doses high enough to increase blood pressure, cocaine prompts sudden tearfulness or a mixed picture of euphoria. Yet a highly unpleasant quality may enter during an especially marked affective release. Cocaine does create a temporary increase of alertness and of feelings of energy. Although it decreases the sense of fatigue, the strength of isolated muscles does not improve when strength is measured directly by handgrip tests.[25]

Cocaine increases the active synaptic levels of DA and NE. It does so by blocking their reuptake back into the presynaptic side of the synapse. In animals, cocaine increases the firing rate of circuits within the reticular formation, and it also causes the low voltage fast EEG activities of arousal.[26]

Dopamine systems are a major target of cocaine. People who seek stimulation from increasing doses of cocaine will soon develop strong, compulsive cravings for it. Can anything temporarily satisfy their craving? Bromocriptine can. How? It is a DA *a*gonist drug. Presumably this DA agonist now acts *directly* on DA receptors. Here, it serves as a kind of substitute for those excess synaptic levels of DA which the person had been "expecting" would be the result of cocaine supplied from the outside. Cocaine also influences opioid mechanisms in ways that could drive the brain further to seek out its stimulant effects.[27]

Zen and the Social Problems of Substance Abuse

The planet is suffering from an enormous cultural problem of substance abuse. It is not a new problem, nor one remote from our own hemisphere. The archeological evidence from *Sophora* seeds unearthed in Texas and Mexico suggests that these seeds had been used to alter consciousness as long ago as 8440 B.C.[28]

What happens after the brain undergoes periods of intense, pleasurable receptor stimulation? The brain, enthralled, develops feeling of craving for more of the same. The person's initial outside stimulus might come from tobacco, food, alcohol, or some other drug. No matter which, this initial episode of substance abuse sets the stage for the next subtly perceived *need*. But suppose the person has been able to avoid overstimulating receptors in the first place. Then there would be no basis for any vulnerable receptors having to signal their compulsive need for extra stimulation later on. One recognizes, in the restraining role of *sila*, that principle commonly known as the "ounce of prevention" (see chapter 17). It is a practical matter. The application of reasonably modest levels of moderation and self-restraint will gradually dampen many of the brain's intrinsic needs to have ever-increasing levels of exciting events stimulating its receptors.

"Substance abuse" is a deceptive term. Persons involved in substance abuse are frequently those already prone to get their kicks from *external* sources. Of course, some of them go on to try Zen too. Zen masters have learned to identify which individuals had been previously overexposed to LSD. Theirs is a "leaf in the wind syndrome." They are hypersuggestible, yield to the faintest impulse, and are unable to distinguish the important from the unimportant.[29]

What about the personality profile of the many other searchers who *do not* keep using drugs? They tend to be more interested in processing their own *internal* private fantasies or thoughts. This personal material seems more appealing to them than anything derived from various drugged or hypnotic states.[30]

External chemical substances are only one way to abuse the nervous system and to promote alternate states. Many societies have used other rigorous means. To help cultivate their "vision quest," the northern Native Americans had long used "fasting, thirsting, self-mutilation, torture, exposures to the elements, sleeplessness, incessant dancing, and other means of bringing on total exhaustion, bleeding, plunging into ice-cold pools, near drowning, lacerations with thorns and animal teeth, and other painful ordeals, as well as a variety of non-hurtful 'triggers,' such as different kinds of rhythmic activity, self-hypnosis, meditation, chanting, and drumming."[28]

The emphasis in this book is on the Zen approach to the Middle Way. This means meditation, not medication. Meditation in moderation, not to excess. Indeed, the major meditative disciplines tend to remain very conservative. The fact is, anything that makes the setting and the experience itself more artificial will later make it more difficult to assimilate this brief state in a positive way into the rest of life's ongoing experiences. I do not endorse or use drugs. But many others have tried both routes. Sooner or later, most abandon LSD. It turns out to be an obstacle, not an aid, to their practice of zazen.[31] Watts, recounting his earlier LSD experiments, went on to entitle his later article: "Ordinary Mind Is the Way."[4] "Ordinary mind" meant a state that was clear, stable, and undistracted by hallucinations. This is the Zen Way.

Moreover, people tend to devalue their drug-induced experiences, and for several reasons: (1) The impression lingers that the moments were contrived, counterfeit, something like an "unearned run." (2) The first, hallucinatory, phase of psychedelics can be unpleasant. This unpleasant tone—in ways not yet fully defined—prevents the full impact of the experience from being either fully registered, clearly perceived, or integrated thereafter in a positive transforming way. (3) Persons who shoot up frequently may have other difficulties, primary or acquired, psychiatric, neurological, or legal. These problems prevent them from integrating with the mainstream of society. (4) There is increasing awareness that drugs, cocaine in particular, can damage the brain or kill. (5) Cultural and religious biases persist against "mind-altering" drugs.

These negative biases may be much more ancient than we think. In the original biblical sense of the Garden of Eden, only the fruit from one particular tree was absolutely forbidden. Eat of that fruit, said the serpent, and "your eyes shall be opened, and ye shall be as gods." Michelangelo's painting, *The Fall of Man*, illustrates that it was only after Adam and Eve ignored this injunction, and ate the apple from this tree of knowledge, that they fell from grace. Apple is metaphor. To theo-botanists, the biblical tale of Genesis was the ultimate warning: do not use hallucinogens that are of plant origin.[32]

But even this caveat can be tempered by some of the findings to be discussed in the next chapter. For, in broad brush strokes, we will develop the theme that drugs like LSD do produce *a series of levels and evolving sequences* of psychedelic experience. Interpreted with due caution, *the later* sequences are clearly relevant to Zen.

And by way of a brief introduction to these later sequences, let us close by citing one report illustrating the kind of religious experience that might supervene if LSD is given to a dying patient.

The patient was a physician. He knew he was on the threshold of death from cancer of the pancreas. He received 200 micrograms of LSD intramuscularly. It took longer than usual before his LSD symptoms began, and he skipped over most of the earlier visual phenomena. Yet this physician-patient then entered a deeply unitive experience. His descriptions of it carried a memorable global feeling, and they sounded "alternately like excerpts from Buddhist texts and accounts of Jewish and Christian mystics."[33]

101

Levels and Sequences of Psychedelic Experience after LSD

The psychedelic experience is neither an easy nor a predictable way to God. Many subjects do not have spiritual elements in their sessions despite many exposures to the drug. Those who do have a mystical experience frequently have to undergo psychological ordeals that are at least as difficult and painful as those associated with various aboriginal rites of passage or rigorous and austere religious disciplines.

S. Grof[1]

For exciting events within the brain, 1943 was a vintage year in Switzerland. Not far from where Hess was stimulating cat brains with electricity, an organic chemist, Albert Hofmann, was busy at his laboratory bench. His goal was to resynthesize one of his earlier derivatives of lysergic acid. Later that day, he found his imagery racing, and felt so restless that he was forced to return home. Puzzled by his agitation, he made a remarkably accurate self-diagnosis: it must have been the molecule he had just made in the laboratory.

Three days later, Hofmann followed up his hunch. He took what he thought would be only a tiny oral dose of this substance: a mere 250 micrograms. During the resulting trip his mental functions became so disrupted that he had to abandon his research protocol. This molecule was the twenty-fifth compound in his series. It was lysergic acid diethylamide, LSD-25.

Not until the late 1960s did LSD ("acid") reach its peak of popularity in the United States. Finally, in the Controlled Substances Act of 1970, it was listed as a prohibited drug. Why? Because it had a high potential for abuse and lacked an accepted medical use. However, that was years too late, for by 1970 the genie was irrevocably out of the bottle. LSD is still very much with us. In 1991 the National Institute on Drug Abuse estimated that among those Americans who were under the age of thirty-five, some 10 million had tried it. Nothing in this book is intended to endorse or to sanction the use of psychedelic drugs. However, a prudent look into the phenomenology of these drugs and the ways they act is germane to Zen and the brain.

So, what were the flower children of the 1960s looking for? And what did they find? At the onset, two points bear emphasis. First, as Grof's opening quote makes clear, not until a person has undergone many drug exposures do experiences arise that may be of sustained, practical "religious" import. Second, the alert reader will note something very interesting in the variability of the following accounts and in table 15: even when different experienced observers administer LSD, they each emphasize rather different phenomena. This evidence suggests that their subjects' reports are open to different interpretations. The reports also suggest that their individual subjects are having different responses—to the *same* dose—at different times.

Masters and Houston based their data on 206 drug sessions, and on interviews they had with another 214 persons.[2] Their subjects had used either LSD-25, or peyote (which contains mescaline). Only 5 percent of their psychedelic

Table 15
Two Views of Psychedelic Experiences: Levels, Sequences, and Mixtures*

Masters and Houston[2]	Grof[7, 8]
1. *Sensory level* A "perceptual feast."	1. *Abstract and aesthetic experiences* Vivid colors and illusions differ when eyes are opened or closed.
2. *Recollective-analytic level* Past experiences, relived.	2. *Psychodynamic experiences* Personal memories, condensed and released with an affective charge. This category has "Freudian" aspects.
3. *Symbolic level* Symbolic mythological and ritual themes. This level includes a pervasive "affective consciousness."	3. *(Existential) experiences of various types* Grof places "cosmic unity" in this phase, noting that it too is experienced differently depending on whether the eyes are open or closed. Some existential experiences, occurring in mixtures, have a "very definite transpersonal flavor." Some culminate in ego death and rebirth. This category has "Rankian" or "Reichian" aspects.
4. *Deep integral level* Authentic religious experiences; not "cosmological mysticism." Includes a "spiritual consciousness," which has the flavor of eternity.	4 *Transpersonal experiences* This somewhat "Jungian" category includes 26 examples, some still within conventional objective reality. Of those others outside it, two examples are (a) "consciousness of the universal mind," and (b) the "supracosmic and metacosmic void." Mixtures occur with existential types which resist classifications.

*Note that these two approaches to classification start out the same but then diverge.

subjects underwent a fundamental, positive, integrative transformation: a mere 11 out of the original 206.

As a parallel with persons who undertake meditative training, *it is noteworthy that many psychedelic subjects tend to pass through a sequence of changes.* Masters and Houston distinguished four of these general levels.

1. *The sensory level.* During this, the subjects undergo a "perceptual feast" of vividly colored, evolving aesthetic images. Especially marked when the eyes are closed, the images (which the authors referred to as "eidetic") usually involve persons, animals, architecture, or landscapes. These appear either as single, unrelated "pictures," or as a sequence of related "pictures." Neither type has much meaning or function for the subject.

2. *The recollective-analytic level.* Next, visual images become more purposive and personalized. Emotion deepens, and boundaries dissolve between consciousness and unconsciousness. Past experiences are relived, and release emotions in the process.

3. *The symbolic level.* In this deeper level, the person now enters into symbolic dramas either as a spectator or as a participant. The themes have common mythological and ritualistic overtones. They include the rites of initiation, those of passage, and those of the eternal return. At the symbolic level, the person's usual forms of consciousness still keep track of what goes on. Even so, there may enter another variation on the theme of consciousness. It is called "affective consciousness." It is the seeping in of a quiet, but powerful, beneficent "atmosphere" or "climate." The subject becomes aware of this pervasive emotional response but has no voluntary control over it. I was once infiltrated by precisely this kind of atmosphere during the later portions of a state of internal absorption (see chapter 119).

4. *The deep integral level.* Only at this level do authentically religious experiences finally arise. On LSD, this experience is an emotionally charged, direct encounter with the ultimate level of reality. It presents a transforming interpretation of the person in the world. It can also wipe out old behavioral constraints. This fourth level can also give rise to yet another type of consciousness. It is called "spiritual consciousness." It occurs in mature, well-developed persons, and addresses the ultimate issue: that person's existence and existence in general. It is a totally new and unfamiliar perspective, carrying the "flavor of eternity." This novel mode of consciousness lies far beyond the person's usual categories of space, time, and existence. Part VII considers another personal experience at this level.

Masters and Houston "guided" their subjects through their drug trips. In the process, these authors also devised positive criteria—as had Zen masters centuries before them—for validating which psychedelic experience was "authentically religious." One notes below how important was the issue of *sequences* in the three major criteria which they set up. For, if the experience was to be validated as authentically religious, their subjects had to pass three hurdles. They would need (1) to have directly encountered the ultimate reality at the fourth, deep integral level; (2) to have passed previously through each of the three prior sequences, while undergoing a major cumulative expansion of personal insights and associations; and (3) to have been thereafter transformed.

The authors' three *exclusion* criteria are also pertinent. Like Zen masters, they rejected (1) *most visual imagery,* on the grounds that it was not accompanied by a true "religious" emotion. Even though some 91 percent of their subjects had visualized temples, churches, or other religious settings, they appreciated their images primarily for their impressive architectural features alone; (2) *experiences of intense empathy,* such as the "euphoria-inducing experience of empathy with a chair." Empathy experiences were impressive, especially when they occurred along with a loss of ego and dissolution of the body image. Religious professionals were particularly prone to mistake the sow's ear of mere empathy experiences for the silk purse of sacramental or authentic religious experiences; (3) *experiences of "cosmological mysticism."* Almost half of the LSD subjects had these ecstatic experiences. They carried a pervasive sense of deep insight into, and identify with, the essential nature and structure of the universe. The subjects described them in terms of energy states or in pantheistic terms. Why did the authors choose *not* to regard them as religious experiences? First, because they did not transform. Second, because they only rarely involved a personal encounter with what was perceived as "Ultimate Being." The authors took the position that the "scientific arcana of cosmological mysticism" was but a "subliminal triumph of the weekly news magazines." They hypothesized that the subject had become familiar, through prior exposure, with the buzzwords and hypotheses out at the new frontiers of science.[2]

Only 3 percent of Masters and Houston's psychedelic subjects (6 out of 206 participants) met their criteria for a subcategory called "Unitary Consciousness." It emerged out of their fourth, deepest integral level, and was empty of all "sensuous or conceptual or other empirical content."[3,4] Who were these six persons? Were they different in other ways?

To begin with, they had older brains. All were over forty years of age, intelligent, well-adjusted, and creative. They were also a highly motivated group, for they had either sought out mystical experiences in previous meditative or spiritual disciplines or had long maintained a major interest in integral levels of consciousness in general. Their prior years of preparation had left them with a "somewhat abstracted attitude." During their first, sensory level on LSD, these few mature subjects showed an especially rich array of psychedelic phenomena. However, they then barely skimmed over the second and third level of experiences. As a result, they arrived rather quickly at the threshold of the fourth, integral level of experience.

At this point, these six subjects then had remarkably stereotyped experiences.[4] The episode usually began with the ego dissolving into "boundless being" amid a perception of extreme light. Categories of time vanished into eternity. The world was transfigured into an undifferentiated unity. Knower, knowledge, and known all became one. Thereafter, the person became more interested in, and more responsive to, the basic phenomena of everyday existence. This latter quality is an essential aspect of Zen transformations. When it becomes permanent, it is no small accomplishment. Nonetheless, when a psychedelic *drug* precipitated this rare kind of acute experience, it *rarely* went on to transform the person in the same radical way as did those other *spontaneous* religious experiences, occurring without the use of drugs, which would also have reached the integral level.

Why weren't these six psychedelic subjects more transformed? The authors speculated: Had their long previous experience already matured them to the point where they finally had less room, as it were, for further transformation? Or, given the fact that these six subjects had been already more advanced in some respects, had they somehow missed the beneficial aspects of working through the earlier levels of their own psychodynamic material? Three other speculations might be added. Had these subjects been deprived of some rigorous psychophysiological benefits, as yet undefined, which might have accrued during previous deep absorptions? (see chapter 152). Were they basically a subset of different personalities (with different brains) to begin with? Did they have a different kind of experience because their brains had gone through the process of aging? (see chapter 153). Whatever the underlying reason(s), by the time these six subjects finally did take a psychedelic drug, it seemed to have given them "the final push off the mystical brink" on which they were already standing.[5]

At this point in the discussion, it may need to be emphasized that on LSD a person may enter a state otherwise typical of internal absorption. Consider the following excellent description by a normal subject who had taken 150 micrograms of LSD.

> There was an awareness of many directions—but all at once . . . There was no longer a "I" or a "me". . . There was just vast, total nothing . . . There was no sound but there was the hearing of no sound. There was nothing to see but there was seeing of this nothing to see. Dualities ceased, there was just a wonderful moving in nothing—empty, still and quite nothing.[6]

Which of these phenomena are typical of absorption? They include the omnidirectional expansion of awareness, the explicit loss of the bodily I and Me, and the striking way that sound and vision drop out from the usual sensate realm (see part VI).

To some, psychedelic mystical experience "*is* mystical experience."[2] Yes and no. Some small *segments* appear authentic. Still, I side with Masters and Houston in concluding as follows: when one takes a critical view of the psychedelic type of experience not in terms of its isolated segments, but in its total context, it differs "diametrically" from that emerging in the Zen meditative context. To cite only three of the reasons why this is so:

1. The trained meditative subject, not exposed to drugs, learns gradually to empty the mind. In contrast, the subject driven by psychedelics is self-propelled into a sustained roller coaster ride, exposed to a heavy barrage of pressing perceptual, affective, and other mental phenomena.

2. The drug experience lasts much longer. Some psychedelic subjects remain in their affect-charged experience at the integral level for from fifteen minutes up to

two hours or more. After this encounter, they don't wish to return to another psychedelic experience in the near future.

3. The drug experience transforms less frequently, and to a lesser degree.

Grof's accounts are of additional interest, because he summarizes seventeen years of experiences giving LSD[7,8] and analyzes almost 5000 records.[1] He specified two techniques for giving LSD.

1. *High-dose psychedelic therapy.* This meant one to three sessions, using "overwhelming" doses, which ranged from 300 to 500 micrograms, by mouth. The goal was to prompt a deeper mystical or religious experience. The patients were lying down, used eyeshades, listened to stereophonic music through headphones, and had minimal verbal contact. This setting is not that of zazen.

But sometimes he conducted a session outdoors, in the mountains or at the seashore. And it turned out that, in one sense, there was a kind of "power" in this natural outdoor setting. We return to this theme subsequently (see chapters 105 and 154). Indeed, on these "externalized" occasions, Grof found that *if* the subject's eyes remained open he would have to reduce the dose below 100 micrograms. Otherwise, his high dose approach soon activated so much unconscious material that it distorted the way the subjects perceived their environment. In even more complex environments, LSD caused such a mishmash of perceptions and *mis*perceptions that there was no possibility of keeping any fruitful introspections on-line. Clearly, this is not the goal of zazen.

2. *Lower-dose psycholytic therapy.* This meant giving LSD at intervals of every one or two weeks, and in doses ranging from 75 to 300 micrograms. These drug sessions were repeated between 15 and 100 times, and averaged around 40.[1]

Over this longitudinal period of months, it became clear that, even though a given patient was taking the same LSD dose each time, each trip was usually very different, both in content, character, and course. Sometimes an LSD session might plunge to become experientially profound, even though this person had skipped over the otherwise typical early visual perceptual changes. Sympathetic and parasympathetic symptoms also varied remarkably, bearing no necessary relationship to the dose. For example, the pupils were usually dilated, but they could be constricted, or could vary between being large and small. Constricted pupils, incidentally, occur in D-sleep, where they are an expression of heightened cholinergic tone in the brain stem.

What hard facts emerge from such observations? Reading between the lines, we begin to understand why *spontaneous* mystical experiences are also so variable. Put simply, the collected evidence suggests that different experiences—spontaneous or drug-induced—will tend to surge up when the person's brain is in slightly different phases, either of its three major physiological cycles (waking, dreaming, or sleeping) or of their transitions (see chapter 77). With regard to dreaming, Grof made an interesting observation. The kind of dreams his subject had *before* the LSD session often *anticipated* the content of the subsequent psychedelic session itself.[9]

In Grof's patients, LSD produced two general categories of effects: (1) enhanced mental processes, and (2) a qualitative *change* in consciousness. This change ran in the direction of a dreamlike state. For these reasons, Grof believed that LSD was only a *non*specific catalyst, one which amplified the person's existing biochemical and physiological processes. He felt that the drug produced "an undifferentiated activation." This activation was the process which facilitated "the emergence of unconscious material from different levels of the personality."[10]

Suppose we agree that the drug LSD is merely a catalyst. But, we're going to go a step further, to conclude that meditation, likewise, *is a catalyst for moments of activation* in the brain. The proposal carries three important implications. One is that both LSD and meditation are *undifferentiated* activators. That they act only by helping to release the latent potentials already there (already described are the brain's ample resources for its arousals and activations; see chapters 36, 37, and 53). Another implication is that each of the two agents can teach us what kinds of optional states and substates the brain is capable of. Finally, it should not surprise us to find that certain *segments* of the meditative and LSD experiences do appear identical, phenomenologically.

Any patient who could endure the ordeals of forty LSD sessions must surely have trusted the therapist. Grof believed that he had built this trusting relationship on one basic premise. This starting point was the larger "worldview." It was the same universal philosophical base from which all forms of mentation ascend to operate freely, without boundaries. Grof also had a strategy. It emphasized living in *this* present moment, free from notions about the past or future. And what if some of his patients lacked those positive feelings which would be able to affirm life's everyday experiences? Then Grof would encourage them to seek these feelings "inside, through a process of deep self-exploration and inner transformation," not through trying to manipulate external circumstances alone.[11] The reader will notice how closely these approaches resemble the procedures which Zen masters have been refining and practicing for centuries.

Grof went on to develop his own versions of the categories of psychedelic experiences (see table 15). They were also four in number. Note again that these four also tended to emerge in a distinctive sequence, even though they did not seem to reflect any linear or stratified system.[12] He chose to emphasize different features, and would give a more psychoanalytic flavor to some of the later ones.

1. *Abstract and aesthetic experiences.* These occur early in each session, at lower or medium LSD dosages. They are seldom present in more advanced sessions. Bizarre optical illusions evolve into "orgies of vision," and synesthesias occur in which music is "seen," colors "tasted."

2. *Psychodynamic experiences.* Grof interpreted these as a relatively specific constellation of condensed memories and related fantasies drawn from different periods in each individual person's life.

3. *Existential experiences of various types.** This is more of a mixture than a category. The subject can undergo dramatic, unbearable pangs of birth, pain, disease,

---

*Some such noncommittal term seems a preferable substitute for Grof's second "perinatal" category, which, as he carefully pointed out, is a word which might imply premises that could only be tentative.

dying, and death. These themes tend to arise during the early high-dosage LSD sessions among more stable, normal subjects who have no serious emotional problems. But when they occur in psychiatric patients, they tend to follow in sequence the previous level of psychodynamic experiences.

There is room here to allude to only one positive form that such an experience can take.[13] Grof originally described it as an "experience of cosmic unity." It was beyond self/other distinctions, and beyond time and space. The person experienced direct insights into the essence of being and existence, insights stamped by strong feelings of certainty. It was also pervaded by an exceptionally strong positive affect and a sacred quality. The sense of peace and bliss could approach "oceanic ecstasy."

It suffices here to emphasize one other important point about vision that we will expand on later (in chapter 139, table 19). Grof found that *his subjects' experiences differed in ways which depended on whether their eyes were closed or opened.* Clearly, this is another reason why psychedelic experience varies. To illustrate: the subject whose *eyes are closed* will experience the tension-free phenomenon of "cosmic unity as an independent, complex, experiential pattern."[14] In contrast, *when this same subject opens the eyes,* there occurs the sense of "merging with the environment" as well as feelings of "unity" with the objects that are being perceived.[15] At this moment, with the eyes open, the world is then seen as a place of indescribable radiance and beauty. Now the subject, imbued "with feelings of complete security," sees no negative aspects either in the world or "in the very structure of the cosmic design." In this perfection, "everything is as it should be."[16]

In chapter 132, we will observe how some aspects of these *open-eyed* LSD experiences of unity do resemble the qualities of "suchness," perfection, and lack of fear which arise during the Zen experience of awakening. Another similarity: some insights which arise in the psychedelic setting are totally foreign to the person's previous traditional religious beliefs. Thus, "a Moslem may get insight into the law of karma and cycles of reincarnation; and a Rabbi may experience a conversion towards Zen Buddhism." Why, then, do the subjects go on to accept such "strange" insights? Because they do *not* seem strange. The subjects interpret them as being completely appropriate and compatible with their own *basic* personality.[17]

One does well to remember how many negative, uncomfortable experiences are included in Grof's third category. One of them is a hellish existence, nonsensical and monstrous. Another presents first as a titanic struggle with unbearable suffering, followed by a "volcanic ecstasy," and major symptomatic complaints. Blinding white light, or golden light, can occur along with an expansion of space.

Grof also describes in frightening terms the "ego death" that finally comes after many repeated LSD sessions. When LSD prompts this phase of personal dissolution, it carries a sense of complete catastrophic annihilation. Grof believes that most persons will finally complete this harrowing process—which implies their going from "ego death" to "rebirth"—*if* they undergo repeated sessions, using high doses of pure LSD, in a setting where they have become active participants in an in-depth exploration of self. When the brighter avenue finally does open, it can lead into the positive elements of "cosmic unity," and then into this following final category of experiences.

> 4. *Transpersonal experiences.* "Transpersonal" experiences mean that the person feels that consciousness expands beyond the usual boundaries of the personal ego, and past the usual limitations of time and space. These experiences do not usually arrive until the subject has undergone many prior separate LSD sessions. In sequence, they tend to follow the second and third categories of experience. Some are more "Jungian" than others.[18] They, too, can occur mixed in with the existential types of the third category.

Two broad subgroups exist within this fourth, transpersonal category. In the first, though consciousness seems to expand, it still retains the usual time and space frameworks of ordinary reality. However, in the second subgroup, the psychedelic experiences escape beyond space-time boundaries. The reader can appreciate this point from the words used to describe two of the latter: "Consciousness of the Universal Mind" and "The Supracosmic and Metacosmic Void."[19]

A major qualification remains. The subjects on LSD may feel certain that they have intuitively grasped the essence of the universe. But have they totally comprehended at that moment its every cause-and-effect relationship? No skeptic would agree. Their insights, in short, do not answer specific questions that can be logically framed. Rather, something else occurs. For as soon as the subjects have stepped outside those former boundaries which had constrained their old concepts of cause and effect, of space and time, they will have then entered *a novel system of reference.* Everything is different herein. Here, the old urgent questions either don't exist, are no longer relevant, or don't need to be asked.[1] As Kobori-roshi had once predicted, "Finally you will stop asking your questions."

Transpersonal LSD sessions are "a continuing philosophical and spiritual search . . . aimed at solving the riddles of personal identity, human existence, and the universal scheme."[20] The search carries the "sense of belonging, meaning, natural spirituality, and synergistic participation."[21] One can say the same, of course, of the Zen Way. The cautious reader, realistically concerned about the complications of LSD as well as its other pros and cons, is well advised to read chapters 3 and 5, and the appendix of Grof's book.[1]

Stimulated by the permissive drug culture of the 1960s and 1970s, many curious people then took LSD, of variable purity, on their own. Terms such as "theo-pharmacology" crept in, along with that bankrupt phrase, "Turn on, tune in, drop out." Alan Watts also took LSD, after having had three earlier "natural and spontaneous" mystical experiences.[22] He felt that his first LSD experiment was an interesting aesthetic and intellectual experience. His next two LSD exposures went deeper than his previous spontaneous experiences. They also had "a peculiar quality of unexpectedness." Watts then distinguished four dominant themes in his subsequent experiences on psychedelics:

1. *A slowing down of time* and a concentration in the present moment.

2. *An awareness of the interdependence of opposites.* He used saints and sinners as an example. Explicitly different, each helps to define the other.

3. *An awareness of relativity:* Innumerable forms and levels of life are all linked in an infinite hierarchy, all being part of the same thing.

4. *An awareness of eternal energy,* conveying the notion that energy lies at the center of all existence, frequently accompanied by an intense white light.

The Self/Other Interface

Psychedelic and spontaneous mystical experiences can each radically modify the self/other boundary. Snyder, a world-renowned neuropharmacologist, described how it felt when LSD evaporated this interface between his self and his non-self. First came a "serene sense of being at one with the universe." ... "All is one, All is one" ... But then this feeling gave way to the terrifying loss of awareness of who he was. During this phase he called out, "Who am I? Where is the world?"[23]

What does the slow, prosaic route of meditative training offer, by way of contrast? It serves two major functions: (1) it familiarizes the meditator with the loss of this self/other boundary; (2) it quiets down, relatively selectively, some fear-generating circuitries deep in the brain. Gradually, in these two ways does the training not only help the meditator steer clear of states which are disruptive and disintegrative but also contributes to the emergence of ongoing *positive* experiences, to those which promote a stable, ongoing reintegration.

Jordan, a teacher of religious studies, tried to express in words the four different ways that LSD radically modified his "self."[24] It could help the reader appreciate how subtle are the properties of these changes if you imagine that you are experiencing the events listed below as immediate realizations, not in the form of your own usual thought-filled conceptualizations.

1. Everything is Self,* including myself.

2. Certain objects or people become quite literally myself, even though the other boundaries of the larger Self remain as before. A strong sense of empathy goes out to these Self-identified people or objects.

3. While remaining essentially myself, this larger Self takes on a more relative existence in relation to others. This larger Self no longer exists as a completely independent entity. "I" and "other" interact interdependently, and with empathy.

4. Self and other give way to "beingness." Beingness goes on in the absence of the universal Self. However, during the process, conscious awareness still continues, and "perhaps more clearly than ever, with all the activities of body, mind, feeling, other humans, stars, sun, sky, earth, etc., continuing on in a complex, boundless flow neither chaotic nor orderly."

---

*In place of this confusing word, Self, as spelled with a capital *S*, the reader may wish to substitute something like "the larger universal principle."

As one reflects over the nature of these curious descriptions by Snyder and Jordan, one begins to appreciate how extraordinary it is to feel that one's basic self/other boundary has been dissolved and transformed into "beingness" (see chapter 145).

Even so, it might seem to the reader that some of the shallower psychedelic quickenings reviewed in recent chapters were only tangential to the substance of Zen. And were hardly relevant to the oceanic Zen described and lived by authentic masters like Rinzai, Hakuin, and Dogen. So, it is time to put the book down for awhile. To let go of it. Let *go* . . .

Besides, next in the offing* is a "miracle," of sorts.

102

The Miracle of Marsh Chapel

We may be trying against insurmountable odds to communicate what is incommunicable and requires to be experienced.

R. Masters and J. Houston[1]

The question now to be addressed is, What effects do psychedelic drugs have, not in some artificial laboratory or other setting, but in religious rituals? In keeping with a new field which seemed already to have mushroomed overnight, Hofmann went on to make his second chemical contribution. He purified psilocybin, and then identified it as the active agent of the special "magic mushroom" which the native tribes of Central America had long used in their religious ceremonies.[2] The chemical structure of psilocybin turned out to resemble serotonin even more so than did his original molecule of LSD-25. A mere four years elapsed before psilocybin would be tested under highly elevated, if not rarified, circumstances. The rituals took place not in some distant jungle but in Boston, no less. The occasion would become known as "The Miracle of Marsh Chapel."

The presiding investigator in 1962 was a psychiatrist who had previously received his Doctor of Divinity degree.[3] His name was Walter Pahnke, and he stated that he had no prior personal experience with psychedelic drugs. He asked the following question: Would a psychedelic drug, added within the framework of a religious service, enhance the "religious" aspects of the mystical state of consciousness?

First, he had to decide which phenomena would be his criteria for such a "mystical" state. He settled on the categories of (1) unity, (2) transcendence of time and space, (3) deeply felt positive mood, (4) sense of sacredness, (5) objectivity and reality, (6) paradoxicality, (7) alleged ineffability, (8) transiency, (9) persisting positive changes in attitude and behavior.

Pahnke then devised a controlled experiment. He chose twenty Christian theological students, none of whom had been exposed before to psilocybin or to related drugs. Only half of the group would receive the active drug. The dose of

---

*Offing. That part of the deep ocean which one can already see by standing on the shore and looking out to sea. *In the offing.* In the near or foreseeable future.

psilocybin was set at thirty milligrams for each of the ten experimental subjects, and at fifteen milligrams for five of his group leaders. The remaining ten control subjects and their other five group leaders would each receive 200 milligrams of nicotinic acid, also by mouth, as a placebo. This dose of nicotinic acid produces flushing of the face, warmth, and tingling. It is an "active" placebo. Its side effects reinforce the power of suggestion, and convince people that they must have taken something. Pahnke and his group leaders then prepared a positive, trusting, religious atmosphere. They selected a special time and place for their experiment, and further enhanced its devotional qualities. They chose Good Friday.

On that Friday, in 1962, their subjects entered Marsh Chapel on the Boston University campus. Here they listened to a two-and-a-half-hour religious service. Pahnke collected his data not only during the experiment but at various times up to six months afterward. It is useful to begin with the kinds of experiences his *control* subjects reported, for these reports convey the flavor of the setting itself and the way it affected the participants.

What the control subjects most commonly experienced was "love." The maximum possible score a person might reach for "love" had been set at 100, and this group of control subjects was rated as having reached 33 percent of this maximum. (A reasonable enough result, given the combination of a chapel service plus a placebo.) The next most frequent finding was the report that the subjects had developed a persistent, *positive* attitude or behavior. This was rated at 31 percent of the maximum. Sacredness was scored at 28 percent. Of only passing note here was the degree to which these same controls rated an experience called "unity." Internal unity was rated at a level four times higher (8%) than was that of external unity (2%).

There was no doubt about which subjects had taken psilocybin. Most commonly, they reported having transcended time and space (84 percent vs. only 6 percent in the controls). Their other highly rated categories included transient experience (79 percent), ineffability (66 percent), objective reality (63 percent), unity (62 percent), paradoxicality (61 percent), deeply felt positive mood (57 percent), and a change in attitude and behavior which persisted after the experiment was over (57 percent).

The psilocybin subjects also rated high on the scale for unity. They reported levels of internal unity (70 percent) almost twice as high as external unity (38 percent). Their deeply felt positive mood was one either of love (57 percent), or of joy, blessedness, and peace (rated as 51 percent). The psilocybin subjects believed they had undergone a persistent positive change as the result of an attitudinal change in *themselves* (57 percent), whereas the control group was rated at only 6 percent in this subcategory. Pahnke considered that psilocybin had played only a facilitating role. He believed that the drug was a necessary ingredient, but was not sufficient in itself to explain the results.

After completing his follow-up interviews, Pahnke concluded that their Marsh Chapel experience had made a profound impact on the lives of eight of the ten subjects who had received psilocybin. The change was especially evident in terms of their religious feeling and thinking. Whatever other qualifications exist on this pioneering experiment, especially noteworthy is the fact that it was conducted in the context of an authentic religious service, not in a laboratory. As a result, the participants could derive special meaning from Marsh Chapel's religious symbols, and the whole Good Friday atmosphere also provided a framework within which they could begin to integrate their experiences.

The Ritual Use of Mescaline

Mescaline is of interest because its chemical structure resembles that of the catecholamines (dopamine and norepinephrine), not that of serotonin. Mescaline is a major active ingredient in the buttons obtained from the peyote plant. Peyote can still be used legally in rituals by the Native American Church and the indians of Mexico.[4] Subjects who remain silent, in solitude and self-absorption, develop more visual hallucinations on mescaline. When their eyes are open, the outer world appears as though seen through "a veil of unreality." Through such a veil, the subjects interpret a given object as being completely different and "unreal," even though it has not otherwise changed its color and shape. Hearing seems sensitized, and time appears to lengthen in a rush of many fantastic thoughts.

On mescaline, some subjects feel that something has been "taken away" from their personality. Others feel something strange is being substituted. In a kind of dual awareness, two separate beings may be present. One is a "fantastic being of delusion and fantasy." The other, seeming intellectual and emotionless, observes the first with extraordinary detachment. Space may extend to the point of infinity; rooms may become huge chambers or seem filled with a strange and unearthly light. A feeling of depression during the first half-hour can then give way to euphoria and elation. Even after the major symptoms and signs of mescaline intoxication disappear, the person remains very restless, highly aroused, unable to sleep, and has no appetite.

Blofeld took mescaline after having studied Buddhism for many years. His initial response was terrifying. Suddenly, his terror subsided. At this moment he also let go of himself, totally surrendered, and entered into an ecstatic experience of undifferentiated unity and unutterable bliss: "I felt as though, after many years of anxious search for the answer to some momentous problem, I was suddenly confronted with a solution so wholly satisfying and so entirely simple that I had to burst out laughing. I was conscious of immense joy and of incredulous amazement at my own stupidity in having taken so long to discover the simple truth."[5] We have discussed this particular laughter, the kind that erupts when old complex mental sets give way, in an earlier chapter (see chapter 99).

After his mescaline experience subsided, Blofeld examined an important issue. What had determined its content? Had he *learned* these things from his previous Buddhist teachers, his studies, and practices? No, he concluded, the drug experience was "much too foreign to my previous understanding of those teachings to have been a subjective illusion based on them." I agree completely with this conclusion, having been astonished by the content of the states I experienced without having taken drugs.

On psychedelics, it is common for the subject to be overtaken by a feeling of great surprise once his or her personal identity finally drops off.[6] One recalls how Watts describes a "peculiar quality of unexpectedness," and notes Blofeld's words of "incredulous amazement." Yet this is but one of many surprising events. For the psychedelic subjects encounter other major changes. These alter their perception of the clarity and size of space, and the speed with which time passes.

Are such striking perceptual changes innocuous? Or, in themselves, could they create affective consequences? It is not widely appreciated that similar perceptual modifications do engender major *secondary* effects. This fact became evident when normal subjects were studied under hypnosis.[7] Suppose you place normal, *non*drugged subjects under hypnosis. You then give them the suggestion that in the *post*hypnotic period they will go on to experience alterations of space, vision, size, or time. More specifically, your posthypnotic suggestions to them further include *space* that has no depth or is expanded in depth; *vision* that is blurred, clear, or distinct; objects that are larger or smaller in *size; time* that is fast, slow, or stopped.

In one of these studies, male subjects were instructed during hypnosis that their perception would later change. Their responses to this subsequent change were contrasted with the responses of hypnotized controls. The controls had *not* been given posthypnotic suggestions. An independent clinical observer then interviewed each subject, unaware of the experimental design.

Seven of the hypnotized subjects had received posthypnotic suggestions that their dimension of visual depth would expand. They developed positive feelings, as well as an enhanced visual awareness of the world. Three in this group were so impressed by how much more orderly the world now seemed that they viewed this event as having religious significance. In contrast, unpleasant symptoms followed the posthypnotic suggestion that space had no depth. These negative symptoms resembled the kind of bad trips that people have on psychedelic drugs. The blinded outside evaluator was led to wonder whether these "no depth" subjects were schizophrenic.

What happened after it was suggested that vision would become clear and distinct? The subjects developed an attention to small details, a preoccupation with the world, and an impression of its beauty. Most subjects also became energized. The suggestion that time would change produced a still different set of posthypnotic phenomena. These subjects became anxious if they were under "fast" time. During "slow" time, they developed depressed feelings. Moreover, changes in body image, withdrawal, depression, and feelings of unreality emerged after it had been suggested to them that time had "stopped."

The powers of "positive thinking," of belief and suggestion are well-known ingredients in religious rituals, whether in chapel, temple, or elsewhere. However, we still know rather little about the physiology of hypnosis, and this ignorance qualifies the interpretations one might draw from the foregoing experiment. Still, the data emphasize how even the *suggestion* that perception is modified can itself go on to be associated with other distinctive symptoms and changes in behavior. So the studies raise an intriguing issue: How much of the phenomena in psychedelic and spontaneous alternate states of consciousness might come about because the brain has shifted the way it *sees* and perceives space and time?

This question serves to preview how important it is to have a better understanding of space and time. Indeed, these two topics will later be discussed in four separate chapters (see chapters 114, 121, 134, and 135).

How Do Psychedelic Drugs Affect Amine Receptors?

It is not easy to establish relationships among psychedelic drugs, neurotransmitters, brain activity and states of consciousness. The brain is complex and inaccessible to delicate experimental manipulation by chemical means.

L. Grinspoon[1]

A true statement. But the normal brain can function well only when its own chemical signals are being delivered by the most delicate means available. This leads us to consider receptors. A receptor is a long chain of many peptides which loops repeatedly in and out of the cell's outer membrane. This microarchitecture enables the receptor to serve as a go-between. Outside, the receptor's first assignment is to recognize the specific chemical configuration of its primary messenger molecule. Then, as this key-into-lock process continues, it will set off two kinds of responses which transduce this message inside the cell. The first responses are of the quick electrical variety. The second are the slow, secondary *metabolic* responses (see chapter 48).

In the preceding chapters of part V, we have observed that both psychedelic drugs and intensive meditative training procedures promote prominent excitatory phenomena. Why do some of these effects closely resemble one another? To begin to understand, it is useful to start with two model receptors for norepinephrine. These tiny "buttons," each shaped to receive a molecule of NE, serve as initial models for the other amine receptors.

Norepinephrine Receptors

The NE beta-receptors are poised to modulate memory, as well as motor and sensory functions. In the human brain, they are most dense in the hippocampus (especially in its CA1 region) where they influence its data-processing functions.[2] What happens elsewhere, say in sensory systems, when NE activates its beta-receptors? First, the next cell *slows*. But this only occurs because beta-receptors suppress its spontaneous background firing activity. For the final result of this brief inhibition will soon be to improve the signal-to-noise ratio of this postsynaptic cell. Now those next waves of other incoming impulses can stimulate the cell into stronger excitatory synaptic responses.

Norepinephrine alpha$_1$-receptors also promote excitation. Their approach is slightly more direct. Usually, the brain's synaptic excitations last for only tens of milliseconds.[3] But excitation lasts for *hundreds of milliseconds* once NE activates its alpha$_1$-receptors. Still, even these long-lasting alpha$_1$ responses will not, in *themselves*, prompt the next nerve cell to fire. For, once again, this target cell must also be receiving other kinds of major excitatory input at the same time. So, when NE acts on its alpha$_1$-receptor, one sees a typical example of a *neuromodulator* system in action. It does not initiate. It *amplifies* some other major *transmitter* function which is already ongoing[4] (see chapter 34).

Serotonin Receptors

The salient impact of many psychedelic drugs falls early on the receptors for norepinephrine, serotonin, and dopamine (see chapter 44). Thereafter, when the first wave of these receptor responses takes over, studies of behavior illustrate that physiological constraints are soon placed on unrestrained excitability. Consider, as one example of this point, the psilocybin which Pahnke had given in Marsh Chapel. Taken by mouth, this drug desynchronizes the human EEG, increases the speed with which the EEG reacts to each single flash of light, and shortens the time it needs to recover after each flash.[5] Yet even at the very moment when the person's EEG is now responding more briskly, the side effects inherent in excessive arousal still *slow* the person's *behavioral* reaction times.

In chemical structure, LSD and psilocybin resemble ST. LSD stops the firing of ST nerve cells in the raphe nuclei. And LSD also causes prominent visual hallucinations. Simple question: Did LSD release these hallucinations because it had blocked the raphe cells from firing? For LSD does act as a direct ST agonist on many different kinds of ST receptors. And some of these ST receptors also reside on raphe cells themselves. There, they act to inhibit their own cell's firing.[6] We have also seen that the discharge rate of raphe cells drops off to its lowest level during desynchronized sleep. Therefore, it might seem as though that simple question has an easy cause-and-effect answer: the sole reason LSD seems to be enhancing REM episodes, *and* hallucinations, is because it acts to stop ST cells from firing (see chapter 100).

Not so fast. This cannot be the final answer. LSD acts in more intricate ways, and ST systems themselves are more complex. Recent evidence suggests that LSD acts not only as an agonist at ST1a receptors but also as an *antagonist* at ST2 receptors.[7,8] Moreover, we now know that even when ST cells of the raphe nuclei do slow down, this slackening need not have any simple direct relationship with LSD-induced behaviors.[9,10]

Other evidence also stands in the way of easy generalizations. Mescaline too, causes hallucinations. But when mescaline is applied locally in the raphe nucleus, it does *not* inhibit ST cell firing there. True, lisuride does block the firing of cells in the dorsal raphe nucleus in animals. But in human subjects lisuride does not cause hallucinations.[11] Repeated doses of LSD in cats still keep slowing the firing rates of their raphe cells. However, these treated cats no longer show their previous behavioral reactions to the drug. Humans who take LSD each day also find that LSD no longer produces its psychic changes after the fourth daily dose.[12]

Moreover, LSD also enhances the actions of norepinephrine. These mechanisms are *indirect*. For example, two things occur when LSD or mescaline is microinjected into the locus ceruleus: (1) each drug inhibits the ongoing spontaneous background firing of these NE cells; (2) each drug causes the NE cells to fire more when they respond to sensory volleys sent up from stimulation of the sciatic nerve down in the leg. Again, the two drugs share the familiar property of increasing the signal-to noise ratio.

But both hallucinogens also share a different kind of action. This one is also *indirect*. For LSD and mescaline also activate ST2 receptors. These ST2 receptors reside on other postsynaptic cells, on cells far distant from the neurons in the locus ceruleus. And present evidence suggests that these ST2 receptors on distant cells play a key role in producing the hallucinations that are caused by various psychedelic drugs.[13] Especially do ST2 receptors cover the particular target nerve cells at higher levels which receive their ST from the ST cells of the dorsal raphe nucleus[14] (see figure 7). Target cells up in the frontal cortex are among these nerve cells rich in ST2 receptors.

But the process does not stop here. It is not limited to those cells which are covered by ST2 receptors. For another set of impulses then returns from such far distant, postsynaptic target cells, and these impulses travel back down to the brain stem. Here again, the result is to make *norepinephrine* cells fire faster in response to sensate stimuli arriving from the outside.[9] Put simply, there are several avenues through which *an initial activation of ST2 receptors can translate, indirectly, into an increased release of NE.*

In primates, dense networks of NE terminals envelop most sensory pathways. So whichever ST mechanism causes more NE to be released can soon go on to influence perceptual functions throughout many vital regions.[15] An increased release of NE in regions such as the pulvinar, lateral posterior thalamic nuclear group, caudal parietal cortex, superior colliculus, and the reticular nucleus of the thalamus could contribute to the remarkable sensate phenomena caused by LSD or mescaline. Neuroimaging studies of primates should soon be able to test these hypotheses.[9]

Could all of the hallucinogens have one action on *second* messengers, or share some other primary receptor mechanism in common? Not likely. For even though LSD does stimulate the enzyme which makes cyclic adenosine monophosphate, mescaline and psilocine do not. And while LSD seems to be linked with some additional properties as a dopamine agonist,[16–18] neither mescaline nor psilocine acts as a direct DA agonist. However, mescaline does release some DA from DA nerve terminals. And by indirect routes, mescaline also suppresses the firing of ST nerve cells, without acting directly on them per se.[19]

So even this brief review shows how many gaps remain in our current understanding of psychedelics. Despite these gaps, the existing facts fully support Trulson who concluded that: "it seems unlikely that a single neurotransmitter system could account for all of the behavior and psychological effects of hallucinogenic drugs in humans."[10] How, then, can we possibly arrive at an abbreviated summary—within the scope of this book—limiting ourselves to four plausible mechanisms by which these drugs produce their effects?

1. First, it seems likely that they create an *elaborate mixture of interactions*, at sites both presynaptic and postsynaptic, among ST, NE, and DA nerve cell systems.

2. This dynamic mixture goes on to modulate chiefly the excitatory properties expressed by the other major transmitter systems.

3. Already, during the initial phase, the above set of events is directly altering the person's perception. And it is setting in motion a secondary metabolic cascade.

Acting in combination, such changes carry the potential to modify mental functions (including the sense of space and time) in unexpected ways.

4. (The latent power of this final mechanism is difficult to fully appreciate when one is resting comfortably, and is in an undrugged state.) The subject's brain develops the sense of being in peril. The drug-induced psychophysiological ordeals finally trigger emergency responses commensurate with the primal fear of death. Ancient circutries deep in the subject's brain set off layers of stress responses within the brain itself.

The next chapter will make clear the steps through which these processes evolve into consciousness.

104

Near-Death Experiences; Far-Death Attitudes

No choice is uninfluenced by the way in which the personality regards its destiny, and the body its death. In the last analysis, it is our conception of death which decides or answers to all the questions that life puts to us. . . . Hence, too, the necessity of preparing for it.

Dag Hammarskjold (1905–1961)[1]

Does our concept of death influence the way we *live?* If Hammarskjold is correct, then it's about time each of us developed some valid concepts about death, and started to prepare for it. Easier said than done.

A century ago, Albert Heim summarized in the following sentences the reports of thirty people who instantly confronted death. Their ordeals were precipitated by long falls from Alpine heights. Having come back from the very brink of death these survivors spoke of having felt, in that moment, a

"calm seriousness, profound acceptance, and a dominant mental quickness and conse of surety. Mental activity became enormous, rising to a hundred-fold velocity or intensity. An overview took in the relationships of events and their probable outcomes with objective clarity. Time became greatly expanded. The individual was not confused, but acted with lightning quickness in full accord with an accurate assessment of the situation. In many cases there also followed a sudden review of the individual's entire past; and, finally, the person falling often heard beautiful music and fell in a superbly blue heaven containing roseate cloudlets."[2]

So, in Heim, the Swiss had another early contributor to our understanding of "peak" experiences, this time of a different kind. Heim was both an alpinist and a geology professor. Like Darwin, he became fascinated by the rapid mental flow which took place during his own descent. Although Heim had taken a longer and more serious fall, he said he "felt no trace of anxiety or pain." In fact, he faced his death "matter-of-factly and without dread. It all had to happen that way; it seemed eminently correct . . . I had the feeling of submission to necessity."[2]

Fortunately, as occurred in Charles Darwin's case earlier, the descent also had a benign outcome. Again, at first, Heim experienced a major rush of thoughts and images pulled out of random memory. In earlier pages, we had referred to these first, simpler moments—those at the Darwinian end of the spectrum—as "near-life" experiences (see chapter 91). The purpose was to distinguish them from this later series of more complicated phenomena which Heim went on to cite in detail.

These latter phenomena have since come to be called "near-death experiences." Now the person faces imminent death. The threat is *real*. The ordeal is unhinging, if not unnerving. The added physiological instabilities thrust extra psychological dimensions into the experience. For example, outer time slows; inner time races; events seem to happen in slow motion. This kind of time warp occurred in most (75 percent) of Noyes and Kletti's survey of 104 survivors.[3] Many of their subjects (64 percent) felt detached. Almost half felt they were detached from their bodies (49 percent). They also experienced a run of old scenes flashing by (36 percent). No narrative continuity linked this revival of memories (see chapter 90).

Some investigators have applied the term "panoramic" when they describe the way these isolated memory segments slip by.[4] However, we need to be clear about how this word is being used in the near-death context. The reports refer to the wide *variety* of snapshots cast up from different decades of the person's historical past. And, in this loose usage, "panoramic" then refers to events in slices of *time*. It does *not* necessarily imply that some wide-angle, visual panorama of total *space* has opened up all around, all at once, such as we will find occurring in the ambient vision of major absorptions (see chapter 116). Indeed, as Heim had specified, "I saw my whole past life take place in many images, as though on a stage at some distance from me."[5] Such vivid mental images can seem as real as are actual, ongoing perceptions.

Only then, after first having passed through this initial sample of replayed memories, do some subjects enter the next phase. It is indeed "another world," conveying qualities difficult to describe. They include a sense of great understanding (37 percent), of harmony or unity (35 percent), and of being in a timeless state, beyond time.

Farther on, we will be considering similar kinds of experience as part of the phenomena of enlightenment (see part VII). So it becomes important to ask, which subjects report having these "mystical extensions" during this later phase of their near-death experiences? With few exceptions they are the persons who at that very moment were later presumed to have had some disorder of their cerebral functioning. That is, they were drowning, oxygen-deprived, in vasomotor shock with low blood pressure, or otherwise seriously ill. In contrast, mystical ingredients did *not* tend to arise in the course of uncomplicated falls. Nor did this mystical phase occur during traumatic accidents *if* the person had no associated head, chest, or other relevant injuries that presented as a surgical emergency.

Powerful inner forces surge up when survival hangs in the balance. Even so, many subjects find their personal resources overwhelmed by inexorable circumstances. At this point they may then undergo what Professor Heim so beautifully expressed as "the feeling of submission to necessity." But note: this is chiefly a *passive* relinquishing of control. This is not some person engaged in a willful, thought-out renunciation of self. It is a process which, because it happens by itself, implies a basic and spontaneous dissolution of the *I-Me-Mine*. And it will be at this point of surrender—of unconditioned and unconditional surrender—that any transient fear is also subsiding by itself. Now, with the self gone from the field of struggle, death is accepted with utter calm.[2] Profound tranquility ensues.

During the perils of their ordeal, the subjects have no sense of being distressed by these depersonalizing symptoms or by the blunting of their own emotions. Rather will they look back subsequently in gratitude at what had been their impressive sense of calm.[3] Moreover, some of this same momentary calmness in the actual face of danger will later become an ongoing fact. Afterward, they recall the incident with dispassion, and tend to be relatively undisturbed by the emotional impact of perils that the rest of us might suppose would cause them frightening dreams and anxieties.

The Gallup survey of near-death experiences included a large number of personal interviews with some fifteen hundred adults.[6] In this survey, two points are of interest to note at the outset. Of those who faced a brink-of-death encounter, how many went on into an alternate dimension of consciousness? Only a minority, about 35 percent. Moreover, most of the *individual* features of each experience they described, as will be cited below, have also been reported by other subjects during many other diverse situations. Did most of these other more ordinary circumstances place the person's life in jeopardy? No. So being close to *actual* death is not the critical factor.

Now, these other situations do include meditative retreats. Meditative settings can be very rigorous but they pose no *real* threat to life. On the other hand, when the meditator finally does reach a deep baseline level of mental calmness and one-pointed clarity, then relatively covert events, including triggers, can prove exciting momentarily. Viewed from sea level, prominent hills rise up like higher mountains. Given this preamble, what cluster of features turned up in the Gallup survey?

1. The out-of-body sensation. This is the feeling that one's witnessing awareness is separated from one's physical body. Nine percent of adults report having had this sensation during their near-death experience.

2. An acute visual perception of one's surroundings and of every event then taking place in it (8 percent). Such a heightened visual sense occurs from a point of view located away from the actual physical position of the person's eyes.

3. Audible noises coming from real people nearby or from some other source (6 percent).

4. Overwhelming peace and loss of pain (11 percent).

5. A blinding, bright light (5 percent).

6. A fast review or reexamination of the person's life (11 percent).

7. A distinctive sensation of being in an entirely different world (11 percent).

8. A feeling that someone special was present (8 percent).

9. A sense of the presence of some kind of tunnel (3 percent).

10. Premonitions about some future event (2 percent).

Let us consider the first two of these further. Out-of-body experiences may last perhaps a half a minute or so. (A few are alleged to last up to half an hour.) Most occur at times of emotional duress and during circumstances *other* than a near-death experience.[7] For example, some persons, while meditating or sleeping, also feel that they have undergone a shift of their center of conscious experience. This center of awareness appears to be displaced outside the limits of their physical body.[8] At these moments, the subjects have the impression that they are floating up high, looking down and seeing their own body. The experience seems real, not a dream.[9]

Most subjects who are undergoing a near-death experience still feel that they retain at least something of their *essential personal self*.[10] This personal self is usually the primary external observer on the scene. It goes on observing the "other" physical self, the one that is detached off in the distance. A number of these subjects are grateful to find that their personal identity seems to be continuing at death.

Sometimes the essential personal self will be projected into the scene. There it is watched by another, double, personal self. The phenomenon of seeing oneself, a kind of mental diplopia, is termed *autoscopy*. What causes autoscopy? It is noteworthy that it can also occur in those epileptic patients whose seizures start in the temporal lobe.[11]

But some subjects go on to dissolve their personal identity. And after this, a series of other phenomena (items not specified on the above list) enter at still later stages of the near-death experience. For example, the next moment may then seem to expand, as it blends into something comparable with a "timeless, spaceless immanence of the universal being in a particular center." In some subjects this sense of merging into a universal being then takes on a higher "quality and grandeur," however short some may interpret its failing to attain "all the amplitude and power of God."[12,13]

One can read both sensate and insightful layers of meaning into the old phrase, "to see the light" (see chapter 85). Recent surveys suggest that the particular persons who report an enhanced sensate perception of light are also the subjects most likely to have been closest to actual death.[14] And the personalities of those who had undergone the experience of light tend subsequently to be the most transformed.[15]

Heim survived to describe the psychic events during his sixty-six-foot alpine fall. But a puzzle remains. Many are grazed by death. Few develop the *full* spectrum of all the major features of the experience. In fact, by more recent estimates, only 22 percent or so of selected cases who go through the ordeal of having a very close call, *not* 35 percent, will develop the near-death experience.[16] Why so few? The discussion in the next chapter will serve as one possible explanation. For it will make the point that abrupt, startling events, *of whatever kind*, will be effective triggers of an alternate state *only if* they strike at a special moment, in a certain person's biological cycle, and in a particular setting. One may wonder in passing, could that tendency which Darwin mentioned—the way he often slipped into episodes of absorption—have somehow set the stage for the mental rush of his near-life experience?

Transformations

Already, one important fact is clear: some near-death experiences later transform the survivor's life. The survivor may literally feel reborn, and sets off on an in-spired search for spiritual values. In these respects, the late phase of a major experience is an awakening. It is an enlightenment, which can mimic an otherwise conventional mystical experience, one which had no *obvious* danger as its pre-lude.[10] Some 64 percent of the persons in one group of 215 near-death subjects said that their prior experience had transformed their whole attitude about mat-ters of life and death.[17] How had their attitude changed? They now benefited from (1) a reduced fear of death, (2) a sense of relative invulnerability, (3) a feeling of having some special importance or destiny, (4) a belief in their having been especially favored by fate or by God, and (5) a strengthened belief in their own continued existence.

A close brush with death heightens general awareness, and it leads the per-son to develop several additional attitudes. These include (1) an appreciation of how precious life is, (2) a feeling of urgency and a reevaluation of priorities, (3) a greater awareness of living in this present moment, and (4) a more accepting attitude toward large-scale natural events. Many of these one may not, in fact, be able to influence realistically.

Not every survivor changes for the better, either remarkably or enduringly. Take, for example, the unexpected results of a questionnaire mailed to those who considered themselves to have had a near-death experience and who had gone on to join the International Association for Near-Death Studies. To the eighty-nine respondents, their own social and material success was still judged almost as important as it was to the control group of 175 other persons who had *not* undergone such experiences. And this particular group of near-death responders did not happen to place any higher values on self-actualization, or on altruism, or on spiritual matters than did their controls.[18]

Deathbed Experiences

Nowadays, the public is well aware of near-death experiences. Given all the pub-licity, it is worth noting that many persons had never been, in fact, so "near" actual death as they might once have been led to believe.[14] But now we come to an irrevocable set of circumstances. These occur at the authentic end of the life cycle. They culminate in the *deathbed* experience.

Most of these terminal patients—the doctor who had cancer, for example—will have had hours if not months to contemplate the absolute finality of their situation. Again, one early result is a heightening of awareness and other mental functions. This was well described by Samuel Johnson, who noted how the mind becomes wonderfully concentrated when hanging looms only a fortnight away. In our era, Levine observes that "many people say they have never been so alive as at the time they are dying."[19]

A great many psychic phenomena can arise during this protracted phase of enhanced terminal alertness. Some of these quickenings now enter in a more subacute form. They are not compressed into seconds, as occurs otherwise in the turmoil of the near-death experience. And now, during episodes of heightened mood, the dying patient's sensorium may become host to hallucinations. These take the form of apparitions, or visions of heaven-like states. Moreover, while asleep, the patients' dream scenarios are also rich in symbolism. Representative examples are to be found in Carl Jung's descriptions of his own hallucinations and dreams which occurred in the hospital after his heart attack (see chapter 138).

It is worth noting an interesting feature of certain more shallow near-terminal phenomena. At least some of these also occur when the patient's mental status is otherwise clear, and when drugs or low blood pressure or fluid and electrolyte imbalance can be excluded. However, sleeplessness from worry can be an obvious contributory cause. And there is much, still at the shallow end of these psychic experiences, which resembles other quickenings that could stem from the way any susceptible brain responds to the stressful impact of knowing that certain death lies ahead. But note: more insightful processes of deepening can also be evolving. We will be addressing these in the next section below.

Many survivors of near-death experiences have been profoundly influenced by the intimate drama inherent in what they have just undergone. So, too, have other witnesses been impressed who had been sitting in vigil at a patient's death-bed. One can understand why these two sets of private experiences—firsthand, and secondhand—have given rise to many public overinterpretations in past centuries. Today, for what it is worth, relatively few scientists accept that life really continues "in another world beyond the grave." Fewer still think that near-death experiences are an "authentic glimpse into the hereafter." But scientists are already a skeptical lot, as Gallup's data suggest: a mere 16 percent of scientists do believe in some kind of a life after death, in contrast to 67 percent of the rest of the population.[16]

Still, gripped by what seems like true death, even neuroscientists observe that their attitudes can shift. When the neurologist Ernst Rodin was under anesthesia, he experienced not only the feeling but the absolute *certainty* that he had died. At that very moment, his death became a complete and total "subjective reality." Only afterward, when he came out of anesthesia, could he then conclude that all these earlier deathly certainties had been an illusion.[20] It is an impressive lesson to learn that one's deepest convictions can be illusions, a lesson important for anyone. And no personal event shatters our mirrors of illusions more than does experiencing the *death of self*.

Far-Death Attitudes and Their Parallels

When all fictions of selfhood melt away, death loses its sting. Some persons begin this educational process earlier in life; others postpone it to life's close. This century has now seen many normal persons, young and old, still in full health, embark on the long meditative path. En route, a series of events begins to distance them from their previous fear of death. They are being led deeply to understand the fact that they, too, are impermanent, as transient as are the leaves on the trees. Growing older, and perhaps wiser, they develop perspectives which might in a sense be called "far-death attitudes." Are these more experienced meditators trying to deny death? Are they merely pushing it farther away? No. They're confronting it, accepting its inevitability, incorporating its reality more dispassionately.

Laboratory tests confirm these changes in attitude. Younger persons whose training has already opened them to alternate states of consciousness are measurably less disturbed by the idea of death than are their controls. Indeed, words related to death prompt only slight physiological responses (in heart rate and skin conductance responses) from Buddhist meditators who have followed Zen or Tibetan traditions. The meditators also had low scores on a scale of death anxiety.[8] When being interviewed about death, the Zen subjects responded to questions briefly but precisely. Their answers suggested that they had already cast off the notion of a personal self. Death remained neither as a current concern nor as something that needed to be worried about far off into the future.

How had they developed such a fearless, "far-death" attitude? It reflected both their prior training in "ego-death," and their actual experiences that the egocentric self had been only an illusion. Moreover, having learned to focus on the "now" of the present moment, these trainees could begin to internalize and to accept whatever might happen in this moment, then move on to the next. And the next . . .

Earlier, we considered nine ways that a beginner who followed the meditative approach could start to dissolve the egocentric self (see chapter 32). In that chapter, the discussion was taking place in the broad context of this particular question: how can healthy people learn to *live* their daily lives at the most vital level of awareness? But now we have come to the endgame. At the end of life, will a completely different question arise? Or, as death draws near, could the very same basic approach of mindful introspection still be fruitful? Can a person *learn how to die a better death?* If so, how does one go about it?

Indeed, some patients do tell us that their terminal illness is their last great teacher. The course they must now pass is required of everyone. It will be the most rigorous of all sesshin. For some individuals, it becomes a kind of last-minute crash course. A raw momentum shatters all sham, and strips life down to its ultimate essentials. For these patients, dying becomes their final opportunity to shed deeply held, but artificial beliefs. Finally, they can work through whatever may come, and live fully in each present moment. Isn't this the essence of meditation, as we have been describing it throughout this book?

In the clarity of this final deepening, many patients then begin to see what life is all about. Some discover how much of their life's earlier suffering, and their current discomfort, is rooted in the fearsome fictions of an *I-Me-Mine*. For a few patients, the process of accessing insights at still deeper levels seems to ease their final moments, and it does help them to die a "better death." The most profound of these insights may take another very few of them so far along the path that they access the wide-open state of Ultimate Being which appears to lie beyond (see part VIII).

The deathbed story of Yaeko Iwasaki, both stirring and authenticated, is one rare example of this development. This twenty-five-year-old Zen Buddhist woman had only five days to live before she succumbed to the complications of diseased heart valves. Yet her total concentration during these last days, while confined to bed, enabled her first to enter kensho, and then to deepen, by degrees, into true enlightenment.[21]

Daily, at many other bedsides—in homes, in hospices, and in clinics around the world—increasing numbers of health professionals are providing a much needed service—close support to dying patients. These trained Bodhisattvas are guiding the terminally ill, preparing them for the rigors—but also for the potential insights—of their final learning experience. To these teacher-guides, an obvious personal parallel exists with the deep changes in attitude that they see emerging in their patients. For they see patients shedding the fear of death, dissolving one pretense after another, facing reality head on, and accepting whatever comes. Many of them are already familiar with this same process, having watched it evolve firsthand. *It has been happening during their own meditative quest.*

And so, in broad outline, may the late-onset learning experiences of a person's final passage start to resemble some of those at the beginning. Indeed, as Levine concludes, "The stages of loss, of dying, clearly parallel the stages of spiritual growth."[22]

A Neurological Perspective

We have been examining a spectrum of phenomena. It extends from near-life to deathbed experiences. Mythologies remain comforting, but it is time to examine any resistances one might have against biological explanations for such experiences. Does it matter what goes on in the brain during these episodes? Yes. Here it does, because our hypotheses are going to evolve along lines which will later help explain why similar phenomena also occur on the path of the Zen Way.

But *states tend to unfold in sequences.* And *their psychophysiologies evolve over time.* So first, in order to address the mechanisms underlying the present spectrum of experiences, we'll need to arrange their phenomena in sequence.

Begin with Darwin's fall. An abrupt descent. The immediate result is a brisk cascade of physiological events. The earliest of these will reflect fast neurotransmission. This phase implies a surge through the ascending systems which release acetylcholine and glutamate. Parallel processing would spurt. From its matrix would leap the impression—not at all incorrect—that the brain's "inner" time has vastly accelerated. This would create the sense that *external* events were unfolding in slow motion and with great clarity. One can also speculate that fresh impulses could enter from the outside world, speed down the parahippocampal gyrus, and rush into the hippocampal formation. There they could find the capacities of hippocampal circuitries already enhanced by high-speed processing, casting off a few random chunks of old memories into slices of time.

This brain has been jolted. Sudden, adverse circumstances will prompt many of its nerve cells to fire excessively. The brain now shifts from its previously slower rate of processing into a new, superfast processing mode. As it does so, some of its deeper functioning networks can be "jostled" temporarily out of phase. And these dissociated systems—split off during dynamic transitions—would then be free to join, briefly, into new physiological configurations. Among the sources for such activated shifts, the connections from the hypothalamus merit brief mention here. Also participating could be several clusters of larger nerve cells lower down in the brain stem, and their higher extensions (see chapters 36, 37, 43, and 62).

What might the hypothalamus, and its connections, contribute to near-death and related experiences? In the 1930s, in the course of surgical operations, the human hypothalamic region was grossly stimulated through electrodes placed against the underlying sphenoid bone. The patients' pupils dilated, their skin flushed, they perspired, and developed a major increase in blood pressure. Then, in addition to anxiety, crying, fear, and sobbing, emerged a phase of greater interest. For then, "several patients saw their lives pass before their eyes, as has been described in drowning."[23] It bears emphasis, however, that the way *fear drops out* of awareness is a characteristic feature of later phases of the usual near-death experience. This means that some of the usual sources of primal fear, such as those in the amygdala, are no longer in operation (see chapters 41 and 136).

A synaptic turmoil occurs during the first seconds of a major near-death experience. It will quickly release, *into the brain,* its biogenic amines and peptides. Impulses racing through the deeper visual pathways could generate a sense of light (see chapter 86). One has no need to invoke special electromagnetic forces, coming from an unspecified source *outside* the body, as the agents which must produce the "loving white light." And other events will be set in motion which extend their influences as low as the medulla. Here, for example, lie such large cells as those of the paraglgantocellular nucleus.[24] What excites them? Not only noxious stimuli in general (see chapter 44). They are also excited when the brain releases its own opioids of the enkephalin type.

It now becomes possible to envision how a sudden drop in blood pressure—shock—could secondarily set off the stress responses inside the brain. For if the injured person's blood pressure were to drop, some large nerve cells in this nucleus would also fire, as part of the usual reflex response set up to raise low blood pressure back up toward normal levels. Within milliseconds, impulses rising from this paragigantocellular nucleus would travel that short distance up to the locus ceruleus. Here, they would prompt its cells to release their norepinephrine throughout the central nervous system. This NE would help set off another major round of the brain's own stress responses (see chapter 53). These intrinsic stress responses influence functions at many levels, including those powerful functions of the hypothalamus.

Our progenitors were survivors. Survival hinged on their capacity to shift into high-velocity processing speeds, leading to that extra burst of action which could dodge dire circumstance. These ancient physiological systems remain our allies. Joining forces with other circuits added later, they are still capable of creating in modern brains the impression that time expands, in the clarity of a fearless present. The person senses "more" seconds, more time for making those skillful last-ditch efforts to escape.

Later still, when every biological life cycle is finally drawing to its inevitable close, there will ensue a flurry of terminal physiological responses. Where do the patients' resulting psychic scenarios come from? They can draw upon the vast imaginative capacities at the core of the primal human psyche, wherein all persons are playwrights, novelists, and dreamers ad lib. Are we required to read something meaningful and symbolic into every such natural event on the final threshold of death? Must it be cast in terms of institutional religion or philosophy, metaphysics or supernatural spirit worlds?

It is time to return to a simpler view of the mystical phenomena which enter into the later sequences of near-death experiences. We have every reason to expect that much of their form and content will be colored by each subject's earlier personal and cultural belief systems. Not surprisingly, cross-cultural studies have revealed the Navajo as then "seeing a great chief in a beautiful field, a Hindu seeing a death messenger coming to take him away, and the Catholic meeting with the Virgin Mary in a great cathedral."[16]

Among the young and old who walk the spiritual path, many are now practicing different forms of meditation, both formal and informal. They will be intrigued by the findings that the alternate states described in this chapter can enter quickly, during *non*meditative circumstances, in subjects who for the most part had never meditated previously and who had not been stimulated by a psychedelic drug. And they will be interested, further, in the evidence that when such experiences do arrive, they too can yield clarity, enhance processing, dissolve fear, and later go on to create major enduring, salutary changes in the personality.

Does the Zen Buddhist aspirant have any particular reason to be drawn into debates about the religious or psychodynamic significance of near-death experiences?[25] From its historical beginnings, Zen has taken a different stance. From its perspective the key question is not, Is there life *after* death? Or does life exist in some *after*life? For too long such controversies have obscured the central, practical issue.

In Zen, the basic point is, How shall we live *this life,* after birth, right now, to its fullest, vitalizing extent? Not living in some daydream. Not seeking some make-believe "virtual reality." But fully living out *this* life, *on-line,* right into its final moments.

105

Triggers

> In the third night of the eighth week, when the meditation ended, the attendant monk came and filled our cups of tea. As the boiling water splashed over my hand, I dropped the cup which fell to the ground and broke with a crash.
>
> Instantly, I cut off my last doubt (about my own Self) and rejoiced at the realization of my cherished aim. I was like someone awakening from a dream.
>
> Master Hsu-yun
> (1839–1959)[1]

Sometimes, a sudden event sets off a mystical or an enlightenment experience. The triggering stimuli can be thoughts, smells, sights, sounds, trauma, or falls. Taste, which enters low in the brain stem, seems an interesting exception.

Zen annals have recorded triggering events for many centuries. Kao-feng abruptly became enlightened when he saw a verse on a portrait.[2] Bankei, 26 years old at the time, was washing his face in a stream when he suddenly smelled the fragrance of plum blossoms. Every attachment and lingering doubt vanished.[3] Tokusan's satori came in darkness. His master had suddenly blown out the candle.[4]

Hakuin's series of awakenings started when he was in his early twenties. When he was 27, he was struck unexpectedly by a wielded broom, and this triggered a major satori which resolved his koan.[5,6] Later, hearing a cricket chirp, Hakuin finally penetrated the lotus sutra at the age of 42.[5] When Ikkyu was 26, he was enlightened by the sound of a crow's caw.[7] The elder Ming reached enlightenment when he heard words spoken by the Sixth Patriarch. Amazed, he then asked the Patriarch if these words carried secret significance. Hui-neng answered: "In what I have shown you nothing is hidden. If you reflect within yourself and recognize your own original face, secrecy is in yourself."[8]

Kyogen (Ch: Hsian-yen) was sweeping one day when his broom dislodged a pebble. *Clack* went the pebble when it went on to strike bamboo. After this satori, he said "At one stroke I forgot all my previous knowledge."[9]

Chiyono, a young widow, was filling her bucket in the stream. Suddenly, the bottom fell out of the bucket, and she had a flash of insight-wisdom. Subsequently, she completed her Buddhist training and was authorized to teach.[10]

Daigu was enlightened by a fall on a hot summer day. He had chosen to sit in zazen in a cooling draft, suspended on a plank across the top of an open well. The plank broke, and he fell head over heels to the bottom of the well shaft.[11]

What has been happening in the inscrutable Orient? None of these examples seem to fit into the proprieties of our orthodox Western religious perspective. How can a religious experience be valid if it hinges on such happenstance? But the trigger does not detract from the awakening. However, triggered, kensho is no trivial event for that person. Moreover, one can't conclude that the triggering event was the sole *basic* cause for the flash of kensho. For Hsu-yun had been meditating day and night with increasing zeal. He was already one-pointed and beyond thoughts when his burned hand lost its hold on the teacup. And it would take many long years before that pebble crack wiped out Kyogen's previous knowledge, years during which he was incubating his frustrations about not reaching enlightenment. Moreover, before Kao-feng focused on that key verse on the portrait, he had become so thoroughly wrapped up in his koan that no irrelevant thought arose. During the previous six days, he had become oblivious to other people, "like an idiot, like an imbecile."[2]

So in the Zen *meditative* context, triggers will be striking deep *after a very long prelude*. These years of preparation, incubation, and struggle tend to escape notice. If, in a sense, the novel event does close some kind of waiting circuit, it is one already high in potential energy. And if that sudden stimulus is the last straw, then it landed on top of a very large bale.

In fact, our Western literature also contains reports of triggers which had occurred before other, less profound mystical experiences.[12] Laski's survey revealed several other situations which had clearly precipitated what she chose to call an "ecstatic interlude."[12] In the group of her Christian contacts, an encounter with art was the most frequent event (30 percent). It was followed next in line by religious settings (17 percent) or by nature (15 percent). Among those of her other subjects who did not believe in religion, the three most frequent events involved sexual love, nature, and art.

Laski observed that the ecstasy associated with childbirth can occur when the baby is placed in the mother's arms, or when the child's first cry is heard. It was not necessarily related to how painful the birth had been. However, it did occur most often when the first child was born, and this delivery is not only a novel event but often the most painful.

Laski also identified "anti-triggers." These factors nullify triggers. The presence of other people was most inhibiting. This observation speaks for how essential it will be for the meditator to set aside the time "to get away from it all," and to "commune with Nature" in solitude. In this regard, we're reminded that the word *monk* stems from the Greek *monakhos,* meaning single or solitary one. Another negative influence was commercialism. Humorous events were not true triggers (although uncontrollable laughter can occur subsequently, as has been noted, during the release of kensho or satori).

When Greeley surveyed subjects who had mystical experiences, their usual triggers included listening to music (49 percent), prayer (48 percent), the beauties of nature (45 percent), and moments of quiet reflection (42 percent). Less common precipitants were childbirth (20 percent) and sexual lovemaking (18 percent).[13]

Do such diverse events share anything in common? What happens when stone clatters against bamboo, when water gushes unexpectedly out of the bottom of a bucket? A sudden, novel stimulus alerts the brain. One can envision an abrupt barrage of stimuli leaping up through specific sensory systems. This prompts a brisk, intense discharge within the brain stem activating system and its higher projections.[14]

Meditation sensitizes the person. Minor examples of the phenomenon are commonplace. After repeated quiet sittings in sesshin for only two or three days, I find that certain sound stimuli evoke an especially penetrating response. Outside the meditation hall is the large wooden board, and it now yields a potent *crack!* when the mallet strikes it. Each blow struck causes a click in my ear. (The reader can experience the same noise by the act of swallowing. One hears it, and feels it. Nothing special; it's only our middle ear muscles tightening our eardrum.) In my case, this *reflex* response to the sound of the crack arises from my brain stem. This click response does not habituate.

Countless crows caw. Why did Ikkyu's brain overrespond at *that* instant to so trivial a stimulus? Again, the several leading possibilities illustrate the basic principle: major striking phenomena occur when a sudden direct increase of excitation overwhelms a decrease in inhibition, or vice versa. So, included among the relevant sequence of events already cited in part III would be the following short list of possible explanations: (1) a decrease in the inhibition from the thalamic reticular nucleus; (2) a decrease in the inhibition normally arising from the lower reticular formation in the pons and medulla; and (3) a simultaneous increase in excitation coming down from the cortex or arising from certain subcortical nuclei.

Perhaps Zen literature does overemphasize the brusque impact of startling sensate events. But this is not to overlook the obvious fact that natural settings contain sublime elements, and these also serve as precipitants. The beauties of nature exert a more gradual triggering effect, generating a subtle power all their own (see chapter 154). Accordingly, we need to consider the possibility that when crucial limbic themes are woven into the matrix of thought, they might *descend* to activate the reticular formation.

This "descending" possibility returns us to Segundo's earlier descriptions of what occurred when he began to stimulate discrete areas of monkey cortex. Previously, the monkey's electrocorticogram had shown the usual slow-wave activity of drowsiness or sleep. "Now it was transformed, immediately and for a sustained period, into one exhibiting the low voltage and fast tracing of wakefulness (EEG arousal or 'desynchronization')."[15] From which cortical sites could he most effectively activate the midbrain reticular formation? From the superior temporal gyrus, the inferior frontal region, and the cingulate gyrus (see chapter 37). Stimulate with electricity any one of these three cortical regions on only *one* *side*. Instantly, impulses descend to the reticular formation, bounce back up, and are then rebroadcast to the cortex in the form of *bilateral* arousal responses. This cortex has aroused itself, on *both* sides.[15]

Suppose you suddenly overstimulate the *midbrain* reticular formation. What happens? Below it, the *medullary* reticular formation reacts with a brisk, inhibitory response. Stimulate the midbrain only gradually, and it prods this medulla into a slower, more graded inhibitory response. But suppose, first, you had already inhibited the lower medulla itself, using procaine. Now, with nothing left to restrain it, the midbrain stimulation is unchecked, and arousal overflows into a major enhanced response up in cortex.[16]

The normal brain stem, then, has its own regulating mechanisms. They prevent excessive excitation from spreading up from the midbrain. Consider, however, what might happen if you had already learned to calm the medulla, as it were, by quiet breathing and by long meditative practices. Given a sudden stimulus, in this setting, one might speculate that an enhanced response could spring more readily from the reticular systems above it. The click response to the crack on the board illustrates this point.

There is another way to stop the medulla from exerting its usual ascending inhibiting influence. It can be blocked one level higher, in the pons. After this, even when the cat is already in D-sleep, it still *reacts* to a face or to a test object as though it were wide awake. The cat has entered a dissociated state, one more example of that curious category of waking-while-dreaming[17] (see chapter 73).

What do unexpected stimuli do to the locus ceruleus? They trigger it into firing a "short burst of impulses followed by a prolonged silence."[18] Both phases are noteworthy, both the burst *and* the long silent pause. For it is indeed a major switch suddenly to alternate between high and low levels of norepinephrine function. And this kind of polar change within NE systems could be the kind that would "facilitate transitions between behavior states."[18] One also recalls, for example, that the drop in NE firing is a characteristic feature of the entry into desynchronized sleep.

Painful stimuli also serve as triggers. Pain signals relay, in part, through acetylcholine pathways. And once pain signals reach the ACH cells of the parabrachial region, they pass on next to the ventromedial hypothalamus, soon to be translated into the cascade of stress responses.[19]

PGO Waves and Startle Responses

When researchers made electrical recordings from animals, they soon discovered that large distinctive waveforms were sweeping into many different brain sites. Because these striking waves were prominent in the *pons*, lateral *g*eniculate nucleus, and *o*ccipital lobes, they received the acronym PGO waves. The first waves occur just as desynchronized sleep starts. As we observed earlier, in part III, two major ACH influences help activate them. One ACH pathway arises from the parabrachial nucleus at the junction between midbrain and pons. The second ACH path comes from the medial pontine reticular formation.[20]

PGO waves reach high amplitudes (200–300 microvolts), and each lasts for a relatively long time: 250 milliseconds. Moreover, during the quarter-second of each PGO wave, the brain briefly opens up its sensate window to the outside world. Now, many visual impulses coming back from the optic tract can sweep through the geniculate nucleus to reach the visual cortex.[21] A series of associated PGO spikes take the lead during arousal, whether the animals are on their ascent to waking from slow-wave sleep or from desynchronized sleep.[22]

Now, it also turns out that serotonin cells of the dorsal raphe nuclei stop firing just before each of these PGO spikes occurs, when the brain is in its normal transition period between S-sleep and D-sleep.[23] Moreover, repeated PGO spikes occur *after* the animal receives a drug like reserpine, which markedly reduces the flow of ST impulses. As each PGO spike then sweeps throughout the cat's brain, the animal briefly becomes alert, and appears startled. This startle reflex can be conceptualized as the expression of an early warning "alerting network." It enables the alerted animal to respond more efficiently to sensory impulses coming in from the outside.[21]

The early phase of the startle circuitry is organized down in the brain stem.[24] Within its higher extensions, in the forebrain above, ST plays its usual tonic—chiefly inhibitory—role. Whereas below it, in the spinal cord, ST exerts a predominantly excitatory effect. What procedure will enhance startle the most, in an experimental animal? The release of opioids directly into the central gray substance. Here, opioid receptors appear to inhibit a separate local system that has been holding startle in check. A brief increase of dopamine will also increase startle responses.

Humans can be startled, of course. But do we also have some version of PGO activity? Or something along the same lines of this impressive activity found in other animals? Surprisingly little is known, considering how important is the question. The silence in the human literature is almost embarrassing. Yet we do show high amplitude waveforms which enter before our eyes move, waves which come before the next phase of fast activity in our EEG. These large waves arise in the central region of the human midbrain.[25] (Apparently not from the site of those key ACH cells tucked away off in the lateral and dorsal aspect of the tegmentum.) And after researchers apply special processing techniques to the human EEG, the data obtained from scalp electrodes suggest the possibility that posterior "PGO-like" spikes could exist.

In the human EEG, such spikes as do emerge reach their higher amplitudes over the *right* parieto-occipital region. Here, they tend to localize nearer to the midline and to the top of the skull than do their counterpart spikes over on the left side.[26] Suppose a sensate trigger does startle the human brain into some form of PGO-like activity. What would happen? The above finding suggests an intriguing possibility: its impact might be greater in the *right* posterior hemisphere. Soon to be placed in evidence are two more reasons to look for an occasional right posterior visual bias in cerebral activation. For such a proposal would be consistent (1) with the fact that a hallucinated leaf appeared in the left side of my vision (see part VI), and (2) with some of the other phenomena of syncretism (as will be discussed in part VII).

How are we, meanwhile, to interpret those impressively large PGO spikes and waves so obvious in animals? They appear to be further expressions of general *activating* mechanisms. As emphasized, these mechanisms emerge along a spectrum. It extends from normal awakening, to alerting, and to desynchronized REM sleep. When similar expressions of PGO activity are projected up to higher levels, they might provide a kind of "copy" signal. This might help translate into the forefront of consciousness a variety of dreamlike phenomena.[20] Perhaps in like manner may the effects of triggers ramify. The results might then open up a person's field of consciousness to some of those vivid qualities and other dreamlike properties that one can experience during certain alternate states.

106

The Surge

When your activity of mind is exhausted and your capacity for feeling comes to a dead end, if something should take place not unlike the cat springing upon the mouse or the mother hen hatching her eggs, then in a flash great livingness surges up.

Master Hakuin (1685–1768)[1]

More and more the surges of everlasting nature enter into me, and I become public and human in my regards and actions.

Ralph Waldo Emerson (1803–1882)[2]

I was lucky to spend my boyhood summers on a farm. Here I watched instincts in action: cats catching mice, and mother hens hatching eggs. And here, too, some sweltering night, one became a spectator at a different kind of rural event. In the heat, more electrical appliances had been turned on. Refrigerators and fans were all working overtime. Suddenly, every room darkened as its electric light bulbs dimmed. Nothing mysterious; the local power plant had simply fallen behind and wasn't delivering enough electricity to keep up with the overload. Moreover, back in that era, rural power systems lacked those smoothly coordinated overlapping networks we take for granted today. So, then, several dark moments after things had run down, a big bolus of extra current arrived. Now, a fresh rush of electricity surged through the local circuits. Light bulbs glowed brighter than normal, some even burned out with the overload. The refrigerator hummed with new vigor, and the fan whirred at high pitch like a quail taking off.

After these few seconds at high intensity, everything phased back toward normal. Then a visitor from the city might undergo a phase of faint embarrassment. Had others in the room also experienced the same phenomenon? Or was it only me? It was as though one sought confirmation that light and sound had really changed, that the brain hadn't created an illusion. And so one cast furtive, sidelong glances, to be reassured that others had also witnessed the event. City folk out for a trip in the summer were the ones most impressed by the phenomenon; year-round residents were inured to it. Nowadays, the power networks and their modern feedback systems rarely release such a surge in their circuitry, but the tendency remains to seek to verify lesser degrees of the experience.

So it is with our usual states of consciousness. They mesh so well with one another that we rarely recognize their transitions. Each time we shift mental gears effortlessly, the smooth overlap is silent tribute to the way sophisticated brain circuits mesh their firing patterns. Yet, during periods of transition, our receptors are undergoing their most rapid *rate of change*. And at these dynamic interfaces between its different modes of awareness our labile brain is most vulnerable to overshoot.

Researchers who study the responses to drugs have become aware of a general rule of thumb. It goes something like this: if you wish an animal to respond more to a drug which *enhances* a function, you give the drug when that function has already dropped down to its physiologically lowest level. So the lower the "initial value" of this activity, the more the animal tends to respond. Suppose, conversely, the animal's level of functional activity was already very high to begin with. Then—with fewer of the same resources remaining—it may respond less to the next added stimulus.[3] When discussing Hakuin's surge of "great livingness," this so-called law of initial value is a useful starting point.

For example, some drugs reduce biogenic amines to very low levels, and cause their corresponding physiological functions to fall to baseline levels, both at the same time. Now the pharmacologists administer the test drug to see if it can restore these lost functions to higher levels. Suppose you first give reserpine to a rat. The rat slowly becomes stuporous, because the drug depletes its available stores of dopamine, norepinephrine, and serotonin. Some twenty hours after reserpine, the rat's brain has become thoroughly deprived of these amines. At this point you inject a very weak dose of levodopa, the precursor to DA and NE.[4] Now, *freshly synthesized* molecules of DA and NE become available, waiting to pour out of their nerve terminals as soon as each impulse arrives. Released into the synaptic gap, these messengers then stimulate the specific receptors sensitive to DA or to NE on the next cell. The resulting leap—from low to high receptor activity—generates an extra-strong physiological reaction. The rat awakens and scurries about. But if you had given this same very low dose of levodopa previously, during the rat's usual waking state, nothing would have happened.

To the degree that prolonged meditative calming invokes the "rest principle," and has already caused low initial levels and a low turnover of some of the brain's messenger molecules, it becomes possible to visualize the next scenario. Because when the next seemingly trivial stimulus arrives, it might be able to trigger an energized surge of "great livingness," and cause an unexpected overshooting of mental functions.

Observe the grappling of two huge sumo wrestlers. Well matched, they arrive at a balanced standoff. Now, even the slightest leverage, deftly applied in the right spot at the right time, moves a major mass not only out of the ring but off the platform. To any arena, the nervous system also brings an array of powerful forces, similarly pitted against one another. They usually shelter us, confining us safely inside one conventional state of consciousness at the expense of others. But again, this delicate physiological balancing act can suddenly give way, and can thrust a person out of the usual transition zone into a highly unusual state.

Out of the depths of dark depression, some patients quickly shift up into mania. Why? One current theory for this "switch process" runs something as follows: when their GABA activity becomes reduced, more substance P is released. Subsequently, this peptide then goes on to excite DA neurons into firing.[5] And then other excitatory messengers might also surge in, potent transmitters such as glutamate or acetylcholine. They, too, could help not only by further driving the DA neurons but also by shifting other functions of the once-inert depressed person up into a manic phase. Brain-damaged patients seem more likely to be tipped into secondary "manic-like" states by any conditions which happen to enhance the functional activity of their DA and NE systems.[6] A person's surge, then, can express *several mechanisms which converge and interact.*

Do surges come *down* from "above" to illuminate alternate states of consciousness? (The previous chapter considered the "descending" route.) Or do they well *up* from "below?" Long ago, Hughlings Jackson pondered similar questions. He concluded that our highest functional activities, the ones which gave rise to our most vivid consciousness, were generally "determined by activities of lower, more organized nervous arrangements . . . Roughly speaking, the highest nervous states are determined from below."[7] Where is "below?" For purposes of this discussion, much of Jackson's "below" could begin in activating systems located as far down as the medulla. Here, one notes, are important ACH cells in the lower ACH column (see chapter 38). Then, could the basic properties of circutries low in the brain stem help explain some of the "otherworldly" qualities of alternate states? Let us begin to speculate on this point, still proceeding from Jackson's hypothesis that physiological events going on down "below" help set in motion many of our "highest level" nervous activities.

Under most ordinary circumstances, we will be awake during all those times when our higher *midbrain* reticular formation is sponsoring its wide range of daytime activations. Indeed, this active midbrain has long been a major source of input for those lesser quickenings which enlarge our everyday perceptions and enhance our readiness to act. So by now, the rest of our *waking* brain is likely to be highly "familiar" in this regard, with the usual way consciousness "feels," in a sense, when its midbrain is being tonically and phasically engaged.

But things are different when the *lower* reticular formation enters the picture. For at what point are we, in our usual twenty-four-hour cycle, when *it* starts to volley its first big sets of fresh signals? Not awake. But in bed, lights out, still wrapped up in the dark cocoon world of S-sleep.[8]

So, if some extra-strong surge did happen to issue from relays starting as low as the *medulla*—and the *person was awake at that particular time*—it could be a novel event, perceived as quite extraordinary. As though something strange and unfamiliar had entered into the field of waking consciousness. Indeed, as these particular impulses rise upward through the *medial* thalamocortical projection system, they might inject fresh qualities of awareness that one rarely experiences, except in dreams.

Why should any events from the lower brain stem, volleying up through the *medial* thalamus—when they ascend during wakeful awareness—be perceived as being so unusual? Because they might have relatively few ties to our higher constructs of self. When, in fact, does the brain elaborate most of its specific sensory input into sophisticated egocentric concepts? Not until after these messages have entered into the more *laterally placed* nuclei of the thalamus (see chapter 59).

Jackson and Hakuin, each in his own way, might find such a curious proposal not too far removed from their own thinking. The scenario envisions our lateral networks of self being bypassed or preempted by medial instinctual pathways, "by activities of lower, more organized nervous arrangements," by impulses that rise up quickly next to the midline core of the brain. Moreover, these same considerations illustrate an important general principle. *An alternate state of consciousness implies that alternative pathways are linking alternative circuitries into unexpected configurations.*

In the foregoing discussion, we have summarized several simplified examples, drawn from both humans and animals, of the way a normal brain is capable of welling up into special moments. Emerson would call them "surges of everlasting nature." Master Hakuin's chosen examples were simple: cat and mouse, and hen and egg. Clearly, he wanted us to know that the artesian events in Zen flowed up with deep instinctual properties.

And yet, our conditioning has always imposed many other added jacksonian layers. These socially useful top-down functions hold unfruitful instincts in abeyance. Still, once the meditator begins to *let go* of some top-down functions, the other circuits deep in the brain stand ready to surge from relative underactivity into hyperactivity. This process opens up the field of awareness to a sequence of novel changes. First to arrive during the early years of meditation is an array of quickened sensate functions. These are born in the depths and the *back* of the brain. Later will come the deep shifts that yield flashing insights. These are drawn much more selectively. It is plausible to attribute the higher-order aspects of insights to the *front* part of the brain, but only as it acts in concert with certain other regions of the association cortex and the limbic system.

We begin the remaining parts of the book by taking up each of these two large topics in turn. But first, it will prove useful to step back, and review how far we have already come in our understanding of Zen and the brain.

First Zen-Brain Mondo

> Be patient toward all that is unsolved in your heart and try to love the questions themselves . . . Live the questions now. Perhaps you will gradually, without noticing it, live along some distant day into the answer.
>
> Rainer Maria Rilke (1875–1926)[1]

In Zen, a mondo is a question asked and replied to. The reply can be far from the answer expected. In this chapter we also use a question-and-answer format, but do so in the conventional way. Here we use it to summarize some major conclusions of parts I through V. I hope this dialogue form will prove useful, and invite correspondence in these matters. But please note: many questions and answers are overstated in a brief, simplistic way. This does not always imply that the questions are valid. Nor does it mean that the answers are unqualified. In fact, many of the replies remain speculative.

What is Zen?

It is a form of Buddhism that emphasizes meditation as a way to enlightenment. This spiritual awakening is called *kensho* or *satori*. It will dissolve the egocentric self and reestablish the sense of a direct relationship with things as they really are, the universal reality principle.

What does Zen training focus on?

The ongoing perception of each moment as *it* really is. This means an awareness stripped of those obscuring layers imposed by our mindless thoughts, self-referent attachments and prior dogma.

Does this imply doing away with my whole personality, and leaving it "blank," as it were?

No. It is true that the Zen approach does address the whole personality, but it transforms chiefly the unfruitful parts of the *I-Me-Mine* complex. It is a process of liberation. It will transform an over-conditioned, self-centered person into a more humane being, one who is *actualized, buoyant,* and compassionate.

What causes cravings? How can one stop them?

In the broadest sense, cravings express a physiological "need." Recent research in substance abuse suggests that craving occurs when activation has been withdrawn from previously overstimulated receptors. Our everyday feelings of "needing" something stem from psychophysiological attachments. These attachments are a root cause of suffering. Meditation contributes to an optimal approach: to a life of moderation which avoids overstimulating such receptors in the first place.

What happens during breathing out?

Breathing *out* quiets down the activity of many nerve cells. Expiration slows the firing of nerve cells in the amygdala and in the nucleus of the solitary tract, for example. Such slowings, taking place in the limbic system and elsewhere, may contribute to the basic calming effect that meditation has, and that chanting has as well.

Why could quieting down the brain during zazen go on to enhance conscious awareness instead of promoting sleep?

Our ordinary waking lives are beehives of distraction, swarming with over-stimulated thoughts and behaviors. Zazen decelerates. Many systems in the brain may operate more effectively at a lower speed. Some of its intuitive functions seem to flow best from settings of undistracted awareness.

In general, barbiturates depress and inhibit behavior. Why does excitation occur when the lower brain stem is inhibited by a local infusion of a barbiturate?

An important principle is involved. Lower brain stem regions normally inhibit the activating mechanisms higher up in the midbrain reticular formation. Remove this usual restraint from below, and it will release some of these higher excitatory mechanisms. This release of prior inhibition is called *disinhibition*.

What causes fine-grained visual perception during sudden quickenings?

The phenomena may reflect the way the cortex develops fast desynchronized activity in response to complex shifts at subcortical levels. For example, the intralaminar nuclei of the thalamus may recruit cortical dendrites more effectively when the functions of other thalamic nuclei are reduced. Similar perceptual changes sometimes occur shortly after LSD is given intravenously.

What could explain an enveloping light?

Acetylcholine nerve cells down in the brain stem normally send volleys of impulses up to influence the visual pathways. The net result of this is that more visual messages now flow through the lateral geniculate nuclei. These moments of enhanced visual transmission occur especially during that transition period between slow-wave sleep and desynchronized sleep. An extra surge of visual excitation could be perceived as light as it goes on next to relay through the superior colliculus, the zona incerta, and the pulvinar of the thalamus. Normally, it will also be within such higher-order projections that we start to develop a subliminal awareness of the space all around us. The experience of an enveloping light could arise when additional impulses, signaling "light," spread throughout this normally subliminal "sense of place."

What are some of the steps through which meditative training could facilitate the entry into states of absorption and kensho?

Meditation changes the rhythms of our two natural, cyclic trends toward desynchronization. Waking is only one of these major states. The other state is desynchronized sleep (D-sleep, also known as REM sleep). Repeated meditation shifts the usual entry times of these two activated states. It also changes their momentum. And while our major physiological trend is to wake up once a day, we also have a lesser tendency to become more awake every 90 minutes or so. Rigorous meditative retreats will change a person's sleep-waking habits, destabilize each of these biorhythms, and open up consciousness to new options.

What else could prompt the brain into sudden surges of enhanced desynchronization?
Stressful circumstances, or triggers that arrive during moments of open detachment. By creating brief physiological instabilities, these sudden events could in a sense jar loose and dissociate some "looser fragments" of adjacent physiological rhythms. And when these coalesce, the person could experience the resulting new constellations of functions as extraordinary states of consciousness.

How else could meditative practice encourage more frequent peak experiences?
It might create more, longer, and deeper detached pauses. Into these, random novel physiological events might thrust up more effectively. As noted above, outside events could provide destabilizing influences. But less obvious events could also intrude along the potential fault lines of internal rhythms. And these two kinds of vectors could converge.

A cluster of acetylcholine nerve cells lies in the dorsolateral part of the pons. What special attributes do these cells have?
They excite the thalamus, stimulating two kinds of ACH receptors. Nicotinic receptors respond with brisk excitatory responses; muscarinic receptors respond more slowly.

What is so special about the large acetylcholine cells farther down in the medulla?
They also excite the thalamus, plus the midbrain reticular formation. They are sentinels which initiate desynchronization. Usually, they fire both during the activating prelude when the sleeping brain rouses up to full wakefulness, and during the transition period when S-sleep leads on to D sleep.

What could cause sudden feelings of relaxation, euphoria, and profound satisfaction?
Humans report similar "positive" feelings during electrical stimulation of the frontal lobe, temporal lobe, and brain stem. Positive feelings might arise when impulses spread into these regions, and into their many connections elsewhere.

Sometimes even a gas mixture of oxygen and carbon dioxide can precipitate religious and mystical states. But the subjects must already be late in their course of a long series of repeated doses of LSD. What does this mean?
Carbon dioxide produces an acidosis that strongly arouses the brain and body. This is a major physiological arousal. Even though the process operates *non*specifically, it does serve as a kind of prolonged triggering event. For it appears to "tip over" the person who happens to be already on the brink of entering one of these alternate states.

Low LSD doses prompt REM episodes to enter earlier than usual. They also thrust micro-REM intrusions into S-sleep. What do these observations signify?

They suggest that the REM mechanisms within desynchronized sleep are targets sensitive to the arousing effects of LSD. They reinforce the view that some kinds of LSD imagery represents dreamlike intrusions. They also remind us that psychedelic drugs tend to enhance functions that, in a sense, are "already there," in the brain, not supernatural imports from "outside."

During stage 1 and stage 2 sleep, a person's normal dreamlike images may lack emotion. But on other occasions certain dream images have potential gaps of meaning filled in by "understanding" and emotion. And these latter images enter at the times when alpha EEG activity coincides with REM episodes. Could some of these normal aspects of sleep imagery help clarify why the average meditator sometimes experiences similar extremes of emotional involvement?

These observations suggest that a drowsy meditator's brain may sometimes draw upon, and express, whatever degree of affective tone might be nearby, and available, in his or her adjacent states of S-sleep and D-sleep.

How else can meditation encourage alternate states?

By promoting more frequent transitional periods, and by training the meditator to remain experientially aware for longer intervals during them.

Does desynchronized sleep really resemble waking?

Yes. D-sleep and waking are each physiologically active brain states. They employ many of the same acetylcholine pathways which ascend from the brain stem to activate functions at successively higher subcortical and cortical levels. On the other hand, norepinephrine and serotonin functions drop during D-sleep.

How could stressful circumstances affect the brain in ways that precipitate alternate states?

Stressful events prompt the brain to release many of its primary and secondary messenger molecules. In particular, stressful events prompt peptide nerve cells within the hypothalamus to send pulses of their corticotropin-releasing factor (CRF), ACTH, and beta-endorphin widely throughout the diencephalon and brain stem.

Brain peptides coexist with other messenger molecules. Which sets of these peptide combinations have the most intriguing implications for Zen and the brain?

CRF has excitatory properties, and it coexists with enkephalins in the hypothalamus. CRF also releases both ACTH and beta-endorphin from the arcuate nucleus of the hypothalamus. Nitric oxide and dynorphin coexist with ACH in the potent activating ACH pathways which rise up from the dorsolateral pons. Substance P also coexists with serotonin in some descending pathways. These can increase the tone of extensor muscles along the spinal column. Cholecystokinin (CCK) levels are relatively high in frontotemporal cortex, where CCK coexists with dopamine.

Enkephalin and dynorphin systems also contain coexisting dopamine. The beta-endorphin system does not. What does the difference imply?

A surge within enkephalin or dynorphin systems could create additional effects secondary to their corelease of dopamine. In contrast, beta-endorphin surges could create their additional effects due to the additional release of ACTH, not dopamine.

What difference does it make if the eyes are open or closed during psychedelic drug-induced experiences of "cosmic unity?"

In each instance, the brain responds differently. When the eyes are closed, the LSD subject perceives the experience as an independent complex pattern. In contrast, with the eyes open, the person may develop a sense of merging with the environment and of becoming one with the objects perceived. Investigators who study alternate state phenomena need to be aware of these differences.

What is special about the cortex of the anterior temporal lobe?

Into it converge both ACH and opioid pathways. Moreover, the temporal tip plays a major role in the complex ways that LSD changes perception.

All along, there has been an emphasis on the way that meditative training encourages the aspirant to pay specific undivided attention to the events of present experience. But what does this imply in psychophysiological terms?

Bare, mindful attention is a mode of clear awareness. It focuses on the concrete realities of *this* present moment. This "now" moment is far removed from our usual thought congestion, and it provides an open, undistracted setting. Into this mode, many lesser insights will enter, cresting on their own little-known intrinsic rhythms. Moreover, the awareness of *this present moment* is a few steps closer to that instant, extraordinary grasp of *things as they really are*, a topic that will be further clarified in part VII.

PART VI

Turning In: The Absorptions

Zen must be understood from the inside, not from the outside.

Daisetz Suzuki (1870–1966)

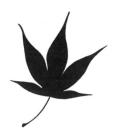

Vacuum Plenum: Kyoto, December 1974

And then some evening their bodies will
become quite comfortable and their minds
quite still. Ah! And for a moment, a bare
moment, they have an intimation of what
Hakuin meant when he sang:
This very place is the Lotus-land,
this body Buddha.
Afterwards, without speaking a word, they
will put on their coats and go home.

Ruth Fuller Sasaki (1883–1967)[1]

It is the evening of December 2, 1974, a typical cool, damp time of the year in Kyoto. The last beautiful, red Japanese maple leaves are now dropping off. Soon we too will be departing to spend the second half of the sabbatical year in Stockholm. Change is in the air.

During the previous months, I have been sitting regularly in zazen two mornings a week at Ryoko-in. Now the major sesshin, called *rohatsu,* is in its second day.[2] Yesterday, I sat in zazen for two hours in the morning from 8 to 10 A.M. Following it came a work period, a lecture, and two more hours of evening zazen. This morning, after another morning of sitting, and an interview with Kobori-roshi, I went back to the university as usual to work in the pharmacology laboratory. This evening, I have returned for two more hours of zazen. This particular evening sitting is being held in another small subtemple of Daitoku-ji nearby. It is called Ryosen-an, and here Ruth Sasaki used to be the abbess.

I have never been in Ryosen-an before. My senses feel open, poised, as I enter its unfamiliar gate in the dark. After two consecutive days of both morning and evening zazen, I am relaxed, concentrated, centered. I feel an unusually strong sense of calm determination and purpose. During the second period of zazen this leads me to consider adopting an even firmer sitting posture, so that I pull the left leg over even more than usual. In this snug half-lotus position I have a more stable base. Yes, but within minutes my left leg tingles uncomfortably. Soon, numbness ascends until my whole lower leg and back of the thigh falls totally asleep. Still, the original calm resolve has one other, more salutary, effect. It leads me consciously to restrain from moving myself, or the leg, for the noise would disturb others in the zendo. So I abandon myself to this numbness, stick it out, accepting the consequences.

When the second sitting ends, perhaps a quarter of an hour later, I lift up the senseless, paralyzed, left leg by hand and massage it for a very long minute. It finally tingles reassuringly. Unusually painful pins and needles take over. These are gradually replaced by enough function so that, still limping, I can enter the kinhin line and barely hobble along for the few remaining minutes of walking zazen.

Disappointing. Just when I think I am getting somewhere, I find that my sitting is flawed! Back on the mat once more for the last sitting of the evening, my former resolve has vanished. *My* will has dissolved during this process of giving in, and of giving myself up to numbness and paralysis. Gone is any sense of striving, pressure, stress, or strain. A passive affective tone now prevails: a settled, relaxed release from purpose. Simple acceptance. . .

Perhaps as a result, at this final sitting, both the position of my legs and the rest of the zazen posture now become natural, balanced, comfortable. I am not sleepy. I feel mentally calm and physically stable. I register these feelings and the next one, but they are my last conscious sensate thoughts for a long interval of time . . .

Noting that this new zendo has more electric light illumination than does our regular zendo, I lower my eyelids slightly, half-closing them to reduce the brightness.

What follows is an abrupt, complete blank. It lasts an indeterminate period of time. Nothing intervenes—no feeling sleepy, no head nodding, no quick trunk movements to catch myself from dropping off. However long this blank period lasts, it does not change my tone or posture. Consciousness drops out. Unknown to me, my body remains erect.

A seamless interval runs between this phase of absolute mental blankness and the next phase. Hyperawareness then turns itself on immediately but *smoothly*, as with a rheostat. The transition period contains no sense of physical, mental, or emotional startle. Instantly I am *extra*–wide-awake, more totally awake than ever before in my life.

A gray indistinct mist engages the top half of seeing, perhaps because my lids are half-open. It blends with a soft, pink color in the bottom half. Neither occasions any surprise, nor does the image which now presents itself to total awareness.

A small red maple leaf is THERE. It has made no entrance, it is simply there. It hangs far up in the top left corner of what is now a black field of vision. Everything stops. The leaf, too, stays motionless, stem pointing down to the left, tip directed diagonally up to the right. Along its edges and veins, sharp contrasts and surface markings are intensified in exquisite fine-grained detail. Its vivid colors glow. They are a stained glass window transilluminated from behind. It all seems *right*, a complete answer satisfying some unasked question.

And the leaf hangs there as a simple bare, detached fact, in an utterly still black void.

It is the sole inhabitant. It and awareness anonymous. For no personal self is in this scene, or observing it. No head, body, arms, legs—no *one* is in the center. Extraordinarily clear perception is going on *by itself*, spontaneously, automatically.

Vanished by now is every ordinary physical and mental constraint that would limit the boundary of a visual field. Total visual awareness is all-encompassing, its focus wide-open to a space which extends 360 degrees in every direction. Its vantage point extends as far up and as far down under as it does forward. It reaches back around to the rear as far as to the right and left sides. And *it stretches out into an infinite distance,* especially in front of its witness, that fully aware nonentity back in its center.

The motoric "looking" aspect of gaze feels steadily fixed on a single, forward-directed hold. In contrast, the sensate events on the receptive side take on global properties. The process of "seeing" is defining itself spontaneously. Seeing *what?* Empty space? No. *Jet blackness, glistening in fine detail and with great immediacy* throughout the entire volume of limitless space.

So this leaf is simply hanging up there in this black, silent, vast anonymous awareness. (If the neurologist were there, he would recognize that the leaf hangs far too high up and to the left to be seen by any person who is using only a "normal" field of vision. But no neurologist is there.) Yet, despite its impossibly remote position, the leaf is still being seen as clearly as though it were placed directly in front of the viewer. Again, neither the enhanced clarity nor the striking colors register as an inconsistency. The leaf is seen and appreciated; it is not thought about, let alone analyzed.

Then the leaf vanishes. It drops out as softly as it came. No forewarning, afterimage, or sense of loss.

With its departure, the sole object in view is the immense open vault. It is a singular expanse. Total awareness perceives it as blacker than black, yet glistening like a huge crystal of obsidian. Moreover, the same clear awareness—as it pervades this semitransparent void—is itself infiltrated from every direction by a subtle, exquisite aesthetic enchantment.

Subsequently, a different sense takes over. A deep, serene atmospheric comfort infuses every dimension of this earlier enchantment. It is the cozy feeling one knows from having been extra-snug indoors during a snowy winter holiday, comforted at the hearth by a warm fire. It is not a caloric heat, nor is any hearthlike visual glow present. It is something far more profound. It is a deep satisfaction, and it also enters unannounced, not in response to something. No overwhelming sense of goodness, no badness, no notions of Heaven or Hell, no great wisdom, no almighty presence, no time, no person is there to share it.

Nor is any sound there. Absolute silence is prevailing ever since the leaf arrived. No trace remains of the usual background hum that accompanies everyday hearing. No distant hiss as from a seashell held to the ear. No faint echoes. It is being in a total soundless vacuum.

The black, timeless, silent void continues. It lingers, then very subtly wanes. Slowly, smoothly, uniformly, everything goes through a diminuendo to return to a person on the mat.

To a person on the mat who is not the same person. Within the residual bliss, the first feeling is a wave of profound gratitude mixed with a sense of awe. No disappointment lingers, no wish to get back inside the experience. Then, over the next several minutes, the detached person is gradually reinfiltrated by some of the usual sensibilities of the *I-Me-Mine* existence. Even so, he-I perceives that there is a striking difference. It is the novel sense of being *fully* alive. It is a mental-physical compound, a blend of some of the initial extraordinary mental clarity plus those physical sensations which go along with one's having entered into a fully erect, alerted posture. For this new feeling, which comes from being extra-upright, has taken over the back of my head, neck, and entire spinal column. Even so, it feels altogether natural, unstrained.

Moreover, getting up from the mat is simple. *Movements perform themselves.* Both legs and the rest of my body feel about a third their usual weight—free, agile, mobilized by a quick liveliness. With senses sharpened, the sound of the final bell penetrates deeply, as do other sounds during the rest of the evening. Yet none so loud as to be unpleasant. Having accepted a ride home later that night with two other friends from the sangha, I find no inclination whatsoever to talk about the experience. It takes on its own, deeper, private, sacred-like quality. Sleep that evening is deep, dreamless, restful.

By the next morning the light body, lively movements, erect posture, sharpened senses, and the residual mental clarity are half-gone. Over that day and the next, everything gradually fades away. Yet several brief traces of each of these return over the following two days, intensified together and lingering for a few seconds each time.

Two mornings after the event, I enter my next sanzen interview with Kobori-roshi. I begin with the innocent remark that during evening zazen I have seen a leaf. Immediately, his face darkens. He shakes his head and utters a brusque, "NO! When you concentrate too hard, you may see things." Muttering in Japanese for many seconds, he then abruptly and summarily dismisses the topic from further discussion. I leave the rest of the interview feeling disappointed, but I have been learning. I remain silent.

Could the inquisitive neurologist in me ever stop wondering: how did all these remarkable events come about? But it would take many weeks for me to be aware that I was overlooking something peculiar. For you would think that I might also have been curious enough to ask: why did *this particular leaf* enter the scene?

109

The Leaf: Coda

Just an old leaf, yet
try to follow its structure—
or count its colors!

J. Hackett[1]

It is a longer story than one might suppose, this account of letting go, of yielding, and of seeing that red Japanese maple leaf in a void of space. Two months have passed. I now have in my hand the latest batch of 35-mm color transparencies. Taken in Japan, they have been processed in the United States and just forwarded to me in the mail to Sweden. I am looking, astounded, at one set of photographs. They do more than remind me about that leaf I had hallucinated while meditating. They *prove* that I had seen it even earlier, and had interacted with it once before.

The photographs reveal that I had already framed the very same Japanese maple leaf in the viewfinder of my camera. The date indicates that I had done so back in November in Kyoto. The transparencies also show that the actual leaf was lying in the identical, diagonal position: its stem pointing down and to the left. Obviously, before the sesshin, the real leaf had made a strong aesthetic impression on me as it lay flat against a damp cobblestone pavement. Moreover, it had made multiple visual impressions on my brain as well, because I had carefully focused three times on this leaf, each at a different exposure, while photographing it from above.

The evidence of the mounted transparencies jogs my memory. Sure, *now* I recall the day and the very spot where I had photographed the real leaf. The date was six or seven weeks before the leaf image reappeared that night in the zendo. Two separate and distinct events. This was odd. Why hadn't I made the connections? Indeed, would I ever have rejoined the associative links between them if I had not later seen the transparencies? I doubt that I would. *The two experiences seemed to have been stored in separate mental compartments.*

Nor does the story end then. Five years later, returning to Kyoto on a trip, I make the pilgrimage to Ryoko-in to pay Kobori-roshi an informal visit. In the course of the conversation, I venture to explore the episode again. This time, in view of the way he had reacted before to the leaf, I consider it prudent to describe all the rest of that early experience at the subtemple of Ryosen-an. Now, the roshi's immediate response is totally accepting. He obviously appreciates hearing about it. He leans forward, listens attentively, nods his head repeatedly, flashing his warm, knowing smile. Choosing not to dwell on any detail, he simply says, "Yes, when I had that, it was like being in a vacuum."

Next, in one graceful gesture, he raises his left arm slightly and then drops it all the way, palm down. It remains down there at his side for several seconds. Then he says: "After blankness, going down, there is . . ." No need for him to finish the sentence. For then, without a word, he simply turns his palm up and this time raises his entire left arm up to shoulder height.

By gesture am I led to understand: going this deep is followed by an especially steep ascent. Moving quickly on, he preempts any further wordy discussion of the topic. This time, by what he *omits,* will I be led to understand: in Zen, this episode of five years ago, however remarkable it may seem to me, is to be regarded as "nothing special."

But there remains much more to be said, certainly in any book about Zen and the brain. Indeed, we now address the specific elements of this experience in the remaining chapters of part VI. Before doing so, we first need to clarify many ambiguities. They're embedded in the use of the word *samadhi.*

110

The Semantics of Samadhi

The time comes when no reflection appears at all. One comes to notice nothing, feel nothing, hear nothing, see nothing . . . But it is not vacant emptiness. Rather it is the purest condition of our existence.

Katsuki Sekida[1]

A slippery topic, samadhi. A word so many-sided that it poses major semantic problems. It suffers in translation, as will anyone who tries to tag it with but one meaning. Some render it as "concentration," others as "absorption," still others as "trance," "stillness," "collectiveness," etc.[2]

The ambiguities date to ancient times. In Sanskrit, samadhi implied a "placing together," a joining of things in the sense of a union.[3] Successive cultural traditions employed the word in different ways. Six different Chinese characters were used to render the term samadhi, three used to convey the sound and three others to confer meaning.

Drawing on ancient yogic practices, the early Indian Buddhists specified some eight levels along the pathway to what they called samadhi.[4] The levels are difficult to visualize in the abstract, and Zen itself will tend to pay rather little formal notice to such divisions. However, they do describe sequences which are still of general interest to us. For example, the first four stages unfold when the meditator concentrates on some object, some material form, or on some related concept. Initially, thoughts cease, whether they are derived from sensations which had internal or external origins. Then, a sustained, one-pointed rapt attention sweeps in to center on the primary object of concentration. It is accompanied by feelings of rapture and of bliss. Clearly, we are on the path referred to as *concentrative* meditation (see chapter 16).

The early texts denote the next four of the phases of samadhi as being "formless levels." During these successively more advanced stages, rapture then fades, respirations slow markedly, bliss fades, and equanimity enters. There arise further refinements of one-pointedness and equanimity. And by this time, all definite body sensations such as bliss or pleasure are lost. Now, infinite space becomes the object of consciousness, followed by an awareness of objectless infinity, and then by an absorption into a void which has "nothingness" as its object. Finally, within the eighth phase, there evolves "neither perception, nor nonperception," accompanied by additional refinements of the feelings of equanimity and of one-pointedness. At such advanced levels, the field of consciousness is empty of distracting thoughts or recognized patterns of association.[5] Higher levels of samadhi become accessible only to subjects who make a full, intense commitment to the concentrative meditation techniques, not to the casual meditator.

The word "samadhi" is currently used in a more restricted sense in Buddhism, where it continues to connote many of the phases, described above, which arise along this general path of concentrative meditation. But in Hinduism generally, the elasticity within the term allows it to be stretched. So that sometimes it also goes on to convey that state of deep concentration in which union or absorption occurs into something closer to the "ultimate" reality.[6]

For our present purposes, samadhi can still imply a bringing together, and a uniting, *if* we regard such a union as implying the way awareness moves toward, blends into, holds on to, and becomes absorbed into *whatever is in its field*. To me, samadhi needs to be qualified in order to find its most appropriate use in the Zen context. I reserve the term for complex states of *extraordinary absorption*. I prefer the general term, absorption. It recommends itself for two reasons: (1) it conveys the way the physical self dissolves when one's attention is enhanced far beyond its ordinary limits; and (2) it implies becoming totally committed—almost *held* it would seem—within one attentional field to the exclusion of others.

Think back to some occasion in ordinary everyday life when a critical event captured your attention. To the angler who fishes with a bobber, one-pointed absorption comes when it plunges out of sight. Only a big fish could yank it this far down! Time evaporates to a standstill during such moments. Well-coordinated movements may go on with rod and reel, but consciousness of the physical self drops far off into the background.

A satisfying activity or hobby can totally engross a person for many minutes or hours. To become playfully lost in a hobby means to submerge oneself so deeply and with such a light touch that no person remains who worries about the project's success or failure. Then the hobbyist is no longer the captive of time.[7] Life then *flows* along joyously. Nishitani puts it succinctly: "You are in samadhi when you are no longer conscious that *you* are thinking" (italics mine).[8] A Japanese word for this state is *yugizammai*, "playing samadhi." It literally means *play-absorption* (see table 10, category VI-A). It bears emphasis that any person who engages in play-absorption must still conduct highly efficient playing behavior out in the real world at large. So when you enter "playing samadhi," you don't lose that acute vision, hearing, or the other requisite sensate functions which would, of course, then make it impossible skillfully to land that fish or to perform any other physical activity.

Even in its simpler everyday forms, samadhi implies an awareness that expands outward in the direction of merging with the object concentrated upon. Examples could be the surgeon whose absorption arises out of close volitional control when he copes with a crisis on the operating table; the spectator who can't help becoming wrapped up in the baseball game when the winning run rounds third base. In such instances, an ongoing *external* event totally captures that person's attention. Some would use the term "positive samadhi" for such situations.[9] For our purposes here, it seems better to preserve this same key distinction by introducing a less elastic term. And *external absorption* seems to be the most appropriate way to describe such moments when the person's eyes are wide-open and seeing, in preference to "external samadhi."[10]

On the other hand, some absorptions are the result of a deep *inward turning*.[10] When the state becomes this internalized, the corresponding descriptive term would be *internal absorption* (see table 10, category VI-B). The central features of a major internal absorption include (1) no spontaneous thought; (2) an intensified, fixed, internalized awareness; (3) an expansion of especially clear awareness into ambient space; (4) the disappearance of the bodily self; (5) a distinctive closing off of all sight and sound; (6) a deep, blissful serenity; and (7) a marked slowing or cessation of respiration.

It is a singular state, this sensate loss, combined with an awareness amplified to brilliant intensity. No such mixture is possible to imagine. A person must have been there and returned. In the interim, a pair of diagrams may assist in our discussion. Suppose we begin by adopting the following premise: that the boundary which separates our ordinary self from the outer world is a mental construct. In this case, our conscious mental field containing these self/other relationships will resemble that diagrammed in figure 15. Then, for contrast, the state of

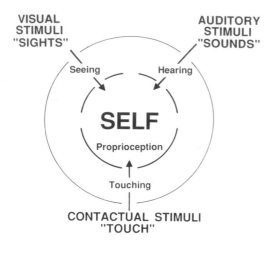

OUTER WORLD

VISUAL STIMULI "SIGHTS"

AUDITORY STIMULI "SOUNDS"

Seeing

Hearing

SELF

Proprioception

Touching

CONTACTUAL STIMULI "TOUCH"

OUTER WORLD

Figure 15   The ordinary mental field
Stimuli enter from the outside world and from internal proprioceptive events. The blend seems to contribute to a central thinking "self." Figure 1 diagrams the kinds of *I-Me-Mine* constructs which further constitute this "self" (see chapter 9).

internal absorption with sensate loss can be represented schematically by the second diagram, figure 16.

Note how much *stops* during internal absorption. The person's mental field lacks sensations of vision, hearing, and touch. Something stops them from entering from the outside world. Absent too are the subtler proprioceptive senses arising from inside the physical self. All that remains is clear awareness expanded to the nth degree throughout a vacuum plenum. The two bars in figure 16 indicate the possibility, soon to be discussed, that synaptic transmission can be blocked in the brain at more than one site.

In the depths of internal absorption, not only does sensate input drop off but no thoughts engage in any of their usual mental reflections. Later, as the person comes out of this internalized moment, sensate perceptions and affect seem to have been rinsed. "You find yourself full of peace and serenity, equipped with strong mental power and dignity. You are intellectually alert and clear, emotionally pure and sensitive."[11]

Meditators usher in their everyday sitting with a prelude of bowing and other meditative rituals. These become semivoluntary preparations, part of their routine for enhancing concentration. But later, in an episode of absorption, what supervenes is an *involuntary* concentration. And the way that it takes over is quite extraordinary. Some authors[1] have concluded that three meditative techniques make it easier to enter into samadhi: (1) becoming totally absorbed in "crawling along" inch by inch from one exhalation to the next; (2) focusing attention on the

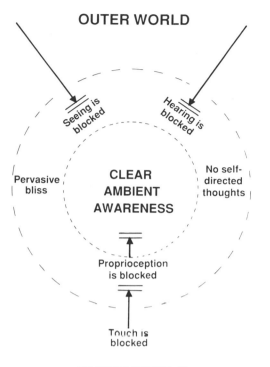

OUTER WORLD

Seeing is blocked

Hearing is blocked

Pervasive bliss

CLEAR AMBIENT AWARENESS

No self-directed thoughts

Proprioception is blocked

Touch is blocked

OUTER WORLD

Figure 16 The mental field of internal absorption with sensate loss (State VI-B)
A major absorption vanishes the bodily self and effaces the ordinary physical boundaries of the *I-Me-Mine*. Here, the dotted lines serve only to indicate its former boundaries. What remains is a witnessed, silent, heightened clear ambient awareness. Note that sensations are blocked. This block shuts off not only the outer world but also proprioceptive information from the head and body. Aside from a pervasive enchantment and bliss, most emotions do not register. This state lacks permanently transforming, major insights unless conjoined with elements of State VII. Contrast with figures 15 and 19.

lower abdomen (the tanden); and (3) closing the eyes (unorthodox for Zen), so as to facilitate looking inward.

D.T. Suzuki describes what happened to him on the fifth day of one particular sesshin. At that time he had entered samadhi and had become totally absorbed in his koan, *Mu*.[12] By then, he had lost every artificial separateness which had previously been implied by the phrase, "being conscious *of*" Mu. Instead, he was "*in Mu*." United with his koan, he was in the union of "samadhi."

Now comes the next phase, a rising up and out from samadhi. It is a sensitive interval, and it can prove critical. In this period of clarity, a sudden stimulus might trigger kensho or satori. To those same persons who, moments before, had been totally absorbed in their koan, being abruptly released from such focused concentration could become an avenue for reaching the threshold of kensho. Indeed, further to illustrate this point, it is important to note what then happened in D.T. Suzuki's own circumstance. For it was when a bell awakened him out of this particular samadhi that he went on to experience satori.

In this, and in numerous other examples, one finds that a period of samadhi can be a prelude to kensho. Most often, it is a separate episode which precedes awakening by weeks, months, or years. But sometimes, it can precede it by seconds. One can then appreciate how, when these two states do evolve back to back, they could have great impact. A stunned novice might later describe the whole episode as one complex evolving event, oblivious to the fact that two categories of events had merged as they had fallen one after the other in sequence.

The simpler episodes of samadhi blend themselves into daily life in other ways. As the more advanced meditators sink deeper, to enter and leave successively deeper periods of absorption, they retain for a longer period thereafter their residues of clear awareness and their light, brisk, fluid behaviors. These qualities will then diffuse out to reinforce that quiet awareness which goes on gratefully appreciating each of the wondrous events that make up the day.

111

The Vacuum Plenum of Absorption: An Agenda of Events to Be Explained

> The vast flood rolls onward,
> But yield yourself
> And it floats you upon it.

Ikkyu (1393–1481)[1]

Let us retrace the several events which took place during that evening in Kyoto. Absorption came as a complete surprise. It awed this meditator, and baffled this neurologist. Nothing prepared me for it; nothing in medical school, specialty training, experience with patients, or bench research. Nothing in my previous reading about Zen, or about the brain either.

A human subject has undergone a curious set of phenomena. He now finds himself cast in the role of being his own guinea pig. What happened to him? At once, our search for answers brings us to the frontiers of neuroscience. Because, as the reasons for the contents of parts III through V now start falling into place, we will be invoking these mechanisms to explain a challenging agenda of events. It runs as follows:

1. Erect posture was maintained, but consciousness totally ceased. Then, out of this blank period, emerged an extraordinary total awareness. Highly selective, it took in certain mental events that were generated internally. Yet it sharply excluded sound and other external events.

2. As it began, the silent hyperawareness floated up a loose fragment of visual recall. It projected an object seen weeks before into a formed visual hallucination: a leaf, rendered in vivid colors and fine-grained detail. The leaf was located impossibly far up and out to the left. It was perceived way up there as clearly as though it were being "seen" straight-ahead.

3. Unlimited space unfolded, encompassing a crystalline, jet blackness.

4. Clear awareness was heightened to the nth degree, and permeated this entire space in all directions. Even so, there was the simultaneous impression that gaze was being held, fixed straight-ahead.

5. Perceptions registered with great immediacy.

6. First, cool enchantment entered. Only later was the experience infiltrated by a different affective tone. It was warm and blissful.

7. Events were witnessed anonymously; no physical or shallow mental concepts of self remained.

8. The experience unfolded in some other world outside time. Still, its events evolved in a temporal sequence. The witness could later identify them and describe them in sequence.

9. Coming out from the episode, a conventional form of consciousness gradually resumed. It retained some of its previous clarity, and carried this new clarity into the subsequent perception of external and internal events.

10. Head and trunk posture then became unusually erect. Movements were lively, infused by a remarkable sense of physical lightness.

11. The experience became indelible, and subtly changed attitudes.

12. An earlier act, that of photographing the leaf, had been forgotten. This forgotten event seemed to have been kept in some mental compartment separate from the visual memory trace of the leaf image that was later hallucinated.

Four other items are also noteworthy. They provide us with antecedent circumstantial evidence:

1. Attention had earlier focused repeatedly on the original leaf through the viewfinder of a camera.

2. The tempo of meditation had increased during the two preceding days, leaving the subject feeling centered, poised.

3. The episode occurred during the last sitting of the evening in a new, unfamiliar setting.

4. Some twenty minutes before this, prolonged compression of the sciatic nerve had occurred. This created an unusually numb, tingling left leg. It was a period of associated mental distress. It was then followed by a yielding. Next came the gap during which consciousness dropped out.

These sixteen items form our agenda. One must become a kind of detective to explain each of them. Most of the clues are in parts III and IV. Building on the framework of the discussions in the other parts, we develop in the following chapters a set of coherent explanations for the way each event fits into the general framework of Zen and the brain.

The Plunge: Blankness, Then Blackness

> By the ceaseless and limitless going out of yourself and out of all things else, you will
> be led in utter pureness, rejecting all and released from all, aloft to the flashing
> forth, beyond all being, of the divine dark.
>
> Pseudo-dionysius[1]

The first phase of this internal absorption was a sudden plunge into the depths.
There was no time to test the water with a toe. First came one kind of "dropping
off of body and mind." Next, its total opposite: the fullest awareness possible.
The two phases of the meditator's situation during such moments have been aptly
described as follows: "How long a time has passed he does not know. Suddenly
he comes back to himself, and feels as if he were at the bottom of the fathomless
depths of the sea. All is silent. All is dark. Was he asleep? No, his mind is wide
awake. An internal strength seems to be welling up within him . . . No joy. No
grief. Whether it is night or day, he does not know."[2]

Why does Zen have the phrase, "the dropping off of body and mind"? And
why did Kobori-roshi drop his arm? Had I simply fallen asleep during the first
blank period? For one possible explanation is ordinary, natural sleep. Still, if this
gap in consciousness consisted of simple S-sleep, then it would be atypical in
several respects. It would also need to be a state so dissociated from the rest of
its usual sleep properties that it could plunge very far down, very fast, without
toppling the meditator, and then abruptly reverse its course.[3] For several reasons,
it seems prudent to remain open to several other optional explanations.

To begin with, we have seen how electrical stimulations can prompt sleep
by *exciting* parts of the brain. These regions include the thalamus and the basal
forebrain. Sleep also occurs when researchers use a chemical stimulant resembling glutamate to excite the thalamus in its mediodorsal nucleus. Many pathways connect this mediodorsal nucleus with other sleep-regulating areas. These
networks could express unusual variations on the basic theme of sleep.[4]

Sometimes, an entranced cat briefly withdraws its focused attention from a
mouse. The unfocused cat seems to be elsewhere. What happens in its brain, at
this instant? Many of the slower eight-per-second rhythms of "nonattention" take
over in its deep medial thalamic nuclei.[5] Primates also show these particular
rhythms of nonattention. It is worth noting that they can be enhanced by increasing serotonin tone only *slightly*. And one way to cause this slight increase in ST is
to give *low* doses of its precursor molecule, 5-hydroxytryptophan (see chapter
44). These eight-per-second rhythms of lapsed attention are quite different from
the other slow waves of ordinary S-sleep. They are very sensitive to a little ST,
whereas ordinary slow waves are not enhanced until the animal receives *higher*
doses of the ST precursor.[5,6]

There are other clinical settings in which human subjects also experience
temporary blackouts. Usually, the subjects are in a phase of being generally hyp-
erresponsive at the time. And yet, into this dominant mode, they also insert long

pauses of *no* conscious mental activity. Such pauses occur, for example, early in schizophrenia. It is then, and under conditions when they are already mentally overloaded, that some patients briefly block out their functions of thinking, ongoing activity, responsiveness, and perceptions. The patients describe this vacant interval as involving much more than the blackout of vision per se. In their words, it resembles "being in a vacuum," and entering "another world." "My mind went blank and everything got switched off."[7]

On balance, the present evidence suggests the interpretation that the blank period which came at the beginning of internal absorption was the clifflike onset of an *unusually amplified, but basically sleeplike, state*. Why, then, did this phase then proceed to envelop the awakened witness within *another world, blacker than black*?

Absolute Blackness

Suppose you enter a lighttight closet and close your eyes. In the dark, you'll still "see" some grayness. Grayness represents the background noise in the visual system. One might think of it as comparable to the faint hum in the background of your hearing. Internalized absorption penetrates beyond this, reaching *absolute blackness*. Absolute blackness is eye-catching, and it commands attention in itself. The Apollo astronauts, in their quest for the moon, looked out and were awestruck by the "blacker-than-black" intensity of outer space. That which permeates the depths of *inner* space casts a spell no less enchanting. In the mystical literature of the West, another term for the black void is "the Divine Darkness." We must be careful about the word "darkness." It is one more metaphor (like "light") which mystics sometimes stretch to include other states.[1]

Suppose, back in that dark closet, you now decide to push your attention to its voluntary limits. You strain your senses to the utmost, trying to hear the faintest noise, attempting to see the faintest glimmer of light. As a result, you may develop a sense that your visual perceptions are so enhanced that they are now penetrating to the brink of seeing "something" definite everywhere, even perhaps at very high resolution. Does this occur in internal absorption? Yes and no. Yes, there does remain the *impression* that visual contrast sensitivities are "tuned up" everywhere, in a kind of "immaculate perception." But when this space becomes vacant of images, the absorbed witness perceives nothing within it, save for the clarity of absolute blackness, glittering at high resolution.

Then, too, there is another curious aspect of absorption. Awareness turns on *spontaneously*. And maximal awareness is already *there*, even though no voluntary effort has been expended. After Kobori-roshi had dropped his arm, he then raised it straight up. A telling gesture. It points to an important property of the *ascending phase* of internal absorption: after that gap during which consciousness first drops out, consciousness then rises. Immediately it becomes witness to heights of processing speed and clarity previously unknown, even to one's most willful attempts at attention (see figure 17). And this happens automatically. No feeling of strain enters in.

The darkness has two other properties. First, it glistens. Hakuin described the gloss on what was seen as being "black like lacquer."[8] The second quality of the blackness is related to the first. To me, it recalled the *glassy transparency* of obsidian. Obsidian exists in a glasslike state. It derives its common name, volcanic glass, from the way the earth's deep core of energy once poured out its molten silicates in a form which could harden quickly into a black glass. Obsidian's glistening transparency requires no mysterious explanation. It happens when common, ordinary molecules of bedrock rearrange their internal structure into an exceptional vitreous configuration.

The brain exemplifies the principle of yin and yang as does no other organ. Excite it unduly, and its layers of inhibitory circuits swing into action. Moreover, a wide variety of norepinephrine and serotonin receptors is available to modulate the amplitude of *each* of these swings in either direction. So one can account for much of the blackness on the following basis: when the back of the brain enters into a phase of excessive excitability and desynchrony, it adjusts by shutting off incoming visual impulses. Now they can no longer be transmitted past the lateral geniculate nuclei. Our normal ascending pathways routinely help perform this same feat during our everyday sleep-waking states. Moreover, other descending pathways from an overexcited cortex can also help to place a cap on the sensate thalamus[9] (see chapter 60). A proprioceptive block in the thalamus might help explain why I felt none of the usual sensory aspects of "attentive strain" (see figure 16). Usually, one feels this sense of straining whenever extra-attentive tension enters into the muscles of the eyes, face, head, and neck.

So, after the first gap in consciousness, the sense is that awareness has leaped far beyond its usual constraints. But this heightened awareness is then quickly countered by a lower tier of offsetting inhibitory responses. Broadly stated, this is the basic reason why, even though the brain's *capacity* for sensate awareness seems so totally amplified, one actually perceives only a black void, a vacuum empty of sound and of bodily self.

Who could have believed such a state existed? Not I.

113

The Hallucinated Leaf

> Why does the eye see a thing more clearly in dreams than the imagination when awake?
>
> Leonardo da Vinci (1452–1519)[1]

It is difficult to focus on a leaf located very close to you, especially when you're using a telephoto lens. You must scrutinize a lot of fine details, pay close attention to edges and veins. Finally, you'll slide the two overlapping leaf images into one sharp focus in the viewfinder. Only then does your brain signal: closure. After you've run through this procedure three times you will have sent many messages along the central, foveal channels of your visual system. You will have performed much concentrated attentive work.

But in the background are the other reasons why you chose the leaf. Japanese maple leaves begin by having a strong aesthetic appeal of their own. Then too, living in Kyoto, one's attitudes are reinforced by the culture. This fallen maple leaf was redolent with *hakanai jinsei,* a phrase expressing the transiency of life. Sometimes the Japanese wish to tinge their special appreciation of nature with the feeling that *all* things are impermanent. In this instance, they use a more specific term. It is *mono-no-aware.* Perhaps sentiments of this kind help explain why I was so attracted to this maple leaf in the first place. No single object in recent months had received so much of my repeated, careful focused attention.

Why would an attentive photographer later hallucinate such a leaf? Research in the neurosciences now presents us with plausible reasons. Consider the properties of a few of the special nerve cells lying far forward on the undersurface of the temporal lobe (see figure 3). These cells help store prototypes of an object previously seen. They seem to file it away into longer-term visual memory.[2] So when a monkey is trying hard to discriminate one visual pattern from another, these special nerve cells are especially active. Some of them (in areas 21 and 22) fire much faster when the monkey finally closes the link between two visual images and generates an association.[3,4]

Other remarkable cells reside in the nearby perirhinal region. This important band of temporal cortex lies between the outer inferotemporal cortex and the inner parahippocampal gyrus. Some perirhinal cells have a major connection with V4 cortex. This link enables them to draw upon those particular visual circuits which are highly sensitive to different colors.[5] Within such networks reside traces of what we humans would call mental representations. As each stimulus event arrives from the outside world, these higher-order circuitries greet it and meld it into the brain's own internal centers of reference.

Moreover, many cells fire vigorously within the interotemporal region when the monkey attends to specific visual details, appears motivated, and seems expectant.[6] Any not-so distant primate relative who had focused repeatedly on a red leaf through the viewfinder of his camera, and who had paid extra attention to the closure of this task, would surely have discharged many of his own inferotemporal and color-coded neurons, and would have laid down lasting visual memory traces in the process.

Sometimes researchers can reactivate memory images in human subjects. How? By delivering electrical stimulations to the medial temporal lobe (see chapters 87 and 88). The images called forth are "vivid hallucinated re-experiences of previous events."[7] Specific scenes are actively played out before the mind's eye, not vague recollections. So the temporal lobe still retains some kind of a card index reference function, no matter how widely dispersed are our memory traces in hologram-like fashion.

What happens when an investigator delivers brief stimuli to *both* of a subject's medial temporal lobes simultaneously? The patient still goes on *perceiving* the events of the moment. Perceiving, yes. But not recognizing, and not remembering. For the stimulation has garbled both recognition and memory functions. In this disorganized state, the subject no longer knows whether an object then being seen is a new one, or some old one that has been seen many times before.[7]

Why had I forgotten that I had photographed the hallucinated leaf? Within the above observations lie two potential explanations for this curious fact: (1)

Perception is relatively durable. It can still go on registering present events, even though certain other compartments of recognition memory are not fully communicating with one another in the medial temporal lobe. (2) When a person loses all sense of a physical self, there remains no central point of reference, no long physical axis that associations can latch on to. This might have rendered it impossible for parts of my brain, after they had quickly scanned my memory bank, to say, in effect, That thing *you* are now seeing is the very same leaf *you* photographed weeks ago, when *your* hands were holding the camera in front of *your* face.

And there might be a third, related explanation. Back when I was photographing the leaf, in my ordinary state, the memory codes which had conferred meaning were going at a relatively slow pace. They would have had to shift into high speed to match the pace of my much faster, state-bound associations during the hallucination (see chapter 58).

This leaf *was* a formed hallucination. It was also the *initial positive* event in a sequence of other phenomena in the second phase of this absorption. For these reasons, it is important to localize its site of origin. Why was it seen on the left side? This indicates that the image was generated within networks in the *right* side of my brain. Recent research shows that we humans do preferentially activate the *right* anterior temporal lobe when we pay selective visual attention to the shape of an object.[8] In the monkey, once visual impulses have first registered back in the primary visual cortex, they then pass through area V4 on their way down to the inferotemporal cortex. V4 is a rich palate, heavily daubed with many potential colors. Not only are these V4 nerve cells remarkably responsive to colors, they also fire extra volleys when a monkey brings extra effort into its attention.[9] In the human brain, the cortical counterpart to V4 is located in the lower medial part of the visual association cortex. In my case, it is reasonable to attribute many of the leaf's color properties to this particular region in and around the right fusiform and lingual gyri (see figure 3).

But there was more to the hallucinated leaf than heightened colors. Its details of line and contour were greatly enhanced over those of the original. Each leaf detail was resolved into ultrafine-grained textures. The image surpassed even the sharpest picture now being promised by advertisements which invite us to buy high-definition TV. In humans, many of the same visual channels that serve us for color vision also help us perceive the form and depth of textures.[10] Then, farther back in cortex, we amplify our sensitivities to spatial contrasts within the parieto-occipital region. Again, this occurs chiefly on the *right* side. So the evidence suggests that several properties of the leaf image had been drawn from visual regions on the right side. Still, the total number of cells involved in the network of the leaf image may have been relatively few. Human cortex can be activated so focally that an EEG recorded from the overlying scalp will easily miss the site.[11]

The size of the real leaf as it was first seen through the viewfinder, its distance from the camera, together with its size in the final 35-mm transparency— all were in correct register with the size of its counterpart hallucinated image. Based on the size of the image, I would guess in retrospect that the leaf image had been projected as though it were hanging about three feet up and out in space. This implies that the image had neither been magnified nor shrunk.[12]

However, only a very special kind of "seeing" could have regenerated such an image. The image was special for four reasons. To begin with, it re-created *only the foreground*. That is, it synthesized only the leaf itself, the object I had especially focused on originally. It excluded the entire background plane, every moist cobblestone and fallen pine needle of it.[13] In the second place, there was the remarkable placement of the image. The leaf picked up as a hallucination was *not centered*, as had been the leaf in the viewfinder. The image was shifted into an impossibly eccentric position. It was placed far beyond the usual boundaries which lid and brow impose on what a person's two eyes can see. (In this respect, the leaf shared some of the same properties as did the rest of the vast space which surrounded it. For both the leaf image and space had been carried beyond the rim of my conventional visual field.) This feature indicates that after the real leaf had first been seen, the placement of its representation had undergone much further processing in the brain.

The third unusual feature was that the leaf simply materialized out of no-where. What kind of process could have regenerated and projected its image? Only functions which operated automatically. I did not call it forth, and there was no other requirement for any "voluntary" directing of attention on my part. And the final property of the "seeing" was its most singular feature: attention did not need to shift in order to *see* any detail of the reimaged leaf! Here it was, *already in sharp focus*, even though it was displaced impossibly far up, and too far off at an angle, to ever be in focus if only my ordinary frontal vision had been in charge of "seeing" it! And so, as it hung way up there, it sponsored no motor impulse which might have corrected my gaze—trying to shift it high up there and off to the left—in order to "see" the leaf.[14] None of these curious visual paradoxes seemed out of place to the witness at the time.

Suppose two groups of patients have large lesions in the same regions. But in one group the lesions are in the right cerebral hemisphere, whereas the other group has the damage on the left side. In *general*, which part of space will both groups of patients be most *in*attentive to? *They will both neglect the farthest edge of opposite space*.[15] Perhaps, then, it is time to start inquiring: would the reverse tend to be true during a *hyper*attentive state? Suppose an extraordinary state of enhanced attention were to exaggerate functions more in the parieto-temporal cortex of one side, say the right. The hypothesis proposed is that when an image is swept up into this unusual state, it might tend to be experienced farther off toward the edge of an expanded *left* visual field.[16]

From the descriptions presented in chapter 87, one can now diagnose most of the features of this leaf. It was a sleep-related hallucination. For the edge of sleep is what is implied by the prefixes *hypna-* and *hypno-* in the words hypnagogic and hypnopompic hallucination. These technical terms are tricky to spell, and difficult to keep separate. But as we now search for the mechanisms which cause absorption, their particular form of sleep-related imagery is highly pertinent. Let us review several facts which clarify this point:

1. Hypnagogic hallucinations occur during the descending transition period. The person is on the way *down*, between waking and S-sleep. Hypnopompic hallucinations are less common, but their images are otherwise identical. They occur when the sleeper is on the way *up*. This is the ascending phase. Sleep is now becoming lighter, on its way up to the waking state. Given a hallucination, these terms simply designate *which of these two possible transition periods* the subject is in at that moment.

2. The critical sequence of events was: a quick descent into a sleeplike gap of consciousness; the rapid ascent up to wakefulness; seeing vaguely through half-closed lids; the entry of the hallucinated leaf at the start of wakeful hyperawareness (see figure 17).

3. The leaf was a specific item, a memory trace laid down weeks earlier during a period of highly focused attention. Only at the *start* of this extraordinarily activated state of consciousness had events tapped into this trace discretely. Only at the start had it been held onto briefly.

4. During our normal transition periods, the major acetylcholine pathways play a key role in the processes of memory and in activating the brain.[17]

5. Other potent activating influences arise from the lateral hypothalamus. They excite both the hippocampus and visual regions as well. So several defined pathways make it possible for states of absorption to sweep up either memory traces from the remote past or ongoing sensate impressions, and then to inject them almost at random into whatever other scenery or spatial matrix prevails in the mental field at the moment (see chapter 43).

6. A dense network of serotonin terminals invests the primary visual cortex, the inferotemporal cortex, the lateral geniculate nucleus, and the intermediate layer of the superior colliculus. Typically, one might expect that ST tone would start lessening late in the evening on the way into the *usual first* transition period. This would be a time when the trendlines of our major activity cycles are on the way down, descending from waking toward sleep. So, in addition to the usual drop in ST, several other sources might contribute to the *disinhibitions* during this descending interval, setting the stage for the entry of brief hallucinatory responses.

7. But more ST can be released as part of the response to earlier stressful circumstances (see chapter 44). Moreover, there are several different subtypes of ST receptors. And one recalls that an early clinical effect of LSD, when the drug is injected intravenously, is the enhancement of fine visual details. The subject then sees items, out at the *edge* of the visual field, becoming as visually impressive and important as objects in the center.[16]

One tenet central to Zen is to empty the theatre of the mind. With no actors on stage, and neither scenery nor props around, the set can become truly empty (and ready for the main event). Operationally, this means that the trainee will learn to enter periods of prolonged meditation, and will learn (usually by example) to downplay the by-products of the vision quest. Are we downplaying this visual hallucination? Hardly. For the purposes of this book it is being cited as evidence of many things. Among them is the fact that when one meditator's brain was undergoing a brief surge of activity, it had not become 100 percent "emptied" of a certain once-impressive leaf. For that evening, the surge of natural events had swept up an incidental item, in the same casual manner as might any brook, when swollen with rain, rise to engulf some fallen leaf on its bank.

One other matter was fully as impressive as the leaf. It was that singular theatre of empty space it hung suspended in.

114

Space

> With a wall all around, a clay bowl is molded; but the use of the bowl will depend on the part of the bowl that is void . . . So advantage is had from whatever is there; but usefulness rises from whatever is not.
>
> Lao Tzu (?604–?531 B.C.E.)[1]

> Can all the sky, can all the World, Within my Brain non lie?
>
> Thomas Traherne (1636–1674)[2]

Space is a weightier subject than one might think. The way the self interrelates within space has long been a central issue in Zen. It was obvious to William James that the way we perceive space was a critical issue for psychology as well. He devoted more pages of his classic textbook to the chapter on space—148 pages—than he did to any other subject.[3] And in those pages, one finds many words describing space placed in italics. For instance, he says we perceive spatiality as taking "the shape of a simple total vastness, in which *primitively* at least, no *order of parts* or of *subdivisions* reigns."[4] Moreover, we sense that its vastness is "*as great in one direction as in any other.*"[5] These italicized phrases suggest that James had once carried on an intimate relationship with space. Indeed, no person who has once entered into the vastness of this spatial relationship is likely thereafter to underestimate how important space is.

How did we build our "*original sensation of space?*" James believed that we brought together those elements of volume, vastness, or extent which arose as the products of our ordinary sensations. Out of these sensations, he said, a "primordial largeness" emerged, one which consciousness could then go on to measure and to subdivide. Only after our brain had finally woven all these elements together would the resulting spatial fabric then become what we think of as the "real space of the objective world."[6]

In order to appreciate what else space involves, it will help to imagine ourselves in a specific situation in space. Start with now. Here we are aware that we are attending to a sensory field which lies *in front* of us. And right here, in front, we are now becoming acutely *conscious* that we are paying attention to a particular line, on a page, in a book. Farther out still is an edge of subliminal awareness, fading in and out.

But beyond these, we also possess an even more subtle implicit awareness. It is absolutely essential to the way we function, yet we are rarely conscious that it exists. Even so, preconsciously, its elements have been keeping track of precisely where this book is in relation to you, its reader. They also registered, preconsciously, the position you occupy at this very moment in the room, building, or outside. Without your even being "aware" of it, these functions of "incidental awareness" have registered the rest of the world *all around*. It will take three words to describe our normal hidden capacity for sensate inferences: *unconscious circumspatial awareness* (see table 16, chapter 116).

Now this covert capacity of spatial awareness is *not* what we usually call our "mind's eye." For what does the mind's eye do? It typically summons up images of people and things *in front* of us. It functions, more or less, under our conscious commands. We can will it to retrieve. When it does project these visual images, they tend to remain passively in front of us. At this point we may say, I can *see* it in my mind's eye.

In contrast, our hidden awareness is *un*conscious and *circum*spatial. It may seem to start out with that property which we refer to by calling it our ordinary "sense of place." But psychological tests suggest that our usual sense of place is already relatively large, and that it does not restrict itself to that limited zone which ordinary frontal vision perceives out in *front* of us. No, our true sense of *space* goes on to encompass a cycloramic field of no less than 360 degrees.[7] Indeed, as our large visual brain goes on to represent this huge space, its scope extends *in back* to encompass a whole "visual world behind the head."

When we speak about "representations" in the brain, we usually tend to think in terms of smaller items, set in static, three-dimensional spatial relationships. A face, a leaf. But when the vast representations involve space itself, they don't just sit there passively. We *use* them. Indeed, this dynamic matrix of polysensory properties serves as the framework we hang onto when we act out our complex behaviors. This process enables the Japanese bicycle repairman, so mindfully intent on fixing my flat tire, to reach up far behind *without looking,* and grasp, instantly, the one tool he needs from his long shelf. And you could access circumspatial awareness in pitch darkness if some emergency occurred, and your survival depended on running down a familiar flight of stairs. So one's circumspatial awareness is utterly practical. Its scope extends usefully not only behind the head but above it, and below the feet.

Does this sound strange? Then consider other examples in daylight. The outfielder moves with the batter's swing at the plate, before he hears the crack of ball on bat. While still sprinting he leaps, makes an impossible backhand catch over his shoulder, tumbles, and comes up with the ball. The harried quarterback releases his pass toward a prearranged empty space. Moments later his wide receiver cuts left and jumps to snatch it from a swirl of moving defenders. Athletes practice for years these repertoires for catching and throwing. Their early sense of place—first localized mostly to the space in front—becomes refined into a huge, imaginary but skill-full volume. Within this circumspace, trajectories and intercepts plot themselves automatically.

However clumsy we may think of ourselves, the rest of us have also defined our space, unknowingly, in ways that help us act within it. Our parietal association cortex has been sending much of its output to the outer surface of our frontal lobe. These two regions help develop options for acting in spatial contexts which are already well structured. In contrast, the inner folds of orbitofrontal cortex have gathered softer, limbic biases mostly from the anterior cingulate gyrus and the temporal lobe. Some of its options unfold as motivations, others as cautions. So actions *might* take place in the space of the world outside. But then again, they might not.[8] Within such ambivalences, amateur athletes sometimes "choke up in the clutch" when driven by fear of failure or lust for fame.

Imagine, for a moment, how it feels when you are seated at your usual breakfast table. There, even after you had closed your eyes, you still wouldn't be able to dislodge the compelling reality of your being physically present in *that* precise spot. And, as James noted, much of that unshakable local sense of place draws upon a host of previous incidental memories. For not only had you been in that same place many times before but subliminal sensate cues had also reinforced that sense of location: the aroma of your coffee; the tinkle of a spoon in a bowl; the taste of cold orange juice.

No laboratory rat depends any less on *his* morning meal. Wherever you deposit him in a complicated maze, he'll finally work his way back to that very same spot where he, too, had found his breakfast before. His hippocampus plays a key role in this spatial working memory. Why are some of its pyramidal cells called "place cells?" Because they fire more *only* when this rat occupies one particular place in the maze.[9] Certain animal strains perform especially well on such tests of working memory. Bred selectively, they now have extra-large mossy fiber terminals in their hippocampus.[10]

You can assist a less-gifted, wayward rat to quickly find its meal. You can set out various cues at different places in his maze environment. The cues can be as diverse as a source of light, a breeze, or a sound stimulus. Each cue causes some place cells to fire. Does it seem as though the rat is "triangulating?" If so, it is not in the conventional visual sense in which one might use this surveying term. Instead, the rat is *integrating* its several types of spatial cues. Indeed, its place cells, being exquisitely *polysensory*, help to specify one stationary point of reference because they can pull together and *associate* several stimuli from such very different modalities as vision, touch, and sound. Still other hippocampal cells fire depending on how *far* the rat moves. These cells provide dynamic, feedback data, and so are called "*dis*place units."

What happens when lesions wipe out a rat's place and displace functions in the hippocampus on both sides? The rat appears disoriented. Sensory cues may still enter the rat's brain, but they aren't being integrated at higher spatial levels. In this respect, experimental disorientation resembles the findings in two human disorders. One occurs after a surgical resection has removed much of the right hippocampus and adjacent temporal cortex. These patients lose their short-term visual memory for where an object is located in space.[11] The other disorder is called transient global amnesia. "Where am I? What day is this?," the patients say, repeatedly. They appear to be experiencing dysfunction in the posterior hippocampus, or in the parahippocampal region which supplies the whole hippocampus with many sensory cues (see chapter 42; figure 3). These are key portions of the larger matrix underlying our normal concepts of place and space. Transient disconnections here can cause a major change in the quality of consciousness.

How did we develop this capacity to be aware, so unconsciously, of the spatial envelope around us? In utero, as yet unborn, our brain stem had no context for the richness of adult three-dimensional space, let alone for the extra dimensions it could reach during the alternate states of maturity. This tiny stem was still largely unconditioned. How could the fetus attach any higher conceptual meanings to a sound, a touch, or a visual stimulus? Yet the brain stem of a newborn baby is no tabula rasa, no blank floppy disk in a computer. It is already channeling stimuli into certain designated regions. These will serve its primitive needs to localize. In this sense, the stem is a floppy disk which has already been formatted. Now ready to record a signal in one specific locus, it has taken that essential first step which will later make it possible *to access and retrieve one specific message.*[12]

After birth, where does the infant's brain begin to elaborate its subliminal grasp of space? Probably in those polysensory nerve cells of the midbrain colliculi and in the pulvinar of the thalamus (see chapters 54 and 61). Later will come the relays up to the large visual association cortex. Here, many other cells are also coded to respond when both sound *and* visual signals come from the one particular locus in space.[13]

Early astronomers devised a simple sky map. It was based on a system of declinations and ascensions. On their sky map, stargazers could localize, in two dimensions, each bright star to a designated point in the heavens. But *flat* maps, based on two coordinates, are of limited use. Suppose you needed to know where our nearest star, alpha centuri is. Is it close to the planets or way out in space? And so, because the later astronomers needed to measure the *depth* of outer space, they came up with the idea of using light years. Now, in this *third* dimension, they could describe its vast distances.

What kinds of spatial coordinates does a person's brain use to grasp that apple on the table? One can put some of them into simple words: right/left, up/down, near/far. Note, however, the initial assumption: "that" apple is going to be out in *front* of the viewer. Not so with unconscious circumspatial awareness. It starts from a different premise. It stands poised to grasp an object *anywhere,* in the total envelope of space around the person.

Human beings soon insert meanings into any object we find set in space. Consider that cluster of lights in the night sky we would name Orion. Does it have a "hunter's belt"? Only by a wild stretch of the imagination. Starting with a few lights, way out in space, we lined them up and transformed them into something relevant to the personal world in which *we* live.

External space is not the sole source of data for our elaborate notions. Having developed the concept of our physical self, we went on to construct an imaginary *internal* plane which divides our whole body into its right and left halves![14]

These internal mental constructions begin in early childhood. Children gradually learn that some objects do have implicit planes of space. No, you can't actually *see* these planes, but they still lie hidden *within*.

Consider how different fruits each turn out to have their own kind of "inner space." Slicing a peach is easy: you can approach a hard peach stone by any globe-girdling route. A grapefruit is difficult. First you need to recognize its poles, then enter its soft pulpy compartments using an equatorial approach. And, already as children, we have also found that individual people have their own internal psychological attributes. So now we have begun to carry our spatial abstractions even further, into the softer realm of the psyche. As Oliver Wendell Homes once phrased it: "The outward forms the inward man reveal;/We guess the pulp before we cut the peel." [15]

Egocentric and Allocentric Cell Systems

The far-ranging cat reveals a further refinement on the theme of place cells. These special cells were discovered deep within the internal medullary lamina of the thalamus (see figure 11). Even though the cells have large receptive fields, they still fire only when stimuli arrive from one stationary location, or when moving stimuli enter this same spot. But the most interesting feature of these cells is their "global" property. It is almost as though the cat brain has on board a global positioning system (GPS). For these GPS cells are sensitive to one particular spot inside what appears to be an *absolute* field of space. [16] Nerve cells with properties such as these are called *allocentric*. This means that they are coded to receive signals from a certain fixed *absolute* place in the *outside* environment. They are *not* registering signals from this site in relation to the position of the viewing animal's head or body.

Now, allocentric nerve cells have also been found in the posterior hippocampus of the monkey. And here, more detailed studies make clear how much they differ from their adjacent *egocentric* neighbors. For these nearby egocentric cells employ a compass needle which inevitably reinforces the sense of self (see chapter 8). They are part of a self positioning system. How does their egocentric "SPS" system of reference operate? It, too, localizes sensory signals from a certain site, but it always points, as its standard of reference, back to the head and body of that particular observing monkey. [17,18]

One may speculate on these findings. However, the hypotheses are not yet testable because current neuroimaging techniques are still too slow and are limited in their degree of resolution. The speculation is that allocentric nerve cells will play a responsible role in reinforcing a sense of unity in alternate states. The corollary is that, simultaneously, egocentric nerve cell functions will be dropping out (see chapter 126). [19]

On the other hand, one can develop other plausible working hypotheses. These help explain how some of our networking functions enable us to "copy" an item—say, a leaf or an apple—and then remember it after we have once seen it "out there" in space. [8] For when human subjects turn their attention outward, and notice things globally, their brain metabolism increases in both the anterior cingulate gyrus and the right prefrontal cortex.[20] This observation is supported by the evidence that humans lose similar attentive functions (to the opposite side of their environment) if their cingulate gyrus has been damaged (see chapter 40).

Moreover, the normal cingulate gyrus does not attend only to external visual stimuli. It also registers painful and other somatosensory signals which are arising *inside* various regions of the body itself. The various lines of evidence suggest two mechanisms by which the cingulate gyrus could intensify our attachments. Perhaps one role for the cingulate gyrus is to become involved when the field of our interest is more outwardly directed, say, at some time when we were, in a sense, "painting" an actual landscape, outdoors, on some canvas held within our "frame" of reference. And then, at other times, the cingulate could be helping us focus on inner events, as our attention turned to touching up our own self-portrait, preoccupied as it usually is with vanities and related internal themes.

Let us now suppose that breakfast is over. We are now in the process of walking out the front door. As usual, our unconscious circumspatial awareness is very active. It is filing away in its card index system set after set of its mundane (but accurate) representations of what we are leaving behind, those incidental and largely visual memories of where the furniture and pictures were. But on rare occasions the veil parts, and our subliminal domain of space opens up. Only then—fully conscious at the time—do we discover this vast spatial capacity, and look out into the remarkable theater it has been able to conceive.

Not a theater-in-the-round. Not a place where the members of the audience face *in* toward a central stage and watch the performance going on in front of them. But a theater completely turned inside out. For now, a fully conscious witness occupies center stage, a nonentity who still sees, all around, the wide-open spectacle of circumspace . . .

115

The Ascent of Charles Lindbergh: Ambient Vision

> There is no limit to my sight—my skull is one great eye, seeing everywhere at once.
> Charles Lindbergh (1902–1974)[1]

When he hauled back on the stick, *The Spirit of St. Louis* barely made its ascent into the air. It was 7:52 on the morning of May 20, 1927. Nineteen hours later, he had reached the point of no return on his epic three-thousand-mile solo flight to Paris. But he was now very sleep deprived, starting his third day without benefit of genuine sleep the night before. The results were beginning to tell. One more hour, and distinctions became blurred: "At times I am not sure whether I am dreaming through life or living through a dream. It seems I've broken down the barrier between the two, and discovered some essential relationship between living and dreaming . . ."

Two more hours, and the next dawn was getting ready to break back at the Long Island airport. There his former biological clock time was the equivalent of 4:52 A.M. At that hour, under other circumstances, he would likely have been in bed, dreaming a major part of the time. Instead, he was above the unforgiving Atlantic, starting his twenty-second hour of constant vigilance at the controls. Even though his eyes remained open, he was dozing off in an unusual way.

> When I fall asleep this way, my eyes are cut off from my ordinary mind as though they were shut, but they become directly connected to this new, extraordinary mind which grows increasingly competent to deal with their impressions . . .
>
> While I am staring at the instruments, during an unearthly age of time, both conscious and asleep, the fuselage behind me becomes filled with ghostly presences—vaguely outlined forms, transparent, moving, riding weightless with me in the plane. I feel no surprise at their coming. There is no suddenness to their appearance. Without turning my head, I see them as clearly as though in my normal field of vision. There is no limit to my sight—my skull is one great eye, seeing everywhere at once.
>
> These phantoms speak with human voices—friendly, vapor-like shapes, without substance, able to vanish or appear at will, to pass in and out through the walls of the fuselage as though no walls were there . . .
>
> I'm not conscious of time's direction . . . All sense of substance leaves, there is no longer weight to my body, no longer hardness to the stick. The feeling of flesh is gone . . . I live in the past, present, and future, here and in different places all at once . . . I'm flying in a plane over the Atlantic Ocean, but I am also living in years now far away.[1]

Twenty-five-year-old Charles Lindbergh was a healthy, strapping specimen. But for several days it had been crucial for him to stay vigilant. Now, sleep-deprived and responding to other stressors, the veils parted. His brain tapped into its innermost recesses. Out of their "one great eye" he could see everywhere at once.

Ambient Vision

One great eye? What *is* this unbounded vision? A useful word to describe it is *ambient*. The word means "surrounding on all sides." Here, we use ambient vision to describe *a person's visual experience of being surrounded by space*.[2] This is not ordinary space. *This space does not end.* It has no equator or other constraining boundary. Nothing encloses its volume and limits it inside some conventional sphere. In one sense, this space represents an enormous, open empty theatre. Inside it, phantom presences *behind* the viewer might take shape. Sometimes, a leaf might even materialize out of thin air.

Ambient vision is an illusion, a global representation which an overactive brain elaborates under rare circumstances. It implies that heightened attentive circuitries are doing more than expanding those functions we are usually conscious of. They are now gaining ready access to other circuitries that were formerly hidden, including the networks which subserve our ordinary circumspatial awareness. Moreover, within the once-covert matrix of this preconscious space, a stressed normal brain will project all sorts of images, including hallucinations (see chapter 89).

Ambient vision creates an indelible impression. And compounding its awesome immensity is the vacancy in its center. Similar events are not limited to solo pilots who have lost sleep and are stressed. Emerson, choosing his words carefully, would say: "I become a transparent eyeball; I am nothing; I see all . . ."[3] What *is* this "nothing?" It too is *vacant* space. *This is where the physical self used to be.*

The poet Baudelaire once had a similar experience while he was deeply immersed in romantic music. Feeling released from the sense of gravity, he entered a delightful state, one which seemed as though he were in the grip of a long daydream. The space he then experienced was "a solitude with an *immense horizon* and widely diffused light; in other words, immensity with no other setting than itself."[4]

Why is immensity of this degree so impressive? Commenting further on Baudelaire's description, Bachelard noted that immensity itself then takes on "a primal intimate value." With this, one can agree. He then goes on to say that, "When the dreamer really experiences the word immense, he sees himself liberated from his cares and thoughts, even from his dreams. He is no longer shut up in his weight, the prisoner of his own being."[4] Our interpretations of absorption will diverge from these. First, the liberation of internal absorption is only partial. The real *psychic emancipation* is different. It begins to occur only with the initial kensho. Second, yes, there can occur in absorption a sense of lightness of the physical body. But this is a separate sensate impression. And ambient vision has not, in its immensity per se, caused the body to feel released from gravity. The lightness of the body is simply one other significant event which becomes evident after ambient vision occurs, and then continues on its own.

The brain tends to fill up empty spaces in perception. Cut off its usual sensory input from an arm or a leg, and it goes on to hallucinate the extremity (see chapter 93). When deprived of a limb at the periphery, the brain re-creates a phantom limb, having drawn on a wealth of the limb's central representations. Why do we populate our own dreams and daydreams with other kinds of elaborate scenarios? Possibly because we are basically image-makers. The floodgates of "image-ination" are poised to open whenever our sensate input drops off. *Ambient space is the expanded stage for the grand and global theatre of a rich imagination.*

During stimulating circumstances, this stage does not stay empty. Soon, scenery and plot are improvised. Central casting easily supplies characters. The temporal lobes, in particular, provide many susceptible links in a person's lifelong chain of subliminal associations. Tugging on these links, the stressed human brain can take off on solo flights of imagination, and it can even fill up a fuselage *behind* the pilot with surrealistic, phantom spirits. Similarly, patients whose eyes have remained closed can gather enough inferences from their surgeons' and nurses' voices to fill in the rest of the details of an entire operating room. In the phenomenon called autoscopy, such patients imagine their body in detail, lying down on the operating table, seeming to witness the whole scene from above.

We need not jump to extrasensory, metaphysical conclusions about any of these descriptions. (Nor, incidentally to those provided by the so-called alien abductees.) Instead, we need only keep three facts in mind: first, how spacious the ambient theatre really is; second, how enormously fertile are the playwright capacities in every brain, for it can create fantastic scripts and embroider them with details drawn from as far back as the remote past and from as far forward as the inconceivable future; third, how heavily overcommitted our brain usually is, and how constantly it calls dress rehearsals for imaginary scenarios which will never take place.

Given a true appreciation of the last two facts in particular, it also becomes easier to understand how a meditator's busy brain might benefit from entering the quiet depths where listening goes on in silence (see chapter 117).

116

The Ambient Vision of Meditative Absorption

> Above, there is not a tile to cover his head; below, there is not an inch of ground for him to stand on . . . This is that state of total empty solidity, without sound and without odor, like a bottomless, clear pool. It is as if every fleck of cloud had been wiped from the vast sky.
>
> Master Hakuin[1]

Considering how much ambient vision implies about the brain, it is curious how little scientific attention it has drawn. Yet many meditators have certainly experienced unbounded circumspatial sight when they entered an episode of internal absorption. Among them was the Chinese monk, Bukko, who migrated to Japan and founded Enkakuji seven centuries ago.[2] When Bukko was twenty-two, sitting in zazen, his koan disappeared along with the consciousness of his body. What remained was only the immensity of space, and no thoughts.

Hakuin, too, had witnessed the immensity of space. He was impressed. In his *Chant in Praise of Zazen*, he exclaims: "How vast is the heaven of boundless samadhi!" In this instance, he was making a specific reference to the way internal absorption extends its visual awareness into an enormous circumspatial field. He was not referring to what we usually perceive consciously: that limited field of vision in front of us. Nor was he talking about our usual, localized latent sense of place.

But on another occasion Hakuin might also have been using a simile to describe the vastness of the distance involved. For then he said, "attain a state of mind in which even though surrounded by crowds of people, it is as if you were alone in a field extending tens of thousands of miles."[3] So we need to note carefully the possibility that a very experienced person might use the *sensate* aspects of ambient vision to serve as a simile or as a loose metaphor for the other more complex kinds of objective *mental* distancing which occur later, in the psychic realm. Here lies a trap for the unwary. It can account for many serious misunderstandings in the literature about what constitutes the form and content of absorption as distinct from insight-wisdom.

This book aims to minimize similar misunderstandings. The main purpose of table 16 is to summarize the properties of our ordinary subtle awareness of the

Table 16
Types of Ordinary and Extraordinary Awareness of Space

Type	Degree of Control	Field	Comment
Unconscious, circumspatial awareness	Automatic, ongoing	The large "sense of place" normally surrounding the person	The hidden, polysensory, integrated registration of space which we access in our usual, everyday activities
Ambient vision	An automatic surge, e.g., in internal absorption	Vast, unbounded space	The experience of a circumspatial awareness in rare states of heightened consciousness
Comprehensive vision	A brief, automatic surge, e.g., in kensho	Space in front, infused with coherent insight-wisdom	Syncretism; the direct experience of all things as *they* really are, in the absence of the personal self

envelope of space all around us. With this preamble, one can begin to appreciate how its properties could be amplified into ambient vision. Later, in part VII and in table 18, we consider at greater length those distinctive features of the different, more advanced psychic domain which here is called simply comprehensive vision.

High in Katmandu is the temple of Bodnath. Two large painted eyes look out into the world from each of the four sides of its tower. Eight eyes. What could they be seeing? There exist several possible levels of interpretation. When I first visited this temple back in 1963, the Nepali told me that they symbolized the all-seeing eyes of Buddha, who always looked with omniscience into the world in every direction at once. But what did this kind of a global outlook really mean? At the time, I had no personal basis for appreciating its nuances. Eleven years later, I experienced ambient vision during internal absorption. Only then could I finally begin to grasp a few of the elementary principles of what might be implied, even to a beginner whose basis for interpretation had been limited to this lower ambient, sensate level.

Ambient vision, restricted to no frontal plane, does encompass the four quadrants. But it doesn't stop there. It sees into vacant space *above and below the witness*. In this respect, the ambient "seeing" then goes on exactly as Hakuin described. It takes off the tile roof. It leaves out every inch of the ground beneath. Moreover, it proceeds inside a circumspace stripped of every anatomical reference to the head and body of the witness in the center.

Some persons might become overly impressed by the way their vision had opened up into ambient space. So much so that they might assume it must represent intuitions that had come from a much higher level: a true glimpse into the ultimate realities of the outer void of cosmic space. From this premise they could be misled into believing that during absorption they had entered into the kind of supranatural *extra*sensory perception that only the "eye of the Buddha" itself could be capable of. Maybe this is the way it seems.

Here we have adopted a more limited interpretation: ambient vision as but an introductory phase on the long meditative journey; as a kind of intensified seeing which rises into consciousness from one's interior capacities, those of the covert sensate realm; as the product of one's natural matrix of circumspatial awareness that had been there all along, and was now highly energized; as an experience which implies only that physiological events have surged through several levels from the midbrain on up.

A mundane conjecture, compared with the cosmic theory, but only slightly less remarkable. For the present interpretation means that the experience is a very special *intra*sensory event. It implies that the human capacity for ambient vision discloses our mature tabula rasa, as it now exists. And that this empty slate is the expression of our adult spatial network shorn of what we had earlier packed it so full of: bodily self; sensate memories of people and things; simple physical attachments and elementary scenarios, all of which our bodies might soon have been ready to act out into behavior.

What could set off such an amplification of one's ordinary, unconscious circumspatial awareness? How could it expand into a person's full consciousness in the form of ambient vision? Maybe it's the other way around. Perhaps *conscious* awareness itself, when *it* becomes amplified enough, will set in motion this kind of seeing. The sequence of events during my episode of absorption supports the latter interpretation. For the ambient vision began as one part of an extraordinary *general* heightening of total awareness. After all, it was an extra–wide-awake visual brain that had briefly sprouted the leaf image far out on one of its many potential arborizations.

Which circuitries normally have properties that could help create ambient space? A few simple examples, taken from the lower processing levels, serve to illustrate the mechanisms which could cause space to "expand." Suppose you stimulate a cat's midbrain reticular formation, or even its paw. This stimulation causes cells in the lateral geniculate nucleus to expand the size of the visually receptive fields that the cat is able to "see" and will respond to.[4]

Farther along in the visual pathways lie sensitive polysensory cells. We now understand why nerve cells that possess these special properties normally help us get a sense of where a stimulus is in space. each single cell can be excited by a visual *or* an auditory *or* a somatesthetic stimulus. And each of these stimuli will be coming from only *one* direction, or from a particular location. Polysensory cells fulfilling these requirements occur at several levels: in the colliculi of the midbrain, the pulvinar of the thalamus, and in the cortex of both the temporal[5,6] and parietal lobes. Most of these regions are parts of the *second* visual system. Moreover, norepinephrine terminals make a salient excitatory contribution to many of them (see table 5). So extra NE released from these nerve endings may help explain how a person's unconscious circumspatial visual awareness could expand to such a large extent during those meditative and other circumstances which share intensity, stress, or pain in common (see chapters 44 and 53).

Put simply, ambient vision suggests that the basic spatial capacities of certain regions become especially activated as part of the same processes which greatly amplify awareness *itself*. At such moments—when the sensitivities of diverse cells are being encouraged collectively—they could confer the sense of being poised to receive stimuli from *all* directions, not from just one. Under these conditions, active "allocentric" nerve cell networks could reinforce the sense that perceptions were being referred to the "outside," not to the "inside."

Prepared though various systems may be, nothing much happens. Strain though they may to perceive more, they generate a spatial matrix which usually remains empty, aside from a brief, stray hallucination. If the visual systems are so stimulated, why don't they see more? What do their circuitries lack? Two things seem to be missing. One is the influx of fresh specific sensate impulses from the outside. The other is the replay of messages which might come from the interior data bank. Block or bypass input from these two sources, and there can be no content to the formless space at hand. The result is absolute blackness.

On your next visit to a planetarium, lean back in the darkness. As your eyes adapt, you will begin to see the distant points of light which it disperses over the inner surface of its otherwise blackened hemisphere. These lights, projected from the compound lens in the center, start taking the form of stars, planets, and constellations like Orion. Sitting quietly, you might then vaguely recall the circumstances of Siddhartha's ultimate awakening: he became enlightened when he saw the first morning star. Nowadays, instruments in many planetariums are so very well programmed that the projectionist can turn back the clock many centuries in response to a visitor's request. Suppose you were to ask, What did the panoramic display of the heavens look like, just before dawn, on some particular morning, say five centuries B.C.E.? In any era, Venus would usually have been the brightest morning star. But beyond this, the atmosphere through which we must search for ancient historical facts becomes too hazy. No one knows the actual date when Siddhartha meditated nightlong, struggled, endured phantoms of his own, saw his morning star, and finally became the historical Buddha.

That programmed instrument at the planetarium can project, equally well, its "memory into the future." Human brains are no less programmed, just less accurate in their distant forecasts. We have a big problem. Any images we project forward are mixtures: a few hard facts plus many soft assumptions, symbolic interpretations, random associations, and preconscious insights. None of these have codes accessible to ordinary language. The result is an inchoate mixture which swirls around in some kind of potential, interactive space.

When talking about this, we sometimes use the term "mental space." It refers, loosely, to that large mental field which involves itself mostly with events which take place in the present tense. Mental space accurately describes, both literally and figuratively, what we do seem to require—a big uncluttered *volume* free of sticky mental cobwebs—whenever we need to process many operations at high speed. When such a mental space *expands*—as it does in internal absorption—the awareness within its vacancy almost tingles with all its preparations for imminent sensate experience. The visual result, in its simpler forms, is a realm glittering with potentials and infused with enchantment to the nth degree. It is perceived as "a great round mirror, black as lacquer."[7]

But this is only a mere, three-dimensional prelude to what a human subject might later be capable of projecting throughout the mental field of inner space.

For when the *Avatsamsaka Sutra* goes on to describe the higher refinements of such phenomena, it will use this arresting image: a spider web–like network throughout a space extending to infinity, filled with colorful gems and crystals, each so reflecting all of the others and resonating so much in tune with all of them that the slightest vibration at any one point communicates itself to every other point. Such a net is also known as "Indra's net," after the Hindu deity of the firmament.[8]

Overtaken by such an awesome experience, some persons might be left with the impression that they had reached the ultimate understanding of universal reality. How else could a witness have tapped into the way atoms gleam and molecular bonds resonate, all the way from the innermost to the outermost levels of the physical universe? Once more, a mundane interpretation suggests itself. It is that such an experience may represent so impressive a release from inhibition that the excited brain goes on to reach exalted heights of processing within its large polysensory matrix of space.

But whereas some forms of ambient perception may take off on solo flights and glisten in pitch-blackness, rarely do they ascend into this highly charged stratosphere, shimmering and vibrating with its synesthesias. Indeed, during internal absorption, no sound penetrates the meditator's space. The silence of this no-sound has its own distinctive features, each full of implications for those prepared to listen.

117

The Sound of Silence

> Every day go into the calm quiet where you really belong, face the other way and turn your gaze back; if you do this over the long years, that which is not illusion will of itself reveal itself before you.
>
> Master Daikaku (1203–1268)[1]

> All final spiritual reference is to the silence beyond sound . . . It can be spoken of as the great silence, or as the void, or as the transcendent absolute.
>
> Joseph Campbell (1904–1987)[2]

Suppose you're a subject whose evoked potentials are being tested. While you are listening through earphones, your brain signals its response as soon as each auditory stimulus arrives (see chapter 64). But what happens if you now decide to focus every bit of your attention on each sound stimulus? By listening more intently, you'll *hear* more, and you will also amplify the height of your brain's evoked potentials.[3]

Consider, on the other hand, the meditator who listens, *totally*, to *absolute silence*. This witness is left with a singular impression: lavish attention—though it is fully deployed spontaneously—hears absolutely nothing.

It is being so poised that you could hear a pin drop . . .

Yet no pin drops.

Acute, temporary, total deafness. Rarely does a neurologist encounter such a condition in a patient, let alone experience it himself. Could it be explained the same way as is that other unusual disorder, loosely called "cortical deafness?"

Genuine cortical deafness is rare.[4] The few cases serve to illustrate the point that, normally, we hear using two major systems.[5] Now this may come as no surprise, because we have already noted that vision also streams through its "first" and "second" systems (see chapter 54; table 5). Similarly, our first hearing system transmits our more conscious auditory perceptions. The second set of auditory pathways services our more reflex responses. How can specialists make the diagnosis of cortical deafness? Only by proving two things: (1) that the higher-level "conscious" system is gone; (2) that the lower "reflex" system remains intact.[6]

Normally, as sound signals stream inward from each ear, they first travel through the cochlear nerve. Next, impulses rise through its nuclei in the pons, then relay up through the inferior colliculi and the medial geniculate nuclei, and finally reach the primary auditory cortex on both sides (see figure 11). Note: all along, these nerve fibers for hearing are crossing back and forth across the midline. So by the time sound messages have reached the auditory cortex, those signals which began in one ear are being represented extensively on *both* sides. These crossings over explain why a patient whose damage is limited, say, to only the left auditory cortex does not become totally deaf. Indeed, no one-sided lesion even raises the hearing threshold above normal.

But suppose some rare disease destroys *both* sides of a patient's primary auditory cortex. You might think that a little hearing would still remain, given the ways some experimental animals behave.[7] However, human cortical deafness is different. Studies now document an unexpected result: patients perceive *no* sounds at all when they sustain *acute*, severe dysfunction of the auditory cortex on both sides.[4,8] Moreover, bilateral lesions do markedly elevate their hearing thresholds for pure tones. One such patient didn't budge, even when the auditory stimuli were increased to deliver loud sounds above 100 decibels. Fortunately, his hearing thresholds dropped to normal levels after his acute condition improved.

Let us go on to offer a simpler explanation for the utter silence of absorption: bilateral *subcortical* dysfunction. For the next obvious level, below cortex, would be one step lower, in the posterior thalamus (see figure 11). To cause deafness, a process here would need to interrupt the function of the medial geniculate bodies on *both* sides. Yet this would stop all of the usual auditory messages from radiating up to the cortex. This proposal is supported by a recent case report indicating that bilateral *sub*cortical deafness is indeed experienced as a *strange silence*. The patient had two separate lesions, four years apart. At the moment when the second lesion occurred, he suddenly "felt that the world around him had become strangely silent." Running water evoked no sound, nor did traffic. Hearing tests performed two days later still showed a major hearing loss ranging from 60 to 100 percent. Lower-pitched sounds were especially lost.[9]

If you return inside that dark quiet closet, and really listen, you can verify the existence of a faint, normal background noise. This tinnitus is a kind of static arising along the hearing pathways, like a very soft white noise. Ordinarily, we pay no attention to its hum or hiss. In contrast, utter silence has *zero* background noise.

So, do we need a complex explanation to account for (a) this meditator's sudden onset of absolute silence; and (b) the way the silence then vanished within a minute or so? Not if we take into account the fact that the silence was accompanied by utter blackness. For the most likely explanation is straightforward. We partake of its mechanisms daily as we shift in and out of desynchronized episodes, whether they are those of D-sleep or of waking. Indeed, it is during these normal transitions that we block sound and light signals from passing through both sets of nuclei which would otherwise mediate our hearing (the medial geniculates) and seeing (the lateral geniculates). Every night, we undergo similar episodes of transient, subcortical deafness and blindness at the level of the thalamus. On these occasions, are we acutely conscious that we have become blind and deaf? No. Nor do we think of ourselves in this manner. And so it is easy to overlook these natural sleep-related mechanisms when we seek to explain why similar phenomena also occur, displaced into some other state, at a time when we happen to be wide-awake.[10]

Notice, however, that hearing does fade—if one preempts it—during the daylight hours. Try shifting into a visual mode, and focusing all your *visual* attention selectively on some object or event in front of you. Soon, many sounds tend to get diluted out. Similarly, during a major internal absorption, even if a few sound signals did escape from being blocked at lower levels, their impact might not register fully in the face of all the other brief hyperactivations which had taken over other parts of the brain.[11]

Owls catch mice, using their superb *exteroceptive* sense to pinpoint the rustle of a distant mouse. We are not nearly so good at localizing external sounds. Still, by integrating and "triangulating," blindfolded humans do manage to localize reasonably well in all three dimensions of space. However, during internal absorption, something unusual happens to these normal abilities. Out there, in its vast silent space, the witness no longer finds those former three-dimensional reference points which used to sense where sound cues might be coming from. And this unique void, this *vacuum* through which no sound is transmitted is as strange and otherworldly to the auditory cortex as it is to the visual cortex.[12]

Subcortical Vestibular "Silence"

Our normal vestibular system is privy to inside information. It is our *interoceptive* counterpart to hearing. Its sensors inform us where our own head and body are positioned in three-dimensional space. But unlike hearing, this vestibular system operates almost entirely sub rosa. Normal consciousness seems to have little need to pay much formal attention to its tacit signals. However, its messages do translate into truly remarkable reflex functions. Even while we move, this system helps keep a big pumpkin of a head nicely balanced on the thin reed of a neck, and maintains our whole body upright with respect to gravity. All automatically.

Now the pathways of this vestibular system tend to run close to and parallel with most hearing pathways. So a few of their ascending signals will be relaying, through the ventral posterior region of the thalamus, on their way up to the temporal cortex. Up here, the primary vestibular cortex lies just in front of its auditory counterpart. A few vestibular messages then go on up to the parietal lobe. Here they blend into that mosaic of refined sensate data which makes us aware of our physical self and the positions of its muscles, joints, and tendons.

The working hypothesis of this chapter predicts that the ascending vestibular system would also be disconnected. Where? Below the temporal cortex and within the thalamus. Note that the level at which such an afferent block is placed would not interrupt the *reflex* functions of the lower vestibular circuits. For these reflex pathways, having already peeled off at lower levels, will still bring their vital vestibular signals into the pons, medulla, and cerebellum. So a disconnection up as high as the thalamus will spare the person's normal *reflex* postural adjustments. These ongoing mechanisms would still keep head and body erect, and would prevent the meditator from toppling over during zazen. However, if you were the person on the mat who had lost all vestibular contributions within the thalamus, you might become aware of a not so subtle deficit: you would no longer have conscious access to any vestibular hints about *where your head and trunk were oriented in three-dimensional space.*

Douglas Harding, an architect, once had a very impressive experience. He "lost" his head. The event was so striking that he wrote a book about it, entitled *On Having No Head.* At the time it happened, he was on a trek high in the Himalayas. He noticed a peculiar quiet, stopped thinking, and developed an awareness of the entire world. What kind of a world was this? It was "utterly free of me. I had lost a head and gained a world. Lighter than air, clearer than glass, altogether released from myself, I was nowhere around."[13]

Even to someone who has experienced such a physical vacancy at a time when his or her oxygen level was normal, the event delivers an impressive reminder: our brain normally receives a great deal of feedback information from head and body. These sensate data are generally *proprioceptive* and specifically *interoceptive.* And these sensory systems are constantly informing us that our head and body do exist. They go further. They specify *where* our head and body are located in space. However, if the relevant nuclei of the thalamus are disconnected temporarily, these physical correlates of self vanish.

It is one thing to "hear" the silence beyond sound. It is another to imagine that the conceptual boundary of such a condition expands from there to include the "transcendent absolute," as Campbell suggests in the opening quotation.[2] Again, we'll need to be careful about how powerful a myth can be when it stretches similes and metaphors. True, we have been referring to an absolute *sensate* silence in internal absorption. But this variety is hardly the ultimate. It is merely the first, impressive hint of those layers of quiet spiritual reference that are yet to come (see chapter 146).

The Loss of the Self in Clear, Held Awareness

All of a sudden he finds his mind and body wiped out of existence . . . This is what is known as "letting go your hold." As you become awakened . . . and regain your breath, it is like drinking water and knowing for yourself that it is cold . . . Joy inexpressible.

Master Hakuin[1]

Common sense constrains the skeptic. If the I really vanishes, and if no-I is left to have an experience, then how could any experience be perceived? The person who first experiences this "letting go" of self knows better than to ask this question. For nothing of the old personalized identity remains inside. Gone is that old impression—*I'm* seeing. Instead, there exists a new operative mode: awareness *is*. Ask a common sense question: *Where* is this new heightened awareness? The strange answer: Focused outward *in all directions* into a vacuum of extrapersonal space.

The skeptic has ample cause for other disbeliefs. How could a subject's pure awareness continue with no thoughts? And, if thoughts are absent, then how could awareness still register all the other ongoing events, and do with such accuracy that the events could later be remembered, defined, and put into words? It may help to resolve these doubts by considering an analogy with another situation. Take, for example, the way we can become absorbed in our favorite symphony (as did Baudelaire). Music, too, doesn't demand that we participate in active verbal thought processes. No. We settle in to listen, and proceed to appreciate the music thoroughly. Even so, music also registers in the brain, leaving enough of its notations in memory to enable us later to sing or whistle it, without thinking.

It is a momentous event when the whole bodily self drops off. How could it happen? Let us take a closer look at the posterior thalamus. Here lies the smallest volume of nervous tissue where sight, hearing, vestibular input, and other vital proprioceptive sensations from the head and body can *all be disconnected at one time* (see figure 11). Our review has specified three physiological mechanisms which can converge to blockade this small region. The first closes down the usual flow of sensory messages up through the thalamus. Nothing bizarre here, because *this normal sensate blockade also goes on within the dynamic architecture of sleep* (see chapter 70). It occurs during the descent from waking into S-sleep *and* during the ascent from S-sleep.

The second way to block sensation is to activate the cortex excessively. For instance, suppose one stimulates, electrically, the small cortical region representing only the area of the face. Exciting this part of the parietal sensory cortex increases the metabolic activity of the reticular nucleus down in the thalamus on the same side.[2] The reticular nucleus then acts as a "cap" (see chapter 60). It applies its powerful GABA inhibition to cause a *drop* of 10 to 30 percent in the metabolic activity of those nearby thalamic nuclei which usually enable sensory impulses to be transmitted higher.

Among the nuclei studied, two are of particular interest in the present context. One is the lateral posterior nucleus.[2] Normally, this nucleus projects the sensate information it receives up to inform the superior parietal association cortex (*LP* in figure 11). The other is the ventral posteromedial nucleus (see figure 11). It relays the sensory information coming up from the head. If you wanted to lose all feeling from the tissues of your head, this would be the nucleus to inhibit.

The research just cited suggests how the reticular nucleus acts to prevent a sensory overload in sensory cortex. When it "tightens the cap," it shuts off incoming impulses that might further overexcite the cortex. Whenever a sensate cortical function itself becomes overactive, this second braking mechanism could cause temporary deafferentation of the thalamus. How would this be perceived? None of the usual kinds of sensations could enter which would otherwise help maintain the construct of the physical self. Of course, activations from other, nonsensory, regions of cortex also stimulate the reticular nucleus (see chapter 60). If several of these desynchronizing events occurred, in separate regions of cortex, the sleep spindles otherwise typically seen in normal drowsiness might not be evident. Indeed, some slower oscillations could be obscured by fast activity if EEGs were being recorded only from the scalp.

A third avenue for blockade rises up from *below*. This pathway comes into operation when the midbrain reticular formation is directly stimulated. At this time, some of the more *anterior* parts of the reticular nucleus also become involved. So now, not only are the lower and posterior tier of sensory relay nuclei inhibited but *also other nuclei farther forward in the thalamus*.[3] It will be of great interest when these two normal processes of primary excitation and secondary inhibition are monitored along the same three avenues, over a twenty-four-hour period, in the brains of animals larger than rats.[2,3] Then the ways in which the reticular nucleus interacts with its neighboring nuclei in the thalamus and basal forebrain can be worked out in fine detail. The results should further clarify how very relevant thalamic mechanisms are to the Zen experience of absorption and enlightenment.

Involuntary Hyperattention

The self is sovereign. It usually maintains some subliminal sense that we are in charge of our own voluntary attentive processes. Not so during absorption; involuntary mechanisms take over. Nothing intentional directs the shift into this heightened global awareness. And it is as vacant of voluntary thoughts as it is of the usual points of spatial reference.

True, the transition into this state is seamless. Yet, in one sense, the brain seems to have responded almost as though it had just been startled. Instantly, the previous baseline, whether it had been one of distant awareness or sleep, turns into a fixed *hold* on attention. Perceptions arrive already sharpened and broadened, automatically. Both gaze and hearing become riveted. The witness is caught up, as a passive spectator, in a highly active process. And whatever might, or might not, show up in this subject's EEG up at the surface, the witness inside will later appreciate that regions deep in the brain must also have helped generate this involuntary hyperattention (see chapters 21 and 37).

Which regions? Let us start with the limbic system. Here, stimulation does exaggerate attentive behaviors. Grastyan gave an interesting name to the resulting response. He called it the "sensory fixation reaction." It developed when he delivered electrical stimuli to the limbic system either in the preoptic area, the fornix, the mammillothalamic tract and hypothalamus, the lateral mammillary nucleus, or in the lateral hypothalamic area. His stimulated animals then attached their attention to any moving object. Indeed, he said, the animal becomes "riveted to it as if it had been a magnet."[4]

Hernandez-Peon observed the same kind of "magnetic" attraction behavior. He chose to use carbachol, an acetylcholine agonist, and to stimulate the septal region near the anterior commissure.[5] Then, even an old cat behaved like a kitten entranced by a piece of string. The cat now focused its gaze upon any object within its visual field, and tracked it with great intensity. A pencil was followed "just as iron filings are attracted to a moving magnet." This phenomenon gave rise to the term "magnetic attention."

It has long been known that the meditator who intensifies the techniques of concentrative meditation is setting the stage for the next shift into absorptions. Why? The studies cited above begin to supply one plausible explanation. Together, they suggest that attention can be captured and held fixed when extra degrees of excitation proceed within the lower anterior portions of the limbic system.

Close at hand is the ergotropic triangle (see chapter 22), followed by the other ascending pathways in the reticular formation and beyond (see chapters 37 and 62). It is to these regions that one also turns to help explain other striking properties of absorption's heightened awareness. As Hakuin once noted, its crystal-clear perception resembles that of a bottomless, clear pool. And to William James, such clearness was a vital quality in itself. What was its critical precondition? Attention.

Attention, said James, augmented the "clearness of all that we perceive or conceive."[6] To him, clearness meant that things had become separate and distinct, one from another, early in perception. It is with this total clarity that the witness looks out into "empty" space during internal absorption, only later to be able to identify three of its properties: (1) perceptions seem fine-grained, detailed; (2) their sharpness penetrates; (3) they impact with special immediacy.

What does immediacy mean? It describes what happens to that interval between the instant a stimulus is first detected and the moment it becomes fully registered in the brain. This interval shrinks. Indeed, because stimuli seem to enter consciousness sooner, it feels almost as though consciousness itself had expanded *its* outer limits. The shortened interval further suggests that immediacy does operate, as James foresaw, in what we now call the *pre*attentive mode (see chapter 63). Put simply, the implication is that immediacy occurs in absorption because the flow of impulses is (1) speeded by massive parallel processing and encounters fewer synaptic delays; (2) takes shortcuts and is relayed by fast neurotransmitters.

This meditator's heightened awareness that evening appeared to be caused by a combination of factors. One mechanism is especially relevant to the cross-legged meditative sitting posture. Compression of nerves in the leg, and of their blood vessels, can cause tingling and other painful sensations to rise up through the large sciatic nerve. In rats, stimulating this same sciatic nerve causes certain key nerve cells in the hypothalamus to fire faster. These are the corticotropin-releasing factor (CRF) cells. When they release CRF, this excitatory peptide sets in motion many of the brain's other intrinsic stress responses[7] (see chapter 53).

Impulses descending from the hypothalamus have only a few millimeters to go before they reach the midbrain (see figure 3). Here are several circuits which might begin to blend a subject's heightened awareness into a large expanse of space. They include, for example, those nerve cells in the colliculi that have large receptive fields, and whose brisk responses are easily amplified to major propor-tions (see chapter 54). And just below the depths of the colliculi resides not only the long cylinder of central gray but also the two main sources of dopamine input (see figure 7). Dopamine from the ventral tegmental area could play an obvious role in energizing the intensity and the effects of concentrative meditation tech-niques (see chapter 44).

Humans find it aggreeable to feel all their senses being placed on keen alert by caffeine. They also search for the thrilling challenges that prompt alertness, and go out of their way to be stimulated by horror movies or roller coaster rides. Both dopamine and norepinephrine play active roles in the heightened awareness that is a critical part of such states of excitement. In this regard, recent studies suggest that the human personality trait of novelty seeking is correlated with the genetic locus for the DA_4 receptor, a dopamine receptor that is concentrated in limbic regions.[8]

This is not to overlook acetylcholine as a major source of the clarity in aware-ness (see chapter 38). For don't we also take pleasure in nicotine, and in the clarity which enters many of our most vivid dreams at 6 or 7 A.M.? But having come out of absorption, something still seems very strange: clear attention has shifted itself *in*voluntarily into a vacancy of utmost clarity, a space so devoid of the physical self, an ambience so abundant in other respects.

119

The Warm Affective Tone

> Exultation is the going of an inland soul to sea.
> Past the houses, past the headlands, into deep eternity!
> Bred as we, among the mountains, can the sailor understand
> The Divine intoxication of the first league out from land?
>
> Emily Dickinson (1830–1886)[1]

Two waves of feeling swept into absorption. First came cool clear enchantment, next a cozy blissful affect. Each phase entered involuntarily. In retrospect, neither

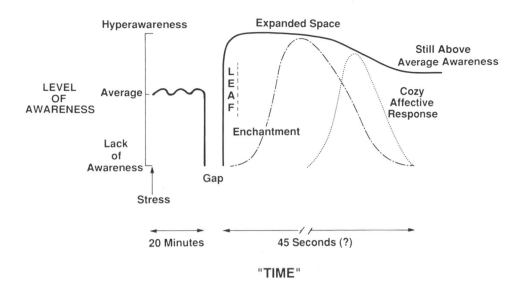

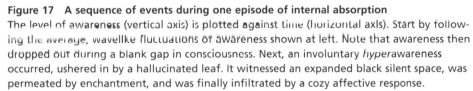

"TIME"

Figure 17   A sequence of events during one episode of internal absorption
The level of awareness (vertical axis) is plotted against time (horizontal axis). Start by following the average, wavelike fluctuations of awareness shown at left. Note that awareness then dropped out during a blank gap in consciousness. Next, an involuntary *hyper*awareness occurred, ushered in by a hallucinated leaf. It witnessed an expanded black silent space, was permeated by enchantment, and was finally infiltrated by a cozy affective response.

feeling seemed attributable solely to the rest of the content of that moment. The sense was of being entranced in general, not of simply being spellbound by a single leaf. For not only was the feeling of enchantment out of all proportion to the leaf's aesthetic qualities but it also continued to infuse the whole space even after the leaf had vanished from it (figure 17).

To this experiant, the second phase of the *plenum*—its cozy, enveloping blissful abundance—resembled the feeling which had entered during his two previous exposures to morphine.[2] Some of the later phenomena of internal absorption may therefore reflect the release of endogenous opioids deep in the brain (see chapter 47). Presumably, when rapture and ecstasy go on to overwhelm a person, they build on some of the same foundations and amplify others.

Opioids yield a complex array of physiological and experiential results. When opioid agonists finally reach their receptors, they *inhibit* the firing of the next nerve cell at most sites in the brain. In this manner (by acting on Mu_2 opiate receptors, for example), opioids could contribute to a drop in respiratory rate during internal absorption.[3] One exception is the hippocampus; here most opioids have direct excitatory actions.

Where could the effects of beta-endorphin enter into a major internal absorption? Among the potential sites are several midline regions, already cited, where electrical stimulations produce a floodtide of positive affect. These sites include the septal nuclei and higher mediofrontal regions. Both are well supplied with endorphin fibers. Moreover, the local release of enkephalins and dynorphin might also contribute to opioid mechanisms. The blissful infiltrating affective tone suggests that a deep pulse of one or more of these opioids could have penetrated chiefly the central and paracentral portions of the subject's brain at several levels.[3] Here they would escape the cast of the inhibitory net of the reticular nucleus.

Enkephalin pathways extend high and low, right and left. They supply regions more or less along the core of the brain, as well as those much farther out toward its surface.[4,5] If enkephalins were to superimpose a few of their basic inhibitory actions during internal absorption, the effect might be to add a fourth component (to those just noted in chapter 118) which would lead to an even more effective sensate block. It turns out that, with regard to this latest opioid mechanism, the cochlear nucleus, the medial geniculate body, and the inferior colliculus receive a rich supply of enkephalin. So the release of extra enkephalin could further block hearing *at the level of the brain stem.*[6]

Poetic license might seem to have ample reason to invoke a kind of "divine intoxication" in the bliss of internal absorption. But it will not be the first league, nor the first trip, out past the headland that reaches deep eternity. Real eternity is not immediately in the offing. It lies far beyond, way over the horizon. Each inland soul must wait patiently, and for some later voyage, to plumb its depths (see part VII, chapters 133 and 135).

120

Motor and Other Residues of Internal Absorption

> Thus, one true samadhi extinguishes evil, purifies karma, and dissolves obstructions.
>
> Master Hakuin's *Chant in Praise of Zazen*

I found my head, neck, and trunk posture were unusually erect when I emerged from internal absorption. An exceptional sense of lightness and freedom of movement prevailed for several days. What do these two features tell us about Zen and the brain?

The pathways responsible for extending the head and neck start at least as high as the nucleus of Cajal. In humans, this nucleus lies high up on either side of the central gray[1,2] (see figure 3). Impulses relaying from this region finally reach motor nerve cells in the spinal cord. When these lower motor nerve cells fire, they contract the splenius capitis and other major muscles along the back of the neck. These contractions arch the cervical spine. One's head and neck now rise into the erect position.[3,4]

Some neurological patients develop a disorder called retrocollis. In this condition there occurs a forcible chronic overactivity of these same extensor neck muscles. Neurosurgeons can relieve their excessive head extension by making discrete lesions of the nucleus of Cajal.[1]

Now, the tone of these long extensor muscles of the spine does stiffen when nerve cells respond to opioids (see chapter 47, topic number 8). And muscle tone also increases in response to other excitatory influences. For example, when one of the raphe nuclei is stimulated low in the medulla, there occurs a very long, *sixty-minute*, release of serotonin (and possibly of the excitatory peptide, thyrotropin-releasing hormone). Such a release could also enhance the firing of the particular motor nerve cells in the spinal cord which extend the whole spinal column by contracting its long axial muscles.[5]

So an increase in the tone of spinal muscles is a plausible explanation for the way the motor residues of internal absorption subsequently extend the neck and the rest of the spine. Could this same spine extension provide any clue pointing to those sources earlier in the episode which had generated my sense of fresh, clear perception? Perhaps, in a general way. For most responses of those same muscles along the spine are organized by way of the reticulospinal tracts. And these motor tracts begin high up, at the level where the reticular formation extends into the hypothalamus and the thalamus. Moreover, the ergotropic triangle is also included in this same general region, at the site where the midbrain merges into the diencephalon (see chapter 43). Simply put, along this same *upper zone of the central reticular core,* the brain is deploying several vital circuits that have the capacity to enhance various dimensions of one's conscious awareness.

Accompanying the extension of the spine, there is a second category of motor residues. It is a blend. The first of its components is a remarkable sense of lightness of the body. The second is a collateral feeling: one's motor capacities are enhanced. Accordingly, such a close partnership of properties could originate in a change in the bias of the subject's proprioceptive systems, or be part of an improvement in strength, or reflect other motor changes in patterning and coordination. All these are testable hypotheses, and they are not mutually exclusive. There is plenty of time—ample minutes and hours *after* a major episode—in which to sort out these issues, using controlled objective laboratory tests. Indeed, Alan Watts mentions how, in one of his spontaneous experiences, his feelings of lightness and of clarity continued for the next eighteen hours after "the weight of my own body disappeared."[6]

Internal absorption has other residues. Coming out of its jet-black silence, the meditator finds that consciousness has undergone a kind of spring housecleaning. This goes beyond a simple "rinsing of the doors of perception." True, sensory signals continue to arrive with freshness and immediacy, and the clear mental landscape seems swept free of cobwebs. But the heightened sensitivities coincide with substantial emotional and "spiritual" overtones. One recognizes the first of these overtones in the form of a restrained, subtle ongoing emotional high lasting several hours or days. And, as for the second, this meditator also felt a lingering sense of reverence and awe. This subtext lent a sacred quality to internal absorption and inhibited my talking about it.

One other interesting personal development of note took place after this episode that evening in Kyoto. Up to that time, photography had been a prominent hobby. Ever since then, photographing things became distinctly less appealing. Why did my interest in photography then seem to drop off? Some of this could be attributed to the mechanical bother of using a camera. It was a distraction. It interfered with my registering the beauty of the present moment. This attitudinal change appeared to be the result of a quiet decision, made at some depth, to attend to the *now* of the moment itself. No more would I try to coerce a scene through a glass lens and frame it, artificially, onto a print or a transparency.

No longer would I later have to file it away someplace. In retrospect, this was the first of many other adjustments. They would enable me to examine carefully, and then to simplify, the way I lived.

The initial major absorption does more than pull aside a veil. It throws open a window, disclosing a surprising new realm. Here, consciousness seems immensely clarified. Following this, the meditator may sense the presence of a kind of primitive understanding, a spurious "wisdom." Not the true deep wisdom of the later insights, but a preliminary variety. It is one which was referred to, in the past, as that of "The Great Perfect Mirror."[7] How does such clarity help to further Zen training? It makes explicit the fact that the aspirant really does possess innate capacities to dissolve obstructions, to change course, and to reexperience the world. It confirms that meditation is the vehicle of change. Now the meditator has the feeling of being on the right track.

But herein dwells another trap. Indeed, the person who clings to this state will be stuck in what is called "stagnant water Zen." In Hakuin's words, "He whose activity does not leave this rank sinks into the poisonous sea."[8] In fact, the transient states of absorption afford but a temporary balm. They resolve none of life's central problems. The experiences can seriously mislead the beginner who lacks a seasoned roshi. Novices may think they have now vanquished the "I," vanished into a "void," and attained the much esteemed "emptiness." But they will be in for their most awesome surprise when kensho finally strikes.

121

The When and Where of Time

> In [that] watch of the night
> Before the moon appears,
> No wonder when we meet
> There is no recognition!
> Still cherished in my heart
> Is the beauty of earlier days.
>
> Master Tozan Ryokai (807–869)[1]

The questions before us now involve time and timing. When does absorption tend to occur? And where does one's sense of time "go" during it?

We begin by noticing when just *any* kind of physiological surge might start. It could start when a subject was either at a low or at a high tide of arousal activity, or in between these two extremes. So, a low-activity surge might thrust up at such times as: during quiet meditation, a quiet pause, a drowsy period, or in the (seemingly quiet) intervals of sensorimotor deprivation. Whereas a high-activity surge might take off in the participant at a religious revival, in a subject whose arousal activity had already been whipped up to a very *high* pitch. In this latter instance, the added surge might reflect more of a kind of overshoot, stirred up by all the extra physical and mental excitement.

But some persons need much more than a brief physiological flurry to shift into an alternate state. In them, the surge will need to be reinforced. That is, whether it starts from a low or a high initial value, it will need to fall *into phase* with the timing of the peaks and valleys of that person's everyday activity cycles and longer biological rhythms (see chapter 77).

The working hypothesis outlined above proposes that all states build on one foundation: *the natural ups and downs of our brain's functional activities.* Then, where do random events fit in, such as the impact of stress, or triggers, or psychedelic drugs? Each is capable of prompting absorptions or major awakenings. But each acts only as a *non*specific precipitant. And it will be most effective only when the brain's biological cycles had also drifted or had been shaken into unusually vulnerable phases. Why does the hypothesis state so many contingencies? Because it will need to explain two things about extraordinary states. First, why they are relatively rare. Second, why they seem, at first glance, to be so unpredictable. But are they, really? Or could internal absorption be more likely to occur at special times?

The most recent translation of Tozan's verses hints that the episode tends to occur at the "beginning of the night, before the moon appears."[1] And the previous opening quotation by Sasaki (see chapter 108) also suggests that the striking stillness of internal absorption could arrive earlier in the evening. During these earlier hours, the average subject is more likely to be staying up and still meditating as opposed to the last watch in the depths of the night.

What transpires in zazen during this first watch of the night, say from 8 P.M. until midnight? Superficially, it might appear that only two states would contend in the brain. One is wakefulness (W), seemingly on the wane; the second is S-sleep, then gathering momentum. But our focus is on *meditators.* We now understand how meditation can introduce many more than two contingencies (see chapter 77) For example, brief segments of D-sleep can also occur early, at sleep onset. And the clues that other active "microstates" have indeed been displaced in this manner are those sleep-related hallucinations which some persons dislodge at the dynamic edges of their transitions.

During this beginning watch of the night, the meditator who nods off may soon awaken. Now, in this drowsy transition, a *hypnopompic* hallucination could occur. This episode of excitation arises on the *ascent* toward renewed waking, because the meditator still remains readily rousable into desynchronized moments of wakefulness. So the more frequently these two cycles for desynchronization converge and overlap, the more likely they are to provide the requisite, stimulating setting for (a) higher background levels of mental arousal; and (b) extra surges of high amplitude awareness. These surges, otherwise unaccountable, will occur because the crests of several covert cycles now come into phase and reinforce one another.

For contrast, let us finally consider the second watch of the night. All the pressures to remain stuck in S-sleep continue to be strong. During these wee hours, from midnight until 4 A.M., the person's tendency toward a wakeful arousal clearly will have descended to its lowest level. Therefore, when S-sleep is maximal, what will have happened to that capacity to reach full awareness, the essence of major absorption? It will be at low tide. (The dip in the large black zone at 2 A.M. in figure 13 illustrates this point.) For these reasons, the least likely time for internal absorption to occur would seem to be during the second watch, in the middle of the night. This hypothesis is testable.

The episode in Kyoto that evening suggests a complementary proposal, more difficult to test at present. This theory predicts that the usual degree of sensate block caused by the reticular nucleus could become especially profound when three mechanisms converged, each capable of enhancing its *inhibitory* effects. One would be an extra fast descent into S-sleep. The second mechanism would be an unusually high degree of generalized cortical activation. This could have been prompted by stressful circumstances (some self-imposed, as it were, from a psyche above; others ascending from the tingling left leg). The third mechanism would be an added degree of focal cortical excitation, itself contributed by the same lateralized process that had generated a formed hallucination.[3]

Of course, we also stand watch during the other twelve daylight hours. No hypothesis that internal absorption is more prone to occur at either end of the night can exclude the likelihood that absorptions could occur during these other hours. For during these mostly wakeful hours, we also shift in and out of similar transition periods, and we can be influenced by meditation or stressful events. For example, normal persons undergo substantial fluctuations in vigilance every 60 to 110 minutes during the daylight hours.[2] (The wavy lines at the left in figure 13 serve to emphasize this point.)

And meditation, performed day or night, not only shifts the times of entry but also changes the tidal momentum of those clusters of linked physiological functions, which we conceptualize as representing our usual ninety-minute and twenty-four-hour cycles (see chapter 77).

These general points, concerning the impacts both of stress and of meditation, are applicable to the way a particular series of events happened to converge before the episode of internal absorption began. The tempo of meditation had intensified for the two previous days during sesshin. That evening's zazen was held in a novel place, the zendo at Ryosen-an at Daitoku-ji. Moreover, twenty minutes before the subject plunged into that first blank gap, he underwent an episode of unusual physical and mental distress. During this stressful period, he remained a neurologist all too aware that his left leg was becoming totally paralyzed. Never before (or since) had the leg been this numb. Sitting through this sciatic nerve paralysis meant two things. First, inner turmoil. Second, a concession of some magnitude.

We have reviewed the steps through which a sequence of stress responses could soon begin to influence a person's brain directly (see chapter 53). In addition, for reasons of timing, one needs to consider the further possibility of a unique *seasonal* convergence. For, in Kyoto, this is the time when the weeks of late autumn are merging into early winter. And now, two *annual* cycles are coming together into their peak conjunction—those regulating brain serotonin, and those releasing glucocorticoids from the adrenal gland (see chapter 77).

How long did the experience last? A person inquires only in retrospect. Inside it, no entity had any valid basis for making an estimation. *Time was not there.* The introductory period was a blank, an absence. This unknowable gap could become evident only subsequently. As for the leaf, a guess would be that it might have stayed up there for five seconds, maybe more than less. How long did its setting last, that enchanted black space? It seemed to linger for perhaps four times longer, say twenty seconds. Only its second half was suffused with bliss. Subsequently, the diminuendo evolved over perhaps another twenty seconds, an equivalent period. If so, then guesswork would suggest that the whole episode unfolded in only *forty-five seconds,* more or less. Figure 17 takes into account the fact that these sequences, otherwise indelible, have uncertain durations.

Where had time gone? (Can time go anyplace? We address this issue later, in chapter 135). It felt as though time had been *preempted.* But factors of sensate deprivation might have contributed to its apparent suspension. For, as William James pointed out, our sense of hearing, if left to itself, gives no reliable basis for subdividing durations of time.[4] Consider, then, the condition of an experiant who has entered into absolute black silence. Now, time sense is doubly deprived, because it has lost both conventional vision and its fallible auditory clues.

Which of the two major states comes first? Absorption or kensho? Let us return to the second line of Master Tozan's verse. Now there are no ambiguities of translation. For when he alludes to "the moon," he does mean kensho (see chapter 138). Therefore, the sense of his verse is that internal absorption will usually occur first in sequence, *before* kensho's "moon" of enlightenment. The fact that absorption tends to precede awakening is in full accord with the sequence in my case, and with the accounts of drug-related experience (see chapter 101). Moreover, as D. T. Suzuki noted, kensho sometimes occurs at the moment when the person is coming out of internal absorption.

The evidence suggests the following conclusion: absorptions are a prelude. Usually, many months or years elapse before enlightenment arrives. But there are occasional exceptions when the interval between the two states may be very short.

122

Gateway to Paradox

> Sitting on a stone,
> a cloud materializes
> in the monk's garment.
> Only later will the moon appear
> in his jug of spring water.
>
> From calligraphy by Kobori-roshi[1]

When does a paradox occur? When elements are valid individually but incompatible together. Absorption baptizes the person in a sea of paradox. A vacuum of space? It holds fullness in abundance. Does it shed even the physical self? Yes, but it is a plenum of intimate and private awareness.

Silent, it hears the *sound* of silence. Pitch-black, it is seen into. Internal absorption harmonizes all such individually incompatible ingredients into one vast clarified perception. From then on—from these heights and depths of sensate experience—each student will know that such irreconcilables can be reconciled.

And in this manner a deep internal samadhi does indeed serve as "an intimation" of insights yet to come, as Ruth Sasaki had described.[2]

Paradoxes are not to be dismissed. Stace observes that our logical theories will themselves break down if they attempt to explain away every contradiction of mystical paradox.[3] For a true paradox is not the result of a poor description by a mistaken mystic. Nor is it a rhetorical flourish used for poetic effect, though each of these certainly occurs. Rather, the core of the paradox expresses actual incongruities: an extraordinary set of events is being juxtaposed, in an extraordinary way, into one experience.

Paradoxes in science are especially fertile fields. It was once thought that D-sleep with REM—an active brain in a sleeping, paralyzed body—was also a paradox. This was at a time when the pioneer sleep researchers lacked all the facts. Many others were also trapped by that fixed mental set which held that none of these individual ingredients "really belonged" together in one state called sleep. But now we know more about how each of the separate properties of D-sleep arises, and this understanding has made paradoxical sleep less puzzling.

Yet our mental functions do operate on two or more planes at any one time. And it is a fact of everyday introspective experience that we can still listen, and taste, both at the same time. So why couldn't two other functional systems also coexist in the forefront of consciousness? Namely, one field of awareness beholding the vacuum, the other field aware of the plenum? Indeed, the research reviewed in parts III and IV helps us understand how several distributed functions, each arising from separate modules and compartments of the brain, could express themselves simultaneously.

Then what is implied when a subject encounters empty space, brimful of awareness, but shorn of intellectual content? Again, perhaps not much more than that a surging stream of heightened, wakeful awareness is flowing quickly down a widened mainstream, and that it has briefly given up those two former side channels which had previously diverted it. Where had awareness been diverted previously? Into the wide fields of exterior sensory experience and convoluted interior thoughts.

Peptides have presented many paradoxes, and it has proved very difficult to assign them a specific role in human brain functions. The blissful state, later in absorption, deserves further study. It could reflect a pulse of endogenous opioids, released along the midline plane as far forward as the cingulate gyrus and septal region. Consider, for example, how far the peptide fibers from the arcuate nucleus distribute their beta-endorphin and ACTH: forward to the lateral septum, preoptic region, interstitial nucleus, and nucleus accumbens, up to the paraventricular nucleus and midline thalamus. Moreover, the arcuate nucleus also has a pathway that *descends* from the hypothalamus. It releases its beta-endorphin in the spinal trigeminal nucleus, the solitary nucleus, the locus ceruleus, and the dorsal horns of the spinal cord. Painful stress is an important trigger, causing these arcuate nerve cells to discharge their beta-endorphin.[4]

Another paradox presented itself when Hokfelt and colleagues found *two* messenger molecules inside one nerve cell.[5] In previous decades, neuroscientists had felt comfortable with a self-evident doctrine: each nerve cell could make only one messenger molecule. Now, the impossibility was a reality: biogenic amines *coexisted* with peptides! Still, the qualification arose: are these two different messengers usually *released* at the very same time? Probably not. Instead, under ordinary conditions—which means *slower* rates of firing—only the *smaller* storage vesicles will usually be releasing their contents into the synapse. And these smaller vesicles contain only the usual messengers, *not* the peptides (see chapter 46). Then where do the larger storage vesicles enter into the picture? *These large vesicles are the sites where peptides coexist with other transmitters.*[5] *So when the brain surges to high firing rates, many nerve cells could release both standard transmitters and peptides from these larger vesicles.* This combination could help explain some of the ecstatic phenomena which occur when absorptions are driven to maximum levels of intensity.

Coexistence is the new doctrine, now widely accepted. It could provide an attractive working hypothesis for some of the infiltrating, affective overtones which occur later during absorption. In addition, once peptide receptors have been activated, they help regulate both the number and the affinity of the nerve cell's other receptors for biogenic amines.[6] Therefore, having certain neuropeptides coreleased during a time of high impulse flow might go on to help some residual memory traces to be laid down in more enduring form. This could contribute to the fact that absorptions remain impressive events, and it might also help leave other residues which linger for several days.

Ineffability

Two conventional notions are commonly held: mystical states are difficult to describe; language is "in the left hemisphere." The two notions might lead the public to conclude that mystical experiences are taking place in the right hemisphere, the side "where language isn't."

Throughout this book we will offer other explanations for ineffability (see chapters 5, 131, 142). Obviously, no experiant has a ready frame of reference to describe an event which suddenly evaporates the previous physical self into hyperawareness. Looking back now, the Kyoto experience was otherworldly. It was something akin to having lived for a lifetime in an old, familiar house, a home where each room was known intimately, but then abruptly being cast, extra–wide-awake, into the patio of an enchanted garden, a place that must always have been there but which had somehow escaped discovery. Yet, if one took into account how vast was this enchanted space, it would surely have to lie in the whole outdoors. At this point, the analogies could turn more toward awakening from a nap out in some high Alpine meadow suffused by warm sunlight, where the rarefied atmosphere was clear, crisp, and soundless . . .

Nonsense, says Zen. These are metaphors one invents later. They can't capture experiential paradox. True . . .

Neuroscientists, undaunted, might venture a few other theories to help explain ineffability. Some patients who sustain a relatively small stroke in the left thalamus have language problems. They can't retrieve words, nor can they register and retain verbal material.[7] Therefore, it is difficult to exclude the possibility that in some ineffable states, those parts of the thalamus usually involved in language are preempted, or are disarticulated from their usual routines, or bypassed. If such were the case, on one or both sides, then some portion of ineffability might imply that the corresponding parts of the person's deeper language functions had been out of the loop in a sense, and were then far removed from the rest of the mainstream flow of the experience.

The old Zen masters were at home with paradox. They knew they couldn't describe everything, even if they had wanted to. And they didn't want to. Even so, they did speak and write. But what did they leave? A legacy of allusions and riddles. It baffles every beginner. Even at best, the words are tangential to what actually goes on. Still, we can count on Hakuin to add a few observations which are highly accurate. We need to pay close attention when he says there is *no tile above and no ground to stand on*. First let the aspirant encounter ambient space. Then, in retrospect, will the impossible truth be known. Hakuin's statement means, quite literally, that perception is arrayed inside a vast space lying above and below the witnessing center (see chapter 116).

Things are not so clear when Hakuin comments from his own high vantage point about Master Tozan's five ranks of Zen progress, for Hakuin then calls them a "torch on the midnight road."[8] Maybe so, yet no Zen beginner can see clearly what internal absorption really is by the flickering torchlight of Tozan's allusive verse. But let us turn back to look again at Tozan's description, the one which serves as the opening quotation for the previous chapter. Some ambiguities might begin to make more sense. For example, what does it imply to be met but not recognized? Could it mean that no bodily self, no physical I, remains which could be recognized by awareness anonymous?

Throughout, we have noted how a few fragments of past experience can get swept up into whatever new state may be coalescing at that moment. Could this observation also help us interpret Tozan's closing phrases, about that beauty which the heart still cherishes? We today may never know what Tozan actually meant in his distant century. Still, a part of me would like to think that the present translations of his verse might have predicted another interesting paradox: the way a red leaf could reenter absorption—a beautiful cherished, fragment of memory—and yet not be recognized as having been the center of attention during an earlier day's walk among the maples in Kyoto . . .

123

Second Zen-Brain Mondo

> The human brain is a world consisting of a number of explored continents and great stretches of unknown territory.
>
> Santiago Ramón y Cajal (1852–1934)[1]

By asking pointed questions of Zen experience, we can begin to focus on great stretches of territory, unknown to the early explorers, and still largely obscured.

How could a meditator's intense attentive focusing become so amplified that it reaches a state of intense absorption?

Higher levels of arousal can create an additional release of the biogenic amines dopamine, norepinephrine, and serotonin. These modulators interact to enhance attentive functions at multiple levels in the brain.

Why could breathing stop briefly in extraordinary states of absorption?

The final, most basic cause could be inhibition, within the medulla, of its usual rhythmic in-and-out respiratory cycle.

Then how could this interruption of breathing coincide with states of clear consciousness?

The mechanisms which ascend to activate heightened levels of awareness could also become linked with other circuits nearby. These could descend to inhibit the breathing cycle down in the medulla. Moreover, some parts of the medulla can inhibit arousal functions at higher levels. As soon as these particular regions of the medulla are themselves inhibited, alerting functions are then released at higher levels.

What could prompt the heightened awareness of internal absorption to occur in the evening, as compared with the morning?

The alertness cycle reaches its peak later than one might think, not until around 9 to 10 P.M. Next comes a dynamic interval, the transition period which usually ushers in the person's drowsy descent into slow-wave sleep. But this trendline of S-sleep is not smooth, nor does it necessarily drop straight down. Indeed, it can be interrupted when *two* kinds of desynchronized microepisodes are thrust into this interval. One is sleep-onset REM. The other is brief awakenings. This dynamic setting is ripe for the entry of a sleep-related hallucination (of the hypnopompic or hypnagogic variety).

Can a sleep-related visual hallucination occur at the start of the night, when a meditator drops off and then awakens suddenly?

Yes it can. In this instance, it could still be termed a hypno*pompic* hallucination. For this technical term simply refers to imagery that has entered during the transition phase on the *ascent* from S-sleep up to waking.

How could meditation promote episodes of absorption?

Meditation destabilizes. In a sense, it loosens some of the physiological bonds which hold each of our ordinary states together. Rigorous meditation dismantles the barriers that separate one state from another. Thereafter, brief desynchronized episodes could slip into such openings, and reach higher physiological peak levels. In addition, the person who intensifies the techniques of concentrative meditation can begin to evoke some of the intrinsic stress responses of the brain. These responses further enhance the mechanisms underlying absorption.

Is internal absorption a lucid dream?

No. "Lucid" means only that the dreamer is aware of dreaming at that moment. Deep internal absorption is characterized by a witnessing center shorn of the physical self. And this nonentity is fully aware, *not* of dreaming, but of being extra–wide-*awake* inside a vacuum. In contrast, some lucid dreamers retain enough self-awareness to be able consciously both to direct their own movements and also to direct events during their dream scenarios.

How can an excessive activation far up in the cortex contribute to a marked reduction of vision, of hearing, and of other sensations from the head and the rest of the body?

An overstimulated cortex goes on to excite the reticular nucleus of the thalamus. The reticular nucleus then blocks sensory impulses so that they can no longer be transmitted up through its underlying thalamic nuclei. This inhibitory "cap" prevents a further excessive excitation of the cortex.

But more recent controlled studies have found that sensory stimuli do cause the brain to generate evoked responses during "meditation," at least as meditation has been broadly defined. Why should future studies show otherwise?

In fact, few studies have focused on those singular instances when ordinary levels of meditation suddenly drop off into *the state of genuine deep internal absorption*. These absorptions are rare. They need to be carefully studied, at the very moment they occur, using modern techniques.

Why are states of internal absorption and kensho so different, yet each so memorable?

It is being proposed that many of their properties arise in association with extra firing activity, along *different* acetylcholine and glutamate pathways, involving different regions of the brain. For example, extra firing of cells along the perforant path could enhance long-term potentiation within the hippocampus. This could help to heighten the subject's ongoing memory of each event. Some peptides may also be released, as part of the basic mechanisms of these states. And peptides could also be triggered *secondarily* by the impact of the strikingly novel content of the new state per se. Chief among the peptides which could help further shape the differences between the states would be corticotropin-releasing factor, ACTH, and the three endogenous opioids: β-endorphin, enkephalins, and dynorphin.

Why did a hallucinated leaf occur in the author's expanded left visual field?

Humans seem physiologically biased to sponsor more visual imagery within the right posterior part of the brain. A tingling left leg might have contributed further to this image-generating propensity of the right side of the brain.

Why does ambient vision perceive such a vast space?

It brings into the foreground of full consciousness all of the person's covert capacity for *un*conscious circumspatial awareness. It had been there, unrecognized, all along.

Part VII

Turning Out: The Awakenings

A perception, sudden as blinking, that subject and object are one, will lead to a deeply mysterious wordless understanding; and by this understanding will you awake to the truth of Zen.

Master Huang-po (died 850)

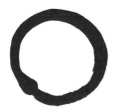

Dimensions of Meaning

In every object there is inexhaustible meaning; the eye sees in it what the eye brings
means of seeing.

Thomas Carlyle (1795–1881)[1]

Living creatures with sentient nervous systems are what make our planet distinctive. But evolved nervous systems do more than perceive. Relentlessly, they confer
meanings on other things. Within a few thousandths of a second after you encounter anything new, your brain endows it with meanings along three major
dimensions.

Evaluation is the first of its operations. Like the others, evaluation has a range
of options spread out between two extremes. Sensitive to gradations, it decides
whether the new thing is good or bad, right or wrong, pleasant or unpleasant.
The second dimension is termed *potency*. It decides whether the new thing is
strong or weak. A third, termed *activity*, settles on meanings along the spectrum
from passive to active.[2] When we add to these three operations the ready bias of
an emotional push or pull, we quickly tip the balance of our scales of meaning in
one direction or another.

Our brain's capacity to grasp instant meaning is a basic, *pre*attentive process.
It is over and done with long before attention itself gets underway. It is also crucial. Which progenitors survived to beget us? Only those who could decide in a
flash that some new object was a threat to life because its features seemed bad,
strong, and active. Each day, our survival still hinges on instant decisions made
along several other dimensions of meaning. One such scale, already cited, is crucial to memory, for it stamps events with a special quality. It labels them as being
either familiar (déjà vu) or unfamiliar (jamais vu). Much of this operation goes
on automatically, deep in our temporal lobes.

Modern brains are thrust into highly complex social situations. And they
cope by adapting very old endowments to solve new problems. As part of our
current techniques for problem-solving, we seem almost to have set up our ancestral criteria for meaning inside a volume of *semantic space*. What is meant by this
term, "semantic space"? To begin with, like those ancient forests and savannahs
in which it evolved, it too has three-dimensional properties. That is, it still distributes those old criteria of evaluation, potency, and activity along three different
"planes." Take for example, certain loaded words, like "kind" or "cruel." Studies
show that everyone regards these contrasting words as occupying three distinctly
opposite spatial coordinates. These run "up, down, and across" in more than a
figurative sense. How do people judge "kind?" It is very *good*, quite *weak*, and
slightly *passive*. "Cruel" lies off in three other directions. It comes out being very
bad, quite *strong*, and slightly *active*. Subjects from different cultures around the
world come to these same value judgments by using such coordinates in their
planes of semantic space.[2]

Do you "think visually"? If so, then even more of your large visual brain may be involved than you are aware of. To illustrate, suppose you wanted to emphasize how important something was. Often, your next words could be very well chosen. You might select such words in an almost literal, spatial sense: speak of valuing some object more "highly"; or write about its always remaining "near and dear." Whereas less important things would drift "out of sight, out of mind," being "lower on the list" of priorities. When we use spatial words in this manner, it suggests that they have become associated with constructs which once evolved within a kind of spatial matrix. We call it *mental space.*

Some system of coordinates within our spatial matrix maintains positions reasonably fixed in relation to one another (see chapter 114). By the time we enter adolescence we will have proceeded to construct elaborately biased spatial systems. Consider how some teenage opinions will already have become so firm as to appear either "high-minded" or "low-down"; and how attitudes may have hardened into those of either a "right-wing" conservative, or of a "left-wing" liberal.

Actually, our semispatial representations began as far back as infancy. For the infant brain was already sensitive to certain harder realities of existence. It could detect abrupt edges, impenetrable barriers, and other literal boundaries in the outside world. Soon, as tiny hands grasped eagerly at anything within our small envelope of space, we began to define many other limits. Indeed, some limits would be forcefully defined for us. Because it was OK to clutch and wave the rattle. But definitely *not* a stray pencil. An emotionally tuned brain was learning that some words—*No! No! Hurt* the baby!—had a sharp affective edge. And when my grandmother would caution me in German, the guttural message was unmistakable.

So our brain, imprinted early with these spatial and emotional metaphors, gradually conditioned itself. It learned to erect sharp emotional and cognitive distinctions which polarized an event. Slowly, on either side of this electrified fence, a proactive conscience developed. It was a subliminal sense, but it conferred strong hints about our *feeling* good or bad each time we came near a situation where we "should" feel good or bad. Soon, rigid mental compartments would harden around abstract distinctions. Issues involving politics or religion became loaded topics, charged with right or wrong. Gradually, tall iron curtains (well-guarded) would divide up our mental space, and lead to internal conflicts. For, in one compartment, warm longings bound fantastic thoughts to emotions. In another, cold loathings pushed thoughts farther apart. Where does Zen fit into the picture, given this necessarily brief overview of developmental psychology?

Iron curtains. Longings and loathings? All these are the everyday grist for the mill of Zen. Where, in every brain, did we sculpture the smooth contours and chisel the sharp edges of each distinction that would prove emotionally meaningful? At many levels. Including, finally, the cerebral cortex. The evidence for such distinctions is easy to find. It shows up, in normal subjects, using the simplest of tests: line drawings of faces, expressing basic human emotions. As we know, the lines representing eyebrows and mouth are especially eloquent. Their slope conveys *facial emotions* which suggest either positive or negative feelings. So it takes only one quick glance, at lines that could turn either up or down, for the observing subject to discern whether the test face is wearing an expression of happiness, grief, or fear.[3] And with each brief decision, it turns out that these subjects' scalp electrodes then go on to show a distinctly different set of electrical potentials. Mere lines, in themselves, could not account for such different brain potentials. What could? Only lines which had been *interpreted,* and given different *emotional meanings.* In much the same way had Pavlov's hungry dogs learned to associate the mere sound of a bell with their being fed (see chapter 74).

These lines of research return us to that old half-forgotten word, *apperception.* It refers to the sensitive process which infuses emotional resonances into each of our perceptions. Apperception quickly scans large networks of associations. There, it detects a clue which links past with present. Something which hints that two experiences have shared emotional or other symbolic ties. But apperception per se provides no simple answers. It does not know which ties, nor does it understand *why* they have been linked together.

Suppose, however, that we need to *untie* some old and very tight psychological knots. To do so, we will need to go back and discover *which* ties lay at the roots of the trouble, and find out *why* we had assigned meaningful weight to these particular links. Only very slowly then, if limited solely to an effort of will, can we access the more rational top layer of our conditioned mental sequences. For our willed conscious thoughts tend to proceed in a serial, linear manner. And even when we grope for meaningful clues in the "subconscious" (at still relatively shallow levels), we find that the clues are faint, and are difficult to keep on-line. Moreover, the more Freudian approaches to self-analysis require even larger blocks of open time, time free of bias and distractions.

What happens in a major flash of insight? A sharp contrast with these slow, willed, thoughtful attempts. And insight also leaps beyond the mere hints of apperception. Instantly, effortlessly, it comprehends profound meanings, illuminating the basic existential issues of life and death. Its communication is direct, authoritative, beyond sound or articulation.

It is during these peak insights that our field of consciousness expands with yet another dimension of meaning. It is the special quality of *salience.* At its nether end, it begins with the trivial. Rising near the midpoint of its scale, salience conveys what William James called a "deepened sense of significance." We feel its presence when we encounter an otherwise simple truth embodied in a maxim, proverb, or formula.[4]

What does it feel like when such a sense of significance deepens and infiltrates one's consciousness? James learned this from personal experience. Indeed, one night he was able to single it out, and to identify it as an almost independent, added-on quality. Earlier that day, he had climbed 5344-foot Mount Marcy in the Adirondacks, and was still invigorated by the trek. For as he lay awake in the moonlight, he remained in a memorable state of "spiritual alertness," filled with an "intense significance of some sort." But he could not assign this "significance" to anything specific. And so, because he could not discover the source of his weighty portent, it remained a mere "boulder of *impression*."[5] We will have occasion later to refer to the same useful distinctions between a boulder of impression and other properties of a flash of insight (see chapter 142).

Yet one may begin to wonder: what happens when the impression itself becomes pervasive and overlaps these other properties? Could it be that the form of a revelation enhances its content? Does something else slip in which makes the whole package more attractive? The advent of fast magnetic resonance imaging (functional MRI) permits neuroscientists to study similar brief segments of mental activity, even those lasting only ten seconds or so. Fast MRI now makes it feasible to focus on the origins of that induced salience which recurs—reproduceably—during segments of the nitrous oxide model response (see chapter 98). For example, while human subjects are inhaling N_2O, they could press a button, signaling that their significant impressions (of this Jamesian variety) had risen to a peak. The brief time-frame within which fast MRI operates could help define which particular regions of the brain are functioning most actively during these special moments.

Anyone who takes lightly the weight of salience can be seriously misled. When peak experiences tap into the potentous end of the scale of salience, the boulder of impression becomes momentous indeed. Then, comprehensive insights strike deep into clear consciousness. Deeper still when the episode strikes spontaneously, and the subject's consciousness is not clouded by drugs. The weighty impression left by major insights becomes an internal reality. It enables insights later to be actualized and to have positive transforming effects in a larger social context.

In our survey of consciousness early in part IV, it was evident that scholars are still debating what consciousness is, and where it arises in the brain. Still, if one proceeds from the foundation of the functional anatomy of the brain, as reviewed in part III, it becomes possible briefly to suggest, in the next paragraph, ways in which some preliminary working models could support the theories about meaning that have been outlined above.

For example, some believe that we develop feelings of significance within those regions of the brain which interconnect the limbic system with the thalamus. As the limbic system curves and plunges deep next to the midline, its borders enclose the rounded contours of the thalamus (see chapter 59). Within the thalamus, certain nuclei are believed to help us shape meaning. They make up the limbic thalamus, so called because these nuclei are richly supplied with "emotionalizing" connections from the limbic system. Among such regions are the mediodorsal, anterior, and lateral dorsal thalamic nuclei. Two other parts of the limbic system itself may further infuse their resonances into meaning.[6] They are the lateral septum and the pathways curving from the cingulate gyrus down into the hippocampus (see figure 6). And all along these networks the brain can reinforce meaning by infusing opioids of its own making.

Reflect back on that large, meaningful operation summarized briefly just above, the one we started to build when we were infants. Our mental development began with an infrastructure of simple basic meanings; it next added layers of more complex attitudes and biased opinions; it finally superimposed a thought world divided by many lighttight bureaucratic compartments. True, we have distributed many of these rigid partitions diffusely among various networks in our brain. But it would be a mistake to conclude that they are merely soft and intangible "thought structures." In fact, they are the source of our most firmly opinionated, hard-edged "shoulds" and "oughts." Take any attitude. Try to let go of it. *Try*. It is very difficult to let go. Is it a basic mindset? Then it *is* set, in concrete. From here, it can bias our snap judgments.

Originally, it started out as a purely practical matter. Humans needed partitions. Partitions helped separate good from bad, right from wrong. Commandments had survival value. It was to cope with life's complexities that societies helped us erect all these "shalts" and "shalt nots." Only later do we discover the consequences. Each longing, each loathing, is a burden. In this particular sense, it makes little difference whether it is desire or disgust which had tied us up in knots. Each exacts a personal price. A classic Zen parable illustrates the point. It is the old story about the two monks and a girl at the river.

The monks were on a pilgrimage when they came to the ford of a river in flood. There, on the bank, they saw a girl dressed in all her finery. She was deeply distressed, because crossing the river in high water would spoil all her clothes. The elder monk bent down, motioned her onto his back, carried her safely across the torrent, and set her down on the far shore. Then the monks continued their own way on foot. At once, the younger monk started to complain: "Surely it is not right to even touch a young woman. It is against all our commandments. How can you go against our rules?" This went on and on. Having endured this for several miles, the old monk finally said: "I carefully followed the commandments. I set her down on the riverbank. Why are you still carrying her?"[7]

125

Authentic Meanings within Wide-Open Boundaries

> Good you say,
> means doing good.
> Bad indeed
> the mind that says so!
>
> Good and bad alike,
> roll them both into one ball,
> wrap it up in paper,
> then toss it out—forget it all!
>
> Master Bankei, circa 1653[1]

The perennial questions are simple: Where do we come from? What are we? Where are we going?[2] Paul Gauguin's brush would add them to one of his Tahiti paintings. Each of us asks, in his or her own way: Does *my* life really have meaning? Does the universe have meaning and purpose? Broadly speaking, our answers fall into one of three categories.[3] *Physicalism* holds that there are only physical entities in the universe, not values. *Idealism* says that values and meaning are implicit in the universe. *Perspectivism* replies that it all depends on your perspective. From the perspective of a pragmatist, what counts is what works.

Within the moment of Zen awakening, however, the flash of insight-wisdom performs an awesome synthesis: it makes the three categories all valid simultaneously. Physical entities are seen into. New dimensions of implicit meaning are revealed. Everything seen works perfectly.

But suppose we were looking at such rare moments from the *outside*, as usual. Then Zen eludes our grasp. The earnest young monk tries to understand what this insight is, asking "What is the basic truth of Buddhism?" His old master replies, "The cyprus tree in the courtyard." Earlier masters uttered many other seemingly zany responses. The monks' questions were reasonable; the answers seem irrelevant. What explains the mismatch?

We are confused, as usual, by our own preconceived notions. We expect that a Zen master's response will fit into the mold of *our* cultural expectations for meaning. When it doesn't fit, we're dissatisfied, and turn to some other belief system which might offer to bring real meaning into our everyday existence. Frankl would base his whole approach to psychotherapy on this universal hunger for meaning.[4]

So when we first encounter Zen, or any other new religion, we're likely to look at it askance, sparing only one eye to scrutinize it critically out of a slit window in the stone wall of our mental edifice. Unfortunately, no one can understand alternate states of consciousness from any such narrow perspective. Zen, in particular, implies a brain open in more directions than one can ever imagine.

On the playing field, we can actually see an outfielder leap high and make an "impossible" backhand catch of a fly ball. This is a spectacular *physical* feat, an act which occurs in full view. Far greater creative leaps are commonplace in the arts, the sciences, and along the mystical way. But these are "mental." They are much less obvious. Yet we know that everyone has a mental repertoire and a capacity for the leaps of a highly creative imagination. What happens during these interior leaps? Trajectories of thought intersect inside a covert "mental space." Whenever the connections occur—during daydreams, reverie, or dreams at night—they tug on the old coordinates of meaning and pull them into new configurations. For these are consummate acts of integration. And their vectors will be drawing at least as much upon deep subcortical networks, including those of the thalamus, as they reach up to engage higher transcortical levels.[5]

What, then, does it imply when a person enters a brief moment of enlightenment? In one metaphoric sense, it does mean a *return*. Not a regression, but a genuine return to the kinds of free passage that adults feel whenever their tight mental boundaries open up. It means being liberated to take associational leaps which reach impossibly beyond those rigid bureaucratic compartments of one's old mental edifice.

To awaken is to access the capacity to begin, let's say, in the northeast corner on the first floor of a more open, neutral, mental structure; then to move quickly down diagonally, to be as grounded in the earth as is the foundation on the southwest side. Finally, and just as quickly, zigzagging far up at another angle to exit through some opening where a roof no longer presses down; free now to leap out and intersect associations from any other adjacent mental edifice at any level.

No barriers to passage en route. No distinctions. No floors, walls, ceilings, windows, or outer shell. Nothing remains to enclose any previous formal mental constructs. What, if anything, are we left with? It is an edifice or brain, built on a more open plan. It is a matrix now configured in a way which supports and encourages the natural flow of life's experiences. In this uncluttered mental space, no longer do old barriers constrict, block, discriminate. Kensho sweeps them all out, along with every sticky cobweb of their former contradictions.

Again, from an outside perspective, such a view of Zen enlightenment seems too far out. Why can't we, or the novice monk, understand it from our ordinary state of consciousness? For one other important reason. Meaning doesn't pass readily from one state to another. Fischer and Landon observe that meaning tends to be determined, at least in part, by that same level of arousal at which it had first been experienced. "It appears meaning on a particular level of arousal is meaningless on another level, and that each level of arousal and hyper-arousal has its own space-time coordinates, information-content, meaning and logic, all of which is relevant to that level."[6] Accordingly, it will not be possible fully to communicate a particular meaning—which is so obvious to one person in one alternate state—to another person in another state. No need to look to research papers for examples. Try to explain to your tired and fussing child how reasonable it is to go to bed.

Fischer and Landon note that an outside observer can ask a simple question, and it will seem entirely appropriate to subjects who, at the time, are still in their ordinary waking state of consciousness. But once they reach the peak of their psychedelic drug experience, these subjects view the same question as the epitome of baby talk: "ridiculous, childish, simply inapplicable, redundant, offensive, and ambiguous."[6] Later, however, after the subjects have recovered from the drug experience, and while again reviewing these very same questions and answers— now in the clear light of ordinary consciousness—they will disagree with what they had said above.[6]

But let us return to our ordinary levels of experience. Start with an appropriate question, and a relevant answer pops up to meet it. Meaning condenses automatically. Why? Because we are processing all the data within a self-centered context. It is a context in which the *I-Me-Mine* composed the rules. Its self-referent programmings are codes which govern which kinds of meaning we will find in the events of everyday life. Then why don't these same standard sets of rules apply at the moment when meaning is emerging out of a major alternate state? *Because then our usual subjective self is absent.* One does not, for example, expect to have BASIC programming rules work if one's personal computer had already been programmed to operate solely in FORTRAN.

To Western eyes and ears, contemporary Zen has become relatively straightforward. These days its teachers are responding with few cypress tree answers to earnest questions. Yet, it is also easy for the rest of us to commit nonsense on occasion. Consider, for example, how permissible it is for anyone to sing in public the nonsense lyrics of the American song, "Oh, Susanna": "It rained all night the day I left, the weather it was dry; the sun so hot, I froze to death, Susanna don't you cry." But a steady diet of such non-meaning? If Tang dynasty Zen was genuinely religious, how could it indulge in so much gibberish?

In this manner do we question the basis of Zen, and keep sympathizing with the young monk. Like him, our programming keeps us listening carefully for any code words that will reveal clear literal meaning at our standard level of comprehension. But the old Zen masters were *de*programmed at this level. They responded with free associations, associations which alluded to *much subtler levels of meaning*. Why? *This was the way they had realized Zen*. And in those days *this was the customary way to demonstrate their realization*. The outsider, baffled then as now by all this, readily concludes that Zen is not only irrational but fraudulent.

It turns out there is some method in the madness. Many of the old masters' spur-of-the-moment responses were highly distilled and remarkably appropriate for the context of their historical era. Peering at these early responses through the mists of history and translations, one begins to find the faint outlines of at least four other common themes.[7]

First, the masters' responses are liberated from conventional thought modes. Second, they deflect all abstract questions. Third, they point students toward the concrete. Finally, they fuse the freest of associations into behavior. In the process, one discovers that the master has either deftly ignored, rebuffed, or demolished the beginner's premise. And he has frequently done so using brisk forms of body English. What do all of his actions say, louder than words? "No! The way lies in a different direction." In fact, during our first meeting at Ryoko-in, Kobori-roshi had forewarned me that his *no* was intended to condition away years of unfruitful patterns of thinking and behavior. So these are some of the reasons why the early Zen dialogues radically negate the logical rules which we had always been led to expect might bring meaning into ordinary speech.

One old Japanese master's comment beautifully illustrates this point. It was Muso Kokushi (1275–1351), who said

> Clear-eyed Zen masters do not equip themselves with a stock of invariable doctrines. They simply seize upon a teaching in response to the moment, giving their tongues free rein. Zen masters do not hole up in any fixed position. When people ask about Zen, the master may answer with the words of Confucius, Mencius, Lao-Tzu or Chuang-Tzu. Or he may expound the teachings of the doctrinal schools. On other occasions he will answer with the popular proverbs, or draw attention to something close at hand. Then again, he may use his stick, shout loudly, raise a finger, or wave a fist. These are the methods of Zen masters, the unfettered vitality of Zen. Those who have not yet reached this realm cannot fathom it through the senses and intellect alone.[8]

Observing several Japanese and Western Zen teachers over the years, I have seen how much they rely on the simplest of teaching methods. Glancing over at the flower in a nearby vase, Joshu Sasaki-roshi invites me: "*Show* me how you manifest your original nature when you look at this flower!" Nothing outlandish or complicated here. No high-technology "virtual reality." Just *do* it. What do such basic techniques accomplish? They encourage students to take their first steps into the real here and now, to establish direct relationships with simple, concrete things. However small these early steps may be, they are a prelude to the later revelation: each thing shares its deeper intrinsic meanings with *all* things.

In this subsequent state, the insight-wisdom of enlightenment, everything rings true to some *absolute*, eternal standard of reality. Ultimate meanings now authenticate themselves at unprecedented levels of value and of portent. Acting in conjunction, their sources in the brain will infuse something deeper into salience than a person's ordinary imprimatur, which merely sanctions. And they will provide something more than a facile solution which simply dissolves all prior sense that opposites had been locked in conflict. No, this experience of insight-wisdom must be receiving its ultimate stamp of authenticity from other sources. Having instantly reconciled the opposites, in a manner that proves both unifying and aesthetically satisfying, it appears to have gone beyond this openly to resonate with humankind's most universal perspectives.

Yet, this is not how we usually operate each day. For our usual daily task is to *close down,* to filter out, and so to dispense with most sensate data. These quick preconscious processes leave behind our slower, more consciously developed meanings. In contrast, insight-wisdom leaps into the foreground of consciousness. Already, its sense of final closure has both met, and satisfied, other filtering criteria. The new criteria are far more elegant than those which serve our everyday humdrum routines. To begin with, they are awesomely *impersonal.* But what else makes them so extraordinary? It is the fact that they already have rendered a unique verdict. They have declared the presence of an *ultimate* degree of significance.

How can this be so? No such conclusion has *ever* been accessed before—at least openly—in any of the subject's prior autobiographical memories. How could meanings be "known" to be authentic if they have not been experienced before? Again, part of the explanation stems from the fact that the egocentric self has dropped out of the picture in the same split second when such authenticity invests meaning. Gone, too, are all its former, self-limiting criteria for meaning. But how then could a selfless brain arrive at so *novel* a conclusion, the one that would label an experience as being both ultimate and authentic? Could a mere three-pound brain possess this natural capacity to generate such qualities and criteria? Or, to explain such depths of universal meaning, must we invoke some kind of an outside agency?

On these key issues, the personal opinions of neuroscientists are divided. They tend to fall also into those same three categories of physicalism, idealism, or perspectivism that we outlined at first. One part of the reason they do so occurs by default. The brain is incredibly complex, and the plethora of research journals are making it seem exponentially more complicated each year. Even large teams of investigators cannot specify today, in a way that will convince all others, how an awakened brain *can* generate such ultimate meanings. But another reason is to be laid at our own doorstep. Why do we stand divided and at odds? Because our words are too imprecise. The terms we use to describe so-called peak experiences have both multiple and ambiguous meanings.

First, we must address these vexing problems caused by words. Then we'll be able to specify the essential differences which separate the properties of the early absorptions from those of the deep awakenings of insight-wisdom. The latter states are the theme now under discussion in part VII.

Word Problems: "Oneness" and "Unity"

The best things can't be told; the second best are misunderstood.
Heinrich Zimmer (1890–1943)[1]

Zen has no words; when you have satori, you have everything.
Master Ta-hui (1089–1163)[2]

Surely, "oneness" ought to be indivisible. But is it? "Unity" should mean only *one* thing. Does it? Within the moment of insight-wisdom, yes. Outside, not so. The problem begins with not being able to communicate from one state into another. But misunderstandings abound for other reasons. One major difficulty, as Stace observed, is that "mystics in general do not distinguish between the introvertive One and the extrovertive One."[3] What do mystics really mean when they say "oneness"? We're left guessing, because we cannot accept all their overvalued metaphors at face value. And the words *we* use further muddle the situation.

Back in 1960, Stace proposed a solution. Split mysticism into only two categories. Let the word "extrovertive" mysticism describe spontaneous experiences which looked out through open senses. Suddenly, a "unifying vision," would transfigure what had formerly been the usual multiplicity in the outside world of objects. What was this kind of seeing? It conveyed the basic knowledge that throughout the universe "all things are One."[4] As a term, "extrovertive" had one temporary advantage: it did emphasize that the person's physical senses were open to receive the world outside. It had a subtle, but major disadvantage: in all innocence, it passed over the fact that other relevant words had long been used to describe similar moments. These "inside" words, already in place, emphasized the interior process, the *in*sight, the *in*tuition, the penultimate quality of the *inter*nal shift. The way enlightenment shifts one's internal perspective is an aspect at least as impressive as is the matter of senses being open to the exterior world.

But by then it was too late. The issue of the interior shift had been preempted, because the proposal of 1960 had also set up a second category of mysticism. It used "introvertive," as the only other contrasting term remaining. This category was intended to describe other experiences which seemed less spontaneous. That is, they tended to be prompted only after the mystics had deliberately cultivated them using techniques of concentrative meditation. For the moment, "introvertive" did appear to have more merit than its counterpart, at least to the degree that the public might use it as an alternative term for internal absorptions. For example, the word did convey the way awareness itself sometimes turned "inward into the mind" and away from external things. There, in pure, inward-focused consciousness, it would perceive a void, a "complete vacuum of particular mental contents."[5] This *vacuum plenum* (an excellent term for its paradox) had no content except itself.[6]

So far, so good. Then Stace concluded that this introvertive category of mysticism perceived, again, the "One." The words "undifferentiated unity," devoid of all multiplicity were used to describe the essence of this introvertive state.[7] The words and the context suggested that the two "ones" might be the same. At this point, all earlier distinctions became blurred. They further parted company with experience when the introvertive experience was described as *non*spatial.[8] The fact is, internal absorption can open up an impressive volume of space; a vast, unmistakable endless vault of it (see chapter 114).

The discrepancy leads one to wonder: could Stace have really meant that there *was* a space, but that it had no fixed points of reference or other items which could serve as landmarks? This could be a plausible reinterpretation, because ambient vision does lack coordinates which might otherwise have served as spatial pegs to fix positions within its vastness. By now the reader's mentation may have begun to bend, to cope with the ambiguities inherent in the two terms, "introvertive" and "extrovertive."

Finally, it turns out that "introvertive" has yet another disadvantage if we limit mysticism to only two categories, and if there are to be no subdivisions. The word does not accurately describe a different type of meditative absorption which tends to probe shallower depths. In such instances, the meditator's awareness becomes intensely focused—this time *outward*—on an external item in the outside world, and then enters into an intense affinity with it. In this particular situation, as attention again becomes highly focused *externally*, it also absorbs and effaces some of the old boundaries previously set up between subject and object. This *outwardly directed* attention then evolves into one more variation on the already blurred theme of "oneness." For such an experience, "external absorption" might seem to be a more expedient descriptive phrase (see table 10).

"Merging" is a useful descriptive term when it is used in the context of the several kinds of absorptions. For they may leave the impression that self and other have *merged*, flowed together, coalesced into an openness. The flavor of much of this seems straightforward. It is something that one might anticipate would happen when sensory impulses are blocked at higher levels. Because at this point, many of the person's self/other boundaries have dissolved. No longer does the central witnessing awareness feel that a proprioceptively informed *physical self* is remaining "inside," isolated from the rest of that other physical world "outside," as it had seemed to be previously.

How do we normally reinforce these notions that each of us exists, as a private physical self, inside that other world outside? One can attribute many self/other constructs to the body image–spatial functions emerging from our parietal lobe and its deeper thalamic networks (see chapters 55 and 93). But suppose absorption nullifies these connections temporarily. Now the witnessing awareness no longer has the basis for experiencing the same old physical dualities of this self/other relationship. Instead, it might perceive vaguely that "something else" had arrived at its former interface in space. What kind of a new "something" could enter, where moments before two sharply divided domains had existed? An impression of "oneness"; a sense that two domains had merged into one vacancy.

The quasi-spatial unifications that occur in absorptions are not rare. They are widely experienced. The context is a familiar one, but infrequently acknowledged. In fact, the mergings resemble the levels of direct experience which one usually reaches only after repeated intensities of rapturous lovemaking. Lovers appreciate how, on such occasions, awareness also enters into one dark, expansive, coextensive embrace. This "little death" has dissolved the boundaries which had previously served so well to separate one physical self from the other.

It would be left to the lay monk Van Ruysbroeck (1293–1381) to bring into print that fitting description: "the dark silence in which all lovers lose themselves."[9] Another accurate descriptive phrase, also applied to this state, calls it the perfectly transparent "crystalline bed." Curious how little open acknowledgment there has been that this state is associated with sexual intercourse.[10]

In common parlance, the two words "oneness" and "unity" have taken on many different shades of meaning. Used this loosely in practice, these terms no longer serve as criteria which distinguish absorptions from major insights. This lax situation makes it imperative to emphasize how the *sensible impression* of unity during major internal absorptions differs from intuition's consummate refinement, the intimate *comprehension* of unity during insight-wisdom. In table 17, yet another attempt is made to distinguish the two.

Internal absorption's keynote is sensate. It changes *sensibilities*. Yes it will engage some subtle interior ones which have emotional properties. But it does so only as part of an intensified awareness which leads to a block of sensations from the outside. In contrast, insight-wisdom strikes at the higher *comprehensibilities*. And those illuminated in its foreground hold no greater interest for us than the others which it drops. For especially does it cut off the psychic roots of longing, loathing, and fear—the root causes of suffering.

Speed is another distinguishing feature. Internal absorptions merge and coalesce more slowly. Insight-wisdom flashes in. One swift stroke of supraordinating vision cuts off every old emotional valence with which the person had set up conceptual distinctions. Absorption's silent blackness has a glistening, crystalline

Table 17
"Unities"

The Unity of Major Internal Absorption	The Unity of Insight-Wisdom
A slower merging and coalescence.	An abrupt supraordinating vision.
Occurs more frequently.	Rare
Has more physical, sensate aspects: it affects *sensibilities*.	A higher conceptual process: it affects *comprehensibilities*.
Lacks long-range transformative potentials.	Has long-range transformative potentials.
The internal sense of a bodily self drops out, along with that of all outside sensate data. A hyperaware consciousness witnesses and then merges into a pervasive, boundless benificence.	The unity is empty of every last extension of the personal psychic and bodily self. It immediately reinterprets the whole outside world.
The witnessing center perceives 1. a vast unbounded space; 2. absolute silence; 3. utter blackness; 4. a plenitude.	Every item seen exists 1. in eternal perfection, in and of itself; 2. with no distinctions from other items, including from the usual opposites in a relationship; 3. integral to the larger coherent whole.

quality. Suso's term, "dazzling," captures this light/dark paradox.[11] Insight-wisdom sees deeply into external things, disclosing what *they* really are: each an authentic integral part of the larger whole. Its coherent view of reality is awesomely simple: it is nothing more, or less, than the eternally true state of affairs when *we* are not intruding. The shift into this profound level of understanding occurs with such astonishing ease that it may seem to have come from without.

Zen has a phrase for this totally transfigured vision. It is called *seeing into one's true nature.* It is also referred to as returning to one's *original self.* The other names are *kensho* or *satori. Kensho's* insight illuminates life's central existential questions. Infinitude is its scope, not that single small, target zone revealed during our shallower "Eureka!" type of intuition. Pure kensho is noetic: a lightening strike of profound intellectual illumination authenticated with utmost clarity.[12] In this respect, it will differ from the kinds of revivalist-type religious conversion experiences which tend to be pervaded by charged, emotionalized connotations.

How do we usually look out into the turning world? From our usual position, *inside,* where our head and body are always pierced by the axis of self (see chapter 8). From such a fixed, viewer-centered perspective, we have little choice but to interpret each event within our own egocentric context. "Egocentric" nerve cells reinforce this notion. What is the consequence of all this ordinary self-referent knowing? It keeps reaffirming that we are inhabiting a dual world. Here the opposites must be I/it and subject/object.

Kensho dissolves this old physiological axis instantly. It strikes off every earlier physical concept *and psychic root* which had given rise to these dichotomies. Now, when subjectivity drops out, all dualities vanish. Perception shifts into a fresh, open, and objective field relationship. "Allocentric" nerve cells could reinforce this alternative vantage point (see chapter 114). Everything that the brain now perceives is seen from this single new coherent perspective. Reality is no longer a matter of "I seeing *my* sights," or of "I feeling *my* feelings." No former monograms exist in this new context. For the world now revealed is not something that can be "owned" personally in any sense, but an infinite domain that is "oned." The Japanese have a word for this. It is *ichinyo.* The term means the many existing as one.

Only in retrospect could the subject consider that this state was an "otherworldly" experience. For inside that moment itself, *prajna's* insight strikes directly into that very same world of the commonplace which had existed a split second before. "All" it does is reinterpret it. The curtains of self, now thrown back, disclose the ultimate simplification: everyday things, as *they* really are, are all integral threads in the rich tapestry of universal perfection.

D. T. Suzuki once illustrated enlightenment. His metaphor was a pail of water. If one follows the traditional Eastern way of looking at things, the water bucket is not merely described as a container, a cylinder bounded at its bottom. Nor does it consist only of all the water inside. It exists both as pail and water set in the context of all the rest of the world outside. Ordinarily, when we lift our pail full of water, we fully expect that it will hold all its contents inside. What is satori like? A master answered, "The bottom of a pail is broken through."[12]

The major distinctions outlined above in the discussion and in the table have been known in the East and West for ages. It was not some minor technical disagreement that had also led the medieval writers in Europe to distinguish two types of mysticism.[13] Back then, Van Ruysbroeck had identified one of these two forms of mysticism, a category which came to be called *epithalamian*. Apropos of his earlier phrase, "the lovers' dark silence," one should again observe that the "thalamic" portion of epithalamian happened to draw on very ancient words for the bridal chamber. It did so long before later anatomists borrowed the word, *thalamus*, and used it to describe a part of the brain.

Then what did the monk have in mind when he set up this initial category? He intended this category to identify a preliminary state, one that would remain limited in scope. For even during the seemingly "peak" moments of this type of mysticism, it was believed that whatever sense of "union" might occur would still be an *incomplete* one. It would be restricted to no more than a mere "relationship" with the divinity principle.[14] Why was absorption to be qualified in this manner? Because it was not the final state of true "oneness." Absorption still retained important distinctions that separated self from other. In this book, we specify these potent lingering distinctions. They have been identified as the *psychic* bonds of the *I-Me-Mine* (see chapter 9).

In contrast, Meister Eckhart and Tauler were emphasizing the other category, called *unitive* mysticism. Here, the union experienced would take the form of a complete "identity" with the ultimate principle.[15] This unity went beyond all distinctions. It reached the unqualified "absolute." So, too, does the insight-wisdom of kensho.[16]

Having gone to some length to present the case that "unities" differ, it is important to reserve one other possibility. These two larger categories, the states of absorption and insight-wisdom, may sometimes occur so closely together that they not only overlap at their edges but occur in mixtures. For example, situations resisting classification would seem especially likely to arise whenever mental processes are driven, repeatedly, to aberrant levels by drugs or by intensely devotional services which become highly arousing.

Confusion seems likely to continue until the descriptions finally clarify other specific points: are the subjects' eyes open and seeing out, open and *not* seeing, or closed? (see chapter 139). And if the subjects *are* seeing out, are they only absorbed in the sensate details of what they see, or have their psychic selves vanished into a total comprehension of the "big picture?" Even then, the semantic muddle seems likely to persist unless we use different words, or until we qualify carefully the ones which reinforce our expectations. Meanwhile, let no one underestimate how readily the ambiguities inherent in "oneness" and "unity" will find their different dimensions of meaning in the subject, the investigator, the scholar, and in the reader at large.

How Often Does Enlightenment Occur?

Of a thousand or ten thousand attempting to
enter by this Gate,
only three or perhaps five pass through.

Master Huang-po[1]

Huang-po had rigorous criteria. In 1975, Greeley published a national survey of 1460 Americans.[2] One questionnaire item was: "Have you ever felt as though you were very close to a powerful, spiritual force that seemed to lift you outside of yourself?" Eighteen percent of the respondents reported that they had such mystical experiences once or twice, and 12 percent said "several times." What does it imply when this many Americans say that they have had more than one powerful uplifting experience? It confirms that such experiences are not rare. It also suggests that they tend to recur.

In one particular subgroup, 43 percent of the subjects reported having mystical experiences.[2] Who were they? People then in their fifties, all of them born during the ten-year period starting around 1914. Was there anything unusual about this generation? For one thing, it had been raised under a set of circumstances that John Burroughs might regard as "adverse". This particular generation had been sobered at the youngest age by the consequences of one or two world wars, by a major depression, by the Korean and Vietnam conflicts, and then by the turbulent 1960s. If its members did not bear the burden of such sufferings firsthand, they could not have escaped being assailed by suffering as it was presented in the new photojournalism. For this generation had seen seemingly kind humans wage cruel wars against one another on an unprecedented scale. Death struck everywhere, not only out on the front lines but in cities far removed and in concentration camps. During the Second World War alone, civilians suffered two thirds of the estimated 50 million casualties. This was a generation of *gravitas*, the first ever that would need to add chapters on poison gas and on radiation sickness to its textbooks of military medicine.

Does profound adversity sensitize a person to existential issues? Several historical reasons lead us to consider this hypothesis valid. Siddhartha Gautama's mother died shortly after he was born. He led a sheltered life as a young child, shielded inside his enclave from the suffering world outside. As a result, he was profoundly shaken when he first encountered out on the streets such harsh realities as a dead man, a beggar, a sick man, and an old man. It was the heavy burden of these life-and-death issues which finally compelled him to begin his quest for enlightenment. In later centuries, many who followed the spiritual path as masters or as laypersons had also struggled through adversity. Their fathers died when Hui-neng and Dogen were both children. Dogen's mother also died when he was seven. Dr. Bucke's parents both died when he was only a few years old.[3]

Hardships enter every era. And though many are called, few go all the way. According to Master Dogen, it would be only one or two, out of several hundred or even a thousand disciples, who became truly enlightened, even after they had trained with a great Zen master. Presumably Dogen was then referring to what we will take up later, in part VIII: to total awakening in its most advanced ongoing form. Elsewhere, he was more inclusive, saying, "A person who gives rise to a real desire and puts his utmost efforts into study under a teacher will surely gain enlightenment . . . Those who have this drive, even if they have little knowledge or are of inferior capacity, even if they are stupid or evil, will without fail gain enlightenment."[4]

In a traditional Rinzai monastery, monks were expected to reach some level of kensho after two or three years of training. Thereafter, it would usually take another ten to fifteen years of training before they fully matured.[5] In confirmation, Kobori-roshi also told me that it would usually take three years "to get through the Gate." Following this he smiled and said "But not into the temple yet." He also estimated that it would require another ten to twelve years before the awakened monk became skillful enough to teach other monks, at least in the rigorous Rinzai tradition.

A famous Chan master of the Sung dynasty, Ta-hui, was said to have experienced eighteen great awakenings and innumerable smaller ones.[6] Hakuin describes some thirteen experiences of awakening, each of differing kinds and degrees, starting when he was twenty-two years old.[7] Neuroscientists need to pay more attention to how mature a brain must be before it reaches its full capacities for awakening.[3] The existing quantitative EEG techniques suggest that the human brain matures in stages. For example, not until we are between seventeen and twenty-one years old will our prefrontal region finally attain its mature adult characteristics, at least by EEG criteria.[8]

A century before Hakuin, 108 nuns attended a training retreat. Thirty-five passed through koan studies.[9] From such random observations does it appear that it will take several years of meditative practice before the first significant awakening occurs. Thereafter, some of the greatest Zen masters will go on to have multiple experiences. These vary in kind and in depths that can be only hinted at in the pages of this book.

128

A Taste of Kensho: London, 1982

> How bright and transparent
> The moonlight of wisdom!
>
> Master Hakuin, Chant in Praise of Zazen

It is the next sabbatical, from 1981 to 1982. My wife and I are spending most of the year in London, at the cradle of British neurology, the National Hospital, Queen Square. I have joined the London Zen Centre led by Irmgard Schloegl, known now by her Buddhist name, Myokyo-ni. Having trained for 12 years in Japan, she is genuinely wise in the ways of Zen and is a most effective teacher. The event now recounted takes place on the second morning of a two-day sesshin in March.

It strikes unexpectedly at 9:00 A.M., on the surface platform of the London subway system. Getting up at home half an hour earlier than usual, I am en route to the sesshin on a peaceful, balmy Sunday morning. I am a little absent-minded, and take the first train available. I wind up at a station where I have never been before. There, I submit to the reality of a slight delay. After the clatter of the departing train recedes, the empty platform is quiet. Waiting at leisure for the next train to Victoria Station, I turn and look away from the tracks, off to the south, in the general direction of the river Thames. This view includes no more than the dingy interior of the station, some grimy buildings in the middle ground, and a bit of open sky above and beyond. I idly survey this ordinary scene, unfocused, no thought in mind.

Instantly, the entire view acquires three qualities*:

- *Absolute Reality*
- *Intrinsic Rightness*
- *Ultimate Perfection*

With no transition, it is all complete. Every detail of the entire scene in front is registered, integrated, and found wholly satisfying, all in itself.

The new scene is set gently, not fixed on hold. It conveys a slightly enhanced sense of immediacy. And despite the other qualities infusing it, *the purely optical aspects of the scene are no different* from the way they were a split second before. The pale-gray sky, no bluer; the light, no brighter; the detail, no finer-grained.

And furthermore, this scene also conveys another sense. It is being viewed directly with all the cool, clinical detachment of a mirror as it witnesses *a landscape bathed in moonlight.*

Yes, there is the paradox of this extraordinary viewing. But there is no viewer. The scene is utterly empty, stripped of every last extension of an *I-Me-Mine*. Vanished in one split second is the familiar sense that *this* person is viewing an ordinary city scene. The new viewing proceeds impersonally, not pausing to register the further paradox that no human subject is "doing" it.

Its vision of profound, implicit, perfect reality continues for a few seconds, perhaps as many as three to five. Then it subtly blends into a second series of lancinating insights.

Within this second wave are three more indivisible themes. They penetrate the experiant, each conveying *Total Understanding* at depths far beyond simple knowledge:

- *This is the eternal state of affairs.* It has always been just this way, remains just so, and will continue just so indefinitely.

---

* Capitals, italics, and lowercase letters are used, in keeping with convention, simply to convey the unique qualities of depth and scope compressed into these interpretations.

- *There is nothing more to do. This train station, in and of itself, and the whole rest of this world are already totally complete and intrinsically valid. They require no further intervention* (on the part of whoever is remotely inferred).*
- *There is nothing whatsoever to fear.*†

These insights penetrate for perhaps another three to five seconds. There is no counting of insights or of seconds.

Then a third wave of pulsing insight-interpretations wells up. It is a natural ferment, a fountain flowing with knowledge-ideas. By this time, some kind of diminutive subjective i seems to exist off in the background, because something vague is responding with faint discriminations. And the following ideas now arrive in sequence:

1. This totally new view of things *can't be conveyed.* It is too extraordinary. No conceptual framework, no words exist to describe the depths and the qualities of these insights. Only someone who went through the same experience could understand.

2. i can't take myself so seriously any longer. Because this particular interior feeling is that of a diminutive i, it is so indicated, using lowercase letters.

3. A wide buffer zone exists before this i gets involved in anything. The zone seems almost to occupy space, because it takes the form of feeling literally distanced from outside events.

These three ideas last for perhaps another three to five seconds. Then two others enter. The second idea is an observation now being made by a growing, self-referent awareness. It discovers that it has a physical center inside the bodily self of that vaguely familiar person who is now standing on the platform.

4. This physical person is feeling *totally released mentally.* Clear, simplified, free of every limitation. Feeling especially *good* inside. Revived and enormously grateful! *Wow!* But it is a big, *silent* exclamation mark. This expansion of capacities remains internalized, does not proceed into overtly exultant behavior. And even though this person is now standing straighter and moving more freely, these two physical feelings are much less obvious than they were just after the earlier absorption in Kyoto, years before.

5. This experience is *Objective* vision. No subject is inside. It lacks all subjective ties.

---

* Up to this point, we have been using the term *experiant* to refer to whatever experiences when the personal self is absent, a witness not "really" there. But there is a qualification in this instance. A distant quasi-person is being ever so remotely inferred. This curious inference is now indicated by placing it within parentheses: ( ).

† Within this transformed perspective of the world, if there had been even the slightest lingering notion of death—and there was none—it would have had no bearing on the existence of whomever might have been remotely inferred above. We began the introductory discussion of this kind of transformation earlier, when considering how near-death experiences evolve into far-death attitudes (see chapter 104).

A thoughtful I then boards the next subway train to go to the sesshin. The feeling is of being awed, deepened, and calmed within a profound ongoing intellectual illumination. The sesshin takes on more resonant meanings and flows along easily to a graceful close.

During the rest of that Sunday, and the next two days, the following interpretations enter as gentle ideas, more or less separate. When I mull them over, they are now at or close to my usual superficial levels of reflective consciousness:

1. An objective Reality exists. In the past, whenever I sensed its presence, I had always considered it at an intellectual level. I had thought of it as "Nature." Now, it is no longer a word, a concept, or a metaphor. It is really *real*, not an "as if." It is both infinite in scope and profoundly intimate. I am one grain of sand in all of it.

2. Such Reality is the basis for all right thinking and right actions. If one were to act always within this perspective, one could do no wrong. Only ignorance and the insinuation of self-centered motives are the root cause of wrong actions.

3. If the subjective I had somehow still remained on that subway platform, it would have beheld the most subjective of potential experiences. But when this subjective I vanishes, an astonishing moonlight of utter objectivity pervades the scene.

4. I can't now step out of this physical body. No decision or effort of will can bring me back inside that rare moment of being granted such a fresh vision of the larger Reality. But I understand now that this Ultimate Reality does exist, and that it is eternal. Understanding this, I take a more distant, objective view of myself in the present world. Graced by the larger perspective, it is easier now to be very critical about my personal inventory, to diagnose the roots of my liabilities, to work out solutions.

Not until Tuesday is it my turn to see Irmgard Schloegl in sanzen. I outline the experience. She listens carefully and nods supportively. After a few pointed questions, she then leans back, smiles in her kindly way, and says, simply, "I'm very happy for you. With no pause for further discussion or congratulation, she promptly adds the following comments and suggestions.

"Now, move on. Leave the experience behind. Don't hold onto it like you were keeping a picture or a photograph. Regard it as you would a scene you'd just glimpsed out of the window of a moving train. There it is; there it goes. Now it is past. Others will come. Do not grasp them tightly. Just take them to indicate that you are on the Way. Most will occur when one least expects them, not during zazen itself. Use their impetus to go forward, not as an occasion to look backward.

"These moments of no-I are not some 'secrets' of the East, and they certainly aren't secrets in Zen. Anyone can read about them in books. Many people have them. Indeed, one can shout their message from the rooftops. No one else seems to pay much attention, for no-I must truly be experienced to be appreciated."

Yes.

What Is My Original Face?

> The elder Wei Ming then bowed deeply to the sixth patriarch and said: "I am like a man drinking water who knows in himself how cool it is."
>
> J. Blofeld[1]

Six months earlier, in London, I had asked Irmgard Schloegl for a second koan. She chose "Original Face." It is based on an old story, whose concluding lines are cited above. As the story begins, the Sixth Patriarch is up on a mountain retreat. The elder monk, Wei Ming, asks him for instruction, and in return receives this quick question: "Before a single thought arises, without thinking of right or wrong, what is your *original face* before your parents were born?"[2]

When Irmgard spoke the words of this koan, I was more bewildered than stunned. The word-thoughts began. What *is* my original face? How could I even *have* a face before my parents were born?

No such thoughts stopped Wei Ming. He became enlightened the very instant the patriarch posed the question. And note carefully those next words of his, at the end of the opening quotation. They preserve a classic record of the cool taste of kensho. It could also be relevant to notice that Wei Ming had finished climbing up the mountain just before he approached the patriarch. While still in this enhanced state of physiological activity, the question may have struck him with telling impact. Mountains do this to people. Sometimes.

Face. Face? Not until *after* the insights on the subway platform could I have realized what "face" implies. The term "face" begins with several levels of meaning, including the delicate one of preserving one's dignity. Do only those in the Orient care about saving face? It would be delusion to think so. In fact, we all fear being embarrassed or insulted. People in every culture spend years constructing a "face," a mask-image of self. Then, of course, they're stuck with the kind of image which must be "saved."

In contrast, during kensho, the experiant awakens to a face*less*, selfless state. Awakening sheds every psychic construct of the old *I-Me-Mine* (see chapter 9). No wonder kensho seems otherworldly when it is looked back on afterward. Yet it is none other than the state inferred in this perennial koan.

Original. Original? What does the word "original" have to do with Zen? In a sense, much of Zen may be thought of as an ongoing celebration. It is a celebration extolling those same perfections in everyday life which one awakens to in the state of one's "Original Face." Yet the phrase itself is but a pale metaphor. And part of the metaphor alludes to the kinds of fresh, unbiased viewpoints we assume that each infant brain might "originally" have had.

That line of reasoning runs as follows: back when we were naive infants, our awareness and actions would have emerged from the basic ground of our direct perceptions. Why do we assume our earliest perceptions had been so direct? Because our brain, such as it then was, had not yet been *conditioned*. Still unsophisticated, it had no big library of experiences to be self-conscious about.

No hidden agenda. So we tend to think that our original infant brain was capable of registering the elemental perfection of some metaphoric Eden. (This was of course, the original Eden. No one had yet decreed that humankind must have gone on to "sin" or had "fallen.")

By now, it will have become clear why these two words, "Original Face," are deceptive. Neither word in the koan is to be taken at face value. Taken together, they don't mean that literal, anatomical face which you can see in a mirror. They refer back to one's "true nature." It is our elemental self, unindoctrinated, lacking all those judgmental attitudes and behaviors which could shame it into feeling embarrassed. Let the experiant awaken suddenly to *this* "Original Face," and no traces would remain of any attachments to roles or possessions. Here, in the silent core of the self, there is no need for "keeping up appearances."

Parents. Where would one's superego have acquired its attitudes about rights and wrongs? Its dutiful "shoulds," and its weighty "should nots"? Trace back these rights and "thou shalts." Follow those wrongs and "shalt nots" to their source. Does one not hear familiar voices and see familiar faces: one's parents, *their* parents, and a long line of other tall authoritarian figures which might stretch back endlessly into human history? But suppose all these role models had never been born? Could anyone else have delivered such admonitions?

Now we're getting closer to the general sense of the koan. For the answer is no. No, there could exist neither rights nor wrongs in a timeless "original" domain. This is a region into which no parental figures had ever been born.

When I first heard the words of this koan, I was listening with my intellect alone. I heard nonsense. But, during the same period, I was also putting much effort into formal group practice, two evenings each week. And with this additional zazen, I was also becoming more concentrated in general, my major preoccupation being the early themes of this book. Yet, I could never reach Hakuin's burning intensity. After four dry months or so, "Original Face" seemed to have gone underground. Was it in the back of my mind? Perhaps so, but on the day kensho struck, I was not consciously aware of addressing this koan in any manner. Nor, in the seconds to hours thereafter, did I connect kensho's insights with any sense that their message had provided a specific "answer" to this koan. Or at least that they were an answer to what I had *mislead myself into thinking* might be the question it posed.

I was badly mistaken. In fact, I had greatly underestimated the koan. Had I really worked hard to penetrate its basic question? No. I had taken its words literally. "Original Face" had not sunk in. Had I even come close to incorporating the profound issues it implied? No. These were two obvious reasons why I did not appreciate immediately that kensho had resolved the sense of this koan. Two other explanations are more subtle. One will be the limitation which confronts any person who would try to translate *state-bound* information out of an alternate state into a form which an ordinary waking state will be able to recognize (see chapter 58).

The second explanation is basic. What had kensho resolved? Nothing less than the central issues of Reality itself. And it had resolved these key issues at levels beyond word-thoughts. So, from this perspective, no *literal* construction of the words in my koan would be of much value to me, or of much help to me either. In previous months the phrases had become but an artificial finger. It could point vaguely up toward the sky perhaps. But certainly not directly *at* the moon.

Then, after the cool draught of kensho, this riddle began to unfold. Over the next few hours and days, the words made sense, the allusions became clear. Now I could finally discern that this second koan, "Original Face," was a highly accurate metaphor. Now I could appreciate why only insight could penetrate its original, *faceless* domain. For here, in the eternity which prevails everywhere before anyone's parents are born, no varieties of conditioning will ever be found.

And another matter has continued to evolve. It is that I appreciate increasingly the true beauty of this koan. As the years pass, I comprehend it from different perspectives. I still use the phrase as a concentration device at the start of zazen.

130

Major Characteristics of Insight-Wisdom in Kensho

> I saw and heard, and knew at last
> The How and Why of all things, past,
> And present, and forevermore.
>
> Edna St. Vincent Millay (1892–1950)[1]

One can now begin to define Zen enlightenment, *kensho*. It is an expanded, *un*self-consciousness. The word *kensho* means seeing into one's true nature. *Ken* is seeing into something; *sho* means one's true nature. It is a term derived from the Chinese, *chien-hsing*, to see the essence.[2]

What is a person's *true* nature? To Sekida, it is the living realization that "You and the external objects of the world are now unified. It is true that they are located outside you, but you and they interpenetrate each other . . . there is no special resistance between you and them."[3]

To many, kensho would serve as a generic term, and it would include a person's *initial* intuitions into the essence of all things. This would still leave room for further awakenings at much deeper levels. The term *satori* is often reserved for these. They come later in sequence and unveil the most complete, universal understanding of reality. Whichever words might be employed, each such insight breaks through the bottom of the personal bucket. The experiant's brain now comprehends *one* large world. No longer are there two old worlds split into self vs. other.

Which characteristics help define kensho? It is fitting to begin a formal list with criteria cited by Daisetz Suzuki.[2] The first eight of those enumerated below follow the general outline of this state (he preferred to call it satori).[4] The next five characteristics are derived from Pahnke.[5] The final five supplementary items represent my rounding out of their lists for the sake of completeness. Subsequent chapters expand on features of special interest.

1. *Beyond rationality.* The subject later cannot explain the episode logically in terms of any previous personal experience.

2. *Intuitive insight.* The insight conveys not only universal knowledge but clarifies issues of personal existence.

3. *Authoritativeness.* Depths of truth are revealed with the very same certainty that attends drinking cold water. No logical argument refutes them.

4. *Affirmation.* The basic mood and tone is strongly positive toward all existence. It remains positive even though the person may later use words to describe certain qualities of the experience which are cast in negative terms.

5. *Sense of the beyond.* The experience may convey a subtle sense that it is rooted elsewhere. (And afterward, it does illustrate the paradox of being both "Reality" and otherworldly.)

6. *Impersonal tone.* Among Buddhists, a sudden enlightenment makes no reference to the image of Buddha, nor to any notion that his person has intervened in any way. In this respect it differs from a few mystical experiences set in a Christian context in which Christ or the Virgin Mary are reported to be present.

7. *Feeling of exaltation.* The experiant feels an infinite expansion of new attributes and capabilities.

8. *Momentariness.* The episode is abrupt in onset and brief.

9. *External unity.* The whole world is experienced as one. The central theme of this unity is that there are no subject/object distinctions, or any other distinctions among parts of the huge whole.

10. *Changes in the boundaries of time and space.* Not only is clock time absent, but a sense of "eternity" pervades the experience. Moreover, a sense of "infinity" is conveyed, because the old mental boundaries drop out that had been previously affiliated with notions that physical space is somehow limited.

11. *Ineffability.* The experience seems impossible to communicate, because it eludes all words and familiar descriptive categories.

12. *Objectivity and reality.* The experience is "realer than real." The true nature of things is seen into, things as they really are.

13. *Subsequent persisting positive changes in attitude and behavior.* The experience changes the way the subjects think about themselves and about the rest of the world, and it transforms their behavior.

Five other features are conjoined. The last two may seem self-evident, but tend to be overlooked.

14. *Perfection.* The world revealed is awesome in its perfection. This gives rise to the sense that it is sacred and is to be revered.

15. *Beyond doing.* There is a distinct disinclination to intervene. Nothing remains to be done in the face of such perfection.

16. *Sense of release.* Fear vanishes. And, as all the other psychic ambivalences of the *I-Me-Mine* drop off, the experiant feels a sense of total mental and physical relief.

17. *Memorable quality.* The experience strikes deep, has great impact, and is highly valued. Some fragments of the whole remain indelible. But though the person

can later dip into the surface of memory by an effort of will, the whole experience itself remains a gift which cannot be duplicated either in thought or in any other kind of mental imagery.

18. *Unimaginable.* The experience is inconceivable in advance. True, internal absorption does provide one shallow intimation of the way the physical self can drop off. But kensho thrusts deeper. The experiant will be astonished by the way it cuts off all the psychic constructs of the *I-Me-Mine* and leaves only objective vision in its place.

These eighteen properties of insight-wisdom become our prime agenda. A few introductory comments are in order. When reality distills to its essence, existence seems enormously simplified. This understanding of simplicity is a singular property. It pervades, complements, and completes the physiological sense of having been totally released. The scope and degree of the entire release is stunning. It is mental, physical, psychological, and behavioral. And to this experiant, it led to what seemed to be the *spontaneous* responses of profound gratitude, humility, and peace. These positive affective tones had welled up, by themselves, in a natural *automatic* reaction to everything the experience was unveiling. Nothing in them felt as though it had been derived from any remotely volitional or intellectual process.

The literature reports that some subjects have then tumbled into laughter and crying, expressing both their associated behavioral activation as well as their sense of release. Others, overcome in silence, have soon begun to change their behaviors and to simplify their lives in rather different forms of activity. Consider the actions of Te-shan (J. Tokusan; 780–865), that ancient sage of the Tang dynasty. In years past, he had always regarded as priceless his scholarly written commentaries on the *Diamond Sutra*. After satori, he burned them all. He had a simple explanation for this act: "However deep your knowledge of abstruse philosophy, it is like a piece of hair placed in the vastness of space; and however important your experience in things worldly, it is like a drop of water thrown into an unfathomable abyss."[6] This degree of enlightenment seems rare, at least among those writers of today, present company included.

Prajna: Insight-Wisdom

All is empty, clear,
revealed effortlessly, naturally.

Neither thinking nor imagination
can ever reach this state.

Master Seng-ts'an,[1] Affirming Faith in Mind

Certain contents issue from a psyche that is more complete than consciousness. They often contain a superior analysis or insight or knowledge which consciousness has not been able to produce. We have a suitable word for such occurrences—intuition.

Carl Jung (1875–1961)[2]

Small intuitions dart in as grace notes to enlighten our everyday lives. Many enter during a subtle pause when consciousness of the outside world has faded away briefly. Perhaps we had become internally preoccupied with something. Perhaps with nothing at all, in which case even less of our former self was still around. On rare occasions, even larger insights fall into place. So easily that we then say afterward, Why didn't I think of that before?

The question answers itself. See what it contains. It holds "I," and "think." Why don't our ordinary thought processes raise deeper insights? Because logical thoughts retrace pathways that are mostly conventional, if not predictable. And too many association loops of the *I-Me-Mine* are entangled in their circuitry. But if you let these self-referent connections drop off, a totally fresh synthesis can emerge.

No wonder Kobori-roshi emphasized *prajna* at our first meeting. Its insight-wisdom comes from an extraordinary leap of intuition. It is a leap which takes place in the presence of full awareness, but in the absence of self and of all other dualities. Effortlessly, it bypasses tortuous detours of formal analysis, a fact suggesting that massive parallel processing systems have snapped into a novel configuration.

Prajna is not as simple to appreciate as one might suppose. So, in the following paragraphs, we are going to proceed slowly, in stages. We begin by using familiar terms, considering first the form of its insight, while reserving its specific existential content for other chapters.

How does prajna transmit its special knowledge? *Wordlessly.* And yet knowing still occurs, intimate knowing of the most comprehensible kind. In our English language, this verb form, "to know," is inadequate to our present task. It does not clarify the fact that a person comes to *know* in different ways. Some foreign languages do a better job. For example, the French begin with their verb, *connaître.* The Germans start with *kennen.* These words stand for a person's ordinary form of knowing, the kind that knows a simple fact. And a variation on this theme of knowing stands ready to recognize an apple. How? Because the real apple will match a pattern laid down in the back half of the brain, an expectation in the temporal lobes in particular.

Then we come to the next higher level of knowing. Here, the corresponding foreign words are *savoir* and *wissen*. They still refer to the kinds of knowing we use in everyday living. But now they specify a certain kind. This particular variety means *understanding, comprehending*.[3] To comprehend is to engage in a highly specialized activity, one which links many association loops throughout much of the brain. When you arrive at this level of knowing, you will understand a lot about different kinds of apples, including perhaps how to grow them in general.

Cognition is one route to such understanding. What is it? Dictionaries give it an intellectual flavor. They limit it to mean the particular *thought*ful process by which we gain knowledge. To illustrate: suppose you want to plant some apple trees. You'll now need to select only those varieties which can survive in your climate zone. Accessing cognition, you'll rely on its series of logical steps. These will lead you through all the mouthwatering options in the nursery catalogues. As each step sifts, it draws on large networks of associations. So, at the end of all your time-consuming deliberations, you'll be left with the sense that you've put a good deal of mental work into your decision-making process.

The two strains of Delicious apples are each rich in flavor. Your choice was the red, not the yellow variety. Was this because you were partial to red? If so, then you may begin to appreciate the subtle inroads of *affection*. It is that pervasive emotional or feeling aspect of our consciousness which serves as a contrast to cognition. During emotional knowing, no willed, logical, wordy steps intervene.

We have now surveyed four attributes that enter into our ordinary levels of knowing: (1) recognition, (2) intuitive understanding, (3) cognition, and (4) affection. They are the preamble. Now we can appreciate the final refinement of knowing. It is rare. It cannot be willed into consciousness. Moreover, it cuts off the usual emotions attached to the psychic self.

This is the domain of *prajna* (J. *hannya*). Its special feature is the quick grasp of unlimited, universal reality which clarifies the vast unity of all things. This profound insight-wisdom flashes in, takes over, proceeds at an extra-fast pace, and conveys no sense of mental effort. In these last few respects only, it might cause a neurologist to wonder: could it faintly resemble a frontal lobe disorder, the kind called forced thinking? The particular patients who undergo forced thinking are having a focal seizure. It starts in the dorsolateral part of the frontal lobe. As a result, they experience brief episodes during which intrusive thoughts rush in.[4] The thoughts are accompanied by a remarkable feeling tone. Its quality is cold and nonemotional. Why? Possibly because the seizure begins out in the forward compartments of the frontal lobe. We have noted that this convex surface of the frontal cortex is relatively far removed from limbic circuits (see table 7, chapter 57). But prajna is different. Defined as supreme intuitive wisdom, its scope is never that narrow. Nor is it that stereotyped, when it recurs in the same person.

Our other ordinary forms of knowing, cited above, splash around at shallower depths. How could it be otherwise? They are always based on a subject: *this*. Hence, they always stand opposed by an object: *that*. In Buddhism, the technical term given to our customary mode of perceiving dualities is *vijnana*. Its scope is always limited to either/or differences. We may insert an ambivalent hedge or two, but vijnana restricts us to dualities. All these distinctions split up our own small private mental field. We glimpse only fragments of the whole.

Kant took a formal inventory of what went on inside this ordinary, divided mental field. He found that our distinctions fell into five general categories.[5] And by using all these divisions we were able to create a sense of structure within our ordinary experience. It will prove instructive to list these Kantian structures. For soon it will become very clear: insight-wisdom cuts each of them off at the roots. The formal categories are:

1. Space and time (Is it here or there, now or then?)
2. Quantity (Is there one, more than one, a universality?)
3. Quality (Is this reality, nothing, or a limitation placed on something?)
4. Relationship (Is this substantial, cause and effect, reciprocal?)
5. Modality (Is something only a possibility, an actuality, a necessity?)

Prajna dismantles the entire framework of these five constraints. In its place, it leaves the impression that consciousness has escaped from the gravity pull of worldly logic and is now operating within the immensity of a universal context.

But is this really *wisdom?* And is it taking place at a sage level, or even at some "cosmic" level? Or could it be the rare expression of brain functions which happen to open up and to link in a novel, instinctive way? Whatever bias shapes our answer, one result is noteworthy: the actions coming directly out of prajna will be swift, sure, and free from error. Indeed, Bankei had emphasized that they don't make "a single mistake." Then are all revelations to be viewed as truly infallible? Certainly not. But let them spring from prajna, and be genuinely emancipated from the *I-Me-Mine*. Now they will make no *self*-centered mistakes.

Each of us spends lifetimes with word-messages embedded in every thought, and all too frequently on our tongue. We forget how intuition strikes. It comes in a lightning-like flash. This *flash* of insight is also the basis for the phrase, *the Thunderbolt Vehicle*, used in connection with the esoteric Buddhism of Tibet. Moreover, prajna's intuitions do more than strike quickly and wordlessly. Having cast off their allegiance to intervening word-thoughts, they strike *directly as conclusions, unique in the way they integrate knowing, feeling, and being.*

The result is an altogether fresh *un*conditioned kind of seeing. What does it perceive? The time-honored affirmations of the *Hsin hsin ming*[1] tell us: a realm with no dualities, indivisible; nothing left out, nothing in excess. Within it, black will *coexist* with white, high with low, front with back. No distinctions remain, either between such items or among them. What can happen when antitheses are equally valid, when stark opposites are reconciled? First, *all things then become equally important*. Second, *their basic interrelationships are understood*. In this big picture, unity prevails.

Within prajna, the old conditioned emotional weightings drop out. So do the formal rules of serial analysis. Saints and sinners? They will coexist, no longer ranked along the old hierarchies imposed by priority or by convention. Instead, the mental field opens up instantly to unique variations on those five former Kantian themes. The result is a new mode. It will comprehend not either and not or. Yet it will understand *both, all, none, and then some.* Insights at such levels open up unimaginable dimensions of meaning, of truth and reality. It would remain for Nils Bohr, the physicist, to prepare us, at least partially, for their mind-bending scope. Bohr said, "The opposite of a true statement is a false statement. But the opposite of a profound truth may be another profound truth."[6]

What does it imply when such understanding strikes with no word-thoughts? The message is that when consciousness shifts into prajna, our usual language connections are being bypassed or preempted. This leads to a plausible hypothesis: prajna does not draw from ordinary language circuits, or at least not from the usual ones out over the left cortical surface which link our receptive and expressive language areas (see figures 2 and 12).

So then, could prajna be drawing on *sub*cortical circuits, including those farther down in the thalamus? If so, perhaps we may then usefully take into account the unusual anatomical fact about the thalamus. As our brain evolved, it seemed almost as though some oversight in the blueprints of the thalamus might have deprived its specific and association nuclei from supplying one of their potential target regions higher up (see notes to chapters 59 and 117). For while these two groups of thalamic nuclei did project many messages up to most other areas of the cortex, *they sent relatively few large fast fibers up to inform the vast bulk of the temporal lobe.* And a prominent role of this temporal lobe is to *receive and decode the patterns of spoken language* (see chapter 56). So almost all of this large lobe would remain in a condition sometimes referred to as *a*thalamic.

What effect could such relative sparing have? In a sense, many of the language-linked networking functions of the temporal lobe would seem to have been left a step or more behind the rest of the cortex. For the fastest input from the thalamus would not be going directly into most temporal lobe circuitries. On the other hand, such an arrangement could leave other temporal circuits relatively free, momentarily, to generate their own lines of interpretation (see figure 11).

Suppose that the critical mass of the insights which first flashed into consciousness had developed in sites elsewhere in the brain not initially devoted to language per se. For example, let us postulate that they had first leaped from interactive circuits linking the front of the thalamus to the frontal lobe. During these early milliseconds, salient meanings would already have entered the forefront of consciousness. And by then they could already be in forms that a somewhat laggard temporal cortex might subsequently find difficult to decode into ordinary word-thoughts.[7]

Buddhists have another apt metaphor for prajna. It is a two-edged sword. When wielded by the bodhisattva Manjusuri, the sword cuts both ways. One edge cuts off prior concepts. The other strikes back at the very context of its *own* interpretations. In this latter sense does the second sword-edge illustrate a less-appreciated, but fundamental asset inherent in certain qualities of the wisdom within prajna. It is a nuance the person only discovers step by step, as a fact of later ongoing experience: *the wisdom is self-negating, self-critical, and self-correcting.*

These special properties constitute part of the silent wisdom of prajna, and bring a sense of proportion to the process as a whole. They enable the person to escape from pride, and to keep evolving toward further levels of maturity and humility.

132

Suchness

> To concentrate your mind on something is not the true purpose of Zen. The true purpose is to see things as they are, to observe things as they are, and to let everything go as it goes.
>
> Master Shunryu Suzuki (1905–1971)[1]

> When the mind does not discriminate,
> all things are as they really are.
>
> Entering the deep mystery of this suchness
> releases us from all our attachments.
>
> Master Seng-ts'an, *Affirming Faith in Mind*

Daisetz T. Suzuki believed *suchness* was "the basis of all religious experience."[2] You might think that by now everyone would know what was meant by something this important. Not so. What's the problem? It is, as Suzuki also noted, that one must personally experience suchness. Only then does one understand what it is. He was absolutely correct.

Before experiencing suchness, the word's opacities eluded me. Indeed, even after having undergone the experience, it still did not dawn on me that this was what was meant by a term I must have glossed over in D. T. Suzuki's writing eight years earlier. Finally, another two years after tasting kensho, I again encountered the term, once more while browsing through Suzuki. Only then did I understand what he had been referring to. (Talk about a laggard brain!) As a mere word on a page, suchness is one more very pale imitation of the real thing.

Real suchness is not a concept. It is an experience beyond reach of the intellect. Is there no way a finger can point, even in the same general direction as this experience? Let us try, first by looking at what seems to be an ordinary pebble. In the early milliseconds, we will have already taken it away from itself. We will have processed its wavelengths and transformed them into a percept framed in our own *personal* terms of reference. Thoughts wandering, as usual, we might even go on to discriminate whether it was a light or heavy pebble, igneous or metamorphic, etc., etc. If its black surface and white quartz veins seemed aesthetically pleasing, we might succumb to the rock hound's powerful impulse (almost primal, it seems) which drives the "collector's need" to take it home. Or if it were flat enough, and we had energies to burn, we might hurl it skipping along the water's surface.

What happened to the stone *itself* in all this? The pebble got lost. For its true suchness is none of these extra, human, layers. It is the stone, seen thoroughly but spared from being processed further. And seen not as *our* object. But *just as it is*, the thing-in-itself, uncomplicated by any of our autobiographical references. In suchness, viewing perceives that very stone, and it relates directly to it. Immediate perception. Uncluttered by any personal reverberations.

So what? What does it add to see things *exactly* as *they* are? Little, at first glance. Little, in terms of the way most Western religious systems might usually formulate their priorities. However, it really does mean seeing into the world as a whole new realm. And, from this fresh vantage point, the illuminating vision enhances the basis of all religions. Why? Because it elevates them to the *same matter-of-fact but sacred status* which infuses everything else in the universe. As Shunryu Suzuki aptly phrased it: "Not to be attached to something is to be aware of its absolute value."[3] Suchness confers this unique, absolute perspective. It operates only when the human scale shrinks.

Primitive humans arrived late in this planet's history. *Homo sapiens* evolved much later still, bringing sundry concepts, labels, dictionaries, and transient pages like this one. Pebbles existed eons before all these other things did. Each pebble existed in its own way, in its *essential namelessness*. In itself, it had no need to prompt any human sensation, to be tagged by some label and fitted into any human scheme of things. Nothing about this basic situation changed simply because our species had arrived. We and the pebble are still integral parts of one and the same ongoing universe. *It is still a universe undivided*. It has never been split up by such artificial distinctions as minutes, first names, rock names, or place names. It *is*, in its suchness. It will still be so even when human beings are no longer around to see it, and to proliferate thoughts about it.

To illustrate further: suppose you consent to take part in a brief harmless experiment. All you're invited to do is to put on a blindfold and to swallow a bland liquid. The liquid will be warm tea, imported from India. You won't know that before you swallow. First, you feel the heat of a liquid, then the wave of taste-aroma from the tea. Next you conclude that it is, indeed, hot tea. But that isn't all. For soon, you'll go on to think and even to verbalize a long string of associations to it. Zen lies in the direction of those early, uncomplicated milliseconds. Then, you and the teacup and the hot tea simply exist in the whole seamless universe.

Zen's home lies in these first milliseconds when poignant experience and behavioral responses flow naturally. The Western world may take note of this, attuned as it is to instant gratifications. Still, it doesn't remain convinced. Could anything worthwhile be this simple? The answer is yes.

For Zen flows in the mainstream of the old minimalist tradition. It conveys a radical, straightforward message: direct experience *is* both simple and worthwhile. Less *is* more. Zen literature abounds in examples of this one absurdly simple fact. Two examples.

One old Zen story, frequently cited herein and elsewhere, describes the novice who comes to study under Sho Zenji, a master in China.[4] He asks his master, "How do I go about entering into the study of Zen?" Will the acolyte be directed to the sacred scriptures? No. Nor to anything complex and abstract. The master's advice is excellent; just listen to a simple, basic sound: the gurgling of a mountain stream.

And there is the other old mondo whose variations we have often referred to: the one where the monk asks master Chao-chou, "Why did the First Patriarch come from the West?" (What is the essence of the matter?) And Chao-chou answers: "The cypress tree in the yard."

Nothing could seem more opaque to the beginner. Or more clear to one of experience. Let the aspirant really see into the cypress tree in all *its* suchness, truly hear the babbling of the brook as *it* really is. Then—when the intimate reality of all things is perceived, just like *that*—this special moment will serve to answer any questions a monk might have.

Even so, in the first year after the taste of kensho, a lingering part of me sometimes returned to wonder: A *train* platform? Why not somewhere more inspirational, like on a mountain? Later my understanding would stay on line and not waver: *one place is just as suitable as any other, and certainly as sacred in the universal sense.* Any setting will do. For kensho is an art appreciation course. The setting remains optically the same. What is different? It has instantly been *seen into* and transformed by new meanings.

The early Zen masters knew this. Eschewing words, they taught by indirection. Chao-chou's "cypress tree" response exemplifies the technique. Not an answer in kind. *But one which points toward what suchness implies.* Any young monk who learns to listen and look into the world of nature will finally get there himself in due course.

Had Chao-chou already seen into the reality of that particular cypress tree? On that day or on some earlier day? Was this response a random expression of a master's advanced stage of ongoing enlightenment? We are not told, nor do we need to know. On another day, he might have responded differently to the same question. No matter. What counts is the *form* of the old master's answer, not its verbal content. For the message is embedded in the form. It points toward the profound insight within suchness: every thing is unique. Every thing shares equally in that vast original, concrete reality of Everything.

Not only are *things* seen into—objects like pebbles and trees—in such a way that their intrinsic nature is revealed. *Persons* are also seen into. This includes both the present self and the erstwhile self. Now the roots of one's biases and firmest convictions are laid bare, as though an obscuring veil of complexity had been cast off. In this manner does suchness, central to insight-wisdom, go on to see *all* things—animate and inanimate—in their original unconceptualized form, stripped of all personal frames of reference, unconditioned by any discriminating characteristics, free from any invidious comparisons with anything else.

In pure form, the viewing is sometimes described as being mirror-like. But this simile alludes only to the way the experiant's perception and insight merge into that single state which sees everything clearly and immediately without distortions. When Hui-neng was still a young monk, he made a simple statement that no "dust" could settle on *this* "mirror." His words were recognized as having risen from the depths of his own direct experience, and they contributed to his being selected as the Sixth Patriarch in China.

Eastern languages had spoken about suchness long before Immanuel Kant. Still, it would take his writings to help bring credence to suchness in the West. We need not agree with this philosopher to the degree that, as will be evident in the following paragraph, he seemed completely to have excluded the possibility that suchness would *ever* occur in human experience. Yet, when Kant focused on what a thing was *in itself*—the *Ding an sich*—it became one of his major contributions to Western thought. When the American poet Wallace Stevens wished to distill into three words the essence of his lifelong search for reality, he would refer to "the Thing Itself" (as opposed to ideas about it).[5]

Kant went so far as to say: "It remains completely unknown to us what objects may be by themselves and apart from the receptivity of our senses. We know nothing but our manner of perceiving; that manner being peculiar to us, and not necessarily shared by every being, though, no doubt, by every human being."[6]

In fact, it was *not* completely unknown before Kant's time (1724–1804). Indeed, in Japanese, the word *sono-mama* had long implied that something could stand as it is, untouched. In Chinese, the expressions *Chi-mo* or *Shi-mo* were used to mean "just so," or "so it is."[7] And an even earlier corresponding word for suchness was *tathata*. In Sanskrit, *tatha* implied "in that manner," "in that way," *thusly*. When *-ta* was added at the end, it implied "-ness".[8] So *tathata* refers, then, to the essential original nature that all things in the universe basically share. This is known as Buddha-nature. And each one of us is always *right in it*, not extrinsic to it.

Following the lead of D. T. Suzuki, the tendency developed to speak about the profound experience of thusness or suchness, and these two words came to be used more or less interchangeably. Gradually, another explicit phrase entered common usage: "things as they really are." So is this what it boils down to? Is this the essence of enlightenment, the basis (as Suzuki said) "of all religious experience?" Then what is it? *It is seeing directly into this true nature, into things as they really are.*

Brief though the experience is, its residues linger. Back in the eighth century, Layman Pang, in one simple statement, conveyed their awesome quality: "How wondrous this, how mysterious!/I carry fuel, I draw water."[9]

Yet it is extraordinarily rare for someone to walk *permanently* in "suchness." Rare to stay so alive every minute of every day, so totally aware of reality in this deeply meaningful way. Indeed, one can appreciate how completely enlightened the Buddha was, because his followers had a very special way to describe him: he was the tath*agata*. They reserved this term for the rare person so thoroughly enlightened that he continually *goes in thusness*—his suchness is ongoing.[10] Part VIII discusses this in more detail.

Perhaps a moment ago you glimpsed what suchness is. Then, the sense of "the way things are" slipped far away again. So this next time try to grant yourself a rare gift borrowed from two movies you've seen. Imagine that you are now viewing things not as an earthbound human. Instead, you are looking from another vantage point. For the moment, you are an E.T., an extraterrestrial humanoid perched far out in the still point of a wheeling galaxy. Suppose further that you too have arrived at that stage of grace which yields an innocent, yet all-knowing comprehension. It is an advanced stage of insight-wisdom. You are aligned with every fundamental principle in the cosmos, in a kind of harmonious interrelationship with "The Force," if you will. As a result, from this perspective you can look down on planet Earth, and perceive any single pebble, or knobby cypress tree, or babbling brook as *it* exists.

Now take away the E.T. humanoid. But let that same universal perspective remain. It still goes on witnessing and comprehending The Way Things Really Are. And, How They Have Always Been.

Is this stretching imagination too far? Something similar actually happened out in space. In February 1971, Edgar Mitchell, the astronaut, was out there on his Apollo XIV expedition, heading for the moon. When he looked back, it was to behold the "breathtaking experience of seeing planet Earth floating in the vastness of space." Incredibly beautiful, the Earth was "a majestic sight—a splendid blue and white jewel suspended against a velvet black sky." His seeing it *thus*— a jewel in black space—triggered a deep insight into the nature of his existence. It was "the sort of insight that radically changes the inner person."[11] This knowledge came to him abruptly, in a form that he would later call "an experiential cognition." It directly informed him that "the universe has meaning and direction."

For millennia, human beings on Earth have experienced that megashift of insight which informed them that they were in the presence of the universal, meaningful reality. Such a "brand-new" perspective is probably the ultimate one the human brain can generate. Some would call it "cosmic consciousness." Yet, even as it is fading toward its afterglow, it leaves the person with a definite impression of surprise: what has just been glimpsed was already there, in the everyday world, all along! Bumps, warts and all . . .

As Greeley would phrase it, each of us already exists in the most fundamental biological way, "at one with the hydrogen-nitrogen-oxygen cycles, the processes of growth and decay, day and night, autumn and spring, sleep and waking, death and rebirth. In the ecstatic interlude, we are taken possession of by that which we already possess."[12] Watts finally came to the same kind of self-evident realization. His took place during the final phase of an LSD session when he was *descending* out of the drug state into his ordinary mental state. Then, he suddenly realized what supreme awakening really is. In fact, it meant that one had simply awakened to the realization of what constitutes so-called ordinary consciousness.[13]

Even such a subsidiary realization presents a totally new point of view. And it will leave any person who had first entered suchness, and then left it, marveling at the way this moment had briefly illuminated, reinterpreted, and vivified the seemingly bare sensate impressions of ordinary life.

On our agenda are several other qualities which kensho blends into its strong sense of things as *they* really are. Next, we explore some of these properties individually, remembering that they are all making an impact together.

Direct Perception of the Eternally Perfect World

We all move on the fringes of eternity and are sometimes granted vistas through the fabric of illusion.

Ansel Adams (1902–1984)[1]

One truth is clear, whatever is, is right.
Know then thyself, presume not God to scan;
the proper study of mankind is man.

Alexander Pope (1688–1744)[2]

Master Bankei had a metaphor for our original nature. He called it the "unborn primary mind." Nowadays, to avoid confusion, we need not take literally, or even too metaphorically, the way he used the term "unborn." Indeed, as Bankei himself went on to explain: "The true Unborn has nothing to do with fundamental principles, and it's beyond becoming or attaining. It's simply being as you are."[3] Being "as you are" means opening up the shutter of one's brain to an illumination so fundamental that it pierces the old "fabric of illusion" and directly grasps perception. Bankei illustrated what he meant in the following manner:

> While you face this way listening to me now, if a sparrow chirps behind you, you don't mistake it for a crow; you don't mistake the sound of a bell for a drum, or hear a man's voice and take it for a woman's . . . You hear and distinguish those different sounds, without making a single mistake, by virtue of the marvelous working of illuminative wisdom . . . The place in which there's no difference between persons in the hearing of those sounds is the Unborn, the Buddha-mind, and it's perfectly equal and absolutely the same in each one of you . . . At the place of the Unborn, before the thought arises, attributes such as "man" and "woman" don't even exist.[4]

So Bankei's "unborn" brain is instant, pure perception. Before a thought arises. Because it is unconditioned, and untangled by personal associations, it defines physiological levels which lie beyond psychodynamic formulations. Its natural functions are primary, beyond notions of good or evil, undistorted by desires or fears. Bankei went a step further. He emphasized that the "unborn" extended beyond perception into reflexive behavior. To illustrate this point he chose another instructive anecdote. It concerned the way two men would behave while walking along a narrow path. "One is a good man and the other an evil man. . . . If a horse or cow approaches from the opposite direction, both men will step aside to let it pass. . . . There isn't the slightest difference between them in performing this act. It shows that the Unborn Buddha-mind is found even in an evil man."[5]

Insight-wisdom includes other subtle properties. Because they are indivisible at impact, and are perceived directly, it will be only afterward that the experiant thinks about associating them with words. In my case, the words were eternity, perfection, and immanence. Now I finally appreciated the truth in Kobori-roshi's statement: Zen is closest to poetry.

Eternity. The glimpse into eternity comes as the most incredible surprise, and it exerts an immensely powerful influence on one's long-range attitudes. It is a realm of the "always so," not only the "just so." *It is a world of ever thusness. It presumes no moment of creation, no creator, no specific creative force.* Indeed, the experiant enters a realm not only unborn but not even conceived. Long ago, Master Dogen may have been alluding to this striking quality when he said that things, just as they are, are already present "in complete form."[6]

Now, in everyday life we place great reliance on a set of standard "fundamental principles." These, Bankei noted, were absent in kensho. One of our old reliables is the principle of cause and effect. We rest comfortably in the common-sense belief that the present physical universe must have been created earlier, and by some creative force. This idea is imbedded in our Judeo-Christian and scientific heritage. Still, let us admit that when we apply seemingly logical principles, it sometimes does create problems. For example, common sense would also lead us to conclude that light could not be both wave and particle. Nor could mass and energy be equivalent. In each case, we wonder: do the physicists really know what's going on?

Perhaps they were only preparing us to be stunned by an even more dramatic mind-bender. This one comes from Stephen Hawking and James Hartle of Cambridge University. One of their mathematical formulas describes our post-Einsteinian cosmos. Their model uses terms which suggest that we are living in a self-contained universe. This means, astonishingly, that the cosmos has never been created. Never created to begin with, it will never be destroyed. So it is, in fact, eternal.[7]

The Orient has long been on speaking terms with this preposterous notion. The title of the ancient book, the *Tao Te Ching,* can be translated as "The Book of the Immanent Way." In it are the following lines:

The Tao is infinite, eternal,
Why is it eternal?
It was never born;
thus it can never die.[8]

The Chinese have a particular phrase, no-birth (*wu sheng*). When it is translated as nonarising or nonexisting, it also expresses something of this same curious quality.[9]

Perfection. This is the second quality investing kensho. Everything is seen as ultimately *right.* Anything that exists is already intrinsically correct. Alexander Pope must have understood this, for he went on to affirm the point in the ringing line: "One truth is clear, whatever is, is right." The implications of this particular line are substantial. In literature, however, Pope's next sentence would be the one most often quoted.

Immanence. This third property of kensho registers at about the same time. The term comes from the Latin, *immanere,* to remain in. Dictionary definitions of immanence describe it as the presence of the ultimate reality principle *embedded entirely within and throughout the whole physical universe*. Immanence goes beyond the second statement of perfection. For it implies that the highest and most sacred principle, Deity if you will, is manifest in all things *right down here*, ourselves included. It is inherent *within this world*. Right under our nose, and *in* our nose. Not up there, on some separate higher level, taking the form of a distant overarching creative principle.

This same, down-to-earth theme was known to some early Christians. The Gnostic Christian sects existed during the first centuries of the Christian era. Their name comes from *gnosis:* the intuitive process of self-knowledge. In their text, the Gnostic Gospel according to Thomas, one finds Jesus making an interesting statement about immanence. Here, he begins by saying that, if the "Kingdom of God" were to be up in the sky or down in the sea, then the birds and the fishes would have been the first to arrive. Instead, he continues, "the Kingdom is inside of you, and it is outside of you . . . spread out upon the earth, and men do not see it."[10] A related word of Hebrew origin further emphasizes the intrinsic quality of immanence. It is Immanuel. It means God with us. When used in the Christian context, it refers to Jesus being God's manifestation *within this* world. Kant was well named. So immanence, being all-inclusive, and with its feet always planted into the ground, stands in sharp contrast with transcendence. Transcendence is a word that has come to acquire several other meanings.

Transcendence, when used theologically, implies that the highest deity principle extends above and beyond this physical world. Does this notion have anything to do with Zen? No. D.T. Suzuki neatly distinguished Zen from such transcendence. He said: "By transcending 'this,' another something is created. In Buddhism, especially in Zen, 'transcending' is not to go out of this thing, but to be in it and yet not in it."[11]

Issues of previous faith aside, the person who directly perceives the immanent perfection of things as they really are, enters that "peace which passeth all understanding." And because this profound peace has evolved in the absence of self, it will know neither time nor fear.

The Construction of Time

In rivers the water that you touch is the last of what has passed and the first of that which comes: So with time present.

Leonardo da Vinci (1452–1519)[1]

...for it is not so much to know the self
as to know it as it is known
by galaxy and cedar cone,
as if birth had never found it
and death could never end it ...

A.R. Ammons (Born 1926)[2]

It was a fact of personal experience that time disappeared during absorption and kensho. Why did time change, in each instance? If we could clarify this, it would help resolve two related issues. First, how we construct time in general. Second, how two sets of mechanisms combine to create these two different states of absorption and kensho.

Time is a construct, an enormously compounded one. The scope of our inquiry will be limited. We need to simplify such issues as processing delays; the critical length of a stimulus; the interval between stimuli; backdating; past, present, and future time; the equivalence of time and distance; the way time flows in one direction; personal time; and time sequencing. Let's look first at how we construct time. Before long, we'll find ourselves on very soft ground.

A child's sense of time is already off to a running start by one year of age, according to Piaget. And notice, during our early months, that each of us is also beginning to build three other vital concepts. They are all interconnected. First, they relate us to space in general. Second and third, they relate us to the other people and objects which soon start filling up that space.[3] Most of the basic operations which then feed into our sense of "time" will themselves take shape in a split second. For example, suppose a peripheral stimulus arrives out on its sensory end organ. The next sixty to seventy milliseconds are taken up by processing delays. It takes this long before our nervous system can integrate the stimulus in purely *neural* terms.[4]

Even then, the peripheral stimulus itself must continue for a while. Otherwise we won't perceive it. Indeed, if one simple stimulus itself doesn't last for more than another sixty to seventy milliseconds, it will seem to be a signal with no apparent duration. Some human studies suggest that the traces from one sensory event must then endure in the brain for at least 500 milliseconds—a long half-second—if this event is to go on to enter *full* consciousness.[5] But meanwhile, our brain isn't ready to acknowledge that it required this much time to generate subjective experience. So what does it do? It arbitrarily backdates the stimulus, and "re-times" its moment of entry. This now gives us the impression that we had felt the stimulus "at once." Whereas, in fact, we didn't really reach the basic neuronal adequacy to "feel" the signal until many milliseconds *after* it had arrived. Clearly, we've built a personal clock so facile that it can shift its own time zones. Neuroscientists are still not clear how the human brain manipulates time in this sleight-of-hand manner.

Perceptions can stand by themselves as bits, the basic units of our experience. And some researchers have estimated that each separate bit lasts between 10 and 100 milliseconds.[6] By merging the edges of these separate perceptual frames, we gain the impression that our ongoing experience has a sense of continuity. The so-called psychological moment is that brief segment of time inside which two separate events are so close together that we still fuse them into one single unit of impression. In normal persons, this interval varies, and it can range from 50 up to 250 milliseconds.[7] In order to have an average number to work with, let us assume that our brain's sensory sampling interval is set to operate at, say, 200 milliseconds.[8] And, if two successive tones each last only one-fifth as long as this, we'll lump them together and "hear" an intermediate tone, fabricated out of thin air. In contrast, patients who have suffered damage to their left cerebral hemispheres need a much wider window of time in order to distinguish two separate sounds. And they may require an interval as long as *600* milliseconds to decide which of the two tones appeared first.

How long is our impression of the *Now?* William James held that the center of our present moment, the "Now" if you will, usually contained a nucleus of "the dozen seconds or less that has just elapsed." One vague fringe will have vanished backward into the past, and the other will be extending off toward the future.[9] He was close. A recent article suggests that people estimate their "Now" to embrace intervals of time lasting anywhere from one, to three, up to fifteen seconds.[10] This leaves plenty of room for subjects to misjudge the durations of their alternate states.

Time as Distance and Sequence

Even though we may try to attach numbers to it, time remains a more elastic construct than we might think. This is only the beginning. Now consider two of the constituents of our sense of time: sequences and distances. Firmly embedded within it, both ingredients tend to equate with time. Start with Lindbergh's solo flight, for example. It involved a sequence: first a takeoff, then a landing. And we can express this epic flight in either of two ways: in its elapsed time of thirty-three and a half hours, *or*, in the distance he covered—some three thousand miles from Long Island to Paris.

In that same year, closer to home, a child could look way up, at the tall "ticktock" which stood in my grandparents' house. And he would have seen hands there, on this grandfather clock, moving slowly from one numeral to the next, measuring time as they spanned distance. Hidden from view was that internal mechanism which made the ticking sound as it swung the pendulum back and forth over an arc of inches. Today, the tick of an atomic clock hinges on the resonant frequency of cesium. Even the quartz crystal in a watch covers a distance, as each of its vibrations also resonates through tiny amplitudes three thousand times each second.

Will it help us to understand that our normal time sense is contingent both on sequences *and* on covert distances? Yes, because this kind of knowledge will leave us better prepared to appreciate kensho. For we are soon going to develop a new hypothesis. It will propose that time evaporates when these two contingencies vanish.

A leaf floats past on the river's surface. Having been swept in upstream, it drifts out of sight downstream. Thoughts do likewise. They are seen to come and go during meditation. So, yes, we do have that capacity to warp time, back and forth. Nevertheless, time still *flows in one direction:* past → present → future. How do we develop this highly subjective notion that time flows in only one direction? We go through the same procedure that Leonardo did, 500 years ago. First we register event A, then register event B a little later. We then reach a *wordless* "recency decision." We base this on our own *personal* time clock. This clock helps decide that, because the signal from event B arrived most *recently,* event A must therefore have happened first, earlier. We have now defined the interval between A and B. And we defined it with reference to our own private internal dateline. So once more another standard line of reference is leading back to the personal self. And once again we have imposed our *own* sense of order on an impression. Note the potential consequences. Every time we do this, we are creating the set of conditions which *will also dismantle our sense of time as soon as our subjective framework of self drops out.*

Milner studied how brain damage affects the way we *sequence* events in time.[11,12] She asked her patients to leaf through two sets of cards. One set of cards had words printed on it. The other set had samples of abstract art. Then—at a given point in each series—she asked the patients to judge: "Among those cards which you leafed through, which cards did you see most recently?"

Patients with left frontal lobe damage showed major defects in the way they time-sequenced the *word* "cards." But those who had right frontal lobe damage had problems pulling *visual* cards into the proper order. Now any normal person must first register the cards, and recognize them, back in the more posterior, sensate, parts of the brain. But thereafter, it will be mostly up to the frontal lobes to help a normal subject impose some *sense of order* on events. This ordering process allowed us to "decide" that event B came *most recently* in sequence, in contrast to event A which had occurred more remotely. Suppose every last one of the sequencing functions of the frontal lobes had been either lost, preempted, or bypassed. What then? Ongoing experience would be stripped of the framework which helps monitor our sequences of time and establish its sense of flow.

Future Time

Of course, Milner's studies focused on the way her subjects constructed a semblance of "time" that had already flowed past, with the aid of "recent" cards or "remote" cards. But one can also look upstream at this river of time. Upstream lies future time. This is the vague domain of "not yet, but someday." Normally the general "forward tilt" of our frontal lobe functions will orient us toward these "forseeable" events floating in from this upriver direction. It is an old clinical observation that frontal lobe lesions do block foresight, our capacity to project consequences off into future time.[13]

In this regard, Ingvar has proposed the term "memory of the future." It describes the ability of the normal brain not only to encode, retain and recall but to be conscious of the fact that it is laying great plans to address future events.[14] Yet these networks rehearse scenarios endlessly, running through one script after another. Our internal dialogues reflect self-centered, worrisome concerns, and cause many distractions, but yield few scenarios of practical use. The low yield of these dialogues is easy to appreciate. Meditators are very familiar with it, as are the subjects who may be trying hard to relax in the artificial setting of a research laboratory. And during such times of poor relaxation, studies show that frontal lobe blood flow increases to values half-again higher than elsewhere in the brain.

Of what consequence is this high traffic flow of intrusive thoughts? It does prevent each of us from being truly alive and focused in the present moment. Aware of this everyday problem, Hui-neng once said, "The ignorant person practices seeking future happiness, and does not practice the Way."[15] Zen practice means staying directly in touch with the flow of the immediate moment, da Vinci's "time present," the *Now*.

Kensho leaves behind many clues. Some of these clues are overt, and are as diagnostic as a fingerprint. Others can be recognized by the deficit they leave. A group of "negative signs" fall into this latter category. They are the functions—which one otherwise expects of the normal brain—that drop out, *silently*, during kensho. Their silence is eloquent. And can be put to practical use. Conan Doyle established an instructive precedent for this kind of "useful absence." We come next to the part of our own detective story which illustrates the hidden value of an eloquent silence. It corresponds with the clue Doyle dropped, for the benefit of his readers, in the tale of "Silver Blaze."

The Dissolution of Time

This truth is unmeasurable
one instant is ten thousand years . . .
Words fail to describe it
for it is neither of the past, present, nor future.

Master Seng-ts'an, *Affirming Faith in Mind*

Nothing hinders the soul's knowledge of God as much as time and space, for time and space are fragments, whereas God is one. Therefore, if the soul were to know God, it must know him above time and outside space.

Meister Eckhart (1260?–1327?)[1]

Time seemed to disappear, in different ways, in kensho and absorption. In each case we want to know: where did time go? For its disappearance is more than a singular absence. It is the kind of silent clue that helps solve a very large problem. As did that clue of the dog who *didn't* bark in the Sherlock Holmes tale.

Part of one's clinical training in medical school is to learn to evaluate our patient's mental status. The critical criterion is: Is this patient oriented to time, place, person, and situation? If not, then something is very abnormal about the state of the brain.

Yet we have just observed how our internal clock runs on flextime. We bend time, in keeping with changes in our internal and external circumstances. For example, as William James had noted, we have "no sense for empty time." This means we cannot tell how long an interval is if it lacks all sensible content. And depressed patients feel that time stands still, arrested in its passage. Time moves again when their depression lifts. Can these phenomena be measured? Tests on humans do show that segments of time that last one or two seconds seem shorter when they are vacant, but seem longer once they are filled with clicks of sound.[2]

And rats, too, can add to our understanding. Researchers can train rats to "learn" certain longer intervals of time. The technique is to withhold food until the end of each such interval. It can then be shown that cholinergic mechanisms influence the way the animals estimate these time intervals. Indeed, higher effective levels of acetylcholine appear to help the rats retain useful memory traces both in their long-term *reference memory* and in their ongoing *working memory* functions.[3] But the experiments also suggest something else: when rats are rushed into storing memories faster, they don't remember well the particular time interval involved. And other drugs that enhance the synaptic functions of dopamine cause the rats' internal clock to speed up.

During such experiments, the animal's brain seems to draw inferences about how much time has elapsed. The experimenter reinforces these inferences by using the stimulus of food. Food then satisfies an appetitive function, hunger. In the process, the animal's brain becomes conditioned. This means that it will link its visceral functions into some "semi–higher-level" notions about time (see chapter 74). As children, we too learned, from hunger pangs and gut rumbles, that an uncomfortably long interval had passed since we ate last. So one begins to wonder: suppose a person's brain were to be cut off briefly from the cues linked to these appetitive drives; assume also that it had been cut off from its other references to the personal self at multiple other levels. What would happen to its constructs of time? Rephrasing the question: when you lose both your physical and psychic self, wouldn't that dissolve personal time sequences? Wouldn't it interrupt cause-and-effect relationships?

Doing-Time

Each person's internal time clock is a very private matter. The "time" of the historian is time in the abstract. Suppose we of the Atlantic community are given three dates: 1776, 1066, and 1492. We are then asked simply to sequence these three years in the order in which they occurred. Our brains reshuffle these numbers, manipulating them in "time," in this abstract historical sense. We wind up with 1066, 1492, 1776. Important years, to be sure, but they remain musty, detached, impersonal. We weren't *there*. But let some memorable event happen to *us* directly, not to Jefferson, or the Normans, or Columbus. Say it was the close call from that car when we were walking across the street at the age of ten. This moment went into our own time frame. It was stamped with our own monogram. It became an event in *our time*.

But "our time" has a vast infrastructure of which full consciousness remains largely ignorant. Why so ignorant? Because, into many levels of *unconscious* behavior, we also wove countless other forgettable things which happened to us. And no matter how forgettably incidental each of these events was, our private time clock still took note of it. In the process, it developed an implicit operational definition: this is what one second means in *motoric terms*. Let us sum up this operation with the phrase *doing-time*.

"Doing-time" keeps track of how much you can actually *do* in a given interval of time. Preconsciously, it factors in more than how fast you can run. It also judges how wide are those next streets to be crossed, and how fast the cars are coming. So the results are twofold. Now the person's estimates of the duration of time become a useful basis for subsequent go/no go decisions. Moreover, these same estimates of doing-time also enlarge our silent notions of self. No longer is it a static physical self. It becomes a dynamic self-in-motion, running at a requisite speed. This self knows how fast it must run that unforgiving distance between two curbstones on either side of the street.

Time is embedded in our memory traces. And some of these traces are almost like tree rings laid down in the trunk of an old bristlecone pine. Earlier memories of grade school seem to cluster into the inner layers. And following after such older associations, we sense that more recent events have arrived, say during the ages from fourteen to seventeen. In any tree, the annual rings run thick and thin. Years of austerity and struggle form the toughest part of the grain. You can't erase these dark, dense traces no matter how you cut the log or sand the board. The human constructs of time, likewise, are very difficult to erase. With each passing year, we incorporate new layers of associations into our grain. A succession of memories reinforces our own physical and psychic image. The result is a very firmly layered construction: *ourselves in our time*. Now suppose some very dramatic event happens, such as kensho. A state which planes off every last ridgeline of the grain of time! Could anyone be more astonished than a neurologist, someone who relies on the criteria of time to assess his patient's mentation?

Now, in this book, we're approaching Zen not to bring us more puzzles and riddles. We're pointing toward Zen because it can also help clarify where time is coming from, and perhaps why time dissolves. Let us now dig further into what happens to time, first while sitting quietly, next during meditation, then during absorption and kensho.

Ordinary, quiet sitting shrinks the estimate of time. Thirty seconds of real time contract so that they seem to last only twenty-six seconds. During zazen, meditators tend to expand their estimates of time. Thirty seconds of real time now seem to last thirty-seven seconds. A meditator's slow respirations could contribute cues which might help stretch time. For instance, when subjects breathe rapidly, they estimate twenty-second-long intervals as having increased to twenty-three seconds. In contrast, breathing slowly further increases the estimate to thirty-five seconds.[4]

Daily life practice hones the meditator's attention. It keeps bringing its focus back—time after time—on the sharp tip of this present moment. Later, when a major absorption finally occurs, attention also shifts into an ultraclear, one-pointed mode which encompasses the absolute NOW. Where is the past? Where is the future? They have simply fallen off the knife edge to either side. In a subject whose attention has been *held* transfixed for seconds in this manner, the data become deeply imprinted. A similar phenomenon occurs during other momentous occasions. Generations of people remember vividly where they were when they first heard of the unexpected death of a president. And the death of a close family member brings home something else. Let's refer to it as the *sands of time*. For the human sense of time remains privately aware that it has finite limitations. It understands, deeply, that life is transient; this is not a rehearsal. *Hakanai jinsei* implies that *our* sands of time will run out, sooner or later.

Streams of these thoughts and countless other undercurrents swirl through our brain. So much so that, under most ordinary circumstances, we accept (as being reasonably accurate) Descarte's statement: "I think, therefore I am." Absorption is different. All thoughts stopped when the writer's brain entered into a long moment of absorption: time seemed mostly *suspended* (see chapter 121). Anyone can experience a somewhat similar time lapse, briefly. Suppose some word or concept on a page totally absorbs your attention. At this moment, the notion drops out that there had been previous pages, or that there will be pages yet to come. So let us begin here (in order to sharpen a later contrast), by representing this absence of time during absorption as

Kensho goes much further. Inside it, there was no sense of my being outside time or beyond time. For such phrases might suggest to the reader that time might still have been lurking around back there somewhere else, serving as a basis for comparison. Instead the impression afterward was that *timelessness had permeated a nonentity.* Can this be possible? Not unless simultaneously, all *personal* time traces had dropped out. Indeed, kensho seemed to have cut off, from the field of conscious awareness, each of time's previous affiliations with the self. When all the old emotional polarities in this circuitry drop out of the picture, they leave a Grand Canyon–sized experiential gap. No word levels in descriptive psychology convey how deep is this chasm.

Just as we have shackled guilt to events in our past, so do we project fears which mortgage the future. Yet suppose this imaginary future time drops out. What happens? All such fearsome event sequences vanish. Moreover, during no-I, no basis remains for estimating how much I *can* do, *should* do, or *must* do in a given period. No meddling impulses arise which would need to invoke these covert functions of doing-time. The timeless moment stands as it is, already perfect.

Each human lifetime, like an airplane flight, takes off on a baby's birth date, soars for a while, then comes in on a final approach for the inevitable landing of some kind. Birth and death. One more pair of opposites. They occupy either end of an autobiographical yardstick. No need for either concept in kensho. It lacks this yardstick, carries no implication of birth or death. Therefore, in a manner of speaking, it does remain "unborn," just as Bankei said, and its timelessness recedes at both ends into the open-endedness of infinity. As a result, the field of consciousness, in kensho, shorn of *I* and all of its time cues, has the sense that

ETERNITY *is*

What is this eternity? No conventional yardsticks of time do it justice. True, every commonsense line of reasoning leads us to believe that the present universe did have a beginning. And the astrophysical data could be interpreted as consistent with at least some kind of creative force, or deity principle if you prefer. On the other hand, alternative views began to be held even at the dawn of Western traditions. Some Greeks believed in a different kind of universe. It was one that had no beginning, end, *or* creator. Parmenides, the pre-Socratic Greek philosopher, concluded that being *is;* that it has no past or future. He would phrase it: "Nor was it, nor will it be, since it is now altogether one, cohesive."[5] Another pre-Socratic Greek, Heraclitus, stated: "No God or man made the present scheme of things, the same for all—instead, it always was and is and will be an always-living fire, being kindled in measures, and being quenched in measures."[6] However thoughtful and imaginative were these pioneer philosophers, one may doubt that intellect alone could have led them to draw such startling conclusions unless deep insights had first paved the way.

A few mystics, having once experienced this timeless state, then become carried away. Convinced that birth and death are forever erased, they hold that there is, in fact, no passage of time at all, that *all* time is an illusion. One doesn't have to be an archeologist who relies on the decay of carbon 14 or some other element to know this is not true. Such false notions are also alien to the visitor at the natural history museum who sees, preserved, the casts of footprints made at Laetoli by our first erect ancestors, 3½ million years ago. Nor can these delusions arise in the vacationer at the Grand Canyon, awed by seeing exposed those layers of geological time reckoned in hundreds of millions of years.

So let us conclude that the mental construct we call "time" does exist, and that its sequences are backed up by rock-solid layers. Then what happens, *inside* kensho, to create so different an impression? As noted in the previous chapter, Piaget's studies showed that children develop several concepts—*all together*—during their first year. These include their initial concepts of time and their personal affiliations with other things inside "their" space. One may hypothesize, then, that when three such integral functions have developed together during the same dynamic period they might be more likely to shatter simultaneously during the impact of insight-wisdom.

Can any other simple analogies help us understand how time dissolves? In Japan, a Zen monk's working clothes include a light cotton garment called a *sa-mugi*. The upper half is basically a loose-fitting blouse. It has a flap that wraps around to close the front, and two square-cut arms sewn onto either side. Soshin-san, a kindly Rinzai nun, once assured me that she could easily sew the pieces together, and to do so would be "no trouble at all." (She had seen that I lacked appropriate garb, then insisted that I purchase some yard cloth, so that she could make me a *samugi* of my own to use for zazen and work!)

Envision our concept of personal time as also cut out of whole cloth. Its fabric is composed of interwoven association networks. Out of the open body of the present moment, one sleeve reaches back into the distance of the past. The opposite arm gropes out into the matrix of future space. In such a garment of "time," the pieces are loosely joined, for only looping circuitries approximate their edges at various levels throughout the brain. And if you were to cut the stitches which hold this fabric together, the semblance of time might drop out of ongoing experience.

Time-Related Circuits

How do we weave the fabric of time? And where could a few scissor cuts cause a whole garment to come apart? Patients develop major defects in estimating time after lesions that damage their mediodorsal thalamus on both sides. They become confused about the hour and date, don't know what season it is, or how old they are.[7] The fornix and its closely related limbic regions also enter into our initial "time-tagging" operations, and they play an important role in our working memory for time. A patient who suffers damage to the fornix can lose memory specifically for recent events.[8] (In the rat, lesions which interrupt the fornix can reduce the rat's memory for *certain* time-related events, yet they spare the workings of that larger "internal clock" which goes on to measure all such events.[9])

A normal person remains well oriented to time, place, and person, keenly appreciating that edges exist along these planes of experience that help define different situations. Things become blurred along these three interfaces in patients who are recovering from surgical operations on their cingulate gyrus. They cannot distinguish between their *own* internal mental events on the one hand, and real happenings in the outside world. Time turns into a jumble of incorrect temporal sequences: they can't recall recent events, and they contaminate the present mental field with memories displaced out of the remote past. In addition, their thoughts and dreams become more vivid.[10]

The clinical deficits cited above occur secondary to acute structural lesions in the thalamus or limbic system. Many of these same deficits stand in contrast to the mental status of a normal person *after* he or she emerges from internal absorption or kensho. After either state, the subject may then recall not only the details, patterns, and sequences of most events which had just occurred but finds them especially memorable. *So most time-tagging operations seem to have been preserved in the medial temporal and fornix regions, at least for the facts of that particular impressive ongoing experience.*

Given that most details of the immediate kensho experience itself do remain in memory, then how are we to account for the temporary dropping out of the rest of the vast bulk of time? One possibility is that its brief absence reflects a selective lack of inclusion of certain prefrontal systems, at least in the way their usual orderly functions had been organizing experience. In the preceding chapter, the case could be made that our frontal lobe functions usually help us restructure sequences of events into different working strategies. Indeed, patients who have large lesions in the prefrontal lobes often lose those cognitive and behavioral functions which project time constructs usefully into the future. Moreover, other patients whose lesions damage the *undersurface* of their forebrain regions tend to lose their memory for time over a broad front. They drop out short-term, long-term, and remote memories.[8] And after frontal and basal forebrain lesions, rats can't *divide* their attention if they are presented with tasks which require that they keep track of the arrival time of more than one stimulus.[11]

In assessing the experiments cited above, one must be careful not to assume that "time" and "memory" mean the same thing in different animals. And it is more difficult still to draw valid analogies between what animals experience and what we humans experience. For yes, patients can't place words or pictures into their proper sequence after damage to various prefrontal regions. Yet, when trained monkeys develop similar sequencing impairments, it will be after lesions of their *dorsolateral* prefrontal cortex. Whereas, when rats show similar time-sequencing defects, it will be after lesions of their *medial* prefrontal cortex.[12] One might interpret such differences as follows. Perhaps when rats normally perform their sequencing tasks, they are relying more on the older, lower, "smell-brain" variety of *limbic*-frontal circuitries. Whereas higher mammals (including humans) normally may be engaging more of their higher-level *parieto*frontal functions.

So it is useful to envision the loose garment we call time as drawing on at *least* these two major components—limbic and parietal—as well as on several others to be sure. For this sense of time is not an abstraction. It is a working garment. Woven out of a variety of sensorimotor networks, it includes a dynamic doing-time which operates within our larger matrix of personal space. And therefore, normally, as part of the stitching which holds all this together at the seams, our sense of time would seem to extend through much of the whole brain, involving regions on both sides that function in an integrated manner.

Timelessness is *letting go* of all this. Through a process of transient disconnections, jammings, or bypassings.

136

The Death of Fear

When you were born, all you had was the unborn Buddha-mind. There wasn't any fear. Your fear is an illusion or figment of thought that you have created on your own after you came into the world.

Master Bankei[1]

Every little yielding to anxiety is a step away from the natural heart of man.

Japanese Proverb[2]

Bad things do happen in life, and people find reasons to fear what is loosely called "bad karma." *Karma* is the subtotal of cause-and-effect relationships. It begins with the events which caused us to be born with certain kinds of DNA. Soon, it includes those events prompted by the particular culture we grew up in, and by the significant people who conditioned us. It goes on to be determined by events which were the product of our own subsequent thoughts and actions, whether we were aware of these or not.

No mysteries here. Nothing occult in how all these forces interact. Nothing arcane in the fact that many processes beyond our control decide who we are as a person, shape how much we can actually change our own futures, and how we can then influence others as a result. What does kensho do? It cuts through the recurrent neurotic patterns in this tangled web of relationships. And by deconditioning the person of the anxieties that had been linked to these patterns, it opens up new capacities for change.

Some people are born anxious and high-strung. Tests show that one baby in five is already highly reactive at only four months of age. When these same overreactive babies are followed up and tested at fourteen and twenty-one months, about 40 percent of them will now be excessively anxious when confronted with unfamiliar people and novel situations.[3] Why? Part III suggests that some answers have deep-seated origins. They begin in the circuits between the amygdala, the central gray, and the hypothalamus. These three subcortical regions create our fearful foundations of consciousness, and project their concerns to the frontal lobes. Of interest are the recent findings in another group of timid infants and children. These subjects seem temperamentally predisposed to restrain their approach behavior. Their hesitation correlates with greater degrees of right frontal lobe EEG activation[4] or lesser degrees of left frontal lobe EEG activation.[5]

Some dogs are especially high-strung. Pointers inherit a DNA pattern which ultimately translates into highly neurotic and fearful behavior. Their brains show high levels of norepinephrine, elevated by two thirds, in the brain stem reticular formation, and low serotonin levels in the septal nuclei.[6] These findings become of interest in relation to one subset of abnormally anxious humans, the adult patients who suffer from panic disorder. Research on these patients suggests that they, too, lack the normal kinds of brain mechanisms which would otherwise prevent their NE system from becoming overactive.[7]

Even the more "stolid" varieties of human DNA often seem no match for our pressurized, threatening times. Relatively few practice meditation for long enough to arrive at the calmness associated with it. People feel anxious in general, estranged from the "natural heart of man." Living most of their lives "off-center," many yield to a "tabloid mentality" and drift toward drugs for relief. In crisis situations, one particular group of "antianxiety" drugs is often prescribed which can afford *temporary* relief of anguish for a week or two.[8] These drugs, in the benzodiazepine class, act by

1. Reducing NE and ST functional activity in the septal-hippocampal system;
2. Decreasing NE activity in the hypothalamus;
3. Reducing DA activity in the prefrontal cortex.

Among these antianxiety prescription drugs, diazepam (Valium) and chlordiazepoxide hydrochloride (Librium) have become all too well-known. How could they relieve anxiety? By acting on special receptors in the brain which secondarily reduce the release of NE. These receptors share the same complex site as do the receptors for GABA, and they nudge the GABA receptors into a conformation which further enhances GABA's inhibitory functions (see chapter 45). Countless numbers of these benzodiazepine-GABA receptors end on NE terminals, both in the hippocampal formation and in cerebral cortex. Here they act to shut down the amount of NE released.[9] A different drug, buspirone, also reduces anxiety. It acts on $ST_{1}A$ receptors, and it slows the firing of ST nerve cells in the dorsal raphe nucleus.[10]

Marihuana is also used to relieve anxiety. Its active ingredient, tetrahydrocannabinol (THC), inhibits a second-messenger system and reduces cyclic adenosine monophosphate (cAMP). This action *against* cAMP resembles the effect of opioids, and opioids are by far the most effective drugs in dissolving anxiety.[11] The receptors for THC are most concentrated in the basal ganglia, hippocampus, cerebellum, and cingulate cortex. And this particular pattern also resembles the distribution of several second-messenger systems. So, it would seem that, given this convergence of the data, the brain stands ready to prescribe at least two very basic home remedies to relieve its own anxieties. One inherent mechanism will reduce the functional activity of certain biogenic amine systems, as noted in the three examples listed above (see chapter 44). The other will reduce the activity within certain cAMP second-messenger systems[12] (see chapter 48).

It causes great anguish to lose contact with one's support group. Observe how a monkey behaves after it has just been isolated from its own social group.[13]

Alone, separated from the troop, it cries out and appears very disturbed. Its separation distress is an eloquent reminder. Who can forget how very unsettling it was to be lost, cut off by a huge physical and psychic gap from one's family and friends?

In monkeys, only certain parts of the brain activate these cries of separation distress. Higher up, they include a broad band of deeper cortex buried along both sides of the midline. The band extends forward from the anterior cingulate gyrus down to the posterior gyrus rectus of the inferior frontal lobe (see figure 3). Something within this region prompts a lonely primate to respond vocally when it feels cut off from meaningful self/other relationships. Yet in kensho, two points bear reemphasis: the self is indeed "lost," but *this* particular form of awakening causes no distress. What do these two facts of experience imply? They confirm that the person's old self/other distinctions have indeed vanished. Had these old dualities still been present, they would have perceived both a lost self *and* a large separation gap, filled with distress.

Humans fear death. We can appreciate, more than do animals, how much stops when living is foreclosed. But we are the ones who created the basis for this fear, as Master Bankei observed. How long must *I* fear what death does to *Me?* Only for so long as *I* grasp hold of *my* life, as being *Mine* to lose. Fear dies in kensho for several reasons. One of them is that kensho absolves each of these three components in the *I-Me-Mine*, and relieves it of its implicit primal fear of loss.

There is a second reason. Kensho is birthless and deathless. At the very instant that it renders time beginningless and endless, neither birth nor death exists. Within such a state of numberlessness, there's no counting of birthday candles nor does any person remain whose sands are numbered. As soon as all links to such concepts vanish together, the experiant can finally enter into what William James once called the "state of assurance."[14] Among its central characteristics, he included "the loss of all the worry, the sense that all is ultimately well with one, the peace, the harmony, *the willingness to be,* even though the outer conditions should remain the same." Similar states of assurance are of widespread occurrence. Thus, an Alaskan *shaman* described the very soul of the universe as having once gently said to him, "be not afraid of the universe."[15]

Religious symbols and rituals speak louder than words. In many statues of Buddha, one observes a particular *mudra,* or position of the hand. In this distinctive *abhayamudra,* the Buddha's right hand faces away from his torso, at waist height. His wrist is flexed in the upright position, and his fingers are close together. In the West such a position might suggest "halt." Not so in Buddhism, where this hand posture is often interpreted in ways that translate into "fear not."

To me, the latter interpretation is too shallow. It tends to leave the impression that the Buddha's gesture indicates "don't be afraid." "Fear not" could merely suggest that he might be trying to reassure the lay onlooker that there was nothing in the Buddhist way to be afraid of. From within kensho, a stronger interpretation suggests itself. It is that the mudra portrays graphically the striking *loss of fear* so central to enlightenment. Indeed, at Borobudur, the huge temple complex in central Java, the Buddha statues all along the north side have been suggesting the existence of this state to Buddhist pilgrims for the past thousand years. The gesture is one of total *fearlessness*.

By now, the reader will have become aware that to enter kensho is not to find trumpets and angels. It is *a place of no. No-I, no* time, *no* fear. Why is this death of fear so significant? Because it sets the stage for the person to undergo that major transformation of attitudes described in chapter 104. And, indeed, with every such liberation from anxiety, the person will be moving one step closer to the natural human heart, just as is hinted in the old Japanese proverb.

137

Emptiness

> Silent! Empty!
> Existing by itself, unchanging,
> Pervading everywhere, inexhaustible,
> It might be called the mother of the world. Its name is unknown:
> I simply call it Tao.
>
> Lao Tzu (Circa 604–531 B.C.E.)[1]

> The outside world of form-and-name and the inner world of thought and feeling are both no more than the construction of mind, and when the mind ceases, the weaving-out of a world of particulars is stopped. This stopping is called emptiness or no birth, but it is not the wiping out of existence, it is on the contrary viewing it truthfully unhampered by discriminative categories.
>
> Daisetz Suzuki[2]

You can't begin to grasp Zen emptiness from the outside. It must be experienced. The emptiness pointed toward in this book means the same as *shunyata,* a Sanskrit word used in early Mahayana Buddhism. And let us quickly point out that in this usage, emptiness is not a concept like nihilism or nothingness. "Nothingness" can mean several other things. Some psychologists even use nothingness to describe a person's feeling *something,* namely loneliness, depression, anxiety, guilt, frustration, anger, boredom, apathy, or anguish.[3] As a result, nothingness has become almost as elastic as samadhi.

Zen emptiness implies *no* mental constructs and none of these feelings. Philosophical considerations aside, it is the absence of the psychic self. It is a vacancy of that discriminative self which had previously consisted of a tangled bundle of concepts and feelings (see figure 1). Emptiness is this old slate wiped clean. Indeed, the visceral level at which I felt this cleansing occur would invite comparisons with the roots of the other term, *catharsis.* Hair-splitting over the centuries led to a situation in which emptiness took on several levels of meanings. In fact, the earliest Buddhist traditions of the *Lankavatara Sutra* list seven different kinds.[4]

So it serves a useful purpose to continue to specify what Zen emptiness is *not.* It is not what beginners experience; not those superficial droppings off during meditation into levels of sinking or of no thinking. Nor does it describe the sensate losses of absorption which open up into the vacuum of a vast spatial void. Instead, foremost among its meanings is the deep *emptying out from consciousness of every former subjective distinction and personal attachment.* Yes, this is a zero state of the personal psyche. But does this state imply that consciousness is lost? No. It means that looking out, from inside the zero of this state, all things will then be perceived objectively, just as *they* really are.

This explanation clarifies why Kobori-roshi viewed "emptiness as Suchness, 'as-it-is-ness.'" He observed that emptiness was all too easily misinterpreted as some kind of "endless void."[5] Emptiness, as Abbot Obora further noted, "does not have the meaning of the void with nothing in it. It means not leaving a trace."[6] So the experience of emptiness is *selective:* it begins as a state in which *only* the I-Me-Mine and all of its intimate related concepts of self-in-the-world are null and void. It is not a blank, inert state of oblivion.

But the various Buddhist schools do not agree that it is quite so simple. Chang found that he needed a three-word phrase: "Illuminating-Void-Suchness" to convey something of its complex properties.[7] This hyphenated phrase implies three simultaneous events: insight illuminates consciousness; attachments drop off; and the essence of all things prevails. At this instant, the forms of all things are empty of all references to self. Now the everyday world (*samsara*) is seen to be the same as Nirvana.

Words become increasingly inadequate at the several deeper levels which scholarship still includes under the rubric of emptiness. Here, we consider only three such subtleties, reserving the next section for a fourth. One of these aspects of emptiness lacks every last trace of the "habit-energy generated by all the erroneous conceptions of beginningless past."[4] What is this lack of all "habit-energy?" It seems to point to more than the dropping out of one's simpler appetitive compulsions and obsessions. To me, it appears to suggest the final loss of some of that curious nuance implied in nondoing, or nonintervention (see chapter 142).

A second aspect is an existential emptiness. This is perceived to be the essential nature of *all things.* They too—not only the self—are understood to be nothing besides appearances. These particular words might appear to begin pointing in the general direction of Ultimate Pure Being (as we discuss later, in part VIII). And a third aspect, perhaps farther off in this general direction, is what sages hint is that rarest refinement of wisdom. It is nothing less than a state of *groundlessness* which lies altogether beyond. The *Heart Sutra* proclaims such unfathomable depths of wisdom as: "gone, gone beyond, gone altogether beyond; awakening, fulfilled!" (see appendix A).

It stretches our everyday intellectual processes too far to ask them to grasp a state which is, simultaneously, both an emptiness *and* the absolute reality of all things. Still, this is the message. For the qualities that will emerge within this ultimate Zen paradox are a blend of profound emptiness and ultimate being. Parts III and IV have revealed how many covert capacities reside in our multifaceted brain. And part VI has described how a vacuum can contain a plenum. Given this background, we should not be too surprised to find that the most objective depths of consciousness can open up to receive, in one mental field, the final essence of Being, distilled from multiple topics.

Impermanence

The "gone beyond" of the *Heart Sutra* can be interpreted as a hint that a separate subtle quality exists. It is a refinement of the second, existential, aspect described above. The word "voidness" is really too opaque to do it justice.[8] But when some authors do use voidness in this manner, it stands for the particular insight that no phenomena exist as *permanent*, independent entities. Consider, for example, how the form of a mountain deceives us. True, the Mont Sainte-Victoire of Cezanne still stands high, a century after he painted it so many times. To climbers and viewers it seems rock-solid, age-old, and independent. But these are human concepts, notions we've elaborated on a human time scale. For in fact any mountain is a huge hunk of matter always in flux. It is countless atoms, coalescing, their energies born eons ago in a star. Often, some other dense massive shape had been near there even earlier, a solid rock that itself had once been raised up, only to be worn down into sand. Mountains go through cycles.

So here stands any such mountain, rising up high before us today. No one would deny that it now exists as a concrete object by every conventional term of reference. But on the geological time scale, it is here only temporarily, as transient as we are. It has no independent, inherent ongoing existence in the dimensions of a beginningless time. So the "voidness" of the mountain implies that, *in the perspective of eternity*, it lacks final autonomous, independent existence. The technical term for this particular intuition is *impermanence*. Note that it would be expected to arise only in association with the insight of eternal timelessness.

The insight of impermanence is another old one that has become incorporated into systems of belief. The aphorism that "nothing endures but change" goes back in the West to the time of Heraclitus (ca 540–480 B.C.E.). Nor was the concept that the godhead was a void some idea restricted to the religious traditions of the Far East. Judaism expressed similar phrases during the thirteenth through sixteenth centuries. In its Kabbalah, the interpretation of the divine, the ultimate godhead implied not only something that was unlimited. It was also a nothingless abyss about which nothing could ever be known. As always, one treads with caution, because all such elastic concepts and phrases suffer in translation, and the words have come to carry different implications in different religions during different historical times.

The Zen roshi of today are usually very aware of the scholarly intricacies of Buddhism, and of their inherent pitfalls. But to any student who might become caught up in the web of such elaborate thought-systems, they would say "Let go."

Emptiness is to be experienced, not thought about.

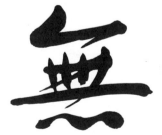

138

Objective Vision: The Lunar View

It is not that something different is seen, but that one sees differently. It is as though the spatial act of seeing were changed by a new dimension.

Carl Jung[1]

Calm and serene in the moonlight,
Lo! A deserted boat on the water,
not tossed by the waves or drawn by the breeze,
bathed in the pale light
of the moon!

Master Dogen[2]

Jung and Dogen describe it well. Expression gropes further: which shorthand phrase might sum up the otherworldly taste of kensho? In my case, the word was *objective*. It popped in within a minute after kensho subsided, and objective *vision* phrased itself during the next few minutes. Expression found no better term: objective meant the sharpest possible contrast with my usual process of vision. At one stroke, kensho exposed a naked truth. What had all my previous years of seeing been? Self-referent, *subjective*.

This new objective vision cut off every old association which linked the *I-Me-Mine* to things that were being seen. And it laid bare a striking paradox. For all things seen were not diminished in any way. Indeed, they embodied perfection in *their* own, original state. Now—with *Me* out of the picture—*they* existed, existentially.

Could analogies ever convey how much one loses when every subjectivity drops out? No, but let us begin. First, let us return to that example, cited earlier, of the warm childhood subjectivities that infuse one's very own house. Consider the underlying feelings of the person who wrote these revealing sentences: "I say Mother. And my thoughts are of you, Oh, House. House of the lovely dark summers of my childhood."[3] Are not both House and child tied to the same apron strings?

Reminisce for a moment. Even to have conjured up the image of standing in front of one's house was to find it permeated with endless sentimental associations. Yet, as soon as each simile and metaphor arose, it interfered with our experiencing this simple structure for what *it* was, *objectively*: just a house in the abstract; not *our* home. What would need to happen before we could experience it *objectively*?

Zen often returns to the analogy of a mirror. A mirror registers faithfully. But it has no lingering, emotional resonances. It remains unaffected. If our perception were to be like that of a mirror, we could catch the reflection of the house instantly, clearly. Simultaneously, we would be able to let go of it, unlike the way a leaf remained in the photographic emulsion of my roll of film, or in my brain. Similarly, the moment of objective vision cuts off all our old private attachments,

Table 18
Contrasting Types of Visual Experience Related to Space

Type	Data Source	Degree of Control	Field	Comment
Conscious recall, reimaging	Internal	Usually willed	Usually smaller and usually in front of the person	This is our usual capacity to summon visual images of people and things
*Sleep-related hallucination**	Internal	An automatic surge	Smaller, usually in front of the person	Vivid images are projected during drowsy transitions between waking and sleeping
Objective vision	External	A major, automatic shift of mental set	The existing field is totally transformed by a comprehensive interpretation	The existing world is seen in *its* suchness, with no personalized attachments

*Sleep-related hallucinations can occur during the descent into sleep (hypnagogic), or during the ascent toward the waking state (hypnopompic) (see chapter 113).

pro and con. How does its seeing proceed? Not merely with an *im*personal tone, but with a tone so *a*personal that it lies beyond all desires and aversions.

Years later, I would find that "objective" was a description not original with me. Hughlings Jackson had also explored the objective/subjective interface. Jung, too, used the word, but he did so in quite a different context. He was not referring to what he actually saw out in the *real* external world in front of him. Instead, he was referring to the quality of the *visions* he saw while he was hanging on the "edge of death" for three weeks following his heart attack in 1944.[4] Table 18 will help distinguish between the internal products of ordinary imaging, of sleep-related hallucinations, and the process of objective vision, the term we are now reserving for the kind of transformed seeing that occurs during kensho.

In 1944, Jung was hospitalized, and in a desperate situation. Depressed during the day, taking codeine, falling asleep toward evening, he would awaken at midnight, to become absorbed by enchanted visions during the next hour. Of these "glorious" hallucinatory experiences, he wrote: "I would never have imagined that any such experience was possible. It was not a product of imagination. The visions and experiences were utterly real; there was nothing subjective about them; they all had a quality of absolute objectivity."[5] Jung later experienced his "objectivity" once again in a dream. He saw his dead wife wearing an expression of being "objectively wise and understanding, without the slightest emotional reaction, as though she were beyond the mist of affects."[6] So, having experienced this kind and level of objectivity in himself, Jung was then able to recognize the presence of objectivity in other persons.

Jung's account demonstrates that one's early levels of objectivity can be impressive in themselves, irrespective of what else may accompany them in the form of hallucinatory phenomena or dreamlike states. But Jung had been a very sick patient, and powerful destabilizing influences were at work. He was not someone who had been entranced into a kind of shallow vision quest. The outside world was at war, and he too had good reasons to fear he might not survive. Being so close to death surely deepened the psychophysiological impact of his whole sickbed experience (see chapter 104).

These deeper levels of adversity carry an objectivity that has the power to transform. And after he drew back from the abyss of his cardiac illness, Jung took a very positive view of his newfound objectivity. "The objectivity which I experienced in this dream and in the visions is part of a completed individuation. It signifies detachment from valuations and from what we call emotional ties." His next point could serve as a rebuttal to any critic who, thinking that Zen detachment was amoral, might therefore regard it as having no redeeming social value. For Jung concluded that the "detached" person did not flee from moral values. Yes, he acknowledged, emotional ties do play an important role in society. But he also observed that such ties "still contain projections, and it is essential to withdraw these projections in order to attain to oneself and to objectivity."

What does kensho's sword strike off? Precisely these *psychic projections* which are the hidden roots of the *Mine* (see figure 1). So during kensho the person is cut off *not* from the process of genuine social bonding itself, but only from the clasp of those pernicious tentacles which cause bondage.

Jung took a positive view of his near-fatal illness. He saw how it had helped him to affirm his own destiny. For, during this existential crisis, he had forged a new, objectified ego. It was made of much tougher stuff than his earlier one. The new ego was the kind "that does not break down when incomprehensible things happen; an ego that endures, that endures the truth, and that is capable of coping with the world and with fate."[7]

Jung believed that his objective insights had other ramifications. They enabled him later to move on and grow into an even more creative phase. As he then became increasingly "individualized," it would also become clearer to his readers that this word then carried no entirely personal, selfish connotations. For he had grown, he said, into "an affirmation of things as they are: an unconditional 'yes' to that which is, without subjective protests—acceptance of the conditions of existence as I see them and understand them, acceptance of my own nature, as I happen to be."[7] Rebounding from his near-fatal illness, Jung saw into reality, and accepted it.

Now to any person threatened by a very adverse situation, these same capacities—first to endure, and above all, to *accept*—are two qualities of inestimable benefit. As part of the long process of character development, the two germinate slowly, in response to undergoing mental anguish and physical suffering. Sometimes, both attributes can emerge from a sickbed. And among meditators, a rigorous retreat soon presents anguish and physical suffering as prominent challenges to be endured.

Back when we were referring to Marsh Chapel, we noted that Pahnke used a sense of "objectivity combined with reality" as one criterion which helped him to define a mystical state.[8] The two words at either end of this phrase are crucial. They inform us that objectivity has a very significant affiliation. Indeed, objective vision is conjoined with a special interpretation. It perceives the *true* state of affairs, Reality itself, not a simple illusion or delusion.

Master Dogen also commented on the several steps through which the aspirant passed on the long road to experiencing the objective world. The steps begin, he said, in the quiet meditative context of no-thought, and then proceed to the letting go of self. In this way, the slow pace of Zen training ensures that the world will increasingly be viewed in the absence of the self and its many entanglements. He summarized the Zen Way in the following manner: "To study the Way of the Buddha is to learn about oneself. To learn about oneself is to forget oneself. To forget oneself is to experience the world as pure object. To experience the world as pure object is to let go of your 'own' body and mind as well as that of 'others'."[9]

Meister Eckhart had also commented on the fact that the mental posture of mystical experience was one of *disinterested* detachment. Having started from the premise of a Christian God, logic then led Eckhart to elaborate the concept somewhat differently. "I put disinterest higher than love . . . Disinterest brings God to me, and I can demonstrate it this way: Everything likes its own habitat best; God's habitat is purity and unity, which are due to disinterest. Therefore, God necessarily gives Himself to the disinterested heart . . ."

He continued: "Being disinterested, a man is sensitive only to God . . . experience must always be an experience of something, but disinterest comes so close to zero that nothing but God is rarified enough to get into it, to enter the disinterested heart. That is why a disinterested person is sensitive to nothing but God."[10]

In this century, Maslow would use the term "B-cognition" to describe that particular detached mode which experiences objectively. The letter *B* stands for Being. It implies that the world is now seen "in its own Being, as an end in itself." This kind of Being-world is not "something to be used or something to be afraid of or something to wish for, or to be reacted to in some other personal, human, self-centered way."[11] Moreover, when the world is perceived in B-cognition it is a world independent not only of the perceiver but of humans in general. Over the course of many centuries, when a Zen trainee enters this same domain, the words used to describe the experience translate into kensho, suchness, and no-I.

When Merrell-Wolf experienced "The Event," he first entered a period of utter satisfaction. This faded into what he would call a state of "High Indifference."[12] High Indifference was a state of silent equilibrium. It was above all affective modes, a movement in consciousness toward objectivity, containing neither bliss nor any perceived need for joy. Within this state, the usual yes/no principles of contradictory opposites did not apply. Instead, all things complemented one another in a way that seemed "natural, normal and proper." He commented later on the paradox implicit in such a detached state. For when "high indifference" was viewed from inside the state itself, it felt absolutely authentic, "completely solid," "dependable." But when it was viewed later from the outside, that is, from one's ordinary state of consciousness, it seemed to be an abstract concept.[13]

The early Chan masters were well aware that kensho had these unsentimental qualities. In that declaration of faith called the *Hsin hsin ming* (see appendix B), the words begin:

The Great Way is not difficult;
just avoid picking and choosing!
Only when you neither love nor hate
does it clearly reveal itself.

Yet to me, the taste of kensho conveyed something more than detachment. It felt *drained* of affect. This other property of objective vision is hinted at in the paintings of Edward Hopper and Giorgio de Chirico: accurate details in a landscape that stands barren, empty of any human quality of warmth. Their paintings seem otherworldly, conveying as little emotionality as a moonscape. The house of one's childhood? It stands deserted. Dogen knew that it was "bathed in the pale light of the moon."

The Lunar View

Hakuin had been there, several times. His chant extolling zazen exclaims, "How bright and transparent the moonlight of wisdom!" Yet he also accurately portrayed the cold vista of its ice field, noting that, "When a person faces the great doubt, before him there is in all directions only a vast and empty land without birth and without death, like a huge plane of ice extending ten thousand miles."[14] Such stark objectivity comes as a rude awakening to anyone whose heart had previously been set on entering, with bells and whistles, some heavenly place, all bathed in warm sunlight. To Van Dusen, who was coming down from a psychedelic state, this was an unpleasant contrast, a most bitter lesson.[15]

The uninitiated might wonder: why doesn't such an ice-cold, unearthly vision always strike a note too arctic for comfort? But first consider the other saving graces blended into this alloy. Kensho is timeless, fearless, deathless, perfect—as well as emotionless.

The moon is the old Zen metaphor for enlightenment. Finally, one appreciates why. *A clear, cold moonlight-like quality bathes the entire scene. Please note: I am not referring to this lunar view as a simile. It is an internal fact of experience.* It pervades the deepest level of comprehension in the large visual brain. The moon symbolism can be found and understood at many levels. One of the best examples is in Zen calligraphy. "Calligraphy is a painting of the mind," goes the old Chinese saying. For the brush becomes a living instrument. It speaks volumes about who is wielding it. Brush strokes do more than express the person's specific state at that very moment; they expose it in a more general way.[16] In the hand of the enlightened person, brushwork transforms into brush*play*. A full circle completes itself in one easy sweep.

The moon circle is called the *enso*. Simple, moonlike; empty of self, complete in itself. After the calligrapher and his audience have each been initiated into kensho, they both will *understand* why this moon circle is such an accurate symbol. In other cultures, the circle also expresses somewhat related spiritual qualities. Cardinal Nicolas of Cusa (1401–1464) used it in the universal sense, referring to that circle "whose circumference is nowhere and whose center is everywhere; the circle of infinite radius . . ."[17]

Kensho's bright moonlight, vacant of self, illuminates the mental landscape with utmost clarity and coherence. Zen will draw a useful distinction between *fully* internalizing such a peak moment of enlightenment and the more common, intermediate, variety of advanced spiritual understanding. The latter, known as the "hazy moon of enlightenment," was well described by Daiun Harada-roshi (1870–1961).[18] Nurtured by regular meditation and daily life practice, it was that ongoing state of consciousness grown so "ripe and pure" that the person had entered—but only "in a hazy way"—into an approximation of "contact with the light of the essential world." And he noted that however useful would be this level of understanding, it would remain a kind of "conceptual" or "proximate Zen."

Late in our century, science and technology came together. In 1969, mankind ascended to the Moon, in "one giant leap."* A full century after that splendid event would be a fitting time for our descendants to reflect upon this first moon landing's larger implications. For the centennial, in 2069, would be an appropriate occasion to look back critically at the *neuro*sciences. A good time to ask tough, unsentimental questions. Had the neurosciences finally met the real challenge? Had *they* realized their full potential, and enabled more people to reach the moon of full enlightenment?

We can be optimistic. Over the sands at Kitty Hawk, back in December 1903, the Wright brothers' first flight traveled only a few hundred yards. Lindbergh would fly east, crossing both shores of that same ocean, less than a quarter-century later. And the first ascent to the moon came a mere forty-two years after that.

But, like Max Planck, we must also be realistic about any of the sciences, and remain as objective as he was about what they can accomplish. For Planck knew that scientific research would always have its limitations. Science, he cautioned, could not solve nature's ultimate mystery. The reason, he said, was that "in the last analysis, we ourselves are part of nature, and therefore part of the mystery that we are trying to solve."[19]

---

* The site was happily named the "Sea of Tranquility."

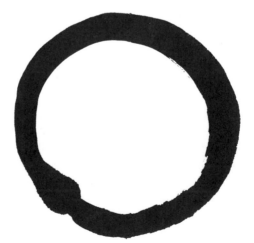

Are There Levels and Sequences of "Nonattainment"?

Patience transforms the mulberry leaf into a robe of silk.

Old Chinese saying

To reach satisfaction in all
desire to possess it in nothing.
To come to the knowledge of all
desire the knowledge of nothing.
To come to possess all
desire the possession of nothing.
To arrive at being all
desire to be nothing.

St. John of the Cross (1542–1591)[1]

Usually, the first kensho reaches only the shallower levels of realization. With it, the explorations begin, not end. And if the seeker had tried to capture such insights, treated them as concepts to "gain," they would not be found. Zen negates all attainment, anyway. So, does it make any sense to talk about "rising" to advanced "levels" when you're on a path which is basically one of subtraction and of *non*differentiation?

It does, but only for our present purposes of wordy analysis. The basic reason for talking about levels goes back to Hess's earlier statement: we can develop only those contents of consciousness which correspond with the way the brain itself is organized. Then what purpose does meditation serve? *It helps uncover capacities already there.* So what does it mean when we observe that the phenomena of the meditative way tend to unfold through a series of relatively distinct phases? It means that each new phase is expressing waves of reorganization within the networks of the brain.

Pointing Toward Nirvana

Given this preamble, it is instructive to examine how the schools of Buddhism in different cultures had approached this issue of levels.[2] The early Indian Buddhists spoke often of *nirvana*. But as Zen passed through China and Japan, the tendency grew to speak less about satori and nirvana. This kind of dodge avoids some semantic pitfalls, but it creates others. For our purposes, it helps to have a conceptual framework in order to relate the classic descriptions of moments of enlightenment, as reported in early Chan and Zen, to the transformations which occur during these states and persist after them. Here we have already discussed the preference for restricting the Zen term *satori* to imply the deeper awakenings which bring about permanent changes. Yet it seems evident that the early Indian Buddhists had originally subsumed many of these same deeper states of enlightenment within what their words described as the several *levels* of Buddhist *Nirvana*.[3]

What did the Sanskrit term *Nirvana* mean to the early Indian Buddhists when they chose to use it in its more general sense? They were not emphasizing visionary or blissful states. Instead, they were referring to the major, permanent *extinctions* of the ego-self, the final blowing out of the hot flame of every yearning and aversion. Moreover, they noted that the aspirant who ardently pursued the path which led through the absorptions might suppress such desires and aversions, but only *transiently.*

Historically, the Indian Buddhists conceived of Nirvana as existing not at one level but at four successive levels. These were accurately regarded as *levels of extinction.* In this usage, Nirvana was a state which could be entered not once, but multiple times. The adept could remain in it for variable periods, the longer the better. These four levels described by the early Buddhists are still informative for anyone today who wonders: through what steps does the human nervous system transform itself?

Extinguished at the first level were unfruitful personality traits and attitudes of greed, lying, or hatred. Jettisoned during the second level was a boatload of positive attractions such as sexual lust, as well as negative aversions toward things previously hated. The result was an even-handed, impartial approach toward anything and everything. After the third level, a still deeper equanimity extended toward all external objects. Now the very notion of hatred was extinguished. Finally, after the fourth level of Nirvana, a saintly attitude prevailed, for now the last self-referent attachment had been extinguished.[3]

Note: this is extinction, not coma. Zen also presents precise parallels of "progress through pruning," or "attainment through extinction," as it were. And it does so even though one might suppose that such notions would be too abstract, thoughtful, and structured. Yet persons of stature in Zen have also spoken about levels, deleting all notions of "gain," and substituting those which stood for *non*attainment. Among them was Master Hakuin who commented on the "Five Ranks" collected earlier by Tozan.[4] Because we have already discussed the topic of the first rank (in chapter 120 in relation to the "samadhi" of "The Great Perfect Mirror"), let us now proceed to consider Hakuin's version of the remaining four degrees of awakening.

1. The "Universal Nature Wisdom." Hakuin describes it as a radiant insight which discards both mind and body. Seeing is objective, self is absent. "It is like two mirrors mutually reflecting one another without even the shadow of an image in between . . . Mind and the objects of mind are one and the same: things and oneself are not two." The universal Buddha-nature of all things is seen into, its suchness revealed through one's very own eyes.

2. The aspirant's "great uncaused compassion" now shines forth effortlessly. Hakuin places its entry earlier in sequence than do most others. Possibly he was referring to compassion's very first appearance in a preliminary form which will later become much more obvious and enduring. Even so, "uncaused" is a very apt trans-

lation. Why? Because it implies that one's native virtues are expressing this kind of compassion *spontaneously* (see chapter 151).

3. "Mutual Integration." At this level, the aspirant reconciles the opposites. Old conflicts, formerly irreconcilable, now coexist in a state of profound *aequinimitas*. To illustrate, Hakuin chose samurai swords for his metaphor. Even "when two blades cross points," he said, "there's no need to withdraw." At this level of maturity the aspirant can not only enter the dirty, noisy, hostile marketplace but thrive there, contributing to the well-being of others. What makes this possible? The enlightened person is now seeing calmly and clearly into the world. From the perspective of this "Marvelous Observing Wisdom," all actions are being executed perfectly, wisely. Compassion enhanced to this degree will fully actualize the bodhisattva principle of helping others. It is a process, he said, like that of a "lotus blooming in the fire."

4. "Unity Attained." This final level implies that all the person's former passions have been extinguished. What remains? Only their "coals and ashes." The traveler on the endless Way can now enter an ongoing phase of "neither being nor non-being."[4] It is *this* final level, the ultimate extinction of all passions, that the Southern Buddhist schools would tend to refer to, in the restrictive sense, using the word "Nirvana."

Increasingly well-known in the West are the Zen pictures and narrative of The Ox and His Herdsman. They present similar progressions, divided into some six to ten stages, depending on the source.[5-7] In reality, they depict the gentling of an unruly, powerful bull. The bull readily represents the brain's inherent energies. The herdsman is the meditating trainee. We observe his passions becoming transformed by degrees.

The reports of psychedelic experiences also have some useful things to teach us about levels and sequences (see chapter 101). But they must be interpreted with great care. Why? First, because psychedelic drugs activate too many receptors, and in unnatural ways. Second, because the varieties of psychedelic experience occur not only in pure form but in mixtures.[8] Still, to have a basis for comparison with the experiences just cited in a meditative context, let us return briefly to where we left off in the psychedelic scene. Immediately, we find that the experiences on drugs illustrate key semantic issues which are important to confront. For example, Grof's comments about some of the experiences called "unity" are going to be particularly interesting. This is because his LSD subjects report having different experiences depending on whether their eyes are open or closed at the time.

One of Grof's varieties was the profoundly blissful "experience of cosmic unity" (a large topic, also discussed earlier in chapters 101 and 126). This was reported as occurring among that group of ecstatic subjects who were receiving higher doses of LSD and were listening to music. When the subjects *closed* their eyes, they experienced their "cosmic unity" as "an independent complex experiential pattern." These word descriptions might suggest that the subjects could tend to be driven more in the direction of the *internal absorptions* at those

Table 19
Differences between Having the Eyes Open and the Eyes Closed

Eyes Open Condition	Eyes Closed Condition
Traditional in Zen (half open)	Not recommended in traditional Zen
Maintains contact with the outside, visual world	Literally shuts off the outside, visual world
Allows more "room" in which to train meditative skills	Allows less "room" for meditative training
May reduce or delay hallucinations and other phenomena of inturned absorption	May facilitate hallucinations and other phenomena of inturned absorption
May help extend awareness, delaying drowsiness and sleep episodes	Facilitates drowsiness and sleep
Is associated with higher amplitude integrated alpha EEG activity when the meditator concentrates on a koan	Is not associated with an increase in alpha EEG amplitude while concentrating on a koan during zazen
Reduces human hippocampal delta and theta EEG activities	Maintains delta and theta EEG activities in the hippocampus
Subjects on LSD tend to develop feelings of merging and of being "at one" with their external environment	LSD subjects tend to experience "unity" more as a complex pattern of experience

particular times when their eyes were closed. In contrast, when the subjects' eyes were open, they tended so to "merge" with their environment that they developed "feelings of unity with perceived objects."[9]

Now, the recommended Zen approach is to keep the eyes *open* with the lids at least half-lowered during meditation. (In actual practice, eyelids droop and meditators do not always heed this orthodox advice.) So what could the LSD "eyes-open" observations imply to persons who chose to meditate but without using drugs? They suggest that keeping the eyes *open* might contribute to the initial sense impression of an affinity with—and perhaps on rare occasions later to the comprehension that the meditators have become at one with—the realities of things actually seen in their outside environment. In previous chapters we have considered several consequences of keeping the eyes open or closed, and they can now be summarized in table 19.

There are too many kinds of transpersonal experiences on LSD to cite here.[10] We will focus on two which seemed to totally escape all the limiting frameworks of time and space (see chapter 101).

1. "Consciousness of the universal mind." This is a profound, ineffable psychedelic experience. The subject now confronts, in all certainty, the ultimate force in the universe. The moment includes qualities of an infinite existence, wisdom and bliss, and answers all questions. (A beginner who could not turn to an experienced counselor for advice might mistake the first "cosmic unity" experience cited above for the arrival of this much more significant later event.)

2. The "supracosmic and metacosmic void." The subject experiences the ultimate source of all existence: primordial emptiness, nothingness, and silence. This ineffable void appears, simultaneously, to be both supraordinate to and to underlie

the world of creation. The episode extends beyond time and space, beyond change, and beyond any dualities such as good or evil, stability or motion. Beyond cause and effect, it can freely interchange with the preceeding "consciousness of the universal mind." If these last two experiences do happen to occur on LSD, they will be the ones likely to motivate the person toward pursuing spiritual matters in everyday life.

Two related issues are worth pointing out. First, only rarely was an LSD session ever associated with this latter ultimate level of "supra-meta" experience. Second, the word "cosmic" has an elastic quality. This can cause much confusion, because it enables "cosmic" to creep into descriptions of both shallower and deeper psychedelic levels.

Van Dusen also described LSD experiences, in a report based on eighteen subjects. Six of these subjects, or one third, came to some level of enlightenment. He lumped all of these into what he loosely termed "satori." In his hands, it took three or more sessions before the so-called satori developed. First there was a "letting go of a personal identity." Then, following this "symbolic death," "satori" came as a sudden, unwilled surprise. All grasping, all effort, blocked it. It was "beyond all our effort but within our giving up." A point to be stressed is that in the nondrug experience of kensho described in chapter 128, *personal identity dropped off spontaneously.* In no active sense was it something to be *let* go of, or to be given up.

Later, off psychedelics, Van Dusen himself had other experiences. These were similar to those on LSD but were of less intensity. He cited one curious advantage of having already used LSD. It was that, once the person had first experienced a large so-called satori on LSD, it was later easier to recognize the lesser "satori" of "simply living." Indeed, it was this particular aspect of LSD which taught Van Dusen what he would describe as his most "bitter lesson." For he discovered that everyday things, exactly as they were, constituted paradise. Here he appears to be describing the experience of suchness. Searching beyond for the divine and the heavenly, he was brought down to earth. He had encountered the striking reality in front of him: "The One beyond time and space and the One of the commonplace were the same." When the commonplace world finally opened up in this manner, he concluded that "the need [*sic*] of the drug draws to a close."[11]

Is what we call Heaven already on Earth? Yes. And to the meditator who has once known kensho, the prospect of living within this immanence wonderfully concentrates the mind (see chapter 133). To the drug user, one may speculate that the prospect of going on to have more experiences induced by LSD might finally be realized as like gilding the lily. Indeed, once the former LSD users (including Watts) had been struck, spontaneously, by the genuine beauty of things as they really are, they no longer felt the same intense "need" to stimulate this experience by artificial means.

Had the former drug users finally decided to stop taking psychedelics solely as the result of a conscious choice, reached by a purely intellectual decision? Or had they grown up as it were, because a series of other events, deep in the brain, had contributed to their loss of taste for LSD? Why do such questions come up? Because our discussion will lead to a set of other explanations why subtle changes in receptors and in brain circuitry could also be responsible for cutting off a person's attachments and cravings at very basic levels. And therefore to other reasons why such changes could extend to include the cutting off of a perceived need for drugs (see chapters 40, 142, and 152).

140

Preludes with Potential: Dark Nights and Depressions

The steep path of self-development is . . . as mournful and gloomy as the path to Hell.

Carl Jung[1]

Mysteriously, in ways difficult to accept by those who have never suffered it, depression comes to resemble physical anguish. Such anguish can become every bit as excruciating as the pain of a fractured limb, migraine or heart attack.

William Styron[2]

Do hills get higher when valleys sink deeper? Periods of depression and despair commonly occur before religious experiences, as was confirmed in Hardy's survey.[3] Indeed, many accounts over the centuries have suggested that the depths of depression can be a prelude to enlightenment. To St. John of the Cross, the aspirant would go through "a dark night of the soul," a preliminary period of intense mental and physical anguish.[4] To Master Han-shan, people appeared like "dead logs."[5] This chapter provides plausible explanations for those dark nights when no moon lights up the steep and slippery path.

Are only certain kinds of people prone to have dark nights on their meditative path? If so, could they (and we) embark on a somewhat different style of meditative practice so as to encourage the preludes of depression to evolve toward the most positive, creative outcomes? We need longitudinal studies to answer these questions. Meanwhile, some reports suggest that the most creative persons are not the ones afflicted by a bipolar manic-depressive disorder. Instead, the creative outcomes tend to occur among their close relatives, in those family members who seem better able to direct their energies more constructively into that fruitful zone between the two polar extremes—the heights so pressured and distracted, the depths so gloomy with blank despair.[6]

Normal people of all ages undergo ups and downs in their biological cycle. Many learn to identify their transient high points and their blahs, especially when the blues go on to last for several days. Some dark thoughts express a specific dissatisfaction; other pessimisms are a disillusion with things in general. The person whose discontents pile up into a large knot may be stimulated to seek relief by adopting a very different set of values.

Those who then choose to take up the meditative path could have several other reasons for manifesting their low spirits. Let us consider some of them in sequence.

1. Too much sitting can be enervating. Overzealous meditation which leads to too much loss of sleep can also contribute to low spirits. Both conditions imply that meditation has been improperly performed, usually for too long. Interim physical work and hard exercise provide the necessary change of pace.

2. Closing the eyes during prolonged meditation may lead to sluggishness and depression in susceptible persons.

3. Beginners get discouraged, because the spiritual search is long and demanding.

4. Insights can have painful consequences. It is difficult to live in the everyday imperfect world. It is hard to give up all of one's old illusions and delusions. Most everyone on the path becomes discouraged sooner or later.

5. Finally, the brain will respond to a rigorous retreat with a variety of stress responses (see chapter 53).

The fifth item leads us to ask: Could some of the stress responses which arise during retreats invoke the same mechanisms which cause nonmeditating people to become clinically depressed during three other conditions of interest? These other situations are (1) our normal brief ups and downs; (2) the terminal depressions which evolve into an open acceptance of dying; and (3) those more pathological forms of depression.

Some answers are now coming in. Recent studies are beginning to clarify the mechanisms underlying several subtypes of depression. One subgroup of patients appears to have a reduced functional level of serotonin activity.[7] Their spinal fluid shows low levels of a breakdown product of serotonin called 5-hydroxyindoleacetic acid. The low functional level of ST activity is believed to render these patients vulnerable to recurrent depressions and suicide attempts. Indeed, most studies do find evidence that brain ST metabolism is reduced in persons who show suicidal behavior.[8,9] Moreover, most depressed patients who had earlier responded successfully to antidepressant drugs will relapse into depression within a few hours after their plasma tryptophan levels are lowered.[10] Note that measures which reduce this precursor, tryptophan, would soon reduce ST levels in the brain (see chapter 44).

Now the ST systems normally hold some norepinephrine activities in check. It follows that an ST *under*activity might then lead, secondarily, to an overactivity of certain noradrenergic functions. Moreover, the breakdown products of dopamine also drop to low levels in the spinal fluid of depressed patients. The levels become almost as low as they are in Parkinson's disease, and they rise as the patients recover. So one factor which might contribute to the slow movements of depressed patients is a reduction in their motoric functions related to dopamine.[11]

Many depressed patients improve after they have been treated with drugs such as the tricyclic antidepressants.[12] But tricyclics do more than increase the synaptic levels of ST and NE. They also have anticholinergic effects. These block the actions of acetylcholine as well. Endless speculation has arisen about what kinds of roles ST, NE, DA, histamine, and ACH play in *causing* depression. Much of this speculation has been based on the fact that, in practice, certain drugs which affect these messengers greatly improve many depressed patients. The reader may find it interesting to note how very specific some researchers have become in weaving biogenic amines into their current hypotheses. For example, some would now postulate that there exist two general types of depression, each of which has a definite profile of NE, ST, and DA.[13,14]

The first type, anxiety depression, is believed to reflect a predominance of *excitatory* activity coming from the locus ceruleus NE, dorsal raphe ST, and meso-cortical DA systems. The second type, anergic depression, is postulated to occur because *inhibitory* activity predominates. It is speculated that this inhibition might arise from separate NE nerve cells farther down in the ventral medulla, from ST activity of the median raphe, and from DA activity within the mesolimbic system.

In contrast, still other evidence suggests that ACH *overactivity* makes the major contribution to the symptoms, signs, and biochemical aspects of depression.[15,16] This is called the "cholinergic overdrive" hypothesis. Indeed, some persons who are prone to melancholy do appear to be supersensitive to cholinergic agents even before their depressions occur.

Endorphins and other peptides are also candidates for some aspects of depression. Clearly, opioids yield positive feelings of pleasure. Therefore, depleting endogenous opioids, or not releasing them, might lead the person to feel that nothing yields pleasure. This anhedonic state of no pleasure is a major complaint in depressed patients. Suppose that low opioid levels earlier had prompted the brain to develop a (compensatory) increase in the number of its opioid receptors (a process called upregulation). Later, a pulse of opioids arrived. When these opioids then activated many of these new receptors, the subject could perceive the experiential impact as extraordinarily effective.

First the lower valley. Then the higher peak. And, as we have noted elsewhere, this principle of compensatory upregulation is not limited to opioids. It applies whenever the brain drops its ST, NE, DA, or other neuromodulators to low levels. Researchers can now measure receptor levels and localize them with the aid of brain mapping techniques. So it is now possible to test the following hypothesis, which centers on this potentially important receptor mechanism: after the earlier phase of an extended dark night, upregulation could help set the stage for a depressed brain to shift up into that rare state which illuminates by the pale light of the moon.

Some patients do shift quickly, from the depths of depression up to hypomania. What causes the shift? Emotional or environmental stresses, or drugs that increase the turnover of biogenic amines.[17] Among such drugs are levodopa, and others that raise amines to higher levels.[18] Still other patients, just before they begin their hypomanic phase, enter a transition period for a number of hours. During this interim period they *spontaneously* reduce their time spent in REM sleep and their total sleep time.[16]

· A new procedure, called "chronotherapy," helps some patients recover from their endogenous depression. It is of interest that they too are *deprived* of sleep, like those meditators who lose sleep during a sesshin. However, in the depressed patients, the sleep loss has already been appreciated to be a mode of "therapy."[19] This therapy proceeds in the following way. Note that it begins by getting the patients up much earlier. The first night, they still go to sleep at their usual time, say 11 P.M. But now they are awakened at 2 A.M. This is five hours earlier than the usual 7 A.M. awakening their biological clock had previously been set for. Next comes a shift in the hour they drop off to sleep. Lights go off at only 6 P.M., so sleep now occurs five hours *earlier* than it did before. The patients then "adjust." Now, having reset their biological clock, they'll awaken when the lights go on again, eight hours later at 2 A.M. The result? *Their mood lifts, later during the next day.* Indeed, in the course of such shifts in their sleep-wake cycle, some 25 to 30 percent of these previously depressed subjects "overshoot," and switch up into a hypomanic or even a manic phase.[20]

In part V we considered the mechanisms underlying surges and quickenings. Now, these patients are presenting us with a specific example of how a delayed overshoot is prompted by a shift in the sleep-wake cycle. What causes the long delay before the depression lifts? Delay raises the possibility that slower metabolic events might be taking place in second-messenger systems (see chapter 48). Among the current candidates are a special class of soluble proteins. These bind guanine nucleotides, and are therefore called G proteins. They are one of the steps in that cascade which starts with the release of glutamate and finally goes on to increase cAMP.[21,22] One other interesting line of evidence suggests that the subjects in the particular subgroup of depressed patients who do respond to sleep deprivation tend to have increased functional activity in the limbic regions of their brain.[23]

Chronotherapy means rescheduling more than a patient's rest-activity and light-dark cycles. It also shifts other major synchronizers. These include mealtimes, caffeine intake, and social activities. When these change, the patient's old biological clock is reset, and a "new" twenty-four-hour day begins. Wouldn't Linnaeus be fascinated if he could see how humans shift *their* personal clocks to "bloom" at different times! (see chapter 77).

More is involved than simply getting out of the old rut. This five-hour phase advance in chronotherapy is a jolt equivalent to the jet-lag of flying east from New York to London. The whole body-brain must shift biochemical and physiological gears in almost a literal sense. So this is a major stressful process of adjustment. And it is in this dynamic setting that the patient's mood becomes elevated as the depression lifts. Two further points are of special note: (1) The type of sleep lost is predominantly D-sleep. It will, however, be made up. (2) Rigorous Zen retreats cause similar kinds of rescheduling. Again, the meditators awaken early, sometimes around 3 or 4 A.M. Many will also advance their formal sleep times (i.e., go to bed earlier), but others stay up late to meditate.

How would meditators be affected during a long retreat if they underwent a well-controlled, *systematic* phase advance, or an equal phase delay, as opposed to *no* change in the setting of their biological clocks? Would the time change make the states of absorption or kensho more likely or less likely to occur? In theory, a phase advance of a kind used in chronotherapy could help the brain uncouple its former cycles, allowing several of their functions to reassemble into more energized alternate states of consciousness. It is time to investigate this carefully.

Some persons' behaviors cycle with the seasons. The more the ambient light, the more active they are, mentally and physically. Full of energy between March and August, they feel more emotional and develop racing thoughts. Only a few weeks later, the darker months begin. Then, light-deprived from September to February, the subjects become so moody and sluggish that they warrant a diagnosis of seasonal affective disorder (SAD), or seasonal depression. If you were a person overly prone to such depression, it would not be appropriate to meditate in the dark or to close your eyes too long. Light treatments (phototherapy) seem to help patients avoid seasonal depression. Some of them improve after receiving bright light during the evening hours from 7 to 9 P.M.[24] Others are helped by exposure to bright light in the morning.[25]

Depression *hurts*. Styron points out that one of its very real constituents is a sense of physical anguish. A reduced activity within ST systems might contribute to depression's prominent symptoms of pain and suffering. Recalling this possibility, the therapeutic effect of imipramine is noteworthy. This drug is known to increase the synaptic levels of ST. And it also helps relieve not only human depression but also a variety of other painful states. Even so, the latest antidepressants—which also enhance the synaptic levels of ST—are not yet considered to be the ideal drugs.[26]

Do the two cerebral hemispheres show different vulnerabilities to depression? This remains moot.[23,27,28] It also remains to be clarified how the increased release of ACTH and cortisol, as evidenced in the blood of many severely depressed patients, relates to their depression. PET scan studies have been performed on patients who have the particular kind of pure monopolar depression that runs in families. These earlier neuroimaging scans suggested that an active amygdala somehow made these patients vulnerable to their basic mood disorder.[29] Subsequent studies, performed in similar patients, showed that one part of the left anterior cingulate gyrus was reduced in volume.[30] This region lies under the anterior bend (the "knee") of the corpus callosum. (Figure 3 represents this region within the crosshatched zone of the cingulate gyrus. It lies above and to the right of the large dot specifying the gyrus rectus.) Other patients have been studied who had other kinds of gross lesions in this ventromedial part of the prefrontal cortex.[31] These patients did not respond appropriately to complex personal and social stimuli, but their primary emotions were not impaired.

To sum up: a broad, dynamic research interface has opened up. Brain mechanisms have now been identified that help to explain certain aspects of depression, of anguish, and of rapid shifts in mood. Relatively simple measures can cause a major shift in the tidal rhythms of our biological clocks. Procedures that reset these clocks will go on to destructure what would otherwise be an orderly rise and fall of our transmitter functions. It will be crucial to focus techniques from these fertile fields of research on selected human subjects who are undergoing long, grueling meditative retreats. Only the results of *multi*disciplinary studies can help clarify why certain persons shift into enlightened states after having endured a very dark night and a gloomy meditative prelude.

Then, someday, will we understand why, as Basho's beautiful haiku once predicted:

> The gloomy storm-clouds crumble, and behold:
> The mountains in the moonlight, clear and cold.[32]

Operational Differences between Absorption
and Insight-Wisdom

> Human values are inherently properties of brain activity, and we invite logical confusion by trying to treat them as if they had an independent existence artificially separated from the functioning brain.
>
> Roger Sperry (1913–1994)[1]

How does absorption differ from kensho? Only after having emerged from kensho does the aspirant truly understand the difference. The distinction is between being wide-awake, and comprehending. Between being rinsed in a cloudburst of warm rain, and being washed away by a flash flood of clear, cool understanding. In either instance, the witness loses the old personal horizon, but loses it in different ways. During internal absorption, the *optical* horizon line dissolves into ambient vision. Lost within this infinity of circumspace is the belt line of one's physical sensibilities. No longer can it establish the physical limits of the self. In contrast, during kensho, the *psychic* boundary line also dissolves. The result is a moonscape, a mental field reduced to absolute psychic zero. But it is a scene empty only of the old warring fictions: self/other, good/bad, right/wrong. Perfect unity prevails.

Back in parts III and IV, we were only temporary reductionists. Our goal then was to become familiar with those physiological functions of the normal brain which contribute most to our states of consciousness. One name given to this larger field as a whole is *psychophysiology*. It is a discipline young in synthesis, so new that some critics still view it as a "presumptuous outsider."[2] To these critics, the formulations we venture to synthesize in this chapter would appear to be those of a presumptuous *insider*. For we are going to draw together lines of evidence which support the following conclusion: different patterns of excitation and inhibition developed in certain regions inside my brain during the experiences of absorption and kensho.

In fact, my presumptions throughout this and the next chapter are nowhere near as definite as they might appear to be. These are the way things seemed to be to one neurologist who set about to review the available brain research during this closing decade of the twentieth century. But the theories do proceed from a bold premise. It is that data already exist—however widely scattered they may be in the literature—which permit one to venture a new working hypothesis for each state. Still, I feel safe in making only one prediction: no final answers will be any less complicated than the tentative outlines sketched out below.

Absorption

The preludes to absorption are of two kinds. One kind involves tonic concentrated attention. The other kind includes phasic events. The latter especially are stressful enough to destabilize the brain's ongoing rhythms. In broad brush strokes, absorption mimics extreme vigilance in its intensity while casting a spell of enchantment. It evolves at a relatively slow pace, and is associated with some of the following mechanisms:

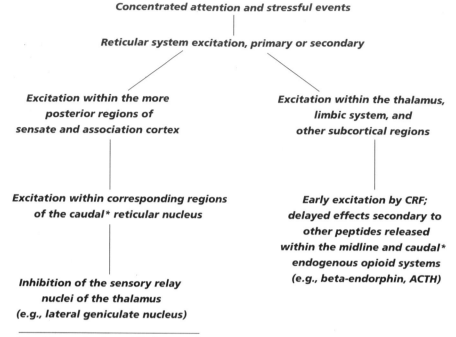

*Caudal, meaning toward the lower end.

The first event in the episode of internal absorption was a brief *lapse* of consciousness (see chapter 108). It was a gap consistent with an interval of robust sleep. This blank interval is interpreted as a preliminary phase. It is a prelude which could contribute to the rebound surge of a widespread, desynchronized excitation. And some of its apparent "blank" properties might even represent the way excitation has covert ways to enhance sleep (as noted in chapter 112). As the excitatory phase neared its peak, the reticular nucleus would already be responding, blocking the brain's fresh visual and other sensate input at levels lower in the thalamus. But excitations were already going on at still higher levels above this sensate block. They would continue to create the impression that the perceptual *capacities* of the visual and auditory systems had been heightened.

Implicit in this theory are several major experiential correlates. One is a hyperawareness so extraordinary that it could generate both a sense of ambient vision and perceive a mislocalized visual hallucination. The fact that bliss seeps only later into the scene could reflect the delayed arrival of a slowly evolving opioid phase. It could have been initiated many seconds earlier when acetylcholine and norepinephrine first stimulated the intrinsic stress responses within the brain itself (see chapter 53). The initial enchantment and the delayed bliss could imply that pulses of CRF, beta-endorphin and ACTH had been released along the deep midline and caudal regions of the brain.

Insight-Wisdom

Kensho is a flash of mental illumination. Comprehension is its keynote. A unique form of comprehension. For only when consciousness is shorn of its entire baggage of self can this special kind of existential comprehension occur. Kensho has a very long prelude of calm, persistent introspection, and of bare attentiveness to the events of daily life. Sometimes it happens when a sharp triggering event impales an open pause.

The quick flash suggests that brisk excitations are flowing through fast pathways. Many of these impulses could leap up through the reticular system both to stimulate its higher ramifications and to pass beyond. Within the resulting insight-wisdom are many different attributes. To explain kensho's patterns of gain and loss, one needs to invoke more *selective* excitations and inhibitions at higher levels. These could occur within such regions as the association cortex of each of the four lobes on both sides, and their counterpart nuclei within the thalamus and the limbic system. Some major themes within the early phase of kensho could then be diagramed as follows:

Sustained bare attention and persistent introspection

Spontaneous (or triggered) excitation, rising up through extensions of the reticular and other arousal systems to higher levels beyond

A. Excitation as it first arose from the brain stem

B. Excitation after it had reached up selectively to involve the association cortex, chiefly in the fronto-temporal regions

Selective excitation within endogenous opioid systems (e.g., enkephalins and dynorphin)

Inhibition within the reticular nucleus

Excitation of corresponding regions of the thalamic reticular nucleus

Disinhibitory release of the more rostral* nuclei of the dorsal thalamus

Inhibition, chiefly within the more rostral* nuclei of the dorsal thalamus (e.g., the medial dorsal nucleus)

Selective effects on other corresponding regions within the cortex and limbic system

*Rostral, meaning toward the upper end.

The lightning-fast flash of kensho could be set off by a deep shift in set-points which then swept up on a "fast track" through the brain's fast-acting glutamate and ACH receptor systems. Note that the reticular activating system could be jolted from *below* by a sensate trigger, as indicated under A. Or it could be excited from *above*, set off by glutamate in a less obvious closure higher up, as in B. In the latter instance, the closure might be associated with some lesser insight or impression near the fringe of thought. If enkephalins and dynorphin had been released beforehand, in response to novelty, their effects could go on to influence many layers of interpretive functions. This could reinforce the sense of being in the presence of ultimate, eternal perfection.

But kensho cuts off as it adds. The total loss of the subjective, psychic self could be correlated with inhibition, by GABA and opioids, not only within the limbic system itself but also throughout its many other projection sites, high and low. For example, among the regions inhibited in the thalamus would be certain nuclei which have strong limbic connections. These include the mediodorsal, anterior, and lateral dorsal nuclei (see figure 11).

The diagram of kensho is more complex than that of absorption. Some of its prerequisite mechanisms are subtle, and their sequences take years to evolve. In the next chapter, we fill in these bare outlines of kensho's profile. But before doing so, it seems worthwhile first to step back and review several points which address themselves to the subtitle of this book (see chapter 32). For the question before us remains: *Through what sequences in the brain does meditation proceed to enlightened states of consciousness?* The thesis we've been proposing is as follows:

1. Enlightened states occur during rare moments when psychophysiological responses converge that are basically intrinsic to the brain.

2. These convergences—syzygies—are likely to happen during the transition periods between otherwise ordinary states, or in response to triggers, or later on during the course of major stressful events that inject a note of peril.

3. Prolonged, regular meditative training confers three major benefits. One is a gradual calming, an "emptying," and moments of no-thought clarity. Another is a less distractible lifestyle. This evolves because the person becomes committed to a simpler, more authentic set of priorities. The third is a tendency to become more focused and more introspective. As a result, when minor intuitions spring up, they can remain on-line longer. Now, good intentions can be translated into decisive acts which can modify unfruitful patterns of behavior.

4. Notwithstanding such sources of increasing stability, the person's brain also remains open to the influence of a series of pauses and physiological shifts. Seemingly random, these arousing events first present themselves in the form of casual "quickenings" involving sensate and affective functions. Later, the scene shifts forward and upward in the brain. There, some events begin to ripen into lesser insights which inspire increasingly comprehensive interpretations.

5. Only after many months or years will a major peak experience of insight-wisdom sometimes surge into the dynamic nuances of such a setting. Will this moment be the culmination of the meditative quest? No. It is the beginning . . .

Reflections on Kensho, Personal and Neurological

In this non-dual world
all is one, nothing left out.

In this unmeasurable truth
one instant is ten thousand years.

Master Seng-ts'an, Affirming Faith in Mind

Zen Master Sengai (1750–1837) was famed for his calligraphy.[1] Once, stroking boldly with only one brushload of ink, he drew three simple symbols. First came the circle, then a triangle, finally a square. They are abstractions, interpretable at many levels, like old rocks rising from the raked gravel at Ryoan-ji in Kyoto.

Some might interpret the symbols as summarizing the relationships of the universe. The circle could stand for the infinite, formless Ultimate Reality of which we are all a part, the *dharmakaya*. The triangle would then refer to the way this universal principle manifests itself throughout all forms. For example, a triad of forms might include one's body, intellect, and spiritual life. Finally, the square seems to remind some logicians that triangles could pair up, back to back. This concept hints at the way opposites fill our ordinary world, where there are two sides to everything: yin has its yang, each "this" implies a "that."

Those who have been struck by kensho can realize the scope of Sengai's insight at many other levels. The calligraphers among them will look directly at the way his ink strokes soaked into the paper. There they will observe how, when the master's brush was first fully loaded with black ink, this ink spread out to fully saturate the circumference of the circle. Then each of Sengai's next brush strokes becomes progressively less intense. Finally, the density of the ink trails off. As it describes the last side of the square, it pales toward gray.

The visual metaphor is accurate. Thin is how the full moon of imminent enlightenment illuminated directly, evolved in seconds, then shaded off to return this person toward the many wan ramifications of his conventional thought processes.

Reflections

Several days after kensho, I appreciated that it might be useful, when discussing it, to distinguish four separate phases within its otherwise seamless interval. Later still came another thought: one could use the word "reflection" to describe these four dynamic phases. But not without allowing the word to evolve in its implications in much the same way that some scholars might wish to coax logical meanings out of the simple black lines which Sengai's brush had once drawn on rice paper (figure 18).

The first way this book used the word *reflection* was the ordinary way (see chapter 10). It is what a mirror does. Similarly, kensho's first phase is mirror-like,

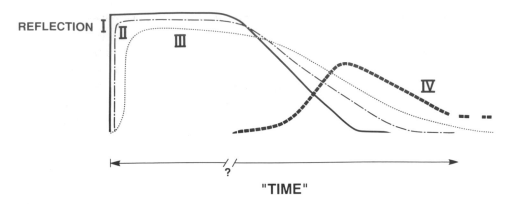

Figure 18 The flashing reflections of kensho
The first two reflections were abrupt in onset and subsided before the last two. The vertical axis indicates intensity; the line of the horizontal axis is interrupted to suggest how impossible it was to estimate time.

all there instantly. No top-down impulse sponsors it, no person injects a self in there, nobody pauses to think over what's going on. It *happens,* spontaneously. One may designate the contents of this phase of kensho as *reflection I.* Reflection I is not merely an abrupt shift which moves consciousness only a short distance. A totally novel interpretation interprets *extra, new meaning* into the matrix of the scene. And so, time and again, we must return to ask, Where does this novelty come from? Why are these new meanings already so salient at their very core?

Now, in common parlance, we also use the word *reflection* in quite a different way. On these occasions, it stands for a *steplike* process, one which "turns over" a sequence of thoughts, and in a quasi-voluntary fashion. We say casually, "on reflection," after we have proceeded, in to-and-fro fashion, through a series of these other *mental* operations. The same plurality is true of *reflections II.* In this case, however, the insights remain wholly *in*voluntary. They are turning over and moving to and fro *by themselves.*

Reflections III is even more interactive. Many of its thought processes are derivative. They seem to be swept up into reverberations which resonate with the overtones of the earlier insights. Not until very late in this third phase does the momentum of reflective thoughts slow down enough to give the sense that some thoughts are responding to a little voluntary steering. This impression of steering suggests that an i-me-mine, a faint trace of the old self, is starting to return in a preliminary form.

Finally, *reflections IV* extends itself, evolving during the first hours and over the next several days. It is a period of enriched, intellectual stimulation. One is mulling over the implications of this direct glimpse into reality, beginning to integrate its messages, seeing how they will influence one's lifestyle. And this part of the process is conducted in full, voluntary thoughtful fashion. It is a kind of "reflective interpretation," as Dumoulin once called it, one which "does not detract from an experience, but rather makes its content and consequences more clear."[2] Yet, even while the person is reviewing what the earlier phases mean, the fourth phase spins off into new generations of lesser intuitions. These pave the way for a very long-range contemplative process. It seems to continue for years.

Obvious examples of the latter are the thoughts which began to form the basis for the essays in this book. The columns in the left side of table 20 summarize the particular insightful reflections in these four categories of personal experience. The last two columns on the right side continue the reflective commentary started in the last chapter. Please note: the first of these right-side headings specifies which brain networks *do* participate. The second specifies which connections do *not*.

What launches a brain into the early flash and flow of such sequences? We have been presenting the case for ingredients which, in the beginning, are fairly standard physiological functions. But having once been shuffled out of their usual context and amplified, some of them will then become free to fall into remarkable recombinations. There is a simple way to develop this thesis further. It is to retrace some of the very same steps we took in an earlier chapter. These steps traced the normal flow of visual messages as they streamed, in their usual manner, through the large visual brain. For the general reader, this could be an opportune time to pause, and to review the visual pathway, as outlined in chapter 54.

Now, to understand *why* kensho visualizes as it does, we will begin by taking up the visual pathway at the stage at which it has already reached the *back* of the brain. From there, we may wander a bit, and backtrack. Still, the overall course will be leading us forward, as before, toward the higher associative levels *in front*.

Have we skipped something? Yes. Kensho does not subtract vision or hearing. So that is why we chose to skip past the lower tier of thalamic nuclei. It was to this region that we have already attributed the sensate loss, so obvious during internal absorption (see figure 11). Therefore, we begin, in reflection I, with sets of uninterrupted sensate impulses which have passed through the thalamic relay nuclei, registered in the back part of the cortex, and are already starting to move forward in much of their usual directions through *various* association pathways.

But *something else has been added to them*. For now, in kensho, there is a new flavor to the whole experience. It hinges on the extraordinary new ways the large visual brain has been receiving input from, and interacting with, other modules high and low (e.g., see chapter 59). What other facts support these conclusions? Some of the evidence collected below is drawn from the experiments of nature that come under a physician's care. These neurological disorders become a useful probe for exploring the nature of Zen enlightenment. Can states of disease help us understand kensho? Yes, for two reasons. First, we can use some of their clinical expressions as contrasts with the properties of kensho. Second, we can turn around other clinical findings, as it were, and consider what might be their potentials in reverse.

Neurological Disorders and Their Relevance to Kensho

Neurological disorders express themselves in two ways. The patient's verbal complaints are the *symptoms*. The *signs* are what the observer finds during the examination. Some signs represent heightened functions: extra-brisk knee jerks, or

Table 20
The Flashing Sequences in Kensho*

Phases	Overall Flavor	Status of the I-Me-Mine	Content of Awareness	Cortical and Subcortical Networks Selectively Participating	Connections Not Selectively Participating
Reflection I	Abrupt, mirror-like, comprehensive viewing	0	Direct perception; comprehending absolute perfect reality	Parieto-occipital regions (syncretism); fast activating ACH networks from brain stem; ? mu opioid enkephalin and endorphin systems (earlier release)	Those involved in generating the discriminating, abstracting *I-Me-Mine*; this includes but is not limited to the following: Amygdala Central gray Nucleus tractus solitarius Anterior cingulate Frontal neocortex
Reflections II	Insightful knowing; understanding at the deepest level of wisdom	0 (i)	Eternally thus; nothing to do, nothing to fear; peace	Prefrontal-temporal lobe; ? hippocampal excitation from enkephalins	
Reflections III	A meld of insights and thoughts	i-me-mine	No words; the experience is indescribable; this person is detached, released, liberated, simplified	Returning toward those involved in usual mentation	Thalamocortical language connections; GABA and other circuitries devoted to constraints and complexities
Reflections IV	Thoughtful mentation has returned	A lesser *I-Me-Mine*	Experiencing reality in this way is the basis of right action; words and superficial labels are seen through	Returned toward those involved in usual mentation	A few inappropriate circuitries have dropped out in the regions cited above

ACH, acetylcholine; GABA, γ-aminobutyric acid.
*A preattentive type of parallel processing accesses consciousness.

convulsions, for example. Others are the signs of deficit. They are the knee jerks which no longer respond to the tap of the reflex hammer. Or the legs that can't shake because they have become completely paralyzed. It is true that one might speak about the exaggerated signs as "positive" signs; just as one might think of the signs of deficit as being "negative." Yet, at the bedside, these polarized words do not carry a pejorative implication. For signs of either type are useful, and are to be regarded objectively. One can view events in kensho in the same manner. As we do so, in this chapter, one begins to appreciate that similar kinds of positive and negative mechanisms also operate in kensho.

A convenient place to begin is with the visual agnosias. These disorders occur in patients who have damage to their posterior temporo-occipital cortex. Freud, who coined the term *agnosia*, pointed out their essential features: seeing stays in; meaning drops out. Which clinical signs help a doctor make this diagnosis? First you verify that the patient can indeed see. For instance, you might ascertain that the patient can clearly see all the details of a wicker chair. But soon you discover something: your patient doesn't recognize what this chair really is. The chair has been *stripped of meaning*, not of the visual lines of its wickerwork.

Rarely, a patient develops a special kind of visual agnosia, called *prosopagnosia*. A stroke or tumor has *undercut* the occipital cortex, usually on both sides. The patient can still see faces clearly, *but cannot proceed to recognize them*. There comes no tug of subjective recognition, even from seeing the face of a parent, a spouse, or a sibling. And a few patients can't even recognize themselves—*their very own faces!*

Another finding seems almost as bizarre. Some of these same patients who have this visual agnosia for faces can't pass a lie detector test.[3] Yes, they *say* they don't recognize another person's face. But a very important study now shows that this statement can be *false*. For when the patients see the face, they also show a meaningful blip on their skin conductance responses. This testimony shows that they really *do* recognize the face. Which to believe, the patient or the test? You believe *both*. For the patients' statements are valid. They are only saying that they don't recognize consciously, even though the equipment shows that they are obviously recognizing the face at *subconscious* levels.

Could this be some kind of lying? Not at all. It's just that covert compartments in the patients' brains are issuing signals which can be picked up by sensitive physiological tests. And these hidden compartments connect only with their *subconscious* awareness. Therefore, these silent recognition functions still go on signaling that the face is still being responded to. But *the lower levels at which this response occurs* are not able to feed back their version of this act of recognition to be acknowledged by the rest of consciousness. So the two "truths" are not in conflict. We can now reconcile the two by adding a little bit more to our understanding of the circuitry of the visual brain.

Which pathways in the brain, when damaged, stop these patients from recognizing a face well-known to them? Their lesions have cut only certain *subcortical* pathways. Most of these are on their way "up" to consciousness; others represent some *transcortical* association links which join regions of cortex. Before their lesions occurred, the patients would normally have used a number of these paths to join smaller visual regions into that larger specific configuration which would have enabled them to recognize this familiar face at higher, *more conscious* levels.

But note also what the patients' lesions have spared. The lesions have not cut the other visual links which normally sponsor their more *reflex* recognitions of faces in *deeper* regions. And these other undamaged nerve cells keep relaying their own messages—still signaling the elementary codes of facial recognition—down through the hypothalamus, down into the autonomic nervous system, and out to where these autonomic responses can be picked up by the lie detector test. It is these two remaining lower sets of spared circuitries which continue to assert, in their regular manner, that the patients had indeed come to a true closure within their more *reflexive* pattern recognition systems. What had happened elsewhere in their conscious brain? It had been deprived of such input. It remained innocent of this unconscious decision.[3]

Now, for contrast, let us consider what it is about the viewing in reflection I which—though it also starts out in much the same way—then goes on to differ from this agnosia for faces. Reflection I also sees. It takes in the whole, optically clear scene. And it also perceives the basic data content of this scene during a moment of full awareness. Why do the resemblances end there? For three major reasons. First, because reflection I enters in a flash. It seems not to have passed through a person's ordinary, relatively slow and thoughtful, cognitive channels. Second, it goes far beyond merely recognizing the *bare* facts of the things that it sees, up at the usual, fully *conscious* level. For it has already infused enough salience into these facts to leave the impression that they constitute reality itself. In this viewer, the sense was that these things *really* are, *as* they are. Finally, reflection I slashes off every deep subjective attachment. Indeed, it left this experiant with the impression of having been completely emptied—drained not only of "my" private visual responses but of *all* other potential resonances of feeling. It was as though that sword of Manjusuri, slashing past bone, had cut off every subliminal visceral *unconscious* link serving that old triad of selfhood, the *I-Me-Mine*.

It could be true that awakening blocks, however briefly, certain responses which would emerge from one's deeper visceral pathways. But *is* it true? There is a way to test the hypothesis. Someday, psychophysiologists could be ready to study the flash of enlightenment. In theory, the person who is then cut off from *all* the sources of subjectivity *and* its deep output circuits will show test findings in a direction *opposite* to that in the facial agnosia patients cited.[3] That is, during major awakenings, the experiant might still retain the basis for recognizing faces and familiar percepts, up at their usual fully conscious level. What would be missing would be some of those specifically correlated deep autonomic responses. These were the ones whose blips had shown previously that these agnosia patients still remained deeply in touch with the *emotional* recognition responses of an *I-Me-Mine*. Put simply, one preliminary shorthand formulation of kensho might then be expressed in the following threefold manner: seeing stays in; *new* meanings are infused; certain old visceral responses drop out.

Patients with visual agnosia have an added complaint. Life without familiar meanings is flat. When they meet well-known friends, they can't relate to them with the same old feelings of intimacy. Many become depressed. Do these same unpleasant symptoms of deficit occur in reflection I? No. True, a cool lunar perspective pervades this first phase. But, on balance, it is a view which conveys no overall sense of loss, no personal distress or other clinical liabilities. Indeed, the things seen are not just clearly identified. They are impregnated with so much significance that they can't be improved on.

We began part VII with two chapters devoted to a (seemingly mundane) topic: *meaning,* and the way it develops at many levels. It is plausible to consider that when input is integrated at several of these levels of meaning—up to, and including, the association cortex—it resonates through our ordinary cognition to yield our larger sense of greater meaningfulness. In kensho, we are postulating that several other things would occur. First, that the brain would amplify only certain of its standard higher associative functions. Second, that it would already have infused them with added salience from its subcortical reservoirs below. The proposal, in its simplest form, is that kensho represents a *unique, selective, multi-level blend of functions.* A blend which conveys the sense that the viewer's *remaining* associative links had finally reached the ultimate peak of their capacities to tie cognitive elements together.

But wait. If the naive brain of a normal subject had never been "there" before, then how could *it* "know" and recognize what ultimate *is?* Can one be sure that an outside "agency" is not at work? A "mind" at large? (see chapter 66).

"Original Salience"

Suppose we begin to answer by returning to simpler visual steps (as outlined in chapter 54). We went through the same steps each time we recognized that the fruit was an apple. We recognized the apple by pulling together the many threads of our *prior* relationships with it. The word explains itself: *re*-cognition. And when the unknown fruit matched all those old patterns in our recognition memory, the apple emerged into consciousness, fleshed out with all its familiar dimensions of meaning.

Reflection I departs from this usual procedure. Its first flash preempts or penetrates far beyond one's old, familiar links of *recognition* memory. For, in the same instant that kensho still sees all things, it sees them in a fresh new light. To understand the nuances of such a shift, let us consider how an apple might set off an ordinary train of thoughts. Running through the person's head who had first glimpsed an apple there might spin off a series of free associations, equivalent to, "I think I recognize the kind of red Delicious apple they grow in the state of Washington." In a flash, kensho would have *condensed* all this. Its version arrives as a direct, self-evident, nonverbal statement: "apple!" Yet it is not a simple *visual* picture, not mere optical viewing. This distillate is already full of the essence of all of an apple's implicit relationships—with all the applesauce and sweet-hard cider of fact. And it is stamped with certainty. The same unshakable certainty that knows each swallow of cold cider on a hot day (see chapter 96).

To help clarify why this first glimpse is so full of universal import, we will need to travel farther forward. This step carries us into the flow of the lower visual function stream (see table 6). And as we proceed into the vast delta of the temporal lobe, we remember something: one of its hallmark functions is summed up by the question, *What?* (see chapter 56). So let us invite this complex temporal lobe to respond to one of its own basic operational questions: *What* could it be seeing during reflection I? From inside reflection I comes the instant response:

ULTIMATE REALITY

But, of course, no person remains inside who could ask this, or any other, rhetorical question during kensho. Moreover, total understanding is already implicit in the first phase. So there would be no pause to ask any *What* questions, because the answer is already *known* and certified. Indeed, in reflection I, not only is the optical viewing fully interpreted but the full scope of these insights has been profoundly authenticated. Does this mean that even this first phase blends *three* major brain functions, not one? Yes. Its threefold properties do consist of [optical viewing + insight + salience]. On the other hand, these three fuse into one coherent unity. The sole reason they are enclosed within brackets above is to signify that no interval of time separates the three indivisibles, nor do any conceptual sequences. Reflection I remains seamless, singular.

But the skeptic will say: You must be kidding. How can the feeling that ultimate reality is being directly perceived constitute *the raw data* of reflection I? Surely, an interpretation must have been involved in order to reach so major a conclusion. Therefore, something else must have come first. You must have guided it, steered it in some way into a kind of secondary intellectualized illusion. Conventional wisdom can only look in from the outside. Given this limited perspective, it has only one obvious conclusion to leap to: my brain must have contained some prior, artificially learned doctrines. Cultural influences must have sponsored and contaminated my interpretations.

Not so. No outside religious or ethical doctrines tinge the intrinsic functions of reflection I. It reveals *innate* neurophysiological capabilities. In Zen, these would be called one's *original self*. These shifts of perspective are not theological or philosophical add-ons. They anticipate all teachings. Of Buddha, Christ, or whoever. As they express themselves, they constitute the basic *inborn* working capacities of every person's brain.

Even later on, during reflections II, most of the insights resonate in ways which still seem primal and secular. Indeed, they also appeared to be beyond any extrinsic doctrines which might previously have seeped into the experiant's brain. And therein, of course, lies the immense pragmatic importance of "original salience" to the way we live every day. Suppose no such basic circuitries existed. Suppose we had no way to insert their message of significance into events of practical importance. Then how could any infant's brain begin to learn to orient toward each of those affirmative attitudes it must gradually develop if it is finally to behave as a mature social animal?

One can envision these small reinforcements of salience as coming by degrees, and as building automatically (see chapters 124 and 125). Into each everyday event which had become *especially meaningful and true* for that developing personality would have been infused a small pulse of salience. And in this manner, step by step, would we be enabled to authenticate what seems *real* for us, and to distinguish this personal truth from non truth. Over the years, from the basic neuronal framework underlying such lesser "fleeting truths," would emerge our capability to arrive at refinements of much larger import (see chapter 98). One aspect of the state of insight-wisdom can be thought of as uncovering one's innate, hardwired capacities for conferring original salience in the absence of the egocentric self.

Syncretism

At this point, a separate neurological condition is instructive. It also helps to illustrate the general thesis that certain neurological disorders, serving us as probes, can help clarify alternate states of consciousness. It too is an agnosia, called *simultagnosia*. What does the entire word mean? It means that the patients can't take in the whole scene simultaneously. If presented with a large forest, they will see only one tree at a time, unable to grasp the *whole* picture.[4] In this syndrome, the brain damage occurs higher up, at the confluence between the parietal and occipital lobes. This particular part of the visual association cortex occupies the upper portions of areas 18 and 19 on both sides[5] (see figure 2).

What causes the piecemeal perception in this disorder? The patients cannot sustain the kind of extensive spatial processing which helps the rest of us perceive the *full* scope of a large visual array. They can't deploy that normal macro mode which distributes attention and pulls together many associative threads into the big picture. So, as a result, the patients lack that gift we take normally for granted: the quick, comprehensive reach into space which grasps a whole configuration and helps bracket its elements into one shared, meaningful interrelationship.

During kensho, could the subject be amplifying certain of these same normal brain mechanisms far beyond their ordinary processing limits? Could this be one way the experiant enhances the conceptual grasp of the whole Big Picture? The kinds of processes embedded in the term *syncretism* help us evaluate this possibility.

The root origins of the word come from Crete. They date from a time when its once-clashing cities came together and finally united into a larger federation. So syncretism already implies that several factions, once highly polarized and at odds with one another, have become totally integrated at a higher level of organization. To clarify what an understanding of syncretism implies for Zen, let us turn to some familiar examples of ambiguous figures which are so often pictured in standard textbooks of psychology. There, as we look at one illustration, we first see black, inward-facing profiles. They are two human faces. An instant later these same profiles serve as the outlines of the white vase that just appeared in the center. Another picture presents the boundaries of a cube, drawn in three dimensions. Sometimes the cube edges project forward, other times backward.

In each of the examples above, we quickly see either one aspect *or* the other. Not both. *Why* not both? Each pattern recognition system seems to be locked into its own rigid compartment. There's no breaking out of these either/or sets. It's always either/or. Duality, locked into opposition.

What would the application of syncretism imply? Seeing *both*. Syncretism in visual processing would amount to a supraordinate act of integration. It would do more than take in all dissenting opposites simultaneously. It would reach beyond their old, dissonant patterns and then infer *a new mode of harmonious interrelationship*. Ancient blood feuds? It will reconcile them. Does something about such totally integrated viewing, without distinctions, seem familiar? A prime example of such syncretism is the *visual* unity in the first two reflections. A particular kind of amplified insight has taken over.

But nothing short of a special kind of insight could unify two discordant qualities, so diametrically opposite, as the sublime and the starkly objective. This is one reason for calling it insight-*wisdom*. Fused into one extraordinary interpretive paradox are both the consummate heights of emotionalized appreciation and the coolest depths of clinical detachment. A mountain peak and an ocean trench. If you can imagine Hillary and Norkay shaking hands with Cousteau, you're getting prepared for the reach of kensho.

The Unified Field of Distributed Functions

Let us suppose, further to illustrate the point above, that the attributes of all things can be assigned into the ancient *yin* and *yang* categories of opposites. So any pair might stand for good and bad, warts and beauty, hot and cold, high and low, whatever. Humans have been conditioned to go one step further. We *polarize our two conceptual extremes*. Therefore, let us represent such symbols as now bearing a charge, either positive (+) or negative (−). What does our usual discriminating brain do whenever it finds these opposite symbols in its ordinary mental field? It picks out their disturbing points of diversity and keeps focusing on them. This leaves us constantly seeing these differences sticking out like a sore thumb, as the following elementary example suggests:

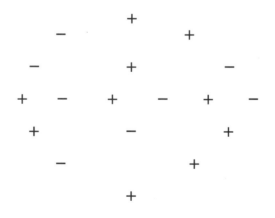

Kensho springs an extraordinary surprise. *Everything coexists, warts and all.* But their *old valences have vanished.* Why? Because every old yardstick has disappeared which had once measured off that emotional distance, say between good and bad or kind and cruel. In one instant, all the old "opposites" are reconciled. Black profiles behold the white vase.

How, then, does a brain drop all its previous sharp contrasts? How can it shift into a state so *un*polarized and accommodating that it blends visual unity, comprehension, *and* affective harmony? At this point, simultagnosia presents a few more helpful clues. True, the patients' deficits only reveal how things start to go "wrong" as soon as local brain functions are disordered. But recall that our plan was to "turn around" such deficits.

In this obverse proposition lies an important consequence. It is the likely possibility that many association networks which feed into and include this parieto-occipital region are indeed the same ones used when we normally conduct our usual orderly, visually unifying, syncretic functions. There is nothing simple about this "ordinary" configuration. For one posterior parietal lobe alone connects with at least *sixty* other identified cortical regions and subcortical nuclei on just that same side of the brain (see chapters 54 and 55). And among these, the right posterior temporal region contributes to this sense of visual closure (see chapter 56).

But we can come to a simplified working hypothesis. It predicts that a process resembling the throw of a kind of *thalamo*cortical master switch could instantly unify a person's mental field in this manner. Indeed, it is plausible that, when their set-points change, certain deeper thalamic and other centralized brain networks, using circuits which normally reach up to integrate the posterior regions of association cortex, can use novel ways both to amplify their functions and to shift instantly into new, shared configurations. The large pulvinar and the lateral posterior nuclei of the thalamus are appropriate subcortical candidates to include in such a syncretic role. Not only do these nuclei interact with this same part of parieto-occipital cortex (as figure 11 illustrates) but they are also poised to contribute to the general sense of salience (see chapter 61).

Neuroimaging studies of normal brains confirm that our simplest psychophysiological functions are already widely distributed. Given the brain's high degree of interconnectedness, it becomes relevant briefly to cite certain findings caused by diffuse head injury. Note: only one particular group of patients is being referred to in this context. These are patients who had suffered only relatively minor degrees of closed head trauma.[6] Still, early in their recovery, tests show two significant problems: (1) the patients can't *divide* attention between two concurrent tasks; (2) they can't *distribute* attention across both their right and left visual fields simultaneously. Fortunately, within three months, many of these head trauma patients will regain the first of these abilities, so that they will relearn to split attention between tasks. But it takes them much longer to relearn to distribute attention across both visual fields in the normal manner.

Attention is a keynote in Zen. Do these problems which occur in this subset of head injury patients have anything to teach us about attention? Trauma does more than contuse the brain locally. It also shears off the fragile threads of nerve fibers throughout many regions diffusely. So the patients' lesions are multifocal, *widely* distributed, and they disconnect many cortical and subcortical sites each from the other. Therefore, even though some of these mild head trauma patients do present difficulties with their visual attention, so called, we must search for other explanations beyond those usual sites, more posterior and deeper, which tend to be among the first to be regarded as "visual" (see chapters 62, 63, and 64). For, in fact, some of these two types of attention deficits could originate in other associative dysfunctions as far forward as the frontal lobes.

Why the *frontal* lobes? Consider the nature of the deficit which occurs in that separate group of patients who have a *single* lesion localized to one frontal lobe. Test *them* with the face/vase type of ambiguous figures. What happens? They're stuck in the white vase. Or they're hung up with two black faces. Their mental set doesn't shift quickly from one option to the other.[7]

So our journey of explanations now seems finally to have led us up to the front of the brain. Here, in the frontal lobes, are many other supraordinate functions, of the kinds that one might expect could enter into syncretism (see chapter 57). For frontal networks would seem capable of helping us solve two critical sets of executive problems. One forward-looking management function will steer us safely through the *Mine*-fields of our old perceptual biases. The other will help us anticipate, with some degree of insight, which particular new qualities are so desirable that any new data will need to possess them in order to be worth paying attention to.

But insight is a soft topic, hard to study. What kind of tests do researchers use when they examine human subjects for the simpler levels of insight? They furnish only a few clues.[8] They base the experimental situation on conventional logic. Therefore, each of their tests still resembles the logical design of a Sherlock Holmes detective story, not the nonrationality of a koan. First, their subjects must quickly spot the key clues. Then they must deploy these clues to intuit their way into the best educated guess.

Now, an educated guess is not a simple matter. It involves scanning a huge data base, while also having on hand suitable strategies and techniques for reading between the lines. For example, Conan Doyle must have been aware of a real dog's uncanny sense of smell. (One estimate is that it is 250 times keener than ours!) And this knowledge enabled Doyle to construct the rest of the fictional plot for his tale of "Silver Blaze." Why didn't the dog bark? Doyle knew that—to a smell-oriented dog—the stolen horse (named Silver Blaze) would still be giving off the same old familiar scent as before. So only mere human beings (not a sensitive dog) would be the ones who could be fooled by a thief who, to disguise the horse *visually*, had covered over its otherwise distinctive white blaze.

Holmes, of course, would not be fooled for long. And some avid detective story readers, engaging their frontal lobes, might also have been able to spot the "nonbarking" clue, then interpret its larger significance. But no sleuth can develop such logical educated guesses after a frontal lobotomy, especially after the left frontal lobe has been removed.[8]

The preceding chapter resorted to two brief working outlines. A set of essential differences separated the diagram of insight-wisdom from that of absorption. These were the steps which emphasized that the *upper*-level sources of kensho's comprehensive, intuitive reach were likely to arise in regions more *rostral*. On the other hand, it was proposed that the *lower*-level mechanisms which affect the sensibilities during absorption would come from regions generally more *caudal*.

Even in so preliminary a sketch, the layers of excitations, inhibitions, and *dis*inhibitions were becoming too complex to represent in one simple diagram. Why? In large part because of the intricate circuitry of the thalamus (see chapters 59, 60, and 61).

Consider, for example, two important points about the function of the reticular nucleus as it "caps" the rest of the thalamus. When the rostral regions of this cap are excited, say by glutamate released from the frontal cortex immediately above, they inhibit the other nearby dorsal nuclei of the thalamus. But suppose these same rostral parts of the reticular nucleus had been themselves *inhibited,* as they indeed are when stimulated from below (see chapter 60). In this instance, the final outcome would be a corresponding *dis*inhibition. The result of this disinhibition would then be to *release* many intrinsic functions of those same mediodorsal and other nearby thalamic nuclei. And their released functions could then reverberate among the circuits of their higher-level counterparts up in the cortex.

Now, the mediodorsal nucleus is poised between the limbic system and the prefrontal cortex (see figure 11). Therefore, in shaping the several frontal lobe contributions to insight-wisdom, its subregions will have pivotal roles to play (see table 7; chapter 58).

In such pairs of observations resides an interesting possibility: different persons might experience slightly different sequences early in kensho. What would decide the difference? It would depend on whether the person's initial subtle stimulus event, or trigger, had shifted set-points while its initial impulse flow was *ascending* through the brain or while it was *descending.* Whichever effect might predominate in a given instance would still find either side of the reticular nucleus competent to play a pivotal *bilateral* role in kensho. For pathways lead out from this reticular cap on *one* side which can shift the functions of other thalamic nuclei on *both* sides.[9] The route these messages travel when they cross the midline from one reticular nucleus to reach the opposite thalamus runs over the subcortical bridge (see chapter 82).

To sum up the evidence considered thus far: kensho's immediate grasp of the total visual scene could arise when certain parieto-occipital *and* frontal sources are unified by their deep thalamic counterparts. But this theory has not yet reconciled a key paradox: how could any person's brain suddenly grasp meanings of the most universal nature, and yet—simultaneously—let go of its most highly prized meanings, those of the tenacious personal self?

Temporal Lobe: Additions and Subtractions

Excitation and inhibition are the two basic categories of physiological processes in the nervous system. Textbooks tend to simplify the two, having first cast them in opposing roles. But it is time once again—as it was on Crete—to take a fresh look at another option. Because the field of consciousness has been totally transformed. A change this major in scope suggests that the effects of excitation and inhibition had *converged* on functions represented at many levels throughout the modular brain. And that now their interactions (which we usually think of as opposing each other) had gone on to strengthen each other exponentially (see chapter 37). Put simply, some modules will then have become more excitable because their corresponding inhibitory systems were reduced, and vice versa.

Let us inquire, now at the level of descriptive psychology: Do some very general properties of consciousness also change in kensho? In its most elementary form, the answer is yes. In general, those properties increase that are affirmative and reinforcing. And, simultaneously, those properties decrease that have aversive aspects or dysfunctional implications.

At this point, it becomes pertinent to recall a finding reviewed earlier (see chapter 41). When monkeys lose the tips of their temporal lobes on both sides, they behave as though they had been cut adrift from their prior emotional connotations. The general thesis proposed here is that some aspects of kensho proceed in a related manner. More specifically, that it briefly *reduces* many of the affective functions which are distributed throughout the anterior temporal cortex, the amygdala, and their multiple close connections.

The resulting deficit could certainly explain why the person loses some affective roots of the psychic self. Formerly, these emotional roots had been tied up in a *subjective* processing mode. This was a mode which could always brand things good or bad, using sharply opposite either/or valences, many of which had been derived from limbic origins. Coming out of kensho, it was finally obvious that my old subjective self had previously constructed a highly biased perspective. What, then, had occurred *during* that flash of insight-wisdom? Something analogous to the earlier diagram of once-polarized symbols. A higher-order perspective had still seen the same field. It had seen an area filled as before with all those former small crossed lines and dashes. But now they existed *in themselves, as impersonal lines.* They had been depolarized, as it were. Stripped of their old divisive charge. They were not plus and minus signs any longer.

So then, where could the *new affirmations* have come from? Has our review of the temporal lobe uncovered other kinds of functions which can help clarify how kensho *adds* such profoundly universal, *positive* resonances even while it *subtracts* the personal self at the same time? It has. For the evidence indicates that the temporal cortex contributes to many higher-level interpretive functions (see chapters 56 and 78). And in its more anterior regions, both acetylcholine and enkephalin connections are becoming very influential. As these ACH and opioid terminals converge on the temporal interpretive cortex, they could be poised to do more than infuse the ordinary hints of salience which reinforce our special moments of everyday living. During rare moments, they might also help raise its levels of significance up to extraordinary new dimensions of meaning.

The insight of immanent perfection begins in reflection I. It continues far into the next phases of kensho, then trails off (see figure 18). Meanwhile, reflections II has flashed in. Like the remaining phases, it has been indicated here in the plural. Why? Because it contains several lancinating insights, sequences which seem to strike in tandem. The insights confer remarkably different kinds of knowledge. As each arrives, its content is already highly branched, *and totally understood*, in complex ways. And underneath these added silent messages, the experiant was also made aware of two deep, diffuse *impressions:* (1) *of having lost every notion of approach behavior;* (2) *of having lost every last ounce of fear.* These dual subtractions were two central facts of experience. We will regard these two extinctions as useful clues. In the next three sections, we trace back the cut ends of each of these losses. They lead us toward what caused them, and where.

Nonintervention

To do, or not to do? Instantly, insight-wisdom resolved any basis for such a soliloquy. In a scene already impregnated with understanding, it first added a soft abstract comment: *there is nothing more to do.* Doing had been undermined along with doing-time.

But then it also dropped a more specific hint. For *inaction.* This, too, was a faint message, a mere tap on the shoulder. For whom? Whose shoulder? Nobody remains. So who would be the recipient of this second, gratuitous, avuncular comment, this gentle advice *not* to act? Could some vaguely *inferred* remote i have otherwise been disposed to approach? Someone whose underlying "habit-energy" might have been ready to insert its impulse to intervene?*

Let us first examine the abstract comment: *nothing more to do.* Emerson had been aware that the brief moment of visual illumination contained tranquility. He said it came from the "knowing that all things go well."[10] And indeed this basic understanding did enter into the flavor of nonintervention. But it arrived as a more exquisitely subtle message, one which went beyond a conclusion that you can't gild a single lily already perfect in itself. For, to this experiant, the first layer of nonintervention counseled: *There's no need to interfere with the grandeur of the whole universal design. All things here do work out very well on their own. What will be, will be.*

In historical perspective, the nuances of this term, *noninterference,* go back a very long way. If one makes allowances for the usual problems in translation, the old Chinese Taoist phrase, *wu-wei,* may have embedded in it two similar subtleties. For sometimes this phrase is translated as "nonassertion, not forcing."[11] And such absolute noninterference with the natural course of events might suggest that the word had a few looser, laisser-faire implications. But wu-wei is more often translated as the principle of *spontaneous, effortless action.* This means that the person's acts have finally become free from all personal motivations or premeditations (see chapter 155). Later, in Japan, Master Bankei had observed that there existed no *shoulds* in our original, unborn state of grace. Being back at the origin implied *that there was no obligation to do something.*

He put it this way: "Notions of what one should do never existed from the start."[12]

No shoulds is a major change from the usual way we live our lives. More recently, when Maslow coined the term "B-cognition," he employed it without making *specific* reference to the broad issue of nonaction as such. Yet he was still referring to that particular kind of viewing which simply sees nature as sufficient unto itself, as "in its own *Being* rather than as something to be used" or to be

---

* Table 20 places this curious potential i, which entered at the end of reflections II, in parentheses: (i).

reacted to.[13] The ancient dictum that Nature is not to be "used" has certainly gathered momentum. It has now come to lie at the core of the modern environmentalist ethic.

For this experiant on the London platform, the two messages of noninterference fused into one gentle reminder: not to micromanage the universal design. And they coincided with something else. Not with discrete idea-messages as such. But with deep *impressions,* as if made by two boulders, in the sense that William James had once used the phrase (see chapter 124). The first impression entered as much more than a feeling that could later be described (in my vocabulary, at least) by a term such as "high indifference." And it was not a specific *dis*interest. The impression, instead, was that roots had been cut off. And not cut off near ground level, but severed at depths beyond all superficial notions about "shoulds," "oughts," or other behavioral obligations. It felt as though the primitive motoric premise had been undermined far underground. *What seemed voided there was the whole motivational disposition to approach.*

Which regions tend normally to sponsor our positive, "forward-leaning" approach behaviors? Among them are the nucleus accumbens and the *medial* aspects of the frontal lobe. But the frontal lobe has its own mechanisms of subtraction. Its flat *orbital* cortex stands ready to inhibit this vertical medial cortex (see table 7). So if some of the operations of certain orbital *restraining* compartments had remained, and had entered consciousness, they might have contributed to the silent messages not to intervene.[14]

No Fear

No fear. Reflections II abolished it. Master Bankei had reminded his own flock that no fear resided in their unborn Buddha-mind. Fear, he said, was only "an illusion or figment of thought."[15] On the London subway platform, the impression was that fear itself had been ousted, as had every trace of defense behavior, its ally (see chapter 52).

Normally, the impressive bulk of fear arises within networks which link our amygdala with the orbitomedial frontal cortex, the anterior cingulate cortex, the central gray, and the hypothalamus. Then what does the death of fear imply? It suggests that aversive valences had dropped out from these limbic regions and their connections. The process feels seismic but silent. The impression is that some deep fracture has quietly shorn off one's visceral roots. This is not the shaving off of a few curled layers of concepts from the cognitive self higher up in the mantle of cortex.

What could cause such a widespread loss of all the overtones of fear? Among the possibilities is a release of opioids (see chapter 47). This could occur both along the links of the aversive chain cited above and also within the limbic thalamus. The opioid hypothesis is testable. But it will be necessary for the investigator to be on the spot promptly to determine (a) the awakened person's pain threshold, to see if it has risen toward levels of analgesia, and (b) the levels of several opioids and of other relevant messengers (including ACTH) in the fluid bathing the brain (see chapters 80 and 81). The technology exists. The needs for advanced planning and precise timing are the limitations.

Earlier we commented on a striking fact: when opioids stimulate mu receptors in the central gray, this causes a *secondary* release of even more opioids a long distance away.[16] This extra release of enkephalins and of beta-endorphin occurs both in the nucleus accumbens and in the amygdala. Accordingly, this phenomenon suggests the possibility that an additional deep layer of opioid mechanisms might supervene. It is one which could reinforce both the message of nonintrusion *and* the accompanying loss of fear.

It is all too easy for a critic outside kensho to be misled. At first glance, one might reason out a thought sequence as follows: the subject had just been convinced that the universe was everlasting; no death could exist in such an infinitude; therefore, this absence of the possibility of death had led to the thoughtful conclusion: there can't be anything left to fear.

Incorrect. Kensho's flash preempts such cause-and-effect logic. Moreover, by reflections II, all the relevant impressions had registered simultaneously, and were fully established: fear, death, and the personal self were all extinguished, snuffed out into the same huge vacancy. Only insight-wisdom creates such a vacancy, not reason.

Dissolution of the Self into Eternity

To address this topic is to continue the dialogue about neurological disorders which began earlier in the second section of this chapter. And our dialogue also continues with the hallmark functions of the temporal lobe. Perhaps when we first discussed this lobe, back in chapter 56, the reader had wondered, Why does this book focus on déjà vu and jamais vu, on déjà vécu and jamais vécu? Because they were two distinct sets of model experiences. They illustrated what is meant by the *interpretive* functions of the temporal lobe.[17]

On that initial occasion, to bring out the contrasts between the experiences, we improvised a purely hypothetical question: *When?* And we directed it earlier at each of these relatively common pairs of experiences. Why not again ask this very same question? Except that this time we will be addressing it to the *quality of viewing* during reflections II. So the issue in this present instance now becomes, Can reflections II also recall *when* it had previously seen the field of items at hand? In other words, inside kensho, can the brain "remember" whether or not it had experienced them in the past?

No answer. For the "when" question, taken out of its former context, is meaningless. No comparable "Yes, once before," or "No, never," answer is possible. Why? One reason is that reflections II retains no personal self as its central reference point. Nobody is inside to judge whether this same field of items had been seen or experienced once before. It is also a nonquestion because *reflections II* was timeless. No clock was ticking off intervals within which an event could be affixed.

Two paragraphs above, it may have seemed only reasonable to take the liberty to pose an artificial question. After all, it had been "answerable" before, at least by persons who were not in kensho at the time. So then is there no simple way to indicate the most basic reason *why* this same "when" question would remain unanswered during *reflections II*? Yes, there is a way. It will seem strange,

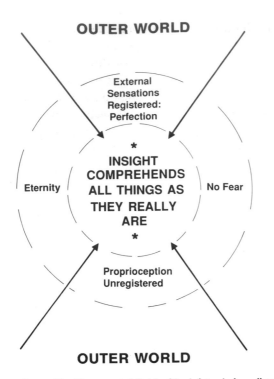

OUTER WORLD

External
Sensations
Registered:
Perfection

*
INSIGHT
COMPREHENDS
ALL THINGS AS
THEY REALLY
ARE
*

Eternity

No Fear

Proprioception
Unregistered

OUTER WORLD

Figure 19   The mental field of insight-wisdom (kensho-satori), State VII
The brain's intuitive capacities reach their peak. At impact, a totally unifying objective vision comprehends the whole outside world, just as it really is. It registers as immanent eternal perfection. Fear vanishes because the entire *I-Me-Mine* drops out at every affective level. Dashed lines serve only to mark the site of former boundaries. Contrast with the mental field of absorption, figure 16.

in print, on this page. Yet the phrase below does allude to the prevailing impression, *inside* kensho, which already would have settled the issue of timing:

ETERNALLY THUS

When the entire *I-Me-Mine* dissolves in kensho, the experiant is aware of this as an impression, at depth. But no idea-messages are in there stimulating discursive thoughts about the weighty personal implications of this impression (figure 19). True, during an earlier major internal absorption, the "self" had also dropped off. But that was only a "little death." On that occasion, it was chiefly the *explicit bodily self* which had vanished (see figure 16). In short, what was absorption? Merely a *dearth of self*, a loss of that physical topography which had previously been established through the sensory channels.

In earlier chapters, we invoked the *back* of the cap of the reticular nucleus to help explain why the sensate framework of this physical self drops out during absorption (e.g., see chapter 118). The theory has a solid factual basis in inhibition. It is plausible to suggest that one mechanism operating in kensho is an extension of this same basic, everyday function of the reticular nucleus. But in this instance the inhibitory cap would need to tighten *much farther forward and also medially.* Only then could the more anterior GABA cells in this nucleus block most of the *limbic* regions of the thalamus from contributing to their old notions of one's *implicit psychic self* (see chapter 141).

It is this cavernous loss of our covert *I-Me-Mine* which constitutes the true *death* of self. It sheds every psychic construct of selfhood: the vain needs for mirror worship, the longings and loathings, those obligatory shoulds and oughts. When all these cognitive and emotionalized properties of the psychic self drop out, ample room remains for a profound state of grace. It enters the mental field of *reflections II* and persists throughout the next phase of *reflections III*.

Deliverance

By *reflections III*, this experiant was feeling totally *released*, liberated, simplified. All knotted legacies from the past had dissolved into tranquility. Nothing remained in the whole mental field that was motivating, that *had* to be planned for; nothing that "should" or "must" be meddled with; nothing threatening to worry about. None of these tangled scenarios, real or imaginary, existed in the field of consciousness. Consider how many networks one usually commits to these activities of planning, obligations and worries! Kensho was deliverance from all such bonds.

Countless persons have tried, for millennia, to put this experience into words. To me, the phrase which still remains most accurate (for several reasons) is "that peace which passeth all understanding." Among Buddhist aspirants, such terms as "Original Face," "The Unborn," the "Buddha-Nature" sow as much confusion as do phrases invoked in other religious traditions. "Lighten up" is perhaps more accurate than enlightenment. Yet all words lure the unwary. We take thought-forms much too literally.

Even in our open societies of today, to be graced by such total freedom would be a remarkable event. But consider how much more dramatic the same deliverance would have been in China and Japan of old. For these were rigidly hierarchical cultures, legendary in how much respect their members paid to age, authority, rank, and tradition. In such structured societies, it speaks volumes about the powerful impact of satori when it so unleashes a monk like Hakuin that he could subsequently strike back at his venerable master. Such freedom of action would be unthinkable in every other circumstance.

Is such an act insolence or irreverence? It would miss the point to think so. Indeed, in the context of kensho-satori, Buddhism reserves a specific technical term for the release from worldly bonds. This freedom from every delusion is called *moksha*. It testifies to an extinction of self so profound that it emancipates the person from all internal and external constraints that these prior delusions had imposed. Reflect back on how many years each of us has also been carefully conditioned to obey and to behave—as subordinate children, students, and employees. Abruptly to lose this yoke! No more do's and don'ts! No shoulds and oughts! Unconditioned consciousness! What a relief!

By its third phase, the rich matrix of awakening is filled with potential paradoxes. Let us review a few of them. Utmost detachment encounters an ultra-unifying vision. A person who does not exist, a no-I who has lost all conscious inclination to act, is still counseled (wordlessly) not to intervene. Marrow drained of prior conditioning openly receives the ultimate principles of existence. An old life vanished, a new reality everywhere. Now all of these elements coexist within *one unified, expanded mental field*. Is paradox evident? Not at this time. Insights and impressions form a coherent whole. Is it any wonder that the awesome unity of kensho escapes words? Or that this unimaginable mixture sometimes gives way to later moments when the subject shifts from laughter to tears?

Perhaps these emotional eruptions will occur especially when the person's arousal level had been high, after much prior tension had been built up, and the tension was abruptly released. On the other hand, long prior meditative training—but under less pressured circumstances—may serve to moderate the swings that biogenic amines add to behavioral arousal. This could channel the emotional charge perhaps along more intuitive avenues. Indeed, in many other instances, when equally profound awakening occurs, it remains dry-eyed and silent but no less awesome in how much it dissolves and reveals.

A few thoughts—ideas which could be defined as *thoughts* at the time— filtered in during the latter part of *reflections III*. Some responded, barely, to steering. It was as though their sponsors had been the first faint traces of a returning i-me-mine. Aside from this, whatever spectator remained was still in absentia, totally objective.

The final phase of *reflections IV* occupied the subsequent minutes and hours of the next day or two. In its diminuendo, kensho's ramifications sank in, infiltrating conventional consciousness. This was a very sobering period. Now I understood. An imperial self? It didn't exist. There was no emperor. That old, disguised *I-Me-Mine* had been seen into, its fictions laid bare. Previously, it had pulled, pushed, and bound every relationship into self-centered constructs. Now that masquerade was over. No mask and no emperor's clothes. A lifetime of old self/ other assumptions had just dropped out of the bottom of the bucket. How irrelevant they seemed in retrospect to the newly emerging self. It had different feelings, concepts, personal insights, and attitudes.

Later the same day, in London, I tried to remember. Back when I was a child, had I ever undergone a release even remotely similar to this present one? Memory retrieved a lesser incident that took place when I was perhaps six years old. It had not seemed so minor at the time. A few tough neighborhood bullies had been picking on the rest of us. Taunted by them, I had become upset. I had let their teasings get under my skin. Finally, a pal told me how to reply. The formula was "Sticks and stones may break my bones, but words can never hurt me." It was magic. Better than any outward security blanket. It worked, especially on me. I calmed down, and I lost every feeling of being oppressed. Once the bullies realized they could no longer get my goat, their teasing stopped.

In such ways do children discover the little coping techniques that bring small-sized liberations. Growing up, one not only learns new approaches but has moments of seeing things in a whole different *light*. Insight-wisdom amplifies these kinds of intuitive "lights" to their ultimate degree. Not until I was an adult did Myokyo-ni help me appreciate the nature of that beast who still responded when teasings and personal insults penetrated his thin skin. It was not a goat after all. It was the powerful bull.[18]

So here was this person who had now understood that things are *themselves*, objectively. A someone who had just understood, on a drab London subway platform, that the universal design needs no meddling on his part. What kinds of thoughts were entering his mental field? Chief among them was *acceptance*. I could now begin to accept realities as *they* are. This was a big change in attitude for a physician inclined to have activist tendencies. To arrive at acceptance, it was necessary first to see things as *they* are. Gradually came the realization of how they happened to become that particular way, and the acceptance that all things are still subject to these inevitable ups and downs of change. At an intellectual level, I had long been comfortable with my role as a transient participant in those cycles of nitrogen and carbon which entered into birth, death, decay, and rebirth. Now this understanding deepened. However, I had never believed that I possessed some kind of "spirit" or "soul" which could later be *literally* reincarnated into the body of another specific person or animal. And none of my reflections encouraged this notion, or any other supernatural ideas.

143

Selective Mechanisms Underlying Kensho

Science prospers exactly in proportion as it is religious; and religion flourishes in exact proportion to the scientific depth and firmness of its bases.

Thomas H. Huxley (1825–1895)[1]

Kensho seems unpredictable. But nowadays, because their scientists have been analyzing many experimental situations, the National Weather Service is starting to predict when lighting might strike. We, too, may someday develop better ways to encourage enlightenment, given a better understanding—and application—of its basic principles. True, awakening flashes in rarely, almost haphazardly. But though its mechanisms may be subtle, it doesn't operate out of total chaos. Chaos is a buzzword currently in fashion. It started as a mathematical term and then slipped readily into biology. As it is used now, the word describes a situation arising in a system so complex that, even if you make a small change in its initial conditions, the resulting ripples go on to create big waves farther downstream, causing a series of tidal changes so major that the whole system finally behaves unpredictably in a nonlinear manner.[2]

The neurosciences today are vast fields so full of hidden complexities that they seem to exhibit their own brand of chaos. But most neuroscientists won't submit easily to the old brands of nihilism under some new guise. Instead, busy as bees, they gather a better data base, repair old theories, devise new testable hypotheses, and try to cope with intricacy by resorting to powerful computer systems. Like the computers of the new breed of climatologists, theirs also hum away, scanning complexity, searching for recurrent cause-and-effect relationships, not mere coincidences.

If kensho doesn't flash out at random, from complete chaos, then where in the brain does it arise, and how? In the previous two chapters, we have been building on some general themes already identified in part III and subsequently (see table 20). Four general processes have emerged, and they now begin to take a more selective form:

1. A brisk conjunction of certain acetylcholine and glutamate activating functions
2. Interactions cosponsored among major thalamic nuclei and their cortical counterparts, both in the frontotemporal and parieto-occipital regions
3. A dropping out of many of the usual temporal lobe, limbic, central gray, and medial orbito-frontal functions
4. A possible enhancement of certain peptide-related functions within these and other specified regions

Caveats are in order. Kensho *is* like lightning, in several respects. Its charge has a longer buildup than one might think. Sometimes a brief hair-raising prelude occurs, *then* a flash. Each of these three requires a multidimensional approach. Within each phase, no single component is going to drop into place simply because one chemical messenger may have acted to change one of its receptors in one small region.

Yet awakening is something more than a single, brief isolated earth-shaking strike. It also has an extended reflective coda. Moreover, in order later to transform, it must set in motion a cascade of psychophysiological and biochemical changes. These will develop a certain momentum (see part VIII). Each ingredient will be contributing to the ongoing total transformation experience, reinforcing other changes at multiple sites.

Consider your favorite symphony. Yes, the higher notes do stand out, way up there in the upper registers of the violin section. But does not the vitality of the music come from the notes and tempo of other instruments in the lower registers as well? No evidence in these pages has so beguiled us with the phrase "higher states of consciousness" that we assign either exclusive or lofty importance to the human cortex. Decisive events also take place in the depths of the brain. When high tide comes in, it will then be events down in the ooze at the bottom where an already taut anchor becomes briefly detached that allow a big wave to lift the boat extra high. Buddhism has a simpler metaphor: "The lotus grows from the mud up." We need to know whether kensho *per se* occurs during breath suspension. If so, this could help clarify some of its levels of origin, and their respective mechanisms (an approach introduced in chapter 22).

In kensho's early phases, only *certain* so-called cortical functions would seem to be involved. Yet these are functions integrally linked with their counterparts down in the subcortex and brain stem (see Table 20). And note how many other *subtractions* had gone on. For insight-wisdom strips consciousness not only of its old, cognitive discriminations. It also frees it from every constraint which might previously have been binding the self to a sorrowful or guilty past, a fearful present, and a worrisome future. During kensho, the full range of cortical language functions also seems to have been left out of its loop. Moreover, language faces an uphill struggle later whenever it tries to articulate kensho's prelinguistic mix of insights, messages, and impressions from one state to another.

Could such a huge new conjunction spring *solely* from either the right or the left side of the brain? Not likely. Consider, for example, how normal subjects respond as they react to items which are so novel that they violate all of the subjects' prior expectations. Under these conditions, *both* sides of the brain contribute their two different strategies to the final outcome.[3]

So then, could kensho's illuminating interpretations arise from everywhere, simultaneously? Is every neuronal light bulb turned on to its maximum? No. The evidence speaks for no primary *global* surge in ordinary parallel processing. Indeed, the normal brain has other ways to process extra volumes of data both selectively and rapidly. It can use fast transmitters, process locally on a relatively massive scale, or take shortcuts through different systems which had been held in reserve, more or less. For example, some impulses might race through the perforant pathway to quickly bypass a potential gridlock of associations taking place elsewhere.

Kensho has more than content. It requires a lengthy introduction: months or years. Then, after a subacute prelude, the shift takes place in a particular acute context. In my case, these last two phases included the reverent tone set by a sesshin, concentrated periods of zazen during the previous day, zazen again that morning, and standing quietly for a brief unfocused moment in a completely unfamiliar train station. One can easily overlook private moments of diastole. And the setting of novelty can contribute a great deal, although there is, as yet, relatively little appreciation of this fact (see chapter 47 and 64). But each factor—diastole and novelty—has important consequences. For instance, certain nerve cells in the basal forebrain will discharge in response to an unfamiliar novel stimulus, irrespective of what value the stimulus has.[4]

In earlier centuries, some monks described preludes of other kinds. One kind was the lengthy period of insensitivity noted three chapters earlier. It was a preamble during which the monk felt withdrawn into a wooden-like or icelike state of depression. We find it further described in the report of the Chan master, Kao-feng (J: Koho).[5] Here was a determined person who could succeed—where I had failed—in becoming totally wrapped up in that koan, "all things return to the One." Indeed, after he had finally fixed it at the very core of his consciousness, no thought stirred which was not relevant to this koan. In his account of the resulting state, he says it was "like being screwed up or glued; however much I tried to shake myself off, it refused to move. Though I was in the midst of a crowd or congregation, I felt as if I were all by myself . . . My one thought covered eternities; so calm was the outside world, so oblivious was I of the existence of other people." He felt like this, "like an idiot," for six days. We can imagine how relieved he was when enlightenment finally struck. For Kao-feng, the trigger was seeing a verse on the portrait of a patriarch.

Rhythms and Triggers

When is kensho most likely to strike? Was it sheer coincidence that my taste of kensho came in the morning? What is morning? It is the time when our peaks and troughs of vigilance are most likely to fluctuate.[6] Each such wave carries the potential—remote though it may be—to break through into a sudden peak experience. Add stressful circumstances, and they can further increase the amplitudes of the morning's physiological oscillations. Next superimpose a trigger, and it could lend an extra jolt to the other sources of morning instability. But even if a trigger does not arrive in the morning, many other underlying cycles are churning around within each day. They present countless other opportunities for functions to come into phase and to summate their effects. Of particular note are our lesser peaks of vigilance which recur every ninety minutes on their individual ultradian rhythm[6] (see figure 13).

Suppose a person, during a retreat, meditates repeatedly during the daytime hours. Then, each period of zazen also thrusts in its own different set of physiological vectors to distort the much more slowly curving profile of the arousal cycle. The net effect could be to shift both the phase entry times and the momentum of the meditator's ninety-minute rhythm. How do the resulting instabilities affect the meditator? They produce shifts into periods of finely held awareness, or swings off toward drowsiness, or moves into varied textures of wakefulness that express zones of transition between the two.

So what is likely to happen, during a stressful retreat, to those persons who meditate repeatedly during the day and who also pursue a koan to reach one-pointed concentration? They may tend to develop higher physiological peaks. These have the potential to rise up sharply from the broad shoulders of other basic rhythms. Now an abrupt triggering event could be the last straw, the closure which completes the pattern of syzygy and precipitates kensho.

Zen has numerous anecdotes about triggers, which are clues to such an interpretation (see chapter 105). They have led us toward one hypothesis: kensho may be prompted by a jolt traveling up through higher extensions of the reticular activating system. Still, many surprising events do this, but nothing else happens. Moreover, most awakenings seem to occur without obvious triggers. So we must probe further, to ask, What special properties do such triggered moments have? And which mechanisms do triggers *share in common* with our other similar, but much more frequent, physiological events?

Again we come back to refocus on the same three basic events that each of us goes through spontaneously under normal, everyday circumstances. They are moments during which one's set-points could change enough to help throw the switch, in a manner of speaking. They are the times when the activating system quickens its discharges, moments when the reticular nucleus of the thalamus is also undergoing its most dynamic shifts. These mundane moments occur during (1) the waking hours, when desynchronizations return every ninety minutes or so; (2) the sleeping hours, when similar trends recur toward low voltage fast EEG activities each time we ascend into desynchronized sleep; and (3) the transition periods. Now drowsiness or sleep yields to desynchronizing arousals, and we glide up into ordinary awakening.

What can happen when some relevant stimulus does strike during the waking state? Or when an internally generated drive does occur as part of D-sleep? In either case, as Steriade and colleagues have recently observed, those thalamic and cortical nerve cells which oscillate at fast frequencies (twenty to forty times a second) are then likely to become "robustly coherent" for short periods of time.[7] A mouse is all it takes to trigger the attentive cat. Then, in Buber's phrase, a "simple magic" links thalamus and cortex into one configuration (see chapter 95).

In my case, as in most others, no overt outside stimulus precipitated kensho. Still, I could have overlooked some ordinary *covert* events which might have superimposed themselves on top of my morning tide of arousal. Such silent conjunctions could also briefly switch a brain out of its major rhythms and cycles into some "robust" new alignment.

Earlier, when we reviewed how fast desynchronizing activity occurred, we found that its contributions arose from different physiological sources. These systems then expressed themselves, at several levels, through several arousal pathways (see chapter 37). So a number of options are available. Within such variety are plausible explanations for why certain activating mechanisms, by reaching up through their higher-order and more rostral ramifications, might prompt kensho. Others, being limited to networks at relatively lower levels, could shape major absorptions (see chapter 141).

Would similar explanations account for the reports that these two states sometimes seem to have occurred back to back? Suppose the two states did happen in tandem, with the elements of absorption leading. Then the sensate changes, infused with blissful emotion, might present first. It would then seem as though they had extended themselves into a mixture which included major insights. Kensho appeared to have struck Daisetz Suzuki when he was coming up out of a brief "samadhi." In the case of Richard Bucke, a complex illuminating experience arrived sometime after midnight at a time when he had already entered a state of quiet, passive enjoyment. He reported his experience as first being ushered in by a flame-colored enveloping cloud and then by immense joyousness.[8] But neither mixtures of states nor the fragments of quickenings need prompt us to lose sight of one basic fact. At the core of kensho's first phase, *reflection I*, is instant, syncretic comprehension, whatever else different brains in their different rhythms might be adding to the amalgam.

Messenger Molecules

Biogenic Amines

Do dopamine, norepinephrine, and serotonin contribute to kensho? (see chapter 44). Our review would suggest that these modulators add rather less to the moment of dry-eyed kensho, on the whole, than they do either to absorptions or to quickenings (see part V). True, in those earlier years when levo-dopa was first given to experimental animals, "awakening" was the term used to describe their energized "behavioral arousal."[9] Later, Oliver Sacks would also use "awakening" to describe some of the other notable ways that certain parkinsonian patients *gradually* change after their brain DA levels are replenished. But levo-dopa treatment does not change these patients' mentation in seconds or minutes. It does so slowly, over a period of many hours to days (as Robert De Niro's performance illustrated in the movie). Only by degrees do the patients develop more physical and mental "energy." Slowly, they also undergo something more, a *qualitative* change: their perceptions, thoughts, feelings, and personal memories are enhanced. Continuing to feel better, their outlook changes. They become less self-concerned, more aware of the "full presence of the world." Incrementally, they add sudden reminiscences which become more vivid, immediate, and highly personal.[10] We now know that the nerve terminals of some DA systems end on frontal and limbic nerve cells (see figure 7). It is reasonable to attribute some of the parkinsonian patients' regenerated mental functions to more DA being released onto these nerve cells.

Still, a DA surge could be one factor contributing to kensho, perhaps more so in younger age groups. Here, the rate of DA turnover is likely to be higher. Extra DA in frontal and limbic regions could further enhance the much greater impact produced there by a primary, and more selective, surge of fast transmitters. Dopamine's metabolic after effects could also linger in second-messenger systems.

Serotonin receptors might play a different kind of modulating role in kensho's unique mode of comprehensive viewing. But with several caveats. The disorganized, disturbing distortions of sensate and affective functions caused by psychedelic drugs are no accurate model for that abrupt thrust of kensho's sharp insights which occurs spontaneously. Moreover, ST has implicit interactions with norepinephrine systems. Even when the psychedelic drugs that mimic ST and NE are given under supervision, the drugged subjects undergo very long, agonized periods and repeated high dosages before their rare deep insights occur (see chapter 101). Such facts suggest that neither ST nor NE, alone or together, determine the abrupt onset and content of kensho per se.

Could ST help *pave* the way, be part of the prelude to kensho? Could it contribute in other modulating ways? For example, it is plausible to think that many of the same nerve cells which have been *primarily* excited *by faster-acting transmitters* in kensho are also responding to some ST, if only to a lesser degree. Indeed, such an excitatory modulatory function is one role served by those ST fibers which release ST onto their ST_2 receptors located on nerve cells up in the frontotemporal region. These ST_2 receptors are the same kind of receptors which can be activated by such ST agonists as LSD (see chapter 103).

Note, however, that these same frontotemporal cells will also be swarming with other receptors for the brain's many other primary messengers. Therefore, it becomes part of our search to ask: What precisely do these same intrinsic frontotemporal nerve cells themselves do? How do their activities contribute to normal consciousness? So this part of the research quest *begins* by clarifying what such cells do; it does not end with the phenomenology of psychedelic drugs which act all over the brain and cause nonspecific stress responses as well. No, in kensho we are postulating that when intrinsic messengers activate their receptors, discretely from within, only certain cells will be *selectively* excited, whereas still others will be inhibited. And the prediction is that both types of cells, those excited and those inhibited, will be acted upon *primarily* by mechanisms much faster and more potent than those usually available to the biogenic amines.

There are implications to speed and potency. *Reflection I* entered as fast as the blink of an eye. Our eyes blink within a mere 200 milliseconds. An onset this abrupt suggests that kensho is expressing (a) fast-acting acetylcholine pathways which exerted their impact first on their *nicotinic* receptors; and (b) fast-acting glutamate pathways.

In this book we have repeatedly emphasized the major potentials of these two systems. Within the early seconds of a surge of ACH, the slower muscarinic ACH receptors also start to phase in (see chapter 38). Their effects continue for another twenty seconds or so. The inestimable time during which kensho evolved seemed to fall within this interval, as best as one could guess. Very long axons issue from some ACH nerve cells down in the parabrachial region. They are long enough to offer an intriguing way for these cells to help unify the brain, forward and aft. For example, among these ACH fibers from the lateral parabrachial cell group, some even reach up to supply the pivotal mediodorsal nucleus of the thalamus. And ACH axons from the medial parabrachial nerve cells also supply the pulvinar. Other neighboring ACH cells extend their axons as far forward as the mediofrontal cortex.

In kensho, not only does the mental field shift quickly into its new interpretation but coherence permeates everything within it. Both observations provide strong evidence for the following two propositions: (1) much of this state of awakening is being integrated within such *centrally located* subcortical regions as the thalamus; (2) the process also extends its reach through large networks using fast parallel processing.

Glutamate can make a critical contribution to the shift of set-points at these very deep central levels. For example, there—in the key suprachiasmatic nucleus—glutamate can phase-advance the circadian clock by stimulating the synthesis of nitric oxide.[11]

Opioids?

Already, in reflection 1, the basic matrix of intact vision is enriched, and by a perspective never seen before. These milliseconds are not necessarily too early for beta-endorphin, enkephalins, and dynorphin *also* to have been released. But they do seem too soon for these opioids then to have gone on to reach the peak and fulfill the range of their *physiological* activities. Too soon, that is, unless the opioids had indeed *already* been released a few seconds earlier, as perhaps they might have been, in response to an *earlier* novel situation. For the reasons indicated, one expects the physiological effects of the opioid and other peptide systems to be a bit delayed, and to rise more slowly to their peaks (see chapter 47). And one also expects that these same actions will fade rather quickly, because such peptide molecules are soon broken down.

On the other hand, many mu opioid receptors exists out near the end of enkephalin circuits in the temporal lobe. Here, they would seem to be available to shape our higher-order perceptual processes. The result could be selectively to modify some of the interpretive capacities of the anterior temporal lobes. Mu receptors are also candidates further to wipe out fear in other regions. They are present in high concentrations in the amygdala and in the orbito-medial cortex of the frontal lobe.[12,13] So mu receptors, responding to a covert earlier event, and acted upon by beta-endorphin and enkephalins, are candidates for contributing climates of additional depth and scope to the resonances of immanence, ultimate perfection, and eternity.

In which directions could consciousness change if one of the very earliest precipitating events were, in fact, a *covert* pulse of enkephalin or dynorphin? These two opioids can excite the hippocampus. Therefore, each might—after a short delay—contribute memorable facets to the resulting experience. Moreover, a brief enkephalin pulse could inhibit the ventral striatum. There, by freezing the action themes of the nucleus accumbens, it might help further shape the deep-seated impression that there was "nothing to do."

Which pathways prompt the brain to release its enkephalins? Today, few circuits are known. Much research remains to be done. In the interim, it seems likely that many nerve cells of very different kinds will be firing rapidly along the leading edge of an extraordinary physiological surge. Such extra-high firing rates could release *both* enkephalins and DA from those nerve cells in which these two messenger molecules coexist. Such a mixture might contribute a spectrum of unconventional qualities both to kensho and to its affiliated alternate states.[14] Enkephalin nerve fibers also end next to ACH terminals in several key regions other than in the anterior temporal lobe. Indeed, within the human thalamus, many metenkephalin terminals supply most of the intralaminar nuclei, not only the posterior nuclei.[15] In such ways could a two-phase surge, one which chiefly releases both ACH and enkephalins from their neighboring terminals, exert an overlapping impact. The results could be potent enough both to help create the initial shift and soon thereafter to permeate subcortical *and* cortical functions.

The way normal subjects respond to anesthetic agents could be providing a relevant clue. Many persons experience a sense of great certainty and meanings of immense significance while under the influence of nitrous oxide gas and other anesthetics (see chapter 98). Sudden strong pulses of beta-endorphin, plus other opioids and peptides, may be released under these circumstances. These messengers appear capable of inducing distinctive kinds of "climate" and "atmosphere." They could help infiltrate such meaningful properties into the frameworks of conscious experience that have been created largely by much faster transmitters.

Waking up to a Great Awakening?

When kensho occurs in the morning, and shortly after the person is introduced into a novel situation, it is again reasonable to wonder, Could extra pulses of β-endorphin also be contributing to it? Chemical measurements show that the level of β-endorphin does reach one of its two morning peaks in human ventricular fluid as early as 6 A.M.[16] But later, just after midnight, our beta-endorphin level drops as far as it has risen, falling to its lowest level at around 1 A.M.[17] From then on, a conscious brain's "night of the soul" could seem dark indeed, given the evidence that both its amine *and* beta-endorphin functions would have dropped to their lowest levels.

But finally we stir, quicken, awaken, and each day is born anew. Is "born again" an empty phrase? Perhaps not. Neither is "awakening." Thoreau understood that "All memorable events . . . transpire in morning time and in a morning atmosphere. The Vedas say, 'All intelligences awake with the morning.'"[18] The Asian lotus (*nelumbo nucifera*) also opens during the morning, from five to six A.M. Its large scented flowers, mostly various shades of pink, growing high up out of the mud, are symbolic of Buddhism at many levels of interpretation.

Mornings soon test us against a set of fresh challenges. The morning hours are therefore an important time to begin to change old habits. Fortunately, in the morning, both corticotropin-releasing factor, beta-endorphin, and ACTH will all be released at about the same time. Having these three peptides come to their peak levels in the morning hours could help make it possible for the brain to reshape two of its vital activities: those of conditioning *and* of deconditioning. Both functions are critical (see chapter 74). Each process helps a brain to change its habits, perhaps to change them so much that the creature can survive to see another sunrise.[19] The particular minutes when we awaken into an early morning period of reverie can open up into fruitful avenues of creative thinking.[20,21]

From his review, Bucke concluded that there was a seasonal influence on the kind of "awakening" known as enlightenment. There appeared to be a tendency for these experiences to occur during the first half of the year, especially around May and June.[22] By then, most of us will already have emerged from our own lesser degrees of relative hibernation and seasonal depression. Now, in the extra sunshine and warmth, we will be renewing our lifestyles with added vigor. We now know that when hibernating animals stir from their icelike state, the nerve cells at the leading edge of this springtime awakening are those in the hippocampus and hypothalamus (see chapter 76). Further research into human biorhythms and cyclic events[11] may help define more precisely why some mornings, and the late spring months, could tend to be more open to states of spiritual renewal.

Meanwhile, in a manner of speaking, awakening continues to be used as an alternative term for enlightenment. Is it an appropriate term? Historically, it seems to be. Certainly the legend that the Buddha came to satori when he glimpsed the first morning star lends an intriguing facet to our ongoing quest to understand the origins of awakening.

Third Zen-Brain Mondo

> It is a secret which every intellectual man quickly learns, that, beyond the energy of his possessed and conscious intellect, he is capable of a new energy (as of an intellect doubled on itself), by abandonment to the nature of things.
>
> Ralph Waldo Emerson, "The Poet." In *Essays:* Second Series

How can long years of meditative training create the setting for short states of enlightenment?

Subjective, self-centered preoccupations fade after years of daily calming. This process clears the meditator's "mental space." Gradually, lesser insights enter, and finally the most objective kind of understanding.

What does "letting go" imply in psychophysiological terms?

It means that certain frontal-limbic activities are no longer required, functions that had previously been consumed by unfruitful plans and elaborate supervisory efforts. Awareness now opens up, released from the burden of conditioning. The person can process ongoing events, free from the biased ways the *I-Me-Mine* had viewed events in the past.

How does internal absorption differ from kensho?

Internal absorption sweeps a witness into heightened interior sensibilities. It blocks exterior sensate impressions and stops those which nourish the roots of the *physical* self. Kensho's flashing insight sees into and comprehends all exterior percepts. Simultaneously, it cuts off the conceptual and affective roots of the *psychic* self.

Why use a koan?

The koan is an artificial concentration device. It puts additional pressure on the meditator. It poses a word question that addresses, tangentially, an existential issue no ordinary thinking processes can answer in words. The meditator incubates the question, usually for months or years. Dammed up behind the koan during this interval is a reservoir of inquiry. Finally, in its burst of insight-wisdom, kensho resolves the basic existential issue. After this, the words of the koan are understood to be a mere finger pointing vaguely toward the moon of enlightenment.

What causes the experiential qualities of direct perception and of immediacy?

These qualities imply that parts of the brain are processing data much more efficiently than usual. They suggest that the brain is enlisting its fast neurotransmitters such as acetylcholine and glutamate, and using them within certain massive, fast parallel processing systems.

What does a novel triggering stimulus do to the brain?

It sets off a variety of activating systems, chiefly those releasing acetylcholine and glutamate. In their higher extensions, these systems prompt an early physiological response from the prefrontal regions in particular. One way this prefrontal response shows up is as a prominent electrical potential, the N200–P300 complex. Novel situations also release beta-endorphin and ACTH, along the deep midline regions of the brain.

Why is the brain especially vulnerable to the impact of a trigger only at certain times?

A trigger represents an abrupt influx of stimulation. It prompts the lower cholinergic and glutamate systems in the brain stem to relay their activations to the cerebrum above. Under ordinary circumstances, our layers of inhibitory GABA and serotonin systems, among several others, suffice to hold these lower excitatory mechanisms in check. But some ascending activating projections may still be able to escape. This occurs especially when the brain happens already to be on the rising tide of one of its less stable transition periods. The advancing tidal edge of desynchronization recurs in cycles. It tends normally to occur at three times: (1) during awakening; (2) recurrently during the waking hours; and (3) recurrently as part of entry into episodes of desynchronized sleep (REM sleep).

Could a release of norepinephrine participate in a triggering event?

Sudden sensory stimuli do prompt norepinephrine nerve cells of the locus ceruleus to fire a short burst of impulses. A relatively long silent pause follows this surge. Alternations between bursts and silence might make it easier for alternate states to slip in, and could also help enhance their content.

Does history provide a conceptual model for enlightenment?

The early astronomers were stuck in a *geocentric* mental set. Earth had to be the center of all the action. Then the Copernican perspective came along and changed all that. Sudden enlightenment works in a similar manner: it gets rid of the old, deluded *ego*centric self. Once this old subjective self-referent perspective vanishes, the experiant finally comprehends the way things *really are*. This objective reality is a brand-new paradigm.

Does time dissolve in a different way in absorptions and kensho?

Absorption replaces time with *NOW*. Time feels suspended, as it does at other moments when one's attention is suddenly amplified and intensely focused into a heightened foreground. Kensho dissolves time into *eternity*. In this timelessness, every time-related concept is cut off from its former roots in the psychic self.

Why is insight-wisdom so far removed from the word-thoughts of our ordinary language?

Insight-wisdom yields instant, syncretic comprehensibilities. These idea-messages and impressions convey *understanding*, but this arrives with no words attached. The brain has many networks for wordless comprehension. They link all four of its lobes with related regions in the subcortex farther below. Here, circuits operate with the most ancient of codes, and some will cross the deep midline bridge more readily than others. The kinds of "word language" found in our dictionaries cannot decipher these codes.

What roles could the reticular nucleus of the thalamus play in kensho?

One example: Its sheet of GABA nerve cells normally inhibits the mediodorsal nucleus of the thalamus. In turn, this mediodorsal nucleus enters into complex relationships with both the overlying frontal lobe and the limbic system. Sudden shifts in the balance between these two thalamic nuclei could therefore infuse novel experiential attributes into many thalamocortical functions.

How might the frontal lobes participate in kensho?

Highly selectively. No simple generalization suffices. Some previous frontal sets and functions drop out. Others, falling instantly into place, seem to express the way the normal "associative fluency" of the prefrontal cortex is able effortlessly to integrate its many affiliated functions throughout the brain. The result is a blend.

Could the large pulvinar contribute to alternate states?

Normally, its cosponsoring functions become most active when the person is fully awake. Perhaps some of its capacities could be reflected in the encompassing vacant plenitude of internal absorption. Subsequently, the pulvinar could also help infuse the heights of salience and coherence into the matrix of insight-wisdom.

Part VIII

Being and Beyond: To the Stage of Ongoing Enlightenment

Even as the traces of enlightenment are wiped out, life with this traceless enlightenment goes on forever and ever.

Master Dogen (1200–1253)

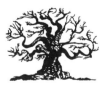

The State of Ultimate Pure Being

Emptiness of the Void (Sunyata) is a term used by Mahayana Buddhism to indicate the Absolute Reality, beyond all characterizing attributes or descriptive adjectives.

D. T. Suzuki[1]

The non-existence of nothingness is the primal nothingness, and so it is the ultimate in all its subtlety.

Yung-chia (665–713)[2]

The path of sudden awakening leads on, beyond the present horizon. Way off "there" lies the "altogether beyond." It is a category of related states. No single term we try to attach to it, such as *Being,* is anything other than a mere approximation. It includes states which neither invite nor require comparisons with fetal, immature, or drugged brain experience.[3] And it goes too deep to be associated with any phantom "spirits" or visions that might earlier have hallucinated their way into the ambient space of the absorptions.

How does it arise? One can only speculate. Keep eroding the *I-Me-Mine* by many years of advanced training, by everyday life practice and episodes of kensho; break free from every clinging vestige of word-thought, body scheme, and psychic self; refine to the nth degree the elemental levels of awareness. Perhaps then what will be left—what would simply *Be*—is the sentient core and connections of the mature brain. There, the basic networks have never lacked for resources; they are merely accustomed to using subliminal codes, an ancient language of atmospheres and impressions. Pre-Sanskrit encoding.

Being taps into the codes for universal relationships. It opens up sublime incomprehensibilities, awesome even to experiants who had formerly thought they might have been living at some advanced ongoing level. Perhaps in its general direction, if not in its destination, a tentative metaphor would invoke that last drop of the larger distillate of what the contemporary Zen monk, Thich Nhat Hanh, chose to call "interbeing."[4] Interbeing is the whole BIG PICTURE. It relates this page of paper back through the pulp to the logger who fed his family by felling the tree, back through the parents who raised him, on through the wheat fields which nourished them all, to the rain clouds and soil and sunshine which made possible all these and everything else.

To Jordan, the hint of Being would come in a form which he termed "beingness."[5] It implied an extraordinary state of conscious awareness that continued in the absence of the universal Self (see chapter 101). For purposes of simplicity, we will also refer to the category of Ultimate Being using the term "State VIII."

It would seem, then, that Pure Being is a state in the direction toward the Ultimate Beyond. Expressed in the depths of this State VIII is the primordial emptiness of the *Heart Sutra,* the Ultimate Nirvana. In its indescribable void will be the extinction of all forms and mental concepts. Gone is any sense that insight-wisdom could ever be something to be attained.

How do we know such a rare "state" really exists? To some persons within the worshiping theistic religions, there might be good reason to doubt that humans could enter a final state which had no specific "holy" resonances coming down from a still higher level. From this "higher principle" perspective, Zen would be as baffling in any era as it once was to the ancient Chinese emperor, Wu. In an old Zen tale, he is said to have asked Bodhidharma: "What is the first principle of [your] holy teaching?" And the monk replied: "Vast emptiness, nothing holy."[6]

The eighth state, Being, seems to go beyond the heights both of ordinary mentation and of affect. Perhaps it would be more accurate to refer to it as "the peace of the depths," instead of as the "peace of the summits." If so, then down "there" would be an emptiness comparable with the kind of total cessation which occurs at absolute zero.[7] Not surprisingly, some persons outside Zen might be as apprehensive about it as they would be about a black hole—too dangerous to get near to, too dense to penetrate, and too distant to be of practical consequence anyway.

Merrell-Wolff reserved the term "pure Being" for that special state of consciousness which had "no subjective or objective element."[8] You might think that when extinction went this far, there would remain no residual properties to which any witness could later attach words. Yet, he continued, it did then seem "As though Space were progressively consuming the whole personal and thinking entity in a wholeness-completion" such that everywhere there was "pure Being." Moreover, even when he had plumbed these deepest depths of darkness and silence, and even after all his "self-consciousness was blown out," he was left with the impression that there remained "a still vaster BEYOND."

Now, a naive question arises. We recall that, during internal absorption, there occurs a kind of inward turning of consciousness. Whereas, during the flash of insight-wisdom the person's vision still sees the external world, but now finds it transformed into a whole new domain of unified reality. So, one asks, is visual perception necessary? Is seeing the details of the external world an absolutely essential part of this next state of Being? Or could even a blindfolded person enter into the essence of Being? One can only speculate. It would be my guess that the kind of "Space" referred to in the lines above does not necessarily imply sight per se. Instead, that it might refer more or less to that level of *insight* which is close to the ultimate refinement of our intuitive faculty. In this instance, it would enable the experiant to draw upon coded associative functions which ramify wordlessly, and sightlessly, throughout many recesses of the large visual brain.

Does Merrell-Wolff's description leave us today any less puzzled than was Wu? We still wonder: what *is* such a state? I stake no claim to prescience in these matters. I confess to have been taken totally by surprise twice before, by all the paradoxes of States VI and VII. My imagination was limited and inaccurate. Yet, everyday imagination can also run too far. Look how generations of interpreters have spun a tissue of images which have further confused the issue of what Nirvana is.[9] Here, we claim no accuracy for the predictions about the form or content of any state(s) beyond the entry level of State VII.

But not to venture any guess would leave us facing a conceptual abyss, and this topic of the eighth state does not merit a nihilistic response. When Naranjo began to address this complex problem, he used a simple diagram.[10] What he was then calling "Being" was located at the ineffable center of four complementary mental states, and it had four arrows pointing to it, as follows:

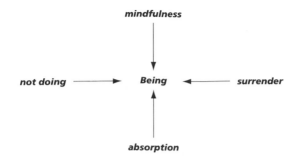

First we need to back up to examine how he had defined "Being." He viewed it as an illuminated knowing which emerged when the ego-self was extinguished, and the depths of emptiness were penetrated. In part VII of this book, however, we had already been saying much the same about the advanced forms of kensho-satori. There we summarized the characteristics of that earlier state of awakening, defined it as categorized by insight-wisdom, and designated it as State VII.* It would seem that Pure Being goes on *from there*. This means that it will plumb further unprecedented, if not incomprehensible, depths, at least in the meditative context when no drugs are involved.

So for our present purposes it seems preferable to modify such a diagram. In the process of first going back one step, let us now take advantage of this fresh opportunity to redefine the general *context* of State VII. By taking this initial step backward, to the previous state of kensho-satori, we can at least clarify what enables *it* to serve as the *prelude* to the next state of Being. Accordingly, what follows below is a gross oversimplification of the context in which State VII occurs. The diagram relabels the center, revises the field, and introduces a potential trigger in the form of a single directed arrow. The trigger could arrive at random or not at all.

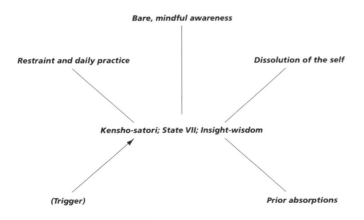

---

* It is only a coincidence that the numbering of the parts of this book now becomes the same as the numbering of the states.[2]

But our original purpose was to try to define Ultimate Pure Being, State VIII. Where did *it* go? Farther on still; altogether beyond. If we keep holding out for something "positive," something *more*, it will surely elude us. It is something *less*, a further subtraction.[7] Indeed, no final list of properties seems to characterize Pure Being. For the purposes of this book, it seems appropriate to do three things: (1) to reaffirm that such a *category* exists, beyond kensho-satori; (2) to suggest that it, too, has depths which shade off, this time into an absolutely "altogether beyond"; and (3) to leave a hint about its ineffable nature.[11]

It might now come as a shock to find that the word God is briefly reentering the discussion. However, to Paul Tillich, "ground of being" served as an optional phrase for the old theistic word, God.[12] What, then, is the extent of this category of Ultimate Pure Being? It lies over our mental horizon, uncapturable by diagrams, let alone by Roman numerals. Whatever remains "out there" will be lying beyond the penultimate comprehensibilities of kensho-satori. Yes, it may begin in a *ground* of being experience. But it will extend toward that "still vaster BEYOND," far off in the direction of those incomprehensibilities which are intrinsic to a paradox that is *groundless*. Off there, in the truly Ultimate Beyond, Pure Being will have rinsed out every molecule of ink from that brush mark of the *enso*. And on the blank paper which remains, there is no trace of a watermark or of any other human symbol.

So what does this leave us with? Is there any suitable way to represent the scope of the eighth state? Perhaps the metaphor of the next, unnumbered page of paper will suffice. Remembering all the while that this is a *state*, and that the person will finally be led back to the everyday earthy ground of interbeing, grateful to see every dandelion blossoming on the lawn, in the sunshine . . .

The Power of Silence

I swear I will never henceforth have to do
with the faith that tells the best!

I will have to do only with that faith that
leaves the best untold.

Walt Whitman (1819–1892)[1]

If I were to demonstrate the Great Matter in strict keeping with the teaching of the
Patriarchal School, I simply couldn't open my mouth.

Master Rinzai[2]

A blank page. The best truths untold. Mouths unopened . . .

Are the advocates of silence engaged in a cop-out? No. It just seems to them that mere words on paper about Buddhist or other experiences of enlightenment are irrelevant. Indeed, among persons most experienced in Zen, few find it necessary even to utter the words *kensho* and *satori*. Elements both of taboo and of personal preference may also enter in. Shunru Suzuki did not use *satori* at all, whereas Daisetz Suzuki regarded it as the "raison d'être of Zen," and used the word frequently.[3]

The orthodox tradition of silence is a very old one. The Greek root *mu*, from which mystic is derived, means silent or mute, and thus unutterable by derivation.[4] Back in ancient China, Tao-sheng (360–434) had said: "Use words to explain thoughts, but silence once thoughts have been absorbed . . . those qualified to seek the truth will grasp the fish and discard the fishing net."[5]

It is a natural hush, this netless silence that both expresses and envelops the most sublime. No one else's words in advance can prepare the aspirant for those profound inner moments when every echo of ordinary discursive word thoughts drops off. Each roshi learns from long experience that students who persist in practicing zazen will awaken, in due course, on their own schedule. Hence, the gist of the old Zen saying: "Better an inch of practice than a foot of preaching."[6] And from the depths of his own understanding Emerson would say: "Do not require a description of the countries toward which you sail. The description does not describe them to you, and tomorrow you arrive there and know them by inhabiting them."[7]

The parsimony of phrasing among the more advanced Zen practitioners reflects a basic neurophysiological fact: the impulse to chatter simply drops away. When *experiencing* the world becomes the operating mode, it replaces talking about it inconsequentially. The meditator learns to avoid being swept up into the pressured jabber of the compulsive talker, or of anyone else whose ververbalizations pass as acceptable forms of social communication. At no time is silence more crucial than during meditative retreats. Then distractions are kept to a minimum so as to help all members of the group become one-pointed. It will be in meditative solitude that one probes most deeply into the layers of self as part of that mindful, introspective search which helps dissolve their fictions.

To preserve the benefits of silence, the ancient Zen masters encouraged dialogue by gesture. Gesture sends rich visual messages. These linger long after tedious word-messages would have been forgotten. Bowing is a powerful gesture. It is an excellent way to practice lowering the sovereign flag of the *I*. Once, a monk asked Rinzai, "What is the essence of Buddhism?" Rinzai's answer was a great *roar.* At this, the monk bowed. Said Rinzai, "That's a man who can hold his own in debate."[8] And in Master Dogen's final year, he too emphasized that the enlightened person would avoid idle talk which could only disturb and distract the mind.[9]

Today, we are battered by decibels, by the sheer noise of what the media offers as "entertainment." No wonder we delight to watch the pure quiet artistry of Chaplin or Keaton in their old silent films. And it is to the mime Marcel Marceau that we will be forever indebted for his telling observation: "You have to understand what is silence, what is the weight of silence, what is the power of silence."[10] This *power* of silence comes from the many levels of understanding within the large auditory brain which do not depend on hearing.

The results of the Andrew Greeley and George Gallup surveys in the mid-1970s suggested that perhaps one out of three persons will feel the power of mystical experiences of some kind or another.[11,12] After they recover, many will want to *know:* What went on? They will be ready for some firm answers, reproduceable results that have originated from reputable brain research.

But hard neuroscience is not comfortable with such soft topics, even in "the Decade of the Brain." And two other aspects of their spiritual quest also disappoint most critical layseekers. The mystical path becomes hard to define, and it is easy to get lost in its noisy thicket of polysyllabic words, arcane concepts, and rituals. Suppose earnest seekers, tiring of pabulum, want a more rigorous approach. If they turn toward Zen, what are their first impressions? High on their list are its evasions and allusions, paradoxes, and nonsense. The public looks for something else. Given the sunshine laws which have raised the public's expectations today, it is surely time to demystify and declassify many aspects of the spiritual path. Silence remains a mixed blessing if religions still keep resorting to it as a coverup for issues which are now best opened up for wider discussion.

On the other hand, mystical experiences seem to have inspired many authors to make voluminous contributions to the literature. This was no less true of Emerson himself, than of Dogen, of D.T. Suzuki, and of countless others representing every religious persuasion. Of course, they might have started out as children with an innately higher pressure toward speaking or writing, or both. Acknowledging this, perhaps there is also something else about the mystical path itself, some impulses that begin to channel the brain of a writer-aspirant toward the solitude in which dwells more *non*spoken forms of self-expression. Diverted from the noise of overt verbalizations, perhaps some inspirations then flow out into literary efforts. Indeed, Alan Watts came to appreciate how his own two earlier mystical experiences had become "the enlivening force of all my work in writing and in philosophy since that time."[13] We do have much to learn about the basic nature of silence. And about the cumulative power of the levels of silence.[14]

But, once again, we'll also need to be careful how we interpret a word as elastic as silence. It has layers of meanings. Similes, metaphors, and other literary devices tend to blur the distinctions between these layers. Consider, for example, what meditators experience in an episode of internal absorption. For one long, blissful moment they will have lost themselves, enchanted in its vast expanse of space. Herein they "hear" the sound of absolute silence, beyond all sound (see chapter 117). This is the early sensate quiet, typical of so-called absolute samadhi. It is merely a faint hint of the depths which silence may reach in the subject who later happens to be penetrated by a major insight into Ultimate Reality. For then, if such an insight does arrive, it can take the form of ineffable messages within an impression of primordial silence. It is noteworthy that the particular nuclei of the brain stem involved in hearing, well-supplied with eukephalin, could be inhibited when they receive an extra-strong pulse of this opioid (see chapter 119). And it is worth pointing out, solely by way of confirmation of the reports of silence among mystics, that a few persons may experience a kind of "void," also described as emptiness and silence, at some time during the course of the most advanced psychedelic states (see chapter 139).

So let us now return to take a second look at some lines which introduced chapter 117, entitled "The Sound of Silence." There, Joseph Campbell would actually seem to have been pointing to a spectrum of phenomena, not only to the usual simple *sensory* connotation of silence, when he chose to write: "All final spiritual reference is to the silence beyond sound." For he then went on to say, "It can be spoken of as the great silence, or as the void, or as the transcendent absolute."[15] And, at this point, his words begin to describe an especially deep level of emptiness, the depths of the authentic void, a state entered by the very few, reserved as a late development on the spiritual path. The few persons who have finally experienced it would not be likely to confuse it with that simpler preliminary silence of absorption cited above, however much that initial sensate silence might once have seemed to be "beyond sound."

Why wouldn't the two "silences" be confused? What have such advanced states of enlightenment finally extinguished and utterly silenced? It is chiefly the central core of that old, wordy egocentric self.[16] That same omnipresent self which, in the past, had always been ready to inject its own psychic language into its every perception. Eleven centuries ago, Huang-po had spoken of the "Stillness beyond all Activity." It came when, with insight, the usual clutter of thought-ideas ceased (see chapter 83). Meanwhile, literary license has frequently gone on to use the one word, "absolute," to describe these two different states, occuring in two very different contexts. This continues to mislead generations of novices, ever ready to believe that when they had first entered the vacuum of their early absolute *sensate* "silence beyond sound" they must have finally arrived at the "transcendent absolute."

The Nobel neuroscientist Walter Hess was in favor of the general closed-mouth approach to the big issues, as was Master Rinzai long before him. Toward the end of his career, Hess suggested that it was appropriate for us to maintain a modest silence, given how ignorant we still were about both the brain and the world in general. We should recognize, he said, that "much exists and evolves in this world which is not accessible to our comprehension, since our cerebral organization is primarily devised so that it secures survival of the individual in its natural surroundings. Over and above this, modest silence is the appropriate attitude."[17]

But Hess's remark about survival begs a basic question. Let us accept the fact that when our progenitors' brains were evolving, it would be under grinding circumstances so harsh that only a lucky few would be fit enough to survive. From such crude beginnings, how could the refinements of enlightened wisdom later emerge? How could ancestral brains, born in times of fierce competition and catastrophe, ever give rise to modern versions of brains such as ours, capable of genuine compassion and altruistic behaviors? These are questions not to silence our neuroscientists and social scientists but to challenge them for many centuries far into the next millennium. Questions we shall return to in chapter 157.

147

Beyond Sudden States of Enlightenment

When your study
Of Buddhism is through
You find you haven't
Anything new.

Master Bankei, Song of Original Mind[1]

When the mind that was in darkness becomes enlightened, it passes away, and with its passing, the thing which we call Enlightenment passes also. Enlightenment exists solely because of delusion and ignorance; if they disappear, so will Enlightenment.

The Teaching of Buddha[2]

There are high-minded, ambitious reasons to aspire to awakening. Who does not share in them, at least in the beginning? The same William James who would not be taken in by "spiritual materialism" had a more tolerant view of those pilgrims who were in "search of the redeemed inward nature." He regarded their quest as the most advanced form of "pure" spiritual self-seeking.[3] Teilhard de Chardin put it somewhat differently, asking, "What is the work of works for man if not to establish, in and by each one of us, an absolutely original center in which the universe reflects itself in a unique and inimitable way?"[4]

Over many years, a very few persistent monks and students—those who undergo multiple awakenings, both gradual and sudden—are led so far beyond all aspirations of the egocentric self that they become fully centered in the universal present moment. As a result, when Zen enlightenment has been completely worked through, it will have passed beyond all the early notions of striving, beyond good works, originalities, uniqueness, and inimitability. By then, sudden brief awakenings will have become matters of fact, transient experiences stripped of institutional religious overtones.

This very word *religion*, when traced back to its original roots, carried so strong a sense of binding that its later derivatives came to mean *ligature. Not until satori also cuts off all such ties can Zen awakening evolve further.* As Hui-neng once phrased it, "If you cherish the notion of purity and cling to it, you turn purity into falsehood . . . And when you claim an achievement by establishing a form to be known as purity . . . you are purity bound."[5] So much for all notions of "purity" that may have arisen when reading the previous chapter.

The Zen way is *self-negating.* Its bonfires consume more than the old verities and vanities. Ultimately, they turn to ashes the whole concept of enlightenment itself. No beginner can believe this. Not until much later come two realizations: (1) only when a brain is still deluded will it "need" to "transcend" its current, less-than-perfect condition; (2) the brain becomes fully awakened to the suchness of the world *when it is totally, continually, and directly in touch with what is going on in the present moment.*

Indeed, after the Buddha's great awakening, he was said to have remained— at every moment thereafter, both coming and going—in the stage of permanent ongoing suchness. He was the *tatagatha* (see chapter 132). A tatagatha is a completely enlightened person who remains fully at home in the natural ongoing flow of Reality itself. To think of someone, in this advanced stage, as being already "There" would be to miss Zen by a mile. *Already Here* is the true meaning. For in this *Here* and *Now,* all distinctions will have vanished between ordinary life and satori. Sacred and profane will have become one. Why? Not because they are merely "thought" to be the same at the level of intellectual knowledge. And not because legend or doctrine says so. But because *they are directly experienced as one and the same,* as they have always been in fact. This is *reality on-line.* Not some hazy, or artificial, or make-believe "virtual reality."

So there is a practical litmus test for complete enlightenment. It is the full, tacit understanding that enlightenment itself is really "nothing special."[6] And whosoever still views his or her enlightenment experiences as "special states" is retaining at least one more layer of attachments. These too will need to be worked through, subtracted and gone beyond. For this reason, the true pilgrim will discover that the path of Zen training has no final destination. Its Way is an endless unfolding. Each successive insight becomes one more point of departure. Each tribulation offers another splendid opportunity to take yet another step on that long journey toward further maturing.

148

The Exceptional Stage of Ongoing Enlightened Traits

> When you are unhindered by bondage or freedom, then this is called liberation of mind and body in all places.
>
> Master Pai-chang Huai-hai (720–814)[1]

The episodes of absorption, kensho, and Pure Being are transient states. For purposes of discussion they are categorized as states VI, VII, and VIII. These moments begin and end. We proceed next to develop a different set of concepts. The first challenge is to find words which describe the *ongoing* transformation just referred to. The next hurdle is to explain how certain transformations can occur and persist *as traits lasting for years*. For the traits that will finally emerge are not simply associated with a very prolonged "plateau experience." "Plateau" only describes a brief, earlier, minor happening. Such an event is not vigorous enough, nor is it sufficiently deep, to create lasting behavioral change (see chapter 5).

I have settled on a long descriptive phrase, "the exceptional *stage* of ongoing, enlightened traits." Why exceptional?" Because even in the monastic context only very few persons reach this rarified altitude let alone continue climbing along its path (see table 11). "Traits," because major dynamic changes have been made, revising the person's old unfruitful attitudes and behaviors.

When we approach this stage, we find three of its aspects interrelated under a single broad theme: *freedom*. We'll need to be especially careful about how we define this word. For this freedom cuts through every contrived ligature that entangles conservative and liberal institutional religions alike. Revealed in its depths will be the liberating core of the religious impulse itself. Why? Because this final transformation will have taken place at basic, psychophysiological levels. Here, there exists as much freedom *from* today's manmade trappings of conventional religion as there is freedom from the licentious entrapments of the self. It is at these basic physiological levels that we will now examine (1) how the freedom originates; (2) what kind of behavior flows out of it; and (3) how that behavior addresses "the opposites."

What is the source of this extraordinary freedom? It must arise from a widely emancipated brain. Why? Because only changes major in scope could then go on to express themselves gracefully in movements, postures, *and attitudes* that remain so liberated both physically and mentally. Unfortunately for clarity, this late stage was another one of the many which got included centuries ago under the rubric of that highly elastic term, *samadhi*. Even so, to Hui-neng it was still the great "eternal samadhi." Here, only the term "eternal" serves to alert us to the fact that he didn't view it as a temporary state. Instead, this was a lasting stage, one marked by a deep *ongoing* realization: the person and the world were in a condition of absolute oneness.[2]

Later, the Soto Zen master Dogen further characterized this stage using the phrase, "Everyday life is enlightenment." For Dogen, the final criterion for becoming supremely enlightened was that the person had entered the "samadhi of self-fulfilling activity," or *jijuyu-zammai*.[3] In the context of Dogen's thought, such a condition implied realizing one's purest, fullest capacities in absolute freedom. And it was this total freedom which expressed one's *original* nature. So here it is, finally, the best definition of what Zen means when it uses the elusive phrase, original nature. To Dogen, one was *born free,* a truth so basic that this memorable phrase is now embedded in our popular music and culture.

How did Dogen recognize when an adult had returned, as it were, to this degree of "original" freedom? He saw that the enlightened person was able to navigate *evenhandedly* between "good" and "bad" alike. Therefore, at this stage, *the awakened person interacts with utmost flexibility among all such opposites.* It is a stage that does not ignore "right" or "wrong." It will not pretend they don't exist. Nor does it hold itself beyond any of the world's other contrasting dualities. It knows the pull of yearnings for good; it feels the push away from the potentially harmful. Its sense of proportion understands the difference between "letting go," and "letting it all hang out." It could not possibly create "new" moralities out of old immoralities. Nowhere does the restraining *sila* of authentic Buddhist Zen afford a clearer contrast with the counterfeit license of "beat Zen."

Sekida observes that the enlightened person enters into a playful, permissive, vigorous liberated interrelationship with the world. This *continues* "on the plane of the normal activity of consciousness, working, talking, even riding in a jolting bus." In previous years, when the meditator had briefly entered into the other, separate moments of absorption, these few seconds had been otherworldly episodes which had left ordinary consciousness far behind. Hence, during the early years of training, the student had available two very different modes of consciousness. One option included acute, transient states and quickenings; the other option included ordinary everyday life. "But now, this is not so."[4] One *stage* of freedom prevails.

Bankei had his first awakening when he was twenty-six years old. What made him different, then, from what he would become later, after he had ripened into greater wisdom? The difference lay in the fact that later in life, "with the perfection and clarity of advanced wisdom, the 'Eye of the Way' becomes clear and bright without a single imperfection of any kind." To arrive at this advanced stage was no easy task; it came about only because he had long cultivated the Way with "total, unswerving devotion." Having gone beyond mere intellectual understanding, Bankei had finally arrived at the stage of living in clear, deep wisdom. Again, there was no room for license in this stage, because his "total freedom" was "fully conversant with the Great Dharma."[5]

Positive things now happen, *with the lightest touch,* to the adept who lives this spontaneously within the flow of events. Is there something supernatural in this degree of actualization? No. Many accounts suggest that the adept's ordinary field of consciousness appears to open up. Perception and action now seem to fuse into a wholly natural-feeling, dynamic unity. So something extraordinary *has* happened. This transformation will enable the person to operate harmoniously, within the world, at a very high level of performance. What is this ongoing, "perfect, clear, advanced wisdom" which Bankei was talking about? And which Hakuin described as a "Marvelous Observing Wisdom" (see chapter 139).

Its symbolic expression is the *urna,* that dot between the eyes in the depictions of the Buddha (see chapter 2). In this book, it will represent properties which emerge from the inside, not the outside, of a three-pound human brain. Although this human brain is a soft biological instrument, it has a singular capacity: it is able both to imagine and to construct tangible metal instruments in its own image. It has helped design many durable products. Three of them can now come to our aid by serving as loose metaphors. For the deeply enlightened brain of the sage seems to deploy a sensitive internal seismograph. Its intuitive functions have been so enhanced that they will pick up subliminal signals long before they turn into rumbles. And this enlightened person of Stage IX stays centered, as though by some internal gyroscope, despite being challenged by the tilt of seemingly impossible circumstances. Finally, there seems almost to be a set of scales, in which the balance comes from an overall sense of proportion. On the pan of one side rests a profound insight into the ultimate and eternal. Weighted evenly on the other side is an earthy good humor which appreciates the intimate fullness of this present moment for all that it contains.

The anonymous sage has become free to operate compassionately from the lowest of profiles. Left behind are all concerns about status, credits, and rank. An old story about Master Hakuin is illustrative. It reveals how remarkable is this capacity finally to enter that stage which accepts, *evenhandedly*, good and bad, triumph and disaster. He was once falsely accused by the parents of a girl who claimed that he had gotten her pregnant. All he said then was, "Is that so?" He even looked after this child for a year, until the young mother finally confessed to having lied about the real father. Her parents then returned to get their grandchild, embarrassed totally and apologizing profusely. One could anticipate that their apologies would have reached heights, and their bows depths, unparalleled outside of Japan. Yet when Hakuin turned the child over to them, he responded only by saying, "Is that so?"[6]

Farther on, the awakened person's attitude evolves into one of total selflessness and wide-open tolerance. There is grateful appreciation, not only for life's simpler essentials but also for each new opportunity to learn by confronting its harsh lessons. If any fruits are forthcoming from the labor, the evolved person remains unattached to them. Hakuin was a critical master, and it is interesting to note the kind words he used when he described this late stage of *living* Zen. It was certainly not that "dead Zen" which he had inveighed against earlier, the one so misapplied that it had tranquilized the person against life. Instead, his next words might almost seem to describe a Taoist sage. "Now you may pass your days in tranquility, drinking tea when there is tea, eating rice when there is rice. If there is nothing further to do, that is all right; if there is something to do, that is all right . . ."[7]

For many generations of students, a series of ten pictures of the herdsman and the bull has served as a traditional visual teaching device. It is an allegory standing for successive phases along the lengthy path to Zen enlightenment.[8] In these sequences, the eighth picture is that empty circle, the *enso*, kensho-satori, the moon of enlightenment. This system of numbering will leave various aspects of the final two pictures to represent, in succession, first, the transient *state* of Pure Being, and last, the ongoing *stage* of enlightened traits (see table 11).

Of these last two pictures, the ninth is entitled *Returning to the Origin, Back to the Source*. Like the empty page resorted to earlier, it shows no traces either of the herdsman or of his bull: merely flowers, rocks, and a blossoming tree. What does it symbolize? Not only the purity of Being, in harmony with Nature in general, but also that basic harmony implicit in our original human nature as well.

The tenth picture is entitled *Entering the Marketplace with Bliss-Bestowing Hands*. We can take it to represent the final, exceptional ongoing stage. The stage is exceptional not only because it is rare. For it is also a distinctive mode of living in the world—helpfully *and effectively*. What makes it so special? Why is the former herdsman smiling and at ease as he enters the hurly-burly of the marketplace? Because he has been liberated from all I-driven impulses to intervene. He now has the sense of being aligned *selflessly* with the world's natural sources of free-flowing energies. And so long as he embodies their simple, artless flow and affinities, his every action will continue to bestow the kinds of bliss that will turn out to be unqualified.

The pictures dramatize both the task and the opportunity facing all students at every step along the Way: "to come home without leaving the world."[9] So deep a transformation reflects an amalgam of trait change, attitude change, and thought change.

149

Simplicity and Stability

> Knowledge is a process of piling up facts; wisdom lies in their simplification.
> Martin Fischer (1879–1962)[1]

The Soto school of Zen is correct. Enlightenment is a gradual ripening, a process of incremental maturation. Very slowly does it reform overall policy, revise daily strategy, and change moment-by-moment tactics. Everyday life *is* enlightenment.

The Rinzai school is correct. Each successive state of sudden enlightenment highlights and redefines anew the human brain's *capacity to change.* Not only in terms of what it can do but also what it can do *without.*

Repeated awakenings and decades of practice can finally bring the exceptional Zen monk into the keenest, most objective, ongoing awareness: *religious realization fully expressed in daily life.* Zen was building up to this rare, unifying mode all along. Not to be tucked away in some rarefied existence, contemplating one's navel, or spinning off increasingly sophisticated abstractions. Instead, to refine one's sensibilities to act within the wondrous immanent present. Right here . . . right now. Living Zen.

What is implied when a sage reaches this advanced stage of ongoing enlightenment? In a figurative sense, the brain's magnetic pole has shifted. New attitudes have fallen into place, realigned along an entire new range of the compass of values. In the following pages, we review a few descriptions of this transformation as they have appeared in the Buddhist literature over the centuries. We then raise the question of its ethical base, and speculate about how such a brain could have changed physiologically.

But first, a word of caution: we will not be talking about the usual Western varieties of temporary, shallow, "born-again" conversions. *Permanent ongoing enlightenment is very rare.* Few indeed are the persons who truly manage to cast off the habitual patterns of a whole earlier lifetime. No single peak experience can permanently eliminate all of a person's ignorant, self-centered perceptions, desires, and aversions. A major problem, as Emerson noted, is that "Our faith comes in moments; our vice is habitual."[2]

Still, the problem is not insurmountable. Myokyo-ni often cited the following Zen story to illustrate how the advanced Zen trainee finally undergoes a profound change of *heart*, not merely a superficial change of thoughts at the level of the intellect.[3]

In order to enter fully into his Zen training, a certain samurai in medieval Japan (the equivalent of a knight) had to leave the lord to whom he had sworn allegiance. Such a change could have come only after a long inner struggle, for to desert one's duty was not permitted under the samurai ethical code. But he did leave, and then trained as a Zen monk for the next ten years in a mountain monastery. Thereafter, he set out on pilgrimage. Unexpectedly, on his path the monk was recognized by another samurai on horseback, a man who was still serving his former lord. This samurai drew his sword quickly and raised it high. Then, deciding not to soil it by striking the monk, he spat contemptuously in the monk's face as he rode on by.

Wiping off the spittle, the monk realized how he would have reacted a decade earlier. Such an insult could only have led to a fight to the death. Deeply moved, he turned and bowed in gratitude toward that mountain monastery where he had received his Zen training. He then composed the following poem:

The mountain is the same old mountain.
The Way is the same as of old.
Truly what has changed
Is my own heart.

A change of heart? What could bring about such a reformation? Only major physiological revisions in the brain. Is the transformed brain emotion*less?* No. It is *stable, balanced, no longer overcome by the ups and downs of the emotions.* Thus did Soyen Shaku, the Zen master whose tour in 1905 introduced Zen to the United States, summarize the fresh attitudes of such an imperturbable brain as a serenity of all the senses, an increased kindness of heart, and a retiring from the field of consciousness of those passions of anger, infatuation, greed, excessive sexuality, and egoism.[4]

Do powerful emotions still intrude? Certainly. But now they penetrate a stable person who dwells in a spirit of equanimity. As a result, anger or desire exert an impact for a moment, not an hour. Or if for an hour, then not for a whole day. Perhaps, in some former social context, the intellect would have raised the old questions such as, How low must I bow? Should I be acting with pride or humility? Now, these conflicts resolve themselves into what Maslow would call "a single complex superordinate unity."[5] More genuine human relationships flow out of the person's sense of deeper kinship with other living and inanimate things. Life does have egregious aspects. These are not denied. But now, because they are seen objectively, they are accepted with fewer subjective dissonances. The potential sword clash of wordly opposites is finally reconciled into the universal, eternal scheme of things. The sky does not fall.

Many people grow, by degrees, as the result of practicing introspection into the troublesome events of their daily lives. The process is not limited to the pilgrims who are on the meditative Way. One raises several children, sees how others' children have been raised, this time from the different vantage point of neighbor, aunt, uncle, or teacher. Finally, one begins to understand the general nature of the interrelationships with one's own children in a much larger interactive context. Whatever wisdom then emerges is the result of participating in the larger dynamic process of caring and parenting. It does not come merely from the passage of time in itself.

Meanwhile, the public looks at Zen through veils of misunderstanding. It views with great skepticism any "born-again" testimonials that may issue from the human potential movement. But long ago in our own country, Emerson had learned what was implied in personal transformation, and some of his knowledge was firsthand. A year before William James was born, Emerson was already speaking of that certain deferential tone, that "wisdom of humanity," which enters when a human being finally and directly encounters the "overarching" spiritual property. Who would finally enter into such an "ineffable" union? It was, he said, those persons who were "lonely and simple." They would be the unsophisticated ones, persons "plain and true," subjects who had dropped off everything "foreign and proud." It would be those who dwelled, he continued, "in the earnest experience of the common day . . ."[6]

In Asia, centuries before, it had been an *accepted practice* to dwell in the earnest experience of the common day. And many observers had also reported that these often solitary, simple people then underwent a series of salutary changes. What words had they used to describe the authentic Zen spirit in its age-old manifestations? Reviewing this vast literature, Harold Stewart, the Kyoto poet, gives us in one paragraph a superb summary of both the form and content of this personal transformation:

> . . . behind an often unprepossessing exterior . . . they rest in compassionate non-attachment and yet display a selfless courage. They delight in silence and solitude, ever quietly contented amid loneliness and poverty. They radiate an unconditional love for children and idiots and old men, for animals and all other beings, sentient and non-sentient, without discrimination. They give their insights suprarational expression through paradox, wordless action, blasphemy, iconoclasm, and obscene humor. They extend a grateful welcome to whatever happens, living always in the present moment, without thought for the morrow. Their unquestioning acceptance of the everyday routine and rigors of monastic discipline, of ceaseless loss and change, of inevitable decay and death; the immediacy and directness of their every thought, word, and act, dealing only with the concrete, the objective, and the particular; their absolute freedom, even from the idea of being free, and above all from moralistic judgements; in the single phrase, their sublime simplicity—these are the principle qualities . . . characteristic of Zen method and attainment.[7]

This is the rare Zen prototype. *It makes no pretensions.* When bleached by the bright, stark moonlight of enlightenment, the purple imperial self fades. Now the natural fabric emerges. To Kobori-roshi, Zen was this "return to the basic simplicity of the undyed fabric." Not so very long ago, we had expected to find many of these same basic virtues exemplified in our kindly neighborhood minister, priest, or rabbi, and sometimes in our family physician: total, selfless commitment to a life of service to others; no distinctions among patients or parishioners in professional attention, neither for economic reasons nor on any battlefield. It is a self-effacing recipe, unlikely to appeal to partisan overachievers of any stripe.

This authentic Zen spirit would be recognized anywhere by an observer who might be inclined to set aside its moments of seemingly blasphemous icono-clasm and obscene humor. At its core is the essence of genuine saintly behavior. So, too, back in medieval Europe, did Saint John of Ruysbroeck (1293–1381) de-vise the following rule of thumb specifying which character traits identified the rare enlightened man of his era, as distinct from other persons: "Whereas the enlightened man, by virtue of the divine light, is simple and stable and free from curious considerations, these others are manifold and restless and full of subtle reasonings and reflections; and they do not taste inward unity, nor the satisfaction which is without images. And by this they may know themselves."[8]

Simple and stable. Key ingredients which identify a bodhisattva, a saint, or a wise old sage in any century. For each of these persons has come to value his or her simplest life experiences, to perceive them directly and resonate with them deeply. These simple people don't need images, don't crave royal purple, or chase other fantasies. Their reality is in the present moment. The time finally came for the same Soyen Shaku to give a Buddhist name to his young pupil, T. Suzuki. He chose Daisetz. It was a sincere compliment. It means "great simplicity."[9]

But our era has now reached increasingly sophisticated heights. Spacecraft fly far past the moon to probe the first light years of outer space. Our self-help literature advertises a Zen you can "use" to drive your car efficiently in traffic. It will enter easily into motorcycle maintenance, lower your golf score, and help you "perform" countless other useful activities. On the other hand, the rare classic prototype person will be practicing Zen Buddhism at a rather different level. This practice doesn't only enter—it *is* everyday life. In a very real sense, the world is now living itself out.

Authentic Zen has always meant inhabiting each present moment in the most natural, direct, and spontaneous way. At such a deeply enhanced level of present awareness, the sage will have shed every layer of conditioned affectation, dropped every self-conscious concern for what current conventions might regard as the "religious" implications of behavior. Ruth Sasaki once distilled this whole Zen approach to life into one sentence. It was "A life lived in full realization of who we really are and what this world we live in really is; a life lived simply, naturally, spontaneously, and awarely; a life dedicated in infinite gratitude to the past, infinite gratitude and service to the present, and infinite responsibility to the future."[10]

Is there room for humility in the Zen prototype? Yes, but not for the ordinary kind, because much of what usually passes for humility still has vestiges of im-modesty. Genuine humility emerges choicelessly, naturally, on its own. It is like internal tranquility. You can't enforce it deliberately by an exercise of thought. Humility begins to stir when spiritual trainees first enlarge their capacity to rec-ognize their own inner failures and resolve to correct them. This particular self-critical faculty grows slowly at first, but finally becomes "crucial to the practical art of spiritual inner development."[11]

Zen simplicity isn't some cookie cutter which clones out each enso in the shape of a round, standardized product. Trainees don't lose their individuality when responding to life's complexities. Nor does simplicity imply the hermit-like retreat of a once-social animal, a recluse who withdraws from making positive contributions to others. It means becoming an organic member of the everyday world, like a sturdy fruit tree whose deep roots have slowly adapted even to the most meager of topsoils.

Observe the many slender branches of some other, wild apple tree that had never been restrained by pruning. Long canes grow in and out in a counterproductive tangle of limbs. Their branches not only bear little fruit but later snap off during any big windstorm. Zen training prunes back the egocentric self. With each cut into the *I-Me-Mine,* those chemical messengers which had once been so inturned, those pathways which had been working at cross-purposes, now become available to flow outward, and to nourish increasingly constructive ends. The result will be a series of sturdy extensions of the basic personality. A human tree: simple, stable, more fruitful.

Looking back from the perspective of this late stage, how are we to visualize the role played by those earlier states of quickening, absorption, and awakening? For these brief episodes were encouraged and manifested by temporary physiological *instabilities.* What kinds of alchemy could enable a succession of these moments to set the stage for the late development of genuine *stability* and simplicity? We address this major puzzle three chapters farther on.

Meanwhile, there remain two other nagging questions to be confronted. First, Does Zen have an ethical foundation? Second, Is it true that genuine compassion can find nourishment and grow after there has occurred so vigorous a pruning, conducted so unsentimentally, of the deep roots and branches of the personality?

150

An Ethical Base of Zen?

Self-nature is without error, disturbance, and ignorance.

Master Hui-neng (638–713)[1]

This teaching spreads Enlightenment as with the Buddha of old, by the transference of truth from one man to another. In the matter of religious discipline, it practices the true method of the wise men of old. Thus, it teaches Enlightenment, in substance as in semblance, and perfects the relationship between master and discipline. In its rules of conduct and discipline, there is no confusion between good and evil.

Master Eisai (1141–1215)[2]

It was a good time to import Chan to Japan. And it was with these words that the Tendai monk, Eisai, made his formal proposal to do so. Soon, the Kamakura period (1192–1333) would degenerate into an era of societal corruption and decline. Why, then, did Eisai believe that his new teachings could repair the frayed ethical fabric of Japanese culture? After all, Zen tends not to state explicit rules of conduct. And in the minds of some outsiders, who see it dropping out distinctions between right and wrong, it seems ethically so neutral as to appear *a*moral. Could anything so iconoclastic have an "ethical" base?

Many centuries later, in our own difficult era, Abraham Maslow would still be speaking to this issue. He concluded that "peak experiences" enable people to grow, this time in the direction of what would now be called "self-actualization."[3] If so, then how could mystics, East and West alike, escape from those twin perils which beset the long mystical path: the one of drifting ill-channeled; the other of being reduced to what Maslow called "the merely-experiential?"[4] It will not do to reply that real mystics must have entered some special inside track, as it were, and that they have become privy to the natural laws of the universe. In fact, some people prefer to believe that Nature manages quite well with no ethical laws at all, as distinct from laws we humans invent on its behalf.

In practice, Zen Buddhism is more ethical than might be supposed. It merely tends not to dwell on it. Some of the reasons date back to those distant centuries when early Zen came of age in the cultural setting of Confucianism. Chan then devised its own set of ten commandments, going on to honor the social compact by professing and by practicing them.[5] But the central fact remains one which I soon realized, and which Hui-neng had enunciated in the opening quotation above: "wrong" actions won't arise when a brain *continues* truly to express the self-nature intrinsic to its kensho experiences. Hui-neng went on to describe the process as follows: "Imperturbable and serene, the ideal man practices no virtue; self-possessed and dispassionate, he commits no sin; calm and silent, he gives up seeing and hearing; even and upright, his mind abides nowhere."[6] Every year, a few monks in many religious disciplines rediscover this phenomenon.

If these words define the "ideal" person, then how long will it take the Zen aspirant to reach this ongoing stage of simplicity and stability? Decades, not months. Decades of Pavlovian unlearning and of reconditioning. In the interim, departures from the ideal are the rule. Neither Zen masters nor their followers can be perfect all of the time. Well may the skeptic ask: Can one practice no virtue but commit no sin? Is it really possible to do so, let alone worthwhile? One answer is that the acts of the awakened person are sel*fless*. The reason they seem to lack "virtue" is that they spring from a genuinely low profile, but one of high awareness. It is a posture lacking all sense of status and pride. It doesn't look around for self-congratulatory pats on the back, nor does it seek outside rewards. Moreover, no aspirant is likely to violate the sacred quality of all things who has once seen into them and shared in their workings. William Wordsworth expressed this utmost sense of respect as follows:

> To every natural form, rock, fruit or flower,
> Even the loose stones that cover the highway,
> I gave a moral life.[7]

Albert Schweitzer's moment of insight infused him with such reverence for all life that it redirected his career into that of a physician-missionary. This same process of discovering things as they *really* are, the moment when true suchness is found to reside everywhere in life, helps channel the Zen aspirant along similar responsible, affirmative lines. As a result, Buddhism does indeed operate within an ethical framework. However, it is one an outsider or a novice can easily overlook, because it is basically *revealed to each person silently* as well as in a series of formal precepts which are elaborated on vocally, in writing, and by example at traditional institutional levels. Aitken-roshi has addressed this specific issue of Zen Buddhist ethics. He includes in his essays the following incisive comment about Zen practice by one of his teachers, Yamada-roshi, who summed it up in one sentence: "The purpose of Zen practice is the perfection of character."[8]

In some Soto Zen temples, an inscribed wooden board stands at the entrance. It says, simply: *Kyakka-sho-ko*. Translated freely this means "Look under your feet."[9] Raising a shoeless foot and peering beneath it, the puzzled visitor or novice finds only a wooden floor, its grain gradually worn smooth over the years. Could there be more to the phrase? Consider how much friction is likely to occur when persons must live together and work at close quarters in a busy monastery, and in a small country bustling with 125 million people. Much courtesy is already implicit in this phrase, even if you first give it the shallow interpretation not to tread on someone else's toes.

Zen has many allusive statements of this kind. They're not instantly as clear to the Westerner as are such phrases as "Do unto others as you would have them do unto you." But some of the statements will also carry a similar message. It can be interpreted along the following lines: Zen is not an anything goes version of the old Taoist expression, *wu wei*. Yes, things do evolve in their own natural rhythms. But ethics begins at home. *First get your own personal house in order*. At the outset, develop a sense of composure. Learn how to relate courteously and effectively to others, and be kind to yourself as well. Do these things first, in all those nitty-gritty matters that come up in everyday life. After *that*, you'll be able truly to attend to the far more complex imponderables that beset the rest of the needy world.

Thus did the young monk, whose shaved head was already bursting with lofty notions about Buddhism, receive the very best, long-range advice when he began by saying to his master: "I have just entered your monastery; please give me instructions." At which old Joshu replied: "Have you had your breakfast?" "Yes, I have," replied the monk. "Then," said Joshu, "wash your bowls."[10] And a contemporary teacher living in an era which invites a more explicit reply might have considered adding: do so *mindfully, in the present moment*. Pirsig adds another current perspective to the larger practical issue, concluding that: "The way to see what looks good and understand the reasons it looks good, and *to be at one with this goodness* as the work proceeds, is to cultivate an inner quietness, a peace of mind so that goodness can shine through."[11]

In our culture, vital living usually implies doing something active to better the world. Self-actualization tends to mean doing more than smelling the flowers and composing poetry. To the early Greek philosophers, true happiness arose not by retreating to live permanently in solitude off on some mountaintop. It came from the full use of all one's powers along lines of excellence. Confirmation of this principle comes from a contemporary study. It was based on the ways adolescent students felt, using samples taken at various times during their everyday activities. When did they feel happiest, the most cognitively efficient and highly motivated? At the particular times when they had raised their sights and were pitting their own highly developed skills against equally high challenges.[12]

Does Zen training stop every impulse to encounter and to improve the world? No, but it invites one to look into the layers of do-goodism as distinct from those of real service. The interrogation begins to open up during moments of introspection: Do *I* have something to prove to myself? Is there something inside *Me* which *I* must make *My* concern to impose on others? Gradually, the long years of probing and training cut off one hidden personal premise after another. Slowly, the person's altruistic priorities redirect themselves toward genuine challenges which become less neurotically driven. In the process, the trainee finds other options. Some of them seem to have been weighed at depths where that wiser, well-oiled set of scales prevails. The Hindu Upanishads have long insisted that a person can remain nonattached in the world but still connected to it, and that nonattachment does not mean indifference or abandonment.[13]

Newborn babies are predisposed to respond when they hear evidence of others' misfortune. Even one- and two-day-old infants will cry when another infant cries.[14] This crying response predominates during the first year. It then yields to more mature, empathic attempts to comfort the victim. Thereafter, people of different temperaments vary widely in what kind of ethical imperatives they have, and in how much time and energy they will devote to becoming involved in the world. Watts observed that we each have finite limits to how much we can improve ourselves, adding that no one should overlook the natural delights of daily living in the frantic effort of trying to become a better person.[15]

Zen has always carried the same positive message: life is to be celebrated as it really is, right here in the present moment. Don't moralize about it and agonize endlessly over its every injustice. *The first reformation remains the internal one.* It starts at the very place where one's own feet stand. Zen practice begins *here*. It focuses on perfecting the character of that driven, *I*-beset person whose feet stand on this very spot. Thereafter, when the natural ethical response does move outward into the world beyond this spot, its reformations will be authentically *selfless*. And this is what will make them so effective.

151

Compassion, the Native Virtue

Zen does not teach to destroy all the impulses, instincts, and affective factors that make up the human heart; it only teaches to clear up our intellectual insight from erroneous discriminations and unjustifiable assertions; for when this is done, the heart knows by itself how to work out its native virtues.

D.T. Suzuki[1]

The feeling of compassion is only possible when there is an understanding that suffering exists in the other.

Asenath Petrie[2]

Each year Americans donate 19 billion hours of volunteer work to causes outside themselves. This does not count the many other instances when someone has made a quick, heroic sacrifice for a total stranger.[3] Still, we inhabit a misanthropic world. How does it regard such a sudden act of Good Samaritan altruism? As being so contrary to self-preservation that it probably has hidden, neurotic motives.

Compassion's primitive, biological roots do not stem from complex, thoughtful sentiments. But neither do they arise at random nor out of sheer ignorance. Perhaps they go as far back as that early highly instinctual interpersonal behavior: the way small fellow creatures huddle together, finding warmth while sharing it. In human societies subsequently, our ordinary levels of compassion tend to be sentimentalized and overvalued. Even with the best of intentions, much of what passes for ordinary compassionate giving still remains self-serving in one hidden way or another. This knowledge once led Kahlil Gibran to observe how "the kindness that gazes upon itself in a mirror turns to stone, and a good deed that calls itself by tender names becomes the parent to a curse."[4]

True ongoing compassion develops slowly. It takes decades of practice before one responds wisely, selflessly. To Kobori-roshi, the process was like the ripening of a persimmon. It too is "sharp and astringent at first, but warmed by the autumn sun it begins to sweeten. Even its coloring gradually mellows. When still high on a branch, hard and green, it can benefit no one. But once it falls to the ground and disintegrates, other lives can partake of it, while its seeds go on to take new life."[5]

If you have ever recoiled from the sharp taste of an unripe persimmon, you'll appreciate his simile. And you may wonder thereafter, how could any chemical process transform so bitter a fruit into a rare delicacy? The fact is, sourness has to phase out in order for sweetness fully to emerge. This elementary lesson, written large on so many pages of Nature's open book, is true of humankind as well: the darker sides of the egocentric self must be transformed if our latent virtues are to prevail.

William James once said about wisdom that it was "the art of knowing what to overlook."[6] Could this be the whole answer to our search for the origins of authentic wisdom? For if this were indeed so, then the reductionist might go on to reach a simplistic conclusion: what we are searching for is only a special pattern of small lesions which have caused the brain to "overlook" certain things. So are we to think of wisdom only as a kind of "negative sign," as the result of many disconnections which led the brain to neglect some things that it formerly overattended to? Or as "subtractions" which caused it to "let go," and to be detached from some of its overactive emotional systems? Or as deficits which led the brain to adopt a kind of "selective forgetting" in its memory system?

Or, on the other hand, could the brain possess some "positive" intrinsic functions which are always there, ready to emerge? In this case, we could also propose the release of a basic process, the potential of which *is affirmative, at its core.*

The Mudra of Natural Compassion

As Suzuki hinted, one first needs to clear out the dense thickets from the apple orchard, get rid of the old errors of perception and false opinions. After this is done, it becomes clear that the young seedlings of compassion are already established in the soil there, ready to grow taller. The ground out of which they arise is the most intimate of all premises: each person's fundamental identity with all other persons and things. In the allegory of the ten oxherding pictures, it will not be until after the old perceptions and attitudes have finally vanished that the enlightened person's behavior now shows him capable of "entering the marketplace with bliss-bestowing hands."[7]

For centuries, various forms of religious art have been expressing the basic principles of *behavioral* neurology.[8] Talented artists became sensitive to the simple facts of body English and to the mudra of natural compassion. Accordingly, they depicted their subjects' postures and gestures as opening up into extension and supination. Arms were shown reaching out gracefully to serve the world, not stiffened into acts which would clutch it in firm embrace or thrust it away in dismissive acts of rejection or revulsion.

There exist, of course, deep psychophysiological counterparts for these motoric expressions of compassion. And there are also precedents stretching back over two thousand years for that socially engaged Buddhism which infuses its traditional compassion and virtues into the daily life of the community. In ancient India, these messages were literally carved into stone in the form of the edicts of its Buddhist emperor, Ashoka. The inscriptions date far back into the third century *before* the Christian era began.[9] Modern versions on the theme are exemplified by the impressive social commitment of the Zen Buddhist monk, Thich Nhat Hanh.[10] Despite the bitter tragedy of Vietnam, his deeds remind us, as do his words, that "The absence of anger is the basis of real happiness, the basis of love and compassion."

From Empathy to Fully Ripened Compassion

So, at the personal level, this very spot where your own feet stand, the process of ripening is inevitably twofold. From the beginning, it means not only the addition of empathy. The really hard part is learning to subtract and rechannel anger. The root origins of this word, *empathy,* reflect the way we start with our own subjective state, and then project it out onto some other person or object. In children, the swelling buds of empathy become evident during their second year. But if this early process is to leaf out and grow into fruitful altruistic behaviors,[11] children will first need to see empathy honored at home. We adults teach them, by our own conduct toward others, that humanity is indeed shared and coextensive.[12] It turns out that most children, by elementary school, are already behaving in ways which exemplify the basic notions of fair play and of how to share with others.[13]

Still later, in adult life, Zen meditation has itself been used to nurture empathy in psychological counselors at the master's degree level.[14] After only four weeks of regular zazen, these student counselors increased their affective sensitivity and their openness to experience. Meditation was most effective among the trainees who had little capacity for empathy to begin with. Yet the nascent stirrings of such empathy are only a prelude. For empathy is limited to the observer's *perceptive,* imaginative side. In itself, empathy carries no direct responsibility to go on actively to improve the situation.

Compassion does have this responsibility. True compassion means we correctly perceive a situation, sense how it would affect us, project our feelings sympathetically toward the other person, *and then reach out selflessly* to respond in the most sensitive, appropriate way. In this manner does fully ripened compassion, subtly informed by the most enlightened wisdom, deliver the milk of human kindness deftly, *non*intrusively.

The technical term for this selfless level of compassion is *karuna*. What else distinguishes it? It is more than mere occupational therapy for the donor. For it operates within the always-so, the eternal, the Universal. It is "in service in the universe," as Martin Buber reminded us. Therefore, at first glance, its true qualities could go unrecognized by the casual critic who might dismiss Zen as being limited to spur-of-the-moment impulsive acts that would simply focus only on the here and now. In fact, this profound compassion taps wellsprings so deep that its flow avoids every added layer of human artifice. Why? *Because the process is automatic.* In Dogo's classic reply one finds the essence of that instinctual quality which makes it so skillful. He was once asked, "How does the Bodhisattva of Compassion use all those many hands and eyes?" He answered wisely: "Like someone asleep, adjusting the pillow in the middle of the night."[15]

Reflect on his answer. One does not perform deliberate acts while asleep. (Nor does a calm sleeper clutch or pound the pillow.) In like manner does this level of fully ripened compassion arise as an *un*premeditated, *un*selfconscious *native virtue*. The instinctual sensitivities embodied in the Bodhisattva of Compassion will encompass all the generations, born and unborn, both of ignorant humans and of innocent animals.

Master Dogen emphasized the positive aspects of the quality we call altruism today. Then, as now, it meant helping other persons, but with absolutely no regard for one's own benefit. Who among us can be the vehicle for such genuine, selfless service to others? Only that server who has first broken free from all self-attachments. But for Dogen, true altruism also meant being neither gullible, unrealistic, nor all sweetness and light. "Going forth with helping hands," yes. Yet acting skillfully, not with the kind of indulgence that works to the disadvantage of the recipient. For Dogen also noted that altruism could express itself in strong actions which might first cause suffering. And other persons, who were blind to the depths of understanding these actions sprang from, could misinterpret such acts as being arbitrary and insensitive. To illustrate, Dogen cited the story of the Zen abbot who had once asked his assistant to beat and drive away a deer that was eating grass in the monastery garden.

The abbot's request met with a vigorous challenge: "Why strike the poor animal and begrudge him the grass? Where is your compassion?" To this, the abbot replied, "You do not yet understand. If we do not chase away the deer, it will soon become too tame. Then, when it approaches an evil person, it will surely be killed. That is why it must be chased away."[16] Is such tough love insensitivity? Or is it skillfully applied compassion, sage enough to take the long view?

Growing up, one encounters a few kind children, and a few cruel bullies, with most other youngsters falling in between. Why, at any age, do bullies act insensitively? Perhaps some of them begin by perceiving differently, or feeling differently. How easy it is for a color-blind person to trample, unknowingly, on small red flowers blooming among the greenery, whereas the rest of us, thanks to normal color vision, will step elsewhere. So if some persons can't develop empathy to the fullest, it might be because they have always been "reducers," not capable of totally sharing the anguish of others' painful experiences[2] (see chapter 80; table 13).

The Chinese use two characters, representing "a passage to the heart," to express the word "caring." In old China and Japan, the early Indian Buddhist principles of compassion and mercy went on to become embodied in the bodhisattva called Quan-Yin (J: Kannon). Now the compassion principle would evolve to reach its ultimate expression. Transformed by the alchemy of supreme enlightenment, it would finally become *dispassionate*. Dispassionate? Is this another Zen paradox? No. It implies only that the *self*less state has lost all selfish passions. Those who chant the *Heart Sutra* (see Appendix A) are celebrating this bodhisattva's highest level of unselfconscious compassion. And they will be extolling this benevolent principle as the essence of Buddhist practice, not as some abstract conceptualization.

In the West, the cultural emphasis now tends to be placed on individuals. We are encouraged to follow our own star, our own "enlightened self-interest." And out of this, we are led to presume, something will (or should) "trickle down" which will also work out to benefit society as a whole. The other side to this coin is the selfishness pervading our "me generations."

The rare sage is different. This sage, who lives within the stage of ongoing enlightenment, sees all beings as one and the same. Now where is the enlightened interest? It will have expanded to equate with that of the whole universe. So what happens finally, after all the old conceptual barriers and highly charged distinctions have vanished? Now, *self = other*. The once-isolated human being has finally entered into the ultimate human equation. And this basic principle, that self indeed equals other, is an equation as fundamental to everyone as $e = mc^2$. Once compassion issues from this ground level of being, the whole person becomes free to relate, ecologically, to the entire environment. Where is the old egocentricity? It has turned inside out. *Ecocentricity* prevails.

Albert Einstein seems to have appreciated this universal *human* equation, for his mental reach extended to regions beyond the abstractions of mathematics. Consider the following sentences in a letter he wrote to a bereaved father. The recipient was a rabbi whose grieving daughter had become inconsolable after her sister had died.

> A human being is a part of the whole, called by us "universe," a part limited in time and space. He experiences himself, his thoughts and feelings, as something separate from the rest—a kind of optical delusion of his consciousness. This delusion is a kind of prison for us, restricting us to our personal decisions and to affection for a few persons nearest to us. Our task must be to free ourselves from this prison by widening our circle of compassion to embrace all living creatures and the whole nature in its beauty.[17]

Zen also focuses on this same "optical delusion of consciousness" in which we have imprisoned ourselves. Was Einstein talking about Zen? Perhaps not directly or deliberately. However, it would be in the same larger sense that Joseph Campbell came to the conclusion that Buddhism was the closest, most valid mythology for this planet. But, while doing so, Campbell became very specific about what constituted the major practical problem. It was that *people could not recognize that all beings are, in fact, Buddha beings, that they are all part of the whole.* So to Campbell, this meant that there was really "nothing to do." Instead, the first task was simply "to know what is." From then on, he said, one could "act in relation to the brotherhood of all these beings."[18]

Earlier we observed how a little gift, arriving unexpectedly, changes a person's behavior (see chapter 79). It doesn't take much. Trivial things like a cookie, a dime, or a note pad will create temporary feeling states. These tend to spread into overtly positive behaviors during the next few hours. The social implications are not trivial. For let us now suppose you had been granted perhaps the most momentous gift of all. Finally, you comprehended what *really is*, that fundamental unity which joined you into a sharing relationship with all things. Would not this sense of interconnectedness help you express the native juices of compassion? And for much longer than a few hours?

152

Etching In and Out

> Any adequate neurophysiology of learning will have to acknowledge this truly remarkable state of affairs: *it is possible to disengage from a functional nervous system what previously has been learned,* while at the same time maintaining full (indeed, enhanced) awareness.
>
> G. Globus[1]

> Excitatory amino acid systems literally have the power to promote the normal development of, or to destroy, many neurons in the mammalian central nervous system.
>
> J. Olney[2]

Etching is an old term. It originated in the process used to prepare a surface for printing. It implies that something must first be *removed*, before something else can occur. Like Zen training, etching proceeds through a series of steps in sequence, no single one of which suffices. First, a hard needle-sharp point digs through the thin surface layer of an acid-resistant resin. Continuing to penetrate, the sharp tip inscribes the desired design into the surface of the underlying copper plate. In the next step, a wash of acid eats into each fine, V-shaped incision cut into the exposed copper. This erodes the shallow cut into a long deep valley. Now it will be capable of retaining printing ink. A layer of ink is then applied to the whole surface. Once the excess ink has been wiped off this broad plateau, the valleys remain the only places still full of ink. Finally, with further pressure, the etched valleys yield their lines of ink, with precision, into each successive sheet of absorbent paper.

Nothing happens unless you first cut out certain discrete regions selectively. Only then do the subsequent intaglio prints yield their crisp black-on-white contrasts. Suppose a highly salient alternate state "etches itself into memory." Is it possible that, somewhere, such a process also removes certain minute parts of the brain? Was Kobori-roshi on the right track when he once placed his arms down into a long V and spoke to me about "a cut in the mind?" (see chapter 25). In this chapter, first we explore the literal implications of this gesture. Later, we venture an additional suggestion—a slower, metabolic mechanism—to explain how the brain of an enlightened sage could become *structurally different* from before, not be merely thinking a few different thoughts.

Another Role for Glutamate

Certain alternate states instantly heighten consciousness. This fact alerts us to the likely possibility that fast-acting excitatory amino acids are among the transmitters released at the time. And so we return, once again, to L-glutamic acid, the most abundant free amino acid in the adult brain (see chapter 45; figure 10). It exists in the form of its sodium salt, glutamate, and is concentrated in temporal cortex, basal ganglia, cerebellum, and amygdala.[3]

When glutamate nerve cells release this fast transmitter onto their receptors, it excites the next nerve cell. So, too, does its related molecule, aspartate (the salt of aspartic acid). The levels of these two amino acids are a thousand times greater in the brain than are those of the biogenic amines. Many lines of evidence suggest that they serve as the major physiological messengers in our everyday *fast*, point-to-point, neurotransmission.[4]* For example, glutamate nerve cells play a vital excitatory role in speeding impulses from cortex to the basal ganglia, in transmitting messages down the perforant path to the hippocampal formation, and in stimulating its CA1 pyramidal cells through collaterals from the CA3 field, to cite only a few of their countless functions (see figure 6).

On the other hand, recent research suggests that the glutamate receptors on the next nerve cell are its vulnerable Achilles' heel. Indeed, when excess glutamate overactivates this postsynaptic nerve cell, *it causes it to die*.[5,6] So, could excitatory amino acids act to "etch" away certain parts of the brain? Not of course in the strict literal sense, as do strong acids which release many hydrogen ions, but etch nonetheless?

Monosodium glutamate provided the first striking evidence that excitotoxins do cause *selective* nerve cell death in the brain. Monosodium glutamate (MSG) is the familiar food additive, in use everyday, and not only in Chinese restaurants. In young laboratory rats, excess MSG destroys, selectively, 80 percent of the nerve cells in the arcuate nucleus of the hypothalamus[7] (see chapters 43 and 47). This key nucleus is the site in the young brain most vulnerable to the excitotoxic effect of excitatory amino acids. Even after researchers inject the excitotoxins at a far-

---

* Amino acid transmitters occur in micromolar concentrations (millionths of a mole).

distant site subcutaneously, these chemical messengers still get into the circulation, hone in on the arcuate target, stimulate it, and destroy it. This fact suggests that arcuate nerve cells are rendered vulnerable to glutamate toxicity because they are coated with glutamate receptors. Our review has prepared us to understand how important the arcuate nucleus is. For example, these very same arcuate cells normally make the two pivotal stress-activated peptides, beta-endorphin and ACTH. And, when stimulated, arcuate cells then release these messengers widely throughout thalamus, hypothalamus, amygdala, and midbrain[8] (see figure 3).

What causes a nerve cell to die an excitotoxic death? The following sequences unfold. First, excess glutamate is released from local nerve terminals. It then activates one or more kinds of its amino acid receptors on the next cell.[9] These receptors depolarize the next nerve cell, open up its membrane channels so that more sodium and calcium flow in, and start a cascade of other changes. This affected nerve cell now fires excessively fast, in a burst of speed. At first, it looks healthy. By the next day after the surge, however, the cell is obviously breaking down. This occurs because the excess calcium which leaks into it is setting off another round of toxic-metabolic and structural changes.[10] Nitric oxide may be a collaborator, actively participating in this local process of delayed cell death (see chapter 98).

A short distance away from the hypothalamus is another important avenue in the limbic system. It is the mossy fiber pathway, another glutamate relay sending excitatory input into the hippocampus[11] (see figure 6). Normally, when messages exit from mossy fiber nerve endings, they stimulate the next cells, the CA3 pyramidal cells, into a burst of firing. But these hippocampal CA3 cells also die if they have been overstimulated by too much input entering from their mossy fiber pathway.[12]

Indeed, CA3 *and* CA1 cells degenerate after 45 minutes of excessive electrical stimulation to the fibers coming down the perforant path. Thereafter, the overstimulated rats show defects in learning and in spatial memory[13] The injection of kainic acid is another experimental technique which enhances cell death. This molecule mimics glutamate, and it overactivates many of glutamate's receptors in the brain. Kainic acid kills even more CA3 cells if, at the same time, stress responses have risen to such a degree that high concentrations of adrenal glucocorticoid hormones have reached the brain.[14] And another way to enhance nerve cell death is to activate serotonin subtype 2 receptors.[15,16]

Many of the nerve cells in the prefrontal cortex normally release glutamate. When these glutamate neurons discharge, a series of excitatory events occur. Some are obviously direct effects. Others are subtle and *indirect*. For when glutamate fibers stimulate the basal ganglia beneath them, they also help, indirectly, to enhance the release of dopamine there.[17] In such primary and secondary ways can glutamate excitation up in cortex go on to doubly energize behavior. Moreover, when a potent derivative of aspartate is released into this prefrontal cortex, it too can cause profound damage to local frontal nerve cells.[18]

One other amino acid pathway can serve as a model. It helps us envision how the death of one of its nerve cells, even though it is localized to one region, could go on from there to have a kind of indirect domino effect on behavior. This particular path projects forward from the hippocampus, and releases its glutamate into the lateral septum[19] (see figure 6). Let us suppose that the cells of this amino acid pathway were to fire excessively, and that this process would cause selective damage to certain lateral septal nerve cells. And suppose that these same septal neurons—the ones which have now been neutralized—had previously been key links in a particular chain of *dys*functional, overemotionalized behavior. (Figure 6 shows a specific segment of one such potential chain. This link connects the lateral septum with the mediodorsal thalamic nucleus, and its relays lead on from there to the orbitofrontal cortex.) Once this dysfunctional circuit—or an equivalent circuit—has been interrupted, its prior contributions to behavioral dysfunction could drop to very low levels. And they might remain neutralized permanently if a sufficient number of other links in the chain had been severed at points throughout the whole network. In such ways could a brief change in state, as this change evolved through successive levels of the limbic system and thalamus, be followed by an enduring change in *trait*.

When the normal hippocampus is already being excited by glutamate, dynorphin further enhances the flow of impulses through CA cells.[20] Moreover, repeated local doses of dynorphin cause CA cells to die. Why? Probably because two things happen. Dynorphin acts on *mu* opioid receptors directly. This reinforces the spontaneous burst firing of CA3 cells.[21] Moreover, as an indirect effect of dynorphin, the local amino acid receptors themselves become activated to an excessive degree.[22,23]

The several studies cited above make it clear that the brain's own excitotoxins can be potent agents, prompting a kind of highly localized "etching" away within certain vital regions. The evidence will be leading us to ask: *which* nerve cells most relevant to the *ongoing* stage of enlightenment could have died an excitotoxic death as a result of a person's having undergone *repeated*, deep extraordinary states of consciousness?

The Issue of Selectivity

Why is selective targeting essential? Because the candidate regions in the brain which would need to be neutralized, like those many other sites which *must be spared*, are already swarming with excitatory amino acid synapses. So that we need to envision two potential primary mechanisms at the local target sites: (1) an especially heightened release of excitotoxic transmitters themselves; (2) some other condition which enhances the sensitivity of their receptors.[6] Along the same lines, two secondary mechanisms might converge on a candidate nerve cell. The cell could be driven into a long burst of firing by a local excess of other excitatory factors (for example, an increase in dynorphin or nitric oxide). Or it could overfire secondary to a dearth of local inhibition (such as might follow from a reduction in GABA functions).

In these four ways could a process of excitotoxic etching be shaped, by local circumstances, to sever certain links within the pathways, say, of both the limbic system and its frontotemporal projection sites. Noteworthy are the observations that local excitotoxic damage can be enhanced secondarily not only by dynor-phin, nitric oxide, and adrenal stress hormones but also by the effects of stimulat-ing ST_2 receptors. For if ST_2 receptors were also to be activated on a given set of target cells, then local etching at that site could become even more profound. It suffices only to note that researchers are currently studying several other normal metabolic products which have excitotoxic side effects.[24,25] These include kynure-nic acid and quinolinic acid. They are normal breakdown products of tryptophan.

However, we are considering an excitotoxic process that must be pinpointed to only certain circuits, and with a neurochemical precision more selective than a surgeon's knife. For instance, it can take rats a longer—not shorter—time to extinguish their learned fearful responses after their medial prefrontal cortex has been lesioned.[26] Still, cumulatively, each *well-placed* tiny lesion could contribute to those much larger patterns of disconnections which could finally become the effective agencies of change.

The hypothesis that repeated surges of alternate states do etch the brain is a testable one. But researchers will need to carefully focus their studies on se-lected brain regions at autopsy to be certain that individual cells and their pro-cesses have dropped out. This is not quite like looking for a needle in a haystack, but it will require electron microscopy and specialized histochemical techniques at very high resolutions. Current studies, still in a preliminary stage, are already attempting to link excess glutamate with such obvious disease states as Hunting-ton's chorea and amyotrophic lateral sclerosis. In these conditions, the shrinkage of the brain or spinal cord is evident to the naked eye.

So the investigations now proposed will have to be highly sophisticated. For one would be searching for certain less obvious kinds of *microscopic* changes in those few genuine sages who had undergone multiple, deep, and transforming enlightenment experiences. In the sages, the shrinkage and fragmentation of indi-vidual nerve cells could be much more subtle and selective than in the patients who die from these diseases.[27] And this kind of a focused research project will require a major commitment: carefully planned and highly sophisticated studies on a well-defined set of human subjects, correlated both during life and post mortem.[28] Goals of this scope are very difficult to meet. To make accurate histolog-ical comparisons, including counts of shrunken nerve cells, researchers must have access to many other brains from well-matched subjects which will serve as ap-propriate controls for nerve cell counts. Twin studies would be ideal.

Target Regions

But suppose everything were ready to go, and you were a researcher right now. Where would you look first? One function this book can serve (beyond encourag-ing such an investigation) is to help generate a list of plausible sites. These will be the potential targets for *one* particular aspect—broadly characterized as *sub-traction*—of the larger transformative process. And this is why, in chapter 7, per-haps to his colleagues' surprise, this neurologist started straightaway to confront the nature of the self and its maladaptions. Soon, however, having peeled back its layers of longings and loathings, we came down to those basic instincts of self-preservation which lay at its core (see chapter 8). Then, in part III, we went on to correlate many of these same vital functions of self-preservation with the functional anatomy of three regions deep in the archaic core of the brain. One can oversimplify, in the following way, the physiological links which connect these three sites:

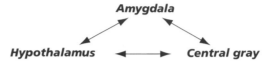

What could *gentle* this imposing triad, if not tame it? Cumulative lesions of two general kinds. First are lesions localized to what might be termed its *input* side. These would stop an inappropriate excess of messages from entering *into* the triad. In this regard, the sea mollusk, *Aplysia,* has already served as one model. The mollusc illustrated, in a generic way, how a nervous system dampens its responses when circuits are shut down on their input side (see chapter 49).

Lesions of the second type would either inactivate the nerve cells within the triad itself, or would disconnect each from the others.[29] Whichever occurred, the result would be finally to shut down the export of dysfunctional messages *from* the triad on its *output* side. Thereafter, those inappropriate levels of messages— which had once signaled turmoil in the visceral core of the self—would no longer escape to exert their maladaptive influences on the rest of the brain.

The early V-shaped cuts into the copper plate are decisive. Their pattern determines what kind of scenes the etched plate will later keep reproducing. Will the etchings be judged beautiful or ugly? In general, whether the etching is by amino acids, or by nitric oxide, or by molecule *X*, cell death has the potential to change a brain for better or for worse. Much would depend on which part of the brain such a process had pinpointed, and on how the localized changes had been performed. Some burnt-out human brains, legacies of the spaced-out drug culture starting in the 1960s, may have been "etched" more at random, and in maladaptive ways.

In contrast, the Zen meditative way presents several potential advantages. It proceeds very slowly, voluntarily, legally. It acts spontaneously from the inside, discretely. Overall, the meditative mental landscape is much calmer, clearer. Nerve cells will have been liberated from much of their usual irrelevant synaptic clutter. In this setting, signal can stand out high, soaring briefly above the background noise. And a sharp, sudden surge through the pathways of self-preservation can penetrate more deeply and into recesses not usually open.

But the advanced meditator is still confronted with that huge old citadel of self. Its high walls are never weakly defended, never eager to surrender its prerogatives, never easily dismantled and reconstructed. Rigid lifestyles resist change. No person becomes permanently, selflessly effective in the world at large simply by having dropped out a few scattered nerve cells. Indeed, it will take decades of working through—wave upon wave of subtle psychophysiological transformations—before the rare person is able to approach the stage of the sage, let alone to enter it and live in it. And the requisite structural subtractions may well be taking place not only at the level of the cell body but also upstream, among its dendrites, and downstream in its axon terminals.

"Additions"

Yes, some dysfunctional circuits might seem to require a total uprooting. Others will benefit more from selective cutting and pruning. Yet, this can't be the whole story. Let's return to all those other key circuits, the countless ones which must remain selectively *spared*. Spared, for several reasons. In the past, many had merely been overdriven, and had wasted energy on that account. In contrast, others had been more or less latent, their potentials not yet recognized. So all the while the vast majority of these two groups of circuits in the brain will first need to be reprogrammed or enlisted. Then their capacities can be rechanneled in full support of the sage's other emergent functions.

In a sense, one might refer to all such newly apparent functions under the remaining broad category. Here it is loosely termed "additions." This is not accurate. Obviously many of them would have always been there, their seeds latent in the brain, carrying the same innate human potentials each of us has to become more creative, adaptive, and affirmative.

And, at this point, we return to specify a final role for glutamate which could otherwise be overlooked. For its versatile receptors can do more than act directly in the service of a nerve cell's fast transmission, and so go on to expose its vulnerable Achilles' heel. Glutamate receptors also help slowly to modify the next cell's membrane excitability properties (see chapter 48). These additional *metabolic* properties of certain glutamate receptors now go by the technical term of *metabotropic*.[30] But all this means is that a surge in glutamate transmission can also set in motion a slower cascade of ripples. These delayed biochemical events, acting through G proteins, have recently been shown to improve both memory and task performance in animals. In this manner glutamate could contribute— in a positive, trophic way—to the seemingly "added" affirmative aspects that transform consciousness as the advanced meditator approaches the stage of ongoing enlightenment.

Someone, perhaps Hakuin, said that it will take five major awakenings before one finally pulls out the last roots of the self. Growing older, each of us becomes intimately familiar with some of the ways the aging process is also changing the very structure of our brains. We turn next to examine the nature of these changes and their cumulative impact.

Aging in the Brain

When your study of Buddhism is through
you find you haven't anything new.
Enlightenment and delusion, too, never existed at the start;
they're ideas that you picked up,
things your parents never taught.

Master Bankei[1]

No longer a kitten,
the cat now pounces on my hand clawlessly . . .

J. Hackett[2]

The kitten, chased by a dog, scrambles frantically far up and out along the higher branches of a tree. There, though it meows at your heartstrings, it still digs its claws into you when you go up on a ladder to bring it down. The older, wiser cat, less paralyzed by fear, climbs safely out of reach, and stays near the trunk. Having verified that the dog has gone, it then backs down carefully, on its own.

But in truth, there is no fool like an old fool, and when one looks over one's own foibles, it is clear that wisdom bears no straight-line relationship with age. Human wisdom ripens on a zigzag path to self-realization. Along the way, adults go through phases not unlike children. Only in retrospect do we fully appreciate how our "passages" had taken us through what Jung would call "the problem of opposites."[3] Problem? The word is an understatement. It is a major task, and painfully difficult, to reassess oneself and others. In fact, any person who would do so must be willing to go to the mat, there to writhe and be thrown by the opposites, time after time.

Yin and yang are *both* martial artists. They twist us inside an arena full of conflicting alternatives. Not until the second half of life, as Jung predicted, do most of us find enough reflective moments "to appreciate the value of the opposite of our former ideals, to perceive the error in our former convictions, to recognize the untruth in our former truth, and to feel how much antagonism and even hatred lay in what, until now, had passed for love."[4]

In short, the passage to adulthood becomes another difficult, long-drawn-out metamorphosis. But does such a normal process involve merely shedding a few cortical layers of discriminative functions? Or does personal growth now take place in deeper, newly discovered dimensions? If the latter, then the beginning of our true maturity implies a twofold agenda: (1) redefining the old premises and priorities; and (2) revising those old affective polarities which had always caused so much discomfort in the past. The older cat still has its claws. Now they remain appropriately sheathed.

Jung used a simple way to describe the complex process. Everyone, he said, had "disposable" psychic energy. Its latent powers lay "dormant in the unconscious." There, they were constantly being used up in attempts to manage each set of contending opposites. But what if one resolved these internal conflicts? Then this psychic energy could be liberated and rechanneled. Now it could revitalize novel regions of the psyche. At least at this descriptive level we can imagine how once-wasted psychic energies might become available for more *selfless* behaviors, including compassion.

Each Zen aspirant has always had to enter the arena of the opposites. One's early steps, through the introspections, are hesitant and proceed at a slow pace. Much later, the sudden flash of insights will illuminate the formerly dark recesses in one's personal landscape. This moonlight exposes the hidden triad of self, the source of the old contending polarities.

Ripening and Pruning

Does wisdom ripen *only* because one modifies a few thoughts, and merely thinks along different lines? Unless we shed this canard, our understanding of the Way of Zen will remain as superficial and fleeting as word-thoughts themselves. During the *lifelong* process of aging, the brain of any species is constantly revising much of its cellular and neurochemical architecture.[5] At *any* age, countless nerve cells are dying because they lose either their presynaptic input or their neurotrophic proteins. The processes of aging in rats, for example, have already caused them to lose—by the time they have reached only a year and a half of age—substantial amounts of norepinephrine in the hypothalamus, of dopamine in the basal ganglia, and of cAMP in the cerebellum.[6] We have already observed how these same two amines, NE and DA, are not merely messenger molecules of the moment. For, in fact, they too can set off a cascade of other messengers. These metabolic ripples can resculpture the architecture and change the responses of the next nerve cells[7] (see chapter 48).

Some persons age gracefully. Their personalities become "mellow." Perhaps at first glance it might seem that these senior citizens had only ripened into equanimity because they had *added* some "positive" qualities. If so, then once we had discovered what these "additions" were, we could begin to clarify how their ingredients might go on to ripen further into some of those rare wisdoms characteristic of a sage.

On the other hand, we may also have gone through the experience of tasting (and remembering) how a persimmon ripens: by degrees. At which point the fact hits home: in order for a whole personality to mellow, some very bitter "negative" qualities must first have to disappear or be transformed. So this leads us back to an earlier general question. It was first raised on the basis of one of William James's comments: does the "mellow wisdom" of these aging oldsters represent some kind of "artful overlooking"? Because if it does, then it would help us if we could pinpoint where and how this process of wisdom occurs in the normal aging human brain.

One conventional place to begin to look is in the human hippocampus. Researchers have the habit of reminding us that our hippocampal nerve cells are dropping out all the time. Some studies estimate that each decade the aging process whittles away about 3 to 4 percent of the neurons in our hippocampal CA1 region.[8] Others' data suggest that about half of our CA1 cells will have dropped out between the ages of forty-seven and eighty-five.[9] If one assumes that the brain has 24 million CA1 cells at age 47, and that only 11 million cells remain at age eighty-five, the implication is that we are losing over 900 nerve cells a day! Yet, what happens as the result of this much hippocampal cell death later in life? It does not appear to have brought everyone into total "transcendence." Nor is it obvious that singling out one CA pathway would be correlated with a total loss of the omni-self (see chapter 142). However, a dwindling number of cells does seem to account for my overlooking where I last placed my glasses. And in other ways this outfall of cells probably does contribute to what many neurologists prefer to call "the benign forgetfulness of advancing years." (Especially when the neurologists are older than forty-seven themselves.)

The aging rat is also forgetful. Yes, its hippocampal granule cells still develop that impressive long-term potentiation, but it doesn't *last* as long (see figure 6). Moreover, fewer responses occur in the collateral pathway which links the rat's CA3 cells to its CA1 cells.[10] Human granule cells can compensate for this by sprouting new connections from some of their mossy fibers.[11]

The aging brain undergoes other structural changes. It loses its receptors for important chemical messengers in *many regions*.[12] For example, neuroimaging studies reveal that the adult human brain loses *half* of its acetylcholine muscarinic receptors in the cortex and striatum during those six decades which extend from the twenties up to the eighties.[13] And its DA_1 and DA_2 receptors also decline in the basal ganglia. This loss of receptors clarifies why levodopa alone is not capable of improving the impaired motor functions of elderly humans.[14,15] In humans, ST_2 receptors show a linear fall in cortex and hippocampus after the age of thirty,[16] and ST_1 agonist drugs also become less effective with age.[17]

On a more cheerful note (from the standpoint of misplaced glasses, at least) are the results which follow the use of certain norepinephrine agonists. The agonists which activate $alpha_2$ NE receptors do improve the "working memory" of an old monkey, helping it to perform better when it needs to remember where an object lies in space.[18] And two drugs that enhance the functional levels of acetylcholine are currently being prescribed for patients with Alzheimer's disease. (Exelon and Arisept).

Aging prunes subtly, but in pervasive ways. It severs a nerve cell's finer dendritic twigs and branches (see figure 4). Collectively, the loss of dendritic twigs and axonal terminals disconnects each cell from the others in its network, slowly sapping the brain's associative powers. Normal adults counter this pruning by sprouting a few new dendrites, at least until they reach the age of eighty years or so.[19] However, relentless dendritic pruning occurs in Alzheimer's disease.

Older persons shorten their REM periods. They also become less sensitive to visual contrasts at the intermediate and higher contrast frequencies.[20] And what of the other minute structural and hormonal changes which make one's brain *physiologically* different as one grows older? Do they have implications for Zen? It seems likely that when an experience of absorption or insight does enter in later decades it might register less intensely, or in a subtly different way, than had it arrived when that same person were younger. Maslow believed that the older person's peak experience did tend to have less of an impression of novelty and of first-time-ness.[21] And the few subjects of Masters and Houston who experienced the state of "Unitary Consciousness" were all over the age of forty (see chapter 101).

In medical school, it is the rare young student who doesn't catch the early symptoms of some fatal illness he or she has just seen or read about. On the neurology wards, medical students tend to contract a malignant brain tumor or amyotrophic lateral sclerosis (Lou Gehrig's disease). How do students finally cope with such dreaded unrealities, as they go on to mature into older physicians? It is a slow process. It isn't easy to shed fears that are centered on self-preservation. Not unlike Zen training, it takes decades before physicians adopt a more practical perspective.

In their later decades, many normal persons seem to have less self to lose. They "loosen up," become more "laid back" and less competitive in their ambitions. They "lighten up," and "need" fewer possessions. Their former hard edges seem smoothed off, less on display. Some older persons become very aware that they have lost these former notions of selfhood. To one author's eighty-five-year-old neighbor, it had become specifically clear that her own sense of self had fallen away during the previous six-year period.[22] I know that mine has too. However, for all of the foregoing reasons, I remain too skeptical to attribute this to my decades of Zen practice per se. It would be interesting to have had a non-Zen twin.

All too soon, one discovers the other results of getting on in years. As presbyopia advances, one reads better at arms' length, telling evidence that the lens in the eye has become more firm. And yet, even while seniors do become more rigid in some of these physical ways, many of them also become increasingly farsighted in another sense. They *add* new, long-range *mental* perspectives. They start to develop what Storr calls a practical "concern with the impersonal."[23] They move on to consider the big picture, the universals. In this way, by adding here and subtracting there, some of them begin to leave very far behind the uncorrected distortions and *I-Me-My-opias* of their youth.

How did we define this maladaptive condition earlier, in chapter 9? As the problem everyone faces. It is that mental shortsightedness which keeps all of us narrowly focused solely on egocentric needs. However, the healthy aging person, in the course of evolving new perspectives, starts moving beyond the clashing swords of the old opposites. Gradually, there arrives an appreciation of the kind of sage advice embodied in the timeless Zen message, which says:

> Conflicts between longing and loathing
> are a disease of the mind.
> Gain and loss, right and wrong
> away with them once and for all!*

---

*Appendix B.

The Celebration of Nature

"I seek the truth," said the young monk. "Where is the entrance to the path of Buddhism?" Master Hsuan-sha replied, "Do you hear the murmuring of that stream?" "Yes," the monk replied. The Master said, "There is the entrance."

Old Zen story[1]

One impulse from a vernal wood
May teach you more of man,
Of moral evil and of good,
Than all the sages can.

William Wordsworth[2]

Sooner or later, as their own aging process unfolds, a time of passage arrives in many persons' lives. Left behind will be those frantic drives of youth which keep one scrambling up through civilization's latest jungle of twigs and branches. A different impulse enters. It is the instinct to turn back, to descend, and to follow the tree of life down to its taproot. A search begins.

Perhaps one is led to such a wordless turning point after having been hit hard by life's tragedies and disappointments; when one senses, as did Siddhartha, how wide a gap separates this present condition from an "ideal" state of affairs. It is a most discomforting realization, whenever it arrives, and the gap creates a yearning to close the distance. At this point, the mature urge to take up a spiritual path becomes as compelling to humans as is their seasonal migration for the salmon and for the V-shaped flocks of Canada geese. A force of nature takes over. A quest begins.

Centuries ago, as they pursued their own earlier quest, the followers and scribes of the ancient sages had begun to litter the path with many artificial thought-forms. Soon, sharp differences in doctrine arose, because different cultures interpreted the journey in very different ways. Still, beyond all the cumbersome rituals and forms of worship, the message of the centuries is that most of the old spiritual paths tend to converge. At the "summit" of a peak experience, the human brain finally comprehends what appears to be the ground of all energies, the integrating principle of the universe. Is not the phenomenon of this closure one more expression of nature as it really is? If our reading of the evidence is to be believed, then latent within each human brain are the innate capacities to integrate its basic rhythms into that unique, coherent configuration.

Is such an event really so special? Or have human longings just made it seem so? Because everything we're made of is held in common with the rest of nature. Water reminds us of this elementary fact. Water makes up most of brain and body, three quarters or so. Sitting indoors, it is easy to lose sight of our commonality. But walk outdoors, listen intently to the murmurings of the stream; or look up into the forest canopy that water made possible: a sunlit cathedral of stained glass leaves, glowing with shades of green in the spring, of red in the fall. Then nothing could be more natural than the basic awareness which comes fully alive when we commune with Nature.

It is genuine communion. We have retracted our steps, come back along the trail to our origin, there to rejoin and revere all the other stardust elements of which everything is made. Now enters that sense of serenity about our true place in the universal scheme of things. Such intimate moments emphasize the truth in D.T. Suzuki's words: "I am in Nature and Nature is in me. Not mere participation in each other, but a fundamental identity between the two."[3]

Nature is our element. We have two major ways to open up to Nature and bring its individual features into focus. The first way is to become intensely aware of the present moment and of its details. The second is that ultra-wide-angle, broadest possible meditation. Through this lens we are led to contemplate the unbelievable miracle we share with all life in general. Therefore, a meditator may begin practice under the impression that it means sitting only indoors, on a cushion. But soon, he or she will be engaged in the time-honored refinements of these two natural processes. Why? Because the formal meditative traditions also tend to follow these same two approaches to awareness: the concentrative and the openly receptive (see chapter 16). *Both avenues come together when each of us enters into a totally unaffected appreciation of our outdoor environment.*

So meditation is not to be viewed as somehow separate from the rest of nature. And the most commonsense explanations underlie the fact that natural, outdoor stimuli are the triggers for peak experiences. Indeed, during their surveys of mystical experiences, Laski[4] and Greeley[5] discovered that *natural* triggers had been the precipitating cause for as many as 20 to 45 percent of the total number of events.

What natural settings had prompted their subjects' experiences? They were induced most commonly by "mountains, hills, and water, by star-lit nights, fine dawns and sunsets, by spring and autumn days, by trees and flowers, by the flight and song of birds, by light and by wind and by the sweet smells of the countryside."[1] Recent physiological and psychological tests confirm a well-known fact. Natural environments do have intrinsic healing properties. Even when videotaped scenes are used, human subjects recover best from the psychic trauma of violence when they view natural settings, not urban scenes.[6]

Back when it was still a young planet, the usual day on Earth exposed its sentient creatures to relatively quieter settings, to simpler events taking place on the ground, in the water, and in the sky. When creatures first began to evolve their primitive nerve networks it would be partly in response to these elemental background conditions. No telephones were jangling at that time; no snarling trail bikes or speedboats or political campaigns had yet disturbed the scene. By the time *Homo sapiens* had arrived, and progressed to reach April of the year 1970, it would be almost an atavistic event when 20 million Americans joined to celebrate Earth Day, in the sense that these millions were simply giving expression to their deepest feelings of spiritual kinship with the natural world!

April 22, 1995 marked our twenty-fifth anniversary of that day. During the intervening quarter-century, increasing numbers of the Earth's inhabitants have taken a very hard look at those earlier short-term attitudes which had once allowed them to so casually exploit nature. Now, it is not only the plant and animal biologists who warn that long-range tradeoffs are implicit in the balance of nature. The groundswell has become increasingly worldwide in scope. Countless other persons have learned the hard way that harsh consequences can foil even their best-intentioned efforts.

Consider the case of DDT, that marvelous insecticide which served as the basis for the Nobel Prize in Physiology or Medicine in 1948. A pernicious molecule, its toxicity lingered in the food chain and finally caused the "silent spring." So many birds' eggs were stilled that DDT would be banned in the United States less than a quarter of a century later. Physicians and patients have also grown skeptical about "new advances," having seen how many drug-resistant bacterial infections occurred after antibiotics had been used incautiously. And yes, big dams do bring electricity. But pitifully few salmon are now able to migrate up our streams. Sooner or later, we too run smack up against the realities of our present world: whenever we grasp out blindly in one direction we'll probably set off some disastrous unforseen consequence in an ecosystem farther down the chain.

The flash of enlightenment illuminates the longest of possible views: an insight into eternity. What drops off in such a sudden awakening? Every former zealous cosmetic impulse to push "progress," at no matter what the cost. Gone is that old pressured yearning for some misguided quick fix. No longer must the natural world always be plundered to serve mankind's own busy image. What kind of alternative perspective does a peak experience present instead? That basic instinct to return *directly* to the world as it is right *now*. To rejoin it, and accept it as it really is, warts and all.

What is the best advice to give a novice whose impulse it is to walk the spiritual path? Each cultural epoch provides its own counsel. *Listen to the murmur of the stream,* said old Master Hsuan-sha, back in ninth-century China. But, if we today were to return to such plain and simple naturalism, or to that of a Thoreau, would not some people regard it almost as though we were abandoning the world and had taken one more kind of a street drug in an attempt to escape from reality? But that isn't really the case. Because when a Zen master prescribes listening, *attentively,* this will always be in the form of a highly practical prescription item. Take this prescription regularly. For an extended period of time. Soon one begins to realize the hidden benefits in moments of attentive meditative contemplation.[2,9] Whether these attentive pauses are performed indoors, or outdoors, they become antidotes for whatever ails one, useful against both the clamoring headlines of the media and the shrill headlines thrust up by one's internal discontents. A similar keen appreciation of nature had long flourished within Western traditions, and did not originate in the East alone. Thus, to Zeno, who founded stoicism, the true goal would be to "live in agreement with nature."[7] And Emerson, too, had followed up by observing how "The intellectual life may be kept clean and healthful, if man will live the life of nature and not import into his mind difficulties which are none of his."[8]

Nature's lessons are our open book. Observe, at leisure, how every breeze may turn over a new page. Passages then leap out from its old and new testaments to reward our mindful inspection at many levels. Rarely, whole pages of the manuscript become illuminated. A sudden flash of insight-wisdom then comprehends the full range of the natural laws. All of their manifestations are accepted without blinking, every seeming passion, delight, and sordid cruelty. None are denied, for all are now understood to be integral parts of the same whole design. At this point, every former bookish intellectual concept about Nature will have vanished, transformed by the awesomely objective insight into what Buddhists have long-called Buddha-nature.

The early Zen Buddhists assimilated a strong nature orientation from the original Chinese Taoists. Later, some seven centuries ago, Daikaku went on to beautifully summarize its many implications when he said, "Realization makes every place a temple."[9] Our true temple is not a computer screen or television set. It is the natural world of field, stream, and vernal woods. Once we genuinely understand how basic are all our affinities with it, we won't despoil its sanctity.

How is it possible for someone to grow in accord with what Emerson had called the "spiritual laws?"[8] To become fully in touch with the entire world; to respect it as a sacred place? It helps, first, to keep reminding oneself, over and over, how to reenter it. The age-old approach is *to fully attend to the here and now.* To focus on simple things like the murmur of the stream. And it doesn't have to be a brook, or the leaves of a tree outside. Even the flow of a kitchen faucet, or the silent appreciation of a houseplant, may serve indoors as well.

But, the beginner protests, What a chore! What purpose does it serve to return to the *now,* time after time throughout each day? One explanation would seem to go something as follows. The present moment is *real;* the past and future are not. In the process of constantly practicing this mindful act of meditation, one seems slowly to enlarge the capacity not only to isolate actual events which are of real significance but also to appreciate each event more calmly, objectively. No longer does the world of distractions then rush past so mindlessly. And no more will one need to grasp hold of things in this world which only invite anguish and confusion.

Imperceptibly, there evolves an enhanced ability to introspect more deeply. Gradually, one begins to see with increasing clarity into relationships, both personal, interpersonal, and universal. As this process of understanding ripens over the years, it appears to tap increasingly into some underground source in the brain. In a sense, it plumbs a year-round spring, one that seems ever ready to become the origin of our authentic spiritual impulses. Finally, major insights tumble out spontaneously. During such natural awakenings, the old shrill egocentric self will have vanished, its voice dissolving into all the rest of the murmuring flow.

Every day then becomes Earth Day.

Expressing Zen in Action

The great end of life is not knowledge but action.

Thomas H. Huxley (1825–1895)[1]

To understand is hard. Once one understands, action is easy.

Sun Yat-sen (1866–1925)[2]

Zen training addresses more than the softer sensibilities. A hard, muscular Zen stretches sinew, makes it supple enough to *change direction*. What creates real change? Only fundamental transformations. Watch the roshi test the depth of his students' kensho. He shatters shallow productions, challenges them with arcane situations: *Where* is one? He wants an immediate motor response. *Now*. Are the students slow to respond? Could their old choreographs be holding them back? If so, then something of the *I-Me-Mine* still lingers, interrupts the flow.

"He who hesitates is lost" is an old saying. Zen implies no hesitation. Could some truth reside in the reverse of the statement? In Zen, is it possible that "he who *doesn't* hesitate has found?" If so, what exactly was found? And did anything also have to be lost? In the simpler terms we have been using, What was added? What was subtracted?

It is the traditional belief that years of Zen training will yield liberated behaviors. Let us first review the major features of such inspired actions. These descriptions will then serve as our springboard for asking, How can fluid movements arise—and flow freely like *tai chi chuan*—in a person whose earlier motor skills had been clumsy at best? Enlightened Zen behaviors are considered to be

1. without initial hesitation;
2. quick in execution;
3. simple but efficient;
4. highly creative, improvisational, yet capable of resolving both the immediate situation and of addressing the big picture as well;
5. expressed from a foundation of poise;
6. liberated from word-thoughts and personal concerns.

An anecdote will illustrate the flavor of Zen actions. The teacher handed one student a fan, and asked him what it was. The disciple returned it, saying: "A fan." The teacher frowned, then handed it to another student, who said nothing. But he scratched his back with the fan, poked the stove with it, opened it, and fanned himself. Finally, having placed a gift on it, he returned it to his teacher. The teacher smiled.[3]

Zen training begins with bowing. After you have lowered the flag of the sovereign I, it becomes easier to bend fully from the waist, not to deliver a casual nod. The Zen trainee's graceful behavior goes on to find its twofold expression:

first in the overlooked art of workaday living; and second in those other activities usually designated as arts, including the martial arts. However, in a sense, the word "arts" is a misnomer. For, in fact, the qualities we are now scrutinizing are the essence of art*less*ness. A better term is "ways."

Each of the several categories of Zen ways is called *do*. The word (pronounced dough) comes from the Chinese *Tao*, meaning way. Each way expresses not technique alone, but going beyond technique and beyond thought. So it is of relatively less importance whether the trainee chooses the way of calligraphy, archery, fencing, or flower arrangement. What matters most is that he or she learns the subtle approaches of "purifying, calming, and focusing the psychophysical apparatus, to obtain to some degree of Zen realization and to express it."[4] On the artistic side, the Zen ways illustrate two ancient Oriental aesthetic preferences. One is for the simple, natural, and quiet (*wabi*). The other is for the mellow patina which comes with advancing age (*sabi*).

The Zen ways do not replace the standard monastic training methods. They provide the meditator with supplementary approaches. And as we now look further into the manner in which the ways are performed, they can help us discover how Zen training influences the brain.

The basic motor impulse is a primal one. It is not too surprising to find that traditional Buddhist mythology honors Samantabhadra, the bodhisattva who personifies great action. Bodhisattvas do resemble real saints, because they serve as exemplars of the highest *qualities* that a religion values. The principles are real, but bodhisattvas are imaginary. What firm evidence exists that Zen training actually does exert a positive influence on motor functions?

One of the Zen ways holds particular interest. It is calligraphy, *sho-do*. Each brush stroke preserves its motor nuances for posterity. The person's many earlier samples of calligraphy can provide an accurate control period, the baseline. From this longitudinal perspective, we can clearly see how Tesshu was transformed after his great awakening took place. The evidence is recorded in black ink, laid down on paper over a century ago. Immediately his brush strokes vibrate with fresh energy. From then on, Tesshu's calligraphy displays increasing refinement until his death eight years later.[5]

Leggett practiced several of the Zen ways, and observed how they incorporated four traditional elements. They consist of (1) inspiration (*Ri*), (2) formal technique (*Ji*), (3) heart (*Shin*), and (4) vital energy (*Ki*).[4] Their motor counterparts are each subtle in translation and hard to pin down, but are powerful in the aggregate.

Start with the term *Ri*. It means to be so in contact with the true, universal nature of the situation that one expresses its beauty and power both naturally and efficiently. *Ri* is inspired by our innate creative wellsprings within. It cannot be taught or imitated.

The word *Ji* refers to particular techniques as such. These methods *can* be taught and observed. Many techniques are imitations, having been handed down from some other person's earlier inspirations of *Ri*. *Shin* refers to the impulse to initiate action. It includes that deeply felt emotional tone which permeates the idea, feelings which were thought in ancient times to come from a person's "heart." It is worth noting that when *Shin* is pure, it retains no trace of selfishness, grasping, fear about the outcome, or inflexibility.

Finally, *Ki* is the proper energetic field involved in the action. *Ki* calmly delivers just the appropriate amount of pure strength in the most coordinated, quick, and efficient way. *Ki* is regarded as having its center down in the *tanden*, whether one is engaged in meditation or the martial arts. This region, a few inches below the navel, is where meditators focus their attention, while breathing in and out. After several rounds of zazen, one may feel a sense of balanced composure and potential strength throughout this region.

For many centuries, the Zen ways have exemplified these same four traditional qualities of action: inspiration, technique, impulsivity, and energy. But a large gap seems to be standing between these old words imported from the Orient and what researchers have newly discovered in this century.[6] Can we bridge this gap? We can begin by teasing out some constituents of these four elusive terms. The next step will be to translate these ingredients into their physiological counterpart functions within certain motor systems of the brain.

Letting Go into the Flow

I think back to my first encounter with Zen. It was in the course of reading *Zen in the Art of Archery*. This book left me puzzled. Later, I came to appreciate how the artless archer does hit the bull's-eye. Not by grasping the bowstring with strong fingers which merely pull. For one's muscles must learn how to *release*, not only contract. It takes years of Zen archery training to develop the subtle skills to *let go* smoothly, passively. In the interim, erratic arrows betray the student's old, self-referent behavior patterns.

Actions inspired by Zen training are focused on just the task at hand, in the present moment. In this absolute Now, no negative legacies from the past project complications into the future. As soon as anxiety drops out of the picture, the imbalances among muscles disappear. Now actions flow swiftly, the result of an artless freedom from those contractions which had formerly interfered with smooth performance. This is freedom within forms, not license in revolt against forms.

Our hang-ups *literally* hang us up. Gradually, most people catch on to this. They discover how counterproductive it is to be constrained by self-inflicted pressures. Professional golfers speak about how the "inner game" enormously influences their "touch." Under the demands of tournament pressure and uneven terrain, they must vary their repertoire from booming 280-yard drives to soft three-foot putts. In every sport, mature pros appreciate how self-scolding attitudes exert a negative influence. I *should* have done it another way. I *ought* to do it this way. Shoulds and oughts; this and that!

Truly enlightened peak performance needs no fictitious alter egos. Is someone still looking down from above, voicing words of scorn or encouragement? These obstacles stand in the way of becoming *one with the action*. No matter how expert an athlete may seem, the John McEnroes who yell at themselves and curse others remain self-centered amateurs who fall short of their own ultimate potential. *Play* remains the operative word. In competitive sports nowadays, whether professional or amateur, a genuine sense of play is rare. When it finally reaches its peak level, the condition called being "in the zone," *athletic performance plays itself* in the flow of a timeless state. Zen celebrates the extension of this zone of the athlete. It extends it into the artless play of *all* our other everyday life activities.

Watch the simple ways in which animals move. They are the essence of the natural actions under discussion. When D.T. Suzuki observed a cat eating food, he noted that "it does not ask whether the food is good or if another cat is eating. It does not make any comparisons, it just goes on eating until it is finished . . . This pure experience is the act itself."[7]

Things get no less miraculous when we examine one of the operations of the human brain. Suppose we choose one of our simpler acts of eating. Let us say that you are hungry, and you see an apple nearby. Leaning forward to pick it up, you've already been *motivated* by hunger signals from your limbic system, and refined your *intentions* to reach for the apple within your frontal lobes and basal ganglia. You've also drawn together many covert layers of *attention.* Now these layers focus (subconsciously) on a particular scenario: your whole body interacting within that vaguely spherical volume of familiar space which is its theatre of action. This means, of course, that before you even begin to reach out, your posterior parietal cortex must already be working in close harmony with its corresponding frontal networks, and with layers of other sensorimotor networks.

Soon, impulses descending through your medial reticulospinal tracts are adjusting the posture of the axial muscles along your spine.[8] Other pathways descend through your lateral reticular formation and red nucleus. They are helping you contract the muscles which move your right shoulder and elbow. And volleys of impulses flowing down from your left motor cortex are starting to shape the fine voluntary finger movements of your right hand.

All along, the existing motor programs in your basal ganglia have been helping to organize each of these two pathways specified above: the descending *reticulospinal* and *corticospinal* systems. In these several basal ganglia, the highest and outermost layer is the large caudate nucleus (see figure 12). It works intimately with your association cortex, regulating the speed and pattern of movements.[9] And, meanwhile, the cerebellum is also helping to compose those individual movements which are now gliding so smoothly to your target. Before you stop to think about it, you have reached the apple, and your fingers have enclosed it.

Of the billions of nerve cells swept into such a simple task, few have actually been in on your final *direct* muscle contractions. These few are called the *lower motor neurons.* Your spinal cord contains a mere 2 or 3 million of them. Onto the dendrites of each cell are converging eight thousand or so synapses. Another two thousand synapses make contact with the body of the cell[10] (see figure 4). Each of these lower motor neurons then serves as the "final common pathway" which directly excites a group of your muscle fibers. So, when this lowest nerve cell finally releases its acetylcholine onto the muscle, the ACH can be viewed as the essence of all the above messages, distilled through innumerable other synapses, receptors, and higher networks. There is a bottom-line message. It is one to humble even the most ardent reductionist: it would be easier to untangle a large bundle of wet confetti than to tease out a single source for any one of our more complex actions.

Somehow, it all works. It works even in humans who have, on hand, vastly more potential behaviors to keep track of than that older, gentler cat who could back down from the tree, finally chew its food calmly and keep its claws sheathed. What accounts for our own very wide range of human behavioral options? Much of it emerges from layers of circuitries partly supervised from the top down.

Up top, in the outer gray mantle of cortex, only an abstraction of convenience would permit anyone to view its motor extensions as separate from their sensory counterparts.[11,12] Consider, for example, how much more efficiently our sensorimotor systems perform when they are being helped by visual input. If you put on a blindfold, and block all vision for only two minutes, this sensory deprivation slows the firing of your muscle units even during simple tasks, and it also dampens other simple reflexes.[13] Similar reductions in motor functions may help explain why some novices find it difficult to sit without wobbling when they close their eyes during meditation.

Moreover, it is well established in Zen traditions that actions proceed from a "total" person. So the goal is not some languid withdrawn meditator whose view of life evolves inside closed lids, but an alert individual who has become increasingly open and responsive to the outside world. In such *openness* and *responsivity* lies an important clue for future investigations into the results of authentic Zen training. For these two properties are leading us back toward *Ri*, *Ji*, *Shin*, and *Ki*, the traditional elements of the Zen ways. And they invite us to consider a "far-reaching proposal" in more than a manner of speaking. As a working hypothesis, the proposal is that *advanced* trainees would have shortened their reaction times, as measured in certain ways. How? Where? Within that large volume which we referred to earlier as unconscious circumspatial awareness (see chapter 114).

Now the basis for such a proposal is not any new data. The historical background dates far back to the samurai swordsman of yesteryear. How did he proceed to develop his most highly advanced level of responsivity? Only by taking up the additional path of long spiritual training. The result was called *Happo Biraki*, a term which means "open on all sides." In feudal Japan, such total awareness was vital. No shield and no parry helped the samurai swordsman ward off blows. His life hinged upon his ability to dodge, and to get in the first, quick two-handed stroke.[14] Skillful means, indeed. Survival, not altruism, was the first objective.

Cortical and Subcortical Layers of Motor Functions

Suppose you're a subject seated in a psychology laboratory. A startling, unexpected flash of light occurs. Your hand starts its *reflexive* jerk a mere twenty-five to fifty milliseconds later. This is an *involuntary* act, so your reaction time is reasonably fast—about as fast as the air bags inflate in some cars. But suppose you become the volunteer subject for a rather different kind of experiment. Your task now is to press a button *only* when you see a light blink on. A contingency.

This uncertainty means that the signal will have to sink in, and pass through several extra layers of circuits. These layers will delay your reaction time for perhaps 150 milliseconds. This preliminary, *voluntary* preparation for action is called *intention*.[15]

Studies of human reaction times suggest that the right hemisphere tends to play a leading role among the many higher processes which prepare both sides of our body to respond behaviorally. And we are now examining the proposal that one result of Zen training is to encourage faster links between attention, implying the readiness to perceive, and activation, the readiness to act. So, one begins to appreciate an unfortunate consequence of the narrow base underlying most current studies of normal actions, at least as they are indexed by the usual kinds of reaction times. For such tests depend heavily on the subject's thoughtful layers of intention, and not only during the phase when they are learning their task.[16]

Now, when a trained person's readiness to act becomes more *involuntary* (the more "Zen-like" it becomes, in a sense), the *less* likely it is to be captured in the confines of the usual laboratory, and to be measured by the standard quasi-voluntary techniques. And conventional methods of biofeedback training don't seem to provide final answers either. At least, the usual human subjects don't necessarily react faster after they have first been trained to remain in alpha EEG rhythms. Indeed, they may take 35 percent longer to react to a sound stimulus than they did initially.[17]

Would any other kinds of approaches seem more appropriate? Suppose you decide to move something simple: your index finger. Actually, your brain may take some 400 milliseconds or so of processing time before it finally makes you aware, *consciously*, that you *had* made this "decision."[18] Researchers uncovered this very long delay—the interval between our unconscious decision and its consciously perceived counterpart—when they began to study the human readiness potential. This is an electrical potential which reaches its peak over the frontal regions. And it peaks there some 350 milliseconds *before* we judge that we are going to initiate a particular act.[19] The act then flashes in seemingly from out of nowhere.

Note the brisk spontaneity implied in this latter motor readiness task. It differs sharply from the requirement imposed during the task cited four paragraphs above. Then, during that contingent response task, you had to *wait* for a light to blink. Instead, the particular subjects whose readiness potentials were being studied were free to move *whenever they felt inclined* to do so. Moreover, after they received further "proactive" training, their frontal readiness potential could arrive as many as 500 to 800 milliseconds sooner than did their conscious awareness that they had made the "decision" to act spontaneously.[19]

Researchers interested in defining the physiological correlates of *Ri* and of the other three old words might find it useful to follow up on the interesting fact that the readiness potential is chiefly expressed over the frontal regions. Its frontal distribution opens up the possibility that more specialized techniques might be able to monitor some of our frontal lobe sets as they intervene to shorten, or to lengthen, our *spontaneous* reaction times (see chapter 57).

Recently, special processing techniques have been used to study the low-voltage, extra-fast 40 cps gamma-wave activity in the human EEG.[20] One of the test groups was composed of those particular normal human subjects who reacted quickly to auditory stimuli. These lively subjects showed complex differences which differentiated them from the other group of slow-responding normals. It would be of interest to extend such techniques to study meditators, and to do so at repeated intervals, over a formal training period of many years. Meanwhile, it seems clear that the more researchers can learn about how the frontal lobes "oversee" action and inaction, the better prepared we will all be to understand how Zen expresses itself in action. Because it is mostly in the *front* of the brain that each impulse to act contends with its opposite bias, not to intervene. Here, every day in society, each of us walks not only on a path but on a most subtle tightrope of behavior (see chapter 142).

A "Promethean Hyperpraxia"

My apologies. The sole reason for introducing this new phrase is to focus attention on an aspect of Zen which has been relatively unappreciated in the literature of the neurosciences.

A person's normal ability to perform skilled movements is called *praxis*. A very few patients, when they lose this ability, do so for reasons which truly justify the diagnosis of *apraxia*. In the hospital, you don't require elaborate equipment to test for a disorder of skilled movements. You can hand an apraxic woman an ordinary comb. She recognizes it at once. Unfortunately, she can't move her hand and arm to show you how she *uses* it. Is she paralyzed? No. A few minutes later, when you contrive to observe her, you see her casually combing her hair, *automatically*. And she is doing so in a perfectly normal fashion!

Well, then, could this be a kind of feigned paralysis? No. Consider what exactly she had lost: it was only her *willed* purposive movements. In particular, she had lost those movements of the top-down variety which had become more "voluntary" as soon as you had specifically asked her to perform them. It will be useful now for the reader to recall the essence of blindsight (see chapter 54) and the fact that facial recognition can still proceed at deep automatic levels in visual agnosia (see chapter 142). These other two disorders help us understand the basic feature of this patient's apraxia, because she is functioning in a similar manner. She has retained her lower-level, spontaneous, *automatic* ability to handle a comb. It was only her higher-level *voluntary* sources for directing this movement that had been damaged. And the location of her lesion in the frontoparietal region would be at a site which would have severed the usual flow of impulses which normally unite these two lobes into one skillful partnership (see chapter 55).

In general, when neurologists examine patients, our mindset is directed toward finding those clues which signal the presence of pathological disorders. Especially are we on the lookout for "negative" signs, searching in the above instance for those particular situations which bring out the patient's temporary inability to use a comb. It may take us time and effort to develop the different set of tests required to identify healthy persons who have amplified their normal functions of praxis. And that isn't all.

Because, in the Zen context, we'll need to focus on the *three* different occasions when forms of behavioral enhancement can occur. The first two occur *acutely,* after either internal absorption or kensho. The third variety arrives more gradually, in the person who moves along the path toward the ongoing enlightened traits. It is difficult to summarize the expressions of these three different varieties in formal scientific terms. If one had to use simple words, one might begin with lightness, psychic release, and harmony.

Consider how animated is the behavior and release of the person who is just coming out of kensho. A kind of "hyperpraxia" prevails. It is a Promethean condition. Motor skills are now unbound, unsuppressed. A mere hint suffices to initiate complex motor sequences. Enhanced behaviors flow perfectly and effortlessly, as though the subject were a skilled mime. Now let the roshi make his inane demands: What does One look like from the back? What is the sound of one hand? Challenge as he may, no test shakes the spontaneity of this moment.

What is implied when a person's abilities are enhanced in this manner? First, that the subject is now using frontoparietal, basal ganglia, and cerebellar systems in a highly integrated, graceful, and efficient manner. Second, that the person's "inner game" is now free from the fetters of previous inhibitory constraints on behavior.

To truly understand Zen in action, we will require a thorough documentation of the basic mechanisms—of both gain and loss, addition and subtraction—which express themselves in lightened movements, hyperpraxias, and liberated behavior. The objective studies necessary will have begun long before by careful recordings of the subject's baseline performance skills. Later, these will be compared with the same person's skills immediately after major absorptions and kensho respectively, and then repeated during subsequent years of follow-up studies as the subject moves further along the path.

Tennis, football, and basketball coaches all know that enthusiasm briefly energizes their teams' normal range of alert, heads-up performance. Athletes do gain something, in general, by getting pumped up, the more so when their activity requires vigorous contractions of large muscle groups. Some *short*-term results of this nature might relate to the way dopamine enhances motor functions and motivation when it is released into such subcortical nuclei as the caudate, putamen, and nucleus accumbens[9] (see figures 7 and 12).

Parkinsonian patients illustrate how much DA can add to performance. Before the patients start treatment, they are slow motion personified. They are also bent into a characteristic posture. It is a posture shifted toward flexion: head bent forward, shoulders rolled forward, back hunched, arms and legs flexed. Later, after levodopa has been started, we see them do more than *move* faster. They gradually "unbend." Their whole posture improves because they return toward their long-forgotten posture of extension. It is the normal, heads-up look of attention: now head and trunk are erect, shoulders are back. If this new look were carried further, what would it finally resemble? The alert, everyday posture of an attentive meditator, well advanced in his or her training.

Given what else we have learned about DA, we can envision DA playing some facile roles in normal motivational arousal and in behavioral activation[9] (see chapters 36 and 37). But in each instance studies show that an energized subject's behavior becomes more efficient only up to a certain point. Beyond that, efficiency drops off. Why? Because the whole motor response, while being excessively activated in general, has not been patterned fully in accord with all the *specialized* skills needed for certain other higher levels of performance.[21] So, in Zen, one is not going to be misled by all those other restless, finger-tapping, gum-chewing, engine-racing activities which might pass, elsewhere in society, for seeming to be on your toes.

Nor does the ongoing awareness of the enlightened person take the form of some headlong or slapdash freedom of movement. Rather is it careful, poised, meticulous behavior, however casual and artless it may appear. Freedom within composure. Master Dogen emphasized this point in his final writings.[22] I saw Kobori-roshi living it.

Two other sets of recent findings converge on the basal ganglia. Each relates to the endogenous gas, *nitric* oxide (see chapter 98). One describes the effect that a glutamate nerve cell (up in frontal cortex, for example) would have where it stimulates its receptors farther down in the basal ganglia. At this point, these lower-level cells can release nitric oxide.[23] Why is this noteworthy? Because it also turns out that the nerve cells in these basal ganglia contain especially high levels of cyclic guanosine monophosphate (GMP) cyclase. And before nitric oxide can be metabolically effective, its local target cells must contain this cyclase enzyme. Diffusing quickly into the next cell, nitric oxide can then set off the next cascade of remodeling reactions. So the glutamate-nitric oxide-cGMP system opens up a number of intriguing ways for a brain to modify its old motor patterns and to adopt a new range of behavioral options (see chapter 152).

How else might a brain fine-tune its advanced levels of motor performance, and do so in ways that are relevant to Zen? Our present scope limits us to two examples. They are chosen simply to illustrate, last but not least, the hidden assets of the *cerebellum.*

The Cerebellar Connection

Recent studies indicate that the cerebellum enters into some quasi-cognitive activities[24] (see figure 2). Deep inside it, the large dentate nucleus plays a crucial motoric role. It relays its covert messages first across to the opposite ventral nuclei of the thalamus. From here their signals ascend to inform the motor and premotor cortex. At first it might seem that this information had only been cast in "negative" terms because these dentate projections do inhibit the thalamic cells next down the line. But, down in the cerebellum, many norepinephrine receptors of the beta type swarm over the dentate cells themselves. So, when NE acts on these beta-receptors, dentate nerve cells will be inhibited. Now they fire more *slowly* than before. The steps in this sequence imply that a localized increase in NE could then translate, through a process of disinhibition, into a release of higher thalamocortical motor functions from their previous cerebellar constraints. Again, the caveat: let NE cause too much activation in general, and it could go on to disorganize more specialized aspects of performance.

Learning and memory involve more than adding something new. They can also mean subtraction. We have been using this term to suggest the process that helps clear the decks so the new function can supersede the old one (see chapter 74). High up in the cerebellar cortex are the big nerve cells called Purkinje cells. They participate in the process of learning new motor skills. During learning, the glutamate receptors which cover these Purkinje cells undergo a curious change.[25] On previous occasions, when glutamate had been released onto its receptors, these large cells would have become excited by it. But now, during motor learning, a local *depression* occurs. Where? At the site of certain of these former glutamate excitations. So that now, as part of motor learning, the big Purkinje cells become *less* excitable than before, even during the first training session. This local "learning" depression can last for as long as ten minutes. Later phases can persist for several hours. This process of long-term depression operates not only in the cerebellum. It also occurs in the hippocampus where, in conjunction with long-term potentiation, the brain can employ it to shape learning and memory along novel, adaptive lines.

156

The Other Side of Zen

> Eastern enlightenment is the full and perfect understanding that the stupidity, vulgarity and hypocrisy of this world is quite all right just as it is . . . This enlightenment is found in Christianity also; it is, "Thy will be done" in infinitely meaningless inanity.
>
> R. Blyth (1898–1964)[1]

> I suspect every European attempt at detachment of being mere liberation from moral considerations.
>
> Carl Jung[2]

Tough words from critics. But the full moon of enlightenment does have its dark side. What else could be said against Zen? To Blyth, Zen had a very weak missionary spirit when compared with Christian standards.[1] He believed it was also possessed of a "certain cold-heartedness"; was individualistic to the point of selfishness, self-reliant to the point of aloofness, and amoral in theory but not in practice. If such were true, had Eisai made the right choice when he decided to import this kind of movement to strengthen his country?

Zen is an easy target. Yes, it did serve to remind every age that Buddhism needed reforms. But Zen too tended to become doctrinaire, and its central message became blurred. Institutional Zen can have all the frailties of any human product, but it redeems its weaknesses in the act of becoming its own severest critic. Rigorous Zen masters of no less stature than Rinzai and Hakuin also condemned it harshly from the inside. Many failings attributed to Zen stem from the way its adherents practice it. True, overzealous sitting may damage the sciatic or peroneal nerves in the leg.[3] But mostly, as in other religions, the problem centers elsewhere: Zen precepts are practiced not too far, but *not far enough*.

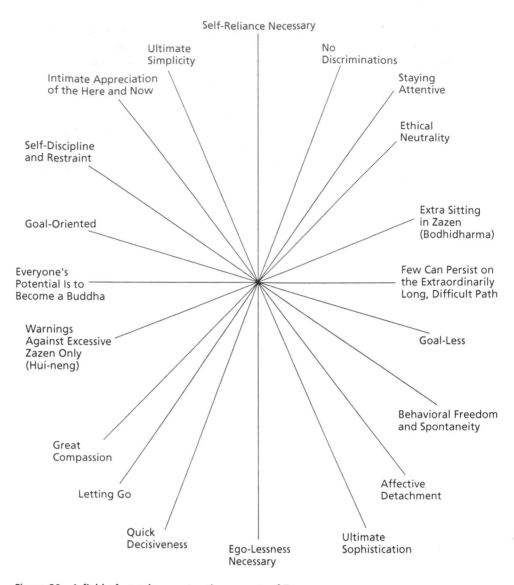

Figure 20 A field of paradox: contrasting aspects of Zen
A trainee encounters many seemingly contradictory elements in Zen. The figure depicts a representative field of these yin-yang characteristics. An inevitable tugging tension exists between each polar pair of opposites. The aspirant learns gradually to reconcile their contrasts and to live spontaneously within this field.

Zen isn't for everyone, probably not for most. Few beginners appreciate how much system lurks behind its paradoxes and its seemingly haphazard training methods. Students soon become doubly confused, for they sense both ambiguities within Zen and flat-out contradictions. We summarize the latter in figure 20, which presents them as diametrical opposites within a field of paradox. For example: how does a person go about being both self-reliant and egoless at the same time? Over the years, the contrasts are reconciled, but they do not necessarily disappear from view.

The encounter with Zen rocks many persons. It evokes reminiscences of the ways Dadaism shocked sensibilities by revolting against conventional attitudes during World War I. Some turn away, hearing about its shouts and blows, its seemingly idiotic answers and irreverent humor. True, over a thousand years ago, masters like Ma-tsu (709–788) were known for shouting at, browbeating, and swatting their trainees. Today, this level of aggression is passé, but the flat stick remains. Why? Its whomp is useful. For one thing, it stings. Moreover, the *whack* of the *kyosaku* sounds loud in the meditator's ears. The two stimuli fuse into one, a concrete example of direct sensory experience. The sting-whack serves as a fine remedy for drowsiness, replacing boredom with attentiveness at those times when something, *anything*, seems preferable to nothing.

Then what of a master's other eccentricities, behaviors that might have found an acceptable niche back in the culture of the Tang dynasty? They would be counterproductive nowadays. But Zen still delivers hard jolts to the intellect, cleverly designed to dislodge the intellectual pretenses of the self. Its training methods have simply become less physical, in keeping with today's gentler versions of Oriental and Western customs.

Cultural expectations are still changing in our lifetime. The 1960s ushered in a widespread mistrust of authoritarian figures, and its momentum went on radically to erode relationships between leaders and led, parents and children, teachers and students. Even before that, I had seen moderation temper the rigorous training of apprentice surgeons whose chiefs were no longer disposed to hurl instruments at them in the operating room. In an era when battered American presidencies may last for merely one short term, the tough old roshi of yesteryear are already an endangered species.

In no era did an authentic, low-profile Zen really need to flaunt its irrationality in order to remain faithful to the tradition of Siddhartha, the founder. Yet, there is a long past history of eccentric Zen behavior, and it continues to give pious monotheists ample reason for concern, whatever their religious background. Think of how many generations have been alarmed when they first heard about that old shocking statement, "Kill the Buddha!" Yet, one's anxieties about the phrase can obscure its real implications, which enter at the most innocuous of levels. The words mean: Don't idolize the *physical* form of a statue of the Buddha. Don't cling to any hallucinated image of him, or to any concept that this historical man exists outside yourself. Open up, instead, to what he taught: a Way to liberate your original nature.

Zen follows up on this age-old theme. What does it still teach its students? To pay total, mindful attention; to attend to the current concrete realities of their physical senses, not to ever-proliferating abstract thoughts. But, then, as the ends of one line in figure 20 illustrate, how does staying attentive fit in with letting go into the vaunted Zen detachment? To call it "nonattachment" will not silence some Christian critics. They may feel that detachment by any name will serve merely to deaden the moral conscience, simply enabling the person "to practice immorality with equilibrium."[4] In fact, this is not what happens. I have had the experience of meeting and sitting in sesshin with four Rinzai and two Soto Zen groups over the last two decades, in Japan, the United States, and England. My experience would not support assertions of immorality or lack of conscience. Compared with other Western religious groups I have known, the mature followers of the Zen Way do tend to have different priorities. But they, too, practice high ethical standards, and they sense how to act with compassion when they enter the hurly-burly of the marketplace.

Spread out before us today is a spiritual supermarket. It teems with alternative altars: EST, psychosynthesis, Silva mind control, TM, Krishna consciousness societies, water tanks, to name a few. When these other options fail, on their own, Zen tends to be tarred with the same brush. At this point, prejudices against the Buddhist Way generalize too far. Yet rarely do such alternative groups come close to the rigorous standards set by authentic Zen monasteries, particularly those in Japan. There, only certain monks will be judged professionally qualified to train others, and some of these select few will have matured through a decade or more of supervised koan studies.

Which neurosurgeon would you chose to operate on your brain? Mine is a very short list. Aspirants are advised to select with great care the personal advisor who will be guiding their psyche. Meanwhile, the neophyte had best steer clear of any form of unseasoned "new-age" mysticism, East or West, that hasn't carefully selected its teachers for many years, over many generations.

No such caveat can ensure that only perfect beings inhabit each *sangha*, the community of Zen practitioners. Lay students of meditation are neither perfect nor content, and totally "happy campers" are rare. Most are younger searchers, still immature, and beset by the turmoil of a stressful urban society. All too soon, the afterglow fades from each hard-sought "experience," exposing anew the raw imperfections of self within the imperfect everyday world. When concentration slips, as it does, the burden of these dual imperfections returns, and it soon leads to marked feelings of disenchantment. Few monks and lay sangha members in any century will approach the same stage of supreme ongoing enlightenment as did the historical Buddha. The rest will be reminded of the ancient truth predicted in Ecclesiastes, that "in much wisdom is much grief; and those who increase knowledge increase sorrow."

But more positive outcomes do develop along the way. Indeed, what happens is that most persons improve substantially. Resistance and indignation, yes. But because the aspirants gradually have less personal dignity at stake, they slowly become less self-righteous than when they began. Lost tempers, yes. But each fuse grows a little longer, and some of the basic causes of anger and fear are being defused. Do emotions still set off a powder charge? Yes, but it is smaller, more efficient, muffled, and has fewer echoes.

Sanghas have been imperfect for centuries. Perhaps as few as 10 percent of the monks were considered to have been "good" monks in Chinese monasteries just before the People's Republic took over.[5] In 1989, a young Rinzai monk in Japan spontaneously mentioned to me this same estimate of only 10 percent "good" monks. However stringent and subjective the criteria of excellence may be, it will take much more than 10 percent to sustain the vitality of any group. In this respect, Zen may sometimes find itself on the long list of other contemporary religious institutions which appear to be slipping out of the public's confidence because some of its individual leaders have not yet been able to set their own personal house in order.

Meanwhile, one does not assume that every person who adopts the garb of a Zen monk and leads a group has become a truly awakened human being. In Japan, many monks simply go on "serving time" in the few training monasteries, waiting until they can take over their father's position as head of a small temple. Relatively few monks will receive the written statement, *inka*, from their own roshi. It is the document certifying that they have been held to their teacher's very highest standards of character and performance for many years. In a world starving for spiritual leadership, inspired roshi are in short supply. Too few are available nowadays who themselves seem to have started on the leadership path with what might be called "the right stuff," who then went on to receive their training from the best roshi in a high-quality training monastery, who passed all the hurdles of daily practice and koan study, and who were finally selected to train others.

In old China, Confucianism provided the sturdy base and the ethical support system for family, secular, and religious life. It served as a useful counterpoise to the detachment implicit in other Taoist influences. If Taoist influences were undiluted, they leaned toward a withdrawn, contemplative mysticism which did not actively stimulate the work ethic. Indeed, Lao-Tzu had once described the person who followed the Way as "like a child, alone, careless, unattached, devoid of ambition."[6] Is there a familiar ring to this laid-back, drop-out status? We recall that a monkey, after having been tamed by lesions in and around the amygdala, also gives up jockeying for position, and soon loses all status in its strongly competitive and hierarchical society.

Authentic Zen training provides a sharp contrast. It emphasizes not only an increasingly competent level of performance but one balanced with a careful, caring mature behavior. In a rigorous Zen sangha no person can survive who remains lazy, careless, and childish. Indeed, it was hard-nosed Master Huai-hai (720–814) who introduced the principle, "a day of no work is a day of no food." On this visceral basis, manual labor became the norm when he founded the first Chan monastery during the Tang dynasty.

Zen masters do not necessarily give up all their own self-indulgent weaknesses. Some still abuse tobacco, alcohol, or food. And, as Roth and Stevens observe, "the majority have high estimations of their own worth," tending to overvalue their own understanding of Buddhism.[7] I have not yet met a Zen teacher who appeared completely free from every last burden of the old egocentric self, the *I-Me-Mine*. But, on the other hand, they each more than made up for their relatively few shortcomings by being exceptional in countless other ways.

The human imperfections within the sangha create troublesome points of friction. Many students seem to expect, quite unrealistically, a utopian group led by Buddha himself. A sensitive relationship exists between a disciple and a rigorous master. The tensions can become especially difficult for someone like Becker, whose atypical view of satori was that it was "nothing more than acceptance of the new value system, an introjection of the master's superego in a final, submissive adaptation to his authoritarian pressures."[8] My experience was totally different. There was no feeling of being coerced into any "adaptation to author-ity." Instead, there was the sense of having been emancipated first by kensho's raw data and then by its spontaneous waves of reflexive interpretations. Moreover, spontaneous awakenings also occur. Some, for example, transpire during a near-death experience. These, too, can transform the subject's life. These spontaneous awakenings require no special interpersonal relationship with an authority figure, nor do they depend on any formal religious context.

The protagonist in Orwell's book, *1984*, after having undergone much brain-washing, is finally described in the concluding, chilling line: "He had won the victory over himself: he loved Big Brother." This is not the style of authentic, self-negating Zen. Its Middle Way has always emphasized self-questioning and independent judgments, not slavish devotion to a master. Zen doctrines, such as they are, are not ideological property. This path suffers from no exclusive hold on truth. What Zen submits for analysis are teachings, not rigid doctrines. If its teachers ultimately become held in high affection, it will be for another reason: no matter at what level they began their own search, they gradually rose above their earlier limitations to become decent, caring, and inspiring mentors.

Does awakening always improve the person? No guarantees lie along the razor-edged spiritual path. The search is a stormy one, as the Grofs observe, for they devote part III and the appendix of their recent book to helpful ways to cope with spiritual emergencies.[9] What can happen if self-imposed restraints and if ongoing mindful practice have not already weakened the *I-Me-Mine?* What if aspirants have not been truly humbled by their alternate state experiences? In every religious persuasion, among those unbalanced persons who lack the crucial supportive foundation, events can take a different turn. These few become dis-torted by the newfound feelings of an exalted state: strength is diverted in the direction of power; invulnerability becomes invincibility; love becomes lust. No odor will smell so bad, said Thoreau, "as that which arises from goodness tainted."[10] The media remind us that zealots lurk on the left or right of every creed and cult, illustrating how far astray the seemingly "religious" may go.

Where does the simple, stable, mature Zen product stand in relation to these unfortunate outcomes? Poised at a distance far removed. It chases no fluttering skirt, crusades under no banner, nor will it hoist a personal flag that must be saluted.

True, some Zen aspirants and perhaps an occasional teacher may profess gold-plated overbeliefs. It is not difficult to slip overboard on tangents of mystical sophistry. But, in general, it is not the Zen sangha that becomes the kind of a problem group headed by a "Perfect Master" who sets out "to save the world."[11] It will usually be some other mystics, those outside Zen, whose imbalance leads them to conclude that they are so much at "one" with the universal "mind" that they have been granted complex powers beyond both common sense and the known physical laws of this universe. A sage roshi, full of infectious common sense, maintains the sangha on an even keel and sets a sound course.

The form of Zen, but not its essence, resembles that of an ancient, gnarled, bonsai tree, handed down reverently from generation to generation. A fine old pot still contains the tree, but its walls now show cracks in several places, and they no longer retain moisture appropriately. What fool would submit this root-bound treasure to a major pruning, let alone think about transplanting it into a new container? Yet the larger concern is not so much for the gnarled old tree of Zen tradition itself. It has stood up well. What is worrisome is the garish character of any new container which would be made from the unnatural plastic products of our modern world. It is a world which today seems turned upside down, having desensitized its inhabitants to lurid headlines and TV, while creating in them fresh yearnings for instant material and other gratifications.

Previous centuries evolved at a slower pace. They allowed sensibilities to be expressed in a more modulated way. This leads us back to the two words evoking the spirit of the old cultural hand-me-downs. One is the term *wabi*, that spare, humble beauty which grows out of a poverty of materials. It would also violate the Japanese aesthetic to disturb the soil around any longstanding relationship that reflects *sabi*, that pleasure in venerable, well-aged things. So special loyalties are already implicit in Japanese culture. They actively resist notions of change.

But on the other hand there is the long view of history. Over the millennia, it reminds us how Buddhism continued to rejuvenate itself. New vitality infused its old core each time it was transplanted—from Dyana, to Chan, to Zen. Moreover, in India, the Upanishads have an even longer tradition, now some three thousand years old. Looking back at that historical record, Radhakrishnan makes an important point when he observes that "Loyalty to our particular tradition means not only concord with the past but also freedom from the past."[12] Even when one scans the decades of this twentieth century, one sees not only how much all religions have changed but how dramatically Japan itself has been transformed. Such changes would have been inconceivable to this young serviceman who first lived there almost half a century ago. Over the same decades, Zen, too, has been slowly accomodating itself, gradually evolving its traditional paradoxes as it continues to spread its influence throughout the world.[13]

157

Still-Evolving Brains in Still-Evolving Societies

Man appears to be the missing link between anthropoid apes and human beings.
Konrad Lorenz (1903–1989)[1]

At each further degree of combination *something* which is irreducible to isolated elements *emerges* in a new order.
Pierre Teilhard de Chardin (1881–1955)[2]

Nature's open book is humbling when we turn back the pages through which we evolved.[3] In the beginning, what was the "word?" For biochemists, it was whatever molecules started to grow in the primordial alphabet soup. Here, nucleic acid bases slowly assembled amino acids into the organic building blocks of life. In seawater, the first living cells merged into multicelled creatures. Needing an integrating core, they gradually evolved a network of nerve cells. Then, hundreds of millions of years ago, cells developed the particular enzymes which could make acetylcholine, norepinephrine, and many other messenger molecules. We still use them to speed impulses from one cell to the next.

The next step, some 600 million years ago, was to build receptors, the tiny targets designed to receive discrete chemical messages.[4] We now know a good deal about one of these. It is the beta-receptor activated by NE, the same kind of NE receptor we just happened to have been discussing in the cerebellum. It is a very long polypeptide, so long that its many loops resemble an overly loose form of stitching. As these loops thread in and out through the cell's outer membrane, they help import NE's message into the target cell.

Something else is very remarkable about this receptor protein. It is similar to rhodopsin. Previously, it had been assumed that rhodopsin occurred only in the eye. After all, wasn't it the visual purple which acted as our retina's receptor pigment? And wasn't this visual purple a light-sensitive protein, of a special kind which enabled even primitive eyes to take the energies from light waves and transduce them into nerve impulses?[5] Yes, on both counts. Then why does the brain's beta-receptor for NE so closely resemble visual purple, sharing with it not only thirty of the same amino acids but also many of rhodopsin's other properties? In fact, these two counterpart proteins—the purple one activated by light and the beta-receptor activated by NE—*both arose from the same source*. Scientists can date their common origin back to one big ancestor protein which they shared hundreds of millions of years ago.

Furthermore, it now turns out that many of our *other* receptors are also similar to rhodopsin. The general family resemblance is so striking that they all can be viewed as members of one large, genetically related group of receptors. The members of this large family include not only the alpha- and beta-receptors for NE but also some receptors activated by acetylcholine (the muscarinic type of ACH receptors), by serotonin (those of ST subtype 1) and by the peptide angiotensin. While turning the pages of nature's history back and forth, one begins to wonder. What are the future implications of our having evolved such a large visual brain? Could some of those ancient receptors, which first started to perceive light rays in our evolutionary past, have now gone on to be linked with states of enlightenment in more than metaphoric ways?

Even our most remote mammalian ancestors were latecomers. Insects had already been swarming over the planet several hundred million years before. Insects need to shed their rigid outer layers. Until its skin cracks and molts, an insect can't proceed to grow larger and develop further. The same transforming process still operates today. Biologists give it the long name, *metamorphosis*. In the first step, the insect brain releases a peptide hormone. This peptide then sets off a whole series of biochemical reactions. These ripple through the cAMP cascade, and at the end they finally release steroid hormones. Only when the steroid hormones *reprogram* other sets of cells can the creature's soft inner body break free from its rigid outer casing. Each successive step in this ancient metabolic mechanism is necessary. Only by acting in concert do they enable the molting insect to expand and mature.[6]

The planet then, as now, was no continuous Taoist idyll. Indeed, the Earth's own layers of history record *seventeen* chaotic planetary crises during the past 650 million years[7] Only two of these were the mass global extinctions of 250 and 65 million years ago that we read about in the daily paper. Which of our primitive ancestors survived? Those few who were able to flee or fight, love or hate, sleep or waken at *just* the most appropriate times.

Each global catastrophe winnowed the field, sparing the most adaptive neural networks. Function followed form, and form followed function. Anatomists point to the pathways radiating to and from our hypothalamus as among the most persistent hard-wired traces of such ancient networks. Darwin reserved a special name for the most basic patterns of adaptive behavior which finally developed. He called them the "indelible stamp" which thereafter testified to our lowly origins.

Food, friend, or foe? The forerunners of our deeper circuits evolved to answer these primal questions. Indeed, this is what *Aplysia's* circuits still do (see chapter 49). But other polarizing pathways also evolved, and they gradually became the visceral roots of our own affective responses (see chapter 78). Behavior now could be shaped by a great range of polar opposites. Unfortunately, many of these charged networks—especially those linking within the triad of the hypothalamus-amygdala-central gray—have long outlasted their earlier biological survival value. Master Bankei's sage wisdom reminds us: that bonfire, so useful in winter, becomes too hot to bear when summertime arrives.

By the time we students had finished biology class, we had learned how each individual embryo first goes through similar stages as did the species as a whole. Ontogeny recapitulates phylogeny. Soon we would be swept up into our own adolescent version of metamorphosis. The steroids from our own endocrine glands took over. Voices cracked and bodies expanded in new regions. We too were on an ascending path: another turbulent series of developmental changes was leading us toward new levels of psycho-social-sexual maturity.

Were still other forces also at work, beyond such routine passages? The Jesuit Teihard de Chardin thought so. He perceived that humankind was also progressing through sequences of *spiritual* development. These spiritual stages, he believed, were a natural consequence of the fact that the human species was still evolving biologically. It is true that we need to be careful about elastic mental constructs like "spiritual" and "soul." Yet evidence recently unearthed shows that even Neanderthal families must have felt the tug of similar sensibilities when they brought flowers to the graveside, and began to engage in simple burial ceremonies.

Long before that—some 5 to 10 million years ago—we primates shared a common ancestor. How do we know we are related to the large family that includes today's chimpanzees and gorillas? Again, the chemical evidence of our proteins serves as the indelible stamp of a common ancestry. Our proteins are about 98 percent identical with theirs.[8] From then on, as recent studies of skulls make clear, the protohuman association cortex kept getting larger. In order to accommodate it, the vault of the primitive skull increased its own size and adjusted its shape. When the toolmakers, *Homo habilis*, arrived some 2 million years ago, they were endowed with cranial capacities of (only) 660 cubic centimeters. Then, between 1 million years ago and 400,000 years ago, *Homo erectus* went on to attain a skull capacity of 1000 cubic centimeters. The gross size of the human brain seems to have stabilized at around 1330 cubic centimeters ever since modern *Homo sapiens* arrived, some 80,000 to 35,000 years ago.[9]

Let us now step back and look over all these comparative observations. In doing so, it seems at least reasonable to correlate the gross size and shape of the Pleistocene brain with the other handmade artifacts found at the archeological sites. For out of the earth's strata have come many devotional artifacts which also increase in their complexity in successive cultural layers. The evidence suggests that hominids have been developing something akin to "spiritual" sensibilities, and adding them to their ever-increasing cognitive skills.

Are we *still* evolving spiritually? How much further will we go? To Teilhard, the answer was: a very long way. He thought of it in terms of the phrase "Omega point." It meant that distant epoch, projected far off into the distant future, when everyone on this planet will finally have evolved. Evolved into what? Into that ultimate central focus which he would call "hyper-personal consciousness."[2] Maybe so. Who knows? Looking back over the obvious trends in the testimony sifted from the earth, it would seem premature to foreclose humankind's capacities in any way. Given the recent rate of change, who is to say that some future Omega descendents might not dig up evidence that we, their progenitors, had started to evolve along new spiritual lines?

But enlightenment for everyone? It sounds like too grandiose a Utopia, especially when we consider how inept human beings seem to be in the face of the harsh realities which confront the planet today. At best, one might hope for a broader secular base in general, for a greater percentage of fully enlightened persons, and certainly for more authentic leaders whose inspiration could light the way. Yet the human species has long shown a second surprising aptitude for improving itself. The process is called *cultural evolution*. It continues currently to civilize billions of humans along many positive, fruitful lines.

Item: Those fierce Vikings of yesteryear who changed into socially concerned Scandinavians in only relatively recent times. Yet suppose our descendants in future centuries could look back critically on all those of us who had lived during the fierce and messy years of this twentieth century. What might they conclude that our citizens lacked the most? One top priority item on any educational list would be a truly user-friendly owner's manual. An ecumenical handbook that spelled out the simple positive things people could do to bring *life's genuine substance*, not more "lifestyles," into their lives. And our descendants might sense our need to have had not only this kind of contemporary *Tao Te Ching*, of ways to live affirmatively, but our need for its precepts to have been put into *actual use* in the workaday world and to have been reinforced by teacher-exemplars at all educational levels, starting in the home.

A tall order. Yet other cultures have also anticipated a better future for humankind. The early Buddhists were especially farsighted about the beneficial effects of biological and cultural evolution. Indeed, they were confident that future generations would develop new fully enlightened religious leaders. In the old city of Nara, there exists today a sublime statue which depicts their long-range faith in graphic form. It is the figure of *Miroku* (Maitrea), the Buddha of the future, and it has remarkably "modern" facial features. One is startled to discover that it was created back in the Japan of the seventh century.

A closer look discloses another curious feature about this Buddha of the future. The statue has *two* protrusions, one on either side of the top of the head *next* to the midline. Why *two*, when the conventional Buddha heads are limited to only one *ushnisha* in the midline? (see chapter 2). Was the remote sculptor sending us some kind of a message? Will evolved brains of the future be twice as enlightened? Or was he hinting that brains might be needing twice as much insight merely to survive the hazards lying in wait in the future? Does a crystal ball predict a future so complex for descendants of the industrial age that they will find it twice as difficult to become fully enlightened in the information age?

Societies reject rapid change. Countless Buddhist scriptures have been burned, and so have martyrs in every religion over the ages. Suppose Teilhard's and others' prophecies do prove correct. If so, then many of our descendents along the way—from right now until that theoretical Omega point—will not have had an easy time of it. They too will have had to survive cataclysms and other rigorous selection pressures. So how realistic is an expectation that fallible human beings will evolve into an Omega race of human*e* beings, *all* Buddha-like in their degree of enlightenment? Given our present deficiencies, could we manage to do so even if we are partners in some benevolent, cosmic design far too grand in scope for our hazy vision ever to foresee?

Many have expressed doubts that the human scenario will have a happy outcome. Buddhists who are now part of the current resurgence of Buddhism can look back only with concern at the ebb in the tides of Buddhism that took place in past centuries, first in India, then in China, Japan, and Southeast Asia. And no pessimist will be easily persuaded that it is always an advantage to have brains slowly increasing in size, shape, and complexity. *Item:* The data showing that violent crimes grew at a rate twelve times faster than did the U.S. population, in only the past generation.[10]

So, in this chapter, let us start to develop a more realistic view, one which considers both our earlier harsh planetary history, and the challenges of our time. Let us doubly qualify this viewpoint at the very beginning. First, by calling it "the *Mu* perspective." Second, by stating that the biological approach which it forsees in continual operation (one might call it the "*Mu* approach") has no finite endpoint, nor does it carry spiritual overtones. Such a matter-of-fact option builds on no pious hopes. It acknowledges that Nature was always "red in tooth and claw," in Tennyson's phrase. Moreover, it is aware that even those bright chimps studied by gentle Jane Goodall at Gombe turned out to be killers of their own kind. Then what kind of a soul-less world could be seen through any such red-streaked glasses except for one flawed by innate inhumanities?

In fact, what *can* be seen is the remarkable capacity empowering each of our creature-ancestors: their capacity to *keep on changing* in response to the stressful challenges of an eternally Darwinian world. This basic capacity to change, to adapt, is an inherent part of our "indelible stamp."

Then why call it *Mu?* For several reasons. (1) It seems more in keeping with the overall spirit of Zen: a word suggesting an ongoing process of becoming, not of having reached some ultimate destination. (2) In this regard, the letter μ (*mu*) is the letter only halfway through the Greek alphabet; Omega is always associated with the end. (3) *Mu* is reminiscent of the koan often given to students who are beginning Zen. It invokes the idea of an arduous struggle over a very long time. (4) *Mu* also stands for micron, one millionth of a meter (μm). It is symbolic of the countless, infinitesimally tiny steps through which nerve cell processes have been reaching out, during evolution and during each of our lives, to establish contact with one another.

Biological evolution has now come to be viewed as a kind of "punctuated equilibrium." It is more of a "hurry-up-and-wait" process than one which keeps moving on at a constant snail's pace. We have observed that Zen meditative training proceeds in much the same way. The major intuitive leaps are relatively uncommon. They punctuate long periods of homeostasis and of glacially slow change.

So let us now take a critical look at the state of awakening, kensho-satori, and reexamine it from the same broad biological perspective. At its core is change. Change means shifting from old to new. What is enlightenment's first crucial contribution? What it *sheds*. What it *subtracts*. It *de*structures, *de*programs and *de*conditions in depth. As a result, the brain becomes less top-heavy; its functions are simplified, revitalized. New systems of adaptive behaviors can develop more readily in such a reorganized brain. Accordingly, one can be cautiously optimistic about this unique capacity of the brain to shift into a wide range of alternate states. For herein resides a potential resource, a resource which could serve as the basis both for our long-range biological survival and for our cultural advancement.

Why could such a capacity contribute to both? Because evolution hasn't stopped. All living things are still on its long shakedown cruise. Selection pressures of various kinds are still pushing DNA back to the drawing boards. They are still forcing our cells to come up with new options in order to cope with the challenges of "adverse surroundings," as John Burroughs' phrased it. Our capacities to endure hardships, to be suddenly alerted by triggers, and to evoke certain latent stress responses intrinsic to the brain—all these have slowly become part of our now deeply ingrained survival responses. And, when nurtured, they are still available to make an indelible contribution to what Isshu-roshi had called "the jewel of spiritual cultivation" and to what Burroughs went on to describe as the "flowering of our spiritual nature."

Advanced alternate states of consciousness exemplify the capacities of the human brain for change. Put simply, they help us cast off our outmoded, hard-shelled, stereotyped behavior patterns. Aided by future variations on this same general theme, some of our adaptable descendants—those whose education had gentled them and made them more flexible—could build on their experiences, become increasingly free to adapt creatively, and so be enabled to survive future crises.

Moreover, at the same time, awakenings could also help them open up to appreciate new *cultural* approaches, and to redesign the increasingly more humane ways of living required to benefit both society as a whole and themselves as contributing members.

All this would proceed millennia by millennia, much too slowly for anyone to appreciate at the time. Let a few more persons multiply who had survived because they had greater capacities for such adaptability, and the resulting series of events might go on slowly to change the ethical and religious climate of the far distant future. Still, from this *Mu* perspective, the basic transforming process would remain a biological one. It would be *an increasing capacity for change*. The *Mu* approach implies a flexibility which would be centered primarily at the operational level of the psychophysiology of the brain.

Biological at its core, the evolutionary process proposed in this qualified hypothesis would continually spin off the related secondary cultural layers. This means that *cultural* evolution would phase in at every step to provide the essential positive and negative social reinforcements. The cultural influences could be of many kinds: spiritual, for example, or environmental or political or economic. The rock edicts of Ashoka remind us that the messages of spiritual leadership can endure and be passed on for millennia.

To judge from the formal polls, most people would prefer to believe that only the workings of some kind of God could conduct such an intricate series of events. If so, the theists can still draw inspiration from the finite perfectibility of an Omega point. Yet they stand in no greater awe at that kind of distant Utopian future than the biologists who would view many of the same events unfolding during the process of the *Mu* approach as the unaimed workings of inexorable natural forces. For the *Mu* perspective is not a directionless angle of vision. It implies as much respect for process as does the former, but is wary about man-made spiritual goals. Meanwhile, opinions aside, the oldest wisdoms of survival still go on, their inheritable capacities slowly transforming our brain and body, almost geological in the way they elude current sentimental categories.

Already, we are the beneficiaries of a civilizing evolutionary process that some observers would date to the river valley cultures starting a mere 8,000 years ago. Recent years have brought forth revolutionary advances in biotechnology. Over the decades, breeders of livestock have become comfortable with the concepts of animal eugenics. But now, hardly a month goes by without some new development in *artificial selection*, involving DNA mapping, "genetic repair," and in vitro fertilization. As the pace accelerates, one begins to get concerned: what new, startling options will soon be opening up?[11] Consider, for example, something not beyond the realm of possibilities. One can at least imagine a new era when some religious group within a culture might decide that it needed to raise and train a new leader. By then, the ancient custom of searching all over for the right baby would long have been given up. It would be viewed as both impractical and too chancy. For this new far-out world would be postmetaphysical, post-Huxleyan, ever braver than before. And by then, "reincarnation" would finally be appreciated as something determined solely by the laws which govern the human genome.

In this far-distant era, it might then be realized that the desired child could best be conceived in a test tube and nurtured in a surrogate mother. Entering into the ever-braver union would be the ovum donated perhaps by a virginal nun, plus the sperm from an exemplary monk, both of whom had been screened and selected on the basis of their outstanding lineage and capacity.[12] It is not necessary for anyone today to buy into this futuristic scenario or to feel comfortable about it. Our task is to take a deep breath and to accept that such a blessed event is now *technically* possible. And not to scoff too quickly. After all, it was only a mere 130 years ago that an obscure Austrian monk started us off on the formal garden path of genetics, while pursuing his hobby of raising hybrid peas and bees. Neither Gregor Mendel nor his superiors could have foreseen such far-out genetic options, given the limited cultural horizon of their day.

During kensho's awakening, does the experiant *actually* grasp Ultimate Reality? Or is the brain in the grip of a powerful illusion? Does such a grasp of silent insights represent only an illusory confluence of rare physiological changes? Perhaps as we step back and consider the following example of the *Mu* approach, we may begin to sense that an option could be opening up between these two extremes, a middle way.

The Symbol of the Urna

In Buddhist iconography, the *urna* is a dot in the middle of the forehead, above and between the eyes. It stands for the levels of enhanced perception that are associated with insight-wisdom. We begin the analogy on the firm ground well-established by the findings of the developmental biologists. They tell us that eons ago, when living creatures first started to reach toward the light, a series of cellular events led to the creation of two tiny dimples. These started in the outer layer of skin, on each side of the primitive head. Each dimple then became a shallow pit. Curving inward further, these unique cells later changed themselves into the early pinhole "eye." Finally they evolved into an eye so specialized that it could focus waves of energy through a flexible lens on visual purple proteins in a light-sensitive retina.

That was only part of it. Simultaneously, two buds of neural tissue had been protruding, micron by micron, from the base of the primitive brain. Groping slowly forward to join each of these specialized patches of skin, these two sprouts would ultimately become the optic nerves. No one was around who could have anticipated this process. No one to marvel at the way that cells from two such different tissues, their tropisms interacting, could gradually transform one another into the earliest functioning eye.

No matter. By then a working, seeing eye had arrived. True, this earliest visual perception was still rather dim and hazy. Yet it was a neurobiological fact. No chemists had to synthesize it; no philosophers or theologians or Zen masters had to speculate about whether it was being directed from some vast outside principle; no neuro-ophthalmologists yet needed to worry about its getting diseased. And for millions of years the original eye went on further to evolve its sophisticated connections and receptor systems. With ever-increasing fidelity it registered and relayed the patterns of light waves reflected into it from things in the outside world.

After all these inherited incremental refinements, what could each creature now perceive? A clear and vastly improved image *of reality*. Yet, back in the remote beginning, no rudimentary forebrain—sensing the far-off presence of that first primitive dimple—had developed enough foresight to direct the destiny of the final results. Nor could it ever have made the incredibly educated guess that its networks would later evolve to such a degree that human beings would someday be granted their added capacities to *en*vision, *im*agine, and *in*tuit.

Only recently, say in the river valley cultures a few thousand years ago, did human brains and complex societies start to adapt even further. Only then did a succession of teachers discover how to employ meditative techniques in the appropriate cultural setting, and to do so in ways that could culminate in *in*sightful transformations at advanced levels. The meditative Way has barely begun to exert its potential cultural influence.

So what? What if a person's brain does continue to refine these innate capacities to awaken into insight-wisdom and then to extend itself into a new mode of living? Let us take the longest possible view of the positive consequences. For each represents a step *forward*. So, too, were the tiny micron steps taken by those early cells and receptor proteins as they slowly assembled themselves, eons before, into a primitive eye and a visual system. And in such infinitesimal steps lies that human potential to evolve toward illumination at more advanced levels. For ours is still a species on an endless journey into an unimaginable future. Each small step that expands our individual and social consciousness may seem as though it were "nothing special." But, as the urna reminds us, it is one small part of a long-range approach which could be bringing us closer to more enlightened perceptions, attitudes and to more humane behavior.

158

Commentary on the Trait Change of Ongoing Enlightenment

> If you think the mind
> That attains enlightenment
> Is "mine"
> Your thoughts will wrestle, one with the other.
>
> Die—then live
> Day and night within the world.
> Once you've done this
> Then you can hold the world right in your hand!
>
> Master Bankei[1]

The writer and the reader of this book have been working on a koan, on a quest to find the wellsprings of genuine simplicity and freedom. Our search has seemed to unfold in living networks all the way from the tip of the frontal lobe down to the spinal cord. Then why does Bankei talk about death? Because "dying to self" is more than a figure of speech. It implies making major changes in the living human brain, bypassing and etching out old circuits of the *I-Me-Mine*.

Do we in the West have precedents for this kind of process? Both Matthew (16:25) and Luke (9:24) speak for that depth of understanding which could say: "Whoever loses his life for my sake will gain it." So this kind of "dying" is not the end. This mortality is the prelude to being "born again." Something to be welcomed, not feared.

In the Zen context, what does it mean when a person loses the dysfunctional self? Above all, it means having shed archaic fears that center on self-preservation. It also implies having substituted wisdom for ignorance. Thereafter, none of the old delusions will trip the emergent policy of compassion. Nor will they be counterproductive to one's other long-range goals. But genuine personal change takes decades. For we have not been talking about only a few short productive experiences, brief states separated by long vacant gaps of many years in between. The training goes on *every day*. It consists of that steady ongoing practice which extends meditative awareness off the sitting cushion and infuses it into everyday living. In this way does a person's daily life practice become a habitual, twofold mode. It serves not only as the ground for personal introspection, skillful behavior and restraint but also as the foundation for one's delight in the bounty of each present moment.

What happens when calm awareness fully engages the here and now of daily living? Fundamental shifts take place whenever a selfless brain does pierce its fantasy life, and perceives the world clearly. Whole new sets of orientation replace those old dreamy thought-castles built on shifting mental sands. Now the person's priorities tilt toward direct, intensified perceptions: into seeing, no longer searching; into hearing, beyond listening; into comprehending, beyond ordinary knowing; into long-range compassion, skillfully performed to help others. The new kind of perception sidesteps lengthy cortical relays and emotionalized consultations. It greets each sense object as *it really is*. The new priorities now flow into appropriate behavior, in swift, sure steps. Gibran distilled the essence of this enriched mode of living into one sentence: "Your daily life is your temple and your religion."[2] What is this daily life practice, so fundamental to the Zen Way? It consists of learning how to be fully alive, at this advanced level of awakening, in the workaday world.

In chapter 149, we outlined some characteristic attitudes and behavior patterns of an enlightened sage who truly lives at this level. A qualification remains. No research project has *proved*, scientifically, that systematic Zen training is alone responsible for producing what was described. On balance, the evidence of the centuries certainly suggests this could be so. But much of it is hearsay, uncontrolled. It could be interpreted otherwise. For one does encounter a few special people, scattered among the grumpy of every generation, who have developed an increasingly tolerant, spiritual, saintly wisdom as they grew older. And they have done so without having contacted any religious establishment.

Could organized religions, including Zen, simply have attracted more of these extraordinary individuals many decades before, entered them into the fold, and then have received undue credit for having assisted them to mature? To settle such questions of sampling artifact, researchers will need to follow many subjects and controls *over decades*. This will mean using sophisticated psychological and psychophysiological tests. It will also mean conducting tests and interviews without having been informed how advanced the subject is on the spiritual path.

Well-established Zen training centers will need to open up and cooperate with legitimate requests for well-planned, rigorous longitudinal studies. Among the investigators who design the studies, both skeptics and believers will be required. Believers are too often uncritical. Skeptics alone, with their biases and "hard" intellect, won't do justice to the subtleties in this sociologically complex arena. As Henri Bergson once explained: "Intelligence is the faculty of manufacturing artificial objects."[3]

It is true that you can develop "positive" mental images that influence your behavior, and that they will also help you modify some responses of your autonomic nervous system. For example, researchers have trained their subjects to imagine a pleasant scene, and in this manner to blot out the arousing imagery which develops in response to an unpleasant situation.[4]

But anger can engulf the person who has been spit at, and the blush of shame also rises from deep in the brain. For this reason, most imagery approaches remain short-term, shallow tactics, not truly comparable with those deep changes of strategies and policies which evolve during long monastic Zen training. These alone would transform a samurai swordsman into a gentler monk.

So the basic issue, which only skillful long-range research can resolve, is: How does a brain change when it shifts its field of focus *away* from the personal, on through the impersonal, and finally beyond into the Universal present moment? This is not a temporary shift into some new mental stance. It means being reprogrammed and transformed by basic psychophysiological postures which *endure*.

As one of the byproducts of such research, it would be of interest to develop ways to identify at a young age, *prospectively*, those persons who do have the potential to mature into our classic ideal of the saintly sage: a next Dali Lama, a future Mother Theresa, or a Krishnamurti in the making, so to speak.

In 1992, Colby and Damon reported the results of a retrospective study of a related question.[5] Using set criteria, they narrowed the field to a select group of twenty-three altruistic Americans. Each of these adults had lived a life of intensely active moral commitment, by virtue of having helped others directly or by reforming society. None had acted this way as the result of having proceeded through some highly logical cognitive process. Nor in this group did it seem that brief peak moments of revelation had been decisive, say of the kind that had once motivated Albert Schweitzer, a "reverence-for-all-life" type. No, these latter-day altruists were empowered by certain longstanding underlying traits of character.

Some years before reading this published report, I had already completed the preceding chapters, and in these had cited certain very well-known attributes of that particular group of Zen adepts who had progressed far along in the course of their monastic training. Briefly to list them, such notable qualities had included swift action, lack of fear, simplicity, stability, the capacity to change, and selfless compassion. So, later in 1994, when I finally read these authors' account, I was struck by several parallels between the two groups.[6]

For Colby and Damon had described their group of American exemplars in the following ways. To generalize, all their subjects had displayed "an unhesitating will to act, a disavowal of fear and doubt, and a simplicity of moral response." Indeed, "risks were ignored and consequences went unweighed."[7] Moreover, these subjects also showed "great capacities for change and growth." And they did so, even though—at the same time—they gave firm evidence of "extraordinary reliability, dependability, and stability in their values and conduct."[8]

One wonders: are the resemblances between the two groups sheer coincidence? Or, in the aggregate, do such qualities become the vital human ingredients which make possible any worthwhile social endeavor? If the latter, then perhaps it is when several key qualities like stability and compassion cluster into a larger critical mass—whether or not they arise out of peak experiences—that they help lead a person out into a life of deep social commitment.

Like long-term meditators, the modern American altruists had enough grit to persist through many vicissitudes. Did some special quality of courage sustain them? No, they disclaimed courage. Had they been supported by an institutional religion (including perhaps even Buddhism), or by a meditative practice? It was true that most had found a religious affiliation which appeared to be supportive. But not all did, and only one altruist was a practicing, meditating member of a Zen community. Buddhism could assume no credit for the group as a whole. Then what factor was common to all? It was a bedrock of faith. Not mere faith in general. But a faith that had drawn on and expressed larger dimensions of *meaning*, intrinsic meanings "above and beyond the self."[9] Faith in *meanings beyond the self* was the foundation of their resolve. In the present book, we have devoted many chapters to the limitations of selfhood and to the origins of meaning. (e.g., chapters 124 and 125 of part VII.)

Altruism is a complex, controversial subject in itself. Yet it is in this general arena, the one where the psychophysiology of an enlightened "no-self" blends into the acts of significant living, that we currently know the least about how a brain transforms its previous traits. Consider the results of primate studies, conducted while monkeys were pursuing their routine, day-to-day activities. As expected, the monkeys do engage parts of their inferotemporal regions when they are in the act of discriminating one object from another. But where do their more *spontaneous* behaviors come from, those skillful impulses that mediate their basic "visual habits?" The origins of such "daily life" habits are more elusive. In no simple way do their covert pathways consult with the monkey's limbic or cognitive visual memory systems.[10] These automatic habit patterns seem to be encoded through many other subcortical circuits which have yet to be identified, let alone deciphered and measured. Future studies must clarify how all this subtle, routine spontaneity comes about, both theirs and ours. And how it both evokes and responds to the larger meanings beyond the self, the ones which connect with the big picture as a whole.

In the interim, we can acknowledge some asymmetries of the hemispheres, including those which enable regions on the left to enter into more "positive" processing of an affirmative type (as noted in chapter 82). Yet it seems unlikely that the higher echelons of our cortical mantle will turn out to be the sole source for all of our higher motives. Perhaps we would be advised to begin searching for their subtle deeper networks in the limbic system, thalamus, basal ganglia, and brain stem. Many of these regions, with pathways crossing over the subcortical bridge, still express the stamp of our lowly origins. Indeed, there will always be multiple levels of interpretation to Master Chi-chen's statement that "The way upward is by descending lower."[11]

In Closing

> There is only one problem: to rediscover that there is a spiritual life, which ranks higher than intelligence and which alone satisfies man. This goes beyond the problem of religion, which is only one form of spiritual life.
>
> Antoine de Saint-Exupéry (1900–1944)[1]

> The radio station WOB, Wisdom of the Buddha, is broadcasting all the time: all we need is a receiving set.
>
> Heinrich Zimmer (1890–1943)[2]

Is Zen an anachronism? Or does the past have a future? If so, then what can a living relic from Tang dynasty China say to us today? Nothing much. Possibly everything. Keep your set tuned to WOB . . .

For Zen celebrates in its unique way the lightning strike of creative intuition. Though these peak moments last only a few seconds, they illuminate existential issues, transfigure the mundane, rinse the person of every self-centered desire and aversion. The deeper each experience penetrates, the more the personality reintegrates itself to set up new priorities. But this process is selective. It is not a delete button that wipes out all of one's previous personal history and memories. Rather does it permit their elements to realign along new motivational interfaces. There they can yield the kind of flexible, adaptive responses which will transform behavior along a higher plane of values.

In the beginning, the person appeared to have started out to walk a path so solitary and inturned that its destination could only seem to be, at best, a lonely variation on the theme of rugged individualism. But as the training slowly evolves, the person returns, more interrelated than ever before, into the larger community of fellow beings.

Today, people ask: Does Zen always work this way? Is it big? Is it growing? The answer is no to each question save the last one. For Zen is certainly growing in the West. But from most utilitarian premises, formalized Zen training is still too time-consuming and arduous to have much practical appeal to the public at large. It remains accessible to relatively few. However, civilizations in earlier centuries, cherishing other values, asked different questions, received different answers. Some answers from the twelfth century still linger in those misty light-blue stoneware bowls, glazed in the Song dynasty, forever luminous in their integrity. Others reside in the unsurpassed serenity of a Japanese garden, or in the concrete allusive quality of a *haiku*. And others will be found in the simplified, stabilized living examples of more humane beings. Theirs is a lineage of spiritual inspiration stretching back more than two thousand years. It testifies to an enduring fact: mankind has been illuminated as the lamp has been handed down from teacher to pupil, the slow, rigorous old-fashioned way.

Where do we, and Zen, go from here? Tides which have always run deep in the history of our species seem to have become more turbulent. Some are coming in, some running out. Humankind still dies from bad diseases, and suffers from the same infirmities of old age which had so distressed the young Siddhartha. Aggressively materialistic societies, East and West, have left in their wake a host of self-indulgent epidemics, spiritual bankruptcies, Elvis sightings, and ecological nightmares. Institutional religions seem to be no match for the lurid disasters we view on TV or for the global scope of others we sense are almost upon us. It is a time for taking stock. Can we really nurture our deepest spiritual impulses, motivate mere humans to become more humane?

Among various tides, those of the neurosciences are surely rushing in at full flood. Vast numbers of leads are converging. They promise to clarify what was only yesterday that black box of a brain. In these pages, having examined these discoveries, what have we found? Complex issues. No single Rosetta stone that finally translates the subtle coded language of the brain into a person's direct experience of extraordinary states of consciousness.

But some models presented in this book do offer plausible ways to interpret the facts at hand. Which of these testable hypotheses may stand for a while? Which others will be of heuristic value only, and which will crumble because they are flat-out wrong? Researchers will answer these questions sooner than we think. Meanwhile, we can't blame too many of our difficulties on Zen. Yes, it *is* hard to make sense of, avoids talking about itself, and indulges in obfuscations. And it is hard to translate the legacy of Asian words into English.

Our real problem starts closer to home. We aren't yet tuned in to receive, and to value, the profound ecumenical meaning of the simplest Zen teachings. Even if the WOB station were to broadcast its messages in plain English, we would still find it hard to believe that they really do imply transforming the brain.

Gulp! I'm not ready for that, we say. No brainwashing for me! My beliefs are mine. I won't let go of my self or allow it to be subverted by some far-out, Eastern religion!

I. Me. Mine. Self. Wandering in the dark, we keep groping for the lost keys which will unlock the door to the kingdom. All the while, the keys lie on the very ground where our own two feet are standing.

Can one change this situation? If so, how? The first step is to diagnose the root of the problem: the egocentric self. Once over this big hurdle, it gradually becomes easier to practice alternative ways of being, knowing, and understanding. At this point, even though Zen goes beyond reasoning, its methods will not be seen to embrace the irrational, in the ways that would worry Bronowski. Instead, they will be seen as steps which cultivate the ascent to insight-wisdom, that loftier function which Saint-Exupéry and Bergson would rank higher than intelligence.

Have we come any closer to understanding Zen? Let's hope so. Still, it keeps slipping in and out of our mental grasp. However, we do get a better feeling for Zen each time we relearn how to approach it. Not by reaching out to catch it in the net of the thoughtful intellect. But by *letting go*. With practice, we find that ethical sensibilities emerge, ones which gradually earn our due respect.

Have we learned anything about meditation? If so, it will not be from applying EEG electrodes to the scalp, but from the deeper act of practicing the meditative mode ourselves and infusing it into the present moment. Finally, each day's practice starts to become life's meditation, by one life, within all life.

As the old millennium closes, the world is inching (a micron at a time) toward a behavioral neurology of religion, a topic slightly more valid and acceptable now than when William James first spoke about it nearly a century ago. Such a field of inquiry is an *experiential neurology* in one sense. At best, one of its branches might be rigorous enough to justify the term, *the meditative sciences* during the next century. The larger discipline of experiential neurology will not abandon the house of the intellect. It will not ignore the firm rules of evidence, nor will it peddle snake-oil, and indulge in false doctrines. It will be correlating the findings from several different brain-mapping techniques.[3] Its sophistocated neuroimaging methods will be focused on very special moments in the lives of many carefully-selected subjects, not from one person, as we have been obliged to do in this book.

An emerging discipline of experiential neurology will include within its broad scope such topics as meditation, preconscious functions, absorptions, and insight-wisdom. Its mission will be to uncover the mechanisms by which each one transforms experience and behavior. The author welcomes correspondence[4] that could help clarify any of these topics, for each is currently undervalued and woefully misunderstood.

Yet, within a few years after this "Decade of the Brain" is finished, one can foresee the vocabulary of this emerging field starting to become as familiar to our citizens as are now such words as cholesterol, DNA, and Alzheimer's disease. For with the advent of the third millennium, investigators will finally be ready to clarify how the human brain does transform itself, and function responsibly in the practical arts of everyday living.

Introduction to the Heart Sutra

The earlier Sanskrit versions of the *Prajna Paramita Sutra* were translated into Chinese as early as the year 172 of the Christian era.[1] In this sutra, Buddhism forged an irrevocable link between the direct experience of emptiness, *sunyata*, and *prajna*, the basic insight of indivisible oneness. Fortunately, the sutra's long early versions were later condensed. In English, the short form can be entitled *The Heart of Great Wisdom Sutra*. It has also been called *The Sutra of the Great Wisdom Gone Beyond*.

The shortened sutra then became so popular and useful that its verses are chanted daily in different tongues all over the Buddhist world. Still, the words of the *Heart Sutra* are not easy to understand by lay readers anywhere, East or West. To make the task easier, the version presented here has again been simplified in the process of condensing it further from the recent English renderings found in Leggett[2] and Schloegl.[3]

In this version, a distillate of all his teachings, the Buddha is explaining to his chief disciple, Shariputra, what it means finally to have become free from suffering as a result of having cast off all delusions.

The reader will note how many things are *absent* during this deepest awakening. There are no hallucinations or other sensate elements. The illusory world of forms has finally been seen into, and found empty of all personal attachments and mental constructs. And among the delusions lost is every last notion that the aspirant might attain some virtuous state in the process of becoming enlightened.

The Buddha chose the Bodhisattva of Compassion to illustrate how much was implied within this advanced level of enlightenment. In Chinese, the important principle of Compassion is embodied in the bodhisattva called Quan-Yin. In Japanese, the name is Kannon. In Japan, other names are also given to this same bodhisattva. They include Kanzeon, referring to one who perceives the sounds of a suffering world; and Kanjizai, implying one who has become free as a result of seeing things as they really are.

The Heart Sutra (The Sutra of the Great Wisdom Gone Beyond)

From the depths of prajna wisdom
The Bodhisattva of Compassion saw into the emptiness
of every construct
And so passed beyond all suffering.

Know then that in such depths
form is only emptiness,
emptiness only form.
Form is emptiness, emptiness is form.

This is true of feelings, perceptions, impulses
and the rest of consciousness.

All these, by their very nature, are emptiness,
being neither born nor dying, stained nor pure,
waxing nor waning.

So in emptiness is there neither form,
feelings, perceptions, impulses or consciousness.
No eye, ear, nose, tongue, body or mind.

No form, sound, smell, taste, touch or object of mind.
No element of sight nor any other element of
consciousness.

No ignorance, no old age or death.
No extinguishing of ignorance, old age or death.
No suffering, no beginning or end, no path.
No wisdom, no attainment.

The Bodhisattva who dwells in this perfect wisdom,
attaining nothing,
is not entrapped by delusive fantasies.
And where there are no such obstacles
there can be no fear.

Now, beyond all delusions,
one reaches ultimate Nirvana.
Having practiced this same Great Wisdom Gone Beyond,
all Buddhas in the past have come to supreme
enlightenment.

Know then that this peerless mantra,
this true mantra of highest wisdom,
unfailingly relieves all suffering.
And so proclaim it:

Gone, gone beyond, gone altogether beyond.
Awakening, fulfilled!
Heart of Great Wisdom!

Selections from Affirmation of Faith in Mind

The *Hsin hsin ming,* a declaration of faith in mind, dates back to the era of the Third Zen Patriarch, Seng-ts'an, who died in 606. It comes down to us as over 140 unrhymed lines of verse, derived from only four Chinese characters a line. For the purpose of this book, only selected verses have been freely rendered from recent translations in this century.[1-3]

It begins by repeatedly observing the harmful polarities in our life:

> The Great Way is not difficult;
> just avoid picking and choosing!
>
> Only when you neither love nor hate
> does it clearly reveal itself.
>
> To see its truth
> be neither for, nor against.
>
> Conflicts between longing and loathing
> are a disease of the mind.
>
> Gain and loss, right and wrong
> away with them once and for all!

It then addresses awakening as follows:

> The Perfect Way, like vast space
> lacks nothing, has nothing in excess.
>
> When the mind does not discriminate
> all things are as they really are.
>
> Entering the deep mystery of this suchness
> releases us from all attachments.
> Viewing all things in their oneness
> we return to our original nature.
>
> This state wherein all relations have ceased
> is indescribable by analogy.
>
> The mind in full accord with the Way
> drops off its selfish preoccupations.
>
> Doubts clear up
> true faith prevails.
>
> All is empty, clear,
> revealed effortlessly, naturally.

Neither thinking nor imagination
can ever reach this state.

This Ultimate reality
retains neither self nor other.

In this non-dual world
all is one, nothing left out.

In this unmeasurable truth
one instant is ten thousand years.

Things do not separate into here, or there
infinity is manifested everywhere.

One thing is everything
all things are One.

If you know only this, then
don't worry about attaining perfect knowledge.

The believing mind is not divided
undivided is the believing mind.

Words fail to describe it
for it is neither of the past, present, nor future.

Appendix C

Suggested Further Reading

Zen has an Oriental flavor. A sampler of the things a Westerner can learn by reading about it would include the following sources:

1. S. Barnet, and W. Burto. *Zen Ink Paintings.* Tokyo, Kodansha, 1982.
2. T. Hoover. *The Zen Experience.* New York, New American Library, 1980.
3. M. Kohn, trans. *The Shambhala Dictionary of Buddhism and Zen.* Boulder, Colo., Shambhala, 1991.
4. N. Ross. *The World of Zen. An East-West Anthology.* New York, Vintage, 1960.

A short list of brief introductions to Buddhist meditative practice in every-day life includes:

1. J. Kabat-Zinn. *Wherever You Go, There You Are. Mindfulness Meditation in Everyday Life.* New York, Hyperion, 1994.
2. Nhat Hanh. *Peace Is Every Step. The Path of Mindfulness in Everyday Life.* New York, Bantam, 1991.
3. I. Scholoegl. *The Zen Way.* London, Sheldon, 1977.
4. S. Suzuki. *Zen Mind, Beginner's Mind.* New York, Weatherhill, 1975.

I hope this book will stimulate the reader to learn about meditation *firsthand.* Should you wish to meditate within the Zen traditions, the following recent works may be of interest:

1. L. Friedman. *Meetings with Remarkable Women. Buddhist Teachers in America.* Boston, Shambhala, 1987.
2. K. Kraft. *Zen: Tradition and Transition.* New York, Grove, 1988.
3. D. Morreale. *Buddhist America. Centers, Retreats, Practices.* Santa Fe, N.M., John Muir, 1988.
4. M. Roth, and J. Stevens. *Zen Guide. Where to Meditate in Japan.* New York, Weatherhill, 1985.
5. H. Tworkov. *Zen in America. Profiles of Five Teachers.* San Francisco, North Point, 1989.

Much still remains to be learned about meditation secondhand. The vast literature is uneven and full of controversy. Recent reviews include:

1. D. Shapiro, and R. Walsh. *Meditation: Classic and Contemporary Perspectives.* New York, Aldine, 1984.

2. M. West, ed. *The Psychology of Meditation.* Oxford, Clarendon Press, 1987.

3. J. White, ed. *What Is Enlightenment? Exploring the Goal of the Spiritual Path.* Los Angeles, Tarcher, 1984.

4. M. Murphy, S. Donovan, and E. Taylor. *The Physical and Psychological Effects of Meditation. A Review of Conremporary Research with a Comprehensive Bibliography 1931–1996. Second Edition.* Sausalito, California, Institute of Noetic Sciences, 1997.

Textbooks providing further background material include:

1. N. Carlson. *Physiology of Behavior,* 4th ed. Boston, Allyn & Bacon, 1991.

2. G. Shepherd. *Neurobiology,* 3rd ed. New York, Oxford University Press, 1994.

Glossary

The nonspecialist will find here simplified descriptions of less familiar terms.

acetylcholine (ACH) A fast neurotransmitter liberated at many brain synapses and at those peripheral cholinergic nerves which innervate muscles.

affect In general use, it refers to the emotional. It also refers to the way emotion is expressed in observable behaviors.

agnosia A failure to recognize what is clearly perceived. Visual agnosia implies that an object, though seen, is not consciously recognized. But note that some other sensory avenue, such as touch, might still permit the person to identify this object.

agonist A drug which acts on specific receptors, and mimics their natural response.

alpha waves An electroencephalographic (EEG) pattern which has a frequency between 8 and 12 cycles per second (cps).

amines Messenger molecules such as dopamine, norepinephrine, and serotonin.

amino acids Most serve as the building blocks for proteins. Some, such as glutamic acid and aspartic acid, also function as excitatory neurotransmitters. Others, like glycine, act as inhibitory neurotransmitters.

amygdala The complex of nuclei, located out near the inner tip of each temporal lobe, which is involved in fear and other emotions.

antagonist A drug which blocks the usual response caused by an agonist.

ascending reticular activating system A network of nerve cells in the brain stem which sponsors arousal functions.

association cortex Regions of the neocortex which confer higher integrative functions. They have no direct sensorimotor function and are particularly well developed in primates.

axon The fiber issuing from the nerve cell which conducts its nerve impulses out toward the terminals.

basal ganglia The paired deep nuclei on either side of the brain concerned with integrating patterns of motor responses. They include the caudate, putamen, globus pallidus, and substantia nigra.

Being As used here, the term refers to an advanced alternate state which reaches silent levels of ultimate comprehension that elude all description.

beta waves Fast brain waves with an EEG frequency between 14 and 30 cps.

Beta-endorphin A large opioid peptide released in the deep midline regions of the brain.

blind sight   Responding to visual stimuli without being consciously able to "see" them, by using the second visual system which projects through the superior colliculus.

bodhisattva (Skt.)   One who postpones reaching full enlightenment but remains dedicated to helping others become enlightened. A saintly person, or embodied principle skillfully applied.

brain stem   The enlarged stalk which lies between the large forebrain and the long spinal cord. It consists of medulla, pons, and midbrain.

central nervous system   The cerebrum, cerebellum, brain stem, and spinal cord.

cerebellum   The brain structure lying behind the brain stem. It is especially involved in sensorimotor coordination and in balance.

cerebrum   The major, forebrain enlargement of the central nervous system. It lies above the midbrain, and contains the outer layer of cortex, as well as deeper structures such as the basal ganglia, thalamus, and limbic system.

cholinergic   A nerve cell or function which uses acetylcholine as its neurotransmitter.

circadian rhythms   Biological rhythms which recur approximately every twenty-four hours.

coexistence   The existence of both peptides and standard neurotransmitters within the same nerve cell. Both may be released when firing rates are high.

coherence   A technical term indicating that the profile of EEG waves in one region resembles that in another. It tends to imply that both regions are yoked at deeper subcortical levels.

colliculi   The four bumps on the roof of the midbrain. The upper two are involved in visual reflexes; the lower two mediate auditory reflex functions.

conditioned reflex   A basic reflex which has been so modified by past experience that it can now be prompted by a new, conditioned stimulus.

cortex   The outer layer of gray matter covering the cerebrum and cerebellum.

dendrites   The branches at the receiving end of each nerve cell. They receive impulses and convey them down to the nerve cell body.

depolarization   The reduction of the charged electrical potential across the nerve cell membrane. When polarization is lost, the cell fires and generates a nerve impulse.

desynchronization   The process of activating regions of the cerebrum. It is associated with arousal, rapid eye movement (REM) sleep (D-sleep) and with low voltage fast EEG activity. Recently it has been appreciated that some fast activities are not as irregular as this word formerly suggested.

diencephalon   The enlarged region just above the brain stem. It includes the thalamus, hypothalamus, subthalamus, pineal body, and habenular nuclei.

disinhibition   The release of an inhibited cell into increased firing, or a release of behavior. In either instance, an inhibitory brake is removed.

dopamine (DA)   A biogenic amine and neuro-messenger. It is released by nerve cells located in the substantia nigra and ventral tegmental area in the midbrain.

downregulation   A decrease in the density of receptors. It "makes up" for their having previously been excessively activated.

eidetic imagery   The exact, detailed revisualization of objects previously seen or imagined.

electrode   A fine metal wire used to detect and transmit the faint traces of brain electrical activity. Stimulating electrodes are also used to deliver electrical stimuli to the brain.

electroencephalogram (EEG)   The recording of the brain's waves of electrical activity. Electrodes are placed on the scalp, in the cortex (electrocorticogram), or even deeper in the brain (depth electrodes).

emotion   A subjective feeling state.

endorphin   see *Beta-endorphin*.

enkephalins   Small opioid peptides made by the brain, of two general types: leuenkephalin and metenkephalin.

enlightenment   Awakening, selfless, to the reality of the unity of all things. In Zen, also known as the states of kensho or satori.

evoked potential   The sum of local brain electrical activity prompted by repeatedly delivering a stimulus at some distance away from the recording site.

excitatory neurotransmitter   A neuro-messenger which, when it activates its receptor on the next cell, causes that cell to become depolarized and to fire faster.

experiant   The one experiencing, even though no sense of self remains at that moment. A useful term, not to be found in dictionaries.

feeling   The subjective experience during emotion.

forebrain   The parts of the cerebral hemispheres and diencephalon which lie above the brain stem.

frontal lobes   The lobes which perform higher executive and associative functions. They lie in front of the sensorimotor cortex in the anterior portion of both cerebral hemispheres.

GABA (gamma-aminobutyric acid)   The major, inhibitory neurotransmitter. It is released by many small interneurons, and by some larger nerve cells.

gamma waves   Fast EEG waves with frequencies between 30 and 50 cps.

glutamate   A major excitatory neurotransmitter. It is the amino acid precursor (glutamic acid) of GABA.

habituation   The process by which a nerve cell, or the nervous system in general, reduces its responses after it receives single stimuli repeated with monotonous regularity.

hallucinations   Sensory perceptions occurring when no appropriate external stimuli are present.

hippocampus   A small region deep in each temporal lobe. It plays a major role in laying down memory traces.

hyperpolarization   An increase in the charge of the original electrical potential across the nerve cell membrane. It makes it more difficult for the cell to fire.

hypnagogic interval   The drowsy interval during the *descent* from waking into sleeping. During this transitional period, hypnagogic hallucinations may occur both in normals and in patients with narcolepsy.

hypnopompic interval   The drowsy interval during the *ascent* from sleeping to waking. The hallucinations during this transitional period are called hypnopompic

hypothalamus   The small, complex, centrally located region lying below the thalamus and above the pituitary gland. It integrates many vital brain and body functions crucial to survival: eating, drinking, blood pressure, etc.

illusions   Misperceptions which begin with some natural stimulus.

inhibitory transmitter   A neuro-messenger which causes the next nerve cell to fire more slowly. It does so by acting on its receptor and causing the cell to become hyperpolarized. GABA is the major inhibitory transmitter.

insight-wisdom   The profound comprehension of the essence of all things.

interneurons   Small nerve cells which have short axons.

kensho   Seeing into the essence of things, insight-wisdom (Ch: Chien-hsing). It is regarded as the beginning of true training, a prelude to the depths of satori.

kinhin   Walking meditation.

koan   An enigmatic statement serving as a concentration device. Insight resolves it, not thought.

lateral geniculate body   The compact region at the base of the thalamus which relays visual messages from the optic tracts back toward the visual cortex.

lesion   A region of local damage to the nervous system. Lesions occur as a result of diseases, such as strokes, which destroy nerve cell bodies and axons. Experimental lesions are also produced by instruments such as a knife, by a local pulse of excess electrical current, or by chemical means, including excitotoxins.

limbic system A series of structures next to the midline on both sides of the brain linked by circuits which generate affective and instinctual responses. It includes the hypothalamus, hippocampus, cingulate gyrus, amygdala, and septal region.

LSD (lysergic acid diethylamide) A hallucinogenic chemical derivative of lysergic acid. It has various other mental effects which reflect its major action on serotonin receptors in the brain.

Mahayana The northern school of Buddhism which gave rise to Zen.

meaning The quality conveyed when the brain links the raw perception of a item to its many related associations. Only certain meanings go on to assume major import (salience).

medulla The lower part of the brain stem lying above the spinal cord. It mediates respiratory, cardiovascular, and other vital functions.

midbrain The upper end of the brain stem.

mood The long-sustained, tidal, emotional feeling tone which markedly influences the way the person perceives the world. Its range extends from elated manic states to depression.

mysticism The ongoing practice of reestablishing, by the deepest of insights, one's direct relationship with the Ultimate Reality principle.

norepinephrine (NE) A biogenic amine neuro-messenger. It is produced especially by the locus ceruleus in the brain stem. At most of its receptors, the first action of NE is predominantly inhibitory.

nucleus A very large collection of nerve cell bodies. They tend to be viewed as an anatomically distinct structure. (It has a second meaning. Each single nerve cell also contains a round nucleus which holds its DNA.)

occipital lobes The lobes at the very back of the cerebrum. They mediate visual functions, and blend anteriorly into the parietal and temporal lobes.

optic nerves and tracts The pathways in the front part of the visual system. They convey impulses from the retina back to the two lateral geniculate nuclei.

paradoxical sleep (also known as desynchronized sleep, D-sleep, or REM sleep) The activated sleep stage during which dreams and rapid eye movements can occur. One paradox is that most other muscles along the long axis of the body are quiet.

parietal lobes The lobes in the back half of the cerebrum which are chiefly involved in integrating higher levels of sensory and attentional functions.

Parkinson's disease A disease of the basal ganglia, usually secondary to a deficiency of dopamine. The patients develop a flexed posture, slowness, rigidity, and tremor.

peptide   A molecule composed of several, linked amino acids. Some peptides act as neuro-messengers and as hormones.

phasic   Pertaining to a brief period of increased nerve cell firing.

pituitary gland   The "master" gland located below the hypothalamus and intimately connected with it. The pituitary gland releases hormones into the bloodstream which regulate the internal environment of the body.

pons   The enlarged portion of the brain stem lying between the midbrain and the medulla.

prajna   (Skt.; J: hannya) The flashing insight-wisdom of enlightenment.

proprioceptive   The kinds of sensations entering from the muscles, joints, tendons, and vestibular system which contribute to one's sense of position and balance.

psychedelics   "Mind-manifesting" drugs such as LSD, psilocybin, and mescaline. They usually have prominent hallucinogenic effects.

rapid eye movement sleep (REM sleep)   (also known as D-sleep or paradoxical sleep) That stage of activated sleep when rapid eye movements and dreams occur.

receptor   A large protein molecule embedded in the membrane of the cell. It is designed to recognize the signal from only a certain specific transmitter, modulator, or hormone, and to transduce its message into the cell.

reticular nucleus   The thin outer layer of GABA nerve cells capping the thalamus. It plays a very important inhibitory role in thalamic functions.

roshi   Venerable teacher; the Japanese pronunciation (rō'shî) of the name of the venerated Chinese teacher, Lao-tzu.

salience   The leaping forth into meaning of the special quality which confers significant import.

samadhi (Skt.)   An extraordinary alternate state of one-pointed absorption. The word has so many other meanings that it tends to imply merely a state.

satori   The term frequently reserved for a deeper, more advanced state of insight-wisdom.

sesshin   An intensive Zen meditative retreat lasting several days; literally, "to collect the mind."

serotonin (ST)   A biogenic amine. It is produced especially by cell bodies in the midline raphe system. ST plays a predominantly inhibitory role. Its longer chemical name is 5-hydroxytryptamine, or 5-HT.

simultagnosia   A patient's inability to grasp the whole scene, although its individual elements are perceived in isolation.

split brain   A brain in which the corpus callosum has been divided surgically. But even after the other smaller (commisural) crossing fiber connections are also cut, the two hemispheres still communicate with each other via their lower "subcortical bridge."

state A temporary condition involving mentation, emotion, or behavior.

striatum Several nuclei of the basal ganglia which mediate motor functions. The caudate and putamen compose the dorsal striatum. The ventral striatum includes the nucleus accumbens.

substantia nigra The paired structures in the midbrain which are rich in dopamine cell bodies and which energize motor functions.

synapse The specialized gap through which the terminals of one cell link with the dendrite, cell body, or terminal of the next cell. The nerve cell on the upstream side is called the presynaptic cell. That on the other side of the gap is called the postsynaptic cell. Neuro-messengers pass quickly across the synaptic gap to activate their receptors on the opposite side. They are then taken back up again and recycled.

synchronization The process of bringing together regions of the cerebrum into regular, rhythmic patterns of firing activity. It is usually associated with a slower EEG, with drowsiness, and slow-wave sleep (S-sleep). However, fast activity can also be rhythmic and synchronized.

syncretism The reconciliation of conflicting opposites into a unity. The origins of the term trace to the way contending Cretan cities finally united into a larger federation.

tachyphrenia A burst of extra-fast mental processing.

tathagata (Skt.) A term originally referring to the Buddha, inferring one who is "thus come." It implies a rare spiritually advanced person who appreciates all things as they really are, as a *permanent* ongoing condition.

temporal lobes The lobes lying deep to each temple. The term includes both the temporal lobe cortex and its deeper, limbic structures such as the parahippocampal gyrus, the hippocampal formation, and the amygdala.

thalamus The deeper nuclear structures positioned behind the basal ganglia and medial to them. They serve largely to integrate sensory and ever more refined messages at a subcortical level. They are also engaged in complex interactions with the cortex.

Theravada The surviving, southern school of Buddhism, still practiced in Southeast Asia.

tonic In a state of sustained firing of nerve cells.

trait A distinctive, ongoing quality of attitude, character, or behavior. Traits are not usually thought of as subject to change. However, they can be transformed by a series of extraordinary, insightful alternate states.

turnover   A term suggesting that more of a given neurotransmitter or modulator is being synthesized, released, used, and broken down. It implies that synaptic activity has increased.

upregulation   An increase in the density of receptors. It compensates for their previously having been underactivated.

ventral tegmental area   A region near the midline in the front of the midbrain. It contains many dopamine cell bodies which project their axons forward through the mesolimbic DA system.

ventricles   Spaces within the brain filled with fluid. They include the large, lateral ventricles within the two cerebral hemispheres; the third ventricle in the midline enclosed by the hypothalamus; and the fourth ventricle behind the brain stem which receives fluid draining from the third ventricle via the small aqueduct.

vipassana   Mindfulness meditation, traditionally associated with the Theravada school.

zazen   Zen meditation in the sitting posture; from the Chinese, *tso-ch'an.*

Zen   A form of Mahayana Buddhism which emphasizes a systematic approach to meditative training and spiritual growth. Its two major schools, Rinzai and Soto, were imported from China and developed in Japan during the twelfth and thirteenth centuries.

zendo   The room used for formal Zen practice.

References and Notes

Preface

1. J. Krishnamurti. Interview with John White. In *What is Enlightenment? Exploring the Goal of the Spiritual Path*, ed. J. White. Los Angeles, Tarcher, 1984, 91.
2. W. James. *The Varieties of Religious Experience*. New York, Longmans, Green, 1925.
3. U.S. Congress *Joint Resolution 174*, 101st Cong., 1989, 69–76.
4. T. Leggett. *The Second Zen Reader*. Rutland, Vt., Tuttle, 1988.

By Way of Introduction

1. D. Thoreau. *Walden*. 1854; Princeton, N. J., Princeton University Press, 1989.
2. W. James. *The Varieties of Religious Experience*. New York, Longmans, Green, 1925.
3. C. Tart. States of consciousness and state specific sciences. *Science* 1972; 176:1203–1210.
4. The first person in this narrative has been introduced once before, in *Chase, Chance, and Creativity. The Lucky Art of Novelty*. N.Y., Columbia University Press, 1978.
5. C. Pierce, in *Zen and American Thought*, ed. V. Ames. Honolulu, University of Hawaii Press, 1962, 143.

Chapter 1   Is There Any Common Ground between Zen Buddhism and the Brain?

1. R. Sperry. Changing priorities. *Annual Review of Neuroscience* 1981; 4:1–15.
2. D. Suzuki. *Zen and Japanese Culture*. Bollingen Series 64. Princeton, N.J., Princeton University Press, 1973.
3. D. Hebb. *Textbook of Psychology*, 2nd ed. Philadelphia, W.B. Saunders, 1966.
4. R. Fischer. A Biochemistry of behavior? *Biological Psychiatry* 1969; 1:107–109.
5. W. James. *A Pluralistic Universe*. Cambridge, Mass., Harvard University Press, 1977.
6. J. Bronowski. *The Ascent of Man*. Boston, Little, Brown, 1973, 437.
7. C. Humphreys, letter to author, 15 June 1980.
8. J. Thomas, T. Hamm, P. Perkins, et al. Animal research at Stanford University. *New England Journal of Medicine* 1988; 318:1630–1632.

Chapter 2   A Brief Outline of Zen History

1. M. Trevor, trans. *The Ox and His Herdsman. A Chinese Zen Text*. Tokyo, Hokuseido Press, 1969.
2. M. Ferguson. *The Aquarian Conspiracy. Personal and Social Transformations in the 1980's*. London, Routledge & Kegan Paul, 1981, 82.
3. H. Dumoulin. *A History of Zen Buddhism*. London, Faber & Faber, 1963.
4. N. Gadjin. The life of the Buddha: An interpretation. *The Eastern Buddhist* 1987; 20(2):1–31.
5. Early Buddhist teachings anticipated the later carbon and nitrogen cycles of the biochemist and the stardust interpretations of the astrophysicist. The teachings viewed all things caught up in the wheel of life as going through recurrent cycles of birth and death. Three features characterized the basic nature of existence. They were called the Three Signs of Being: (1) All things are impermanent and in a state of flux. (2) All things are imperfect, unsatisfactory, and cause suffering. (3) One's personal self is likewise insubstantial, and does not endure.
6. Hu Shih [*sic*]. The development of Zen Buddhism in China. In *Anthology of Zen*, ed. W. Briggs. New York, Grove Press, 1961, 7–30.
7. Lao-Tzu, in B. Stevenson, ed., *The Home Book of Quotations*, 10th ed., New York, Dodd, Mead, 1967, 147.
8. N. Kobori. The ripening persimmon. *Parabola* 1985; 10:72–79.
9. G. Chang. *The Practice of Zen*. New York, Perennial Library, Harper & Row, 1959.
10. D. Suzuki. *Studies in Zen*. New York, Delta, 1955, 13.
11. H. Varley. *Japanese Culture, A Short History*. New York, Praeger, 1973, 73.

12. C. Prebish. Reflections on the transmission of Buddhism to America. In *Understanding the New Religions,* eds. J. Neddleman & G. Baker. New York, Seabury Press, 1978.
13. R. Ellwood. *Alternative Altars.* Chicago, University of Chicago Press, 1979.
14. R. Fields. *How the Swans Came to the Lake. A Narrative History of Buddhism in America.* Boulder, Colo., Shambahala, 1981.

Chapter 3   But What Is Zen?

1. J. Hackett. *The Zen Haiku and Other Zen Poems of J.W. Hackett.* Tokyo, Japan Publications, 1983.
2. D. Suzuki. *Studies in Zen.* New York. Delta, 1955, 28.
3. D. Suzuki. *The Training of the Zen Buddhist Monk.* New York, University Books, 1965, 54.
4. K. Sekida. *Zen Training. Methods and Philosophy.* New York, Weatherhill, 1975, 230.

Chapter 4   Mysticism, Zen, Religion, and Neuroscience

1. E. O'Brien. *Varieties of Mystic Experience.* New York, Holt, Rinehart & Winston, 1964.
2. R. Masters and J. Houston. *The Varieties of Psychedelic Experience.* New York, Holt, Rinehart & Winston, 1966.
3. S. Johnson. In S. Bent, *Familiar Short Sayings of Great Men.* Houghton Mifflin, Boston, 1987, 311.
4. William James. *The Varieties of Religious Experience.* New York, Longmans, Green, 1925, 313.
5. E. Underhill. *Mysticism.* New York, Dutton, 1961, 71.
6. H. Dumoulin. *A History of Zen Buddhism.* Boston, Beacon Press, 1969, 4, 13.
7. C. Keller. Mystical literature. In *Mysticism and Philosophical Analysis,* ed. S. Katz. London, Sheldon, 1978, 79.
8. W. Kaufmann. *Critique of Religion and Philosophy.* New York, Torchbook, Harper & Row, 1972.
9. W. Johnston. *The Still Point. Reflections on Zen and Christian Mysticism.* New York, Fordham University Press, 1970.
10. E. Herrigel. *The Method of Zen.* New York, Vintage, 1974, 14.
11. D. Suzuki. *Studies in Zen.* New York, Delta, 1955, 21.
12. *Ibid.,* 11.
13. *Ibid.,* 74.
14. *Ibid.,* 76.
15. *Ibid.,* 84.
16. James, *op. cit.,* 31.
17. T. Luckman and C. Geertz, cited in A. Greeley, *The Sociology of the Paranormal. A Reconnaissance.* Sage Research Paper, vol. 3, series 90-023, Beverly Hills, Calif., 1975, 56.
18. J. Austin. *Chase, Chance and Creativity. The Lucky Art of Novelty.* New York, Columbia University Press, 1978, 166.
19. Greeley, *op. cit.*
20. A. Schweitzer. *The Mysticism of Paul the Apostle.* New York, Macmillan, 1960.
21. A. Greeley. *Ecstasy, A Way of Knowing.* Englewood Cliffs, N.J., Prentice-Hall, 1974.
22. R. Sasaki. Zen: A method for religious awakening, Quoted in N. Ross, *The World of Zen. An East-West Anthology.* New York, Vintage, 1960, 18.
23. R. Sperry. Changing Priorities. *Annual Review of Neuroscience* 1981; 4:1–15.

Chapter 5   Western Perspectives on Mystical Experiences

1. A. Greeley. *Ecstasy, A Way of Knowing.* Englewood Cliffs, N.J., Prentice-Hall, 1974.
2. W. James. *The Varieties of Religious Experience.* New York, Longmans, Green, 1925, 31.
3. E. Underhill. *Mysticism.* New York, Dutton, 1961.
4. W. Johnston. *The Still Point. Reflections on Zen and Christian Mysticism.* New York, Fordham University Press, 1970.
5. R. Bucke. *Cosmic Consciousness: A Study in the Evolution of the Human Mind.* New York, Dutton, 1962.
6. *Gallup Opinion Index Report,* no. 145, 53–55, 1977–78.

7. A. Greeley. *The Sociology of the Paranormal. A Reconnaissance.* Sage Research Paper, vol. 3, series 90-023, Beverly Hills, Calif., 1975.

8. A. Maslow. The "core-religious" or "transcendent" experience. In *The Highest State of Consciousness,* ed. J. White. Garden City, N.Y., Anchor, 1972, 352–364.

9. A. Hardy. *The Spiritual Nature of Man; A Study of Contemporary Religious Experience.* Oxford, Oxford University Press, 1979; 127.

10. W. Wilson. Mental health benefits of religious salvation. *Diseases of the Nervous System* 1972; 33:382–386.

11. L. Bourque and K. Back. Language, society and subjective experience. *Sociometry* 1971; 34:1–21.

12. J. Campbell. *The Masks of God: Creative Mythology.* New York, Viking, 1968, 67–68, 350–351.

13. P. Moore. Mystical experience, mystical doctrine, mystical technique. In *Mysticism and Philosophical Analysis,* ed. S. Katz. London, Sheldon, 1978, 101–131.

14. S. Katz. Language, epistemology, and mysticism. In *Mysticism and Philosophical Analysis,* ed. S. Katz. London, Sheldon, 1978, 22–74.

15. A. Watts. This is it. In *The Highest State of Consciousness,* ed. J. White. Garden City, N.Y., Anchor/Doubleday, 1972, 436–451.

16. M. Laski. *Ecstasy. A Study of Some Secular and Religious Experiences.* New York, Greenwood Press, 1968. "Intensity" experiences are not usually described as building up to a climax.

17. R. Gimello. Mysticism and meditation. In *Mysticism and Philosophical Analysis,* ed. S. Katz., London, Sheldon, 1978, 170–199.

18. W. Kaufmann. *Critique of Religion and Philosophy.* New York, Harper & Row Torchbook, 1972.

19. A. Deikman. Deautomatization and the mystic experience. *Psychiatry* 1966; 29:324–338.

20. A. Deikman. The missing center. In *Alternate States of Consciousness,* ed. N. Zinberg. New York, Free Press, 1977, 230–241.

21. A. Maslow. *Religions, Values and Peak Experiences.* New York, Viking, 1970.

22. Greeley, *op. cit.,* 74.

23. A. Maslow. Theory Z. *Journal of Transpersonal Psychology* 1969; 1:31–47.

24. J. Davis, L. Lockwood, and C. Wright. "Reasons for not reporting peak experience." *Journal of Humanistic Psychology* 1991; 31:86–94.

Chapter 6   Is Mysticism a Kind of Schizophrenia in Disguise?

1. B. Evans, ed. *Dictionary of Quotations.* New York, Delacorte, 1968, 225.

2. W. James. *The Varieties of Religious Experience.* New York, Longmans, Green, 1925, 326.

3. *Ibid,* 198–201.

4. D. Forrest. Nonsense and sense in schizophrenic language. *Schizophrenia Bulletin* 1976; 2:286–301.

5. M. Ron and I. Harvey. The brain in schizophrenia. *Journal of Neurology, Neurosurgery and Psychiatry* 1990; 53:725–726.

6. A. Rossi, P. Stratta, L. D'Albenzio, et al. Reduced temporal lobe areas in schizophrenia. *Biological Psychiatry* 1990; 27:61–68.

7. R. Suddath, G. Christison, E. Torrey, et al. Anatomical abnormalities in the brains of monozygotic twins discordant for schizophrenia. *New England Journal of Medicine* 1990; 322:789–794.

8. P. Flor-Henry and J. Stevens. The telemetered EEG findings in schizophrenia (letters). *Journal of Neurology, Neurosurgery and Psychiatry* 1983; 46:287–288.

9. I. Mefford, K. Roth, H. Agren, et al. Enhancement of dopamine metabolism in rat brain frontal cortex: A common effect of chronically administered antipsychotic drugs. *Brain Research* 1988; 475:380–384.

10. E. Edwards, C. Ashby, and R. Wang. The effect of typical and atypical antipsychotic drugs on the stimulation of phosphoinositide hydrolysis produced by the $5-HT_3$ receptor agonist 2-methyl-serotonin. *Brain Research* 1991; 545:276–278.

11. R. Fischer. Cartography of inner space. In *Hallucinations, Behavior, Experience, and Theory,* eds. R. Siegel and L. West. New York, Wiley, 1975, 197–239. The larger universal referred

to was designated as the "Self." The word is spelled with a capital *S,* following the conventions of Indian philosophical thought. The purpose in doing so is simply to indicate that it is something beyond our private, small self.

12. K. Wapnick. Mysticism and schizophrenia. *Journal of Transpersonal Psychology* 1969; 1:42–68.

Chapter 7   The Semantics of Self

1. A. Deikman. The missing center. In *Alternate States of Consciousness,* ed. N. Zinberg. New York, Free Press, 1977, 230–241.

2. C. Jung. *Psychology and Religion: West and East,* vol 11. Bollingen Series 20. New York, Pantheon, 1958, 484.

3. S. Freud. The dissection of the psychical personality. In *The Standard Edition of the Complete Psychological Works of Sigmund Freud,* vol 22, ed. J. Strachey. London, Hogarth Press, 1964, 57–80.

4. From the beginning, the *id* was an impersonal it. Nietzsche had used the German word *Es,* meaning "it," to refer to whatever was impersonal in our nature. When Freud's works were translated, *Es* was changed into the corresponding Latin word, *id.* A word creates semantic problems when it stands both for something impersonal and for something quite different, which compels us to behave in ways that are felt passionately.

5. R. Aitken. Zen practice and psychotherapy. *Journal of Transpersonal Psychiatry* 1982; 14:161–170.

Chapter 8   Constructing Our Self

1. M. Gazzaniga. The role of language for conscious experience: Observations from split-brain man. In *Progress in Brain Research. Motivation, Motor and Sensory Processes of the Brain,* vol 54, eds. H. Kornhuber and L. Deecke. Amsterdam, Elsevie/North-Holland, 1980, 689–696.

2. R. Dietrich, W. Bradley, E. Zaragoza, et al. MR evaluation of early myelination patterns in normal and developmentally delayed infants. *American Journal of Neuroradiology* 1988; 9:69–76.

3. A. Gesell. *The First Five Years of Life: A Guide to the Study of the Pre-School Child.* Harper & Row, New York, 1940.

4. J. Anderson. The development of self-recognition: A review. *Developmental Psychobiology* 1984; 17:35–49.

5. M. Hoffman. Developmental synthesis of affect and cognition and its implications for altruistic motivation. *Developmental Psychology* 1975; 11:607–622.

6. A. Galaburda. Commissural transmission: Maturational changes in humans. *Science* 1978; 200.1409–1411. The left hemisphere is more verbal; the right more nonverbal.

7. W. James. *The Principles of Psychology,* vol 1. Holt, New York, 1918.

8. K. Wilber. *No Boundary.* Whole Mind Series. Los Angeles, Center Publications, 1979.

9. J. Droogleever-Fortuyn. On the organization of spatial behavior. *Human Neurobiology* 1982; 1:145–151.

10. J. Simpson. The accessory optic system. *Annual Review of Neuroscience* 1984; 7:13–41.

11. B. Strehler. Where is the self? A neuroanatomical theory of consciousness. *Synapse* 1991; 7:44–91.

12. D. Perrett, M. Oram, M. Harries, et al. Viewer-centered and object-centered coding of heads in the macaque temporal cortex. *Experimental Brain Research* 1991; 86:159–173.

13. Some speculate that it represents these "selves" in a manner likened to that of a hologram wherein separate bits of data distribute themselves throughout the whole image, and the whole image is contained in each bit as well. See, for example, R. Miller. *Meaning and Purpose in the Intact Brain.* Oxford, Clarendon Press, 1981.

14. D. Rubin, ed. *Autobiographical Memory.* New York, Cambridge University Press, 1986.

15. R. Calvanio, P. Petrone, and D. Levine. Left visual spatial neglect is both environment-centered and body-centered. *Neurology* 1987; 37:1179–1183.

16. D. Williams. Man's temporal lobe. *Brain* 1968; 91:639–654.

Chapter 9   Some ABCs of the *I-Me-Mine*

1. Hashida. Shobogenzo shakui. In *The Buddhist Tradition in India, China and Japan*, ed. W. de Bary. New York, Vintage, 1972, 371.
2. A popular saying attributed to Walt Kelly's character, Pogo, in the King Features comic strip.
3. I am indebted to Irmgard Schloegl for her original stimulus in emphasizing the central importance of the "I." The present construct of an italicized *I-Me-Mine* evolved in response to the need to separately identify its major elements in operational terms.
4. K. Wilber. *No Boundary*. Whole Mind Series. Los Angeles, Center Publications, 1979.
5. See Appendix B, Selections from *Affirmation of Faith in Mind*.

Chapter 10   The Zen Mirror: Beyond Narcissism and Depersonalization

1. F. Bacon, from *Novum Organum* (1620), in C. Curtis and F. Greenslet, eds., *The Practical Cogitator*, Boston, Houghton Mifflin, 1953, 15.
2. Zenrin Kushu, in *The World of Zen. An East-West Anthology*, ed. N. Ross. New York, Vintage, 1960, 258.
3. Hui Hai, in J. Blofeld, *The Zen Teachings of Hui Hai on Sudden Illumination*. London, Rider, 1962, 51.
4. R. Satow. Pop narcissism. *Psychology Today* 1979; 13 (October). 14–17.
5. Some psychoanalytic theories view the mystical experience as a welling up of residual "primary" narcissism. This is conceptualized as a return to that early passive-receptive mode which we once used to relate to our intrauterine or infantile world. See, for example, P. Horton: The mystical experience: substance of an illusion. *Journal of the American Psychoanalytic Association* 1974; 22, 364–380. Yet the central nervous system is still incompletely developed in newborns, let alone in the unborn fetus. The hard-wiring is barely there, let alone the soft-wiring. Such theories stretch credulity too far whenever they use the primitive, fragmentary abilities, experiences, or memories of this immature circuitry—other than, of course, in highly metaphoric descriptions—to explain how peak experiences later arise in and then transform the behavior of an *adult* brain.
6. J. Silverman. On the sensory bases of transcendental states of consciousness. In *Psychiatry and Mysticism*, ed. S. Dean. Chicago, Nelson-Hall, 1975, 365–398.
7. J. Cattell and J. Cattell. Depersonalization: Psychological and social perspectives. In *American Handbook of Psychiatry*, 2nd ed. vol. 3, *Adult Clinical Psychiatry*. eds. S. Arieti and E. Brody. New York, Basic Books, 1974, 766–799.
8. J. Nemiah. Depersonalization neurosis. In *Comprehensive Textbook of Psychiatry II*, 2nd ed., vol 1, eds. A. Freedman, H. Kaplan, and B. Sadock. Baltimore, William & Wilkins, 1975, 1268–1273.
9. M. Ferguson. *The Aquarian Conspiracy. Personal and Social Transformations in the 1980's*. London, Routledge & Kegan Paul, 1981.

Chapter 11   Where Does Zen Think It's Coming From?

1. R. Sperry. Brain bisection and mechanisms of consciousness. In *Brain and Conscious Experience*, ed. J. Eccles. New York, Springer-Verlag, 1966, 298–313.
2. H. Stewart, trans. *A Chime of Windbells*. Rutland, Vt., Tuttle. This is a translation of a haiku poem.
3. R. Siu. Zen and science—"No-knowledge." In *The World of Zen. An East-West Anthology*, ed. N. Ross. New York, Vintage, 1969, 308–317.
4. T. Izutsu. *Toward a Philosophy of Zen Buddhism*. Publication 26. Tehran, Imperial Iranian Academy of Philosophy, 1977.

Chapter 12   What Is Meditation?

1. Soyen Shaku came to the United States in 1893, the first Rinzai Zen master to do so. He cautioned that hallucinatory visionary states had nothing to do with realizing the religious life. See Soyen Shaku. The practice of dhyana. In *Anthology of Zen*, ed. W. Briggs. New York, Grove Press, 1961, 266–273.

2. J. Wu. *The Golden Age of Zen.* Taipei, United Publishing Center, 1975, 250; distributed by Paragon Book Gallery. New York, N.Y.
3. S. Suzuki. *Zen Mind, Beginner's Mind.* Tokyo, Weatherhill, 1975, 35.
4. H. Benson. The relaxation response: History, physiologic basis and clinical usefulness. *Acta Medica Scandinavica, Supplementum* 1982; 660:231–237.
5. H-J. Kim. *Dogen Kigen—Mystical Realist.* Tucson, University of Arizona Press, 1975, 72.
6. K. Graf von Durckheim. *Hara. The Vital Centre of Man.* London, Mandala, Unwin, 1977.
7. K. Wilber. *No Boundary.* Whole Mind Series. Los Angeles, Center Publications, 1979, 150.
8. H. Jarrell. *International Meditation Bibliography, 1950–1982.* London, Scarecrow Press, 1985.
9. M. Murphy, S. Donovan, and E. Taylor. *The Physical and Psychological Effects of Meditation. A Review of Contemporary Research with a Comprehensive Bibliography 1931–1996. Second Edition.* Sausalito, California, Institute of Noetic Sciences, 1997.

Chapter 13   Ryoko-in, Kyoto 1974

1. From *Affirming Faith in Mind,* as condensed in Appendix B.
2. J. Austin and S. Takaori. Studies of connections between locus coeruleus and cerebral cortex. *Japanese Journal of Pharmacology* 1976; 26:145–160.
3. T. Leggett. *Zen and the Ways.* Boulder, Colo., Shambhala, 1978.

Chapter 14   Zazen at Ryoko-in

1. This centuries-old Japanese poem has several levels of poetic interpretation. What makes it unique is the way it expresses the many characters of the Hiragana alphabet.
2. A simplified version of the sutra is in Appendix A.
3. D. Suzuki. *The Training of the Zen Buddhist Monk.* New York, University Books, 1965, 33.

Chapter 15   Attention

1. W. James. *The Principles of Psychology,* vol. 1. New York, Holt, 1918, 424.
2. R. Rafal and M. Posner. Deficits in human visual spatial attention following thalamic lesions. *Proceedings of the National Academy of Sciences of the United States of America* 1987; 84:7349–7353.
3. A. Reeves and G. Sperling. Attention gating in short-term visual memory. *Psychology Review* 1986; 93:180–206.
4. M. Arguin, Y. Joanette, and P. Cavanagh. Comparing the cerebral hemispheres on the speed of spatial shifts of visual attention: Evidence from serial search. *Neuropsychology* 1990; 28:773–736.
5. J. Silverman. On the sensory bases of transcendental states of consciousness. In *Psychiatry and Mysticism,* ed. S. Dean. Chicago, Nelson-Hall, 1975, 365–398.
6. James, *op. cit.,* 126.
7. Part III clarifies how the reticular formation interconnects with higher attentional mechanisms.
8. R. Watson, K. Heilman, B. Miller, et al. Neglect after mesencephalic reticular formation lesions. *Neurology* 1975; 25:294–298.

Chapter 16   The Attentive Art of Meditation

1. Dhiravamsa. *The Way of Non-Attachment. The Practice of Insight Meditation.* New York, Schocken, 1977, 33.
2. D. Shapiro. *Meditation: Self-Regulation Strategy and Altered State of Consciousness.* New York, Aldine, 1980, 14.
3. M. Washburn. Observations relevant to a unified theory of meditation. *Journal of Transpersonal Psychology* 1978; 10:45–65.
4. R. Ornstein. *The Psychology of Consciousness.* W.H. Freeman, San Francisco.
5. Ishiguro Zen changes its meditative techniques on each of five successive days. During the first day, numbers are counted from one to ten. During the second to the fourth day, the sound *Mu* is pronounced more emphatically each day. During the fifth day, all muscles are strained to the utmost and then relaxed. This is repeated many times. Finally one

sits, alert, in zazen. See Y. Akishige. *Psychological Studies on Zen I.* Tokyo, Komazawa University Press, 1977.

6. J. Campbell. *The Inner Reaches of Outer Space.* New York, A. van der Marck, 1985, 74–75.
7. J. Ortega y Gasset. *Meditations on Hunting.* New York, Scribner's, 1985, 130, 132.

Chapter 17   Restraint and Renunciation

1. H. Thoreau. *Walden.* N. J., Princeton University Press. 1854; Princeton, 1989.
2. P. Carrington. Meditation as an access to altered states of consciousness. In *Handbook of States of Consciousness,* eds. B. Wolman and M. Ullman. New York, Van Nostrand Reinhold, 1986, 487–523.
3. D. Suzuki. *The Training of the Zen Buddhist Monk.* New York, University Books, 1965.
4. W. Johnston. All and nothing. St. John of the Cross and the Christian-Buddhist dialogue. *The Eastern Buddhist* 1986; 21(2):124–142.
5. R. Masaunaga. *A Primer of Soto Zen.* Honolulu, University of Hawaii Press, 1971, 56.
6. I. Miura and R. Sasaki. *Zen Dust. The History of the Koan and Koan Study in Rinzai (Lin-Chi) Zen.* Kyoto, The First Zen Institute of America in Japan, 1966, 74.

Chapter 18   Zen Meditative Techniques and Skills

1. W. James. *The Principles of Psychology,* vol 1. New York, Holt, 1918, 402.
2. K. Sekida. *Zen Training. Methods and Philosophy.* New York, Weatherhill, 1975.
3. N. Waddell, trans. Dogen's Hokyo-ki. Part II. *The Eastern Buddhist* 1978; 11:66–84.

Chapter 19   Physiological Changes During Meditation

1. J. Davidson. The physiology of meditation and mystical states of consciousness. *Perspectives in Biology and Medicine* 1976; 19:345–379.
2. R. Woolfolk. Psychophysiological correlates of meditation. *Archives of General Psychiatry* 1975; 32:1326–1333.
3. M. Schuman. The psychophysiological model of meditation and altered states of consciousness: A critical review. In *The Psychobiology of Consciousness,* eds. J. Davidson and R. Davidson. New York, Plenum Press, 1980, 333–378.
4. D. Shapiro. *Meditation: Self-Regulation Strategy and Altered State of Consciousness.* New York, Aldine, 1980.
5. H. Benson. The relaxation response: History, physiologic basis and clinical usefulness. *Acta Medica Scandinavica Supplementum* 1982; 660:231–237.
6. D. Holmes. Meditation and somatic arousal: A review of the experimental evidence. *American Psychologist* 1984; 39:1–10.
7. D. Holmes. The influence of meditation versus rest on physiological arousal: A second examination. In *The Psychology of Meditation,* ed. M. West. Oxford, Clarendon Press, 1987, 81–103.
8. M. Delmonte. Biochemical indices associated with meditation practice: A literature review. *Neuroscience and Biobehavioral Reviews* 1985; 9:557–561.
9. R. Sudsuang, V. Chentanez, and K. Veluvan. Effect of Buddhist meditation on serum cortisol and total protein levels, blood pressure, pulse rate, lung volume and reaction time. *Physiology and Behavior* 1991; 50:543–548.
10. H. Jarrell. *International Meditation Bibliography. 1950–1982.* Philadelphia, American Theological Library Association, 1985.
11. J. Hoffman, H. Benson, P. Arns, et al. Reduced sympathetic nervous system responsivity associated with the relaxation response. *Science* 1982; 215:190–192.
12. M. Dillbeck and D. Orme-Johnson. Physiological differences between transcendental meditation and rest. *American Psychologist* 1987; 42:879–881.
13. D. Brown, M. Forte, and M. Dysart. Visual sensitivity and mindfulness meditation. *Perceptual and Motor Skills* 1984; 58:775–784.
14. M. Forte, D. Brown, and M. Dysart. Through the looking glass: Phenomenological reports of advanced meditators at visual threshold. *Imagination, Cognition and Personality* 1984–85; 4:323–338.

15. H. Benson. The relaxation response: Its subjective and objective Historical precedents and Physiology. *Trends in Neuroscience* 1983 (July); 6:281–284.

16. G. Boals. Toward a cognitive reconceptualization of meditation. *Journal of Transpersonal Psychology* 1978; 10:143–182.

17. Y. Akishige. *Psychological Studies on Zen I.* Tokyo, Komazawa University Press, 1977.

18. P. Fenwick, S. Donaldson, L. Gillis, et al. Metabolic and EEG changes during transcendental meditation: An explanation. *Biological Psychology* 1977; 5:101–118. A recent study was performed on three Tibetan Buddhist monks during their specialized meditation techniques. Both increases and decreases occurred in oxygen consumption. These were not correlated with changes in the patterns of EEG activity. However, the EEG did tend to show an increase in right-sided beta-wave activity. See H. Benson, M. Malhotra, R. Goldman, et al. Three case reports of the metabolic and electroencephalographic changes during advanced Buddhist meditation techniques. *Behavioral Medicine* 1990 (summer); 90–95.

19. J. O'Halloran, R. Jevning, A. Wilson, et al. Hormonal control in a state of decreased activation: Potentiation of arginine vasopressin secretion. *Physiology and Behavior* 1985; 35:591–595.

20. R. Pekala. The phenomenology of meditation. In *The Psychology of Meditation*, ed. M. West. Oxford, Clarendon Press, 1987, 59–80. Introspection itself sensitizes subjects to unusual forms of alternate states. This phenomenon is called "introspective sensitization."

21. D. Dinges. Napping patterns and effects in human adults. In *Sleep and Alertness*, eds. D. Dinges and R. Broughton. New York, Raven Press, 1989, 171–204.

22. S. Campbell and J. Zulley. Ultradian components of human sleep/wake patterns during disentrainment. *Experimental Brain Research* 1985; 12(suppl.):234–255.

23. J. Taub, P. Tanguay, and R. Rosa. Effects of afternoon naps on physiological variables, performance and self-reported activation. *Biological Psychology* 1977; 5:191–210.

24. R. Pagano, R. Rose, R. Stivers, et al. Sleep during transcendental meditation. *Science* 1976; 191:308–309.

25. R. Wallace Letter: TM: Meditation or sleep? Reply by R. Pagano, R. Rose, and S. Warrenburg. *Science* 1976; 193:718–720.

26. B. Glueck and C. Stroebel. Biofeedback and meditation in the treatment of psychiatric illness. *Comprehensive Psychiatry* 1975; 16:303–321.

27. D. Orme-Johnson and J. Farrow, eds. *Scientific Research on the Transcendental Meditation Program.* Vol 1, *Collected Papers.* New York, Maharishi European Research University Press, 1977.

28. R. Wallace. *The Maharishi Technology of the United Field: The Neurophysiology of Enlightenment.* Fairfield, Iowa, MIU Neuroscience Press, 1986, 70–72.

29. K. Pelletier. The effects of the transcendental meditation program on perceptual style: Increased field Independence. In *Scientific Research on the Transcendental Meditation Progam,* eds. D. Orme-Johnson and J. Farrow, Vol 1, Collected Papers. New York, Maharishi European Research University Press, 1977.

30. C. Sandman. Cardiac afferent influences on consciousness. In *Consciousness and Self-Regulation*, vol. 4, eds. R. Davidson, G. Schwartz, and D. Shapiro. New York, Plenum Press, 1986, 55–85.

31. J. Glaser, J. Brind, J. Vogelman, et al. Elevated serum dehydroepiandrosterone sulfate levels in practitioners of the transcendental meditation (TM) and TM-Sidhi programs. *Journal of Behavioral Medicine* 1992; 15:327–341.

Chapter 20   Brain Waves and Their Limitations

1. B. Brown. *New Mind—New Body. Bio-Feedback: New Directions for the Mind.* New York, Harper & Row, 1974.

2. T. Mulholland. The concept of attention and the electroencephalographic alpha rhythm. In *Attention in Neurophysiology*, eds. C. Evans and T. Mulholland. London, Butterworths, 1969, 100–127.

3. D. Lehmann and M. Koukkou. Classes of spontaneous private experiences, and ongoing human EEG activity. In *Rhythmic EEG Activities and Cortical Functioning*, eds. G.

Pfurtscheller, P. Buser, F. Lopes da Silva, et al. Developments in Neuroscience, vol. 10. Amsterdam, Elsevier/North Holland, 1980, 289–297.

4. T. Mulholland and S. Runnals. Increased occurrence of EEG alpha during increased attention. *Journal of Psychology* 1962; 54:317–330.

5. A. Williams. Facilitation of the alpha rhythm of the electroencephalogram. *Journal of Experimental Psychology* 1940; 26:413–422.

6. H. Jasper. Neurochemical mediators of specific and nonspecific cortical activation. In C. Evans and T. Mulholland, eds., *Attention in Neurophysiology,* London, Butterworths, 1969, 377–395.

7. W. Penfield and W. Jasper. *Epilepsy and the Functional Anatomy of the Human Brain.* Boston, Little, Brown, 1954, 189–190.

8. O. Creutzfeldt, G. Grünewald, O. Simonova, et al. Changes of the basic rhythms of the EEG during the performance of mental and visuomotor tasks. In C. Evans and T. Mulholland, eds., *Attention in Neurophysiology.* London, Butterworths, 1969, 148–168.

9. H. Legewie, O. Simonova, and D. Creutzfeldt. EEG changes during performance of various tasks under open- and closed-eye conditions. *Electroencephalography and Clinical Neurophysiology* 1969; 27:470–479.

10. J. Hare, B. Timmons, J. Roberts, et al. EEG alpha-biofeedback training: An experimental technique for the management of anxiety. *Journal of Medical Engineering and Technology* 1982; 6:19–24.

11. M. Hashimoto, H. Mukasa, S. Yamada, et al. Frontal midline theta activity and platelet MAO in human subjects. *Biological Psychiatry* 1988; 23:31–43.

12. A. Tebecis, K. Provins, R. Farnbach, et al. Hypnosis and the EEG. *Journal of Nervous and Mental Disease* 1975; 161:1–17.

13. W. Adey. Spectral analysis of EEG data from animals and man during alerting, orienting and discriminative responses. In C. Evans and T. Mulholland, eds., *Attention in Neurophysiology.* London, Butterworths, 1969, 194–229.

14. C. Guilleminault, M. Billiard, J. Montplaisir, et al. Altered states of consciousness in disorders of daytime sleepiness. *Journal of the Neurological Sciences* 1975; 26:377–393.

15. J. O'Hanlon and J. Beatty. Concurrence of electroencephalographic and performance changes during a simulated radar watch and some implications for the arousal theory of vigilance. In *Vigilance. Theory, Operational Performance, and Physiological Correlate,* ed. R. Mackie. New York, Plenum Press, 1977, 189–201.

16. H. Jokeit and S. Makeig. Different event-related patterns of gamma-band power in brainwaves of fast- and slow-reacting subjects. *Proceedings of the National Academy of Sciences of the United States of America* 1994; 91:6339–6343.

17. F. Morrell. Electrical signs of sensory coding. In *The Neurosciences. A Study Program,* eds. G. Quarton, T. Melnechuk and F. Schmitt. New York, Rockefeller University Press, 1967, 452–469.

18. R. Thatcher, E. John. *Foundations of Cognitive Processes.* Vol. 1 of *Functional Neuroscience.* Hillsdale, N.J., Erlbaum, 1977.

19. W. Freeman. Searching for signal and noise in the chaos of brain waves. In *The Ubiquity of Chaos,* ed. S. Krassner. Washington, DC., American Association for the Advancement of Science, 1990, 47–55.

20. T. Ohmoto, Y. Mimura, Y. Baba, et al. Thalamic control of spontaneous alpha-rhythm and evoked responses. *Applied Neurophysiology* 1978; 41:188–192.

Chapter 21   The EEG in Meditation

1. C. Brown, R. Fischer, A. Wagman, et al. The EEG in meditation and therapeutic touch healing. *Journal of Altered States of Consciousness* 1977–78; 3:169–180.

2. A. Tebécis. A controlled study of the EEG during transcendental meditation: Comparison with hypnosis. *Folia Psychiatrica Neurologica et Japonica* 1975; 29:305–313.

3. P. Fenwick. Meditation and the EEG. In *The Psychology of Meditation,* ed. M. West. Oxford, Clarendon Press, 1987, 104–117.

4. F. Griffith. Meditation research: Its personal and social implications. In *Frontiers of Consciousness*, ed. J. White. New York, Julian Press, 1985, 119–137.

5. T. Suzuki. *An EEG Study on My Zazen: With and Without Mental Effort*. Paper presented at International EEG Congress. Kyoto, Japan, 1981. Abstract D10.08.

6. M. Schuman. The psychophysiological model of meditation and altered states of consciousness: A critical review. In *The Psychobiology of Consciousness*, eds. J. Davidson and R. Davidson. New York, Plenum Press, 1980, 333–378.

7. Y. Akishige. *Psychological Studies on Zen I*, vol. 1. Tokyo, Komazawa University Press, 1977.

8. *Ibid.*, vol 2.

9. D. Kiefer. EEG alpha feedback and subjective states of consciousness: A subject's introspective overview. In *Frontiers of Consciousness*, ed. J. White. New York, Julian Press, 1985, 94–113.

10. K. Badawi, R. Wallace, D. Orme-Johnson, et al. Electrophysiologic characteristics of respiratory suspension periods occurring during the practice of the transcendental meditation program. *Psychosomatic Medicine* 1984; 46:267–276.

11. P. Levine. The coherence spectral array (COSPAR) and its application to the study of spatial ordering in the EEG. *Proceedings of the San Diego Biomedical Symposia* 1976; 15:237–247.

12. J. Banquet. Spectral Analysis of the EEG in meditation. *Electroencephalography and Clinical Neurophysiology* 1973; 35:143–151.

13. T. Hirai. Personal communication of studies on Reverend Ashibe, 1985.

14. N. Das and H. Gastaut. Variations de l'activité électrique du cerveau, du cœur et des muscles squelettiques au cours de la méditation et de l'extase yogique. *Electroencephalography and Clinical Neurophysiology* 1955; 6(suppl.):211–219.

15. B. Anand, G. Chhina, and B. Singh. Some aspects of electro-encephalographic studies in yogis. *Electroencephalography and Clinical Neurophysiology* 1961; 13:452–456.

16. B. Anand, G. Chhina, and B. Singh. Studies on Shri Ramanand Yogi during his stay in an air-tight box. *Indian Journal of Medical Research* 1961; 49:82–89.

17. B. Taneli and W. Krahne. EEG changes of transcendental meditation practitioners. *Advances in Biological Psychiatry* 1987; 16:41–71.

18. J. Paty, P. Brenot, J. Tignol, et al. Activités évoquées cérébrales (variation contingente negative et potentials évoques) et états de conscience modifies (relaxation sophronique, méditation trancendantale). *Annales Médico-Psychologiques* 1978; 136:143–169.

19. S. Warrenburg, R. Pagano, M. Woods, et al. A comparison of somatic relaxation and EEG activity in classical progressive relaxation and transcendental meditation. *Journal of Behavioral Medicine* 1980; 3:73–93.

20. P. Fenwick, S. Donaldson, L. Gillis, et al. Metabolic and EEG changes during transcendental meditation: An explanation. *Biological Psychology* 1977; 5:101–118.

21. D. Stigsby, J. Rodenberg, and H. Moth. Electroencephalographic findings during mantra meditation (transcendental meditation): A controlled quantitative study of experienced meditators. *Electroencephalography and Clinical Neurophysiology* 1981; 51:434–442.

22. B. Elson, P. Hauri, and D. Cunis. Physiological changes in yoga meditation. *Psychophysiology* 1977; 14:52–57.

23. R. Pagano and S. Warrenburg. Meditation: In search of a unique effect. In *Consciousness and Self Regulation*, vol. 3. eds. R. Davidson, G. Schwarz, and D. Shapiro. New York, Plenum Press, 1983, 153–205.

24. J. Bennett and J. Trinder. Hemispheric laterality and cognitive style associated with transcendental meditation. *Psychophysiology* 1977; 14:293–296.

25. R. Pagano. Recent research in the physiology of meditation. In *Brain and Behavior*, eds. G. Adam, I. Meszaros, and E. Banyai. *Advances in Physiological Sciences*, vol. 17. Budapest, Pergamon, 1981, 443–451.

Chapter 22   Breathing In; Breathing Out

1. M. Schuman. The psychophysiological model of meditation and altered states of consciousness: A critical review. In *The Psychobiology of Consciousness*, eds. J. Davidson and R. Davidson. New York, Plenum Press, 1980; 333–378.

2. S. Block, M. Lemeignan, and N. Aguilera. Specific respiratory patterns distinguish among human basic emotions. *International Journal of Psychophysiology* 1991; 11:141–154.

3. C. VonEuler. Brainstem mechanisms for generation and control of breathing pattern. In *Handbook of Physiology.* Sec. 3, *The Respiratory System,* vol. 2, pt. 1, eds. A. Fishman, N. Cherniak, and J. Widdicombe. Bethesda, Md., American Physiological Society, 1986, 1–67.

4. R. Shannon and D. Freeman. Nucleus retroambigualis respiratory neurons: Responses to intercostal and abdominal muscle afferents. *Respiration Physiology* 1981; 45:357–375.

5. I. Homma, A. Isobe, M. Iwase, et al. Two different types of apnea induced by focal cold block of ventral medulla in rabbits. *Neuroscience Letters* 1988; 87:41–45.

6. J. Bogousslavsky, R. Khurana, J. Deruaz, et al. Respiratory failure and unilateral caudal brainstem infarction. *Annals of Neurology* 1990; 28:668–673.

7. R. Frysinger and R. Harper. Cardiac and respiratory correlations with unit discharge in human amygdala and hippocampus. *Electroencephalography and Clinical Neurophysiology* 1989; 72:463–470.

8. K. Ohtsuka, K. Asakura, H. Kawasaki, et al. Respiratory fluctuations of the human pupil. *Experimental Brain Research* 1988; 71:215–217.

9. J. Horne and M. Whitehead. Ultradian and other rhythms in human respiration rate. *Experientia* 1976; 32:1165–1167.

10. Y. Akishige. *Psychological Studies on Zen,* vol. 1. Tokyo, Komazawa University Press, 1977, 75.

11. *Ibid.,* vol. 2, 308.

12. *Ibid.,* vol. 1, 125.

13. J. Orem and A. Netick. Behavioral control of breathing in the cat. *Brain Research* 1986; 366:238–253.

14. F. Gault and R. Leaton. Electrical activity of the olfactory system. *Electroencephalography and Clinical Neurophysiology* 1963; 15:299–304.

15. J. Farrow and J. Hebert. Breath suspension during the transcendental meditation technique. *Psychiatric Medicine* 1982; 44:133–153. Respiration also ceased for a long 100 seconds in one expert meditator who felt her "breathing taken over by the mantra" as part of a "near-Samadhi experience." The first change in this particular instance was a substantial decrease in skin resistance. It occurred before the preliminary increase in the heart rate and respiratory rate. The EEG did not change. The authors emphasize that the expert subjects in their study had been practicing a tantric form of active meditation for three hours a day. They were also struggling to achieve union with the object they were concentrating on. See J. Corby, W. Roth, V. Zarcone, et al. Psychophysiological correlates of the practice of tantric yoga meditation. *Archives of General Psychiatry* 1978; 35:571–577.

16. F. Travis and R. Wallace: Autonomic markers during respiratory suspensions; possible markers of transcendental consciousness. *Psychophysiology* 1997; 34:39–46.

17. R. Ogilvie and R. Wilkinson. The detection of sleep onset: Behavioral and physiological convergence. *Psychophysiology* 1984; 21:510–520.

18. K. Badawi, R. Wallace, D. Orme-Johnson, et al. Electrophysiologic characteristics of respiratory suspension periods occurring during the practice of the transcendental meditation program. *Psychosomatic Medicine* 1984; 46:267–276.

19. N. Wolkove, H. Kreisman, D. Darragh, et al. Effect of transcendental meditation on breathing and respiratory control. *Journal of Applied Physiology* 1984; 56:607–612.

20. A. Hugelin. Does the respiratory rhythm originate from a reticular oscillator in the waking state? In *The Reticular Formation Revisited,* eds. J. Hobson and M. Brazier. International Brain Research Organization Monograph Series, vol. 6. New York, Raven Press, 1980, 261–274.

21. S. Long and J. Duffin. The neuronal determinants of respiratory rhythm. *Progress in Neurobiology* 1986; 27:101–182.

22. A. Miller, K. Ezure, and I. Suzuki. Control of abdominal muscles by brainstem respiratory neurons in the cat. *Journal of Neurophysiology* 1985; 54:155–167.

23. J. Zhang, R. Harper, and R. Frysinger. Respiratory modulation of neuronal discharge in the central nucleus of the amygdala during sleep and waking states. *Experimental Neurology* 1986; 91:193–207.

24. J. Zhang, R. Harper, and H. Ni. Cryogenic blockade of the central nucleus of the amygdala attenuates aversively conditioned blood pressure and respiratory responses. *Brain Research* 1986; 386:136–145.

25. K. McCaul, S. Solomon, and D. Holmes. Effects of paced respiration and expectations on physiological and psychological responses to threat. *Journal of Personality and Social Psychology* 1979; 37:564–571.

26. J. Hedner. Neuropharmacological aspects of central respiratory regulation. An experimental study in the rat. *Acta Physiologica Scandinavica Supplementum* 1983; 524:1–109.

27. M. Yeadon and I. Kitchen. Opioids and respiration. *Progress in Neurobiology* 1989; 33:1–16.

28. C. Richard and R. Stremel. Involvement of the raphe in the respiratory effects of gigantocellular area activation. *Brain Research Bulletin* 1990; 25:19–23.

29. D. McGinty. Physiological equilibrium and the control of sleep states. In *Brain Mechanisms of Sleep*, eds. D. McGinty, R. Drucker-Colin, A. Morrison, et al. New York, Raven Press, 1985.

30. W. Hess. *Hypothalamus and Thalamus*. Stuttgart, Thieme, 1969.

31. E. Spiegel and H. Wycis. Stimulation of the brain stem and basal ganglia in man. In *Electrical Stimulation of the Brain*, ed. D. Sheer. Austin, University of Texas Press, 1961, 487–497. It is of interest that the hypothalamus projects to this anterior thalamic nucleus via the mammillothalamic tract (see figure 6).

32. J. Siegfried and M. Wiesendanger. Respiratory alterations produced by thalamic stimulation during stereotaxic operations. *Confinia Neurologica* 1967; 29:220–223.

Chapter 23   The Effects of Sensorimotor Deprivation

1. D. Suzuki. *Manual of Zen Buddhism*. New York, Grove Press, 1960, 127–144.

2. V. Block, M. Valat, and J. -C. Roy. Influences des afférences musculaires sur le tonus réticulaire. *Journal de Physiologie (Paris)* 1965; 57:561–562.

3. J. Zubek. *Sensory Deprivation: Fifteen Years of Research*. New York, Appleton-Century-Crofts, 1969.

4. A. Rossi. General methodological considerations. In *Sensory Deprivation: Fifteen Years of Research*, ed. J. Zubek. New York, Appleton-Century-Crofts, 1969, 16–43.

5. P. Suedfeld. Changes in intellectual performance and in susceptibility to influence. In *Sensory Deprivation: Fifteen Years of Research*, ed. J. Zubek. New York, Appleton-Century-Crofts, 1969, 126–166.

6. J. Zubek. Sensory and perceptual motor effects. In *Sensory Deprivation: Fifteen Years of Research*, ed. J. Zubek. New York, Appleton-Century-Crofts, 1969, 207–253.

7. F. Jeffrey. Working in isolation: States that alter consensus. In *Handbook of States of Consciousness*, eds. B. Wolman and M. Ullman. New York, Van Nostrand Reinhold, 1986, 249–285.

8. D. Schacter. The hypnagogic state: A critical review of the literature. *Psychological Bulletin* 1976; 83:452–481.

9. S. Freedman, H. Grunebaum, F. Stare, et al. Imagery in sensory deprivation. In *Hallucinations*, ed. L. West. New York, Grune & Stratton, 1962, 108–117.

10. J. Zubek. Physiological and biochemical effects. In *Sensory Deprivation: Fifteen Years of Research*, ed. J. Zubek. New York, Appleton-Century-Crofts, 1969, 254–258.

11. J. Mazziota, M. Phelps, R. Carson, et al. Tomographic mapping of human cerebral metabolism: Sensory deprivation. *Annals of Neurology* 1982; 12:435–444.

12. J. Mazziotta, M. Phelps, and D. Kuhl. Human cerebral metabolism studied during limitations of sensory inputs (abstract). *Annals of Neurology* 1981; 10(abstract 15):76.

13. Given the results in other subjects, the greater metabolic activity on the right side in the author's PET scan (see figure 12) is not likely to be attributed solely to his having vision and hearing blocked.

14. Researchers have introduced one other major variation on the theme of sensorimotor deprivation by swinging blindfolded subjects in a large pendulum in various directions over a two to twenty-minute period. The subjects lose their spatial referents, their sense of time, and develop a wide variety of other alternate state phenomena. They may pay "visits" to other worlds, and have religious and other mystical-type experiences. See J. Houston. The Psychenaut Program: An exploration into some human potentials. *Journal of Creative Behavior* 1973; 7:253–278.

15. N. Thoa, Y. Tizabi, and D. Jacobowitz. The effect of isolation on catecholamine concentration and turnover in discrete areas of the rat brain. *Brain Research* 1977; 131:259–269.

Chapter 24   Monks and Clicks: Habituation

1. D. Becker and D. Shapiro. Physiological responses to clicks during Zen, yoga, and TM meditation. *Psychophysiology* 1981; 18:694–699.

2. T. Hirai. *Psychophysiology of Zen*. Tokyo, Igaku Shoin, 1974.

3. W. Keidel, W. Neff, and M. Abeles, eds. Auditory system. In *Handbook of Sensory Physiology*, vol. 5. Berlin, Springer-Verlag, 1975, 2.

4. B. Anand, G. Chhina, and B. Singh. Some aspects of electroencephalographic studies in yogis. *Electroencephalograph and Clinical Neurophysiology* 1961; 13:452–456.

5. B. Anand, G. Chhina, and B. Singh. Studies on Shri Ramanand Yogi during his stay in an air-tight box. *Indian Journal of Medical Research* 1961; 49:82–89.

6. J. Banquet. Spectral analysis of the EEG in meditation. *Electroencephalography and Clinical Neurophysiology* 1973; 35:143–151.

7. A. Kasamatsu and T. Hirai. An electroencephalographic study on the Zen meditation (zazen). *Folia Psychiatrica et Neurologica Japonica* 1966; 20:315–336.

8. L. Johnson and A. Lubin. The orienting reflex during waking and sleeping. *Electroencephalography and Clinical Neurophysiology* 1967; 22:11–21.

9. L. Johnson, R. Townsend, and M. Wilson. Habituation during sleeping and waking. *Psychophysiology* 1975; 12:574–584.

10. J. Paty, P. Brenot, J. Tignol, et al. Activités evoqueés cérébrales (variation contingente negative et potentials evoques) et états de conscience modifies. *Annales Medico-Psychologique* 1978; 136:143–169.

11. All parts of the brain do not habituate equally. Nerve cells in parts of the midbrain show no habituation when sound signals are repeated in random order. See M. LeMoal and M. Olds. Peripheral auditory input to the midbrain limbic area and related structures. *Brain Research* 1979; 167:1–17.

Chapter 25   The Koan and Sanzen: Kyoto 1974

1. R. Sasaki, Y. Iriya, and D. Fraser. *The Recorded Sayings of Layman P'ang*. New York, Weatherhill, 1971, 87.

2. I. Miura and R. Saski. *Zen Dust. The History of the Koan and Koan Study in Rinzai (Lin-Chi) Zen*. Kyoto, The First Zen Institute of America in Japan, 1966.

Chapter 26   A Quest for Non-Answers: Mondo and Koan

1. G. -C. Chang. *The Practice of Zen*. New York, Harper, 1959, 94–95.

2. J. Sasaki. *Buddha is the Center of Gravity*. San Cristobal, N.M., Lama Foundation, 1974, 88.

3. N. Kobori. The ripening persimmon. An interview with Kobori Nanrei Roshi. *Parabola* 1985; 10:72–79.

4. W. Kaufmann. *Critique of Religion and Philosophy*. New York, Harper & Row Torchbook, 1972, 366.

5. This is Trudy Dixon's apt contemporary description of her teacher, the late Shunryu Suzuki. See S. Suzuki. *Zen Mind; Beginner's Mind*. New York, Weatherhill, 1970, 18.

6. D. Suzuki. *Essays in Zen Buddhism*, ed. C. Humphreys. New York, Weiser, 1971, 107.

7. G. -C. Chang. Comment in *Essays in Zen Buddhism*, ed. C. Humphreys. New York, Weiser, 1959, 76–77.

8. T. Leggett. *Zen and the Ways*. Boulder, Colo., Shambhala, 1978.
9. A. Stunkard. Some interpersonal aspects of an oriental religion. *Psychiatry* 1951; 14:419–431.
10. D. Suzuki. *The Training of the Zen Buddhist Monk*. New York, University Books, 1965, xxi.
11. P. Yampolsky. *The Zen Master Hakuin*. New York, Columbia University Press, 1971.
12. E. Nishimura. The meaning of Zen practice. *Japanese Religions* 1975; 8:3–17.
13. I. Miura and R. Sasaki. *The Zen Koan: Its History and Use in Rinzai Zen*. New York, Harcourt Brace & World, 1965, 28.
14. Y. Hoffman. *The Sound of the One Hand*. New York, Basic Books, 1975.
15. H. Dumoulin. *A History of Zen Buddhism*. Boston, Beacon Press, 1963, 107.
16. D. Perkins. *The Mind's Best Work*. Cambridge, Mass., Harvard University Press, 1981.
17. Miura and Sasaki, *op. cit.*, 49. The student who reaches this point can be said to understand the undifferentiated realm of the dharmakaya.
18. D. Suzuki. *Essays in Zen Buddhism*. First Series. New York, Grove Press, 1949.
19. N. Waddell, trans. and ed. *The Unborn: The Life and Teaching of Zen Master Bankei 1622–1693*. San Francisco, North Point Press, 1984, 129. This question is also rendered as: "What is this that thus comes?"
20. D. Suzuki. *Living by Zen*. London, Rider, 1972, 179.
21. Miura and Sasaki, *op. cit.*, 13.
22. J. Austin. *Chase, Chance, and Creativity. The Lucky Art of Novelty*. New York, Columbia University Press, 1978, 187.
23. Leggett, *op. cit.*, 67.
24. D. Suzuki, *Essays*, 249–252.
25. W. DeBary. *The Buddhist Tradition in India, China and Japan*. New York, Vintage, 1972, 390.
26. Miura and Sasaki, *op. cit.*, 46.
27. H. -J. Kim. *Dogen Kigen—Mystical Realist*. Tucson, University of Arizona Press, 1975, 101–102.
28. T. Suzuki. *An EEG Study on My Zazen: With and Without Mental Effort*. International EEG Congress. Kyoto, Japan, 1981, abstract D10.08.
29. R.C. Gur, R.E. Gur, B. Skolnick, et al. Effects of task difficulty on regional cerebral blood flow: Relationships with anxiety and performance. *Psychophysiology* 1988; 25:392–399.
30. Miura and Sasaki, *op. cit.*, xi.

Chapter 27   The Roshi

1. Quoted in Linscott, R., ed, *Selected Poems and Letters of Emily Dickinson*. Garden City, N.Y., Doubleday, 1959. From a letter to Thomas Higginson, her "preceptor."
2. N. Waddell, trans. and ed. *The Unborn. The Life and Teaching of Zen Master Bankei 1622–1693*. San Francisco, North Point Press, 1984, 140.
3. C. Jung. *Psychology and Religion. West and East*, vol. 11. Bollingen Series 20. New York, Pantheon, 1958, 553.
4. J. Sasaki. *Buddha is the Center of Gravity*. San Cristobal, N.M., Lama Foundation, 1974, 43.
5. I. Schloegl (Myokyo-ni). Lecture at London Zen Center, 1982.
6. D. Richards. *The Wit of Peter Ustinov*. London, Frewin, 1969, 107.
7. Waddell, *op. cit.*, 140.
8. Y. Akishinge. *Psychological Studies on Zen*, vol. 1. Tokyo, Komazawa University Press, 1977, 18.
9. P. Haskel. *Bankei Zen*. New York, Grove Press, 1984, 59–60.
10. H. -J. Kim. *Dogen Kigen—Mystical Realist*. Tucson, University of Arizona Press, 1975, 301.
11. F. FitzGerald. A reporter at large: Rajneeshpuram—Part 2. *The New Yorker*, 29 September 1986, 83–125.
12. A. Maslow. *Religions, Values and Peak Experiences*. New York, Viking, 1970.
13. L. Friedman. *Meetings with Remarkable Women. Buddhist Teachers in American*. Boston, Shambhala, 1987.

Chapter 28   The Mindful, Introspective Path toward Insight

1. Dhiravamsa. *The Way of Non-Attachment. The Practice of Insight Meditation.* New York, Schocken, 1977, 109.
2. D. Goleman. The Buddha on meditation and states of consciousness. Part I: The teachings. *Journal of Transpersonal Psychology* 1972; 4:1–44.
3. W. King. *A Thousand Lives Away.* Cambridge, Mass., Harvard University Press, 1964.
4. R. Gimello. Mysticism and meditation. In *Mysticism and Philosophical Analysis*, ed. S. Katz. London, Sheldon, 1978, 170–179.
5. J. Kornfield. Intensive insight meditation: A phenomenological study. *Journal of Transpersonal Psychology* 1979; 11:41–58.
6. J. Goldstein. *The Experience of Insight: A Natural Unfolding.* Santa Cruz, Calif., Unity Press, 1976.
7. N. Zinberg, ed. *Alternate States of Consciousness.* New York, Free Press, 1977.
8. S. Freud. Recommendations for physicians on the psychoanalytic method of treatment. In *Sigmund Freud. Collected Papers*, vol. 2, ed. E. Jones. New York, Basic Books, 1959, 324.
9. Gimello, *op. cit.*, 170–179.
10. K. Wilber. *No Boundary.* Whole Mind Series. Los Angeles, Center Publications, 1979.
11. A. Deikman. Deautomatization and the mystic experience. *Psychiatry* 1966; 29:324–338.
12. P. Yampolsky. *The Platform Sutra of the Sixth Patriarch.* New York, Columbia University Press, 1967, 169.
13. I. Miura and R. Sasaki. *Zen Dust. The History of the Koan and Koan Study in Rinzai (Lin-Chi) Zen.* Kyoto, The First Zen Institute of America in Japan, 1966, 42.

Chapter 29   Inkblots, Blind Spots, and High Spots

1. C. Jung. *Psychology and Religion: West and East*, 2nd ed., vol. 11. Bollingen Series 20. Princeton, N.J., Princeton University Press, 1969, 484.
2. S. Freud, from Reflections on War and Death, cited in C. Curtis and F. Greenslet eds., *The Practical Cogitator.* Boston, Houghton Mifflin, 1953, 40.
3. S. Warrenberg and R. Pagano. Meditation and hemispheric specialization: Absorbed attention in long-term adherents. *Imagination, Cognition and Personality* 1982; 2:211–229.
4. R. Pagano and S. Warrenburg. Meditation: In search of a unique effect. In *Consciousness and Self Regulation*, vol. 3, eds. R. Davidson, G. Schwarz, and D. Shapiro. New York, Plenum Press, 1983, 153–205.
5. J. Smith. Personality correlates of continuation and outcome in meditation and erect sitting control treatments. *Journal of Consulting and Clinical Psychology* 1978; 46:272–279.
6. J. Kagan. The shy and the sociable. *Harvard Medical Alumni Bulletin* 1990–91; 21–23.
7. D. Davies, G. Hockey, and A. Taylor. Varied auditory stimulation, temperament differences and vigilance performance. *British Journal of Psychology* 1969; 60:453–457.
8. K. Thatcher, W. Wiederholt, and R. Fischer. An electroencephalographic analysis of personality-dependent performance under psilocybin. *Agents and Actions* 1971; 2:21–26.
9. H. Barr and R. Langs. *LSD: Personality and Experience.* New York, Wiley-Interscience, 1972.
10. A. Greeley. *The Sociology of the Paranormal. A Reconnaissance*, Sage Research Paper, vol. 3. Series 90-023, Beverly Hills, Calif.
11. E. Maupin. Individual differences in response to a Zen meditation exercise. *Journal of Consulting and Clinical Psychology* 1965; 29:139–145.
12. D. Brown and J. Engler. A Rorschach study of the states of mindfulness meditation. In *Meditation: Classic and Contemporary Perspectives*, eds. D. Shapiro and R. Walsh. New York, Aldine, 1984, 232–262.
13. *Ibid.*, 255.
14. J. Hart. Beyond psychotherapy—A programmatic essay on the applied psychology of the future. In *Biofeedback and Self-Control*, eds. T. Barber, L. DiCara, J. Kamiya, et al. Chicago, Aldine-Atherton, 1970, 43–75.
15. H. Hunt. A cognitive psychology of mystical and altered-state experience. *Perceptual and Motor Skills* 1984; 58:467–513.

16. C. Jung. *Modern Man in Search of a Soul.* New York, Harcourt, Brace & World, 1955, 264.
17. C. Jung. *Memories, Dreams, Reflections,* ed. A. Jaffe. New York, Pantheon, 1962, 196–197.
18. *Ibid.,* 395–396.
19. Jung, *Psychology and Religion,* 507.
20. P. Hartocollis. Aggression and mysticism. *Menninger Perspective* 1976–77 (winter); 4–12.
21. E. Shimano and R. Douglas. On research in Zen. *American Journal of Psychiatry* 1975; 132:1300–1302.
22. A. Maslow. Theory Z. *Journal of Transpersonal Psychology* 1969; 1:31–47.

Chapter 30   Sesshin and Teisho at Ryoko-in, 1974

1. N. Kobori. A dialogue. A discussion between One and Zero. *The Eastern Buddhist* 1957; 8:43–49.

Chapter 31   Sesshin

1. J. Sasaki. *Buddha is the Center of Gravity.* San Cristobal, N.M., Lama Foundation, 1974, 65.
2. R. Thayer. *The Biopsychology of Mood and Arousal.* New York, Oxford University Press, 1989.
3. Orthodox Zen in Japan tends to discourage contrived vocalizations. Various vocal automatisms occur in Gilles de la Tourette syndrome, a condition sometimes associated with heightened dopamine receptor activity.
4. N. Zinberg. The study of consciousness states. In *Alternate States of Consciousness,* ed. N. Zinberg. New York, Free Press, 1977, 1–36.

Chapter 32   The Meditative Approach to the Dissolution of the Self

1. I. Schloegl. *The Zen Way.* London, Sheldon Press, 1977.
2. N. Maclean. *A River Runs Through It.* Chicago, University of Chicago Press, 1976, 61.
3. M. Washburn. Observations relevant to a unified theory of meditation. *Journal of Transpersonal Psychology* 1978; 10:45–65.
4. W. James. *The Varieties of Religious Experience.* New York, Mentor/New American, 1958.
5. J. Engler. Therapeutic aims in psychotherapy and meditation: Developmental stages in the representation of the self. *Journal of Transpersonal Psychology* 1984; 16:25–61.
6. Words have their uses. *Accepting, altruistic, aware,* and *actualizing* remind us that the awakened I has positive connotations. *Buoyant* and *beatified* emphasize that the *Me,* too, can be acted upon for the better. The *Mine,* as well, can learn not only to *concede* its grip but to mutate its impulses so far beyond those of common charity that they approach uncommon *compassion* (see chapter 150).

Chapter 33   Brain In Overview: The Large of It

1. W. Hess. *The Biology of the Mind.* Chicago, University of Chicago Press, 1964.

Chapter 34   Brain in Overview: The Small of It

1. W. Waters and D. Wright. Maintenance and habituation of the phasic orienting response to competing stimuli in selective attention. In *The Orienting Reflex in Humans,* eds. H. Kimmel, E. Van Olst, and J. Orlebeke. Hillsdale, N.J., Erlbaum, 1979, 101–121.
2. N. Osborne. Communication between neurones: Current concepts. *Neurochemistry International* 1981; 3:3–16.
3. D. Calne. Neurotransmitters, neuromodulators, and neurohormones. *Neurology* 1979; 29:1517–1521.
4. G. Siggins and F. Bloom. Modulation of unit activity by chemically coded neurons. In *Brain Mechanisms and Perceptual Awareness,* eds. O. Pompeiano and C. Ajmone-Marsan. New York, Raven Press, 1981, 431–448.
5. Some chemical substances act in more than one way. Biogenic amines such as dopamine act mostly as neuromodulators, sometimes as neurotransmitters. Neuropeptides sometimes act as neuromodulators, at other times as neurohormones.

6.   M. Herkenham and S. McLean. Mismatches between receptor and transmitter localization in the brain. In *Quantitative Receptor Autoradiography,* eds. C. Boast, E. Snowhill, and C. Alter. New York, Liss, 1986, 137–171. Specific receptors are distributed in patterns which do not necessarily correlate well with levels of their own messenger molecules. This fact invites much caution in trying to make final interpretations of brain function when only anatomical patterns, or chemical levels, are available.

7.   S. Foote and J. Morrison. Extrathalamic modulation of cortical function. *Annual Review of Neuroscience* 1987; 10:67–95.

8.   What else can one say in this book about glia, the countless other cells which help support and nourish the nerve cells? Only that they are the bodhisattvas of the brain, essential to the outcome but remaining low in profile.

Chapter 35   Brain in Overview: Coordinated Networks Synthesizing Higher Functions

1.   W. Brain. *Clinical Neurology,* 2nd ed. London, Oxford University Press 1964, 365.

2.   H. Leiner, A. Leiner, and R. Dow. The human cerebro-cerebellar system: Its computing, cognitive, and language skills. *Behavioral Brain Research* 1991; 44:113–128.

3.   M. Mesulam. Large-scale neurocognitive networks and distributed processing for attention, language, and memory. *Annals of Neurology* 1990; 28:597–613.

Chapter 36   The Orienting Reflex and Activation

1.   J. Burroughs. *A Sharp Lookout. Selected Nature Essays of John Burroughs,* ed. F. Bergon. Washington, D.C., Smithsonian Institution Press, 1987.

2.   H. Kimmel, E. VanOlst, and J. Orlebeke, eds. *The Orienting Reflex in Humans.* Hillsdale, N.J., Erlbaum, 1979.

3.   H. Kimmel. Prologue. What is the orienting reflex? In *The Orienting Reflex in Humans,* eds. H. Kimmel, E. VanOlst, and J. Orlebeke. Hillside, N.J., Erlbaum, xi–xiv.

4.   K. Pribram and D. McGuinness. Arousal, activation, and effort in the control of attention. *Psychological Review* 1975; 82:116–149.

5.   C. Vanderwolf. The electrocorticogram in relation to physiology and behavior: A new analysis. *Electroencephalography and Clinical Neurophysiology* 1992; 82:165–175.

6.   J. Lacey. Somatic response patterning and stress: Some revisions of activation theory. In *Psychological Stress,* eds. M. Appley and R. Trumbull. New York, Appleton-Century-Crofts, 1967, 14–42.

7.   D. Wolgin. Motivation, activation, and behavioral integration. In *The Expression of Knowledge,* eds. R. Isaacson and N. Spear. New York, Plenum Press, 1982, 243–290.

Chapter 37   Arousal Pathways in the Reticular Formation and Beyond

1.   G. Moruzzi and H. Magoun. Brainstem reticular formation and activation of the EEG. *Electroencephalography and Clinical Neurophysiology* 1949; 1:455–473.

2.   M. Scheibel and A. Scheibel. Anatomical basis of attention mechanisms in vertebrate brains. In *The Neurosciences. A Study Program,* eds. G. Quarton, T. Melnechuk, and F. Schmitt. New York, Rockefeller University Press, 1967, 577–602.

3.   G. Alema, L. Perria, G. Rosadini, et al. Functional inactivation of the human brain stem related to the level of consciousness. *Journal of Neurosurgery* 1966; 24:629–639. The barbiturate was injected into the vertebral artery.

4.   R. Naquet, M. Denavit, and D. Albe-Fessard. Comparaison entre le rôle du subthalamus et celui des differentes structures bulbomésencéphaliques dans le maintien de la vigilance. *Electroencephalography and Clinical Neurophysiology* 1966; 20:149–164.

5.   R. Vertes. An analysis of ascending brainstem systems involved in hippocampal synchronization and desynchronization. *Journal of Neurophysiology* 1981; 46:1140–1159.

6.   J. Schlag and F. Chaillet. Thalamic mechanisms involved in cortical desynchronization and recruiting responses. *Electroencephalography and Clinical Neurophysiology* 1963; 15:39–62.

7. P. Dean, M. Simkins, I. Hetherington, et al. Tectal induction of cortical arousal: Evidence implicating multiple output pathways. *Brain Research Bulletin* 1991; 26:1–10.

8. J. Skinner and C. Yingling. Central gating mechanisms that regulate event-related potentials and behavior. In *Progress in Clinical Neurophysiology*. Vol. 1, *Attention, Voluntary Contraction and Event-Related Cerebral Potentials*, ed. J. Desmedt. Basel, Karger, 1977, 30–69.

9. F. Gonzalez-Lima and H. Scheich. Ascending reticular activating system in the rat: A 2-deoxyglucose study. *Brain Research* 1985; 344:70–88. The several nuclei activated are distributed along an extensive dorsal (upper) pathway which relies on acetylcholine to transmit its nerve impulses. The several nuclei inhibited tend to be supplied by a second category of acetylcholine fibers. These fibers run in the ventral (lower) cholinergic pathway. Presumably, as the reticular nucleus of the thalamus enters in, it would help inhibit the metabolism of other regions.

10. B. Angrist. Clinical effects of central nervous system stimulants: A selective update. In *Brain Reward Systems and Abuse*, eds. J. Engel and L. Oreland. New York, Raven Press, 1987, 109–127.

11. H. Jasper. Unspecific thalamocortical relations. In *Handbook of Physiology*. Sec. 1, *Neurophysiology*, vol. 2, ed. J. Field, Washington, D.C., American Physiological Society, 1960, 1307–1321.

12. M. Steriade. Mechanisms underlying cortical activation: Neuronal organization and properties of midbrain reticular core and intralaminar thalamic nuclei. In *Brain Mechanisms and Perceptual Awareness*, eds. O. Pompeiano and C. Ajmone-Marsan. New York, Raven Press, 1981, 327–377.

13. A. Kitsikis and M. Steriade. Immediate behavioral effects of kainic acid injections into the midbrain reticular core. *Behavioural Brain Research* 1981; 3:361–380. Kainate (kainic acid) is a potent excitatory analog of glutamate, the excitatory amino acid transmitter.

14. H. Santibanez. Specific and unspecific activation of the brain. Drives and antidrives. In *Psychophysiology: Memory, Motivation, and Event-Related Potentials*, eds. R. Sinz and M. Rosenzweig. Jena, Germany, Fischer, 1983, 231–236.

15. W. Winters, K. Mori, M. Wallach, et al. Reticular multiple unit activity during a progression of states induced by CNS excitants III. *Electroencephalography and Clinical Neurophysiology* 1969; 27:5; 514–522.

16. J. Candy and B. Key. A presynaptic site of action within the mesencephalic reticular formation for (+) amphetamine-induced electrocortical desynchronization. *British Journal of Pharmacology*, 1977; 61:331–338.

17. K. Shellenberger and J. Gordon. Regional role of catecholamines in alpha methyl-*m*-tyrosine–induced electroencephalographic arousal. *Experimental Neurology* 1975; 49:370–385.

18. D. Brooks and M. Gershon. Amine repletion in the reserpinized cat: Effect upon PGO waves and REM sleep. *Electroencephalography and Clinical Neurophysiology* 1977; 42:35–47. Some of the exaggerated response to levodopa reflects the fact that reserpine has also lowered serotonin levels.

19. J. Villablanca. Independent forebrain and brainstem controls for arousal and sleep. *Behavioral and Brain Sciences* 1981; 4:494–514. To help keep such disquieting findings in perspective, it is useful to reflect on one fact: the striking progress we take for granted which has helped critically ill patients survive is the result of pioneering research in animals.

20. J. Nielson and G. Thompson. *The Engrammes of Psychiatry*. Springfield, Ill., Thomas, 1947.

21. S. Feldman and H. Waller. Dissociation of electrocortical activation and behavioral arousal. Nature 1962; 196:1320–1322.

22. M. Demetrescu, M. Demetrescu, and F. Iosi. The tonic control of cortical responsiveness by inhibitory and facilitatory diffuse influences. *Electroencephalography and Clinical Neurophysiology* 1965; 18:1–24.

23. M. Denayer, M. Sallanon, C. Buda, et al. Neurotoxic lesion of the mesencephalic reticular formation and/or the posterior hypothalamus does not alter waking in the cat. *Brain*

Research 1991; 539:287–303. Cats may not depend as much as we humans do on being activated from higher anatomical levels in order to remain awake and functioning.

24. H. Matsumoto, Y. Morita, H. Seno, et al. Arousal mechanism from sleep in cats II: A brain electro-stimulation study. *Japanese Journal of Psychiatry and Neurology* 1986; 40:243–244.

25. J. Wright and G. Ihaka. A preliminary mathematical model for lateral hypothalamic regulation of electrocortical activity. *Electroencephalography and Clinical Neurophysiology* 1981; 52:107–115.

26. C. Saper. Diffuse cortical projection systems: Anatomical organization and role in cortical function. In *Handbook of Physiology.* Sec. 1, *The Nervous System,* vol. 5, *Higher Functions of the Brain,* pt. 1, eds. V. Mountcastle and F. Plum. Bethesda, Md., American Physiological Society, 1987, 169–210. The anterior cells in the lateral hypothalamus use GABA, and are probably inhibitory.

27. J. Wright and M. Craggs. Arousal and intracranial self-stimulation in split-brain monkeys. *Experimental Neurology* 1977; 55:295–303.

28. R. Hassler, G. Ore, G. Dieckmann, et al. Behavioral and EEG arousal induced by stimulation of unspecific projection systems in a patient with post-traumatic apallic syndrome. *Electroencephalography and Clinical Neurophysiology* 1969; 27:3;306–310.

29. T. Tsubokawa, T. Yamamoto, Y. Katayama, et al. Deep brain stimulation in a persistent vegetative state: Follow-up results and criteria for selection of candidates. *Brain Injury* 1990; 4:315–327. The ventral anterior and intralaminar nuclei are both nonspecific thalamic nuclei which exert their influences diffusely.

30. J. Segundo, R. Naquet, and P. Buser. Effects of cortical stimulation on electrocortical activity in monkeys. *Journal of Neurophysiology* 1955; 18:236–245.

31. K. Chow and W. Randall (1964): Learning and retention in cats with lesions in reticular formation. *Psychonomic Science* 1964; 1:259–260.

32. K. Pribram and D. McGuinness. Arousal, activation, and effort in the control of attention. *Psychological Review* 1975; 82:2:116–149.

Chapter 38   Acetylcholine Systems

1. A. Karczmar. Exploitable aspects of central cholinergic functions, particularly with respect to the EEG, motor, analgesic and mental functions. In *Cholinergic Mechanisms and Psychopharmacology,* ed. D. Jendon. New York, Plenum Press, 1978, 679–708.

2. N. Woolf, J. Harrison, and J. Buchwald. Cholinergic neurons of the feline pontomesencephalon. II. Ascending anatomical projections. *Brain Research* 1990; 520:55–72.

3. S. Vincent, K. Satoh, D. Armstrong, et al. Neuropeptides and NADPH diaphorase activity in the ascending cholinergic reticular system of the rat. *Neuroscience* 1986; 17:167–182.

4. P. McGeer, H. Kimura, E. McGeer, et al. Cholinergic systems in the CNS. In *Neurotransmitter Interaction and Compartmentation,* ed. H. Bradford. New York, Plenum Press, 1982, 253–289.

5. M. -M. Mesulam, E. Mufson, A. Levey, et al. Cholinergic innervation of cortex by the basal forebrain: Cytochemistry and cortical connections of the septal area, diagonal band nuclei, nucleus basalis (substantia innominata), and hypothalamus in the rhesus monkey. *Journal of Comparative Neurology* 1983; 214:170–197.

6. N. Wolf and L. Butcher. Cholinergic systems in the rat brain: III. Projections from the pontomesencephalic tegmentum to the thalamus, tectum, basal ganglia, and basal forebrain. *Brain Research Bulletin* 1986; 16:603–617.

7. The dorsal lateral tegmental acetycholine cells are designated CH 6, where CH stands for cholinergic; the pedunculopontine tegmental ACH cells are designated CH 5. CH 8 nerve cells of the parabigeminal nucleus supply most of the ACH to the superior colliculus. See M. Steriade, D. Paré, A. Parent, et al. Projections of cholinergic and non-cholinergic neurons of the brainstem core to relay and associational thalamic nuclei in the cat and macaque monkey. *Neuroscience* 1988; 25:47–67; M. Steriade, P. Gloor, R. Llinas, et al. Basic mechanisms of cerebral rhythmic activities. *Electroencephalography and Clinical Neurophysiology* 1990; 76:481–508.

8. M. Steriade, D. Paré, S. Datta, et al. Different cellular types in the mesopontine cholinergic nuclei related to ponto-geniculo-occipital waves. *Journal of Neuroscience* 1990; 10:2560–2579.

9. K. Semba, P. Reiner, and H. Fibiger. Single cholinergic mesopontine tegmental neurons project to both the pontine reticular formation and the thalamus in the rat. *Neuroscience* 1990; 38:643–654.

10. M. Steriade, P. Curro-Dossi, D. Paré, et al. Fast oscillations (20–40 Hz) in thalamocortical systems and their potentiation by mesopontine cholinergic nuclei in the cat. *Proceedings of the National Academy of Sciences of the United States of America* 1991; 88:4396–4400.

11. S. Datta, R. Curro-Dossi, D. Paré, et al. Substantia nigra reticulata neurons during sleep-waking states: Relation with ponto-geniculo-occipital waves. *Brain Research* 1991; 566:344–347.

12. M. Fodor, T. Görcs, and S. Palkovits. Immunohistochemical study on the distribution of neuropeptides within the pontine tegmentum—Particularly the parabrachial nuclei and the locus coeruleus of the human brain. *Neuroscience* 1992; 46:891–908. The human parabrachial nucleus shows no evidence of substance P.

13. V. Dawson, T. Dawson, E. London, et al. Nitric oxide mediates glutamate neurotoxicity in primary cortical cultures. *Proceedings of the National Academy of Sciences of the United States of America* 1991; 88:6368–6371.

14. B. Hope, G. Micheal, K. Knigge, et al. Neuronal NADPH diaphorase is a nitric oxide synthase. *Proceedings of the National Academy of Sciences of the United States of America* 1991; 88:2811–2814.

15. In some animal species, a third of the acetylcholine nerve cells in the dorsolateral pons may also contain the excitatory peptide, substance P. See S. Vincent, K. Satoh, D. Armstrong, et al. Substance P in the ascending cholinergic reticular system. *Nature* 1983; 306:688–691.

16. M. Steriade, K. Sakai, and M. Jouvet. Bulbo-thalamic neurons related to thalamo-cortical activation processes during paradoxical sleep. *Experimental Brain Research* 1984; 54:463–475.

17. V. Bigl, H. Wenk, U. Meyer, H. -J. Luth. Cholinergic mechanisms in the visual system of rat. In *The Cholinergic Synapse,* ed. S. Tucek. Progress in Brain Research, vol. 49. Amsterdam, Elsevier, 472.

18. K. Sakai. Anatomical and physiological basis of paradoxical sleep. In *Brain Mechanisms of Sleep,* eds. D. McGinty, R. Drucker-Colin, A. Morrison, et al. New York, Raven Press, 1985, 111–137.

19. N. Woolf and I. Butcher. The cholinergic basal forebrain as a cognitive machine. In *Activation to Acquisition. Functional Aspects of the Basal Forebrain Cholinergic System,* ed. F. Richardson, Boston, Birkhäuser, 1991, 347–380.

20. N. Ulfig, E. Braak, T. Ohm, et al. Vasopressinergic neurons in the magnocellular nuclei of the human basal forebrain. *Brain Research* 1990; 530:176–180.

21. L. Detari and C. Vanderwolf. Activity of identified cortically projecting and other basal forebrain neurons during large slow waves and cortical activation in anaesthetized rats. *Brain Research* 1987; 437:1–8.

22. G. Buzsaki, R. Bickford, G. Ponomareff, et al. Nucleus basalis and thalamic control of neocortical activity in the freely moving rat. *Journal of Neuroscience* 1988; 8:4007–4026.

23. M. Herkenham and W. Nauta. Efferent connections of the habenular nuclei in the rat. *Journal of Comparative Neurology* 1979; 187:19–48.

24. R. Wang and G. Aghajanian. Physiological evidence for habenula as a major link between forebrain and midbrain raphe. *Science* 1977; 197:89–91.

25. O. Phillipson and C. Pycock. Dopamine neurons of the ventral tegmentum project to both medial and lateral habenula. *Experimental Brain Research* 1982; 45:89–94.

26. S. Cohen and R. Melzack. Habenular stimulation produces analgesia in the formalin test. *Neuroscience Letters* 1986; 70:165–169. The nucleus has high levels of β-endorphin, as does the interpeduncular nucleus which it projects to. Even though the habenular nucleus,

when stimulated, does reduce the responses to chronic pain, it does so by mechanisms which do not appear to involve opioids.

27. D. Brown. Slow cholinergic excitation—A mechanism for increasing neuronal excitability. *Trends in Neurosciences* 1983; 6:302–307. Acetylcholine does more than activate muscarinic excitatory functions. It inhibits GABA nerve cells which had been holding them in check. This permits the next, postsynaptic cell, now disinhibited, to respond longer when glutamate stimulates it.

28. Other ACH actions are more complex. When ACH acts on those of its muscarinic receptors which cover presynaptic terminals, they shut down the amount of DA, NE, and ST released from these terminals. (See F. Hery. Control of the release of newly synthesized ^{3}H-5-hydroxytryptamine by nicotinic and muscarinic receptors in rat hypothalamic slices. *Archives of Pharmacology* 1977; 296:91–97.) In contrast, DA and NE tend to suppress the excitatory actions of ACH in cortex. (See T. Reader and H. Jasper. Interactions between monoamines and other transmitters in cerebral cortex. In *Monoamine Innervation of Cerebral Cortex*. eds. L. Descarries, T. Reader, and H. Jasper. New York, Liss, 1984, 195–225.)

29. R. Dossi, D. Pare, and M. Steriade. Short-lasting nicotinic and long-lasting muscarinic depolarizing responses of thalamocortical neurons to stimulation of mesopontine cholinergic nuclei. *Journal of Neurophysiology* 1991; 65:393–406. Another drug, prostigmine, also increases beta EEG activity. It increases the effective levels of ACH molecules at the synapse by preventing their breakdown.

30. Y. Stern, L. Millen, and S. Fahn. Long-term effects of high-dose anticholinergic medications. *Neurology* 1988; 38(suppl. 1):248.

31. D. Warburton. Neurochemical basis of consciousness. In *Chemical Influences on Behavior,* eds. K. Brown and S. Cooper. London, Academic Press, 1979, 421–462.

32. D. Weiner, A. Levey, and M. Brann. Expression of muscarinic acetylcholine and dopamine receptor mRNAs in rat basal ganglia. *Proceedings of the National Academy of Sciences of the United States of America* 1990; 87:7050–7054. Muscarinic receptors are designated *M*.

33. D. Paré and M. Steriade. Control of the mammillothalamic axis by brainstem cholinergic laterodorsal tegmental afferents: Possible involvement in mnemonic processes. In *Brain Cholinergic Systems,* eds. M. Steriade and D. Biesold. New York, Oxford University Press, 1990, 337–354.

34. J. Hemmingfield, E. London, and J. Jaffe. Nicotine reward: Studies of abuse liability and physical dependence potential. In *Brain Reward Systems,* eds. J. Engel and L. Oreland. New York, Raven Press, 1987, 147–164.

35. D. McGehee, M. Heath, S. Gelber, et al. Nicotine enhancement of fast excitatory synaptic transmission in CNS by presynaptic receptors. *Science* 1995; 269:1692–1696. This enhancement occurs in the interpeduncular nucleus.

Chapter 39   The Septum and Pleasure

1. R. Heath. Pleasure response of human subjects to direct stimulation of the brain: Physiologic and psychodynamic considerations. In *The Role of Pleasure in Behavior,* ed. R. Heath. New York, Harper & Row, 1964, 219–243. The term "septal region" is used advisedly. Contemporary research requires a much more precise anatomical proof of which site was stimulated than was provided by these early reports.

2. S. Iversen. Cortical monoamines and behavior. In *Monoamine Innervation of Cerebral Cortex,* eds. L. Descarries, T. Reader, and H. Jasper. New York, Liss, 1984, 321–349.

3. P. MacLean. Brain evolution relating to family, play, and the separation call. *Archives of General Psychiatry* 1985; 42:405–417.

4. Problems defining the elastic limits of limbic structures have led one experienced neuroanatomist to conclude that "the use of the terms 'limbic lobe' and 'limbic system' should be abandoned." See A. Brodal. *Neurological Anatomy In Relation to Clinical Medicine,* 3rd ed. New York, Oxford University Press, 1981, 690.

5. In technical language the septal region lies between the frontal horns of the lateral ventricles and in front of the anterior commissure. The term "ventral striatum" is used in-

creasingly to distinguish its nucleus accumbens from the other closely related *motor* functions of the dorsal striatum. See L. Heimer, R. Switzer, and G. VanHoesen. Ventral striatum and ventral pallidum. Components of the motor system? *Trends in Neurosciences* 1981; 5:83–87.

6. A. Brodal. *Neurological Anatomy in Relation to Clinical Medicine,* 3rd ed. New York, Oxford University Press, 1981, 663–667.

7. F. Moroni, D. Malthe-Sorenssen, D. Cheney, et al. Modulation of ACH turnover in the septal-hippocampal pathway by electrical stimulation and lesioning. *Brain Research* 1978; 150:333–341.

8. J. Delgado. Free behavior and brain stimulation. *International Review of Neurobiology* 1964; 6:349–449.

9. Heath, *op. cit.,* 224.

10. H. King. Psychological effects of excitation in the limbic system. In *Electrical Stimulation of the Brain,* ed. D. Sheer. Austin, University of Texas Press, 1961, 477–486.

11. R. Heath. Pleasure and brain activity in man. Deep and surface electroencephalograms during orgasm. *Journal of Nervous and Mental Disease* 1972; 154:3–18. Human subjects' committees nowadays would not approve such research.

12. G. Remillard, F. Andermann, G. Testa, et al. Sexual ictal manifestations predominate in women with temporal lobe epilepsy: A finding suggesting sexual dimorphism in the human brain. *Neurology* 1983; 33:323–330.

Chapter 40   The Attachments of the Cingulate Gyrus

1. D. Pandya, G. VanHoesen, and V. Domesick. A cingulo-amygdaloid projection in the rhesus monkey. *Brain Research* 1973; 61:369–373.

2. L. Laitinen. Emotional responses to subcortical electrical stimulation in psychiatric patients. *Clinical Neurology and Neurosurgery* 1979; 81:148–157.

3. H. Ballantine, A. Bouckoms, E. Thomas, et al. Treatment of psychiatric illness by sterotactic cingulotomy. *Biological Psychiatry* 1987; 22:7; 807–819.

4. R. Gariano and P. Groves. Burst firing induced in midbrain dopamine neurons by stimulation of the medial prefrontal and anterior cingulate cortices. *Brain Research* 1988; 462:194–198.

5. R. Cohen, V. MacCrae, K. Phillips, et al. Neurobehavioral consequences of bilateral medial cingulotomy. *Neurology* 1990; 40(suppl. 1):171.

6. C. Porro and G. Carli. Immobilization and restraint effects on pain reactions in animals. *Pain* 1988; 32:289–307. The monkey's higher-level vocalizations are called "learned cooing."

7. V. Balasubramaniam, T. Kanaka, and P. Ramanujam. Sterotaxic cingulumotomy for drug addiction. *Neurology (India)* 1973; 21:63–66. The volume of each lesion is about the same as that of a cube measuring eight or nine millimeters on each side.

8. T. Kanaka and V. Balasubramaniam. Sterotactic cingulumotomy for drug addiction. *Applied Neurophysiology* 1978; 41:86–92.

9. S. Kwon, S. Nadeau, and K. Heilman. Retrosplenial cortex: Possible role in habituation of the orienting response. *Journal of Neuroscience* 1990; 10:3559–3563.

10. J. Olney, J. Labruyere, and M. Price. Pathological changes induced in cerebrocortical neurons by phencyclidine and related drugs. *Science* 1989; 244:1360–1362.

11. K. Daffner, G. Ahern, S. Weintraub, et al. Dissociated neglect behavior following sequential strokes in the right hemisphere. *Annals of Neurology* 1990; 28:97–101.

12. G. Cadoret and A. Smith. Input-output properties of hand-related cells in the ventral cingulate cortex in the monkey. *Journal of Neurophysiology* 1995; 73:2584–2590.

13. C. Kitt, S. Mitchell, M. DeLong, et al. Fiber pathways of basal forebrain cholinergic neurons in monkeys. *Brain Research* 1987; 406:192–206.

14. The major pathway leading up to the anterior thalamic nucleus from hippocampal sites proceeds first to the hypothalamus. From there it ascends as the large mammillothalamic tract, also known as the bundle of Vicq d'Azyr (see figure 6). More research is necessary

to clarify its ordinary functions. We may then have a better idea of what this ascending path contributes to extraordinary states when it carries either more, or fewer, impulses than usual.

Chapter 41   The Amygdala and Fear

1. D. Thomas. *Oxford Dictionary of Quotations*, 3rd ed. Oxford, Oxford University Press, 1979.
2. King said this in the year he died. Chapters 136, 142 and 148 consider the striking experience of freedom that arrives when all fear vanishes.
3. J. DeOlmos. Amygdala. In *The Human Nervous System*, ed. G. Paxinos. San Diego, Academic Press, 1990; 583–710.
4. G. Roberts, P. Woodhams, J. Polack, et al. Distribution of neuropeptides in the limbic system of the rat: The amygdaloid complex. *Neuroscience* 1982; 7:99–131. Dopamine, norepinephrine, and serotonin terminals are also well represented in the amygdala.
5. M. Mesulam, L. Volicer, J. Marquis, et al. Systematic regional differences in the cholinergic innervation of the primate cerebral cortex. Distribution of the enzyme activities and some behavioral implications. *Annals of Neurology* 1986; 19:144–151. The so-called paralimbic regions, which have the highest levels of acetylcholine innervation, include the parahippocampal, insular, temporopolar, and caudal orbitofrontal regions, but not the cingulate gyrus.
6. R. Adamec. Individual differences in temporal lobe sensory processing of threatening stimuli in the cat. *Physiology and Behavior* 1991; 49:455–564.
7. J. Carlsen and L. Heimer. The basolateral amygdaloid complex as a cortical-like structure. *Brain Research* 1988; 441:377–380.
8. S. Iversen. Recent advances in the anatomy and chemistry of the limbic system. In *Psychopharmacology of the Limbic System*, eds. M. Trimble and E. Zarifian. Oxford, Oxford University Press, 1984, 1–16.
9. T. Robinson and P. Beart. Excitant amino acid projections from rat amygdala and thalamus to nucleus accumbens. *Brain Research Bulletin* 1988; 20:467–471.
10. J. Herbert. Behavior and the limbic system with particular reference to sexual and aggressive interactions. In *Psychopharmacology of the Limbic System*, eds. M. Trimble and M. Zarifian. Oxford, Oxford University Press, 1984, 51–67.
11. L. Dunn and B. Everitt. Double dissociations of the effects of amygdala and insular cortex lesions on conditioned taste aversion, passive avoidance and neophobia in the rat using the excitotoxin ibotenic acid. *Behavioral Neuroscience* 1988; 102:3–23.
12. J. Koolhaas. The corticomedial amygdala and the behavioral change due to defeat. In *Modulation of Sensorimotor Activity During Alterations in Behavioral States*, ed. R. Bandler. New York, Liss, 1984, 341–349.
13. R. Kesner, R. Walser, and G. Winzenried. Central but not basolateral amygdala mediates memory for positive affective experiences. *Behavioral Brain Research* 1989; 33:189–195.
14. T. Gray, M. Carney, and D. Magnuson. Direct projections from the central amygdaloid nucleus to the hypo-thalamic paraventricular nucleus: Possible role in stress-induced adrenocorticotropin release. *Neuroendocrinology* 1989; 50:433–446.
15. L. Cahill and J. McGaugh. Amygdaloid complex lesions differentially affect retention of tasks using appetitive and aversive reinforcement. *Behavioral Neuroscience* 1990; 104:532–543.
16. J. LeDoux, P. Cicchetti, A. Xagoraris, et al. The lateral amygdaloid nucleus: Sensory interface of the amygdala. *Journal of Neuroscience* 1990; 10:1062–1069.
17. J. LeDoux, A. Sakaguchi, and D. Reis. Subcortical efferent projections of the medial (geniculate) nucleus mediate emotional responses conditioned to acoustic stimuli. *Journal of Neuroscience* 1984; 4:683–698.
18. J. LeDoux and C. Farb. Neurons of the acoustic thalamus that project to the amygdala contain glutamate. *Neuroscience Letters* 1991; 134:145–149. The limbic system quickly broadcasts its messages to the upper brainstem, only a few synapses away, without having to

consult "higher-level" connections. Its three major pathways to the midbrain are the medial forebrain bundle, the stria medullaris, and the mammillotegmental tract.[8]

19. J. Hitchcock and M. Davis. Lesions of the amygdala, but not of the cerebellum or red nucleus, block conditioned fear as measured with the potentiated startle paradigm. *Behavioral Neuroscience* 1986; 100:11–22. Antianxiety drugs in the benzodiazepine group act by enhancing the activity of GABA receptors.

20. H. Nishijo, T. Ono, and H. Nishino. Topographic distribution of modality-specific amygdalar neurons in alert monkey. *Journal of Neuroscience* 1988; 8:3556–3569.

21. J. Zhang, R. Harper, and H. Ni. Cryogenic blockade of the central nucleus of the amygdala attenuates aversively conditioned blood pressure and respiratory, responses. *Brain Research* 1986; 386:136–145. The nucleus is inactivated by cooling it.

22. Adult animals can be conditioned into developing the "frozen-with-fear" response. When they do so, they use excitatory amino acids in the process. See J. Kim, J. DeCola, J. Landeira-Fernandez, et al. N-Methyl-D-aspartate receptor antagonist AVP blocks acquisition but not expression of fear conditioning. *Behavioral Neuroscience* 1991; 105:126–133.

23. M. Brutus, S. Zuabi, and A. Siegel. Effects of d-ala-metenkephalinamide microinjections placed into the bed nucleus of the stria terminalis upon affective defense behavior in the cat. *Brain Research* 1988; 473:147–152.

24. M. Shaikh, C. Lu, and A. Siegel. An enkephalinergic mechanism involved in amygdaloid suppression of affective defense behavior elicited from the midbrain periaqueductal gray in the cat. *Brain Research* 1991; 559:109–117.

25. J. Zhang, R. Harper, and R. Frysinger. Respiratory modulation of neuronal discharge in the central nucleus of the amygdala during sleep and waking states. *Experimental Neurology* 1986; 91:193–207.

26. J. Flynn, H. Vanegas, W. Foote, et al. Neural mechanisms involved in a cat's attack on a rat. In *The Neural Control of Behavior*, eds. R. Whalen, R. Thompson, M. Verzeano, et al. New York, Academic Press, 1970, 135–173. The aggressive attack is prompted by stimulating around the site where the fornix enters the hypothalamus.

27. H. Maeda and S. Maki. Dopaminergic facilitation of recovery from amygdaloid lesions which affect hypothalamic defensive attack in cats. *Brain Research* 1986; 363:135–140.

28. R. Doty. Some anatomical substrates of emotion and their bihemispheric coordination. In *Emotions and the Dual Brain. Experimental Brain Research Series 18*, eds. G. Gainotti and C. Caltagirone. Berlin, Springer-Verlag, 1989, 56–82.

29. J. Horel, E. Keating, and L. Misantone. Partial Klüver-Bucy syndrome produced by destroying temporal neocortex or amygdala. *Brain Research* 1975; 94:347–359.

30. M. Fukuda, T. Ono, and K. Nakamura. Functional relations among inferotemporal cortex, amygdala, and lateral hypothalamus in monkey operant feeding behavior. *Journal of Neurophysiology* 1987; 57:1060–1077.

31. E. Halgren, C. Wilson, N. Squires, et al. Dynamics of the hippocampal contribution to memory: Stimulation and recording studies in humans. In *Neurobiology of the Hippocampus*, ed. M. Siefert. New York, Academic Press, 1983, 529–572.

32. R. McLachlan and W. Blume. Isolated fear in complex partial status epilepticus. *Annals of Neurology* 1979; 8:639–641.

33. B. Eichelman. The limbic system and aggression in humans. *Neuroscience and Biobehavioral Reviews* 1983; 7:391–394.

34. Some evidence suggests that humans who have large lesions of the amygdala become calmer and more indifferent. Still, a major problem remains in evaluating the effect of amygdalectomy per se, because removal of the adjacent perirhinal cortex contributes to this behavioral change. See J. Aggleton. The functional effects of amygdala lesions in humans: A comparison with findings from monkeys. In *Amygdala. Neurobiological Aspects of Emotion, Memory, and Mental Dysfunction*, ed. J. Aggleton. New York, Wiley-Liss, 1992, 485–503.

35. D. Tranel and H. Damasio. Intact electrodermal skin conductance responses after bilateral amygdala damage. *Neuropsychologia* 1989; 27:381–390.

36. D. Tranel and B. Hyman. Neuropsychological correlates of bilateral amygdala damage. *Archives of Neurology* 1990; 47:349–355. We need many more multidisciplinary studies to sort out all the complex circuitries which generate human fear and aggression.

37. J. Stevens, V. Mark, F. Ervin, et al. Deep temporal stimulation in man. Long-latency, long-lasting psychological changes. *Archives of Neurology* 1969; 21:157–169. The long-latency, long-lasting psychological changes are intriguing. They raise the possibility that other mechanisms are associated, such as second messengers, long-term potentiation, etc.

38. A. McGregor and J. Herbert. Differential effects of excitotoxic basolateral and cortico-medial lesions of the amygdala on the behavioral and endocrine responses to either sexual or aggression-promoting stimuli in the male rat. *Brain Research* 1992; 574:9–20.

Chapter 42   Remembrances and the Hippocampus

1. G. VanHoesen. The parahippocampal gyrus. New observations regarding its cortical connections in the monkey. *Trends in Neurosciences* 1982; 5:345–350.

2. Each time these sites are referred to as CA1, CA2, CA3, and CA4, they continue to reflect this old cornu Ammonis terminology.

3. V. Braitenberg. Anatomical basis for divergence, convergence, and integration in the cerebral cortex. In *Sensory Functions*, eds. E. Grastyan and P. Molnar. Advances in Physiological Science, vol. 16. Pergamon, Budapest, 1981, 411–419.

4. D. Amaral and M. Campbell. Transmitter systems in the primate dentate gyrus. *Human Neurobiology* 1986; 5:169–180.

5. P. VandenHooff, I. Urban, and D. deWied. Vasopressin maintains long-term potentiation in rat lateral septum slices. *Brain Research* 1989; 505:181–186.

6. B. Gustafsson and H. Wigström. Physiological mechanisms underlying long-term potentiation. *Trends in Neurosciences* 1988; 11:156–162. Long-term potentiation was first studied in isolated blocks of hippocampal tissue.

7. C. Pavlides, Y. Greenstein, M. Grudman, et al. Long-term potentiation in the dentate gyrus is induced preferentially on the positive phase of θ-rhythm. *Brain Research* 1988; 439:383–387.

8. V. Staubli and G. Lynch. Stable hippocampal long-term potentiation elicited by "theta" pattern stimulation. *Brain Research* 1987; 435:227–234.

9. Potentiation in actively behaving animals is a complex matter. We need more multidisciplinary studies in primates to know how messages flow within this whole region and what all the implications are. See C. Bramham and B. Srebro. Synaptic plasticity in the hippocampus is modified by behavioral state. *Brain Research* 1989; 493:74–86; W. Abraham and G. Goddard. Asymmetric relationships between homosynaptic long-term potentiation and heterosynaptic long-term depression. *Nature* 1993; 305:717–179; V. Staubli and G. Lynch. Stable depression of potentiated synaptic responses in the hippocampus with 1–5 Hz stimulation. *Brain Research* 1990; 513:113–118.

10. T. Radil-Weiss. Evidence for a system inhibiting reticulo-septo-hippocampal activity. In *The Reticular Formation Revisited*, eds. J. Hobson and M. Brazier. International Brain Research Organization Monograph Series, vol 6. New York, Raven Press, 1980, 405–413.

11. J. Rawlins. Some neurophysiological properties of the septo-hippocampal system. In *Psychopharmacology of the Limbic System*, eds. M. Trimble and E. Zarifan. Oxford, Oxford University Press, 1984, 17–50.

12. C. Vanderwolf, L-W. Leung, and R. Cooley. Pathways through cingulate, neo-and entorhinal cortices mediate atropine-resistant hippocampal rhythmical slow activity. *Brain Research* 1985; 347:58–73.

13. O. Vinogradova, E. Brazhnik, V. Kitchigina, et al. Acetylcholine, theta-rhythm and activity of hippocampal neurons in the rabbit—IV. Sensory stimulation. *Neuroscience* 1993; 53:993–1007.

14. T. Robinson. Hippocampal rhythmic slow activity (RSA: theta): A critical analysis of selected studies and discussion of possible species-differences. *Brain Research. Brain Research Reviews* 1980; 2:69–101.

15. D. Arnolds, F. Lopes da Silva, J. Aitink, et al. The spectral properties of hippocampal EEG related to behavior in man. *Electroencephalography and Clinical Neurophysiology* 1980; 50:324–328.

16. K. Meador, M. Thompson, D. Loring, et al. Behavioral state-specific changes in human hippocampal theta activity. *Neurology* 1991; 41:869–872.

17. J. Arezzo, C. Tenke, and H. Vaughan. Movement-related potentials within the hippocampal formation of the monkey. *Brain Research* 1987; 401:79–86.

18. C. Olmstead and J. Villablanca. Hippocampal theta rhythm persists in the permanently isolated forebrain of the cat. *Brain Research Bulletin* 1977; 2:93–100.

19. H. Anchel and D. Lindsley. Differentiation of two reticulo-hypothalamic systems regulating hippocampal activity. *Electroencephalography and Clinical Neurophysiology* 1972; 32:209–226. The stimulation site is in the body of the midbrain, called the tegmentum.

20. A. Macader, L. Chalupa, and D. Lindsley. Differentiation of brainstem loci which affect hippocampal and neocortical electrical activity. *Experimental Neurology* 1974; 43:499–514.

21. R. Vertes. Brain stem generation of the hippocampal EEG. *Progress in Neurobiology* 1982; 19:159–186. Some of the effects of stimuli may arise from raphe cells other than those which release serotonin.

22. L. Leung. Fast (beta) rhythms in the hippocampus: A review. *Hippocampus* 1992; 2:93–98. In previous decades, it was the custom to refer to low voltage fast beta activity as being *de*synchronized. This term was used because it tended to replace the much more rhythmic-appearing, synchronized alpha or theta activity. More recently, it has been appreciated that fast activities at 40 cps can arise locally in many sites in the brain. Some of these are indeed too rhythmic to warrant the term "desynchronized." And others, as they become paroxysmal, can reach amplitudes rather too high to be called "low voltage."

23. E. Grastyán. The hippocampus and higher nervous activity. In *Transactions of the Second Conference on the Central Nervous System and Behavior*, ed. M. Brazier. New York, Josiah Macy Jr. Foundation, 1959, 119–205.

24. M. Steriade, N. Ropert, A. Kitsikis, et al. Ascending activating neuronal networks in midbrain reticular core and related rostral systems. In *The Reticular Formation Revisited, eds.* J. Hobson and M. Brazier. International Brain Research Organization Monograph Series, vol. 6. New York, Raven Press, 125–167.

25. R. Heath and D. Gallant. Activity of the human brain during emotional thought. In *The Role of Pleasure in Behavior*, ed. R. Heath. New York, Harper & Row, 1964, 83–106.

26. K. Huh, K. Meador, G. Lee, et al. Human Hippocampal EEG: Effects of behavioral activation. *Neurology* 1990; 40:1177–1181.

27. H. Wieser and G. Mazzola. Do the right and left hippocampi independently distinguish musical consonances and dissonances? *Electroencephalography and Clinical Neurophysiology* 1985; 61:S153. The barbershop comment is a personal note.

28. A. Mandell. Toward a psychobiology of transcendence: God in the brain. In *The Psychobiology of Consciousness*, eds. J. Davidson and R. Davidson. New York, Plenum Press, 1980, 379–464.

29. D. Amaral. Memory: Anatomical organization of candidate brain regions. In *Handbook of Physiology*, eds. V. Mountcastle and F. Plum. Sec. I, *The Nervous System*, vol. 5, pt. 1. Bethesda, Md., American Physiological Society. 1987, 211–294.

30. J. Eccles. Mechanisms of learning in complex systems. In *Handbook of Physiology*, eds. V. Mountcastle and F. Plum. Sec. 1, *The Nervous System*, vol. 5. pt. 1. Bethesda, Md., American Physiological Society, 1987, 137–167. Other less processed messages can peel off earlier, to be shunted up to the septal nuclei or over to the mammillary complex.

31. G. Lynch and M. Baudry. Structure-function relationships in the organization of memory. In *Perspectives in Memory Research*, ed. M. Gazzaniga. Cambridge, Mass., The MIT Press, 1988, 23–91.

32. D. Terrian, R. Gannon, and M. Rea. Glutamate is the endogenous amino acid selectively released by rat hippocampal mossy fiber synaptosomes concomitantly with prodynorphin-derived peptides. *Neurochemical Research* 1990; 15:1–5.

33. L. Stein and J. Belluzi. Cellular investigations of behavioral reinforcement. *Neuroscience and Biobehavioral Reviews* 1989; 13:69–80.

34. B. Derrick, S. Weinberger, and J. Martinez. Opioid receptors are involved in an NMDA receptor-independent mechanism of LTP induction at hippocampal mossy fiber-CA3 synapses. *Brain Research Bulletin* 1991; 27:219–223.

35. K. Stevens, G. Shiotsu, and L. Stein. Hippocampal μ-receptors mediate opioid reinforcement in the CA3 Region. *Brain Research* 1991; 545:8–16.

36. R. Gannon and D. Terrain. U-50, 488H inhibits dynorphin and glutamate from guinea pig hippocampal mossy fiber terminals. *Brain Research* 1991; 548:242–247.

37. E. Rolls. Theoretical and neurophysiological analysis of the functions of the primate hippocampus in memory. In *The Brain*. Cold Spring Harbor Symposia on Quantitative Biology, vol. 55. Plainview, N.Y., Cold Spring Harbor Laboratory Press, 1990, 995–1006.

38. S. Zola-Morgan, L. Squire, and G. Amaral. Human amnesia and the medial temporal region: Enduring memory impairment following a bilateral lesion limited to field CA1 of the hippocampus. *Journal of Neuroscience*, 1986; 6:2950–2967.

39. E. Bertram, E. Lothman, and N. Lenn. The hippocampus in experimental chronic epilepsy: A morphometric analysis. *Annals of Neurology* 1990; 27:43–48.

40. K. Krnjevic. Acetylcholine as modulator of amino-acid–mediated synaptic transmission. In *The Role of Peptides and Amino Acids as Neurotransmitters*, eds. J. Lombardini and A. Kenny. New York, Liss, 1981, 127–141.

41. J. Halliwell and P. Adams. Voltage-clamp analysis of muscarinic excitation in hippocampal neurons. *Brain Research* 1982; 250:71–92.

42. C. Bramham, M. Errington, and T. Bliss. Naloxone blocks the induction of long-term potentiation in the lateral but not the medial perforant pathway in the anaesthetized rat. *Brain Research* 1988; 449:352–356.

43. J. Neumaier and C. Chavkin. Release of endogenous opioid peptides displaces [³H] diprenorphine binding in rat hippocampal slices. *Brain Research* 1989; 493:292–302.

44. B. Gähwiler. The action of neuropeptides on the bioelectric activity of hippocampal neurons. In *Neurobiology of the Hippocampus*, ed. W. Seifert. New York, Academic Press, 1983, 157–173.

45. M. Segal. The noradrenergic innervation of the hippocampus. In *The Reticular Formation Revisited*, eds. J. Hobson and M. Brazier. International Brain Research Organization Monograph Series, vol. 6. New York, Raven Press, 1980, 415–425.

46. R. Nicoll, D. Madison, and B. Lancaster. Noradrenergic modulation of neuronal excitability in mammalian hippocampus. In *Psychopharmacology: The Third Generation of Progress*, ed. H. Meltzer. New York, Raven Press, 1987, 105–112.

47. J. Palacios, D. Hoyer, and R. Cortes. α_1-Adrenoceptors in the mammalian brain: Similar pharmacology but different distribution in rodents and primates. *Brain Research* 419:65–75.

48. T. Dunwiddie, M. Taylor, L. Heginbotham, et al. Long-term increases in excitability in the CA1 region of rat hippocampus induced by β-adrenergic stimulation: Possible mediation by cAMP. *Journal of Neuroscience* 12:506–517.

49. S. Brunel and C. deMontigny. Diurnal rhythms in the responsiveness of hippocampal pyramidal neurons to serotonin, norepinephrine, gamma-butyric acid and acetylcholine. *Brain Research Bulletin* 1987; 18:205–212.

50. P. Kalen. Hippocampal noradrenaline and serotonin release over 24 hours as measured by the dialysis technique in freely moving rats. *European Journal of Neuroscience* 1989; 1:181.

51. W. Penfield. *The Mystery of the Mind*. Princeton, N.J., Princeton University Press, 1975.

52. C. Torda. *Memory and Dreams. A Modern Physics Approach*. Chicago, Walters, 1980.

53. T. Teyler and P. Discenna. The topological anatomy of the hippocampus: A clue to its function. *Brain Research Bulletin* 1984; 12:711–719.

54. L. Thompson and P. Best. Place cells and silent cells in the hippocampus of freely-behaving rats. *Journal of Neuroscience* 1989; 9:2382–2390.

55. J. Feigenbaum and E. Rolls. Allocentric and egocentric spatial information processing in the hippocampal formation of the behaving primate. *Psychobiology* 1991; 19:21–40.

56. H. Altman, H. Normil, M. Galloway, et al. Enhanced spatial discrimination learning in rats following 5,7-DHT–induced serotonergic deafferentation of the hippocampus. *Brain Research* 1990; 518:61–66.

57. S. Zola-Morgan, L. Squire, D. Amaral, et al. Lesions of perirhinal and parahippocampal cortex that spare the amygdala and hippocampal formation produce severe memory impairment. *Journal of Neuroscience* 1989; 9:4355–4370.

58. D. VonCramon, N. Hebel, and U. Schuri. Verbal memory and learning in unilateral posterior cerebral infarction. *Brain* 1988; 111:1061–1077.

59. Human patients, unlike animals, can usually describe the mental aspects of their experience. Some patients with memory disorders tell us that a flood of *irrelevant* items intrudes when they try to retrieve a specific memory. This prevents them from addressing one memory and then manipulating it in an organized manner. Some aspects of this disability may hinge on the way a *normal* person's working memory functions are partly directed by the frontal lobes as they interact with the rest of the memory circuitry. See L. Weiskrantz. A comparison of hippocampal pathology in man and other animals. In *Functions of the Septo-Hippocampal System. Ciba Foundation Symposium* 1978; 58:373–406.

60. B. Hyman, G. VanHoesen, A. Damasio, et al. Alzheimer's disease: Cell-specific pathology isolates the hippocampal formation. *Science* 1984; 225:1168–1170.

61. But what if a patient who has an acute retrograde memory loss does not get better with time? What if this patient's memories of the recent past remain very defective? Then a careful case history will usually uncover the true situation: that even back during the earliest acute phase of the illness, the patient still had a major (but overlooked) loss of ongoing memories. And that this ongoing loss at this early stage was still, *proportionately,* more severe than was the retrograde loss.

62. Cases this important would benefit from being studied during life with polygraphic and functional imaging techniques. Postmortem studies in these patients, and in similar patients who have more restricted cortical lesions, are essential to verify the full extent of the damage. See N. Kapur, D. Ellison, M. Smith, et al. Focal retrograde amnesia following bilateral temporal lobe pathology. *Brain* 1992; 115:73–85; H. Markowitsch, P. Calabrese, J. Liess, et al. Retrograde amnesia after traumatic injury of the frontal-temporal cortex. *Journal of Neurology, Neurosurgery and Psychiatry* 1993; 56:988–992.

63. C. Fisher and R. Adams. Transient global amnesia. *Acta Neurologica* 1964; 40–83, (suppl. 9). The retrograde memory loss is minor in degree, limited to those events during the last several minutes or hours just before their acute amnesia started.

64. *Hypermnesia* is a term already used in psychology (see D. Payne. Hypermnesia and reminiscence in recall. A historical and empirical review. *Psychological Bulletin* 1987; 101:5–27). For this reason it seems preferable to use a different word such as "supermnesia."

Chapter 43 Visceral Drives and the Hypothalamus

1. P. Haskel. *Bankei Zen.* New York, Grove Press, 1984. The quotation is from *Song of Original Mind.*

2. Seng-ts'an in *Affirmation of Faith in Mind,* discussed in Appendix B.

3. F. Netter. *Nervous System. Anatomy and Physiology.* vol, 1, pt. 1. Ciba Publications, West Caldwell, New Jersey.

4. P. Morgane. Introduction to psychophysiology of motivation [organization of the cortico-limbic-reticular axis in regulating hypothalamic activity]. In *Brain and Behavior,* eds. G. Adam, I. Meszaros, and E. Banyai. Advances in Physiological Science, vol. 17. Budapest, Pergamon, 1981, 325–332.

5. J. Huston and A. Borbély. Operant conditioning in forebrain ablated rats by use of rewarding hypothalamic stimulation. *Brain Research* 1973; 50:467–472. "Forebrain" refers to the upper of the three embryonic bulges in the primitive neural tube. Midbrain is next. Hindbrain is lowest.

6. W. Hess. *Hypothalamus and Thalamus.* Stuttgart, Thieme, 1969.

7. M. Fukuda, T. Ono, and K. Nakamura. Functional relations among inferotemporal cortex, amygdala, and lateral hypothalamus in monkey operant feeding behavior. *Journal of Neurophysiology* 1987, 57:1060–1077.

8. T. Ono and K. Nakamura. Learning and integration of rewarding and aversive stimuli in the rat lateral hypothalamus. *Brain Research* 1985; 346:368–373.

9. S. Aou, Y. Oomura, C. Woody, et al. Effects of behaviorally rewarding hypothalamic electrical stimulation on intracellularly recorded neuronal activity in the motor cortex of awake monkeys. *Brain Research* 1988; 439:31–38.

10. E. Valenstein. Channeling of responses elicited by hypothalamic stimulation. *Journal of Psychiatric Research* 1971; 8:335–344.

11. J. Coleman and D. Lindsley. Hippocampal electrical correlates of free behavior and behavior induced by stimulation of two hypothalamic-hippocampal systems in the cat. *Experimental Neurology* 1975; 49:506–528.

12. D. Lindsley and C. Wilson. Brainstem-hypothalamic systems influencing hippocampal activity and behavior. In *The Hippocampus,* vol. 2, eds. R. Isaacson and K. Pribram. New York, Plenum Press, 1975, 247–278. The reduced visual evoked potential is attributable to the way the reticular nucleus of the thalamus counteracts excessive excitation.

13. C. Wilson, B. Motter, and D. Lindsley. Influences of hypothalamic stimulation upon septal and hippocampal electrical activity in the cat. *Brain Research* 1976; 107:55–68.

14. J. Coleman and D. Lindsley. Behavioral and hippocampal electrical changes during operant learning in cats and effects of stimulating two hypothalamic-hippocampal systems. *Electroencephalography and Clinical Neurophysiology* 1977; 42:309–331.

15. J. Stellar and E. Stellar. *The Neurobiology of Motivation and Reward.* New York, Springer-Verlag, 1985.

16. R. Szymusiak, T. Iriye, and D. McGinty. Sleep-waking discharge of neurons in the posterior lateral hypothalamic area of cats. *Brain Research Bulletin* 1989; 23:111–120.

17. K. Sano. Sedative stereoencephalotomy: Fornicotomy, upper mesencephalic reticulotomy and postero-medial hypothalamotomy. In *Progress in Brain Research.* Vol. 21B. *Correlative Neurosciences Part B. Clinical Studies,* eds. T. Tokizane and J. Schadé. Amsterdam, Elsevier, 1966, 1966, 350–372. In technical terms, the sides of the triangle extend to the midpoint of a line drawn between the crossing fibers of the anterior and posterior commissures.

18. K. Sano, Y. Mayanagi, H. Sekino, et al. Results of stimulation and destruction of the posterior hypothalamus in man. *Journal of Neurosurgery* 1970; 33:689–707.

19. W. Nauta and V. Domesick. Neural associations of the limbic system. In *The Neural Basis of Behavior,* ed. A. Beckman. Lancaster, England, MTP Press, 1982, 175–206.

20. K. Sano. Intralaminar thalamotomy (thalamolaminotomy) and posteromedial hypothalamotamy in the treatment of intractable pain. Basel, Karger, *In Progress in Neurological Surgery,* vol. 8. 1977, 50–103.

21. T. Watanabe, Y. Taguchi, S. Shiosaka, et al. Distribution of the histaminergic neuron system in the central nervous system of rats: A fluorescent immunohistochemical analysis with histidine decarboxylase as a marker. *Brain Research* 1984; 295:13–25.

22. F. Wouterlood, H. Steinbusch, P. Luiten, et al. Projection from the prefrontal cortex to histaminergic cell groups in the posterior hypothalamic region of the rat. *Brain Research* 1987; 406:330–336.

23. H. Wada, N. Inagaki, A. Yamatodani, et al. Is the histaminergic neuron system a regulatory center for whole-brain activity? *Trends in Neurosciences* 1991; 14:415–418.

24. P. Lomax and M. Ary. The hypothalamus in narcotic dependence and withdrawal. In *Current Studies of Hypothalamic Function,* vol 2, eds. W. Veale and K. Lederis. Basel, Karger, 1978; 149–162.

25. C. Erickson. Functional relationships among central neurotransmitters. *Reviews of Neuroscience* 1978; 3:1–34.

26. B. Jacobs. Physiological theories of sleep: From the hypothalamus to serotonin. In *Current Studies of Hypothalamic Function,* vol. 2, eds. W. Veale and K. Lederis, Basel, Karger, 1978, 138–148.

27. M. Herkenham and S. McLean. Mismatches between receptor and transmitter localization in the brain. In *Quantitative Receptor Autoradiography,* eds. C. Boast, E. Snowhill, and C. Altar. New York, Liss, 1986, 137–171. The opioid receptors are chiefly of the mu and delta type.

28. J.-T. Pan, L.-M. Kow, and D. Pfaff. Single-unit activity of hypothalamic arcuate neurons in brain tissue slices. *Neuroendocrinology* 1986; 43:189–196.

29. K. Jorgenson, L.-M. Kow, and D. Pfaff. Histamine excites arcuate neurons in vitro through H_1 receptors. *Brain Research* 1989; 502:171–179.

30. B. Everitt, B. Meister, T. Hökfelt, et al. The hypothalamic arcuate nucleus–median eminence complex: Immunohistochemistry of Transmitters, peptides and DARPP-32 with special reference to coexistence in dopamine neurons. *Brain Research. Brain Research Reviews* 1986; 11:97–155.

31. Q. Wang, L. Mao, and J. Han. The arcuate nucleus of hypothalamus mediates low but not high frequency electroacupuncture in rats. *Brain Research* 1990; 513:60–66.

32. C. Takeshige, W.-H. Zhao, and S.-Y. Gvo. Convergence from the preoptic area and arcuate nucleus to the median eminence in acupuncture and nonaccupuncture point stimulation analgesia. *Brain Research Bulletin* 1991; 26:771–778.

33. O. Smith, J. DeVito, and C. Astley. The hypothalamus in emotional behavior and associated cardio-vascular correlates. In *Changing Concepts of the Nervous System,* eds. A. Morrison and P. Strick. New York, Academic Press, 1982, 569–584.

34. R. Michael, H. Rees, and R. Bousall. Sites in the male primate brain at which testosterone acts as an androgen. *Brain Research* 1989; 502:11–20. It will take decades to sort out the mechanisms through which these hormonally responsive circutries interact in contributing to the kinder, gentler behavior of the sage (see chapters 148 and 149).

35. C. Lisciotto and J. Morrell. Androgen-concentrating neurons of the forebrain project to the midbrain in rats. *Brain Research* 1990; 516:107–112.

36. In addition, around 12,000 catecholamine nerve cell bodies also make their home in the hypothalamus. These cells are larger and more numerous in humans than in many other mammals.[36] See H. Su, Z.-C. Peng, and Y.-W. Li. Distribution of catecholamine-containing cell bodies in the human diencephalon. *Brain Research* 1987, 409.367–370.

37. G. Reznikoff, S. Manaker, H. Rhodes, et al. Localization and quantification of beta-adrenergic receptors in human brain. *Neurology* 1986; 36:1067–1073.

38. J. Austin, E. Connole, D. Kett, et al. Studies in aging of the brain V. Reduced norepinephrine, dopamine and cyclic AMP in rat brain with advancing age. *Age* 1978; 1:121–124.

39. C. Decavel and A. Van denPol. GABA: A dominant neurotransmitter in the hypothalamus. *Journal of Comparative Neurology* 1990; 302:1019–1037.

40. J. Liu, K. Sakai, G. Vanni-Mercier, et al. A critical role of the posterior hypothalamus in the mechanisms of wakefulness determined by microinjection of muscimol in freely moving cats. *Brain Research* 1989; 479:225–240.

41. S. Shammah-Lagnado. Afferent connections of the zona incerta: A horseradish peroxidase study in the rat. *Neuroscience* 1985; 15:109–134.

42. C. Legg. Visual discrimination impairments after lesions in zona incerta or lateral terminal nucleus of accessory optic tract. *Brain Research* 1979; 177:461–478.

Chapter 44   Biogenic Amines: Three Systems

1. K. Gale. Neurotransmitter interactions in the basal ganglia: "GABA-GABAcology" versus "DA-DAism." In *Dynamics of Neurotransmitter Function,* ed. I. Hanin. New York, Raven Press, 1984, 189–209.

2. P. McGeer, J. Eccles, and E. McGeer. *Molecular Neurobiology of the Mammalian Brain.* New York, Plenum Press, 1978.

3. S. Fahn, R. Libsch, and R. Cutler. Monoamines in the human neostriatum: Topographic distribution in normals and in Parkinson's disease and their role in akinesia, rigidity, chorea, and tremor. *Journal of Neurological Science* 1971; 14:427–455.

4. S. Loughlin and J. Fallon. Substantia nigra and ventral tegmental area projections to cortex: Topography and collateralization. *Neuroscience* 1984; 11:425–435.

5. R. Roth and M. Nowycky. Non-striatal dopaminergic neurons: Role of presynaptic receptors in the modulation of transmitter synthesis. In *Advances in Biochemical Psychopharmacology* eds. E. Costa and G. Gessa, New York, Raven Press 1977; 16:465–470.

6. S. Foote. Extrathalamic modulation of cortical function. *Annual Review of Neuroscience* 1987; 10:67–95.

7. B. Jacobs, G. Steinfels, and R. Stracker. Dopaminergic unit activity in freely moving animals: A review. In *Catecholamines Part B. Neuropharmacology and Central Nervous System. Theoretical Aspects*, eds. E. Usdin, A. Carlsson, A. Dahlström, et al. New York, Liss, 1984, 393–399. DA nerve cells are sometimes excited before they slow down.

8. B. Jacobs. Single unit activity of brain monoamine-containing neurons in freely moving animals. In *Neurochemical Analysis of the Conscious Brain*, eds. R. Myers and P. Knott. *Annals of the New York Academy of Sciences* 1986; 473:70–79.

9. G. Steinfels, J. Heym, R. Strecker, et al. Behavioral correlates of dopaminergic unit activity in freely moving cats. *Brain Research* 1983; 258:217–228.

10. W. Schultz and R. Romo. Responses of nigrostriatal dopamine neurons to high-intensity somatosensory stimulation in the anaesthetized monkey. *Journal of Neurophysiology* 1987; 57:201–217.

11. A. Freeman and B. Bunney. Activity of A_9 and A_{10} dopaminergic neurons in unrestrained rats: Further characterization and effects of apomorphine and cholecystokinin. *Brain Research* 1987; 405:46–55.

12. G. Blanc, D. Hervé, H. Simon, et al. Response to stress of mesocortico-frontal dopaminergic neurones in rats after long-term isolation. *Nature* 1980; 284:265–267.

13. J. Glowinski, M. Giorguieff, and A. Cheramy. Regulatory processes involved in the control of the activity of nigrostriatal dopaminergic neurons. In *The Reticular Formation Revisited*, eds. J. Hobson and M. Brazier. International Brain Research Organization Monograph Series, vol 6. New York, Raven Press, 1980, 285–301.

14. A. Nieoullon, L. Kerkerian, and N. Dusticier. Presynaptic controls in the neostriatum: Reciprocal interactions between the nigrostriatal dopaminergic neurons and the corticostriatal glutamatergic pathway. *Experimental Brain Research* 1983; (suppl. 7) 54–65.

15. J. Keyser, G. Ebinger, and G. Vauquelin. Evidence for a widespread dopaminergic innervation of the human cerebral neocortex. *Neuroscience Letters* 1989; 104:281–285.

16. E. Ongini and M. Caporali. Different effects of dopamine D-1 and D-2 receptor agonists on EEG activity and behavior in the rabbit. *Neuropharmacology* 1987; 26:355–360.

17. In *human* cortex, DA_1 receptors do not appear to trigger the cell's second-messenger system into producing cyclic AMP (see J. DeKeyser, P. Herregodts, and G. Ebinger. The mesoneocortical dopamine neuron system. *Neurology* 1990; 40:1660–1662). This finding contrasts with the results in animals (see A. Akaike, Y. Ohno, M. Sasa, et al. Excitatory and inhibitory effects of dopamine on neuronal activity of the caudate nucleus neurons in vitro. *Brain Research* 1987; 418:262–272).

18. J. Gorrel, B. Czarnecki, and S. Hubbell. Functional antagonism of D-1 and D-2 dopaminergic mechanisms affecting striatal acetylcholine release. *Life Sciences* 1986; 38:2247–2254.

19. M. Jalilian-Tehrani, G. Karakiulakis, C. Leblond, et al. Androgen-induced sexual dimorphism in high-affinity dopamine binding in the rat brain transcends the hypothalamic-limbic region. *British Journal of Pharmacology* 1982; 75:37–48.

20. T. Crow. Neurotransmitter enzymes and receptors in post-mortem brain in schizophrenia: Evidence that an increase in D_2 dopamine receptors is associated with the type I syndrome. In *Transmitter Biochemistry of Human Brain Tissue*, eds. P. Riederer and E. Usdin. London, Macmillan, 1981, 85–96.

21. U. Rinne, J. Rinne, J. Rinne, et al. Brain receptor changes in Parkinson's disease in relation to the disease process and treatment. *Journal of Neural Transmission* 1983; (suppl. 18):279–286.

22. S. Kish, M. Mamelak, C. Slimovitch, et al. Brain neurotransmitter changes in human narcolepsy. *Neurology* 1992; 42:229–234.

23. D. Hommer, G. Stoner, J. Crawley, et al. Cholecystokinin-dopamine coexistence: Electrophysiological actions corresponding to cholecystokinin receptor subtype. *Journal of Neuroscience* 1986; 6:3039–3043.

24. C. Yim and G. Mogenson. Electrophysiological evidence of modulatory interaction between dopamine and cholecystokinin in the nucleus accumbens. *Brain Research* 1991; 541:12–20.

25. R. Piolti, I. Appollomio, E. Cocco, et al. Treatment of Parkinson's disease with proglumide, a CCK antagonist. *Neurology* 1991; 41:749–750.

26. G. DiChiara and A. Imperato. Preferential stimulation of dopamine release in the nucleus accumbens by opiates, alcohol and barbituates: Studies with transcerebral dialysis in freely moving rats. In *Neurochemical Analysis of the Conscious Brain,* eds. R. Myers and P. Knott. *Annals of the New York Academy of Sciences* 1986; 473:367–381.

27. D. Neill and J. Herndon. Anatomical specificity within rat striatum for the dopaminergic modulation of DLR responding and activity. *Brain Research* 1978; 153:529–538.

28. H. Van Praag, G. Asmis, R. Kahn, et al. Monoamines and abnormal behavior. *British Journal of Psychiatry* 1990; 157:723–734.

29. M. Mintz, R. Tomer, H. Radwan, et al. A comparison of levodopa treatment and task demands on visual evoked potentials in hemiparkinsonism. *Psychiatric Research* 1982; 6:245–251.

30. R. King, I. Mefford, C. Wang, et al. CSF dopamine levels correlate with extraversion in depressed patients. *Psychiatry Research* 1986; 19:305–310.

31. S. Subrahmanyam and K. Porkodi. Yoga—Its probable role in maintaining and restoring normal health. *Yoga Review* 1981; 1:119–130.

32. D. German, B. Walker, K. Manaye, et al. The Human locus coeruleus: Computer reconstruction of cellular distribution. *Journal of Neuroscience* 1988; 8:1776–1788.

33. K. Baker, I. Tork, J. Hornung, et al. The human locus coeruleus complex: An immunohistochemical and three dimensional reconstruction study. *Experimental Brain Research* 1989; 77:257–270.

34. J. Korf, B. Bunney, and G. Aghajanian. Noradrenergic neurons: Morphine inhibition of spontaneous activity. *European Journal of Pharmacology* 1974; 25:165–169. Some of the endogenous opioid could arrive when the arcuate nucleus is stimulated. See H. Strahlendorf, J. Strahlendorf, and C. Barnes: Stimulation of hypothalamic arcuate nucleus inhibits locus coeruleus unit activity: Evidence for endorphin mediation. In *The Role of Peptides and Amino Acids as Neurotransmitters,* eds. J. Tombardini and A. Kenny. *Progress in Clinical and Biological Research* 1981; 68:161–169.

35. B. Jacobs. Single unit activity of locus coeruleus neurons in behaving animals. *Progress in Neurobiology* 1986; 27:183–194.

36. G. Duncan, R. Kaldas, K. Mitra, et al. High activity neurons in the reticular formation of the medulla oblongata: A high-resolution autoradiographic 2-deoxyglucose study. *Neuroscience* 1990; 35:593–600.

37. G. Aston-Jones, M. Ennis, V. Pieribone, et al. The brain nucleus locus coeruleus: Restricted afferent control of a broad efferent network. *Science* 1986; 234:734–737.

38. In such studies it is necessary to deliver a discrete electrical stimulus which itself does not spread so far that it excites adjacent nerve cells.

39. R. Oades. The role of noradrenaline in timing and dopamine in switching between signals in the CNS. *Neuroscience and Biobehavioral Reviews* 1985; 9:261–282.

40. V. Kumar, S. Datta, G. Chhina, et al. Alpha adrenergic systems in medial preoptic area involved in sleep-wakefulness in rats. *Brain Research Bulletin* 1986; 16:463–468.

41. L. Heginbotham and T. Dunwiddie. Long-term increases in the evoked population spike in the CA1 region of rat hippocampus induced by β-adrenergic receptor activation. *Journal of Neuroscience* 1991; 11:2519–2527.

42. G. Buzsaki, B. Kennedy, V. Solt, et al. Noradrenergic control of thalamic oscillation: The Role of alpha$_2$ receptors. *European Journal of Neuroscience* 1991; 3:222–229.

43. A. Washton and R. Risnick. Outpatient opiate detoxification with clonidine. *Journal of Clinical Psychiatry* 43:39–41. The norepinephrine agonist, clonidine, activates α_2-*auto*receptors on NE nerve cells of the locus ceruleus.

44. D. Nutt. Altered central alpha$_2$ adrenoceptor sensitivity in panic disorder. *Archives of General Psychiatry* 1989; 46:165–169.

45. N. Selden, T. Robbins, and B. Everitt. Enhanced behavioral conditioning to context and impaired behavioral and neuroendocrine responses to conditioned stimuli following ceruleocortical noradrenergic lesions: Support for an attentional hypothesis of central noradrenergic function. *Journal of Neuroscience* 1990; 10:531–539.

46. J. Panksepp. The Neurochemistry of Behavior. *Annual Review of Psychology* 1986; 37:77–107.

47. P. Reiner. Correlational analysis of central noradrenergic neuronal activity and sympathetic tone in behaving cats. *Brain Research* 1986; 378:86–96.

48. R. Moore. The reticular formation: Monoamine neuron systems. In *The Reticular Formation Revisited*, vol 6, eds. J. Hobson and M. Brazier. International Brain Research Organization Monograph Series, vol. 6. New York, Raven Press, 1980; 67–81.

49. R. Moore. The anatomy of central serotonin neuron systems in the rat brain. In *Serotonin Neurotransmission and Behavior*, eds. B. Jacobs and A. Gelperin. Cambridge, Mass., The MIT Press, 1981; 37–71.

50. G. Aghajanian and C. Vandermaelen. Specific systems of the reticular core: Serotonin. In *Handbook of Physiology. The Nervous System*, vol 4, eds. V. Mountcastle, F. Bloom, and S. Geiger. Bethesda, Md., American Physiological Society, 1986, 237–256.

51. J. Parnavelas and G. Papadopoulos. The monoaminergic innervation of the cerebral cortex is not diffuse and nonspecific. *Trends in Neurosciences* 1989; 12:315–319.

52. G. Aghajanian, J. Sprouse, and K. Rasmussen. Physiology of the midbrain serotonin system. In *Psychopharmacology: The Third Generation of Progress*, ed. H. Meltzer. New York, Raven Press, 1987; 141–149.

53. J. Baraban and G. Aghajanian. Suppression of firing activity of 5-HT neurons in the dorsal raphé by alpha-adrenoceptor antagonists. *Neuropharmacology* 1980; 19:355–363.

54. B. Jacobs. Single unit activity of brain monoaminergic neurons in freely moving animals: A brief review. In R. Bandler, ed., *Modulation of Sensorimotor Activity During Alterations in Behavioral States. Neurology and Neurobiology*, vol. 12. New York, Liss, 1984, 99–120.

55. R. Bowker. Evidence for the co-localization of somatostatin and methionine enkephalin-like immunoreactivities in raphé and gigantocellularis nuclei. *Neuroscience Letters.* 1987; 81:75–81.

56. T. Hokfelt, B. Meister, T. Melander, et al. Coexistence of classical transmitters and peptides with special reference to the arcuate nucleus–median eminence complex. In *Hypothalamic Dysfunction in Neuropsychiatric Disorders*, eds. D. Nerozzi, F. Goodwin, and E. Costa. New York, Raven Press, 1987; 21–34. Studies of peripheral nerves suggest that classic neurotransmitters might be released at lower rates of neuronal activity from small storage vesicles. In contrast, both peptides and neurotransmitters might be released from the larger vesicles at times of higher impulse flow.

57. J. Pujol, P. Keane, A. McRae, et al. Biochemical evidence for serotonergic control of the locus coeruleus. In *Interactions Between Putative Neurotransmitters in the Brain*, eds. S. Garattini, J. Pujol, and R. Samanin. New York, Raven Press, 1978, 401–410.

58. M. Piercey, J. Lum, and J. Palmer. Effects of MDMA ("ecstasy") on firing rates of serotonergic, dopaminergic, and noradrenergic neurons in the rat. *Brain Research* 1990; 526:203–206.

59. G. Telegdy and I. Vermes. Effect of adrenocortical hormones on activity of the serotonergic system in limbic structures in rats. *Neuroendocrinology* 1975; 18:16–26.

60. J. Gillin, D. Horwitz, and R. Wyatt. Pharmacologic studies of narcolepsy involving serotonin, acetylcholine, and monoamine oxidase. In *Narcolepsy*, vol. 3, eds. C. Guilleminault, W. Dement, and P. Passouant. New York, Spectrum, 1976, 585–604.

61. P. Whitaker-Azmitia and S. Peroutka. The neuropharmacology of serotonin. *Annals of the New York Academy of Sciences* 1990; 600.

62. G. Aghajanian. The modulatory role of serotonin at multiple receptors in brain. In *Serotonin Neurotransmission and Behavior,* eds. B. Jacobs, and A. Gelperin. Cambridge, Mass., The MIT Press, 1981, 156–185.

63. F. Crespi, J. Garratt, A. Sleight, et al. In vivo evidence that 5-hydroxytryptamine (5-HT) neuronal firing and release are not necessarily correlated with 5-HT metabolism. *Neuroscience* 1990; 35:139–144.

64. S. Montgomery and N. Fineberg. Is there a relationship between serotonin receptor subtypes and selectivity of response in specific psychiatric illnesses? *British Journal of Psychiatry* 1989; 155(suppl. 8):63–70.

65. In general, when ST activates its postsynaptic ST_1 and ST_2 receptors, they are relatively weak generators of the cascade of second messengers. On occasion, the lipid phosphatidyl inositol could play a minor role as an accessory messenger. See N. Buckholtz, D. Zhou, D. Freedman, et al. Lysergic acid diethylamide (LSD) administration selectively downregulates serotonin$_2$ receptors in rat brain. *Neuropsychopharmacology* 1990; 3:137–148.

66. L. Tecott and D. Julius. A new wave of serotonin receptors. *Current Opinion in Neurobiology* 1993; 3:310–315. At last count, as many as seven different types had been described.

67. P. Fan. Cannabinoid agonists inhibit the activation of $5HT_3$ receptors in rat nodose ganglion neurons. *Journal of Neurophysiology* 1995; 73:907–910.

68. R. Araneda and R. Andrade. 5-Hydroxytryptamine$_2$ and 5-hydroxytryptamine$_{1A}$ receptors mediate opposing responses on membrane excitability in rat association cortex. *Neuroscience* 1991; 40:399–412.

69. H. Van Praag and S. De Haan. Depression vulnerability and 5-hydroxytryptophan prophylaxis. *Psychiatric Research* 1980; 3:75–83. See also chapter 140.

70. P. Goldman-Rakic, M. Lidow, and D. Gallagher. Overlap of dopaminergic, adrenergic, and serotonergic receptors and complementarity of their subtypes in primate prefrontal cortex. *Journal of Neuroscience* 1990; 10:2125–2138.

71. I. McKeith, E. Marshall, I. Ferrier, et al. 5-HT receptor binding in post-mortem brain from patients with affective disorder. *Journal of Affective Disorders* 1987; 13:67–74. Median raphe fiber systems end mostly on the other receptors of the ST_1 type, chiefly in the basal ganglia and in the hippocampus.

72. J. Mann, V. Arango, P. Marzuk, et al. Evidence for the 5-HT hypothesis of suicide. *British Journal of Psychiatry* 155 (suppl. 8):7–14. ST levels are reduced along with those of its breakdown product.

73. M. Raleigh, G. Brammer, T. McGuire, et al. Dominent social status facilitates the behavioral effects of serotonin agonists. *Brain Research* 1985; 348:274–282.

74. M. Raleigh, M. McGuire, G. Brammer, et al. Serotonergic mechanisms promote dominance acquisition in adult male vervet monkeys. *Brain Research* 1991; 559:181–190.

75. N. Popova, N. Voitenko, A. Kulikov, et al. Evidence for the involvement of central serotonin in mechanism of domestication of silver fox. *Pharmacology, Biochemistry and Behavior* 1991; 40:751–756.

76. J. Higley, P. Mehlman, D. Taub, et al. Cerebrospinal fluid monoamine and adrenal correlates of aggression in free-ranging rhesus monkeys. *Archives of General Psychiatry* 1992; 49:436–441. In this study, the synaptic turnover of ST was assessed indirectly. A metabolite of ST, 5-hydroxyindoleacetic acid, served as the index.

77. Of this breed a friend once said: "If only all of *us* had the same kindly disposition as golden retrievers, humanity would be a lot better off."

78. Having said this, the reader must be warned that major hazards are implicit in unsupervised drug use. Certain "sleep preparations" on the over-the-counter market, containing the ST precursor, L-tryptophan, caused a crippling neuromuscular disorder: the eosinophilia-myalgia syndrome. Moreover, the designer drug, MPTP, causes a severe form of parkinsonism.

Chapter 45   GABA and Inhibition

1. W. Koella. GABA systems and behavior. In *Amino Acid Neurotransmitters*, eds. F. DeFendis and P. Mandel. *Advances in Biochemistry and Psychopharmacology* 1981; 29:11–21.

2. G. Johnston. GABA receptors. In *The Role of Peptides and Amino Acids as Neurotransmitters*, eds. J. Lombardini and A. Kenny. New York, Liss, 1981, 1–17.

3. M. Erecinska and I. Silver. Metabolism and role of glutamate in mammalian brain. *Progress in Neurobiology* 1990; 35:245–296.

4. GABA$_A$ receptors on the next, postsynaptic, cell act by permitting chloride ions to flow into it. This hyperpolarizes the next cell, makes it more difficult to discharge, and thus slows its rate of firing. Rarely, GABA might briefly excite before it causes its usual profound, long-lasting inhibition. See B. Alger and R. Nicoll. Pharmacological evidence for two kinds of GABA receptors on rat hippocampal pyramidal cells studied *in vitro*. *Journal of Physiology* 1982; 328:125–141; M. Avoli and P. Perreault. A GABAergic depolarizing potential in the hippocampus disclosed by the convulsant 4-aminopyrine. *Brain Research* 1987; 400:191–195.

5. A few GABA cells are larger and longer, including some found in the posterior hypothalamus which widely supply the cortex. See S. Vincent, T. Hökfelt, L. Skirboll, et al. Hypothalamic γ-aminobutyric acid neurons project to the neocortex. *Science* 1983; 220:1309–1310.

6. J. Palacios, J. Wamsley, M. Zarbin, et al. Gaba and glycine receptors in rat brain: Auto radiographic localization. In *Amino Acid Neurotransmitters*, eds. F. DeFendis and P. Mandel. *Advances in Biochemistry and Psychopharmacology* 1981; 29:445–451.

7. E. Roberts, T. Chase, and D. Tower. *GABA in Nervous System Function*. New York, Raven Press, 1976.

8. P. Mandel, L. Ciesielski, M. Maitre, et al. Inhibitory amino acids, aggressiveness, and convulsions. In *Amino Acid Neurotransmitters*, eds. F. DeFendis and P. Mandel. *Advances in Biochemistry and Psychopharmacology* 1981; 29:1–9.

9. A. Merriam. Emotional arousal–induced transient global amnesia. *Neuropsychiatry, Neuropsychology, and Behavioral Neurology* 1988; 1:73–78.

10. J. McGaugh, C. Castellano, and J. Brioni. Picrotoxin enhances latent extinction of conditioned fear. *Behavioral Neuroscience* 1990; 104:264–267.

11. N. Kalin, S. Shelton, and C. Barksdale. Separation distress in infant rhesus monkeys: Effects of diazepam and RO 15-1788. *Brain Research.* 1987; 408:192–198. ACTH is the peptide released from the stressed brain and pituitary gland that causes the adrenal cortex to release its stress hormones.

Chapter 46   Peptides

1. U. Von Euler, C.A. Marsan, and W. Traczyk. Introduction. In *Neuropeptides and Neuronal Transmission*. IBRO Monographs, vol 7. New York, Raven Press, 1980, 1–4.

2. D. Krieger. Brain peptides: What, where, and why? *Science* 1983; 222:975–985.

3. J. Belluzzi and L. Stein. Facilitation of long-term memory by brain endorphins. In *Endogenous Peptides and Learning and Memory Processes*, eds. J. Martinez, R. Jensen, and R. Messing. New York, Academic Press, 1981, 291–302.

4. R. Moss and C. Dudley. The challenge of studying the behavioral effects of neuropeptides. In *Drugs, Neurotransmitters, and Behavior*, eds. L. Iversen, S. Iversen, and S. Snyder. Handbook of Psychopharmacology, vol. 18. New York, Plenum Press, 1984, 397–454.

5. T. Hökfelt. Neuropeptides in perspective. The last ten years. *Neuron* 1991; 7:867–879.

6. C. Neal, J. Swaun, and S. Newman. The colocalization of substance P and prodynorphin immunoreactivity in neurons of the medial preoptic area, bed nucleus of the stria terminalis, and medial nucleus of the amygdala of the Syrian hamster. *Brain Research* 1989; 496:1–13.

7. H. Taquet, F. Javoy-Agid, A. Mauborgne, et al. Biochemical mapping of cholecystokinin-, substance P-, metenkephalin-, leuenkephalin- and dynorphin A (1–8)–like immunoreactivities in the human cerebral cortex. *Neuroscience* 1988; 27:871–883.

8. F. Bloom. Whither neuropeptides? In *Neuropeptides in Neurologic and Psychiatric Disease,* vol. 64, eds. J. Martin and J. Barchas. Research Publications Association for Research in Nervous and Mental Disease. New York, Raven Press, 1986, 335–349.

9. E. Audinat, J-M. Hermel, and F. Crepel. Neurotensin-induced excitation of neurons of the rat's frontal cortex studied intracellulary in vitro. *Experimental Brain Research* 1989; 78:358–368.

10. R. Buijs. Vasopressinergic and oxytocinergic pathways, synapses and central release. In *Neuroendocrinology of Vasopressin, Corticoliberin and Opiomelanocortins,* eds. A. Baertschi and J. Dreifuss. London, Academic Press, 1982, 51–60. Excitatory responses to vasopressin occur at concentrations of 10^{-9} molar.

11. B. Beckwith, T. Petros, P. Bergloff, et al. Vasopressin analogue (DDAVP) facilitates recall of narrative prose. *Behavioral Neuroscience* 1987; 101:429–432.

12. C. Nemeroff and A. Dunn, eds. *Peptides, Hormones, and Behavior.* Jamaica, New York, SP Medical and Scientific Books, 1984.

13. A. Gaillard. ACTH analogs and human performance. In *Endogenous Peptides and Learning and Memory Processes,* eds. J. Martinez, R. Jensen, and R. Messing. New York, Academic Press, 1981, 181–196.

14. J. Sagen and A. Routtenberg. Specific anatomical and synaptic sites of neuropeptide action in memory formation. In *Endogenous Peptides and Learning and Memory Processes,* eds. J. Martinez, R. Jensen, and R. Messing. New York, Academic Press, 1981, 541–561.

15. C. Sandman, A. Kastin, and A. Schally. Neuropeptide influences on the central nervous system: A psychobiological perspective. In *Neuroendocrine Regulation and Altered Behavior,* eds. P. Hrdina and R. Singhal. London, Croom Helm, 1981, 4–27.

16. F. Marrosu, G. Gessa, M. Giagheddu, et al. Corticotropin-releasing factor (CRF) increases paradoxical sleep (PS) rebound in PS-deprived rats. *Brain Research* 1990; 515:315–318.

17. S. Pretel and D. Piekut. Coexistence of corticotropin-releasing factor and enkephalin in the paraventricular nucleus of the rat. *Journal of Comparative Neurology* 1990; 294:192–201. Other dense clusters of CRF nerve cells occur in the central nucleus of the amygdala and in the bed nucleus of the stria terminalis, which serves as one output pathway of the amygdala. See P. Sawchenko and L. Swanson. Organization of CRF immunoreactive cells and fibers in rat brain: Immuno-histochemical studies. In *Corticotropin-Releasing Factor: Basic and Clinical Studies of a Neuropeptide,* eds. E. DeSouza and C. Nemeroff. Boca Raton, Fla., CRC Press, 1990, 29–51.

18. K. Hargreaves, G. Mueller, R. Dubuer, et al. Corticotropin-releasing factor (CRF) produces analgesia in humans and rats. *Brain Research* 1987; 422:154–157. When CRF is injected into the *systemic* blood circulation of human subjects, it reduces pain, increases β-endorphin levels in the blood for an hour and a half, and increases adrenal cortisol levels. No anxiety occurs, nor does the injection lead to increased blood levels of epinephrine or norepinephrine.

Chapter 47   The Brain's Own Opioids

1. T. Sydenham. In *The Pharmacological Basis of Therapeutics,* eds. L. Goodman and A. Gilman. New York, Macmillan, 1975, 245.

2. E. Snow, in, G. Seldes, ed., *The Great Quotations.* New York, Pocket Books, 1967, 828.

3. H. Pollard, C. Llorens, J. Bonnet, et al. Opiate receptors on mesolimbic dopaminergic neurons. *Neuroscience Letters* 1977; 7:295–299.

4. P. Rada, G. Mark, E. Pothos, et al. Systemic morphine simultaneously decreases extracellular acetylcholine and increases dopamine in the nucleus accumbens of freely moving rats. *Neuropharmacology* 30:1133–1136.

5. J. Hughes, A. Beaumont, J. Fuentes, et al. Opioid peptides: Aspects of their origin, release and metabolism. *Journal of Experimental Biology* 1980; 89:239–255.

6. H. Khachaturian, M. Lewis, M. Shäfer, S. et al. Anatomy of the CNS opioid systems. *Trends in Neurosciences* 1985; 8:111–119. Figure 2 of this article illustrates the anatomical differences among the three systems. A *very* few β-endorphin terminals supply GABA cells

in the cingulate and frontal cortex. See H.-G. Bernstein, H. Henning, N. Seliger, et al. Remarkable β-endorphinergic innervation of human cerebral cortex as revealed by immunohistochemistry. *Neuroscience Letters* 1996; 215:33–36.

7. B. Everitt, B. Meister, T. Hokfelt, et al. The hypothalamic arcuate nucleus–median eminence complex: Immunohistochemistry of transmitters, peptides and DARPP-32 with special reference to coexistence in dopamine neurons. *Brain Research* 1986; 396:97–155.

8. L. Stinus, A. Kelley, and M. Winnock. Neuropeptides and limbic system function. In *Psychopharmacology of the Limbic System*, eds. M. Trimble and E. Zarifan. Oxford, Oxford University Press, 1984, 209–225.

9. S. McLean, R. Rothman, and M. Herkenham. Autoradiographic localization of μ- and δ-opiate receptors in the forebrain of the Rat. *Brain Research* 1986; 378:49–60.

10. R. Nicoll, G. Siggins, N. Ling, et al. Neuronal actions of endorphins and enkephalins among brain regions: A comparative microiontophoretic study. *Proceeding of the National Academy of Sciences of the United States of America* 1977; 74:2584–2588.

11. H. Moises and J. Walker. Electrophysiological effects of dynorphin peptides on hippocampal pyramidal cells in rat. *European Journal of Pharmacology* 1985; 108:85–98.

12. G. Pasternak. Multiple morphine and enkephalin receptors: Biochemical and pharmacological aspects. In *Stress-Induced Analgesia*, ed. D. Kelly. *Annals of the New York Academy of Sciences* 1986; 467:130–139.

13. B. Wolozin, S. Nishimura, and G. Pasternak. The binding of κ- and δ-opiates in rat brain. *Journal of Neuroscience* 1982; 2:708–713.

14. A. Cross, C. Hille, and P. Slater. Subtraction autoradiography of opiate receptor subtypes in human brain. *Brain Research* 1987; 418:343–348.

15. M. Lewis, M. Mishkin, E. Bragin, et al. Opiate receptor gradients in monkey cerebral cortex: Correspondence with sensory processing hierarchies. *Science* 1981; 211:1166–1169.

16. S. Wise and M. Herkenham. Opiate receptor distribution in the cerebral cortex of the rhesus monkey. *Science* 1982; 218:387–388.

17. E. London, E. Broussolle, J. Links, et al. Morphine-induced metabolic changes in human brain. *Archives of General Psychiatry* 1990; 47:73–81.

18. A. Dunn. Neurochemical effects of behaviorally active peptides: ACTH and vasopressin. *Neuronal Plasticity and Memory Formation*, eds. H. Matthies and C-A Marsan. New York, Raven Press, 1982, 113–122.

19. Opiate antagonists like naloxone also have other effects. For example, they amplify some acetylcholine functions. In contrast, opiate agonists tend to reduce many cholinergic activities. See D. Walker, T. McGlynn, C. Grey, et al. Naloxone modulates the behavioral effects of cholinergic agonists and antagonists. *Psychopharmacology (Berlin)* 1991; 105:57–62.

20. N. Kalin, S. Shelton, and C. Barksdale. Opiate modulation of separation-induced distress in non-human primates. *Brain Research* 1988; 440:285–292.

21. H. Beecher. Relationship of significance of wound to the pain experienced. *JAMA* 1956; 161:1609–1613.

22. H. Beecher. *Measurement of Subjective Responses*. New York, Oxford University Press, 1959.

23. Y. Tong, H. Zhao, F. Labrie, et al. Regulation of pro-opiomelanocortin messenger ribonucleic acid content by sex steroids in the arcuate nucleus of the female rat brain. *Neuroscience Letters* 1990; 112:104–108.

24. S. Roosevelt, A. Wolfsen, and W. Odell. Modulation of brain endorphin-opiate receptor by glucocorticoids (abstract). *Clinical Research* 1979; 27:75a.

25. E. Hahn and J. Fishman. Changes in rat brain opiate receptor content upon castration and testosterone replacement. *Biochemical and Biophysical Research Communications* 1979; 90:819–823.

26. R. Bodnar, C. Williams, S. Lee, et al. Role of μ-opiate receptors in supraspinal opiate analgesia: A microinjection study. *Brain Research* 1988; 447:25–34.

27. R. Tasker. Identification of pain processing systems by electrical stimulation of the brain. *Human Neurobiology* 1982; 1:261–272. The parafascicular nucleus is one of the deep medial nuclei of the thalamus.

28. K. Amano, T. Tanikawa, H. Kawamura, et al. Endorphins and pain relief. *Applied Neurophysiology* 1982; 45:123–135. It is to be noted that the stress of the prior surgery is superimposed on the effect of the brain stimulation.

29. Y. Hosobuchi. Periaqueductal gray stimulation in humans produces analgesia accompanied by elevation of β-endorphin and ACTH in ventricular CSF. In *The Role of Endorphins in Neuropsychiatry*, ed. H. Emrich. *Modern Problems of Pharmacopsychiatry* 1981; 17:109–122. The lack of euphoria and of depressed respirations suggests that pain has been relieved at a site(s) different from where these two other functions are represented.

30. A placebo injection can relieve some patients who have chronic pain problems. They show increased evidence of an endorphin-like molecule in their lumbar spinal fluid at the time. (See J. Lipman, B. Miller, K. Mays, et al. Peak β-endorphin concentration in cerebrospinal fluid: Reduced in chronic pain patients and increased during the placebo response. *Psychopharmacology (Berlin)* 1990; 102:112–116.) It will take many more careful studies to sort out whether the changes reported in the spinal fluid levels of substance P, enkephalin, and dynorphin in other patients can be meaningfully interpreted as factors which are related to the cause of *their* pain problems. (See H. Vaeroy, F. Nyberg, and L. Terenius. No evidence for endorphin deficiency in fibromyalgia following investigation of cerebrospinal fluid (CSF) dynorphin A and met-enkephalin-Arg[6]-Phe[7]. *Pain* 1991; 46:139–143.)

31. However, stimulating the central gray does not go on to increase the *blood* levels of ACTH or adrenal cortisol, nor does it release enkephalins.[29] These facts suggest that when discrete brain stimulation is delivered at a site well away from the hypothalamus it does not necessarily spread its direct effects over to the pituitary gland and then trigger the release of pituitary hormones into the blood.

32. O. Sakurada, L. Sokoloff, and Y. Jacquet. Local cerebral glucose utilization following injection of β-endorphin into periaqueductal gray matter in the rat. *Brain Research* 1978; 153:403–407. We do not know what the *immediate* metabolic effect of the β-endorphin was, because the method used tells us only the total of *all* the brain's metabolic activities during the whole two- to three-hour period *after* the injection.

33. J. McCulloch, P. Kelly, and A. VanDelft. Neuroanatomical basis for the action of a behaviorally active ACTH[4-9] analogue. *European Journal of Pharmacology* 1982; 78:151–158.

34. A. Riley, D. Zellner, and H. Duncan. The role of endorphins in animal learning and behavior. *Neuroscience and Biobehavioral Reviews* 1980; 4:69–76.

35. M. Janal, E. Colt, W. Clark, et al. Pain sensitivity, mood and plasma endocrine levels in man following long-distance running: Effects of naloxone. *Pain* 1984; 19:13–25. A popular notion is that a surge of endorphins from the pituitary enters the bloodstream, and then goes to the runners' brains to make them "feel good." Chapter 53 presents a more likely alternative route.

36. T. McIntosh. Altered plasma dynamics of β-endorphin and postoperative psychosis. In *Central and Peripheral Endorphins: Basic and Clinical Aspects*, eds. E. Müller and A. Genazzani. New York, Raven Press, 1984, 289–293.

37. E. Meyer, D. Morris, D. Brase, et al. Naltrexone therapy of apnea in children with elevated cerebrospinal fluid β-endorphin. *Annals of Neurology* 1990; 27:75–80.

38. B. Siegfried, C. Netto, and I. Izquierdo. Exposure to novelty induces naltrexone-reversible analgesia in rats. *Behavioral Neuroscience* 1987; 101:436–438.

39. I. Izquierdo and J. McGaugh. Effect of a novel experience prior to training or testing on retention of an inhibitory avoidance response in mice: Involvement of an opioid system. *Behavioral and Neural Biology* 1985; 44:228–238.

40. I. Izquierdo and C. Netto. The brain β-endorphin system and behavior: The modulation of consecutively and simultaneously processed memories. *Behavioral and Neural Biology* 44:249–265. The fornix also carries acetylcholine fibers in the reverse direction, from the medial septal nucleus to the hippocampus, as shown in figure 5. One awaits the results of *selective* experimental lesions of the fornix in primates.

41. T. Yanigita. Self-administration studies on psychological dependence. *Trends in Pharmacological Sciences* 1980; 2:161–164.

42. C. Schuster and T. Thompson. Self administration of and behavioral dependence on drugs. *Annual Review of Pharmacology* 1969; 9:483–502.

43. R. Esposito. Cognitive-affective integration: Some recent trends from a neurobiological perspective. In *Memory Consolidation; Psychobiology of Cognition,* eds. H. Weingartner and E. Parker. Hillsdale, N.J., Erlbaum, 1984, 15–63.

44. C. Broekkamp, A. Phillips, and A. Coals. Stimulant effects of enkephalin microinjection into the dopaminergic A-10 area. *Nature* 1979; 278:560–562.

45. F. Jenck, A. Gratton, and R. Wise. Opioid receptor subtypes associated with ventral tegmental facilitation of lateral hypothalamic brain stimulation reward. *Brain Research* 1987; 423:34–38.

46. M. Bozarth and R. Wise. Neural substrates of opiate reinforcement. *Progress in Neuropsychopharmacology and Biological Psychiatry* 1983; 7:569–575.

47. X. Yuan, S. Madamba, and G. Siggins. Opioid peptides reduce synaptic transmission in the nucleus accumbens. *Neuroscience Letters* 1992; 134:223–228.

48. B. Diamond and R. Borison. Enkephalins and nigrostriatal function. *Neurology* 1978; 28:1085–1088.

49. U. Rinne, J. O. Rinne, J. K. Rinne, et al. Brain receptor changes in Parkinson's disease in relation to the disease process and treatment. *Journal of Neural Transmission* 1983; 18(suppl.):279–286.

50. L. Leger, Y. Charnay, J. Chayvialle, et al. Localization of substance P and enkephalin-like immunoreactivity in relation to catecholamine-containing cell bodies in the cat dorsolateral pontine tegmentum: An immunofluorescence study. *Neuroscience* 1983; 8:525–546.

51. D. Millhorn, T. Hokfelt, A. Verhofstad, et al. Individual cells in the raphé nuclei of the medulla oblongata in rat that contain immunoreactivities for both serotonin and enkephalin project to the spinal cord. *Experimental Brain Research* 1989; 75:536–542.

52. J. Wiesner, S. Henriksen, and F. Bloom. Opioid enhancement of perforant path transmission: Effect of an enkephalin analog on inhibition and facilitation in the dentate gyrus. *Brain Research* 1986; 399:404–408.

53. S. Fujii, E. Senba, H. Kiyama, et al. Mammillothalamic enkephalinergic pathway in the rat: An immunocytochemical analysis. *Brain Research* 1987; 401:1–8.

54. M. Yamano and M. Tohyama. Afferent and efferent enkephalinergic systems of the tegmental nuclei of Gudden in the rat: An immunocytochemical study. *Brain Research* 1987; 408:22–30.

55. A. Dickenson, A. Sullivan, C. Feeney, et al. Evidence that endogenous enkephalins produce δ-opiate receptor mediated neuronal inhibitions in rat dorsal horn. *Neuroscience Letters* 1986; 72:179–182.

56. C. Schindler, I. Gormezano, and J. Harvey. Effects of drugs on classical conditioning. In *Behavioral Pharmacology: The Current Status,* eds. L. Seiden and R. Balster. New York, Liss, 1985, 55–71.

57. M. Gallagher, M. Meagher, and E. Bostock. Effects of opiate manipulations on latent inhibition in rabbits: Sensitivity of the medial septal region to intracranial treatments. *Behavioral Neuroscience* 1987; 101:315–324. Injecting the opioid agonist levorphanol into the medial septal region weakens the ongoing inhibition which had formerly held conditioned responses in check. However, it does not interfere with retaining habituation over the long term.

58. J. Walker, H. Moises, D. Coy, et al. Nonopiate effects of dynorphin and Des-Tyr-dynorphin. *Science* 1982; 218:1136–1138.

59. B. Herman, F. Leslie, and A. Goldstein. Behavioral effects and in vivo degradation of intraventricularly administered dynorphin-(1–13) and D-ALA²-dynorphin-(1–11) in rats. *Life Sciences* 1980; 27:883–892. Some dynorphin nerve cells lie in large nerve cells of the paraventricular nucleus, near the third ventricle.

60. R. Caudle and L. Isaac. A novel interaction between Dynorphin-(1–13) and an *N*-methyl-D-aspartate site. *Brain Research* 1988; 443:329–332.

Chapter 48   Ripples in the Next Cell: Second and Third Messengers

1. B. Weiss, L. Greenberg, and M. Clark. Physiological and pharmacological modulation of the β-adrenergic receptor–linked adenylate cyclase system: Supersensitivity and subsensitivity. In *Dynamics of Neurotransmitter Function*, ed. I. Hanin. New York, Raven Press, 1984, 319–329.

2. P. Worley, J. Baraban, and S. Snyder. Beyond receptors: Multiple second-messenger systems in brain. *Annals of Neurology* 1987; 21:217–229. When fast transmission *excites* (depolarizes) the next cell, it opens up its pores to the inflow of positively charged cations like calcium and sodium. But other fast transmitters like GABA *inhibit* (*hyper*polarize) the next cell. They open up its membrane channels to anions like chloride. However, the slower transmitters and modulators are coupled with other specific proteins, called G proteins. They act to transduce signals from membrane receptors into *metabolic* events. These return, only much later, to affect ion flow through the membrane. For example, the biogenic amines influence the flux of potassium ions in this indirect manner.

3. J. Reynolds, A. Baskys, and P. Carlen. The effects of serotonin on N-methyl-D-aspartate and synaptically evoked depolarizations in rat neocortical neurons. *Brain Research* 1988; 456:286–292.

4. R. Miller. Protein kinase C: A key regulator of neuronal excitability? *Trends in Neurosciences* 1986; 9:538–541.

5. J. Schwartz. Cyclic AMP–mediated modulation of gene expression. In *Dynamics of Neurotransmitter Function*, ed. I. Hanin. New York, Raven Press, 1984, 253–263.

6. Cyclic AMP stands for cyclic 3′, 5′-adenosine monophosphate. The brain also has the option of using a different messenger system. It transduces those signals which act on some of its acetylcholine, glutamate, and α-norepinephrine subtypes of receptors. This other "metabotropic" system also works slowly, using inositol lipids in its metabolic cascade. See S. Fisher, A. Heacock, and B. Agranoff. Inositol lipids and signal transduction in the nervous system: An update. *Journal of Neurochemistry* 1992; 58:18–38.

7. There are other ways to hold adenyl cyclase in check. They include activating such different receptors as: mu and delta opioid, α_2 NE, $GABA_B$, ACH muscarinic, dopaminergic (DA_2), and other hormone receptors. See E. Stone. Central cyclic-AMP–linked noradrenergic receptors: New findings on properties as related to the actions of stress. *Neuroscience and Biobehavioral Reviews* 1987; 11:391–398.

8. H. Wagner, G. Palmer, and J. Davis. Sensitivity of noradrenergically mediated cyclic AMP responses in the brain. In *Neuropharmacology of Cyclic Nucleotides*, ed. G. Palmer. Baltimore, Urban & Schwarzenberg, 1979, 152–172.

9. G. Drummond. *Cyclic Nucleotides in the Nervous System*. New York, Raven Press, 1984.

10. A. Batchelor and J. Garthwaite. Frequency detection and temporally dispersed synaptic signal association through a metabotropic glutamate receptor pathway. *Nature* 1997; 385:74–77.

Chapter 49   The *Aplysia* Withdraws

1. W. James. *The Principles of Psychology*, vol 2. 2. New York, Holt, 1918, 369.

2. C. Bailey and E. Kandel. Molecular approaches to the study of short-term and long-term memory. In *Functions of the Brain*, ed. C. Coen. Oxford, Clarendon Press, 1985, 98–129.

3. R. Thompson, S. Berry, P. Rinaldi, et al. Habituation and the orienting reflex: The dual-process theory revisited. In *The Orienting Reflex in Humans*, eds. H. Kimmel, E. VanOlst, and J. Orlebeke. Hillsdale, N.J., Erlbaum, 1979, 21–60. The two processes may even coexist. When they do, the resultant response becomes a vector which combines the two. Sensitization leads; its early increased response is followed by a slow decrease.

4. H. Ursin, K. Wester, and R. Ursin. Habituation to electrical stimulation of the brain in unanesthetized cats. Electroencephalography and Clinical Neurophysiology 1967; 23:41–49.

5. K. Wester. Sensitization and habituation of the intracerebrally evoked orienting response. *Physiology and Behavior* 1972; 9:643–647.

6. M. Davis. Habituation and sensitization of a startle-like response elicited by electrical stimulation at different points in the acoustic startle circuit. In *Sensory Functions,* eds. E. Grastyan, and P. Molnar. *Advances in Physiology and Science,* vol 16. Budapest, Pergamon, 1981, 67–78.

7. J. Wright and M. Craggs. Arousal and intracranial self-stimulation in split-brain monkeys. *Experimental Neurology* 1977; 55:295–303.

8. K. Wester, T. Sagvolden, S. Saunders, et al. Habituation characteristics and reinforcing effects of brainstem stimulation in unanesthetized cats. *Brain Research* 1977; 79:363–374.

9. K. Pribram. The orienting reaction: Key to brain representational mechanisms. In *The Orienting Reflex in Humans,* eds. H. Kimmel, E. VanOlst, and J. Orlebeck, Hillsdale, N.J., Erlbaum, 1979, 3–20.

10. L. Johnson, R. Townsend, and M. Wilson. Habituation during sleeping and waking. *Psychophysiology* 1975; 12:574–584.

11. J. O'Gorman. Individual differences in habituation of human physiological responses: A review of theory, method, and findings in the study of personality correlates in non-clinical populations. *Biological Psychology* 1977; 5:257–318. The indices of arousal include the EEG, skin conductance responses, heart rate responses, and plethysmographic measurements of how much blood flows to the fingers.

12. L. Johnson and A. Lubin. The orienting reflex during waking and sleeping. *Electroencephalography and Clinical Neurophysiology* 1967; 22:11–21.

13. During heightened arousal, a human subject's vasomotor responses do habituate more rapidly if they are tested by using a plethysmograph. However, arousal *slows* the rate of habituation if skin conductance is measured. See B. Goldwater. Effects of arousal on habituation of electrodermal vs. vasomotor responses. *Psychophysiology* 1987; 24:2; 142–150.

14. See chapter 24 for other considerations of the issues.

Chapter 50   Matters of Taste

1. J. Thurber, in A. Adams, ed., *The Home Book of Humorous Quotations.* New York, Dodd, Mead, 1969, 41.

2. M. Carpenter. *Human Neuroanatomy,* 7th ed. Baltimore, Williams & Wilkins, 1976.

3. K. Berkley and S. Scofield. Relays from the spinal cord and solitary nucleus through the parabrachial nucleus to the forebrain in the cat. *Brain Research* 1990; 529:333–338.

4. S. Ivanova and J. Bures. Acquisition of conditioned taste aversion in rats is prevented by tetrodotoxin blockade of a small midbrain region centered around the parabrachial nuclei. *Physiology and Behavior* 1990; 48:543–549.

5. K. Touzani and L. Velley. Ibotenic acid lesion of the lateral hypothalamus increases preference and aversion thresholds for saccharin and alters the morphine modulation of taste. *Pharmacology, Biochemistry and Behavior* 1990; 36:585–591.

6. R. Yirmiya, I. Lieblich, and J. Liebeskind. Reduced saccharin preference in CXBK (opioid receptor-deficient) mice. *Brain Research* 438:339–342.

7. J. Dum, C. Gramsch, and A. Herz. Activation of hypothalamic β-endorphin pools by reward induced by highly palatable food. *Pharmacology, Biochemistry and Behavior* 1983; 18:443–447. Chocolate does not change the turnover of dynorphin.

8. K. Touzani, A. Ferssiwi, and L. Velley. Localization of lateral hypothalamic neurons projecting to the medial part of the parabrachial area of the rat. *Neuroscience Letters* 1990; 114:17–21.

9. N. Alessi, P. Quinlan, and H. Khachaturian. MSG effects on β-endorphin and alpha-MSH in the hypothalamus and caudal medulla. *Peptides* 1988; 9:689–695.

10. Y. Oomura and S. Aou. Catecholaminergic, cholinergic, and opioidergic involvement in monkey amygdala during food intake. In *Vision, Memory and the Temporal Lobe,* eds. E. Iwai and M. Mishkin. New York, Elsevier, 1990, 219–244.

11. J. Steiner. Human facial expressions in response to tast and smell stimulation. *Advances in Child Development and Behavior* 1979; 13:257–295.

12. N. Fox and R. Davidson. Taste-elicited changes in facial signs of emotions and the asymmetry of brain electrical activity in human newborns. *Neuropsychologia* 1986; 24:417–422.

Chapter 51   The Mouse in Victory and Defeat

1. H. Longfellow, in *Hoyt's New Cyclopedia of Practical Quotations*. New York, Funk & Wagnalls, 1964, 101.
2. G. Teskey, M. Kavaliers, and M. Hirst. Social conflict activates opioid analgesic and ingestive behaviors in male mice. *Life Sciences* 1984; 35:303–315.
3. M. Kavaliers. Aggression and defeat-induced opioid analgesia displayed by mice are modified by calcium channel antagonists and agonists. *Neuroscience Letters* 1987; 74:107–111.
4. K. Miczek, M. Thompson, and L. Schuster. Analgesia following defeat in an aggressive encounter: Development of tolerance and changes in opioid receptors. In *Stress-Induced Analgesia*, ed. D. Kelly. *Annals of the New York Academy of Sciences* 1986; 467:14–29. The acquired cross-tolerance to morphine lasts up to a week even if the mouse has been defeated only once.
5. K. Miczek and M. Thompson. Analgesia resulting from defeat in a social confrontation: The role of endogenous opioids in brain. In *Modulation of Sensorimotor Activity During Alterations in Behavioral States*, ed. R. Bandler. New York, Liss, 1984, 431–456.
6. L. Miller, M. Thompson, D. Greenblatt, et al. Rapid increase in brain benzodiazepine receptor binding following defeat stress in mice. *Brain Research* 1987; 414:395–400.
7. J. Diaz and M. Asai. Dominant mice show much lower concentrations of methionine-enkephalin in brain tissue than subordinates: Cause or effect? *Behavioural Brain Research* 1990; 39:275–280.
8. Scientists have much to learn from careful studies focused on certain strains of animals that show well-defined behavioral traits. For example, further research might help to clarify whether genetically determined lower baseline enkephalin levels in the basal ganglia would enhance the expression of those motoric patterns which went on to favor more energized, aggressive, and dominating activities.

Chapter 52   The Central Gray: Offense, Defense, and Loss of Pain

1. R. Bandler. Identification of hypothalamic and midbrain periaqueductal grey neurones mediating aggressive and defensive behavior by intracerebral microinjections of excitatory amino acids. In *Modulation of Sensorimotor Activity During Alterations in Behavioral States*, ed. R. Bandler. New York, Liss, 1984, 369–391.
2. J. Flynn. Neural aspects of attack behavior in cats. *Annals of the New York Academy of Sciences* 1969; 159:1008–1012.
3. J. LeDoux. Emotion. Part 1. In *Handbook of Physiology*, Sec. I: *The Nervous System*. Vol. 5, *Higher Functions of the Brain*, eds. V. Mountcastle and F. Plum Bethesda, Md., American Physiological Society, 1987, 415–459.
4. R. Bandler and P. Carrive. Integrated defense reaction elicited by excitatory amino acid microinjection in the midbrain periaqueductal gray region of the unrestrained cat. *Brain Research* 1980; 439:95–106.
5. M. Shaikh, J. Barrett, and A. Siegel. The pathways mediating affective defense and quiet biting attack behavior from the midbrain central gray of the cat. *Brain Research* 1987; 437:9–25. One pathway critical for affective defense runs up from the central gray to the ventral medial hypothalamus and thalamus.
6. C. Pott, S. Kramer, and A. Siegel. Central gray modulation of affective defense is differentially sensitive to naloxone. *Physiology and Behavior* 1987; 40:207–213.
7. M. Millan, A. Czlonkowski, M. Millon, et al. Activation of periaqueductal grey pools of β-endorphin by analgetic electrical stimulation in freely moving rats. *Brain Research* 1987; 407:199–203.
8. Q.-P. Ma, Y.-S. Shi, and J.-S. Han. Naloxone blocks opioid peptide release in accumbens and amygdala elicited by morphine injected into periaqueductal gray. *Brain Research Bulletin* 1992; 28:351–354.

9. I am mindful of, and sympathetic with, the acute discomfort many persons feel when they read about humans causing pain. The references cited in this book, reflecting the information available on library shelves all over the world, report the techniques used to produce (and study) suffering in humans and animals. There, one can also read countless articles which detail the other methods researchers use to produce cancer, heart disease, etc. It can be appreciated that the goal is not merely to describe, but to create, with the intent ultimately to relieve. No researcher can condone unnecessary suffering. But if one takes the long view of Buddhism itself, it becomes clear that we must understand the root causes of suffering if we are ultimately to relieve suffering in all its forms.

10. P. Schmitt, G. DiScala, F. Jenck, et al. Periventricular structures, Elaboration of aversive effects and processing of sensory information. In *Modulation of Sensorimotor Activity During Alterations in Behavioral States*, ed. R. Bandler. New York, Liss, 1984, 393–414.

11. F. Graeff, M. Brandao, E. Audi, et al. Modulation of the brain aversive system by gabaergic and serotonergic systems. *Behavioural Brain Research* 1986; 22:173–180.

12. F. Jenck, P. Schmitt, and P. Karli. Morphine Injected into the periaqueductal gray attenuates brain stimulation–induced effects: An intensity discrimination study. *Brain Research* 178:274–284.

13. B. Nashold, N. Wilson, and G. Slaughter. Sensations evoked by stimulation in the midbrain of man. *Journal of Neurosurgery* 1969; 30:14–24.

14. J. Moreau and H. Fields. Evidence for GABA involvement in midbrain control of medullary neurons that modulate nociceptive transmission. *Brain Research* 1986; 397:37–46. When opioids are injected into the rostral dorsal central gray, they appear to inhibit a system which *ascends* from there. This system normally promotes aversive escape behavior in response to stimulation of the brain itself. In contrast, microinjections of opioids into the ventral-caudal part of the central gray appear to dampen the responses to other painful stimuli coming in from the periphery. Here, opioids activate another system, one which then *descends* to dampen pain transmission at lower levels within the spinal cord.

15. A. Beitz, J. Clements, M. Mullett, et al. Differential origin of brainstem serotonergic projections to the midbrain periaqueductal gray and superior colliculus of the rat. *Journal of Comparative Neurology* 1986; 250:498–509. The ventral part of the central gray receives its serotonin input mainly from the raphe magnus nucleus. Dorsal regions receive their ST input from other raphe nuclei.

16. M. Moss, E. Glazer, and A. Basbaum. The peptidergic organization of the cat periaqueductal gray. I. The distribution of immunoreactive enkephalin-containing neurons and terminals. *Journal of Neuroscience* 1983; 3:603–616.

17. A. Depaulis, M. Morgan, and J. Liebeskind. GABAergic modulation of the analgesic effect of morphine microinjected in the ventral periaqueductal gray matter of the rat. *Brain Research* 1987; 436:223–228. The sequence involves both local GABA neurons, the disinhibition of still other inhibitor systems, and finally the direct blocking of pain perceptions. See also chapters 80 and 81.

18. R. Ross. Paralysis of downward gaze. *Neurology* 1986; 36:1540–1541.

19. C. Larson. On the relation of PAG neurons to laryngeal and respiratory muscles during vocalization in the monkey. *Brain Research* 552:77–86.

20. F. Skultety. Experimental mutism in dogs. *Archives of Neurology* 1962; 6:235–241.

Chapter 53   The Third Route: Stress Responses within The Brain

1. M. Isshu and R. Sasaki. *The Zen Koan: Its History and Use in Rinzai Zen.* Kyoto, The First Zen Institute of America in Japan, 1965, 40.

2. A. Dunn and N. Kramarcy. Neurochemical responses in stress: Relationships between the hypothalamic-pituitary-adrenal and catecholamine systems. In *Handbook of Psychopharmacology. Drugs, Neurotransmitters and Behavior,* vol. 18. eds. L. Iversen, S. Iversen, and S. Snyder. New York, Plenum Press, 1984, 455–515.

3. J. Logothetis, I. Milonas, and S. Bostantzopoulou. Sleep deprivation as a method of EEG activation. *European Neurology* 1986; 25:suppl. 2:134–140.

4. W. Orr, H. Hoffman, and F. Hegge. Ultradian rhythms in extended performance. *Aerospace Medicine* 1974; 45:995–1000.

5. G. Gilad, V. Gilad, R. Wyatt, et al. Region-selective stress-induced increase of glutamate uptake and release in rat forebrain. *Brain Research* 1990; 525:335–338.

6. G. Curzon, P. Hutson, G. Kennett, et al. Monitoring dopamine metabolism in the brain of the freely moving rat. In *Neurochemical Analysis of the Conscious Brain*, eds. R. Myers and P. Knott. *Annals of the New York Academy of Sciences* 1986; 473:224–238.

7. H. Takayama, K. Mizukawa, Z. Ota, et al. Regional responses of rat brain muscarinic cholinergic receptors to immobilization stress. *Brain Research* 1987; 436:291–295. The increase reflects chiefly an increase in the binding affinity of each receptor for acetylcholine, not an increased number of ACH receptors.

8. S. Antelman and L. Chiodo. Stress: Its effects on interactions among biogenic amines and role in the induction and treatment of disease. In *Handbook of Psychopharmacology, Drugs, Neurotransmitters, and Behavior*, vol. 18, eds. L. Iversen, S. Iversen, and S. Snyder. New York, Plenum Press, 1984, 279–341.

9. M. D'Angio, A. Serrano, J. Rivy, et al. Tail-pinch stress increases extracellular DOPAC levels (as measured by in vivo voltametry) in the rat nucleus accumbens but not frontal cortex: Antagonisms by diazepam and zolpidem. *Brain Research* 409:169–174.

10. W. Fratta, M. Collu, and M. Martellotta. Stress-induced insomnia: Opioid-dopamine interactions. *European Journal of Pharmacology* 1987; 142:437–440.

11. M. Demontis, P. Fadda, and P. Devoto. Sleep deprivation increases dopamine D_1 receptor antagonist [^{3}H] SCH 23390 binding and dopamine-stimulated adenylate cyclase in the rat limbic system. *Neuroscience Letters* 1987; 117:224–227.

12. A. Caggiula, S. Antelman, E. Aul, et al. Prior stress attenuates the analgesic response but sensitizes the corticosterone and cortical dopamine responses to stress 10 days later. *Psychopharmacology* 1989; 99:233–237.

13. S. Antelman, S. Knopf, D. Kocan, et al. One stressful event blocks multiple actions of diazepam for up to at least a month. *Brain Research* 1988; 445:380–385.

14. S. Antelman, A. Caggiula, D. Kocan, et al. One experience with "lower" or "higher" intensity stressors, respectively, enhances or diminishes responsiveness to haloperidol weeks later: Implications for understanding drug variability. *Brain Research* 1991; 566:276–283.

15. H. Anisman. Neurochemical consequences of stress. In *The Expression of Knowledge*, eds. R. Isaacson and N. Spear. New York, Plenum Press, 1982, 291–337.

16. N. Harary and C. Kellogg. The relationship of benzodiazepine binding sites to the norepinephrine projection in the hypothalamus of the adult rat. *Brain Research* 1989; 492:293–299.

17. T. Miyauchi, S. Dworkin, C. Co, et al. Specific effects of punishment on biogenic monoamine turnover in discrete rat brain regions. *Brain Research* 1988; 454:40–50. The raphe nuclei are among the effective sites tested.

18. G. Ixart, G. Barbanel, B. Conte-Devolx, et al. Evidence for basal and stress-induced release of corticotropin releasing factor in the push-pull cannulated median eminence of conscious free-moving rats. *Neuroscience Letters* 1987; 74:85–89. The ether-induced rise of CRF prompts the pituitary into releasing its ACTH. This causes a 20-fold increase in ACTH levels in blood.

19. M. Jones and B. Gillham. Factors involved in the regulation of adrenocorticotropic hormone/β-lipotropic hormone. *Physiological Reviews* 1988; 68:743–818. The precise optimum time for the release of ACTH and β-endorphin into the human brain remains to be determined.

20. S. Leibowitz, S. Diaz, and D. Tempel. Norepinephrine in the paraventricular nucleus stimulates corticosterone release. *Brain Research* 1989; 496:219–227.

21. G. Bishop. Neuromodulatory effects of corticotropin releasing factor on cerebellar Purkinje cells: An *in vivo* study in the cat. *Neuroscience* 1990; 39:251–257.

22. B. Applebaum and S. Holtzman. Stress-induced changes in the analgesic and thermic effects of morphine administered centrally. *Brain Research* 1985; 358:303–308.

23. M. Karteszi, M. Palkovits, J. Kiss, et al. Lack of correlation between hypothalamic serotonin and the ether-induced ACTH secretion in adrenalectomized rats. *Neuroendocrinology* 1981; 32:7–14.

24. G. Telegdy and I. Vermes. Changes induced by stress in activity of the serotoninergic system in limbic brain structures. In *Catecholamines and Stress,* ed. E. Usdin. Oxford, Pergamon Press, 1976, 145–156.

25. B. McEwen and R. Brinton. Neuroendocrine aspects of adaptation. In *Neuropeptides and Brain Function,* eds. E. de Kloet, V. Wiegant, and D. de Wied. Progress in Brain Research, vol. 72. Amsterdam, Elsevier, 1987, 11–26.

26. G. Telegdy and G. Kovacs. Role of monoamines in mediating the action of hormones on learning and memory. In *Brain Mechanisms in Memory and Learning: From the Single Neuron to Man,* ed. M. Brazier. New York, Raven Press, 1979, 249–268.

27. B. McEwen. Stressful experience, brain, and emotions: Developmental, genetic, and hormonal influences. In *The Cognitive Neurosciences,* ed. M. Gazzaniga. Cambridge, Mass., The MIT Press, 1979, 1117–1135.

28. G. Gallup Jr. *Adventures in Immortality.* New York, McGraw-Hill, 1982.

Chapter 54   The Large Visual Brain

1. Chisoku, in A. Adams, ed., *The Home Book of Humorous Quotations.* New York, Dodd, Mead, 1969, 123.

2. A. Ames, in M. Strauss, ed., *Familiar Medical Quotations.* Boston, Little, Brown, 1968, 548.

3. P. Schiller. Input and output specificity of striate cortex. In *Brain Mechanisms and Perceptual Awareness,* eds. O. Pompeiano and C. Ajmone-Marsan. New York, Raven Press, 1981, 21–36.

4. M. Berkley and J. Sprague. The role of the geniculocortical system in spatial vision. In *Analysis of Visual Behavior,* eds. D. Ingle, M. Goodale, and R. Mansfield. Cambridge, Mass., The MIT Press, 1982, 525–547.

5. P. Bishop. Processing of visual information within the retinostriate system. In *Handbook of Neurophysiology.* Sec. 1, *The Nervous System.* Vol. 3, *Sensory Processes,* pt 1. eds. J. Brookhart and V. Mountcastle. Bethesda, Md., American Physiological Society, 1984, 341–424.

6. S. Sherman. Parallel pathways in the cat's geniculocortical system: W- , X- , and Y-cells. In *Changing Concepts of the Nervous System,* eds. A. Morrison and P. Strick. New York, Academic Press, 1982, 337–359.

7. J. Stone. *Parallel Processing in the Visual System.* New York, Plenum Press, 1983.

8. J. Zihl and D. VonCramon. The Contribution of the "second" visual system to directed visual attention in man. *Brain* 1979; 102:835–856.

9. J. Morrison and S. Foote. Noradrenergic and serotonergic innervation of cortical, thalamic and tectal visual structures in Old and New World monkeys. *Journal of Comparative Neurology* 1986; 243:117–138.

10. M. Huerta and J. Harting. Connectional organization of the superior colliculus. *Trends in Neurosciences* 1984; 7:286–289.

11. A. Scheibel. The problem of selective attention: A possible structural substrate. In *Brain Mechanisms and Perceptual Awareness,* eds. O. Pompeiano and C. Ajmone-Marsan. New York, Raven Press, 1981, 319–326.

12. E. Knudsen. Synthesis of a neural map of auditory space in the owl. In *Dynamic Aspects of Neocortical Function,* eds. G. Edelman, W. Gall, and W. Cowan. Wiley, New York, 1984, 375–396.

13. M. Meredith and B. Stein. Visual, auditory, and somatosensory convergence on cells in superior colliculus results in multisensory integration. *Journal of Neurophysiology* 1986; 56:640–662.

14. E. Jones. The anatomy of extrageniculostriate visual mechanisms. In *The Neurosciences: Third Study Program,* eds. F. Schmitt and F. Worden. Cambridge, Mass., The MIT Press, 1974, 215–227.

15. The operation also removes the entire neocortex and hippocampus on the same side. The purpose is to remove the many sources of excitable scar tissue on that side of the brain which had previously caused an uncontrollable seizure disorder. The "blindness" following a left-sided removal occurs in the right halves of vision of each eye. See M. Perenin and M. Jeannerod. Visual function within the hemianopic field following early cerebral hemidecortication in man. I. Spatial localization. *Neuropsychologia* 1978; 16:1–13.

16. G. Celesia, D. Bushnell, S. Toleikis, et al. Cortical blindness and residual vision. *Neurology* 1991; 41:862–869.

17. Taking out the visual cortex also produces a secondary degenerative change in the lateral geniculate nucleus on that same side. However, the operation spares the axons of the second visual system. They still pass directly through the degenerated lateral geniculate, and do not need to pause there for a synaptic relay. This strengthens the evidence that the patients' blind sight abilities do originate in their *second* visual system. See O. Meienberg. Sparing of the temporal crescent in homonymous hemianopia and its significance for visual orientation. *Neuroophthalmology* 1981; 2:129–134; S. Benton, I. Levy, and M. Swash. Vision in the temporal crescent in occipital infarction. *Brain* 1980; 103:83–87.

18. R. DeValois, D. Albrecht, and L. Thorell. Spatial frequency selectivity of cells in macaque visual cortex. *Vision Research* 1982; 22:545–559.

19. R. Tusa. Visual cortex: Multiple areas and multiple functions. In *Changing Concepts of the Nervous System,* eds. A. Morrison and P. Strick. New York, Academic Press, 1982; 235–259.

20. R. DeValois, E. Yund, and N. Hepler. The orientation and direction selectivity of cells in macaque visual cortex. *Vision Research* 1982; 22:531–544.

21. G. Ahlsen, K. Grant, and S. Lindstrom. Monosynaptic excitation of principal cells in the lateral geniculate nucleus by cortifugal fibers. *Brain Research* 1982; 234:454–458.

22. J. Allman, F. Miezin, and E. McGuinness. Direction and velocity-specific responses from beyond the classical receptive field in the middle temporal visual area (MT). *Perception* 1985; 14:105–126. The auditory system also employs inhibitory surrounds. The barn owl's highly developed surround system enables it to shut off an ongoing first sound in its central auditory field and to enhance a second sound, such as a mouse's squeak off at the periphery.

23. D. VanEssen and J. Maunsell. Hierarchical organization and functional streams in the visual cortex. *Trends in Neurosciences* 1983; 6:370–375.

24. C. Gross. Contribution of striate cortex and the superior colliculus to visual function in area MT, the superior temporal polysensory area and inferior temporal cortex. *Neuropsychologia* 1991; 29:497–515.

25. J. Sprague, H. Hughes, and G. Berlucchi. Cortical mechanisms in pattern and form perception. In *Brain Mechanisms and Perceptual Awareness,* eds. O. Pompeiano and C. Ajmone-Marsan. New York, Raven Press, 1981, 107–132.

Chapter 55   Where Is It? The Parietal Lobe Pathway

1. H. Thoreau, *Walden.* 1854; Princeton, N.J., Princeton University Press, 1989.

2. E. DeRenzi. *Disorders of Space, Exploration and Cognition.* New York, Wiley, 1982.

3. M. Mishkin, L. Ungerlieder, and K. Macko. Object vision and spatial vision: Two cortical pathways. *Trends in Neurosciences* 1983; 6:414–417.

4. D. Bellas, R. Novelly, B. Eskenazi, et al. Unilateral displacement in the olfactory sense: A manifestation of the unilateral neglect syndrome. *Cortex* 1988; 24:267–275.

5. "Lobule" means a small lobe. In humans, the inferior parietal lobule includes the angular and supramarginal gyri (areas 39 and 40 of Brodmann) and parts of area 7 as well. Humans and monkeys are not comparable, anatomically. Only in approximation does the parietal lobule of nonhuman primates correspond to the human area 7. Yet the monkey *superior* parietal lobule does tend to correspond with area 5 of the human. See M. Jeannerod. *The Neural and Behavioral Organization of Goal-Directed Movements.* Oxford, Clarendon Press, 1988, 231.

6. Researchers usually use moving stimuli when they test animals for the particular parietal neurons which respond to visual events. These stimuli travel over long distances (100 degrees, for example). Therefore, the results of most animal experiments only hint at the subtleties involved when humans attend to, perceive, and discriminate *stationary* objects located farther away in moving or unmoving space. Readers interested in the complex anatomy and physiology of different areas within the posterior parietal lobe can find these topics reviewed in R. Anderson. Visual and eye movement functions of the posterior parietal cortex. *Annual Review of Neuroscience* 1989; 12:377–403.

7. We do not pay attention to space evenly. We disperse it over a gradient. Patients who damage their right parietotemporal region lose most of their attentiveness at the periphery of their visual space farthest off to their left. (See S. Rapcsak, R. Watson, and K. Heilman. Hemispace-visual field interactions in visual extinction. *Journal of Neurology, Neurosurgery and Psychiatry* 1987; 50:1117–1124.) Curving over this outer edge is a thin temporal crescent of vision. The left crescent enters through the left eye and then relays over to be "seen" by the deep, right, occipital cortex. Pathways yet to be defined connect the right and left crescents with the rest of our attentional circuitry.

8. R. Anderson. Inferior parietal lobule function in spatial perception and visuomotor integration. In *Physiology Sec. 1, The Nervous System*, vol 5. *Higher Functions of the Brain*, pt. 2. Eds. V. Mountcastle and F. Plum. Bethesda, Md., American Physiological Society, 1987, 483–518.

9. B. Motter and V. Mountcastle. The functional properties of the light-sensitive neurons of the posterior parietal cortex studied in waking monkeys: Foveal sparing and opponent vector organization. *Journal of Neuroscience* 1981; 1:3–26.

10. S. Kobayashi, K. Mukuno, S. Ishikawa, et al. Hemispheric lateralization of spatial contrast sensitivity. *Annals of Neurology* 1985; 17:141–145.

11. E. Bisiach and C. Luzzatti. Unilateral neglect of representational space. *Cortex* 1978; 14:129–133.

12. E. Bisiach, C. Luzzatti, and D. Perani. Unilateral neglect, representational schema and consciousness. *Brain* 1979; 102:609–618.

Chapter 56   What Is It? The Temporal Lobe Pathway

1. M. Mishkin, L. Ungerlieder, and K. Macko. Object vision and spatial vision: Two cortical pathways. *Trends in Neurosciences* 1983; 6:414–417.

2. E. Iwai and M. Mishkin, eds. *Vision, Memory and the Temporal Lobe*. New York, Elsevier, 1990.

3. D. VanEssen and J. Maunsell. Hierarchical organization and functional streams in the visual cortex. *Trends in Neurosciences* 1983; 6:370–375.

4. E. Iwai and M. Yukie. Amygdalofugal and amygdalopetal connections with modality-specific visual cortical areas in macaques. *Journal of Comparative Neurology* 1987; 261:362–387.

5. R. Desimone, S. Schein, J. Moran, et al. Contour, color and shape analysis beyond the striate cortex. *Vision Research* 1985; 441–452. For purposes of comparison with the visual field "seen" by a single nerve cell, the horizon stretches 180 degrees from right to left in front of us. Starting from the midpoint of this horizon, it will be 90 degrees to a point directly overhead.

6. D. Braitman. Activity of neurons in monkey posterior temporal cortex during multidimensional visual discrimination tasks. *Brain Research* 1984; 307:17–28.

7. S. Zeki. Representation of colours in the cerebral cortex. *Nature* 1980; 284:412–418.

8. P. Haenny and P. Schiller. State dependent activity in monkey visual cortex. I. Single cell activity in V1 and V4 on visual tasks. *Experimental Brain Research* 1988; 69:225–244.

9. In humans, parts of the fusiform and lingual gyri (see figure 3) appear to serve as the homolog of many of the color functions of V-4 in the monkey. See M. Rizzo, M. Nawrot, R. Blake, et al. A human visual disorder resembling area V4 dysfunction in the monkey. *Neurology* 1992; 42:1175–1180.

10. J. Davidoff. Hemispheric sensitivity differences in the perception of color. *Quarterly Journal of Experimental Psychology* 1976; 28:387–394.

11. J. Doyon and B. Milner. Right temporal-lobe contribution to global visual processing. *Neuropsychologia* 1991; 29:343–360.

12. B. Milner. Right temporal-lobe contribution to visual perception and visual memory. In *Vision, Memory and the Temporal Lobe,* eds. E. Iwai and M. Mishkin. New York, Elsevier, 1990, 43–53.

13. C. Gross, D. Bender, and C. Rocha-Miranda. Visual receptive fields of neurons in inferotemporal cortex of the monkey. *Science* 1969; 166:1303–1306.

14. C. Gross, R. Desimone, T. Albright, et al. Inferior temporal cortex as a visual integration area. In *Cortical Integration,* eds. F. Reinoso-Suarez and C. Ajmone-Marsan, New York, Raven Press, 1984, 291–315.

15. J. Fuster and J. Jervey. Inferotemporal neurons distinguish and retain behaviorally relevant features of visual stimuli. *Science* 1981; 212:952–955.

16. G. Baylis, E. Rolls, and C. Leonard. Functional subdivisions of the temporal lobe neocortex. *Journal of Neuroscience* 1987; 7:330–342.

17. P. Dean. Visual behavior in monkeys with inferotemporal lesions. In *Analysis of Visual Behavior,* eds. D. Ingle, M. Goodale, and R. Mansfield. Cambridge, Mass., The MIT Press, 1982, 587–628.

18. E. Iwai. Visual memory in the temporal lobe of the monkey. *Advances in Neurological Science (Tokyo)* 1988; 32:583–597.

19. Y. Miyashita. Associative representation of the visual long-term memory in the neurons of the primate temporal cortex. In *Vision, Memory and the Temporal Lobe,* eds. E. Iwai and M. Mishkin. New York, Elsevier, 1990, 75–87.

20. B. Jones and M. Mishkin. Limbic lesions and the problems of stimulus-reinforcement associations. *Experimental Neurology* 1972; 36:362–377.

21. D. Perrett, A. Mistlin, and A. Chitty. Visual neurones responsive to faces. *Trends in Neurosciences* 1987; 10:9; 358–364. Several other visual regions participate in the processes of recognizing faces.

22. C. Bruce, R. Desimone, and C. Gross. Both striate cortex and superior colliculus contribute to visual properties of neurons in superior temporal polysensory area of macaque monkey. *Journal of Neurophysiology* 1986; 55:1057–1075.

23. S. Mullen and W. Penfield. Illusions of comparative interpretation and emotion. *Archives of Neurology and Psychiatry* 1959; 81:269–284.

24. H. Suo and D. Linszen. The déjà vu experience: Remembrance of things past? *American Journal of Psychiatry* 1990; 147:1587–1595.

25. G. Fink, H. Markowitsch, M. Reinkemeier, et al. Cerebral representation of one's own past; Neural networks involved in autobiographical memory. *Journal of Neuroscience* 1996; 16:4275–4282.

Chapter 57 What Should I Do About It? The Frontal Lobes

1. R. Emerson. Experience. In *The Complete Writings of Ralph Waldo Emerson. Second Series.* New York, Wise, 1929.

2. S. Batchelor. In G. Rabten, ed., *Echoes of Voidness.* London, Wisdom Publications, 1983, 12–13.

3. J. Droogleaver-Fortuyn. On the neurology of perception. *Clinical Neurology and Neurosurgery* 1979; 81:2; 97–107.

4. H. Edinger, A. Siegel, and R. Troiano. Effect of stimulation of prefrontal cortex and amygdala on diencephalic neurons. *Brain Research* 1975; 97:17–31.

5. F. Lhermitte. Human autonomy and the frontal lobes. Pt 2, Patient behavior in complex and social situations: The "environmental dependency syndrome." *Annals of Neurology* 1986; 19:335–343.

6. M-M. Mesulam. Frontal cortex and behavior. *Annals of Neurology* 1986; 19:320–325.

7. K. Waterman, S. Purves, B. Kosaka, et al. An epileptic syndrome caused by mesial frontal lobe seizure foci. *Neurology* 1987; 37:577–582.

8. M. Verfaellie, D. Bowers, and K. Heilman. Hemispheric asymmetries in mediating intention, but not selective attention. *Neuropsychologia* 1988; 26:521–531.

9. A. Damasio. The frontal lobes. In *Clinical Neuropsychology,* 2nd ed., eds. K. Heilman and E. Valenstein. New York, Oxford University Press. 1985, 339–375.

10. D. Cook and R. Kesner. Caudate nucleus and memory for egocentric localization. *Behavioral and Neural Biology* 1988; 49:332–343.

11. D. Stuss and D. Benson. *The Frontal Lobes.* New York, Raven Press, 1986, 238–249.

12. C. Sem-Jacobsen. Electrical stimulation and self-stimulation in man with chronic implanted electrodes: Interpretation and pitfalls of results. In *Brain-Stimulation Reward,* eds. A. Wanquier and E. Rolls. Amsterdam, North Holland, 1976, 505–520. The stimuli were delivered to the frontal lobe on either the right or left side. It will be important to identify the particular sites in the frontal lobes that sponsor such moods, and to define which pathways are used to convey their impulses to other parts of the brain.

13. For example, it will take years to confirm and to clarify what precisely is implied by the finding that serotonin turnover is normally higher in the right midfrontal cortex. See M. Arato, E. Frecska, D. MacCrimmon, et al. Serotonergic interhemispheric asymmetry: Neurochemical and pharmaco-EEG evidence. *Progress in Neuropsychopharmacology and Biological Psychiatry* 1991; 15:759–764.

14. M. Posner, S. Petersen, P. Fox, et al. Localization of cognitive operations in the human brain. *Science* 1988; 240:1627–1631.

15. R. Knight. Electrophysiology in behavioral neurology. In *Principles of Behavioral Neurology,* ed. M-M. Mesulam, Philadelphia, F. A. Davis, 1985, 327–346. The P-300 potential is discussed further in chapter 64.

16. J. Fuster. *The Prefrontal Cortex,* 2nd ed. New York, Raven Press, 1989, 133.

17. A. Luria. The Human Brain and Conscious Activity. In *Consciousness and Self-Regulation,* vol. 2, eds. G. Schwartz and D. Shapiro. New York, Plenum Press, 1–35.

18. A. Shimamura. Memory and amnesia. *Western Journal of Medicine* 1990; 152:177–178.

19. J. Skinner and G. King. Electrogenesis of event-related slow potentials in the cerebral cortex of conscious animals. In *Rhythmic EEG Activities and Cortical Functioning,* ed. G. Pfurtscheller. Amsterdam, Elsevier, 1980, 21–32.

20. H. Kaneyuki, H. Yokoo, A. Tsuda, et al. Psychological stress increases dopamine turnover selectively in mesoprefrontal dopamine neurons of rats: Reversal by diazepam. *Brain Research* 1991; 557:154–161.

21. Why is it still so difficult, today, to predict the results? Because, in *primates,* a dense dopamine input enters not only the dorsolateral and medial prefrontal regions but also the anterior cingulate region. This means that DA innervates primate cortex in those regions over the front of the brain that are served not only by the medial dorsal but also by the *anterior* thalamic nuclei. (See D. Lewis, S. Foote, M. Goldstein, et al. The dopaminergic innervation of monkey prefrontal cortex: A tyrosine hydroxylase immunohistochemical study. *Brain Research* 1988; 44:225–243.) If researchers stimulate the mediodorsal thalamus itself, it will excite cells in the medial prefrontal cortex. On the other hand, stimulating the ventral tegmental DA area blocks these particular mediofrontal cells from being excited by the mediodorsal thalamus. It also inhibits the spontaneous activity of these frontal cells, and it reduces their firing in response to minimal noxious stimuli.

22. On the other hand, because norepinephrine increases the signal-to-noise ratio, its pattern of effects could be setting the stage for triggering stimuli to activate the prefrontal cortex.[24]. For, in contrast to the results in the dopamine system, locus ceruleus stimulation blocks only the *spontaneous* activity of many prefrontal cells. It does not block the way they fire more in response to noxious stimuli nor does it block their being excited by the mediodorsal thalamus. (See J. Mautz, C. Milla, J. Glowinski, et al. Differential effects of ascending neurons containing dopamine and noradrenaline in the control of spontaneous

activity and of evoked responses in the rat prefrontal cortex. *Neuroscience* 1988; 27:517–526.)

23. T. Brozoski, R. Brown, H. Rosvold, et al. Cognitive defecit caused by regional depletion of dopamine in prefrontal cortex of rhesus monkey. *Science* 1979; 205:929–932.

24. T. Sawaguchi, M. Matsumura, and K. Kubota. Catecholamine effects on neuronal activity related to a delayed response task in monkey prefrontal cortex. *Journal of Neurophysiology* 1990; 63:1385–1400.

25. J. Downes. Impaired extra-dimensional shift performance in medicated and unmedicated Parkinson's disease: Evidence for a specific attentional dysfunction. *Neuropsychologia* 1989; 27:1329–1343.

26. D. Stuss. Disturbance of self-awareness after frontal system damage. In *Awareness of Deficit After Brain Injury,* eds. G. Prigatano and D. Schacter. Oxford, Oxford University Press, 1991, 63–83.

Chapter 58   Ripples in Larger Systems: Laying Down and Retrieving Memories

1. R. Gerard. Physiology and psychiatry. *American Journal of Psychiatry* 1949; 106:161–173.

2. E. Parker and H. Weingartner. Retrograde facilitation of human memory by drugs. In *Memory Consolidation,* eds. H. Weingartner and E. Parker. Hillsdale, N.J., Erlbaum, 1984, 231–251. The biochemical aspects of memory "traces" are beyond the scope of the present inquiry.

3. H. Fujisaki. Outline of the nature and structure of the human memory. In *Integrative Control Functions of the Brain,* vol. 3, ed. M. Ito. Tokyo, Kodansha-Elsevier/North-Holland, 1980, 393–394.

4. L. Squire, N. Cohen, and L. Nadel. The medial temporal region and memory consolidation: A new hypothesis. In *Memory Consolidation,* eds. Weingartner, H. and E. Parker. Hillsdale, N.J. Erlbaum, 1984, 185–210. We can declare a fact. Hence, memory for facts is also termed "declarative memory." Learning a *procedure* has little to do with the medial temporal lobe. Our personal autobiographical memories are also termed "episodic."

5. E. Halgren and C. Wilson. Recall defects produced by after discharges in the human hippocampal formation and amygdala. *Electroencephalography and Clinical Neurophysiology* 1985; 61:375–380.

6. D. VonCramon, N. Hebel, and U. Schuri. A contribution to the anatomical basis of thalamic amnesia. *Brain* 1985; 108:993–1008.

7. M. Kritchevsky, N. Graff-Radford, and A. Damasio. Normal memory after damage to medial thalamus. *Archives of Neurology* 1987; 44:959–962.

8. G. Winocur, S. Oxbury, R. Roberts, et al. Amnesia in a patient with bilateral lesions to the thalamus. *Neuropsychologia* 1984; 22:123–143.

9. J. Eccles. An instruction-selection hypothesis of cerebral learning. In *Cerebral Correlates of Conscious Experience,* eds. P. Buser, and A. Rougeul-Buser. Amsterdam, North-Holland, 1978, 155–175.

10. R. Kesner. A neural system analysis of memory storage and retrieval. *Psychological Bulletin* 1973; 80:177–203. Suppose items are laid down during a state of high arousal. If tested for after only a short delay, we may recall them poorly. Yet, most of these items can still be recalled a long time later. In contrast, items processed during low arousal states tend to stick better, and tend to be recalled a *short* time later. However, they are recalled poorly after a long delay.

11. R. Fisher and G. Landon. On the arousal state–dependent recall of "subconscious" experience: Stateboundness. *British Journal of Psychiatry* 1972; 120:159–172.

12. K. Ho., P. Kileny, D. Paccioretti, et al. Neurologic, audiologic and electrophysiologic sequelae of bilateral temporal lobe lesions. *Archives of Neurology* 1987; 44:982–987.

13. I. Izquierdo. The effect of an exposure to novel and non-novel videotaped material in retrieval in two memory tests. *Neuropsychologia* 1987; 25:995–998. In humans, it is not yet clear how much the natural surges in the release of β-endorphin participate in the processes by which novelty enhances memory.

14. J. Belluzzi and L. Stein. Facilitation of long-term memory by brain endorphins. In *Endogenous Peptides and Learning and Memory Processes* eds. J. Martinez, R. Jensen, and R. Messing. New York, Academic Press, 1981, 291–302. After morphine or enkephalin is injected in *higher* doses in the cerebral ventricles, the rat will then avoid stepping down on an electrified grid where it would otherwise have received a shock. On the other hand, at *lower* opioid dose levels, when doses are given just *after* the training period, the training does not express itself in this highly practical, procedural learning type of behavior.[14] Perhaps (one suggestion goes) the higher opioid dose is acting directly as an agonist on *post*synaptic opioid receptors. In contrast, the low opioid dose might affect *pre*synaptic receptors. In this way, it might inhibit the release of the brain's own endogenous opioids.

15. M. Jones, I. Kilpatrick, O. and Phillipon. Dopamine function in the prefrontal cortex of the rat is sensitive to a reduction of tonic GABA-mediated inhibition in the thalamic mediodorsal nucleus. *Experimental Brain Research* 1988; 69:623–634.

16. As discussed in the next two chapters, a tightened GABA cap from its overlying reticular nucleus acts to hold the medioldorsal nucleus in check. Yet novel or arousing stimuli can block this inhibition from the reticular nucleus.

17. When dopamine alone is supplied, as in parkinsonian patients who are given levo-dopa, the functions which improve fall into the delayed verbal memory category. Immediate memory task performance does not improve. See E. Mohr, G. Fabbrini, S. Ruggieri, et al. Cognitive concomitants of dopamine system stimulation in parkinsonian patients. *Journal of Neurology, Neurosurgery and Psychiatry* 1987; 50:1192–1196.

Chapter 59   The Thalamus

1. H. James, in *The Oxford Dictionary of Quotations*. Oxford, Oxford University Press, 1979, 271. The quotation comes from James' "The Art of Fiction," a chapter in *Partial Portraits*, 1888.

2. A. Walker. *The Primate Thalamus*. Chicago, University of Chicago Press, 1938.

3. E. Jones. *The Thalamus*. New York, Plenum Press, 1985.

4. The thalamus is more than a way station up to cortex. The fine anatomical details of the thalamus define an immense system which could influence, *pre*consciously, the way we feel *and* behave, as well as perceive. Its midline nuclei project to the limbic system. Its more posterior intralaminar nuclei project over to the striatum and back down to the upper brain stem. See M. Steriade. The excitatory-inhibitory response sequence in thalamic and neocortical cells: State-regulated changes and regulatory systems. In *Dynamic Aspects of Neocortical Function,* eds. G. Edelman, W. Gall, W. Cowan. New York, Wiley, 1984, 107–157.

5. D. Paré, M. Steriade, M. Deschenes, et al.: Prolonged enhancement of anterior thalamic synaptic responsiveness by stimulation of a brain-stem cholinergic group. *Journal of Neuroscience* 1990; 10:20–33.

6. E. Jones. Organization of the thalamocortical complex and its relation to sensory processes. In *Handbook of Physiology*. Sec. 1, *The Nervous System*. Vol. 3, *Sensory Processes*, pt. 1, eds. J. Brookhart and V. Mountcastle. Bethesda, American Physiological Society, 1984, 149–212. Taste sensation also ascends from our brain stem to enter its own specific relay nuclei near the other four.

7. Most of the specific sensate messages arising from one side of our head and body are crossed over by the time they arrive in the thalamus. So, too, are the messages that enter from our visual and auditory environment. This means that sensate stimuli from one side of the environment are represented within their respective thalamic nuclei on the opposite side of the brain.

8. J. Bartlett, R. Doty, J. Pecci-Saavedra, et al. Mesencephalic control of lateral geniculate nucleus in primates. III. Modifications with state of alertness. *Experimental Brain Research* 1973; 18:214–224.

9. W. Singer. Control of thalamic transmission by corticofugal and ascending reticular pathways in the visual system. *Physiology Reviews* 1977; 57:386–420.

10. M. Yoshida, M. Sasa, and S. Takaori. Serotonin-mediated inhibition from dorsal raphe nucleus of neurons in dorsal lateral geniculate and thalamic reticular nuclei. *Brain Research* 1984; 290:95–105.

11. A. Oke, R. Keller, I. Medford, et al. Lateralization of norepinephrine in human thalamus. *Science* 1978; 200:1411–1413.

12. J. Morrison and S. Foote. Noradrenergic and serotoninergic innervation of cortical, thalamic, and tectal visual structures in Old and New World monkeys. *Journal of Comparative Neurology* 1986; 243:117–138.

13. T. Sandson, K. Daffner, and P. Carvalho. Frontal lobe dysfunction following infarction of the left-sided medial thalamus. *Archives of Neurology* 1991; 48:1300–1303.

14. L. Glenn, J. Hada, J. Roy, et al. Anterograde tracer and field potential analysis of the neocortical layer I projection from nucleus ventralis medialis of the thalamus in cat. *Neuroscience* 1982; 7:1861–1877.

15. N. Graff-Radford, D. Tranel, G. VanHoesen, et al. Diencephalic amnesia. *Brain* 1990; 113:1–25.

16. H. Jasper. Unspecific thalamocortical relations. In *Handbook of Physiology.* Sec. 1, *Neurophysiology,* vol. 2, ed. J. Field, Washington, D.C., American Physiological Society, 1960, 1307–1321.

17. It has been found that *slow,* repetitive stimulation of the medial thalamus produces spindles and slow-wave sleep, whereas higher frequencies cause arousal. This complicates any notion that recruiting itself must imply either EEG arousal or behavioral arousal. We still do not understand how all the thalamic circuitry translates into human experience.

18. It is a singular anatomical fact that most of our temporal lobe cortex receives *relatively* few large fiber projections coming up from the *specific* thalamic nuclei. Indeed, the temporal cortex used to be called an "athalamic cortex." (See C. Noback and R. Demarest. *The Human Nervous System,* 3rd ed. New York, McGraw-Hill, 1981, 434.) In contrast, at least when looked at under the light microscope, the rest of our sensate cortex is obviously well supplied by major, direct activating projections which rise up to it from the sensory parts of the thalamus.

19. D. Paré, Y. Smith, A. Parent, et al. Projections of brainstem core cholinergic and noncholinergic neurons of cat to intralaminar and reticular thalamic nuclei. *Neuroscience* 1988; 25:69–86.

20. M. Steriade, R. Curro Dossi, and D. Contreras. Electrophysiological properties of intralaminar thalamocortical cells discharging rhythmic (~40 Hz) spike bursts at ~1000 Hz during waking and rapid eye movement sleep. *Neuroscience* 1993; 56:1–9.

21. R. Llinas and H. Ribary. Coherent 40-Hz oscillation characterizes dream state in humans *Proceedings of the National Academy of Sciences of the United States of America* 1993; 90:2078–2081.

Chapter 60   The Reticular Nucleus

1. R. Dingledine and J. Kelly. Brainstem stimulation and the acetylcholine-evoked inhibition of neurones in the feline nucleus reticularis thalami. *Journal of Physiology* 1977; 271:135–154.

2. M. Steriade and P. Wyzinski. Cortically elicited activities in thalamic reticularis neurons. *Brain Research* 1972; 42:514–520.

3. G. Barrionuevo, O. Benoit, and P. Tempier. Evidence for two types of firing pattern during the sleep-waking cycle in the reticular thalamic nucleus of the cat. *Experimental Neurology* 1981; 72:486–501.

4. E. Jones. The thalamus. In *Chemical Neuroanatomy,* ed. P. Emson. New York, Raven Press, 1983, 257–293.

5. M. Steriade, L. Domich, G. Oakson, et al. The deafferented reticular thalamic nucleus generates spindle rhythmicity. *Journal of Neurophysiology* 1987; 57:260–273.

6. K. Kultas-Ilinsky, H. Yi, and I. Ilinsky. Nucleus reticularis thalami input to the anterior thalamic nuclei in the monkey: A light and electron microscopic study. *Neuroscience Letters* 1995; 186:25–28. Physiological studies are required to confirm this point.

7. K. Sano, M. Yoshioka, M. Ogashiwa, et al. Autonomic, somatomotor and electroencephalographic responses upon stimulation of the hypothalamus and rostral brainstem in man. *Confinia Neurologica* 1967; 29:257–261. It is difficult to be certain that electrodes are actually stimulating just the reticular nucleus, so thin is its cap save in the frontal pole. Stimulating unanesthetized patients in what was then considered to be their reticular nucleus was associated with rhythmic, slow, 2- to 3-cps delta activity in all EEG leads, more prominent frontally when the stimulation rates were rapid.

8. F. Crick. Function of the thalamic reticular complex: The searchlight hypothesis. *Proceedings of the National Academy of Sciences of the United States of America* 1984; 81:4586–4590.

9. A. Scheibel. The problem of selective attention: A possible structural substrate. In *Brain Mechanisms and Perceptual Awareness*, eds. O. Pompeiano and C. Ajmone-Marsan. New York, Raven Press, 1981, 319–326.

10. B. Pollin and R. Rokyta. Somatotopic organization of nucleus reticularis thalami in chronic awake cats and monkeys. *Brain Research* 1982; 250:211–221. How can the reticular nucleus make discrete changes in the sensate flow through the thalamus? Each sector sends its GABA fibers back down to inhibit, reciprocally, the same underlying thalamic nucleus which originally sent it collateral messages.

11. C. Yingling and J. Skinner. Selective regulation of thalamic sensory relay nuclei by nucleus reticularis thalami. *Electroencephalography and Clinical Neurophysiology* 1976; 41:476–482.

12. J. Schlag and M. Waszak. Electrophysiological properties of units of the thalamic reticular complex. *Experimental Neurology* 1971; 32:1; 79–97.

13. J. Sharp, M. Gonzales, M. Morton, et al. Decreases of cortical and thalamic glucose metabolism produced by parietal cortex stimulation in the rat. *Brain Research* 1988; 438:357–362.

14. A. Levey, A. Hallanger, and B. Wainer. Cholinergic nucleus basalis neurons may influence the cortex via the thalamus. *Neuroscience Letters* 1987; 74:7–13.

15. M. Steriade, A. Parent, D. Pare, et al. Cholinergic and non-cholinergic neurons of cat basal forebrain project to reticular and mediodorsal thalamic nuclei. *Brain Research* 1987; 408:372–376.

16. C. Yingling. Cognition, action, and mechanisms of EEG asymmetry. In *Rhythmic EEG Activities and Cortical Functioning*, ed. G. Pfurtscheller, Amsterdam, Elsevier, 1980, 79–89.

17. J. Kelly, J. Dodd, and R. Dingledine. Acetylcholine as an excitatory and inhibitory transmitter in the mammalian central nervous system. In *The Cholinergic Synapse*, ed. S. Tucek. Progress in Brain Research, vol. 49. Amsterdam, Elsevier, 1979, 253–266. Acetylcholine acts on its muscarinic receptors to inhibit reticular nucleus cells.

18. D. Pinault and M. Deschenes. Control of 40-Hz firing of reticular thalamic cells by neurotransmitters. *Neuroscience* 1992; 51:259–268.

19. G. Winocur, S. Oxbury, R. Roberts, et al. Amnesia in a patient with bilateral lesions to the thalamus. *Neuropsychologia* 1984; 22:123–143.

20. A very "tight" cap could block all sensation, save for the sense of smell.

21. However, some of these unconscious sensate activities can still participate in such phenomena as blind sight or "deaf hearing."

22. The reticular nucleus is capable, however, of inhibiting the lateral hypothalamus. This inhibition could dampen appetitive reflex functions involved in feeding and other ingestive behaviors. See F. Barone, J.-T. Cheng, and M. Wayner. Reticular thalamic inhibitory input to lateral hypothalamic neurons: A functional and histochemical determination. *Brain Research Bulletin* 1994; 33:575–582.

Chapter 61   The Pulvinar

1. J. Allman, F. Miezin, and E. McGuinness. Direction and velocity-specific responses from beyond the classical receptive field in the middle temporal visual area (MT). *Perception* 1985; 14:105–126.

2. R. Passingham, C. Heywood, and P. Nixon. Reorganization in the human brain as illustrated by the thalamus. *Brain, Behavior and Evolution* 1986; 29:68–76.

3. D. Robinson and S. Peterson. Posterior parietal cortex of the awake monkey: Visual responses and their modulation by behavior. In *Cortical Integration,* eds. F. Reinoso-Suarez and C. Ajmone-Marsan. New York, Raven Press, 1984, 279–290.

4. D. LaBerge and M. Buchsbaum. Positron emission tomographic activity during an attention task. *Journal of Neuroscience* 1990; 10:613–619.

5. D. Amaral. Memory: Anatomical organization of candidate brain regions. In *Handbook of Physiology,* Sec. 1, *The Nervous System,* vol 4, pt. 1. eds. Mountcastle and F. Plum. Bethesda, Md., American Physiological Society, 1987, 211–294.

6. F. Lopes Da Silva, J. Vos, J. Mooibroek, et al. Partial coherence analysis of thalamic and cortical alpha rhythms in dog. A contribution towards a general model of the cortical organization of rhythmic activity. In *Rhythmic EEG Activities and Cortical Functioning,* eds. G. Pfurtscheller, P. Buser, F. Lopes Da Silva, et al. Developments in Neuroscience, vol 10. Amsterdam, Elsevier/North-Holland, 1980.

7. M. Trachtenberg and J. Siegfried. Pulvinar contribution to oculomotor and cortical EEG activities. In *The Pulvinar-LP Complex,* eds. I. Cooper, M. Riklan, and P. Rakic. Springfield, Ill., Thomas, 1974, 118–137.

8. R. Gattass, E. Oswaldo-Cruz, and A. Sousa. Visual receptive fields of units in the pulvinar of cebus monkey. *Brain Research* 1979; 160:413–430.

9. L. Benevento and J. Miller. Visual responses of single neurons in the caudal lateral pulvinar of the macaque monkey. *Journal of Neuroscience* 1981; 1:1268–1278.

10. V. Fosse and F. Fonnum. Biochemical evidence for glutamate and/or aspartate as neurotransmitters in fibers from the visual cortex to the lateral posterior thalamic nucleus (pulvinar) in rats. *Brain Research* 1987; 400:219–224.

11. A. Lysakowski, G. Standage, and L. Benevento. Histochemical and architectomic differentiation of zones of pretectal and collicular inputs to the pulvinar and dorsal lateral geniculate nuclei in the macaque. *Journal of Comparative Neurology* 1986; 250:431–448.

12. M. Steriade, D. Paré, A. Parent, et al. Projections of cholinergic and non-cholinergic neurons of the brainstem core to relay and associational thalamic nuclei in the cat and macaque monkey. *Neuroscience* 1988; 25:47–67.

13. A. Oke, R. Keller, I. Medford, et al. Lateralization of norepinephrine in human thalamus. *Science* 1978; 200:1411–1413. A noteworthy point in reading chapter 94.

14. M. Steriade. The excitatory-inhibitory response sequence in thalamic and neocortical cells: State-regulated changes and regulatory systems. In *Dynamic Aspects of Neocortical Function,* eds. G. Edelman, W. Gall, W. Cowan. Wiley, New York, 1984, 107–157.

15. S. Foote and J. Morrison. Extrathalamic modulation of cortical function. *Annual Review of Neuroscience* 1987; 10:67–95.

16. S. Peterson, D. Robinson, and J. Morris. Contributions of the pulvinar to visual spatial attention. *Neuropsychologia* 1987; 25:97–105.

17. D. Robinson and S. Petersen. The pulvinar and visual salience. *Trends in Neurosciences* 1992; 15:127–132.

Chapter 62   Higher Mechanisms of Attention

1. Daito Kokushi. Final admonitions, quoted in J. Stevens, *The Sword of No-Sword.* Boulder, Colo., Shambhala, 1984, 43.

2. M-M. Mesulam and N. Geschwind. On the possible role of neocortex and its limbic connections in the process of attention and schizophrenia: Clinical cases of inattention in man and experimental anatomy in monkey. *Journal of Psychiatric Research* 1978; 14:249–259.

3. D. LaBerge. Thalamic and cortical mechanisms of attention suggested by recent positron emission tomographic experiments. *Journal of Cognitive Neuroscience* 1990; 2:358–372.

4. R. Cohen, W. Semple, M. Gross, et al. Functional localization of sustained attention: Comparison to sensory stimulation in the absence of instruction. *Neuropsychiatry, Neuropsychology and Behavioral Neurology* 1988; 1:3–20.

5. A. Wilkins, T. Shallice, and R. McCarthy. Frontal lesions and sustained attention. *Neuropsychologia* 1987; 25:359–365.

6. D. Woods and R. Knight. Electrophysiologic evidence of increased distractibility after dorsolateral prefrontal lesions. *Neurology* 1986; 36:212–216.

7. P. Roland. Cortical regulation of selective attention in man. A regional cerebral blood flow study. *Journal of Neurophysiology* 1982; 48:1059–1078.

8. R. Deuel and R. Collins. The functional anatomy of frontal lobe neglect in the monkey: Behavioral and quantitative 2-deoxyglucose studies. *Annals of Neurology* 1984; 15:521–529.

9. S. Nagel-Leiby, H. Buchtel, and K. Welch. Right-frontal and parietal-lobe contributions to the process of directed visual attention and orientation (abstract). *Journal of Clinical and Experimental Neuropsychology* 1987; 9:80.

10. Some studies suggest that, in monkeys, the cortex along both banks of the groove of the superior temporal sulcus can be more critical for directing attention to the opposite side of the environment than is area 7 of the parietal cortex. See R. Watson, E. Valenstein, A. Day, et al. Ablation of area 7 or cortex around the superior temporal sulcus and neglect. *Neurology* 1985; 35(suppl. 1):179.

11. H. Neville and D. Lawson. Attention to central and peripheral visual space in a movement detection task: An event-related potential and behavioral study I. Normal hearing adults. *Brain Research* 1987; 405:253–267.

12. E. Beck, R. Dustman, and M. Sakai. Electrophysiological correlates of selective attention. In *Attention in Neurophysiology,* eds. C. Evans and T. Mulholland. London, Butterworths, 1969, 396–416.

13. M. Verfaellie, D. Bowers, and K. Heilman. Hemispheric asymmetries in mediating intention, but not selective attention. *Neuropsychologia* 1988; 26:521–531.

14. M. Verfaellie and K. Heilman. Hemispheric asymmetries in attentional control: Implications for hand preference in sensorimotor tasks. *Brain and Cognition* 1990; 14:70–80.

15. V. Mountcastle. Functional properties of the light-sensitive neurons of the posterior parietal cortex and their regulation by state controls: Influence on excitability of interested fixation and the angle of gaze. In *Brain Mechanisms and Perceptual Awareness,* eds. O. Pompeiano and C. Ajmone-Marson. New York, Raven Press, 1981, 67–99.

16. V. Mountcastle, B. Motter, M. Steinmetz, et al. Looking and seeing: The visual functions of the parietal lobe. In *Dynamic Aspects of Neocortical Function,* eds. G. Edelman, W. Gall, and W. Cowan. New York, Wiley, 1984, 159–193.

17. M. Bushnell, M. Goldberg, and D. Robinson. Behavioral enhancement of visual responses in monkey cerebral cortex. I Modulation in posterior parietal cortex related to selective visual attention. *Journal of Neurophysiology* 1981; 46:755–772.

18. V. Mountcastle, B. Motter, M. Steinmetz, et al. Common and differential effects of attentive fixation on the excitability of parietal and prestriate (V-4) cortical visual neurons in the macaque monkey. *Journal of Neuroscience* 1987; 7:2239–2255.

19. J. Moran and R. Desimone. Selective attention gates visual processing in the extrastriate cortex. *Science* 1985; 229:782–784.

20. Area PG has a wide variety of connections which can help it set up its "representations." These regions include the primary visual cortex, the deeper superior colliculus, the frontal lobe, the whole cingulate gyrus—especially its posterior part—and the opposite parietal lobe. The monkey's inferior parietal lobule is also "well connected" with the basal forebrain and the lateral hypothalamus. See M. Mesulam. A cortical network for directed attention and unilateral neglect. *Annals of Neurology* 1981; 10:4; 309–325.

21. R. Anderson, G. Essick, and R. Siegel. Encoding of spatial location by posterior parietal neurons. *Science* 1985; 230:456–458.

22. R. Rafal and M. Posner. Deficits in human visual spatial attention following thalamic lesions. *Proceedings of the National Academy of Sciences of the United States of America* 1987; 84:7349–7353.

Chapter 63   Looking and Seeing Preattentively

1. P. Pepe. *The Wit and Wisdom of Yogi Berra.* Westport, Conn., Meckler, 1988, 185.

2. D. Guitton, H. Buchtel, and R. Douglas. Frontal lobe lesions in man cause difficulties in

suppressing reflexive glances and in generating goal-directed saccades. *Experimental Brain Research* 1985; 58:455–472.

3. Many other regions help couple gaze with vision, looking with seeing. They include the supplementary region for eye movements, located over the upper, inner portion of each frontal lobe. See J. Schlag and M. Schlag-Rey. Role of central thalamus and supplementary eye field in voluntary control of gaze in space. *Bulletin of the Tokyo Metropolitan Institute for Neuroscience* 1986, suppl. 17–31.

4. R. Anderson. Inferior parietal lobule function in spatial perception and visuomotor integration. In *Handbook of Physiology*. Sec. 1, *The Nervous System*. Vol. 5, *Higher Functions of the Brain*, pt. 2, eds. V. Mountcastle, and F. Plum. Bethesda, Md. American Physiological Society, 1987, 483–518.

5. R. Jung. Perception, consciousness and visual attention. In *Cerebral Correlates of Conscious Experience*, eds. P. Buser and A. Rougeul-Buser. Amsterdam, North-Holland, 1978, 15–36.

6. D. Broadbent. The hidden preattentive processes. *American Psychologist*, February 1977, 109–118.

7. R. Shiffrin and W. Schneider. Controlled and automatic human information processing: II. Perceptual learning, automatic attending, and a general theory. *Psychological Review* 1977; 84:127–190.

8. S. Hillyard. Electrophysiology of human selective attention. *Trends in Neurosciences* 1985; 8:400–405.

9. B. Julesz. Toward an axiomatic theory of preattentive vision. In *Dynamic Aspects of Neocortical Function*, eds. G. Edelman, W. Gall, and W. Cowan. New York, Wiley, 1984, 585–612.

10. L. Fehmi, J. Adkins, and D. Lindsley. Electrophysiological correlates of visual perceptual masking in monkeys. *Experimental Brain Research*, 1969; 7:299–316.

11. A. Hurlbert and T. Poggio. Spotlight on attention. *Trends in Neurosciences* 1985; 8:309–11.

12. S. Ullman. Visual routines. *Cognition* 1984; 18:97–159.

13. A. Deikman. Bimodal consciousness. *Archives of General Psychiatry* 1971; 25:481–489.

Chapter 64   Laboratory Correlates of Awareness, Attention, Novelty, and Surprise

1. N. Hawthorne, from *The House of the Seven Gables*, in ed. L. Roberts, *Hoyt's New Cyclopedia of Practical Quotations*. New York, Funk & Wagnalls, 1940, 218.

2. K. Nagata, K. Fukushima, J. Nunomura, et al. Functional anatomy of human central auditory system: Cerebral blood flow responses to verbal and non-verbal auditory atimulation. *Neurosciences* 1990; 16:225–230.

3. R. Cohen, W. Semple, M. Gross, et al. Functional localization of sustained attention: Comparison to sensory stimulation in the absence of instruction. *Neuropsychiatry, Neuropsychology and Behavioral Neurology* 1988; 1:3–20. The tone was presented at sixty-seven, seventy-five, or eighty-six decibels.

4. H. Herzog, V. Lele, T. Kuwert, et al. Changed pattern of regional glucose metabolism during yoga meditative relaxation. *Neuropsychobiology* 1990–91; 23:182–187.

5. R. Knight. Electrophysiology in Behavioral Neurology. In *Principles of Behavioral Neurology*, ed. M. Mesulam. Philadelphia, F.A. Davis, 1985, 327–346.

6. M. Brazier. Responses in non-specific systems as studied by averaging techniques. In *Brain Mechanisms*, eds. G. Moruzzi, A. Fessard, and H. Jasper. Amsterdam, Elsevier, 1963, 349–366. The intralaminar nucleus cited is the central median nucleus.

7. M. Oakley and R. Eason. Subcortical gating in the human visual system during spatial selective attention. *International Journal of Psychophysiology* 1990; 9:105–120.

8. In cats, the amount of acetylcholine input that arrives in the hippocampus helps determine the P-300 potential. See J. Harrison, J. Buchwald, K. Kaga, et al. "Cat P300" disappears after septal lesions. *Electroencephalography and Clinical Neurophysiology* 1988; 69:55–64.

9. Late potentials are given the name *endogenous*. This term serves to indicate that late potentials are more an index of the properties of the brain itself than of the stimulus. A negative wave, the N-200, frequently comes just before the P-300 wave and forms with it an

N-200–P-300 complex. See U. Okada, L. Kaufman, and S. Williamson. The hippocampal formation as a source of the slow endogenous potentials. *Electroencephalography and Clinical Neurophysiology* 1983; 55:417–426; R. Neshige and H. Luders. Identification of a negative bitemporal component (N300) of the event-related potentials demonstrated by noncephalic recordings. *Neurology* 1988; 38:1803–1805.

10. M. Onofrj, T. Fulgente, D. Nobilio, et al. P3 recordings in patients with bilateral temporal lobe lesions. *Neurology* 1992; 42:1762–1767.

11. For the sake of this supposition, assume also that you have become a meditator thoroughly adapted to whatever experimental conditions you have been placed in.

Chapter 65   Biological Theories: What Causes Mystical Experiences? How Does Meditation Act?

1. E. Gelhorn. The emotions and the ergotropic and trophotropic systems. *Psycholische Forschung* 1970; 34:48–94.
2. R. Isaacson. Neural systems of the limbic brain and behavioral inhibition. In *Inhibition and Learning*, eds. R. Boakes and M. Halliday. London, Academic Press, 1972, 497–528.
3. E. Gelhorn and W. Kiely. Mystical states of consciousness: Neurophysiological and clinical aspects. *Journal of Nervous and Mental Disease* 1972; 154:399–405.
4. G. Mills and K. Cambell. A critique of Gelhorn and Kiely's Mystical States of Consciousness. *Journal of Nervous and Mental Disease* 1974; 159:191–195.
5. W. Kiely. Critique of Mystical States: A reply. *Journal of Nervous and Mental Disease* 1974; 159:196–197.
6. R. Fischer. Cartography of inner space. In *Hallucinations, Behavior, Experience, and Theory*, eds. R. Siegel and L. West. New York, Wiley, 1975, 197–239.
7. J. Davidson. The physiology of meditation and mystical states of consciousness. *Perspectives in Biology and Medicine* 1976; 19:345–379.
8. A. Mandel. Toward a psychobiology of transcendence: God in the brain. In *The Psychobiology of Consciousness*, eds. J. Davidson and R. Davidson. New York, Plenum Press, 1980, 379–464.
9. *Ibid.*, 432.
10. D. Shapiro. *Meditation: Self-Regulation Strategy and Altered State of Consciousness*. New York, Aldine, 1980, 229–230.
11. B. Russell, from Skeptical Essays, in G. Seldes, ed., *The Great Quotations*, New York, Pocket Books, 296.
12. WW Website: http://www.wrcc.sage.dri.edu/longrang.html
13. One recent set of theories just arrived (too late to insert into page proofs) that will benefit from being submitted to functional MRI testing. See E. d'Aquili and A. Newberg. Religious and mystical states: a neuropsychological model. *Zygon* 1993; 28:177–199.

Chapter 66   Problems with Words: "Mind"

1. Lewis Carroll, *Through the Looking Glass.*
2. Shakespeare, *Romeo and Juliet.*
3. T. Leggett. *Zen and the Ways.* Boulder, Colo., Shambhala, 1978.
4. J. Eccles. A critical appraisal of mind-brain theories. In *Cerebral Correlates of Conscious Experience*, eds. P. Buser and P. A. Rougeul-Buser. Amsterdam, North-Holland, 1978, 347–355.
5. T. Hoover. *The Zen Experience.* New York, New American Library, 1980, 64.
6. W. James. *The Varieties of Religious Experience.* New York, Longmans, Green, 1925, 31.

Chapter 67   Ordinary Forms of Conscious Awareness

1. G. Ehrensvard. In *Scientific Quotations: The Harvest of a Quiet Eye*, ed. M. Ebison. New York, Crane, Russak, 1977, 50.
2. P. Gloor. Consciousness as a neurological concept in epileptology: A critical review. *Epilepsia* 1986; 27(suppl. 2): 14–26.
3. R. Blacher. Awareness during surgery. *Anesthesiology* 1984; 61:1–2.

4. C. Marsh. A framework for describing subjective states of consciousness. In *Alternate States of Consciousness*, ed. N. Zinberg. New York, Free Press, 1977, 121–144.

5. D. Lehmann, H. Ozaki, and I. Pal. EEG alpha map series: Brain micro-states by space-oriented adaptive segmentation. *Electroencephalography and Clinical Neurophysiology* 1987; 67:271–288.

6. B. Libet. Timing of cerebral processes relative to concomitant conscious experiences in man. In *Brain and Behavior*, eds. G. Adam, I. Meszaros, and E. Banyai. Advances in Physiological Science, vol 17. Budapest, Pergamon, 1981, 313–317.

7. O. Simon, H. Schulz, W. Rassman. The definition of waking stages on the basis of continuous polygraphic recordings in normal subjects. *Electroencephalography and Clinical Neurophysiology* 1977; 42:48–56.

8. E. Walker. Consciousness and quantum theory. In *Psychic Exploration, a Challenge for Science*, ed. E. Mitchell. New York, Capricorn, Putnam's, 1976, 544–568.

9. R. Penrose. "Shadows of the mind," a preview and interview. *Journal of Consciousness Studies* 1994; 1:17–24.

Chapter 68 Variations on the Theme of Consciousness

1. Mikhail Gorbachev, quoted in: *Denver Post*, 4 May, 1992.

2. S. Krippner. Altered states of consciousness. In *The Highest State of Consciousness*, ed. J. White. Garden City, N.Y., Anchor/Doubleday, 1972, 1–5.

3. To keep the tables simple, the present outline expands on various aspects of meditation in part II, and treats "quickenings" as important enough to consider in part V. Here they will be viewed as fragments, preludes, and incomplete expressions of other states. The tables do not include those ordinary, relatively common moments of clear awareness and of lesser insights which also take place both inside and outside the meditative period. Nor do we include here prolonged states of rapturous ecstasy, atypical varieties of experience, or others which fall outside the mainstream of conventional Zen experience.

4. D. Shapiro. *Meditation: Self-Regulation Strategy and Altered State of Consciousness*. New York, Aldine, 1980.

5. D. Keifer. Intermeditation notes: Reports from inner space. In *Frontiers of Consciousness*, ed. J. White. New York, Julian Press, 1985, 1138–1153.

Chapter 69 Alternate States of Consciousness: Avenues of Entry

1. C. Tart. A systems approach to altered states of consciousness. In *The Psychobiology of Consciousness*, eds. J. Davidson and R. Davidson. New York, Plenum Press, 1980, 243–269.

2. C. Tart. States of consciousness and state specific sciences. *Science* 1972; 176:1203–1210.

3. C. Tart. *States of Consciousness*. New York, Dutton, 1975.

4. C. Tart. Putting the pieces together: A conceptual framework for understanding discrete states of consciousness. In *Alternate States of Consciousness*, ed. N. Zinberg. New York, Free Press, 1977, 158–219.

5. N. Zinberg. The study of consciousness states, problems and progress. In *Alternate States of Consciousness*, ed. N. Zinberg. New York, Free Press, 1977, 1–36.

6. J. Silverman. On the sensory bases of transcendental states of consciousness. In *Psychiatry and Mysticism*, ed. S. Dean. Chicago, Nelson-Hall, 1975, 365–398.

7. A. Ludwig. Altered states of consciousness. *Archives of General Psychiatry* 1966; 15:225–234.

8. A. Ludwig and W. Lyle. Tension induction and the hyperalert trance. *Journal of Abnormal Psychology* 1964; 69:70–76.

Chapter 70 The Architecture of Sleep

1. W. Dement and M. Mitler. An introduction to sleep. In *Basic Sleep Mechanisms*, eds. O. Petre-Quadens and J. Schlage. New York, Academic Press, 1974, 271–296.

2. R. McCarley. Mechanisms and models of behavioral state control. Chairman's overview of part V. In *The Reticular Formation Revisited*, eds. J. Hobson and M. Brazier. International Brain Research Organization Monograph Series, vol 6. New York, Raven Press, 1980, 375–403.

3. D. Welch, G. Richardson, and W. Dement. A circadian rhythm of hippocampal theta activity in the mouse. *Physiology and Behavior* 1985; 35:533–538.

4. D. Foulkes and G. Vogel. Mental activity at sleep onset. *Journal of Abnormal Psychology* 1965; 70:231–243. These dream reports are low in actual content.

5. W. Zimmerman. Sleep mentation and auditory awakening thresholds. *Psychophysiology* 1970; 6:540–549.

6. J. Santamaria and K. Chiappa. *The EEG of Drowsiness.* New York, Demos, 1987.

7. T. Budzynski. Clinical applications of non–drug-induced states. In *Handbook of States of Consciousness,* eds. B. Wolman and M. Ullman. New York, Van Nostrand Reinhold, 1986, 428–460.

8. M. Steriade, N. Ropert, A. Kitsikis, et al. Ascending activating neuronal networks in midbrain reticular core and related rostral systems. In *The Reticular Formation Revisited,* eds. J. Hobson and M. Brazier. International Brain Research Organization Monograph Series, vol. 6. New York, Raven Press, 1980, 125–167.

9. M. Steriade, K. Sakai, and M. Jouvet. Bulbo-thalamic neurons related to thalamo-cortical activation processes during paradoxical sleep. *Experimental Brain Research* 1984; 54:463–475.

10. M. Jouvet. Neurophysiology of the states of sleep. In *The Neurosciences. A Study Program,* eds. G. Quarton, T. Melnechuck, and F. Schmitt. New York, Rockefeller University Press, 1967, 529–544.

11. P. Ramm and B. Frost. Cerebral and local cerebral metabolism in the cat during slow wave and REM sleep. *Brain Research* 1986; 365:112–124.

12. W. Hess. The sleep syndrome as elicited by diencephalic stimulation. In *Biological Order and Brain Organization. Selected Works of W. R. Hess,* ed. K. Abert. Berlin, Springer-Verlag, 1981, 131–169.

13. Messages from the nearby suprachiasmatic nucleus of the hypothalamus are modulated there by melatonin, a byproduct of serotonin. They then go on to influence the normal sleep-waking rhythms generated up in the basal forebrain. See Y. Hanada and H. Kawamura. Sleep-waking electrocorticographic rhythms in chronic cerveau isolé rats. *Physiology and Behavior* 1981; 26:725–728.

14. P. Dell and J.-J. Puizillout. Experimental reflex narcolepsy in the cat. In *Narcolepsy,* vol 3, eds. C. Guilleminault, W. Dement, and P. Passonaut. New York, Spectrum, 1976, 451–472.

15. W. Koella. The central nervous control of sleep. In *The Hypothalamus,* eds. W. Haymaker, E. Anderson, and W. Nauta. Springfield, Ill., Thomas, 1969, 622–644. In general, it is assumed that lower frequency stimuli may be more "physiological."

16. M. Sterman and M. Shouse. Sleep "centers" in the brain: The preoptic basal forebrain area revisited. In *Brain Mechanisms of Sleep,* eds. D. McGinty, R. Drucker-Colin, A. Morrison, et al. New York, Raven Press, 1985, 277–299.

17. R. Szymusiak and D. McGinty. Sleep-waking discharge of basal forebrain projection neurons in cats. *Brain Research Bulletin* 1989; 224:423–430.

18. D. Schneider-Helmert and G. Schoenenberger. Effects of DSIP in man. *Neuropsychobiology* 1983; 9:197–206.

19. S. Feldman and A. Kastin. Localization of neurons containing immunoreactive delta sleep-inducing peptide in the rat brain: An immunocytochemical study. *Neuroscience* 1984; 11:303–317.

20. W. Koella. Organization of Sleep. In *Brain Mechanisms of Sleep,* eds. D. McGinty, R. Drucker-Colin, A. Morrison, et al. New York, Raven Press, 1985, 399–426.

21. G. Benedek, F. Obal, F. Bari, et al. The effect of atropine on the hypnogenic action of basal forebrain stimulation. In *Sleep 1980,* ed. W. Koella. Basel, Karger, 1981. Electrical stimulation is effective at high or low frequencies.

22. F. Bremer. Existence of a mutual tonic inhibitory interaction between the pre-optic hypnogenic structure and the midbrain reticular formation. *Brain Research* 1975; 96:71–75.

23. C. Gottesmann. What the cerveau isolé preparation tells us nowadays about sleep-wake mechanisms. *Neuroscience and Biobehavioral Reviews* 1988; 12:39–48. Because the forebrain

has been "isolated" surgically, its hemispheres and basal nuclei having been detached from the stalklike brain stem, the result is called the *cerveau isolé*. It will be especially important to study the W→S and S→D transition periods in primates. We need to determine what turns on and off, not only the sensate block but also the other inhibitions which the reticular nucleus imposes on the many other nuclei of the thalamus.

Chapter 71   Desynchronized Sleep

1. Franklin P. Adams, in A. Adams ed., *The Handbook of Humorous Quotations*, New York, Dodd, Mead, 1969, 94.

2. R. Vertes. Brainstem control of the events of REM sleep. *Progress in Neurobiology* 22:241–288.

3. R. Llinás and D. Paré. Of dreaming and wakefulness. *Neuroscience* 1991; 44:521–535. But as chapter 70 explains, fundamental differences also exist. For example, during waking consciousness, our brain has ready access to a set of outside stimuli from an *actual* apple—conveying information about its shape, color, smell, and context. For a recent review of how biogenic amines and coherent neuronal oscillations contribute to "binding" these stimuli together into one enlivened percept, see D. Kahn, E. Pace-Schott, and J. Hobson. Consciousness in waking and dreaming: The roles of neuronal oscillation and neuromodulation in determining similarities and differences. *Neuroscience* 1997; 78:13–38.

4. M. Steriade, K. Sakai, and M. Jouvet. Bulbo-thalamic neurons related to thalamo-cortical activation processes during paradoxical sleep. *Experimental Brain Research* 1984; 54:463–475.

5. M. Chase. The motor functions of the reticular formation are multifaceted and state-determined. In *The Reticular Formation Revisited*, eds. J. Hobson and M. Brazier. International Brain Research Organization Monograph Series, vol 6. New York, Raven Press, 1980, 449–472.

6. The brief muscle twitches during D-sleep come from the lower end of the pons and from some giant cells in the reticular formation. D-sleep also shows variations in blood pressure, pulse rate, and breathing, plus other widely distributed activating waves (called ponto-geniculo occipital [PGO] waves in animals). These several phenomena arise from other circuitries still more laterally placed in the pons.[2]

7. R. Drucker-Colin, R. Aguilar-Roblero, and G. Arankowsky-Sandoval. Sleep factors released from brain of unrestrained cats: A critical appraisal. In *Neurochemical Analysis of the Conscious Brain*, eds. R. Myers and P. Knott. *Annals of the New York Academy of Sciences* 1986; 473:449–460.

8. N. Sitaram, W. Mendelson, R. Wyatt, et al. The time-dependent induction of REM sleep and arousal by physostigmine infusion during normal human sleep. *Brain Research* 1977; 122:562–567.

9. M. Trulson and T. Crisp. Tolerance develops to LSD while the drug is exerting its maximal behavioral effects: Implications for the neural bases of tolerance. *European Journal of Pharmacology* 1983; 96:317–320.

10. O. Pompeiano. Mechanisms of sensorimotor integration during sleep. In *Progress in Physiological Psychology*, vol 3, eds. E. Stellar and J. Sprague. New York, Academic Press, 1970, 1–179.

11. W. Goff, T. Allison, A. Shapiro, et al. Cerebral somatosensory responses evoked during sleep in man. *Electroencephalography and Clinical Neurophysiology* 1966; 21:1–9.

12. J. Hobson and R. McCarley. The brain as a dream-state generator: An activation-synthesis hypothesis of the dream process. *American Journal of Psychology* 1977; 134:1335–1346.

13. M. Steriade, A. Kitsikis, and G. Oakson. Selectively REM-related increased firing rates of cortical association interneurons during sleep: Possible implications for learning. In *Brain Mechanisms in Memory and Learning: From the Single Neuron to Man*, ed. M. Brazier. New York, Raven Press, 1979, 47–52.

14. P. Ramm and B. Frost. Cerebral and local cerebral metabolism in the cat during slow wave and REM sleep. *Brain Research* 1986; 365:112–124. Further metabolic and physiologi-

cal studies in primates could help determine how active the pulvinar remains during brief transitional states.

15. R. Lydic, H. Baghdoyan, L. Hibbard, et al. Regional brain glucose metabolism is altered during rapid eye movement sleep in the cat: A preliminary study. *Journal of Comparative Neurology* 1991; 304:517–520.

16. E. Clarke. *Visions, A Study of False Sight*. Cambridge, Mass., Houghton, Osgood, The Riverside Press, 1980.

17. J. Meyer, Y. Ishikawa, T. Hata, et al. Cerebral blood flow in normal and abnormal sleep and dreaming. *Brain and Cognition* 1987; 6:266–294. Recent PET studies show that the anterior cingulate gyrus is frequently activated, whereas asymmetrical contributions arise from regions such as the right parietal operculum and the left amygdaloid complex. See P. Maquet, J.-M. Peters, J. Aerts, et al. Functional neuroanatomy of human rapid-eye-movement sleep and dreaming. *Nature* 1996; 383:163–166.

18. P. Parmeggiani. Homeostatic regulation during sleep: Facts and hypotheses. In *Brain Mechanisms of Sleep*, eds. D. McGinty, R. Drucker-Colin, E. Morrison, et al. New York, Raven Press, 1985, 385–397. Trends toward vasodilation of similar origin may play a role in the phenomena of skin warming reported in Tibetan meditative traditions.

19. M. Steriade, N. Ropert, A. Kitsikis, et al. Ascending activating neuronal networks in midbrain reticular core and related rostral systems. In *The Reticular Formation Revisited*, eds. J. Hobson and M. Brazier. International Brain Research Organization Monograph Series, vol. 6. New York, Raven Press, 1980, 125–167. In humans, the EEG recorded from scalp electrodes shows only a relatively unimpressive mixture of frequencies, at lower voltages, during D-sleep.

20. M. Steriade. Mechanisms underlying cortical activation: Neuronal organization and properties of midbrain reticular core and intralaminar thalamic nuclei. In *Brain Mechanisms and Perceptual Awareness*, O. Pompeiano and C. Ajmone-Marsan. New York, Raven Press, 1981, 327–377.

21. L. Glenn, J. Hada, J. Roy, et al. Anterograde tracer and field potential analysis of the neocortical layer. I. Projection from nucleus ventralis medialis of the thalamus in cat. *Neuroscience* 1982; 7:1861–1877.

22. One other, lower, pathway remains through which fibers from the large acetylcholine cells of the medulla could also activate the cortex. It relays through the zona incerta, to the posterior hypothalamus, and thence on up to cortex. Other activating pathways can also influence the cortex indirectly. Those from the midbrain can relay through the basal forebrain, and proceed through circuits which modulate the activity of both the reticular and mediodorsal thalamic nuclei. See M. Steriade, A. Parent, D. Paré, et al. Cholinergic and non-cholinergic neurons of cat basal forebrain project to reticular and mediodorsal thalamic nuclei. *Brain Research* 1987; 408:372–376.

23. A. Rosina and M. Mancia. Electrophysiological and behavioral changes following selective and reversible inactivation of lower brain-stem structures in chronic cats. *Electroencephalography and Clinical Neurophysiology* 1966; 21:157–167.

24. O. Petre-Quadens and J. Schlag, eds. *Basic Sleep Mechanisms*. New York, Academic Press, 1974.

25. W. Koella, ed. *Sleep. Circadian Rhythms, Dreams, Noise and Sleep Neurophysiology, Therapy.* Basel, Karger, 1980.

26. G. Vogel. Mentation reported from naps of narcoleptics. In *Narcolepsy*, eds. C. Guilleminault and P. Passouant. Advances in Sleep Research, vol 3. New York, Spectrum, 1976, 161–168.

27. E. Weitzman, C. Czeisler, J. Zimmerman, et al. Biological rhythms in man: Relationship of sleep-wake, cortisol, growth hormone, and temperature during temporal isolation. *Advances in Biochemical Psychopharmacology* 1981; 28:475–499.

28. J. Muzio, H. Roffwarg, and E. Kaufman. Alterations in the nocturnal sleep cycle resulting from LSD. *Electroencephalography and Clinical Neurophysiology* 1966; 21:313–324.

29. H. Schulz and R. Lund. On the origin of early REM episodes in the sleep of depressed patients: A comparison of three hypotheses. *Psychiatric Research* 1985; 16:65–77.

30. Various other techniques promote more and longer REM episodes. They include (a) rocking movements which first stimulate the vestibular system and then increase the firing of the reticular activating system; (b) noises or touching the skin of the neck; and (c) a high carbohydrate supper. For (a) see O. Pompeiano. The generation of rhythmic discharges during bursts of REM. In *Abnormal Neuronal Discharges,* eds. N. Chalazontic and M. Boisson. New York, Raven Press, 1978, 75–89.); for (b) see G. Arankowsky-Sandoval, R. Aguilar-Roblero, O. Prospero-Garcia, et al. Rapid eye movement (REM) sleep and ponto-geniculo-occipital (PGO) spike density are increased by somatic stimulation. *Brain Research* 1987; 400:155–158.); for (c) see F. Phillips, C. Chen, A. Crisp, et al. Isocaloric diet changes and electroencephalographic sleep. *Lancet* 1975; 2:723–725.

31. M. deBarros-Ferreira and G. Lairy. Ambiguous sleep in narcolepsy. In *Narcolepsy,* eds. C. Guilleminault, W. Dement, and P. Passouant. Advances in Sleep Research, vol 3. New York, Spectrum, 1976, 57–75.

32. D. Raynal. Polygraphic aspects of narcolepsy. In *Narcolepsy,* eds. C. Guilleminault, W. Dement, and P. Passouant. Advances in Sleep Research, vol 3. New York, Spectrum, 1976, 671–684.

33. W. Dement. Daytime sleepiness and sleep "attacks." In *Narcolepsy,* eds. C. Guilleminault, W. Dement, and P. Passouant. Advance in Sleep Research, vol. 3. New York, Spectrum, 1976, 17–42. In the laboratory, patients with narcolepsy fall asleep four times faster than do control subjects.

34. J. Moses, D. Hord, A. Lubin, et al. Dynamics of nap sleep during a 40 hour period. *Electroencephalography and Clinical Neurophysiology* 1975; 39:627–633.

35. H. Gordon, B. Frooman, and P. Lavie. Shift in cognitive asymmetries between wakings from REM and NREM sleep. *Neuropsychologia* 1982; 20:99–103.

36. G. Berlucchi. Callosal activity in unrestrained, unanesthetized cats. *Archives Italienne de Biologie* 1965; 103:623–634.

37. F. Crick and G. Mitchison. The function of dream sleep. *Nature* 1983; 304:111–114.

38. C. Smith. Sleep states and learning: A review of the animal literature. *Neuroscience and Biobehavioral Reviews* 1985; 9:157–168.

39. C. Smith and P. Wong. Paradoxical sleep increases predict successful learning in a complex operant task. *Behavioral Neuroscience* 1991; 105:282–288.

40. S. Steiner and S. Ellman. Relation between REM sleep and intracranial self-stimulation. *Science* 1972; 177:1122–1124.

41. R. Broughton. Biorhythmic variations in consciousness and psychological functions. *Canadian Psychological Review* 1975; 16:217–239.

42. The bodhisattva who embodies, throughout the cosmos, the Buddhist ideal of compassion is called Kuan Yin in Chinese, Kannon in Japanese, and Avalokiteshwara in Sanskrit (see Appendix A).

Chapter 72   Other Perspectives in Dreams

1. M. Ullman and N. Zimmerman. *Working with Dreams.* Los Angeles, Tarcher, 1979, 200.

2. J. Hobson and R. McCarley. The brain as a dream-state generator: An activation-synthesis hypothesis of the dream process. *American Journal of Psychology* 1977; 134:1335–1346.

3. S. LaBerge. *Lucid Dreaming.* Los Angeles, Tarcher, 1985.

4. C. Marsh. A framework for describing subjective states of consciousness. In *Alternate States of Consciousness,* ed. N. Zinberg. New York, Free Press, 1977, 121–144.

5. H. Hunt. Forms of dreaming. *Perceptual and Motor Skills* 1982; 54:559–633.

6. M. Greenberg and M. Farah. The laterality of dreaming. *Brain and Cognition* 1986; 5:307–321.

7. P. Madsen, S. Holm, S. Vorstrup, et al. Human regional blood flow during rapid-eye-movement sleep. *Journal of Cerebral Blood Flow and Metabolism* 1991; 11:502–507.

8. N. Kerr and D. Foulkes. Right hemispheric mediation of dream visualization: A case study. *Cortex* 1981; 17:603–610. When tested while awake, the patient had also lost the ability to mentally "unfold" or to "rotate" imaginary figures in his mind's eye.

9. Again, thoughtlike mentation is not unique to D-sleep; it also occurs during S-sleep, but tends not to be remembered. Broughton places this kind of thoughtlike mentation during S-sleep, together with our logical, conscious forms of *daytime* thought, at one pole of our 90- to 100-minute biological rhythm. At the opposite pole would be REM dreaming at night or daydreaming while awake. See R. Broughton. Biorhythmic variations in consciousness and psychological functions. *Canadian Psychological Review* 1975; 16:217–239.

10. H. Dumoulin. *A History of Zen Buddhism*. London, Faber & Faber, 1963, 254.

Chapter 73   Lucid Dreaming

1. S. LaBerge. *Lucid Dreaming*. Los Angeles, Tarcher, 1985. LaBerge was a passive observer in only three of his lucid dreams. Out-of-body experiences occurred in only 1 percent of his lucid dreams.

2. S. LaBerge. Lucid dreaming as a learnable skill: A case study. *Perceptual and Motor Skills* 1980; 51:1039–1042.

3. By convention, the hallucinatory phenomena which occur when one ascends from sleep toward waking are called "hypnopompic." Those which occur as one drops off into sleep are called "hypnagogic" (see also chapter 87).

4. P. Fenwick, M. Schatzman, A. Worsley, et al. Lucid dreaming: Correspondence between dreamed and actual events in one subject during REM sleep. *Biological Psychology* 1984; 18:243–252.

5. S. LaBerge, L. Nagel, W. Dement, V. Lucid dreaming verified by volitional communications during REM sleep. *Perceptual and Motor Skills* 1981; 52:727–732.

6. R. Ogilvie, H. Hunt, P. Tyson, et al. Lucid dreaming and alpha activity: A preliminary report. *Perceptual and Motor Skills* 1982; 55:795–808.

7. P. Tyson, R. Ogilvie, and H. Hunt. Lucid, prelucid, and nonlucid dreams related to the amount of EEG alpha activity during REM sleep. *Psychophysiology* 1984; 4:442–451.

Chapter 74   Conditioning: Learning and Unlearning

1. I. Pavlov, in W. Sargant ed., *Battle for The Mind*. Garden City, N.Y., Doubleday, 1957, 43. After the flood, Pavlov's surviving dogs also became inhibited and showed other altered behaviors. At first, they seemed to respond as much to weak as to strong stimuli. Next, they responded even more actively to weak stimuli than to strong stimuli. Finally, some dogs reversed the "sign" of their previously established conditioned reflexes and behavior patterns. That is, they switched over from positive responses to negative ones, and vice versa.

2. S. Mitchell, trans. *Tao Te Ching*. New York, Harper & Row, 1988, 48.

3. G. Berlucchi and H. Buchtel. Some trends in the neurological study of learning. In *Handbook of Psychophysiology*, ed. M. Gazzaniga. New York, Academic Press, 1975, 481–498.

4. M. Olds. Short-term changes in the firing pattern of hypothalamic neurons during Pavlovian conditioning. *Brain Research* 1973; 58:95–116.

5. C. Schindler, I. Gormezano, and J. Harvey. Effects of morphine, ethylketocyclazocine, U-50, 488H and naloxone on the acquisition of a classically conditioned response in the rabbit. *Journal of Pharmacology and Experimental Therapeutics* 1987; 243:1010–1017.

6. J. Moore. Brain processes and conditioning. In *Mechanisms of Learning and Motivation*, eds. A. Dickinson and R. Boakes. Hillsdale, N.J., Erlbaum, 1979, 111–142.

7. R. Thompson. Are memory traces localized or distributed? *Neuropsychologia* 1991; 29:571–582.

8. M. Segal and F. Bloom. The action of norepinephrine in the rat hippocampus. IV. The effects of locus coeruleus stimulation on evoked hippocampal unit activity. *Brain Research* 1976; 107:513–525.

9. A. Riley, D. Zellner, and H. Duncan. The role of endorphins in animal learning and behavior. *Neuroscience and Biobehavioral Reviews* 1980; 4:69–76.

10. Extinction is not a unitary process of behavior. Several mechanisms are embedded in it. These include selective inattention, inhibition of response, the block of nonreward, and

secondary reinforcement. Therefore, it is difficult to draw conclusions about the effect(s) of any drug on extinction if that drug acts at many sites. Consider, for example, the complex effects of three peptides: ACTH and vasopressin slow the rate of extinction, whereas oxytocin hastens it. See J. Brons and C. Woody. Long-term changes in excitability of cortical neurons after Pavlovian conditioning and extinction. *Journal of Neurophysiology* 1980; 44:605–615.

11. S. Mason. The neurochemistry and pharmacology of extinction behavior. *Neuroscience and Biobehavioral Reviews* 1983; 7:3; 325–348.

12. M. Decker, T. Gill, and J. McGaugh. Concurrent muscarinic and β-adrenergic blockade in rats impairs place-learning in a water maze and retention of inhibitory avoidance. *Brain Research* 1990; 513:81–85.

13. R. Douglas. Pavlovian conditioning and the brain. In *Inhibition and Learning*, eds. R. Boakes and M. Halliday. London, Academic Press, 1972, 529–553. In animals, the neocortex is not responsible for the simpler forms of conditioned inhibition of the blink reflex. See J. Moore, C. Yeo, D. Oakley, et al. Conditioned inhibition of the nictitating membrane response in decorticate rabbits. *Behavioral Brain Research* 1980; 1:397–409.

14. B. Everitt, K. Morris, A. O'Brien, et al. The basolateral amygdala-ventral striatal system and conditioned place preference. *Neuroscience* 1991; 42:1–18.

15. W. Brewer. There is no convincing evidence for operant classical conditioning in adult humans. In *Cognition and the Symbolic Processes*, eds. W. Weima and D. Palermo. New York, Wiley, 1974, 1–42.

16. F. Wilson and E. Rolls. Learning and memory is reflected in the responses of reinforcement-related neurons in the primate basal forebrain. *Journal of Neuroscience* 10:1024–1267. Lesions made in the forebrain transiently interfere with an animal's ability to retain its previously learned visual discriminations. The lesions also create long-lasting deficits in mental agility and in the ability to inhibit responses. See A. Roberts, T. Robbins, B. Everitt, et al. The effects of excitotoxic lesions of the basal forebrain on the acquisition, retention and serial reversal of visual discriminations in marmosets. *Neuroscience* 1990; 34:311–329.

17. E. Kandel and J. Schwartz. Molecular biology of learning: Modulation of transmitter release. *Science* 1982; 218:433–443.

18. D. Mahajan and T. Desiraju. Alterations of dendritic branching and spine densities of hippocampal CA3 pyramidal neurons induced by operant conditioning in the phase of brain growth spurt. *Experimental Neurology* 1988; 100:1–15.

19. M. Gabriel, C. Cuppernell, J. Shenker, et al. Mamillothalamic tract transection blocks anterior thalamic training–induced neuronal plasticity and impairs discriminative avoidance behavior in rabbits. *Journal of Neuroscience* 1995; 15:1437–1445.

20. I. Schloegl. Lecture, Zen Centre, London, 1982.

Chapter 75   Other Ways to Change Behavior

1. J. Delgado. Neuronal constellations in aggressive behavior. In *Aggression and Violence: A Psychobiological and Clinical Approach*, St. Vincent edn., eds. I. Valzelli and I. Morgese. Milan, Mario Negri Institute of Pharmacologic Research, 1981, 82–98. Drug solutions do diffuse in the brain. Hence, the volumes injected must be kept small if drug effects are to remain discretely localized.

2. C. Sem-Jacobsen and A. Torkildsen. Depth recording and electrical stimulation in the human brain. In *Electrical Studies on the Un-Anaesthetized Brain*, eds. E. Ramey and D. O'Doherty. New York, Hoeber, 1960, 275–290.

3. E. Wasserman, Y. Gomita, and C. Gallistel. Pimozide blocks reinforcement but not priming from MFB stimulation in the rat. *Pharmacology, Biochemistry and Behavior* 1982; 17:783–787.

4. As is usual in research, the later speculations tend to become more conservative. Animal observations reemphasize that we can never be certain what animals experience. They also illustrate how important it will be to develop further that branch of the neurosciences

within neurology which focuses on *human experience*. One name for this field might be "experiential neurology." (see final section, entitled In Closing) This could help distinguish it from behavioral neurology, a name still laden with motoric implications.

5. Other recent studies have suggested that *non*dopamine systems are also activated in parallel with the DA nerve cells of the mesolimbic DA system during stimulation of the median forebrain bundle. See C. Gallistel, Y. Gomita, E. Yadin, et al. Forebrain origins and terminations of the medial forebrain bundle metabolically activated by rewarding stimulation, or by reward-blocking doses of pimozide. *Journal of Neuroscience* 1985; 5:1246–1261.

6. L. Porrino. Cerebral metabolic changes associated with activation of reward systems. In *Brain Reward Systems and Abuse*, eds. J. Engel and L. Oreland. New York, Raven Press, 1987, 51–60. The stimulant-type drugs are amphetamine and methylphenidate.

7. Another approach is to reversibly cool small sites in the brain.

8. R. Watson, B. Miller, and K. Heilman. Evoked potential in neglect. *Archives of Neurology* 1977; 34:224–227.

9. R. Michael. Neurological mechanisms and the control of sexual behavior. In *The Scientific Basis of Medicine*. Annual Reviews. London, Athlone Press, 1965, 316–333.

Chapter 76 The Awakening from Hibernation

1. Raphael DuBois, in E. Satinoff. Hibernation and the central nervous system. In *Progress in Physiological Psychology*, vol 3, eds. E. Stellar and J. Sprague. New York, Academic Press, 1970, 207–236.

2. A. Beckman and T. Stanton. Properties of the CNS during the state of hibernation. In *The Neural Basis of Behavior*. Lancaster, England, MTP Press, 1982, 19–45.

3. N. Popova and N. Voitenko. Brain serotonin metabolism in hibernation. *Pharmacology, Biochemistry and Behavior* 1981; 14:773–777.

4. M. Steriade and R. Llinás. The functional states of the thalamus and the associated neuronal interplay. *Physiological Reviews* 1988; 68:649–742.

5. A. Belousov, O. Vinogradova, and P. Pakhotin. Paradoxical state-dependent excitability of the medial septal neurons in brain slices of ground squirrel, *Citellus undulatus*. *Neuroscience* 1990; 38:599–608.

6. A. Beckman. Hypothalamic and midbrain function during hibernation. In *Current Studies of Hypothalamic Function*, vol 2, eds. W. Veale and K. Lederis. Basel, Karger, 1978, 29–43.

7. The four hypothalamic nuclei most activated are the suprachiasmatic, paraventricular, ventromedial and medial preoptic nuclei. See T. Kilduff, J. Miller, C. Radeke, et al. 14C-2-Deoxyglucose uptake in the ground squirrel brain during entrance to and arousal from hibernation. *Journal of Neuroscience* 1990; 10:2463–2475.

8. T. Stanton, A. Winokur, and A. Beckman. Reversal of natural CNS depression by TRH action in the hippocampus. *Brain Research* 1980; 181:470–475. Only one-thousandth as much TRH still evokes complete arousal, but now it starts a little later, after sixty-nine minutes. The potency of TRH is particularly impressive because TRH was injected as the animal was descending into hibernation. This descending phase is usually the most difficult time to waken the animals.

9. P. Kalivas and A. Horita. Involvement of the septohippocampal system in TRH antagonism of pentobarbital narcosis. In *Thyrotropin-Releasing Hormone*. eds. E. Griffiths and G. Bennett. New York., Raven Press, 1983, 283–290. TRH injections do not arouse when made into the preoptic or anterior hypothalamic region or cortex.

10. D. Heal, C. Pycock, M. Youdim, et al. Actions of TRH and its analogues on the mesolimbic dopamine system. In *Thyrotropin-Releasing Hormone*, eds. E. Griffiths and G. Bennett. New York, Raven Press, 1983, 271–282.

11. S. Manaker, T. Rainbow, and A. Winokur. Thyrotropin-releasing hormone (TRH) receptors: Localization in rat and human central nervous system. In *Quantitative Receptor Autoradiography*, eds. C. Boast, E. Snowhill, and C. Altar. New York, Alan R. Liss, 1986, 103–135.

12. A. Beckman, R. Dean, and J. Wamsley. Hippocampal and cortical opioid receptor binding: Changes related to the hibernation state. *Brain Research* 1986; 386:223–231.

13. A. Beckman. Functional aspects of brain opioid peptide systems in hibernation. In *Living in the Cold,* ed. H. Heller. Amsterdam, Elsevier, 1986; 225–234.

14. V. Popov and L. Bocharova. Hibernation-induced structural changes in synaptic contacts between mossy fibers and hippocampal pyramidal neurons. *Neuroscience* 1992; 48:53–62.

Chapter 77   Tidal Rhythms and Biological Clocks

1. R. Thatcher and E. John. *Foundations of Cognitive Processes.* Functional Neuroscience, vol 1. Hillsdale, N.J., Erlbaum, 1977, 82.

2. R. Broughton. Biorhythmic variations in consciousness and psychological functions. *Canadian Psychological Review* 1975; 16:217–239.

3. E. Weitzman, C. Czeisler, J. Zimmerman, et al. Biological rhythms in man: Relationships of sleep-wake, cortisol, growth hormone, and temperature during temporal isolation. *Advances in Biochemical Psychopharmacology* 1981; 28:475–499.

4. H. Schulz. Sleep onset REM episodes in depression. In *Sleep, 1980,* ed. W. Koella. Basel, Karger, 1981, 72–79.

5. W. Dement and A. Rechtschaffen. Narcolepsy: Polygraphic aspects, experimental and theoretical considerations. In *The Abnormalities of Sleep in Man,* eds. H. Gastaut et al. Bologna, Gaggi, 1968, 147–164.

6. E. Souetre, E. Salvati, D. Pringuey, et al. Antidepressant effects of the sleep/wake cycle phase advance. *Journal of Affective Disorders* 1987; 12:41–46.

7. L. Lamberg. *The American Medical Association Guide to Better Sleep.* New York, Random House, 1984.

8. T. Wehr and A. Wirz-Justice. Internal coincidence model for sleep deprivation and depression. In *Sleep 1980,* ed. W. Koella. Basel, Karger, 1981, 26–33.

9. Some shorter ultradian rhythms may consist more of a "sleepiness" rhythm than one of arousal and alertness. See P. Lavie. Ultradian rhythms: Gates of sleep and wakefulness. *Experimental Brain Research* 1985; (suppl. 12): 148–164.

10. D. Kripke, D. Mullaney, and P. Fleck. Ultradian rhythms during sustained performance. *Experimental Brain Research* 1985; (suppl. 12): 201–216.

11. Some researchers speculate that there exists yet another basic cycle. This one alternates between periods of rest and activity. For this reason it is referred to as the basic rest/activity cycle, or BRAC. According to this view, our nighttime REM episodes express *this* fundamental activity cycle each time they interrupt S-sleep every 90 to 110 minutes or so. Further studies are necessary to verify the following two reports of other recurrent daytime phenomena. R. Klein and R. Armitage. Rhythms in human performance: 1 1/2-hour oscillations in cognitive style. *Science* 1979; 204:1326–1328; and H. Gordon and D. Stoffer. Ultradian rhythms of right and left hemisphere function. *International Journal of Neuroscience* 1989; 47:57–65.

12. M. Gillberg and T. Akerstedt. Sleep deprivation in normals—Some psychological and biochemical data from three studies. In *Sleep 1980,* ed. W. Koella. Basel, Karger, 1981, 16–22. T_3 is triiodothyronine; T_4 is thyoxine.

13. M. Bertini, C. Violani, P. Zoccolotti, et al. Right cerebral activation in REM sleep: Evidence from a unilateral tactile recognition test. *Psychophysiology* 1984; 21:418–423. Initially, when the subjects were still wide-awake, their left hands (read: right hemisphere) were superior in recognizing objects by touch. However, when the subjects were later awakened from REM sleep, their abilities to recognize objects with the left hand had improved still further. In contrast, wakings from slow-wave sleep showed no differences in tactile performance between the two hands (read: hemispheres).

14. D. Kripke. Biological rhythm disturbances might cause narcolepsy. In *Narcolepsy,* eds. C. Guilleminault, W. Dement, and P. Passonant. Advances in Sleep Research, vol 3. New York, Spectrum, 1976, 475–483.

15. F. Halberg, M. Engeli, C. Hamburger, et al. Spectral resolution of low-frequency, small amplitude rhythms in excreted 17-ketosteroid: Probable androgen-induced circaseptan desynchronization. *Acta Endocrinologica (Copenhagen)* 1965; (suppl. 103): 1–54.

16. S. Binkley, M. Tome, D. Crawford, et al. Human daily rhythms measured for one year. *Physiology and Behavior* 1990; 48:293–298.

17. M. Eastwood, J. Whitton, P. Kramer, et al. Infradian rhythms. *Archives of General Psychiatry* 1985; 42:295–299.

18. P. Mueller and R. Davies. Seasonal affective disorders: Seasonal energy syndrome? (letter, with reply by N. Rosenthal) *Archives of General Psychiatry* 1986; 43:188–189.

19. M. Kafka, A. Wirz-Justice, and D. Naher. Circadian and seasonal rhythms in α- and β-adrenergic receptors in rat brain. *Brain Research* 1981; 207:409–419.

20. A. Carlson, L. Svennerholm, and B. Winblad. Seasonal and circadian monoamine variations in human brains examined postmortem. *Acta Psychiatrica Scandinavica Supplementum* 1980; 280:75–85.

21. Some of the serotonin data may find dental correlates. Pain sensitivities were tested using a cold stimulus. The pain threshold was lowest in the early morning and highest in the early afternoon. See L. Pollmann and P. Harris. Rhythmic changes in pain sensitivity in teeth. *International Journal of Chronobiology* 1978; 5:459–464.

Chapter 78   The Roots of Our Emotions

1. S. Schachter and J. Singer. Cognitive, social and phsysiological determinants of emotional state. *Psychological Review* 1962; 69:379–399.

2. J. Laird and C. Bresler. William James and the mechanisms of emotional experience. *Personality and Social Psychology Bulletin* 1990; 16:636–651.

3. R. Levenson, P. Ekman, and W. Friesen. Voluntary facial action generates emotion-specific autonomic nervous system activity. *Psychophysiology* 1990; 27:363–384.

4. P. Adelmann and R. Zajonc. Facial efference and the experience of emotion. *Annual Review of Psychology* 1989; 40:249–280.

5. J. Ledoux. Emotion. In *Handbook of Physiology*. Sec. 1, *The Nervous System*. Vol. 5, *Higher Functions of the Brain*, prt. 1, eds. V. Mountcastle and F. Plum. Bethesda, Md., American Physiological Society, 1987, 419–459.

6. R. Zajonc. Feeling and thinking: Preferences need no inferences. *American Psychologist* 1980; 35:151–175.

7. J. Iwata, J. LeDoux, M. Meeley, et al. Intrinsic neurons in the amygdaloid field projected to by the medial geniculate body mediate emotional responses conditioned to acoustic stimuli. *Brain Research* 1986; 383:195–214.

8. Schachter and Singer, *op. cit.*

9. D. Williams. The structure of emotions reflected in epileptic experiences. *Brain* 1956; 79:29–67.

10. *Ibid.*, cases 31, 32, and 35.

11. J. Jackson: On right- or left-sided spasm at the onset of epileptic paroxysms, and on crude sensation warnings, and elaborate mental states. *Brain* 1880; 3:192–206.

12. W. Wittling and M. Pflüger. Neuroendocrine hemisphere asymmetries: Salivary cortisol secretion during lateralized viewing of emotion-related and neutral films. *Brain and Cognition* 1990; 14:243–265.

13. G. Lee, D. Loring, and K. Meader. Hemispheric specialization for emotional expression: A reexamination of results from intracarotid administration of sodium amobarbital. *Brain and Cognition* 1990; 12:267–280.

14. L. Benowitz, D. Bear, R. Rosenthal, et al. Hemispheric specialization in nonverbal communication. *Cortex* 1983; 19:5–11. Studies of split-brain patients suggest that the right hemisphere may be less sensitive in interpreting the way other persons move the rest of their body parts.

15. P. Rozin and A. Fallon. A perspective on disgust. *Psychological Review* 1987; 94:23–41.

16. S. Ogata. The story of Zen philosophy. In *Anthology of Zen,* ed. W. Briggs. New York, Grove Press, 1961, 158. This saying in one of its more literal interpretations is that "the passions are the Buddha-nature, and the Buddha-nature includes the passions." The statement might refer to the experiential content at deeper levels of transformation. By then, the insightful vision has become so comprehensive and is so stripped of self that it sees

into every passionate emotion of greed, anger, and fear. Moreover, it accepts them totally, unjudgmentally, as the natural, integral part of the energies permeating the whole of reality. (See also chapter 154.)

17. I. Schloegl. Lecture, Zen Centre, London, 1982.

Chapter 79   The Spread of Positive Feeling States

1. The Dalai Lama of Tibet. *Awaking the Mind, Lightening the Heart.* San Francisco, Harper, 1995, 44.
2. E. Underhill. *Mysticism.* New York, Dutton, 1961, 264.
3. A. Isen and P. Levin. Effect of feeling good on helping: Cookies and kindness. *Journal of Personal and Social Psychology* 1972; 21:384–388.
4. A. Isen, T. Shalker, M. Clark, et al. Affect, accessibility of material in memory, and behavior: A cognitive loop? *Journal of Personal and Social Psychology* 1978; 36:1–12.
5. A. Isen and T. Shalker. The effect of feeling state on evaluation of positive, neutral, and negative stimuli: When you "accentuate the positive," do you "eliminate the negative?" *Social Psychology Quarterly* 1982; 45:58–63.
6. A. Isen and B. Means. The influence of positive affect on decision-making strategy. *Social Cognition* 1982; 2:18–31.
7. T. Desiraju.: Electrophysiology of the frontal granular cortex III. The cingulate-prefrontal relation in primate. *Brain Research* 109:473–485.

Chapter 80   Pain and the Relief of Pain

1. B. Fuller, *Denver Post,* 2 July 1983, p. 3A.
2. M. Berthier, S. Starkstein, and R. Leiguarda. Asymbolia for pain: A sensory limbic disconnection syndrome. *Annals of Neurology* 1988; 24:41–49. Pain is represented at higher levels in those regions of cortex buried in the insula and parietal operculum.
3. Fast pain relays through the ventroposterolateral nucleus of the thalamus and beyond. Slow pain gets off to its slow start in the so-called slow pain fibers out in the peripheral nerves of the arms and legs. There its impulses travel at a rate of only about two to six feet per second. Slow pain also climbs more slowly in the central nervous system, because there it has to relay up through multiple synapses in the reticular formation and central gray. Now its route takes it both to the limbic system, to the intralaminar nuclei of the thalamus, and to the cortex beyond.
4. L. Watkins and D. Mayer. Organization of endogenous opiate and nonopiate pain control systems. *Science* 1982; 216:1185–1192. We still have much to learn about each system.
5. Signals from this front paw first activate serotonin nerve cells in the medulla, which release their serotonin down onto endogenous opioid nerve cells in the spinal cord. These opioid cells, in turn, release their opioids into the dorsal horn. Here they stop the impulses from entering the cord and from going on to mediate pain.
6. Even so, noxious stimulation of the hind paws does cause much more metenkephalin to be released in the gigantocellular reticular nucleus of the brain stem. A dipeptide, released by pain impulses, secondarily stimulates many enkephalin neurons to release their pain-relieving opioids. See Y. Kuraishi, M. Sugimoto, and H. Takagi. Noxious stimulus–induced release of met-enkephalin from the nucleus reticularis gigantocellularis of the rat. Presented at International Narcotic Research Conference, Kyoto, Japan, 26–30 July 1981, abstract P-27, 95; H. Takagi. Novel endogenous analgesic peptides, kyotorphin and neo-kyotorphin. In *Current Topics in Pain Research and Therapy,* eds. T. Yokota and R. Dubner. Amsterdam, Excerpta Medica, 1983, 125–135.
7. D. Bowsher. Ability to lie on bed of nails not due to endogenous opioids. *Lancet* 1980; 1(8180):1132.
8. Y. Hosobuchi. Periaqueductal gray stimulation in humans produces analgesia accompanied by elevation of β-endorphin and ACTH in ventricular CSF. In *The Role of Endorphins in Neuropsychiatry,* ed. H. Emrich. Modern Problems in Pharmacopsychiatry, vol. 17. Basel, Karger 1981, 109–122.

9. A. Petrie. *Individuality in Pain and Suffering,* 2nd ed. Chicago, University of Chicago Press, 1978.

Chapter 81 Suffering and the Relief of Suffering

1. P. Haskel. *Bankei Zen.* New York, Grove Press, 1984, 59–60.
2. I. Schloegel. Towards wholeness. Zen Traces 1982; 4(March):4–11.
3. H. Warren. *Buddhism in Translations.* New York, Atheneum, 1976, 117–122. The Buddha's practical advice is found in the Lesser Malunkyaputta sermon.
4. Dhiravamsa. *The Way of Non-Attachment. The Practice of Insight Meditation.* New York, Schocken, 1977, 33. Ultimately the desire for enlightenment itself is seen into, and worked through.
5. R. Sin, cited in C. Murphy. Coming to Grief. *Atlantic,* 1991, 268:20–22.
6. D. Suzuki: In F. Franck. The Buddha does not know, he sees. *The Eastern Buddhist* 1987; 20:100–104.
7. H. Beecher. Relationship of significance of wound to the pain experienced. *JAMA* 1956; 161:1609–1613.
8. H. Beecher. *Measurement of Subjective Responses.* New York, Oxford University Press, 1959.
9. W. Mills and J. Farrow. The transcendental meditation technique and acute experimental pain. *Psychosomatic Medicine* 1981; 43:157–164.
10. A. Weil. The marriage of the sun and the moon. In *Alternate States of Consciousness,* ed. N. Zinberg, New York, Free Press, 1977, 37–52.
11. P. Ebersole and J. Flores. Positive impact of life crises. *Journal of Social Behavior and Personality* 1989; 4:463–469.
12. Red Pine: *The Zen Teaching of Bodhidharma.* North Point Press. San Francisco. 1989.
13. S. Asahina. A message to Sokei-An's Zen students. In *Anthology of Zen,* ed. W. Briggs. New York, Grove Press, 1961, 37–41.

Chapter 82 Bridging the Two Hemispheres

1. J. Sergent. Furtive excursions into bicameral minds. *Brain* 1990; 113:537–568.
2. J. Ledoux, D. Wilson, and M. Gazzaniga. A divided mind: Observations on the conscious properties of the separated hemispheres. *Annals of Neurology* 1977; 2:417–421.
3. L. Ellenberg and R. Sperry. Lateralized division of attention in the commissurotomized and intact brain. *Neuropsychologia* 1980; 18:411–418.
4. R. Efron. *The Decline and Fall of Hemispheric Specialization.* Hillsdale, N.J., Erlbaum, 1990.
5. M. Gazzaniga and J. LeDoux. *The Integrated Mind.* New York, Plenum Press, 1978.
6. G. Gainotti. The meaning of emotional disturbances resulting from unilateral brain injury. In *Emotions and the Dual Brain,* eds. G. Gainotti, and C. Caltagirone. *Experimental Brain Research* 1989; series 18:147–167.
7. D. Zaidel. Hemi-field asymmetries in memory for incongruous scenes. *Cortex* 1988; 24:231–244.
8. E. Phelps and M. Gazzaniga. Hemispheric differences in mnemonic processing: The effects of left hemispheric interpretation. *Neuropsychologia* 1992; 30:293–297.
9. N. Etcoff. The neuropsychology of emotional expression. In *Advances in Clinical Neuropsychology,* vol 3. eds. G. Goldstein, and R. Tarter. New York, Plenum Press, 1986, 127–179.
10. W. Penfield. Speech, perception and the uncommitted cortex. In *Brain and Conscious Experience,* ed. J. Eccles. New York, Springer-Verlag, 1966, 221. Flashbacks occurred in 40 out of 432 patients whose brains were stimulated.
11. E. Altenmuller. Cortical DC-potentials as electrophysiological correlates of hemispheric dominance of higher cognitive functions. *International Journal of Neuroscience* 1989; 47:1–14.
12. Some authors speculate that dysphoric moods, fear, and sadness originate more in the right hemisphere, whereas euphoria and anger, and possibly a paranoid mood start over on the left side. (See P. Flor-Henry. *Cerebral Basis of Psychopathology.* Boston, John Wright PSG, 1983.) There is a different way to interpret the link between the right hemisphere and dysphoric moods. It is to postulate that emotionally "negative" stimuli preferentially activate the right side. Once this right side is activated negatively, then the processing of

subsequent stimuli would proceed through a negatively toned emotional bias. (See M. Otto, R. Yeo, and M. Dougher. Right hemisphere involvement in depression: Toward a neuropsychological theory of negative affective experiences. *Biological Psychiatry* 1987; 22:1201–1215.

13. M. Gazzaniga, J. Holtzman, and C. Smylie. Speech without conscious awareness. *Neurology* 1987; 37:682–685.

14. R. Sperry, E. Zaidel, and D. Zaidel. Self recognition and social awareness in the disconnected minor hemisphere. *Neuropsychologia* 1979; 17:153–166. Some persons are born without a corpus callosum, and they appear to be normal. In the rest of us, it remains to be shown how much the subcortical bridge operates during our everyday sensorimotor and insightful functions. Some might argue that the "bridge" functions more as a compensatory mechanism, one which takes on an adaptive role in those few patients in whom the corpus callosum happens to have been cut later in life.

15. A. Cronin-Golomb. Subcortical transfer of cognitive information in subjects with complete forebrain commissurotomy. *Cortex* 1986; 22:499–519.

16. L. Goldstein and S. Harnad. Quantitated EEG correlates of normal and abnormal interhemispheric relations. In *Language and Hemispheric Specialization in Man: Cerebral Event-Related Potentials*, ed. J. Desmedt. Progress in Clinical Neurophysiology, vol. 3. Basel, Karger, 1977, 161–171. In the male patient, the simple act of counting out numbers was enough to cause him to shift his dominant activity over to the left temporal lobe.

17. H. Cohen, R. Rosen, and L. Goldstein. Electroencephalographic laterality changes during human sexual orgasm. *Archives of Sexual Behavior* 1976; 5:189–199.

18. Some evidence suggests that during times of "sympathetic dominance," the erectile tissue vasoconstricts along one side of our two nasal passages. More air then flows through this more widely opened nostril. Parasympathetic dominance is said to cause the reverse changes. Many, but not all, subjects shift their "nasal cycles" back and forth, from one side to the other, every two to four hours or so. Though a more "integrated EEG" is reported to occur in the hemisphere opposite the more open nostril, much more work needs to be done to confirm and to clarify the basis of these findings. See D. Werntz, R. Bickford, F. Bloom, et al. Alternating cerebral hemispheric activity and the lateralization of autonomic nervous function. *Human Neurobiology* 1983; 2:39–43.

19. P. Gott, E. Hughes, and K. Whipple. Voluntary control of two lateralized conscious states: Validation by electrical and behavioral studies. *Neuropsychologia* 1984; 22:65–72.

20. K. Heilman and T. Van den Abell. Right hemisphere dominance for attention: The mechanism underlying hemispheric asymmetries of inattention (neglect). *Neurology* 1980; 30:327–330.

21. E. Altenmuller, R. Jung, T. Winker, et al. Premotor programming and cortical processing in the cerebral cortex. Electro-physiological correlates of hemispheric dominance. *Brain, Behavioral and Evolution* 1989; 33:141–146.

22. H. Ehrlichman, J. Autrobus, and M. Wiener. EEG asymmetry and sleep mentation during REM and NREM. *Brain and Cognition* 1985; 4:477–485.

23. R. Davidson and N. Fox. Frontal brain asymmetry predicts infants' response to maternal separation. *Journal of Abnormal Psychology* 98:127–131.

24. G. Ahern and G. Schwartz. Differential lateralization for positive and negative emotion in the human brain: EEG spectral analysis. *Neuropsychologia* 1985; 23:745–755.

25. G. Lee, D. Loring, J. Dahl, et al. Hemispheric specialization for emotional expression. *Neuropsychiatry, Neuropsychology, and Behavioral Neurology* 1993; 6:143–148. The patients reacted with laughter, or elevations of mood, 30 seconds after amobarbital was injected into the right carotid artery. This would have inactivated the front three quarters of the right hemisphere. "Sad crying" occurred much earlier, at 6 seconds. This happened *only* when a *left*-sided injection had caused dysfunction within corresponding parts of the left hemisphere.

26. H. Ehrlichman and M. Wiener. EEG asymmetry during covert mental activity. *Psychophysiology* 1980; 17:228–235.

27. J. Earle. Cerebral laterality and meditation: A review of the literature. *Journal of Transpersonal Psychology* 1981; 13:155–173.

28. D. Van Lancker. Personal relevance and the human right hemisphere. *Brain and Cognition* 1991; 17:64–92.

29. J. Bennett and J. Trinder. Hemispheric laterality and cognitive style associated with transcendental meditation. *Psychophysiology* 1977; 14:293–296.

30. R. Pagano and L. Frumkin. The effect of transcendental mediation on right hemispheric functioning. *Biofeedback and Self Regulation* 1977; 2:407–415.

31. D. Treffert. The idiot savant: A review of the syndrome. *American Journal of Psychiatry* 1988; 145:563–572. Dustin Hoffman portrayed their paradoxes in the 1988 film, *Rainman*. The so-called idiot savants possess certain prodigious mental skills which stand out in stark contrast against the low background of their many other mental disabilities. Functional MRI scans, other neuroimaging techniques, and post-mortem studies are awaited on many savants, because they do not all seem to represent the same disorder.

Chapter 83   The Pregnant Meditative Pause

1. Huang-po in J. Blofeld. *The Zen Teaching of Huang-po. On the Transmission of Mind.* New York, Grove Press, Huang-po was a teacher of Lin-chi (J. Rinzai).

2. J. Sinclair. *The Rest Principle. A Neurophysiological Theory of Behavior.* Hillsdale, N.J., Erlbaum, Alpha methylparatyrosine is used to block dopamine synthesis.

3. D. McCormick and D. Prince. Noradrenergic modulation of firing pattern in guinea pig and cat thalamic neurons, in vitro. *Journal of Neurophysiology* 1988; 59:978–996. Norepinephrine acts on its α_1-receptors in the visual relay cells of the lateral geniculate nucleus.

4. M. Csikszentmihalyi and R. Larson. Validity and reliability of the experience-sampling method. *Journal of Nervous and Mental Disease* 1987; 175:526–536.

Chapter 84   Side Effects of Meditation: Makyo

1. John Keats, in *Oxford Dictionary of Quotations*, 3rd ed. New York, Oxford University Press, 1980, 292.

2. D. Suzuki. *Studies in Zen.* New York, Delta, 1955, 43.

3. H. Hunt and C. Chefurka. A test of the psychedelic model of altered states of consciousness. *Archives of General Psychiatry* 1976; 33:867–876.

4. A. Greeley. *The Sociology of the Paranormal. A Reconnaissance.* Sage Research Paper, vol 3, series 90-023. Beverly Hills, Calif. 1975.

5. N. Waddell. Dogen's Hokyo-ki, pt. 2. *The Eastern Buddhist* 1978; 11:66–84.

6. J. Kornfield. Intensive insight meditation: A phenomenological study. *Journal of Transpersonal Psychology* 1979; 11:41–58.

7. D. McGinty and J. Siegel. Sleep states. In *Motivation,* eds. E. Satinoff and P. Teitelbaum. Handbook of Behavioral Neurobiology, vol. 6. New York, Plenum Press, 1983, 105–181.

8. P. Ramm and B. Frost. Cerebral and local cerebral metabolism in the cat during slow wave and REM sleep. *Brain Research* 1986; 365:112–124.

9. C. Tart. A psychologist's experience with T.M. *Journal of Transpersonal Psychology* 1971; 3:135–140.

10. R. Walsh. Initial meditative experiences, pt. 1. *Journal of Transpersonal Psychology* 1977; 9:151–192.

11. R. Walsh. Initial mediative experiences, pt. 2. *Journal of Transpersonal Psychology* 1978; 10:1–28.

12. M. Epstein and J. Lieff. Psychiatric complications of meditation practice. In *Transformations of Consciousness,* eds. K. Wilber, J. Engler, and D. Brown. Boston, New Science, 1986, 53–63.

13. L. Otis. Adverse effects of transcendental meditation. In *Meditation: Classic and Contemporary Perspectives,* eds. D. Shapiro and R. Walsh. New York, Aldine, 1984, 201–208. *Zen and the Brain* views Zen in the larger context of research reports drawn from other meditative traditions. But this is not to equate Zen with TM or with any other approach.

14. A. Deikman. *The Observing Self. Mysticism and Psychotherapy.* Boston, Beacon Press, 1982.
15. T. Cleary. *Sayings and Doings of Pai-Chang.* Los Angeles, Center Publications, 1978, 103.
16. G. Rabten. *Echoes of Voidness.* London, Wisdom Publications, 1983, 12–13.
17. J. Engler. Therapeutic aims in psychotherapy and meditation: Developmental states in the representation of the self. *Journal of Transpersonal Psychology* 1984; 16:25–61.
18. The quickenings cited did not seem to follow a predictable sequence over the years. But in broad outline the sensate events came before the episode of emotionalized awareness.

Chapter 86   Bright Lights and Blank Vision

1. R. Tasker, L. Organ, and P. Hawrylyshyn. Visual phenomena evoked by electrical stimulation of the human brain stem. *Applied Neurophysiology* 1980; 43:89–95.
2. M. Livingstone and D. Hubel. Effects of sleep and arousal on the processing of visual information in the cat. *Nature* 1981; 291:554–561.
3. J. Hirsch, A. Fourment, and E. Marc. Sleep-related variations of membrane potential in the lateral geniculate body relay neurons of the cat. *Brain Research* 259:308–312. Similar clusters of discharges occur during ponto-geniculo-occipital waves.
4. B. Cohen, M. Feldman, and S. Diamond. Effects of eye movement, brain stem stimulation, and alertness on transmission through lateral geniculate body of monkey. *Journal of Neurophysiology* 1969; 32:583–594.
5. M. Steriade and R. Llinas. The functional states of the thalamus and the associated neuronal interplay. *Physiological Reviews* 1988; 68:649–742.
6. B. Hu, M. Steriade, and M. Deschenes. The effects of brainstem peribrachial stimulation on neurons of the lateral geniculate nucleus. *Neuroscience* 1989; 31:13–24.
7. R. Dossi, D. Paré, and M. Steriade. Short-lasting nicotinic and long-lasting muscarinic depolarizing responses of thalamocortical neurons to stimulation of mesopontine cholinergic nuclei. *Journal of Neurophysiology* 1991; 65:393–406.
8. M. Demetrescu, M. Demetrescu, and F. Iosi. The tonic control of cortical responsiveness by inhibitory and facilitatory diffuse influences. *Electroencephalography and Clinical Neurophysiology* 1965; 18:1–24.
9. W. Cohen. Spatial and textural characteristics of the ganzfeld. *American Journal of Psychology* 1957; 70:403–410.
10. K. Martin. The lateral geniculate nucleus strikes back. *Trends in Neurosciences* 11:192–194.
11. R. Woolfolk. Psychophysiological correlates of meditation. *Archives of General Psychiatry* 1975; 32:1326–1333.
12. M. Rizzo and R. Hurtig. Looking but not seeing: Attention, perception, and eye movements in simultanagnosia. *Neurology* 1987; 37:1642–1648. Areas 18 and 19 are involved. Chapter 142 considers the syncretic properties of this region.
13. W. James. *The Principles of Psychology,* vol 1. New York, Holt, 1918, 620.
14. A. Arduni. The tonic discharge of the retina and its central effects. In *Brain Mechanisms,* eds. G. Moruzzi, A. Fessard, and H. Jasper. Amsterdam, Elsevier, 1963, 184–203.
15. H. Jasper. Pathophysiological studies of brain mechanisms in different states of consciousness. In *Brain and Conscious Experience,* ed. J. Eccles. New York, Springer-Verlag, 1966, 256–282.
16. It disappears when the involved eye is closed. This light-dark phenomenon recurs every few weeks and can involve either eye.
17. J. Brunette and G. Lafond. ERG responses of rods and cones during dark adaptation. *Canadian Journal of Ophthalmology* 1978; 13:186–189.
18. Apart from the process of adaptation per se, it would be of interest to sort out the several other mechanisms involved, but this is not an easy task.

Chapter 87   Faces in the Fire: Illusions and Hallucinations

1. L. Roberts. Activation and interference of cortical functions. In *Electrical Stimulation of the Brain,* ed. D. Sheer. Austin, University of Texas Press, 1961, 533–553.
2. K. Dewhurst. *Hughlings Jackson on Psychiatry.* Oxford, Sandford, 1982, 131.

3. *Ibid.*, 82.

4. D. Williams. The structure of emotions reflected in epileptic experiences. *Brain* 1956; 79:29–67.

5. S. Freedman, H. Grunebaum, F. Stare, et al. Imagery in sensory deprivation. In *Hallucinations*, ed. L. West. New York, Grune & Stratton, 1962, 108–117.

6. F. Galton. (1951): *Inquiries into Human Faculty and Its Development.* London, The Eugenics Society, 112–128.

7. R. Masters and J. Houston. *The Varieties of Psychedelic Experience.* New York, Holt, Rinehart & Winston, 1966.

8. The unusual spelling of hypnagogic arises from its Greek roots: *hypn*, relating to sleep; *agōgos*, leading. Hence, leading to sleep, or on the way toward sleep.

9. M. Partinen and P. Putkonen. Sleep habits and sleep disorders in 2,537 young Finnish males. In *Sleep 1980*, ed. W. Koella, Basel, Karger, 1981, 383–385.

10. W. Dement and M. Mitler. An introduction to sleep. In *Basic Sleep Mechanisms*, eds. O. Petre-Quadens and J. Schlage, New York, Academic Press, 1974, 271–296.

11. V. Zarcone. Narcolepsy. *New England Journal of Medicine* 1973; 288:1156–1166.

12. M. Ribstein. Hypnagogic hallucinations. In *Narcolepsy*, eds. D. Guilleminault, W. Dement, and P. Passonant. Advances in Sleep Research, vol. 3. New York, Spectrum, 1976, 145–160.

13. P. McKellar and L. Simpson. Between wakefulness and sleep. *British Journal of Psychology* 1954; 45:266–276.

14. D. Schacter. The hypnagogic state: A critical review of the literature. *Psychological Bulletin* 1976; 83:452–481. Auditory hallucinations also occur.

15. D. Foulkes and G. Vogel. Mental activity at sleep onset. *Journal of Abnormal Psychology* 1965; 70:231–243.

16. D. Raynal. Polygraphic aspects of narcolepsy. In *Narcolepsy*, eds. D. Guilleminault, W. Dement, and P. Passonant. Advances in Sleep Research, vol. 3. New York, Spectrum, 1976, 671–684.

17. W. Dement. Daytime sleepiness and sleep "attacks." In *Narcolepsy*, eds. D. Guilleminault, W. Dement, and P. Passonant. Advances in Sleep Research, vol. 3. New York, Spectrum 1976, 17–42.

18. Hypnopompic also has Greek roots. *Hypno* relates to sleep; *pompien*, to send away. Hence, in the process of sending away sleep and becoming awake.

19. T. McDonnell, ed. *A Thomas Merton Reader. False Mysticism.* New York, Harcourt, Brace, 1962, 466–471.

20. S. Mullen and W. Penfield. Illusions of comparative interpretation and emotion. *Archives of Neurology and Psychiatry* 1959; 81:269–284.

21. W. Penfield and P. Perot. The brain's record of auditory and visual experience. *Brain* 1963; 86:595–696. Patients who have epilepsy, schizophrenia, and other disorders have a lower threshold for stimulus-induced hallucinations.

22. J. Adams and B. Rutkin. Visual responses to subcortical stimulation in the visual and limbic system. *Confinia Neurologica* 1970; 32:158–164.

23. M. Horowitz, J. Adams, and B. Rutkin. Visual imagery on brain stimulation. *Archives of General Psychiatry* 19:469–486.

24. E. Halgren. Mental phenomena induced by stimulation of the limbic system. *Human Neurobiology* 1982; 1:251–260.

25. K. Kooi and R. Marshall. *Visual Evoked Potentials in Central Disorders of the Visual System.* Hagerstown, Md., Harper & Row, 1979.

26. H. Bracha, F. Cabrera Jr., C. Karson, et al. Lateralization of visual hallucinations in chronic schizophrenia. *Biological Psychiatry* 1985; 20:1132–1136.

27. J. Morihisa and F. Duffy. Focal cortical arousal in the schizophrenias. In *Topographic Mapping of Brain Electrical Activity*, ed. F. Duffy. Boston, Butterworths, 1986, 371–379.

28. F. Lepore. Spontaneous visual phenomena with visual loss. *Neurology* 1990; 40:444–447. These hallucinations are not seizures.

29. L. Daniell. The non-competitive N-methyl-D-aspartate antagonists, MK-801, phencyclidine and ketamine, increase the potency of general anesthetics. *Pharmacology, Biochemistry and Behavior* 1990; 36:111–115.

30. C. Whitty and W. Lewin. Vivid day-dreaming. An unusual form of confusion following anterior cingulectomy. *Brain* 1957; 80:72–76.

Chapter 88   Stimulating Human Brains

1. E. Valenstein. *Brain Control*. New York, Wiley, 1973, 180.

2. S. Obrador and G. Dierssen. Mental changes induced by subcortical stimulation and therapeutic Lesions. *Confinia Neurologica* 1967; 29:168.

3. P. Gloor. Experiential phenomena of temporal lobe epilepsy. *Brain* 1990; 113:1673–1694.

4. E. Halgren. Mental phenomena induced by stimulation of the limbic system. *Human Neurobiology* 1:251–260. Brain stimulations are a necessary part of the surgical approach to a severe seizure disorder. They help the neurosurgeon to define the normal anatomy, and to decide which part of the brain is so abnormal that the patient will do better if it is removed.

5. C. Sem-Jacobsen and A. Torkildsen. Depth recording and electrical stimulation in the human brain. In *Electrical Studies on the Unanesthetized Brain*, eds. E. Ramey and D. O'Doherty, New York, Hoeber, 1960, 275–290.

Chapter 89   The Ins and Outs of Imagery

1. D. Hume, from *A Treatise on Human Nature*, cited in S. Kosslyn. *Image and Mind*. Cambridge, Mass., Harvard University Press, 1980.

2. R. Finke. Theories relating mental imagery to perception. *Psychological Bulletin* 1985; 98:236–259.

3. J. Barrett and H. Ehrlichman. Bilateral hemispheric alpha activity during visual imagery. *Neuropsychologia* 1982; 20:703–708.

4. G. Goldenberg, I. Podreka, F. Uhl, et al. Cerebral correlates of imagining colours, faces and a map I. SPECT of regional cerebral blood flow. *Neuropsychologia* 1989; 27:1315–1328.

5. M. Farah. The laterality of mental image generation: A test with normal subjects. *Neuropsychologia* 1986; 24:541–551.

6. C. Biggins, B. Turetsky, and G. Fein. The cerebral laterality of mental image generation in normal subjects. *Psychophysiology* 1990; 27:57–67.

7. P. Rappelsberger and H. Petsche. Probability mapping: Power and coherence analyses of cognitive processes. *Brain Topography* 1988; 1:46–54.

8. S. Segal and V. Fusella. Effects of imaging on signal-to-noise ratio; with varying signal conditions. *British Journal of Psychology* 1969; 60:459–464.

9. J. Bumgartner and C. Epstein. Voluntary alteration of visual evoked potentials. *Annals of Neurology* 1982; 12:475–478. The amplitude and the latency of the potentials changed.

10. M. Schatzman. *The Story of Ruth*. New York, Putnam's, 1980.

11. The auditory hallucinations of schizophrenic patients delay the auditory evoked potential just as much as do external sounds. See J. Tiihonen, R. Hari, H. Naukkarinen, et al. Modified activity of the human auditory cortex during auditory hallucinations. *American Journal of Psychiatry* 1992; 149:255–257.

12. R. Frick. A dissociation of conscious visual imagery and visual short-term memory. *Neuropsychologia* 1987; 25:707–712.

13. An oversimplified hypothesis for regenerating images proposes that we mostly redirect many of the original avenues of information flow. See D. Pandya and E. Yeterian. Proposed neural circuitry for spatial memory in the primate brain. *Neuropsychologia* 1984; 11:109–122.

14. B. Brown. Effect of LSD on visually evoked responses to color in visualizer and nonvisualizer subjects. *Electroencephalography and Clinical Neurophysiology* 1969; 27:356–363. In this respect, nonvisualizers resemble patients who have temporal lobe damage.

Chapter 90   The Tachistoscope

1. D. Burr. Motion smear. *Nature* 1980; 284:164–165.
2. J. Santamaria and K. Chiappa. *The EEG of Drowsiness*. New York, Demos, 1987.
3. R. Noyes. The experience of dying. *Psychiatry* 1972; 35:174–184.

Chapter 91   The Descent of Charles Darwin: Computer Parallels

1. F. Darwin, ed. *The Autobiography of Charles Darwin*. New York, Dover, 1958, 8–9.
2. Because many different types of nerve cells are damaged in this disorder, it is not possible to assign the patient's slow mentation solely to a deficit of their dopamine or norepinephrine systems. See R. Mayeux, Y. Stern, M. Sano, et al. Clinical and biochemical correlates of bradyphrenia in Parkinson's disease. *Neurology* 1987; 37:1130–1134.
3. D. Freeman. Street smarts. *Popular Mechanics*, November 1991, 33–36. Prometheus is an acronym formed by: *pro*gramme for *E*uropean *t*raffic with *h*ighest *e*fficiency and *u*nprecedented *s*afety.
4. P. Elmer-Dewitt. Machines from the lunatic fringe. *Time*, 11 November 1991, 74–75.
5. W. Nauta and M. Feirtag. *Fundamental Neuroanatomy*. New York, W.H. Freeman, 1986. The numbers vary among different authors in different texts.
6. V. Mountcastle. Some neural mechanisms for directed experience. In *Cerebral Correlates of Conscious Experience*, eds. P. Buser and A. Rougeul-Buser. Amsterdam, North-Holland, 1978, 37–51.
7. W. Milberg and M. Albert. The speed of constituent mental operations and its relationship to neuronal representation: An hypothesis. In *Perspectives on Cognitive Neuroscience*, eds. R. Lister and H. Weingartner. New York, Oxford University Press, 1991, 368–383.

Chapter 92   Bytes of Memory

1. Of course, none of these observations were quantitated during the chant itself.
2. W. Penfield and H. Jasper. *Epilepsy and the Functional Anatomy of the Human Brain*. Boston, Little, Brown, 1954, 468–469.
3. H. Coslett, D. Bowers, M. Verfaellie, et al. Frontal verbal amnesia. Phonological amnesia. *Archives of Neurology* 1991; 48:949–955.
4. W. Milberg and M. Albert. The speed of constituent mental operations and its relationship to neuronal representation: An hypothesis. In *Perspectives on Cognitive Neuroscience*, eds. R. Lister and H. Weingartner. New York, Oxford University Press, 1991, 368–383.

Chapter 93   Where Is The Phantom Limb?

1. C. Bell, cited in T. Furukawa. Charles Bell's description of the phantom phenomenon in 1830. *Neurology* 1990; 40:1830.
2. P. Bromage and R. Melzack. Phantom limbs and the body schema. *Canadian Journal of Anaesthesia* 1974; 21:267–274.
3. R. Melzack. Phantom limbs and the concept of a neuromatrix. *Trends in Neurosciences* 1990; 13:88–92.
4. P. Wall. Pain and no pain. In *Functions of the Brain*, ed. C. Coen. Oxford, Clarendon Press, 1985, 44–66.
5. The technical term for this active *denial* of ownership of body parts is *anosognosia*.

Chapter 94   The Feel of Two Hands

1. D. Suzuki. *Zen and Japanese Culture*. Bollingen Series 64. Princeton, N.J., Princeton University Press, 1973, 16.
2. The episode took place in London, in July 1982.
3. J. Chapin and D. Woodward. Modulation of sensory responsiveness of single somatosensory cortical cells during movement and arousal behaviors. *Experimental Neurology* 1981; 72:164–178.
4. A. Starr and L. Cohen. "Gating" of somatosensory evoked potentials begins before the onset of voluntary movement in man. *Brain Research* 1985; 348:183–186.

5. H. Sakata. The parietal association cortex: Neurophysiology. In *Scientific Basis of Clinical Neurology*, eds. M. Swash and C. Kennard. Edinburgh, Churchill Livingstone, 1985, 225–236.

6. R. Metherate, N. Tremblay, and R. Dykes. The effects of acetylcholine on response properties of cat somatosensory cortical neurons. *Journal of Neurophysiology* 1988; 59:1231–1252.

7. T. Hicks. *Development, Organization, and Processing in Somatosensory Pathways. Functional Properties of Neurons Mediated by GABA in Cat Somatosensory Cortex Under Barbiturate and Urethane Anaesthesia*, eds. M. Rowe and W. Willis. New York, Liss, 1985, 265–276.

8. J.-I. Oka, E. Jang, and T. Hicks. Benzodiazepine receptor involvement in the control of receptive field size and responsiveness in primary somatosensory cortex. *Brain Research* 1986; 376:194–198.

9. R. Metherate, N. Tremblay, and R. Dykes. Transient and prolonged effects of acetylcholine on responsiveness of cat somatosensory cortical neurons. *Journal of Neurophysiology* 1988; 59:1253–1276.

10. I had risen that morning earlier than usual. Perhaps the episode reflected the crest of an especially high wave thrown up on that morning's rising tide of events. In humans, endorphin levels are among those messengers which peak in the morning. And in rats, various opioids and ACTH molecules do set off grooming behaviors. See W. Gispen, V. Wiegant, A. Bradbury, et al. Induction of excessive grooming in the rat by fragments of lipotropin. *Nature* 1976; 264:794–795. But humans aren't rats, and we will not tend to wash in the morning solely because our β-endorphin levels then happen to be high.

11. B. Waterhouse, H. Moises, H. Yeh, et al. Norepinephrine enhancement of inhibitory synaptic mechanisms in cerebellum and cerebral cortex. *Journal of Pharmacology and Experimental Therapeutics* 1982; 221:495–506.

Chapter 95   The Attentive Cat

1. Martin Buber, cited in D. Suzuki. *Sengai the Zen Master.* London, Faber & Faber, 1971. Pet owners, knowing their dogs and cats *are* Buddha-nature, can be troubled by the koan *Mu*, which they interpret as negating this premise.

2. J. Bouyer, C. Tilquin, and A. Rougeul. Thalamic rhythms in cat during quiet wakefulness and immobility. *Electroencephalography and Clinical Neurophysiology* 1983; 55:180–187.

3. J. Bouyer, M. Montaron, J. Vahnee, et al. Anatomical localization of cortical beta rhythms in cat. *Neuroscience* 1987; 22:863–869. When monkeys are poised to transform their sensory input into a vigorous motor command, they also develop similar fast rhythms in their parietal association cortex. The region activated in the monkey corresponds with area 5A in human cortex.

4. The brain also deploys a separate, *intralaminar* thalamic nucleus to excite the parietal association cortex. A noteworthy feature of this central lateral nucleus is that its responses are further enhanced by attention, arousal, or pain. See B. Rydenhag, B. Olausson, B. Shyn, et al. Localized responses in the midsuprasylvian gyrus of the cat following stimulation of the central lateral nucleus in thalamus. *Experimental Brain Research* 1986; 62:11–24.

5. A. Rougeul-Buser. Monoamines, cortical rhythms and attentive behavior in cat. In *Modulation of Sensorimotor Activity During Alterations in Behavioral States*, ed. R. Baudler. New York, Liss, 1984, 139–149.

6. M. F. Montaron, J. Bouyer, A. Rougeul, et al. Ventral mesencephalic tegmentum controls electrocortical beta rhythms and associated attentive behavior in the cat. *Behavioral Brain Research* 1982; 6:129–145.

7. M. Montaron and P. Buser. Relationships between nucleus medialis dorsalis, pericruciate cortex, ventral tegmental area and nucleus accumbens in cat: An electrophysiological study. *Experimental Brain Research* 1988; 69:559–566. More recently, the fast activity *above* 30 cps has been called *gamma* activity.

8. W. Klemm. Electroencephalographic behavioral dissociations during animal hypnosis. *Electroencephalography and Clinical Neurophysiology* 1966; 21:365–372.

9. J. Chapin and D. Woodward. Modulation of sensory responsiveness of single somatosensory cortical cells during movement and arousal behaviors. *Experimental Neurology* 1981; 72:164–178.

Chapter 96 Emotionalized Awareness without Sensate Loss

1. J. Ray. In B. Stevenson, ed. *The Home Book of Quotations*. New York, Crown, 1967.
2. The episode occurred during a Dai Sesshin at Jemez Springs, New Mexico in 1989.
3. The basic core of these minutes of joyful, tearful purification seems to fit best into the category of State V (see chapter 68, table 10). It is also reminiscent of Laski's "Adamic" subtype of experience (see chapter 5). In point of sequence, this separate "moist-eyed" episode came seven years after the taste of kensho. Had it occurred earlier and coincided with kensho, it could have infused a strong sense of unity into the texture of that experience, prolonging it and making it even more memorable. I had not been fasting during this retreat, and there were no hunger pangs before the episode began.

Chapter 97 Seizures, Religious Experience, and Patterns of Behavior

1. A. Gupta, P. Jeavons, R. Hughes, et al. Aura in temporal lobe epilepsy: Clinical and electroencephalographic correlation. *Journal of Neurology, Neurosurgery and Psychiatry* 1983; 46:1079–1083.
2. H. Gastaut. Fyodor Mikhailovitch Dostoevsky's involuntary contribution to the symptomatology and prognosis of epilepsy. *Epilepsia* 1978; 19:186–201.
3. F. Cirignotta, C. Todesco, and E. Lugaresi. Temporal lobe epilepsy with ecstatic seizures (so-called Dostoevsky epilepsy). *Epilepsia* 1980; 21:705–710.
4. M. Persinger. Striking EEG profiles from single episodes of glossolalia and transcendental meditation. *Perceptual and Motor Skills* 1984; 58:127–133.
5. M-M. Mesulam. Dissociative states with abnormal temporal lobe EEG: Multiple personality and the illusion of possession. *Archives of Neurology* 1981; 38:176–181.
6. K. Dewhurst and A. Beard. Sudden religious conversion in temporal lobe epilepsy. *British Journal of Psychiatry* 1970; 117:497–507.
7. D. Bear, K. Levin, D. Blumer, et al. Interictal behavior in hospitalized temporal lobe epileptics: Relationship to idiopathic psychiatric syndromes. *Journal of Neurology, Neurosurgery and Psychiatry* 1982; 45:481–488.
8. B. Hermann and P. Riel. Interictal personality and behavioral traits in temporal lobe and generalized epilepsy. *Cortex* 1981; 17:125–128.
9. L. Willmore, K. Heilman, E. Fennell, et al. Effect of chronic seizures of religiosity. In *Program of the American Neurological Association*, 1980, abstract 24, 97.
10. E. Rodin and S. Schmaltz. The Bear-Fedio personality inventory and temporal lobe epilepsy. *Neurology* 1984; 34:591–596.
11. C. Dodrill and L. Batzel. Interictal behavioral features of patients with epilepsy. *Epilepsia* 1986; 27(suppl. 2):S64–S76.
12. D. Tucker, R. Novelly, and P. Walker. Hyperreligiosity in temporal lobe epilepsy: Redefining the relationship. *Journal of Nervous and Mental Disease* 1987; 175:181–184.
13. J. Frost, H. Mayberg, R. Fisher, et al. Mu-opiate receptors measured by positron emission tomography are increased in temporal lobe epilepsy. *Annals of Neurology* 1988; 23:231–237.
14. D. Hodoba. Paradoxic sleep facilitation by interictal epileptic activity of right temporal origin. *Biological Psychiatry* 1986; 21:1267–1278.
15. A. Walker and D. Blumer. The localization of sex in the brain. In *Cerebral Localization*, eds. K. Zulch, O. Creutzfeldt, and G. Galbraith. New York, Springer-Verlag, 1975, 184–199.
16. P. Flor-Henry. Epilepsy and psychopathology. In *Recent Advances in Clinical Psychiatry*, 2nd ed., ed. K. Granville-Grossman. Edinburgh, Churchill, Livingston, 1976, 262–295. During orgasm in normals, the left side shows the greater activity.
17. We have no reason to exclude the possibility that, in a few rare patients with seizures, their focal neuronal seizure disorders could not spread (in a disorganized manner) into

some of the same deep pathways that are also activated in alternate states of consciousness.

Chapter 98 The Fleeting "Truths" of Nitrous Oxide

1. W. James. In *Laughing Gas (Nitrous Oxide)*, eds. M. Shedlin, D. Wallechinsky, and S. Salyer. And/Or Press, 1973.

2. W. James. *The Varieties of Religious Experience.* New York, Mentor/New American, 1958, 198.

3. M. Shedlin, D. Wallechinsky, and S. Salyer, eds. *Laughing Gas (Nitrous Oxide).* And/Or Press, 1973.

4. James, *The Varieties of Religious Experience,* 298.

5. B. Fink. Diffusion anoxia. *Anesthesiology* 1955; 16:511.

6. W. Lopez. The effects of nitrous oxide. In *Laughing Gas (Nitrus Oxide)*, eds. M. Shedlin, D. Wallechinsky, and S. Salyer. And/Or Press, 1973, 20–28. N_2O does not depress vasomotor, cough, respiratory, or vomiting mechanisms, or cause major changes in intracranial pressure.

7. T. Yamamura. Fast oscillatory EEG activity induced by analgesic concentrations of nitrous oxide in man. *Anesthesia and Analgesia* 1981; 60:283–288.

8. In a recent report, 50 percent N_2O was said to increase human frontal cortical blood flow about 37 percent. The observation is, however, qualified and needs to be repeated under different conditions. One hundred percent O_2 was breathed during the prior control period. This much O_2 could have artificially lowered cerebral blood flow during the control period. See G. Deutsch and S. Samra. Effects of nitrous oxide on global and regional cortical blood flow. *Stroke* 1990; 21:1293–1298.

9. J. McCulloch. Mapping functional alterations in the CNS with [^{14}C] deoxyglucose. In *Handbook of Psychopharmacology,* eds. L. Iversen, S. Iversen, and S. Snyder. New Techniques in Psychopharmacology, vol. 15. New York, 1982, Plenum Press, 321–410.

10. M. Ingvar and B. Siesjö. Effect of nitrous oxide on local cerebral glucose utilization in rats. *Journal of Cerebral Blood Flow and Metabolism* 1982; 2:481–486.

11. G. Crosby. The local metabolic effects of somatosensory stimulation in the central nervous system of rats given pentobarbital or nitrous oxide. *Anesthesiology* 1983; 58:38–43.

12. R. Quock and J. Mueller. Protection by U-50, 488H against β-chlornaltrexamine antagonism of nitrous oxide antinociception in mice. *Brain Research* 1991; 549:162–164.

13. M. Gillman. Analgesic (subanesthetic) nitrous oxide interacts with the endogenous opioid system: A review of the literature. *Life Sciences* 1986; 39:1209–1221.

14. J. Zuniga, S. Joseph, and K. Knigge. The effects of nitrous oxide on the secretory activity of pro-opiomelanocortin peptides from basal hypothalamic cells attached to Cytodex beads in a superfusion in vitro system. *Brain Research* 1987; 420:66–72.

15. J. Zuniga, S. Joseph, and K. Knigge. The effects of nitrous oxide on the central endogenous pro-opiomelanocortin system in the rat. *Brain Research* 1987; 420:57–65.

16. J. Zuniga, S. Joseph, and K. Kingge. Nitrous oxide analgesia: Partial antagonism by naloxone and total reversal after periaqueductal gray lesions in the rat. *European Journal of Pharmacology* 1987; 142:51–60.

17. R. Quock and L. Graczak. Influence of narcotic antagonist drugs upon nitrous oxide analgesia in mice. *Brain Research* 1988; 440:35–41. The reason for considering dynorphin stems from the observation that an antagonist drug which reduces N_2O analgesia is also a (relatively) selective blocker of kappa opioid receptors.[11]

18. B. Fowler, B. Kelso, J. Landolt, et al. The effects of nitrous oxide on P300 and reaction time. *Electroencephalography and Clinical Neurophysiology* 1988; 69:171–178.

19. R. Sandyk. Analgesic nitrous oxide in alcohol withdrawal. The role of melatonin. *International Journal of Neuroscience* 1991; 56:201–205.

20. D. Koblin, B. Tomerson, and F. Waldman. Disruption of folate and vitamin B-12 metabolism in aged rats following exposure to nitrous oxide. *Anesthesiology* 1990; 73:506–512.

21. S. Vishnubhakat and H. Beresford. Reversible myeloneuropathy of nitrous oxide abuse: Serial electrophysiological studies. *Muscle and Nerve* 1991; 14:22–26.

22. D. Bredt, P. Hwang, and S. Snyder.: Localization of nitric oxide synthase indicating a neural role for nitric oxide. *Nature* 1990; 347:768–770. The nerve cells which make NO˙ are among those relatively resistant to anoxia. This property could enable them to participate in the later phases of near-death phenomena.

23. A. McDonald, D. Payne, and F. Mascagni. Identification of putative nitric oxide producing neurons in the rat amygdala using NADPH-diaphorase histochemistry. *Neuroscience* 1993; 52:97–106.

24. S. Vincent and H. Kimura.: Histochemical mapping of nitric oxide synthase in the rat brain. *Neuroscience* 1992; 46:755–784. Some acetylcholine cells in the mesopontine region also contain other (atrio) peptides. These can act on the *in*soluble form of the enzyme which makes cyclic guanosine monophosphate (cGMP). Therefore these cells have a second way to enhance the metabolic effects of cGMP.

25. T. McCall and P. Vallance. Nitric oxide takes centre-stage with newly defined roles. *Trends in Pharmacological Science* 1992; 13:1–6.

26. D. Linden and J. Connor. Long-term depression of glutamate currents in cultured cerebellar Purkinge neurons does not require nitric oxide signalling. *European Journal of Neuroscience* 1992; 4:10–15.

27. H-C. Pape and R. Mager. Nitric oxide controls oscillatory activity in thalamocortical neurons. *Neuron* 1992; 9:441–448.

28. E. Schuman and D. Madison. Nitric oxide and synaptic function. *Annual Review of Neuroscience* 1994; 17:153–183.

29. T. Nguyen, D. Brunson, C. Crespi, et al. DNA damage and mutation in human cells exposed to nitric oxide in vitro. *Proceedings of the National Academy of Sciences of the United States of America* 1992; 89:3030–3034.

30. B. Heinzel, M. John, P. Klatt, et al. Ca²⁺/calmodulin–dependent formation of hydrogen peroxide by brain nitric oxide synthase. *Biochemical Journal* 1992; 281:627–630.

31. S. Vincent. Nitric oxide: A radical neurotransmitter in the central nervous system. *Progress in Neurobiology* 1994; 42:129–160.

Chapter 99   The Roots of Laughter

1. J. Thurber. *Lanterns and Lances*. London, Hamish Hamilton, 1961.

2. O. Petre-Quadens. Sleep in the human newborn. In *Basic Sleep Mechanisms*, eds. O. Petre-Quadens and J. Schlag. New York, Academic Press, 1974, 355–380.

3. A. Pasi, P. Kulling, D. Voellmy, et al. Beta-endorphin in the brainstem and the cerebellum of the human infant. *Physiology and Behavior* 1989; 46:13–16.

4. S. Duclos, J. Laird, E. Schneider, et al. Emotion-specific effects of facial expressions and postures on emotional experiences. *Journal of Personal and Social Psychology* 1989; 57:100–108.

5. At this late date, we will never know to what degree the behavior of Kanzan's (Hanshan's) happy lunatic friend, the legendary Jittoku, may also have expressed elements of mental deficiency or tendencies toward hebephrenic schizophrenia.

6. D. Suzuki. *Sengai, the Zen Master*. New York, New York Graphic Society, 1971, 94.

7. C. Hyers. *Zen and the Comic Spirit*. Philadelphia, Westminster, 1973, 127.

8. R. Boston. *An anatomy of Laughter*. London, Collins, 1974.

9. K. Kraft. Muso Kokushi's *Dialogues in a Dream*. Selections. *The Eastern Buddhist* 1981; 14:74–93.

10. D. Suzuki. *Essays in Zen Buddhism*, Second Series 1958, ed. C. Humphries. New York, Weiser, 1970, 26–27.

11. P. Kapleau. *The Three Pillars of Zen: Teaching, Practice, and Enlightenment*. Boston, Beacon Press, 1967, 204–207.

12. Suzuki, *Sengai*, 1.

13. W. Kaufmann. *Critique of Religion and Philosophy*. New York, Harper & Row Torchbook, 1972.

14. R. Ironside. Disorders of laughter due to brain lesions. *Brain* 1956; 79:589–609.

15. C. Sem-Jacobsen. Electrical stimulation and self-stimulation in man with chronic implanted electrodes: Interpretation and pitfalls of results. In *Brain-Stimulation Reward*, eds. A. Wauquier and E. Rolls. Amsterdam, North Holland, 1976, 505–520.

16. R. Hassler. Interaction of reticular activating system for vigilance and the truncothalamic and pallidal systems for directing awareness and attention under striatal control. In *Cerebral Correlates of Conscious Experience* eds. P. Buser and A. Rougeul-Buser, Amsterdam, North-Holland, 1978, 111–129.

17. T. Hurwitz, J. Wada, B. Kosaka, et al. Cerebral organization of affect suggested by temporal lobe seizures. *Neurology* 1985; 35:1335–1337.

18. G. Pearlson and R. Robinson. Lateralization of emotional or behavioral responses in intact and hemisphere-damaged humans and rats. In *The Expression of Knowledge*, eds. R. Isaacson and N. Spear. New York, Plenum Press, 1982, 339–390.

19. B. Aaronson and H. Osmond, eds. *Psychedelics. The Uses and Implications of Hallucinogenic Drugs*. London, Hogarth, 1971, 29.

20. S. Schachter and L. Wheeler. Epinephrine, chlorpromazine, and amusement. *Journal of Abnormal Psychology* 1962; 65:121–128.

21. D. Gilbert. *The Upside Down Circle: Zen Laughter*. Nevada City, Calif., Blue Dolphin, 1988.

Chapter 100   How Do Psychedelic and Certain Other Drugs Affect the Brain?

1. L. Grinspoon and J. Bakalar. *Psychedelic Drugs Reconsidered*. New York, Basic Books, 1979.

2. D. Freedman. LSD: The bridge from human to animal. In *Hallucinogens: Neurochemical, Behavioral, and Clinical Perspectives*, ed. B. Jacobs. New York, Raven Press, 1983, 203–226.

3. R. Masters and J. Houston. *The Varieties of Psychedelic Experience*. New York, Holt, Rinehart & Winston, 1966.

4. A. Watts. "Ordinary mind is the way." The *Eastern Buddhist* 1971; 4:134–137.

5. E. Bliss, L. Clark, and C. West. Studies of sleep deprivation—Relationship to schizophrenia. *Archives of Neurology and Psychiatry* 1959; 81:348–359. In calculating dosages, 1 kilogram equals 2.2 lb.

6. S. Grof. *Realms of the Human Unconscious. Observations from LSD Research*. New York, Dutton, 1976.

7. J. Pollard, L. Uhr, and E. Stern. *Drugs and Phantasy. The Effects of LSD, Psilocybin, and Sernyl on College Students*. Boston, Little, Brown. 1965. The term "sensory deprivation" is quoted for two reasons. First, because all sensation was not removed. Second, other elements in the experimental setting did not fit this description. The subjects were healthy college students, surrounded by white noise, presented with a homogeneous milky visual field, and loosely strapped to a foam rubber pad with their hands in cotton mitts. They were also encouraged to speak into a tape recorder, and the whole study was cast in the artifice of an "experimental" mode. Because the subjects were permitted to talk, it would be difficult to equate their artificial setting with that used by Grof or others who played music in the background. The more artificial the laboratory setting, the more it tends to interfere with subjects going on fully to develop either psychedelic states or nondrug meditative states as well.

8. E. Serafetinides. The significance of the temporal lobes and of hemispheric dominance in the production of the LSD-25 symptomatology in man: A study of epileptic patients before and after temporal lobectomy. *Neuropsychologia* 1965; 3:69–79. The LSD dosages were one microgram per kilogram.

9. R. Monroe, R. Heath, W. Mickle, et al. Correlation of rhinencephalic electrograms with behavior. *Electroencephalography and Clinical Neurolophysiology* 1957; 9:623–642.

10. Ram Dass. Lecture at the Maryland Psychiatric Research Center, pt. 1. *Journal of Transpersonal Psychology* 1973; 5:75–103.

11. M. Baldwin, S. Lewis, and S. Bach. The effects of lysergic acid after cerebral ablation. *Neurology* 1959; 9:469–474. The LSD dose was sixty micrograms per kilogram. Most drugs are given to animals in a higher dosage per kilo than the dosage given to humans.

12. S. Snyder. *Drugs and the Brain*. New York, Scientific American Library, 1986.

13. S. Grof and J. Halifax. *The Human Encounter with Death*. New York, Dutton 1977, 184–188.

14. S. Grof. *LSD Psychotherapy*. Pomona, Calif., Hunter House, 1994.

15. D. Freedman. Hallucinogenic drug research—If so, so what?: Symposium summary and commentary. *Pharmacology, Biochemistry, and Behavior* 1986; 24:407–415.

16. J. Muzio, H. Roffwarg, and E. Kaufman. Alterations in the nocturnal sleep cycle resulting from LSD. *Electroencephalography and Clinical Neurophysiology*. 1966; 21:313–324. In most instances when the literature refers to "REM sleep," it includes periods of D-sleep with occasional REM episodes. In this study, the low LSD doses which enhanced human REM episodes ranged between 0.13 and 0.73 micrograms per kilogram.

17. J. Silverman. A paradigm for the study of altered states of consciousness. *British Journal of Psychiatry* 1968; 14:1201–1218.

18. P. Bradley and J. Elkes. The effects of some drugs on the electrical activity of the brain. *Brain* 1957; 80:77–117. The LSD dose cited was thirty micrograms per kilogram. Monkeys given mescaline showed paroxysmal activity in their cortical, as well as in their septal and hippocampal regions.

19. P. Brawley and J. Duffield. The pharmacology of hallucinogens. *Pharmacological Reviews* 1972; 24:31–66.

20. Simpler mechanisms have been proposed to account for the ways LSD changes *motor* behaviors in lower animals. They do not necessarily clarify how LSD affects the complex mental functions of humans and other higher primates in whom hallucinations play the most prominent role.[19] See M. Davis. Neurochemical modulation of sensory-motor reactivity: Acoustic and tactile startle reflexes. *Neuroscience and Biobehavioral Reviews* 1980; 4:241–263; and M. Davis, J. Kehne, R. Commissaris, et al. Effects of hallucinogens on unconditioned behaviors in animals. In *Hallucinogens: Neurochemical, Behavioral, and Clinical Perspectives*, ed. B. Jacobs. New York, Raven Press, 1983, 35–75.

21. E. Ellinwood. Amphetamine psychosis: I. Description of the individuals and the process. *Journal of Nervous and Mental Disease* 1967; 144:273–283.

22. G. Ricaurte, K. Finnegan, I. Irwin, et al. Aminergic metabolites in cerebrospinal fluid of humans previously exposed to MDMA: Preliminary observations. *Annals of the New York Academy of Science*. 1990; 600:699–710.

23. J. Meehan: U.S. allies appear to harden stand on drug money. *International Herald Tribune* October 13, 1988, 1. (The figure cited was 120 billion dollars a year.)

24. R. Post and N. Contel. Human and animal studies of cocaine: Implications for development of behavioral pathology. In *Stimulants: Neurochemical, Behavioral, and Clinical Perspectives;* Creese, I. ed. Raven Press, New York, 1983, 169–203.

25. R. Resnick, R. Kestenbaum, and L. Schwartz. Acute systemic effects of cocaine in man: A controlled study of intranasal and intravenous routes of administration. In *Cocaine and Other Stimulants;* M. Kilbery and E. Ellinwood, eds. New York; Plenum; 1977.

26. C. Van Dyke and R. Byck. Cocaine 1884–1974. In M. Kilbey, and E. Ellinwood, eds. Ibid; 1977, 1–30.

27. A Houdi, M. Bardo, and G. VanLoon. Opioid mediation of cocaine-induced hyperactivity and reinforcement. *Brain Research* 1989, 497:195–198.

28. P. Furst "High" states in culture-historical perspective. In N. Zinberg, ed. Ibid., 1977, 69–70.

29. R. Aitken: LSD and the new American Zen student. *Eastern Buddhist*. October 1971, 4:2,141–144.

30. J. Singer. Ongoing thought: The normative baseline for alternate states of consciousness. In *Alternate States of Consciousness*, ed. N. Zinberg, New York, Free Press, 1977, 89–120.

31. R. Jordan. Psychedelics and Zen: Some reflections. *The Eastern Buddhist* 1971; 4(2):138–140.

32. W. Kaufmann. *Critique of Religion and Philosophy.* New York, Harper & Row Torchbook, 1972, 366.

33. S. Grof and J. Halifax, *The Human Encounter with Death*, 67.

Chapter 101   Levels and Sequences of Psychedelic Experience After LSD

1. S. Grof. *LSD Psychotherapy.* Pomona, Calif., Hunter House, 1994, 270.

2. R. Masters and J. Houston. *The Varieties of Psychedelic Experience.* New York, Holt, Rinehart & Winston, 1966.

3. *Ibid.*, 302.

4. Their usage of "introvertive" in the drug context does not appear entirely consonant with Stace's earlier use of the same term. It illustrates the semantic pitfalls associated with the words "introvertive" and "extrovertive" (see also chapter 126).

5. Masters and Houston, *op. cit.*, 312. We are not informed whether these subjects' eyes were open or closed, what dose of which drug they took, or precisely how many drug exposures they had undergone.

6. W. Van Dusen. LSD and the enlightenment of Zen. *Psychologia* 1961; 4:11–16.

7. S. Grof. Varieties of transpersonal experiences: observations from LSD psychotherapy. In *Psychiatry and Mysticism*, ed. S. Dean. Chicago, Nelson Hall, 1975, 311–345.

8. S. Grof. *Realms of the Human Unconscious. Observations from LSD Research.* New York, Dutton, 1976.

9. S. Grof, *LSD Psychotherapy*, 235.

10. Grof, *Realms of the Human Unconscious*, 32.

11. Grof, *LSD Psychotherapy*, 125.

12. *Ibid.*, 219.

13. Grof, *Realms of the Human Unconscious*, 105–107.

14. Grof, Varieties of transpersonal experiences, 317.

15. Grof, *Realms of the Human Unconscious*, 106.

16. *Ibid.*, 107.

17. Grof, *LSD Psychotherapy*, 127.

18. *Ibid.*, 119.

19. Grof, *Realms of the Human Unconscious*, 203–205.

20. Grof, *LSD Psychotherapy*, 227.

21. *Ibid.*, 241–242.

22. A. Watts. *Does It Matter?* New York, Vintage, 1971.

23. S. Snyder. *Drugs and the Brain.* New York, Scientific American Library, 1986, 181.

24. G. Jordan. LSD and mystical experiences. In *The Highest State of Consciousness*, ed. J. White. Garden City, N.Y., Anchor/Doubleday, 1972, 278–294.

Chapter 102   The Miracle of Marsh Chapel

1. R. Masters and J. Houston. *The Varieties of Psychedelic Experience.* New York, Holt, Rinehart & Winston, 1966.

2. Mushrooms are talented and make a variety of molecules. The wild mushroom *Amanita muscaria* has low levels of three psychoactive agents: muscarine (the acetylcholine agonist), psilocybin (the serotonin agonist), and muscimole (the $GABA_A$ agonist). Its major toxicity comes from high levels of potent plant toxins. However, high doses of pure muscimole itself can cause delirium, coma, and amnesia (See L. Grinspoon and J. Balakar. Psychedelic drugs reconsidered. New York, Basic Books, 1979.) Despite these considerations, some have contended that the "soma" referred to in the ancient Hindu Vedas could have been *A. muscaria*. (See R. Wasson). Fly agaric and man. In *Ethnopharmacologic Search for Psychoactive Drugs*, eds. D. Effron, B. Holmstedt, and N. Kline. New York, Raven Press, 1979, 405–414.

3. W. Pahnke. Drugs and mysticism. In *The Highest State of Consciousness*, ed. J. White. Garden City, N.Y., Anchor/Doubleday, 1972, 257–277.

4. G. Stockings. A clinical study of the mescaline psychosis, with special reference to the mechanism of the genesis of schizophrenic and other psychotic states. *Journal of Mental Science* 1940; 86:29–47.

5. J. Blofeld. Consciousness, energy, bliss. In *The Ecstatic Adventure*, ed. R. Metzner. New York, Macmillan, 1968, 131.

6. W. VanDusen. LSD and the enlightenment of Zen. *Psychologia* 1961, 4:11–16.

7. B. Aaronson. Some hypnotic analogues to the psychedelic state. In *Psychedelics. The Uses and Implications of Hallucinogenic Drugs*, eds. B. Aaronson and H. Osmond. London, Hogarth, 1971, 279–295.

Chapter 103   How Do Psychedelic Drugs Affect Amine Receptors?

1. L. Grinspoon and J. Bakalar. *Psychedelic Drugs Reconsidered*. New York, Basic Books, 1979.

2. G. Reznikoff, S. Manaker, C. Rhodes, et al. Localization and quantification of β-adrenergic receptors in human brain. *Neurology* 1986; 36:1067–1073.

3. G. Aghajanian. The physiology of central α- and β-adrenoceptors. In *Catecholamines Part B: Neuropharmacology and Central Nervous System—Theoretical Aspects*, eds. E. Usdin, A. Carlsson, A. Dahlström, et al. New York, Liss, 1984, 85–92. The key regions tested for their α-receptors include the cortex, lateral geniculate nucleus, and the dorsal raphe nucleus.

4. Slower chemical (metabotropic) changes also occur after norepinephrine α_1-receptors are activated. A phosphated lipid splits off and two second messengers are generated: inositol triphosphate and diacylglycerol.

5. R. Thatcher and E. John. *Foundations of Cognitive Processes*. Functional Neuroscience, vol. 1. Hillsdale, N.J., Erlbaum, 1977. Reaction times are slowed with the eyes either open or closed.

6. These particular receptors are called "autoreceptors." Sensitive to serotonin, they lie out on the *dendrites* of ST nerve cells themselves. Normally, when raphe cells fire, some of their own ST leaks out to reach the autoreceptors. These ST receptors then provide the negative feedback which inhibits further raphe cell firing.

7. D. Nash, P. Sanberg, and A. Norman. LSD: Interactions with serotonin receptor subtypes in the brain (abstract). *Neurology* 1988; 38(suppl. 1): 179.

8. P. Pierce and S. Peroutka. *d*-Lysergic acid diethylamide differentially affects the dual actions of 5-hydroxytryptamine on cortical neurons. *Neuropharmacology* 1990; 29:705–712. The discovery first of ST_3, next of four more ST receptors illustrates how the whole topic of receptors is currently an ever-expanding one.

9. In the pons, when LSD or mescaline acts on ST_2 receptors, the facial motor cells fire faster in response to additional amounts of either ST or NE. See K. Rasmussen and G. Aghajanian. Effect of hallucinogens on spontaneous and sensory-evoked locus coeruleus unit activity in the rat: Reversal by selective 5-HT$_2$ antagonists. *Brain Research* 1986; 385:395–400.

10. M. Trulson. Dissociations between the effects of hallucinogens on behavior and raphé unit activity in behaving cats. *Pharmacology, Biochemistry, and Behavior* 1986; 24:351–357.

11. M. Rogawski and G. Aghajanian. Response of central monoaminergic neurons to lisuride: Comparison with LSD. *Life Sciences* 1979; 24:1289–1298.

12. B. Jacobs and M. Trulson. Mechanisms of action of LSD. *American Scientist* 1979; 67:396–404. The lower dosages of LSD referred to were one microgram per kilo.

13. R. Glennon, M. Titeler, and J. McKenney. Evidence for 5-HT involvement in the mechanism of action of hallucinogenic agents. *Life Sciences* 1984; 35:2505–2511. The ST_2 receptors employ cyclic guanosine monophosphate as their second messengers (see chapter 103). This *guanine* nucleotide (c-GMP) is the same second messenger that is increased by nitric oxide (see chapter 98). Accordingly, ST_2 receptor stimulation could have similar long-range implications for transforming the brain.

14. I. McKeith, E. Marshall, I. Ferrier, et al. 5-HT receptor binding in post-mortem brain from patients with affective disorder. *Journal of Affective Disorders* 1987; 13:67–74.

15. J. Morrison and S. Foote. Noradrenergic and serotoninergic innervation of cortical, thalamic, and tectal visual structures in Old and New World monkeys. *Journal of Comparative Neurology* 1986; 243:117–138.

16. D. Nichols. Structural correlation between apomorphine and LSD: Involvement of dopamine as well as serotonin in the actions of hallucinogens. *Journal of Theoretical Biology* 1976; 59:167–177.

17. B. Jacobs and M. Trulson. The role of serotonin in the action of hallucinogenic drugs. In *Serotonin Neurotransmission and Behavior*, eds. B. Jacobs and A. Gelperin, Cambridge, Mass., The MIT Press, 1981, 366–400.

18. B. Jacobs. Post-synaptic serotonergic action of hallucinogens. In *Hallucinogens: Neurochemical, Behavioral, and Clinical Perspectives*, ed. B. Jacobs. New York, Raven Press, 1984, 183–202.

19. G. Aghajanian. The modulatory role of serotonin at multiple receptors in brain. In *Serotonin Neurotransmission and Behavior*, eds. B. Jacobs and A. Gelperin. Cambridge, Mass., The MIT Press, 1981, 156–185.

Chapter 104   Near-Death Experiences; Far-Death Attitudes

1. D. Hammarskjold, quoted in. K. Osis and E. Haraldsson, eds. *At the Hour of Death*. New York, Avon, 1977, 1.

2. R. Noyes. The experience of dying. *Psychiatry* 1972; 35:174–184.

3. R. Noyes and R. Kletti. Depersonalization in the face of life-threatening danger: A description. *Psychiatry* 1976, 39:19–27.

4. R. Noyes and R. Kletti. Panoramic memory: A response to the threat of death. *Omega* 1977; 8:181–194.

5. S. Grof and J. Halifax. *The Human Encounter with Death*. New York, Dutton, 1977, 133–134.

6. G. Gallup Jr. *Adventures in Immortality*. New York, McGraw-Hill, 1982. By definition, near-death experiences are described by those who survived to tell the tale. [Subjects who don't survive may have had a higher incidence of such experiences before they died.]

7. G. Gabbard, S. Twemlow, and F. Jones. Do "near-death experiences" occur only near death? *Journal of Nervous and Mental Disease* 1981; 169:374–377.

8. C. Garfield. Consciousness alteration and fear of death. *Journal of Transpersonal Psychology* 1975; 7:147–175.

9. C. Tart. Out-of-the-body experiences. In Mitchell, E. *Psychic Exploration. A Challenge for Science*, ed. J. White. New York, Capricorn-Putnam's, 1976, 349–373.

10. K. Ring. *Heading Toward Omega*. New York, Morrow, 1984.

11. O. Devinsky, E. Feldman, K. Burrowes, et al. Autoscopic phenomena with seizures. *Archives of Neurology* 1989; 46:1080–1088.

12. K. Ring. The nature of personal identity in the near-death experience: Paul Brunton and the ancient tradition. *Anabiosis* 1984 (spring); 4:3–20.

13. The word "being" always needs to be evaluated with care. We are already using the same word, "being" not in the near-death context, to define "Ultimate Being." In this latter instance, it refers to a distinctive advanced alternate state of consciousness (see table 11 and chapter 145).

14. J. Owens, E. Cook, and I. Stevenson. Features of "Near-death experience" in relation to whether or not patients were near death. *Lancet* 1990; 336:1175–1177. Like Charles Darwin, most patients in this group, approximately 86 percent, had also remembered having their cognitive functions speeded up and expanded in scope.

15. Chapter 86 discussed alternative explanations which avoid the assumption that special electromagnetic forces, coming from a source outside the body, are involved in producing the "loving white light." See M. Morse and P. Perry. *Transformed by the Light*. New York, Villiard, 1992.

16. G. Roberts and J. Owen. The near-death experience. *British Journal of Psychiatry* 1988; 153:607–617.

17. R. Noyes. Attitude changes following near-death experiences. *Psychiatry* 1980; 43:234–241.

18. B. Greyson. Near-death experiences and personal values. *American Journal of Psychiatry* 1983; 140:618–620. Could the sample be representative? One may wonder whether those persons who prefer not to join organizations or who do not respond because they wish to keep their experiences private would answer differently.

19. S. Levine. *Who Dies? An Investigation of Conscious Living and Conscious Dying.* New York, Doubleday, 1982, 59.

20. E. Rodin. The reality of death experiences. A personal perspective. *Journal of Nervous and Mental Disease* 1980; 168:259–263.

21. P. Kapleau. *The Three Pillars of Zen.* Boston, Beacon Press, 1967, 269–291.

22. Levine, *op. cit.,* 234.

23. R. Grinker and H. Serota. Studies on corticohypothalamic relations in the cat and man. *Journal of Neurophysiology* 1938; 1:573–589. This report stems from a permissive era and this kind of stimulation would not be permitted today.

24. H. Takagi. The nucleus reticularis paragigantocellularis as a site of analgesic action of morphine and enkephalin. *Trends in Pharmacological Science* 1980; 3:182–184.

25. B. Greyson. The psychodynamics of near-death experiences. *Journal of Nervous and Mental Disease* 1983; 171:376–381.

Chapter 105   Triggers

1. Hsu Yun. *Empty Cloud: The Autobiography of the Chinese Zen Master Hsu Yun,* trans. Upasaka Lu K'uan Yu (Charles Luk). Rochester, N.Y., Empty Cloud Press, 1974, 25. Master Hsu-yun was 56 years old at the time.

2. D. Suzuki. *Essays in Zen Buddhism.* First Series. New York, Grove Press, 1949, 249.

3. N. Waddell, trans. and ed. *The Unborn: The Life and Teaching of Zen Master Bankei 1622–1693.* San Francisco, North Point Press, 1984. As indicated in chapter 94, rubbing movements of the hands, in themselves, have physiological consequences.

4. N. Senzaki. A lecture on meditation. In *Anthology of Zen,* ed. W. Briggs. New York, Grove Press, 1961, 281–288.

5. P. Yampolsky. *The Zen Master Hakuin.* New York, Columbia University Press, 1971, 120.

6. T. Leggett. *The Second Zen Reader.* Rutland, Vt., Tuttle, 1988, 175.

7. J. Covell. *Zen's Core: Ikkyu's Freedom.* Elizabeth, N.J., Hollym International, 1980.

8. Suzuki, *op. cit.,* 210.

9. *Ibid.,* 240.

10. T. Leggett. *Zen and the Ways.* Boulder, Colo., Shambhala, 1978, 81.

11. Waddell, *op. cit.,* 29.

12. M. Laski. *Ecstasy, A Study of Some Secular and Religious Experiences.* New York, Greenwood, 1968. Chapter 5 suggests that many of these interludes were not kensho-level awakenings, but examples of other alternate states.

13. A. Greeley. *The Sociology of the Paranormal. A Reconnaissance.* Sage Research Paper, vol 3, series 90-023. Beverly Hills, Calif., 1975.

14. M. Steriade, N. Ropert, A. Kitsikis, et al. Ascending activating neuronal networks in midbrain reticular core and related rostral systems. In *The Reticular Formation Revisited,* eds. J. Hobson and M. Brazier. International Brain Research Organization Monograph Series, vol. 6. New York, Raven Press, 1980, 125–167.

15. J. Segundo, R. Naquet, and P. Buser. Effects of cortical stimulation on electrocortical activity in monkeys. *Journal of Neurophysiology* 1955; 18:236–245. The list of critical regions *secondarily* aroused on both sides includes the tips of the temporal lobes and the sensorimotor cortex, as well as the superior temporal gyrus, the lateral frontal regions, the superior temporal gyrus, and the cingulate gyrus.

16. M. Bonvallet and V. Block. Bulbar control of cortical arousal. *Science* 1961; 133:1133–1134.

17. A. Morrison. Central activity states: Overview. In *The Neural Basis of Behavior.* Laurel, Md., Spectrum, 1982, 3–17.

18. G. Aston-Jones and F. Bloom. Norepinephrine-containing locus coeruleus neurons in behaving rats exhibit pronounced responses to non-noxious environmental stimuli. *Journal of Neuroscience* 1981; 1:887–900.

19. H. Bester, L. Menendez, J. Besson, et al. Spino(trigemino)parabrachiohypothalamic pathway: Electrophysiological evidence for an involvement in pain processes. *Journal of Neurophysiology* 1995; 73:568–585.

20. M. Steriade and R. Llinas. The functional states of the thalamus and the associated neuronal interplay. *Physiological Reviews* 1988; 68:649–742.

21. R. Bowker. Waking PGO waves: Largest amplitudes occur only during alerting reactions, not high arousal levels. In *Modulation of Sensorimotor Activity During Alterations in Behavioral States*, ed. R. Bandler. New York, Liss, 1984, 179–199.

22. L. Kaufman and A. Morrison. Spontaneous and elicited PGO spikes in rats. *Brain Research* 1981; 214:61–72.

23. A. Morrison. Relationships between phenomena of paradoxical sleep and their counterparts in wakefulness. *Acta Neurobiologica Experimentalis (Warszawa)* 1979; 39:567–583.

24. M. Davis. Neurochemical modulation of sensory-motor reactivity: Acoustic and tactile startle reflexes. *Neuroscience and Biobehavioral Reviews* 1980; 4:241–263.

25. W. Wilson and B. Nashold. The sleep rhythms of subcortical nuclei: Some observations in man. *Biological Psychiatry* 1969; 1:289–296.

26. R. McCarley, J. Winkelman, and F. Duffy. Human cerebral potentials associated with REM sleep rapid eye movements: Links to PGO waves and waking potentials. *Brain Research* 274:359–364. Many more studies are required.

Chapter 106   The Surge

1. M. Isshu and R. Sasaki. *The Zen Koan: Its History and Use in Rinzai Zen.* Kyoto, The First Zen Institute of America in Japan, 1965, 40.

2. R. Emerson. The over-soul, in *Emerson's Essays.* New York, Perennial Library, Harper & Row, 1926, 210.

3. J. Wilder. *Stimulus and Response: The Law of Initial Value.* Bristol, England, Wright, 1967.

4. J. Austin, L. Nygren, and K. Fuxe. A system for measuring the noradrenaline receptor contribution to the flexor reflex. *Medical Biology* 1976; 54:352–363.

5. S. Antelman and L. Chiodo. Stress: Its effect on interactions among biogenic amines and role in the induction and treatment of disease. In *Handbook of Psychopharmacology.* Vol. 18, *Drugs, Neurotransmitters, and Behavior,* eds. L. Iversen, S. Iversen, and S. Snyder. New York, Plenum Press, 1984, 279–341.

6. S. Bakchine, L. Lacomblez, N. Benoit, et al. Manic-like state after bilateral orbitofrontal and right temporoparietal injury: Efficacy of clonidine. *Neurology* 1989; 39:777–781.

7. J. Taylor, ed. *Selected Writings of John Hughlings Jackson.* London, Hodder and Stoughton, 1931–32, 73.

8. M. Steriade. The excitatory-inhibitory response sequence in thalamic and neocortical cells: State-regulated changes and regulatory systems. In *Dynamic Aspects of Neocortical Function,* eds. G. Edelman, W. Gall, W. Cowan, et al. New York, Wiley, 1984, 107–157.

Chapter 107   First Zen-Brain Mondo

1. R. Rilke. *Letters to a Young Poet,* ed. D. Herter. New York, Norton, 1934–35, no. 4.

Chapter 108   Vacuum Plenum: Kyoto, December 1974

1. R. Sasaki. Why Zen Buddhism appeals to American people. In *Anthology of Zen,* ed. W. Briggs. New York, Grove Press, 1961, 224.

2. The rohatsu sesshin commemorates the Buddha's supreme enlightenment, the culmination of his long meditative quest. One wonders: how different would Christianity have become if the early Christians had given more systematic attention to the significance of those formative forty days and nights which Jesus spent in solitude in the desert?

Chapter 109   The Leaf: Coda

1. J. Hackett. *The Zen Haiku and Other Zen Poems of J. W. Hackett.* Tokyo, Japan Publications, 1983, 13.

Chapter 110   The Semantics of Samadhi

1. K. Sekida. *Zen Training. Methods and Philosophy.* New York, Weatherhill, 1975, 94.
2. J. Whiteman. The mystical way and habitualization of mystical states. In *Handbook of States of Consciousness,* eds. B. Wolman and M. Ullman. New York, Van Nostrand Reinhold, 1986, 613–659.
3. Chapter 126 considers other semantic problems that surround the issues of union, unities, and oneness. Fragments of oneness can arise as quickenings.
4. D. Goleman. The Buddha on meditation and states of consciousness. Pt. 1: The teachings. *Journal of Transpersonal Psychology* 1972; 4:1–44. A recent review by the same author includes a section on the psychology of meditation. See D. Goleman. *The Meditative Mind. The Varieties of Meditative Experience.* Los Angeles, Tarcher, 1988.
5. D. Brown and J. Engler. A Rorschach study of the stages of mindfulness meditation. In *Meditation: Classic and Contemporary Perspectives,* eds. D. Shapiro and R. Walsh. New York, Aldine, 1984, 232–262.
6. S. Prabhavananda. The yoga of meditation. In *Vedanta for the Western World,* ed. C. Isherwood. New York, Viking Press, 1960, 80–88. In the yoga tradition, samadhi begins with absorption into an identity with the object of meditation.
7. M. Csikszentmihalyi. *Beyond Boredom and Anxiety.* San Francisco, Jossey-Bass, 1975.
8. K. Nishitani. Personal communication, Kyoto, Japan, 16 September 1981.
9. Sekida, *Zen Training,* 62.
10. *Ibid.,* 91–97.
11. *Ibid.,* 95.
12. D. T. Suzuki. *The Training of the Zen Buddhist Monk.* New York, University Books, 1965.

Chapter 111   The Vacuum Plenum of Absorption: An Agenda of Events to be Explained

1. J. Covell. *Zen's Core: Ikkyu's Freedom.* Elizabeth, N.J., Hollym International, 1980, 119.

Chapter 112   The Plunge: Blankness, Then Blackness

1. E. O'Brien. *Varieties of Mystic Experience.* New York, Holt, Rinehart & Winston, 1964, 79. The quotation is chosen to illustrate how matters get confused when writers and translators mix metaphors. "Divine dark" usually implies internal absorption. Yet "flashing" and "release" are two words usually associated with more advanced states of insight. Pseudo-dionysius is the name given to an actual author whose identity is still unknown. This author's later writings had mistakenly been attributed for centuries to Saint Dionysius, a first-century Christian.
2. K. Sekida. *Zen Training. Methods and Philosophy.* New York, Weatherhill, 1975, 232.
3. It is true that the thalamus undergoes its major drop in metabolism during the deeper phases of slow-wave sleep. But this drop in metabolism takes much longer to evolve than did the plunge described. See P. Maquet, D. Dive, E. Salmon, et al. Cerebral glucose utilization during stage 2 sleep in man. *Brain Research* 1992; 571:149–153.
4. G. Marini, I. Gritti, and M. Mancia. Ibotenic acid lesions of the thalamic medialis dorsalis nucleus in the cat: Effects on the sleep-waking cycle. *Neuroscience Letters* 1988; 89:259–264. Ibotenic acid mimics the receptor-stimulating properties of the brain's own excitatory amino acid transmitters, glutamate and aspartate. We need to have a detailed understanding of how the reticular nucleus of the thalamus responds to overexcitation of the mediodorsal nucleus. In cats, adenosine has sleep-promoting actions.[7] At present, we do not know what might be the effects in human subjects of abrupt, brief fluctuations of adenosine in the basal forebrain.
5. A. Rougeul-Buser. Monoamines, cortical rhythms and attentive behavior in cat. In *Modulation of Sensorimotor Activity During Alterations in Behavioral States,* ed. R. Bandler. New York, Liss, 1984, 139–149. These nuclei include those of the central-median-parafascicularis complex.
6. R. Ursin, B. Bjorvatu, L. Sommerfelt, et al. Increased waking as well as increased synchronization following administration of selective 5-HT uptake inhibitors to rats. *Behavioral Brain Research* 1989; 34:117–130. A pulse of melatonin, by hastening the onset of sleep,

might also play some role in enhancing the kind of "blank" phase that can usher in internal absorption.

7. As a model of interest in this regard, molecules of adenosine per se have intriguing *biphasic* effects. Adenosine's physiological actions on its receptors are different from the structural role it serves as the core for adenosine triphosphate (ATP, the basic unit of energy metabolism) and for cyclic AMP. When adenosine is released into the basal forebrain, S-sleep soon occurs, followed by the prompt appearance of D-sleep (see C. Portas, M. Thakkar, D. Rainme, et al. Role of adenosine in behavioral state modulation: A microdialysis study in the freely moving cat. *Neuroscience* 1997; 79:225–235.)

8. I. Miura and R. Sasaki. *The Zen Koan: Its History and Use in Rinzai Zen.* New York, Harcourt Brace & World, 1965, 63–72.

9. J. Sharp, M. Gonzales, M. Morton, et al. Decreases of cortical and thalamic glucose metabolism produced by parietal cortex stimulation in the rat. *Brain Research* 1988; 438:357–362.

Chapter 113 The Hallucinated Leaf

1. Leonardo da Vinci, in M. Strauss, ed., *Familiar Medical Quotations,* Boston, Little, Brown, 1968, 118.

2. L. Weiskrantz. Visual prototypes, memory, and the inferotemporal cortex. In *Vision, Memory and the Temporal Lobe,* eds. E. Iwai and M. Mishkin. New York, Elsevier, 1990, 13–28.

3. Y. Miyashita. Associative representation of the visual long-term memory in the neurons of the primate temporal cortex. In *Vision, Memory and the Temporal Lobe,* eds. E. Iwai and M. Mishkin. New York, Elsevier, 1990, 75–87.

4. B. Richmond and T. Sato. Enhancement of inferior temporal neurons during visual discrimination. *Journal of Neurophysiology* 1987; 58:1292–1306.

5. O. Creutzfeldt. Neuronal activity in the temporo-basal cortex and the lateral temporal lobe of man during memory tasks and other cognitive-behavioral situations. Presented at Fourth Tokyo Metropolitan Institute for Neurosciences International Symposium: Vision, Memory, and Temporal Lobe, abstracts II, Tokyo, 16–17 March 1989.

6. H. Spitzer and B. Richmond. Task difficulty: Ignoring, attending to, and discriminating a visual stimulus yield progressively more activity in inferior temporal neurons. *Experimental Brain Research* 1991; 83:340–348.

7. E. Halgren, C. Wilson, N. Squires, et al. Dynamics of the hippocampal contribution to memory: Stimulation and recording studies in humans. In *Neurobiology of the Hippocampus,* ed. W. Siefert. New York, Academic Press, 1983, 529–572.

8. M. Corbetta, F. Miezin, S. Dobmeyer, et al. Selective and divided attention during visual discriminations of shape, color and speed: Functional anatomy by positron emission tomography. *Journal of Neuroscience* 1991; 11:2382–2402.

9. J. Spitzer, R. Desimone, and J. Moran. Increased attention enhances both behavioral and neuronal performance. *Science* 1988; 240:338–340.

10. P. Schiller and N. Logothetis. The color-opponent and broad-band channels of the primate visual system. *Trends in Neurosciences* 1990; 13:392–398.

11. F. Morrell. Electrical signs of sensory coding. In *The Neurosciences. A Study Program,* eds. G. Quarton, T. Melnechuk, and F. Schmitt. New York, Rockefeller University Press, 1967, 452–469.

12. Sometimes, when seizures arise in this general region, objects appear enlarged (macropsia) or shrunken (micropsia).

13. I had not concentrated on these. This exclusion of the background took the leaf out of its context, and the editing could have contributed to the reasons why I did not recognize the leaf by itself.

14. P. Schiller. The superior colliculus and visual function. In *Handbook of Physiology.* Sec. 1, *The Nervous System* Vol. 3, *Sensory Processes,* pt. 1, eds. J. Brookhart and V. Mountcastle. Bethesda, Md., American Physiological Society, 1984, 457–505.

15. The larger question concerns the degree of attention in general, not only blindness per se. See S. Rapcsak, R. Watson, K. Heilman. Hemispace-visual field interactions in visual extinction. *Journal of Neurology, Neurosurgery and Psychiatry* 1987; 50:1117–1124.

16. Why were all details of the leaf seen so clearly? In fact, its image was projected "too far out" in the periphery even to have been *seen* by my normal vision, let alone to have been seen clearly! One speculative explanation will require a stretch of the imagination. (Here is the obvious place to introduce the hypothesis, although the full background for this stretch hypothesis will be presented in the next chapter.) For it suggests that, during the early excitatory phase of internal absorption, the attentive focus of a person's own sense of place might "expand" asymmetrically. And in this manner it will displace the site of a retrieved memory image far beyond the usual limits of the temporal crescent. To begin to understand this notion, it may help to conceptualize our *normal* attentive focus as analogous to a highly sensitive site on the inside of a small rubber balloon. Now suppose this balloon of visual attention were to become blown up to huge proportions. At this point, that original locus of apparent attention could drift far off toward the more sensitive temporal edge of circumspace.

17. Several other kinds of hallucinations during meditation can be interpreted as variations on the themes of early dream images. Most current interpretations suggest that many such images represent fragments of old memory traces which have been reactivated during the REM periods of desynchronized sleep. See E. Hennevin and B. Hars. Post-learning paradoxical sleep: A critical period when new memory is reactivated? In *Brain Plasticity, Learning, and Memory,* eds. B. Will, P. Schmitt, and J. Dalrymple-Alford. New York, Plenum Press, 1985, 193–203.

Chapter 114   Space

1. E. O'Brien. *Varieties of Mystic Experience.* New York, Holt, Rinehart & Winston, 1964, 316–317.

2. T. Trahern, quoted in R. Miller. *Meaning and Purpose in the Intact Brain.* Oxford, Clarendon Press, 1981, vi.

3. W. James. *Principles of Psychology,* vol 2. Chapter 22. New York, Holt, 1918.

4. *Ibid.,* 145.

5. *Ibid.,* 136.

6. *Ibid.,* 136–145.

7. F. Attneave and P. Farrar. The visual world behind the head. *American Journal of Psychology* 90:549–563.

8. D. Pandya and E. Yeterian. Proposed neural circuitry for spatial memory in the primate brain. *Neuropsychologia* 1984; 22:109–122.

9. L. Thompson and P. Best. Place cells and silent cells in the hippocampus of freely-behaving rats. *Journal of Neuroscience* 1989; 9:2382–2390.

10. H. Schwegler, W. Crusio, and I. Brust. Hippocampal mossy fibers and radial-maze learning in the mouse: A correlation with spatial working memory but not with non-spatial reference memory. *Neuroscience* 1990; 34:293–298.

11. B. Milner. Right temporal-lobe contribution to visual perception and visual memory. In *Vision, Memory and the Temporal Lobe,* eds. E. Iwai and M. Mishkin. New York, Elsevier, 1990, 43–53.

12. Currently, a disk is formatted by dividing it into some forty concentric, circular tracks, and then interposing nine pie-shaped sectors, which extend radially from the center hole to the outside edge. When data are stored and card-indexed in this fashion, they can later be retrieved.

13. F. Morrell. Electrical signs of sensory coding. In *The Neurosciences. A Study Program,* eds. G. Quarton, T. Melnechuk, and F. Schmitt. New York, Rockefeller University Press, 1967, 452–469.

14. E. Bisiach, E. Capitani, and E. Porta. Two basic properties of space representation in the brain: Evidence from unilateral neglect. *Journal of Neurology, Neurosurgery and Psychiatry* 1985; 48:141–144.

15. Oliver Wendell Holmes, in *The Home Book of Humorous Quotations,* ed. A. Adams. New York, Dodd, Mead, 1969, 25.

16. J. Schlag, M. Schlag-Rey, C. Peck, et al. Visual responses of thalamic neurons depending on the direction of gaze and the position of targets in space. *Experimental Brain Research* 1980; 40:170–184.

17. T. Ono, K. Nakamura, M. Fukuda, et al. Place recognition responses of neurons in monkey hippocampus. *Neuroscience Letters* 1991; 121:194–198.

18. Cézanne, painting a still life, knew that even when he got up and moved, the apple and the pear still seemed to stay on the table in their original position. They did so not only in absolute space but also in relationship to each other. This sense that our perceptual phenomena are stable is technically called "space constancy." It implies that our brain keeps readjusting its higher-order "seeing."[16]

19. The hypothesis has heuristic value. One hopes that it will stimulate neuroscientists to hone in on the mechanisms that turn each of these two sets of cells on and off. Given this information, we will be better able to evaluate how much each contributes when the self/other boundary vanishes during alternate states.

20. M. Corbetta, F. Miezin, S. Dobmeyer, et al. Selective and divided attention during visual discriminations of shape, color, and speed: Functional anatomy by positron emission tomography. *Journal of Neuroscience* 1991; 11:2382–2402.

Chapter 115   The Ascent of Charles Lindbergh: Ambient Vision

1. C. Lindbergh. *The Spirit of St. Louis.* New York, Scribner's, 1995, 389–391.

2. The discussion so far has indicated that our everyday vision falls into focal and peripheral categories. We use *focal* vision when we constrict our visual field to handle an object directly *in front* of us. It is true that, in the past, Trevarthen had once applied the term "ambient" while referring to the processes which function out at the margin of our ordinary form of *peripheral* vision (see S. Benton, I. Levy, and M. Swash. The temporal crescent in occipital infarction. *Brain* 1980; 103:83–97). In that particular context, he was using "ambient" to mean that the person was orienting in a more *reflexive* way to an object which was *off at the far edge* of the usual, *normal-sized, frontal* visual field. Therefore, this marginal region of vision was still located largely in *front* of the viewer, and merely off to either edge. Earlier we established that the "second" visual pathway enables us to catch such quick glimpses of items which are off at this peripheral edge of our normal frontal vision (see table 5). And we also noted, in contrast, that focal vision illustrated the functions of the "first" visual pathway. This book emphasizes a different kind of vision. It choses to employ "ambient" more in keeping with the basic dictionary definition. Ambient is a good word. It seems especially appropriate to be used in its larger sense to describe the *extraordinary* seeing of *unbounded* space, not merely the periphery of ordinary frontal vision. So ambient vision, as we are now using it, perceives *circum-space*, that space which has expanded so far beyond every margin of the witness's usual frontal vision that it now encompasses a 360-degree field in *all* directions.

3. *The Collected Works of Ralph Waldo Emerson.* Vol. 1, *Nature, Addresses, and Lectures.* Cambridge, Mass., Belknap Press, Harvard University Press, Critics of Emerson's description seem not to have taken into account how accurate it is.

4. G. Bachelard. *The Poetics of Space.* Boston, Beacon Press, 1969, 165.

Chapter 116   The Ambient Vision of Meditative Absorption

1. I. Miura and R. Sasaki. *The Zen Koan: Its History and Use in Rinzai Zen.* New York, Harcourt Brace & World, 1965, 63–72.

2. T. Leggett. *Zen and the Ways.* Boulder, Colo., Shambhala, 1978, 95. Later, Bukko was again in deep zazen when two pieces of wood clacked together in the customary temple signal. At the *CRACK* he again experienced a vast expanse of space. His eyes were closed, but his limitless interior space then contained "everything."

3. P. Yampolsky. *The Zen Master Hakuin.* New York, Columbia University Press, 1971, 59.

4. M. Meulders and J. Godfraind. Influence du réveil d'origine réticulaire sur l'étendue des champs visuels des neurones de la région genouillée chez le chat avec cerveau intact ou avec cerveau isolé. *Experimental Brain Research* 1969; 9:201–220.

5. K. Hikosaka, E. Iwai, H. Saito, et al. Polysensory properties of neurons in the anterior bank of the caudal superior temporal sulcus of the macaque monkey. *Journal of Neurophysiology* 1988; 60:1615–1637.

6. T. Ono. Responses of single neurons in monkey amygdala and hippocampus during object and directions discrimination. Presented at Fourth Tokyo Metropolitan Institute for Neurosciences International Symposium: Vision, Memory, and Temporal Lobe, abstracts 9. Tokyo, 16–17 March 1989.

7. R. Kita and K. Nagaya. How altruism is cultivated in Zen. In *Anthology of Zen,* ed. W. Briggs. New York, Grove Press, 1961, 45–69.

8. In such ways have the particular personal experiences of ancient mystics entered into the general vocabulary of religion and mythology.

Chapter 117   The Sound of Silence

1. T. Leggett. *Zen and the Ways.* Boulder, Colo., Shambhala, 1978, 95.

2. J. Campbell. *Power of Myth.* New York, Doubleday, 1988, 98.

3. T. Picton and S. Hillyard. Human auditory evoked potentials. II. Effects of attention. *Electroencephalography and Clinical Neurophysiology* 1974; 36:191–199.

4. K. Ho, P. Kileny, D. Paccioretti, et al. Neurologic, audiologic and electrophysiologic sequelae of bilateral temporal lobe lesions. *Archives of Neurology* 1987; 44:982–987.

5. W. Webster and L. Aitken. Central auditory processing. In *Handbook of Psychophysiology,* ed. M. Gazzaniga. New York, Academic Press, 1975, 325–364.

6. This means that (a) the patient shows no higher behavioral response to sounds; but (b) the lower hearing pathways are intact from the middle ear up through the brain stem and into the thalamus; and (c) other evidence localizes the site of the dysfunction high up in the primary auditory cortex, in Heschl's gyrus, area 41. It lies in the upper, outer part of each temporal lobe (see figure 11).

7. W. Keidel and W. Neff, eds. *Auditory System.* Handbook of Physiology, vol. 5(2). Berlin, Springer-Verlag, 1975.

8. W. Neff, I. Diamond, and J. Casseday. Behavioral studies of auditory discrimination: Central nervous system. In *Auditory System,* eds. W. Keidel and W. Neff. Handbook of Physiology, vol. 5(2). Berlin, Springer-Verlag, 1975, 307–400.

9. N. Motomura, A. Yamadori, E. Mori, et al. Auditory agnosia: Analysis of a case with bilateral subcortical lesions. *Brain* 1986; 109:379–391.

10. There remain several lesser ways to inhibit sounds. None seem likely to account for more than a portion of the absolute silence of absorption. The reader is referred to J. Desmedt. Physiological studies of the efferent recurrent auditory system. In *Auditory System,* eds. W. Keidel and W. Neff. Handbook of Physiology, vol. 5(2). Berlin, Springer-Verlag, 1975, 219–246; A. Starr. Influence of motor activity on click-evoked responses in the auditory pathway of waking cats. *Experimental Neurology* 1964; 10:191–204; W. Winters, K. Mori, C. Spooner, et al. Correlation of reticular and cochlear multiple unit activity with evoked responses during wakefulness and sleep. *Electroencephalography and Clinical Neurophysiology* 1967; 23:539–545; I. Rapin, H. Schimmel, and M. Cohen. Reliability in detecting the auditory evoked response (AER) for audiometry in sleeping subjects. *Electroencephalography and Clinical Neurophysiology* 1972; 32:521–528.

11. Once again, there is the curious fact that few projections rise up directly from the specific sensory nuclei of the thalamus to supply our so-called athalamic temporal lobe cortex. The exceptions, of course, are the primary auditory and vestibular pathways just cited. These ascend from the medial geniculate region up to the small region centered in Heschl's gyrus. (See C. Noback and R. Demarest. *The Human Nervous System,* 3rd ed. New York, McGraw-Hill, 1981, 434.) What survival value does this arrangement have? Neuroanatomists and neurophysiologists do not have the answers. This particular design does, however, leave the interpretive cortex of the temporal lobe *relatively* free from being instantly distracted by huge volumes of early sensate data. Only after this information has first been preprocessed will the temporal cortex receive it.

12. There is one type of normal auditory evoked response called the "middle latency response." Recorded from the scalp, its components reflect the activity produced by those sound impulses which finally do reach up as high as the region of Heschl's gyrus. The theory proposed here for the silence of internal absorption could be tested objectively. This response should drop out during an episode of acute absolute silence. Note that it also drops out acutely in patients who suffer an acute bilateral deafness caused by discrete dysfunctions within Heschl's gyrus (or by lesions which block all impulses from rising up to this gyrus.)[4]

13. D. Harding. *On Having No Head: A Contribution to Zen in the West.* London, The Buddhist Society, 1961. The stress, hypoxia, and exhilaration associated with exercise high in the Himalaya Mountains could have combined to produce this experience, as is discussed in the next chapter.

Chapter 118   The Loss of the Self in Clear, Held Awareness

1. D. Suzuki. *Essays in Zen Buddhism.* Second Series, ed. C. Humphreys. New York, Weiser, 1958, 107.

2. J. Sharp, M. Gonzales, M. Morton, et al. Decreases of cortical and thalamic glucose metabolism produced by parietal cortex stimulation in the rat. *Brain Research* 1988; 438:357–362.

3. F. Gonzalez-Lima and H. Scheich. Ascending reticular activating system in the rat: A 2-deoxyglucose study. *Brain Research* 1985; 344:70–88. This line of research again raises the important questions which need to be resolved: (a) Does the reticular nucleus inhibit the vast bulk of the *front* part of the thalamus (including the mediodorsal nucleus) to the same degree that it is known to inhibit the smaller sensory relay nuclei?; (b) how does this translate into experience and behavior?

4. E. Grastyan. The hippocampus and higher nervous activity. In *Transactions of the Second Conference on The Central Nervous System and Behavior,* ed. M. Brazier. New York, Josia Macy Jr Foundation, 1959, 119–205.

5. R. Hernandez-Peon and G. Chavez Ibarra. Sleep induced by electrical or chemical stimulation of the forebrain. *Electroencephalography and Clinical Neurophysiology* 1963; 24(suppl.):188.

6. W. James. *The Principles of Psychology,* vol 1. New York, Holt, 1918, 426.

7. D. Saphier and S. Feldman. Iontophoresis of cortisol inhibits responses of identified paraventricular nucleus neurones to sciatic nerve stimulation. *Brain Research* 1990; 535:159–162.

8. R. Ebstein, O. Novick, R. Umanski, et al. Dopamine D4 Receptor (D4DR). Exon III polymorphism associated with the human personality trait of novelty seeking. *Nature Genetics* 1996; 12:78–80.

Chapter 119   The Warm Affective Tone

1. Emily Dickinson, in *Emily Dickinson, Great American Poets Series,* ed. G. Moore. New York, Potter, 1986.

2. Receptors differ strikingly in the way they are distributed in the brains of different species. This means that a given subset of mu opioid receptors, for example, is likely to enter in a rather different way into the higher ramifications of *human* experience than this same subset does even in other primates.

3. I was not counting how slowly I breathed either while experiencing the effects of morphine or during absorption. Research cited earlier suggests that respirations might be suppressed during a major episode of internal absorption (see chapter 22). The hypothesis that respirations are also suppressed during the states of insight-wisdom (State VII) and Ultimate Being (VIII) is testable.

4. Among its effects, metenkephalin is also capable of turning *off* β-endorphin by inhibiting its nerve cells in the arcuate nucleus. See R. Zhang, S. Hisano, M. Chikamori-Aoyama, et al. Synaptic association between enkephalin-containing axon terminals and pro-opiomelanocortin-containing neurons in the arcuate nucleus of rat hypothalamus. *Neuroscience Letters* 1987; 82:151–156.

5. For future reference in subsequent chapters, let us note that many other enkephalin endings elsewhere are poised to affect sensory experiences by (1) markedly slowing the firing rate of the locus ceruleus; (2) reducing the sensory input from the vagus nerve into the nucleus of the solitary tract; (3) preventing somatosensory signals coming from the body from entering the spinal cord; and (4) blocking much of the somatic sensation coming from the head from entering into the brain stem through the fifth cranial nerve. See M. Kuhar. Opioid peptides and receptors in the rat brain stem. In *The Reticular Formation Revisited*, eds. J. Hobson and M. Brazier. International Brain Research Organization Monograph Series, vol. 6. New York, Raven Press, 1980, 317–328.

6. This opioid mechanism could contribute to some of the absolute sensate silence of internal absorption (State VI), although it might play its most obvious role in certain more advanced states of insight-wisdom (State VII) and Ultimate Being (State VIII) (see chapter 146).

Chapter 120 Motor and Other Residues of Internal Absorption

1. K. Sano, H. Sekino, Y. Tsukamoto, et al. Stimulation and destruction of the region of the interstitial nucleus in cases of torticollis and see-saw nystagmus. *Confinia Neurologica* 1972; 34:331–338. The interstitial nucleus of Cajal is located below the small white band of crossing fibers termed the posterior commissure.

2. K. Fukushima, J. Fukushima, and T. Terashima. The pathways responsible for the characteristic head posture produced by lesions of the interstitial nucleus of Cajal in the cat. Experimental *Brain Research* 1987; 68:88–102. The descending pathway runs through the reticular formation of the pons and the reticulospinal system.

3. K. Sano, M. Yoshioka, M. Ogashiwa, et al. Central mechanisms of neck movements in the human brain stem. *Confinia Neurologica* 1967; 29:107–111.

4. Stimulating in and around the red nucleus of the midbrain also causes muscle contractions in the back of the neck. Still higher levels of the neck extension pathways may reside in the diencephalon in the inner portion of Forel's field H. See T. Isa, T. Itouji, and S. Sasaki. Excitatory pathways from Forel's field H to head elevator motoneurons in the cat. *Neuroscience Letters* 1988; 90:89–94.

5. E. Brodin, B. Linderoth, M. Going, et al. In vivo release of serotonin in cat dorsal vagal complex and cervical ventral horn induced by electrical stimulation of the medullary raphe nuclei. *Brain Research* 1990; 535:227–236. The ST nucleus cited is the raphe obscurus.

6. A. Watts. Psychotherapy and liberation. In *The Highest State of Consciousness*, ed. J. White. Garden City, N.Y., Anchor/Doubleday, 1972, 195–203.

7. I. Miura and R. Sasaki. *The Zen Koan: Its History and Use in Rinzai Zen*. New York, Harcourt Brace & World, 1965, 29.

8. *Ibid.*, 68.

Chapter 121 The When and Where of Time

1. The first line of Tozan's original verse has been open to different interpretations. The ambiguity might be traceable to differences between what the Chinese words for the different hours of the "watch" implied back in Tung-shan's days (807–869), as opposed to what they mean in our own era. Cleary's translation places this "watch" at the beginning of the night. Both his version and that of Miura and Sasaki continue to refer to this as the "third" watch. See T. Cleary. *Kensho. The Heart of Zen*. Boston, Shambhala, 1997, 72; I. Miura and R. Sasaki. *The Zen Koan: Its History and Use in Rinzai Zen*. New York, Harcourt Brace & World, 1965, 67.

2. M. Okawa, M. Matousek, and I. Petersen. Spontaneous vigilance fluctuations in the daytime. *Psychophysiology* 1984; 21:207–211.

3. Chapter 44 describes the roles that norepinephrine plays in enhancing excitability and in promoting S-sleep. I have not had a similar hypnagogic or hypnopompic hallucination at any time before or since while falling asleep in bed at night, while awakening in the morning, or while going in and out of naps.

4. W. James. *Principles of Psychology*, vol. 2. New York, Holt, 1918, 611.

Chapter 122   Gateway to Paradox

1. Calligraphy given to the author in 1988. Its ten kanji characters may date back to old China. They were only subsequently collected into anthologies such as the *Zenrin-ga-kusho*. In some Zen centers, similar verses have served as "capping phrases" (see chapter 26). Can a cloud appear in one's sleeve? Can a moon enter water? No, but meaning resonates at many levels within these paradoxes. Our present purposes are more broadly instructional than literary, and it best serves the former to translate the lines freely. In doing so, the first sentence hints that adversity—the sheer discomfort of sitting on a hard stone—might precipitate internal absorption (see part VI). And that therefore, with the physical self now lost, a stray cloud can easily enter the empty space in this vacant garment. A free interpretation of the metaphors of the second sentence suggests that not until a later phase—when kensho's moonlight finally bathes the scene—will its insight illuminate the deepest sources of one's origin (see chapter 138).

2. Opening quotation of chapter 108. (R. Sasaki, quoted in W. Briggs, ed., *Anthology of Zen*. New York, Grove Press, 1961, 224.

3. W. Stace. *Mysticism and Philosophy*. Philadelphia, J.B. Lippincott, 1960.

4. R. Zhang, S. Hisano, M. Chikamori-Aoyama, et al. Synaptic association between enkephalin-containing axon terminals and pro-opiomelanocortin-containing neurons in the arcuate nucleus of rat hypothalamus. *Neuroscience Letters* 1987; 82:151–156. Painful stress releases enough CRF and substance P to trigger the release of β-endorphin from arcuate nerve cells.

5. T. Hokfelt, B. Meister, T. Melander, et al. Coexistence of classical transmitters and peptides with special reference to the arcuate nucleus–median eminence complex. In *Hypothalamic Dysfunction in Neuropsychiatric Disorders*, eds. D. Nerozzi, F. Goodwin, and E. Costa. New York, Raven Press, 1987, 21–34.

6. L. Agnati, K. Fuxe, F. Benfenati, et al. Postsynaptic effects of neuropeptide comodulators at central monoamine synapses. In *Catecholamines Part B: Neuropharmacology and Central Nervous System Theoretical Aspects*, eds. E. Usdin, A. Carlsson, and A. Dahlström, et al. New York, Liss, 1984, 191–198.

7. E. Mori, A. Yamadori, and Y. Mitani. Left thalamic infarction and disturbance of visual memory. *Annals of Neurology* 1986; 20:671–676.

8. I. Miura and R. Sasaki. *The Zen Koan: Its History and Use in Rinzai Zen*. New York, Harcourt Brace & World, 1965, 63–72.

Chapter 123   Second Zen-Brain Mondo

1. Santiago Ramón y Cajal, in M. Strauss, ed., *Familiar Medical Quotations*. Boston, Little Brown, 1968, 46. Cajal pioneered the histological basis of the neurosciences.

Chapter 124   Dimensions of Meaning

1. Thomas Carlyle, in *Hoyt's New Cyclopedia of Practical Quotations Drawn from the Speech and Literature of All Nations*. New York, Funk & Wagnalls, 1964, 247.

2. C. Osgood. Exploration in semantic space: A personal diary. *Journal of Social Issues* 1971; 27:5–64.

3. R. Vanderploeg, W. Brown, and J. Marsh. Judgements of emotions in words and faces: ERP correlates. *International Journal of Psychophysiology* 1987; 5:193–205.

4. W. James. *The Varieties of Religious Experience*. New York, Longmans, Green, 1925, 382.

5. H. James, III, ed. *The Letters of William James*, vol. 2. Boston, Atlantic Monthly Press, 1920, 76–77.

6. M. Gabriel, Y. Kubota, and V. Shenker. Limbic-circuit interactions during learning. In *Information Processing by the Brain*. ed. H. Markowitsch. Toronto, Huber, 1988, 39–63.

7. I. Schloegl. *The Wisdom of the Zen Masters*. London, Sheldon Press, 1975, 39.

Chapter 125   Authentic Meanings within Wide-Open Boundaries

1. Bankei, by attribution, in "Song of Original Mind," cited in P. Haskel. *Bankei Zen*. New York, Grove Press, 1984, 125–132.

2. Paul Gauguin. The inscription on the painting reads *D'ou venons nous / Que sommes nous / Ou allons nous* [*sic*], 1897.
3. William Rhodes. Personal communication, 1985.
4. V. Frankl. *Man's Search for Meaning*. New York, Washington Square Press, 1965.
5. J. Austin. *Chase, Chance, and Creativity. The Lucky Art of Novelty*. New York, Columbia University Press, 1978.
6. R. Fischer and G. Landon. On the arousal state–dependent recall of "subconscious" experience: Stateboundness. *British Journal of Psychiatry* 1972; 120:159–172.
7. In fact, the underlying themes within the master's own ad-lib responses resemble those themes which he will be searching for in his students' responses when he challenges the way they have resolved their koan (see chapter 26).
8. K. Kraft. Muso Kokuski's *Dialogues in a Dream*. Selections. *The Eastern Buddhist*. 1981; 14:75–93.

Chapter 126   Word Problems: "Oneness" and "Unity"

1. H. Zimmer, cited in J. Campbell, *The Inner Reaches of Outer Space*. New York, A. van der Marck, 1985, 21.
2. Ta-hui, cited in D. T. Suzuki, *Essays in Zen Buddhism*. Second Series, ed. C. Humphreys. New York, Grove Press, 1971, 31.
3. W. Stace. *Mysticism and Philosophy*. Philadelphia, J.B. Lippincott, 1960, 67.
4. *Ibid.*, 61.
5. *Ibid.*, 86.
6. *Ibid.*, 161.
7. *Ibid.*, 87.
8. *Ibid.*, 131.
9. *Ibid.*, 163.
10. J. Campbell. *The Masks of God: Creative Mythology*. New York, Viking, 1968, 65.
11. Stace, *op. cit.*, 256.
12. D. T. Suzuki. *Essays in Zen Buddhism*. First Series. New York, Grove Press, 1949, 229.
13. Campbell, *op. cit.*, 585. In the East, the tranquil path toward the one-pointedness of the absorptions is called *Samatha*. The path to insight-wisdom is called *Vipassana*.
14. This state, with its lingering sense of duality, may correspond with the so-called *sa-vikalpa samadhi*, a Sanskrit term. See M. Jain and K. Jain. The science of yoga, a study in perspective. *Perspectives in Biology and Medicine* 1973; 17:93–102.
15. This highest state of non-dual union may correspond with the term, *nir-vikalpa samadhi*, used in Vedanta. Again, one notes that samadhi has been used to describe dissimilar events.
16. The kinds of unity reported in psychedelic states are discussed further elsewhere. See J. Austin. Dimensions of meaning. A Zen/brain perspective. *Ultimate Reality and Meaning* 1992; 15:60–76.

Chapter 127   How Often Does Enlightenment Occur?

1. J. Blofeld. *The Zen Teaching of Huang Po. On the Transmission of Mind*. New York, Grove Press, 1958, 65.
2. A. Greeley. *The Sociology of the Paranormal. A Reconnaissance*. Sage Research Paper, vol. 3, series 90-023. Beverly Hills, Calif., The study was conducted in 1973. The subjects ranged in age from their teens into their seventies and were interviewed for an hour or so.
3. R. Bucke. *Cosmic Consciousness. A Study in the Evolution of the Human Mind*. New York, Dutton, 1962, 7.
4. R. Masunaga. *A Primer of Soto Zen*. Honolulu, University of Hawaii Press, 1971, 39. Redemption in Buddhism, as in other faiths, can come to evil persons and to those of low IQ.
5. I. Miura and R. Sasaki. *The Zen Koan: Its History and Use in Rinzai Zen*. New York, Harcourt Brace & World, 1965, 29.

6. P. Yampolsky. *The Zen Master Hakuin.* New York, Columbia University Press, 1971, 14.
7. W. deBary. *The Buddhist Tradition in India, China and Japan.* New York, Vintage, 1972, 381–388.
8. W. Hudspeth and K. Pribram. Psychophysiological indices of cerebral maturation. *International Journal of Psychophysiology* 1992; 12:19–29.
9. T. Leggett. *Zen and the Ways.* Boulder, Colo., Shambhala, 1978, 95.

Chapter 129   What Is My Original Face?

1. J. Blofeld. *The Zen Teaching of Huang Po.* New York, Grove Press, 1958, 65.
2. P. Yampolsky. *The Platform Sutra of the Sixth Patriarch.* New York, Columbia University Press, 1967, 110.

Chapter 130   Major Characteristics of Insight-Wisdom in Kensho

1. Edna Saint Vincent Millay, from "Renascence," in C. Aiken, ed., *Twentieth-Century American Poetry.* New York, Modern Library, 1944, 242–247.
2. D. Suzuki. *Essays in Zen Buddhism.* Second Series, ed. C. Humphreys. 1958, 30–36.
3. K. Sekida. *Zen Training. Methods and Philosophy.* New York, Weatherhill, 1975, 233.
4. In this book, it is convenient to refer to the gradient of the states of insight-wisdom as *kensho-satori*, and to reserve satori for the most transforming of this range of awakenings.
5. W. Pahnke. Drugs and mysticism. In *The Highest State of Consciousness*, ed. J. White. Garden City, N.Y., Anchor/Doubleday, 1972, 257–277.
6. D. Suzuki. *Essays in Zen Buddhism.* First Series. London, Rider, n.d., 245.

Chapter 131   Prajna: Insight-Wisdom

1. Appendix B contains a shortened version of *Affirmation of Faith in Mind*.
2. C. Jung. *Psychology and Religion: West and East*, 2nd ed., vol. 11. Bollingen Series 20. Princeton, N.J., Princeton University Press, 1969, 41.
3. B. Bryson. *The Mother Tongue. English and How It Got That Way.* New York, Morrow, 1990.
4. J. Bancaud and J. Talairach. Clinical semiology of frontal lobe seizures. In *Frontal Lobe Seizures and Epilepsies*, eds. P. Chauvel, A. Delgado-Escueta, E. Halgren, et al. New York, Raven Press, 1990, 3–58.
5. J. Campbell. *Masks of God: Creative Mythology.* New York, Viking, 1968, 582.
6. N. Bohr, cited in J. Berryman, *Delusions, Etc.* New York, Farrar, Straus & Giroux, 1972, 33.
7. Neither of these considerations removes the possibility that kensho influences some association nuclei of the thalamus at the functional interface between memory and language. For example, disorders of the left medioldorsal nucleus interfere with a patient's memory for verbal material. See L. Speedie and K. Heilman. Amnestic disturbance following infarction of the left dorsomedial nucleus of the thalamus. *Neuropsychologia* 1982; 20:597–604.

Chapter 132   Suchness

1. S. Suzuki. *Zen Mind, Beginner's Mind.* New York, Weatherhill, 1975, 33.
2. D. Suzuki. *Studies in Zen.* New York, Delta, 1955, 141.
3. S. Suzuki, *op. cit.*, 66.
4. C. Jung. *Psychology and Religion: West and East*, 2nd ed., vol. 11. Bollingen Series 20. Princeton, N.J., Princeton University Press, 1969, 539. In most versions, the master is Hsuan-sha (Gensha, in Japanese). He is also remembered because he became enlightened when he stubbed his toe against a stone.
5. J. Miller and K. Farley, eds. *Heritage of American Literature.* Vol 2. San Diego, Calif., Harcourt Brace Jovanovich, 1991, 883.
6. Immanuel Kant. *The Critique of Pure Reason*, vol. 2, trans. 1881; London, Macmillan, 37. Kant was saying that we can know about objects of our experience as phenomena, in the form in which they appear to use. But he was maintaining that things in themselves, which he called *noumena*, were unknowable.

7. D. Suzuki, *ibid.*, 141.
8. E. Wood. *Zen Dictionary*. Rutland, Vt., Tuttle, 1957, 138.
9. D. Suzuki. *Zen and Japanese Culture*. Bollingen Series 64. Princeton, N.J., Princeton University Press, 1973, 16.
10. A. Watts. *The Way of Zen*. New York, Vintage, 1957, 67.
11. E. Mitchell. Introduction: From outer space to inner space. In *Psychic Exploration. A Challenge for Science*, ed. J. White. New York, Capricorn Putnam's, 1976, 25–50.
12. A. Greeley. *Ecstasy, A Way of Knowing*. Englewood Cliffs, N.J., Prentice-Hall, 1974, 66.
13. A. Watts. Ordinary mind is the way. *The Eastern Buddhist* 1971; 4:134–137.

Chapter 133   Direct Perception of the Eternally Perfect World

1. A. Adams, in A. Adams and M. Alinder, *Ansel Adams: An Autobiography*. New York, New York Graphic Society, 1985, 382.
2. A. Pope, *An Epistle on Man*, epistle I. 1, line 267.
3. N. Waddell, trans. and ed. *The Unborn. The Life and Teaching of Zen Master Bankei 1622–1693*. San Francisco, North Point Press, 1984, 129.
4. *Ibid.*, 88.
5. *Ibid.*, 91.
6. T. Kasulis. *Zen Action. Zen Person*. Honolulu, University Press of Hawaii, 1981, 83–86. Dogen referred to it in his writings about *Genjo-koan*, a term implying that "everyday life is enlightenment."
7. S. Hawking and J. Hartle. Profile on Stephen Hawking, *Time*, 8 February 1988, 60.
8. S. Mitchell, trans. *Tao Te Ching*. New York, Harper & Row, 1988, 7.
9. G. Chang. *The Practice of Zen*. New York, Perennial Library, Harper & Row, 1959, 221.
10. E. Pagels. *The Gnostic Gospels*. New York, Random House, 1979, 128–129. In 1945, a large jar was found near Nag-Hammadi in Egypt. It contained many Gnostic writings which had been translated from the earlier Greek texts dating back to around the year 140 of the Christian era. Jesus spoke in Aramaic. We do not know what his exact words were. Nor do we know the exact words spoken by Siddhartha before him.
11. D. Suzuki and W. King. Conversations with D. T. Suzuki. *The Eastern Buddhist*, n.s. 1988; 21(spring):82–100. In this context, being "not in it" is not double talk. It can be interpreted as referring to nonattachment.

Chapter 134   The Construction of Time

1. Leonardo da Vinci, cited in C. Curtis and F. Greenslet, eds., *The Practical Cogitator*. Boston, Houghton Mifflin, 1953, 556.
2. A. Ammons. *Selected Poems, Expanded Edition*. New York, Norton, 1986, 11.
3. J. Piaget. *The Construction of Reality in the Child*. New York, Ballantine, 1971, 338.
4. R. Efron. The duration of the present. In *Interdisciplinary Perspectives of Time*, ed. R. Fischer. *Annals of the New York Academy of Sciences* 1967; 138:713–729.
5. B. Libet. Timing of cerebral processes relative to concomitant conscious experiences in man. In *Brain and Behavior*, eds. G. Adam, I. Meszaros, and E. Banyai. Advances in Physiological Science, vol. 17. Budapest, Pergamon, 1981, 313–317.
6. H. Lehmann. Time and psychopathology. In *Interdisciplinary Perspectives of Time*, ed. R. Fischer. *Annals of the New York Academy of Sciences* 1967; 138:798–821.
7. R. Miller. *Meaning and Purpose in the Intact Brain*. Oxford, Clarendon Press, 1981.
8. R. Thatcher and E. John. *Foundations of Cognitive Processes*. Functional Neuroscience, vol. 1. Hillsdale, N.J., Erlbaum, 1977, 79. In actuality, as the authors explain, a single auditory stimulus must last for at least 120 to 170 milliseconds in order for it to remain completely distinct and unblended. And stimuli processed by the visual system must last for between 120 and 240 milliseconds.
9. W. James. *The Principles of Psychology*. New York, Holt, 1890, 613.
10. J. Brown. Psychology of time awareness. *Brain and Cognition* 1990; 14:144–164.
11. B. Milner. Interhemispheric differences in the localization of psychological processes in man. *British Medical Bulletin* 1971; 27:272–277.

12. B. Milner, P. Corsi, and G. Leonard. Frontal-lobe contribution to recency judgements. *Neuropsychologia* 1981; 29:601–618.

13. Recently, studies have been designed to show how subcortical connections also enter into the ways we encode time relationships. See A. Parkin, M. Leng, and N. Hunkin. Differential sensitivity to context in diencephalic and temporal lobe amnesia. *Cortex* 1990; 26:373–380.

14. D. Ingvar. "Memory of the Future": An essay on the temporal organization of conscious awareness. *Human Neurobiology* 1985; 4:127–136.

15. P. Yampolsky. *The Platform Sutra of the Sixth Patriarch*. New York, Columbia University Press, 1967, 154.

Chapter 135   The Dissolution of Time

1. R. Blakney. *Meister Eckhart*. New York, Harper Bros., 1941, 131.

2. W. James. *The Principles of Psychology*. New York, Holt, 1890, 618–619. James also observed that "time filled with varied and interesting experiences seems short in passing, but long as we look back."

3. W. Meck and R. Church. Cholinergic modulation of the content of temporal memory. *Behavioral Neuroscience* 1987; 101:457–464. Rats can be given physostigmine, a drug which increases their effective level of acetylcholine.

4. Y. Akishige. *Psychological Studies on Zen 2*. Tokyo, Komazawa University Press, 1977, 381.

5. S. Austin. *Parmenides, Being, Bounds, and Logic*. New Haven, Conn., Yale University Press, 1986, 163.

6. I am also indebted to Professor Scott Austin for this quotation from Heraclitus.

7. E. Armstrong. Limbic thalamus: Anterior and mediodorsal nuclei. In *The Human Nervous System*, ed. G. Paxinos. San Diego, Academic Press, 1990, 469–481.

8. D. Bowers, M. Verfaellie, and S. Rapscyk. Different forms of temporal amnesia following basal-forebrain vs. retrosplenial-fornix lesions in man. *Journal of Clinical and Experimental Neuropsychology* 1987; 9:15.

9. D. Olton, W. Meck, and R. Church. Separation of hippocampal and amygdaloid involvement in temporal memory dysfunctions. *Brain Research* 1987; 404:180–188.

10. C. Whitty and W. Lewin. A Korsakoff syndrome in the post-cingulectomy confusional state. *Brain* 1960; 83:648–653.

11. D. Alton, G. Wenk, R. Church, et al. Attention and the frontal cortex as examined by simultaneous temporal processing. *Neuropsychologia* 1988; 26:307–318.

12. R. Kesner and T. Holbrook. Dissociation of item and order: Spatial memory in rats following medial prefrontal cortex lesions. *Neuropsychologia* 1987; 25:653–664.

Chapter 136   The Death of Fear

1. N. Waddell, trans. and ed. *The Unborn: The Life and Teaching of Zen Master Bankei 1622–1693*. San Francisco, North Point Press, 1984, 126.

2. Quoted in M. Strauss, ed., *Familiar Medical Quotations*. Boston, Little, Brown, 1968, 21.

3. J. Kagan. The shy and the sociable. *Harvard Medical Alumni Bulletin* 1990–91, 21–33.

4. S. Calkins, N. Fox, and T. Marshall. Behavioral and physiological antecedents of inhibited and uninhibited behavior. *Child Development* 1996; 67:523–540.

5. N. Fox, K. Rubin, S. Calkins, et al. Frontal activation asymmetry and social competence at four years of age. *Child Development* 1995; 66:1770–1784. Researchers can only guess *why* their subjects (young or old) are not actively entering into a social encounter, and how their subjects' EEG relates to such behavior.

6. G. Gurguis, E. Klein, I. Mefford, et al. Biogenic amines distribution in the brain of nervous and normal pointer dogs. *Neuropsychopharmacology* 1990; 3:297–303.

7. D. Nutt. Altered central α_2 adrenoceptor sensitivity in panic disorder. *Archives of General Psychiatry* 1989; 46:165–169.

8. J. Gray. *The Neuropsychology of Anxiety: An Enquiry into the Functions of the Septo-hippocampal System*. New York, Oxford University Press, 1981, 295.

9. M. Novas, J. Medina, and E. DeRobertis. Benzodiazepine receptors in the rat hippocampal formation: Action of catecholaminergic, serotonergic and commissural denervation. *Neuroscience* 1983; 8:459–465.

10. J. Witkin, R. Mansbach, J. Barrett, et al. Behavioral studies with anxiolytic drugs IV. Serotonergic involvement in the effects of buspirone on punished behavior of pigeons. *Journal of Pharmacology and Experimental Therapeutics* 1987; 243:970–977. Buspirone acts at other receptor sites as well.

11. A. Howlett, M. Bidant-Russell, W. Devane, et al. The cannabinoid receptor: Biochemical, anatomical and behavioral characterization. *Trends in Neurosciences* 1990; 13:420–423. Drugs related to delta THC cause analgesia, catalepsy, inhibit locomotion, and lower body temperature. Further studies are necessary to assess how endogenous cannabinoids might be involved in some aspects of kensho or other alternate states.

12. M. Herkenham, A. Lynn, M. Little, et al. Cannabinoid receptor localization in brain. *Proceedings of the National Academy of Sciences of the United States of America* 1990; 87:1932–1936. Cannabinoids also act on ion channels and have other complex interactions.

13. P. MacLean and J. Newman. Role of midline frontolimbic cortex in production of the isolation call of squirrel monkeys. *Brain Research* 1988; 450:111–123.

14. W. James. *The Varieties of Religious Experience.* New York, Longmans, Green, 1925, 247.

15. J. Campbell. *Myths to Live By.* New York, Bantam, 1980, 212.

Chapter 137   Emptiness

1. Lao-tzu, from the *Tao Te Ching,* in B. Stevenson, ed., *The Home Book of Quotations,* 10th ed. New York, Dodd-Mead, 1967, 147.

2. D. Suzuki. *Studies in the Lankavatara Sutra.* London, Routledge & Kegan Paul, 1930, 297.

3. W. Kraft. *A Psychology of Nothingness.* Philadelphia, Westminster Press, 1974.

4. D. Suzuki. *The Lankavatara Sutra.* London, Routledge & Kegan Paul, 1932, 66.

5. N. Kobori. A Dialogue, a discussion between One and Zero. *The Eastern Buddhist* 1957; 8:43–49.

6. T. Leggett. *The Second Zen Reader.* Rutland, Vt., Tuttle, 1988, 20.

7. G. Chang. *The Practice of Zen.* New York, Perennial, Harper & Row, 1970, 46.

8. G. Rabten. *Echoes of Voidness.* London, Wisdom Publications, 1983, 12–13.

Chapter 138   Objective Vision: The Lunar View

1. C. Jung. *Psychology and Religion. West and East,* vol. 11. Bollingen Series 20. New York, Pantheon, 1958, 546.

2. M. Anesaki. *History of Japanese Religion.* Rutland, Vt., Tuttle, 1963, 208.

3. G. Bachelard. *The Poetics of Space.* Boston, Beacon Press, 1969, 165. The writer of these lines was 45 years old.

4. C. Jung. *Memories, Dreams, Reflections,* ed. A. Jaffe. New York, Pantheon, 1962, 196–197. Jung did not describe most of his visions as dreams.

5. *Ibid.,* 295. It is noteworthy how this keen sense of their objectivity precluded even Jung from regarding the visions as vivid products of his own imagination.

6. *Ibid.,* 296.

7. *Ibid.,* 297.

8. W. Pahnke. Drugs and mysticism. In *The Highest State of Consciousness,* ed. J. White. Garden City, N.Y., Anchor/Doubleday, 1972, 257–277.

9. W. deBary. *The Buddhist Tradition in India, China and Japan.* New York, Vintage, 1972, 371.

10. Meister Eckhart. Quoted in S. Ogata, *Zen for the West.* New York, Dial, 1959, 18–19.

11. A. Maslow. The "core-religious" or "transcendent," experience. In *The Highest State of Consciousness,* ed. J. White. Garden City, N.Y., Anchor/Doubleday, 1972, 359.

12. F. Merrell-Wolff. *Consciousness Without an Object.* New York, Julian Press, 1973.

13. F. Merrell-Wolff. *Pathways Through to Space.* New York, Julian Press, 1973.

14. P. Yampolsky. *The Zen Master Hakuin.* New York, Columbia University Press, 1971, 145. The "great doubt" has several interpretations. A period of deep, existential questioning is

one. It can also be interpreted as the "great unknown" which, in kensho, one finally faces up to and resolves.

15. W. Van Dusen. LSD and the enlightenment of Zen. *Psychologia* 1961; 4:11–16.

16. O. Sogen and K. Terayama. *Zen and the Art of Calligraphy,* trans. J. Stevens. London, Routledge & Kegan Paul, 1983.

17. J. Campbell. *Masks of God: Creative Mythology.* New York, Viking, 1980, 582.

18. H. Maezumi and B. Glassman. *The Hazy Moon of Enlightenment.* Los Angeles, Center Publications, 1977, 15–16.

19. Max Planck, quoted in M. Strauss, ed., *Familiar Medical Quotations.* Boston, Little, Brown, 1968, 521. Planck lived from 1858 to 1947.

Chapter 139   Are There Levels and Sequences of "Nonattainment?"

1. W. Johnston. All and nothing. St. John of the Cross and the Christian-Buddhist dialogue. *The Eastern Buddhist* 1988; 21:124–142.

2. There are many different schools of Buddhism. The Tibetan traditions describe numerous discrete successive levels, many of which result from the emphasis upon concentrative meditative techniques. Yet these are said to culminate in insight into the essence of things. See D. Brown. A model for the levels of concentrative meditation. *International Journal of Clinical and Experimental Hypnosis* 1977; 25:236–273.

3. D. Goleman. The Buddha on meditation and states of consciousness. Pt. 1: The teachings. *Journal of Transpersonal Psychology* 1972; 4:1–44.

4. I. Miura and R. Sasaki. *The Zen Koan: Its History and Use in Rinzai Zen.* New York, Harcourt Brace & World, 1965, 67–72. The first rank is quoted in chapter 121.

5. W. Rahula. *Zen and the Taming of the Bull.* London, Fraser, 1978.

6. D. Suzuki. *Manual of Zen Buddhism.* New York, Grove Press, 1960.

7. Myokyo-ni [Irmgard Schloegl]. *Gentling the Bull. The Ten Bull Pictures. A Spiritual Journey.* London, Zen Centre, n.d. In some early Chinese versions, the bull underwent a change from black toward white. The change is symbolic. A doctrinal interpretation might be that the "white hairs" were only those native virtues which had simply been there all along.

8. S. Grof. *Realms of the Human Unconscious. Observations from LSD Research.* Dutton, New York 1976, 157.

9. *Ibid.,* 106. "Cosmic unity" tends to enter at Grof's third level. It occurs before such other experiences as ancestral memories or archtypal experiences. However, there are ambiguities of classification within this third level, because it necessarily includes a mixture of experiences. Therefore, some psychedelic events included within this third level could be interpreted as consistent *either* with (a) states that were actually more advanced than absorptions; (b) mixtures of absorptions and of "higher" states; (c) misdescriptions prompted by the pressured pace of the drug-induced state.

10. S. Grof. Varieties of transpersonal experiences: observations from LSD psychotherapy. In *Psychiatry and Mysticism,* ed. S. Dean. Chicago, Nelson-Hall, 1975; 311–345.

11. W. Van Dusen. LSD and the enlightenment of zen. *Psychologia* 1961; 4:11–16. The subjects' LSD dosages ranged between 50 and 200 micrograms. Two of the subjects were said to have come to "satori" previously without having used LSD.

Chapter 140   Preludes with Potential: Dark Nights and Depressions

1. C. Jung. *Psychology and Religion: West and East,* 2nd ed., vol. 11. Bollingen Series 20. Princeton, N.J., Princeton University Press, 1958, 553.

2. W. Styron. *International Herald Tribune,* Letters to the Editor, 20 December, 1988, 5.

3. A. Hardy. *The Spiritual Nature of Man. A Study of Contemporary Religious Experience.* Oxford, Oxford University Press, 28; 91–92.

4. E. Underhill. *Mysticism.* New York, Dutton, 1961.

5. G. Chang. *The Practice of Zen.* New York, Perennial, Harper & Row, 1959, 130. This Hanshan is *not* the layman poet of the seventh century.

6. D. Kinney and R. Richards. Creativity and manic depressive illness. *Science* 1986; 234:529.

7. C. Dackis and M. Gold. The serotonin subtype of depression. In *Advances in Psychopharmacology: Predicting and Improving Treatment Response,* ed. M. Gold. Boca Raton, Fla., CRC Press, 1984, 107–120.

8. H. Van Praag. Central monoamine metabolism in depressions I. Serotonin and related compounds. *Comprehensive Psychiatry* 1980; 21:30–43.

9. H. Van Praag. Biological suicide research: Outcome and limitations. *Biological Psychiatry* 1986; 21:1305–1323.

10. P. Delgado, D. Charney, L. Price, et al. Serotonin function and the mechanism of antidepressant action. *Archives of General Psychiatry* 1990; 47:411–418.

11. H. Van Praag. Central monoamine metabolism in depression. II Catecholamines and related compounds. *Comprehensive Psychiatry* 1980; 21:44–54. This phenomenon needs to be separated into its primary and secondary components. Inert patients who don't move at all could reduce, secondarily, their dopamine turnover.

12. The first improvement is delayed for many days. This suggests that slow metabolic adjustments have modified the synaptic excitabilities of many nerve cells.

13. F. Lechin, B. van der Dijs, J. Amat, et al. Central neuronal pathways involved in anxiety behavior: Experimental findings. *Research Communications in Psychology, Psychiatry, and Behavior* 1986; 11:113–143.

14. *Ibid.,* 149–192.

15. S. Dilsaver. Cholinergic mechanisms in depression. *Brain Research. Brain Research Reviews* 1986; 11:285–316.

16. R. Tandon and J. Greden. Cholinergic hyperactivity and negative schizophrenic symptoms. *Archives of General Psychiatry* 1989; 46:745–753. The "negative" symptoms in schizophrenia which are being compared with depression include flattening of affect, slowing, and social withdrawal.

17. W. Bunney, F. Goodwin, and D. Murphy. The "switch process" in manic-depressive illness. III Theoretical implications. *Archives of General Psychiatry* 1972; 27:312–317.

18. Among the latter drugs are those which energize because they inhibit the enzyme monoamine oxidase. Normally, this enzyme will be breaking down the biogenic amines (norepinephrine, dopamine, serotonin, and epinephrine) and limiting their effects.

19. E. Souetre, E. Salvati, D. Pringuey, et al. Antidepressant effects of the sleep/wake cycle phase advance. *Journal of Affective Disorders* 1987; 12:41–46.

20. J. Wu and W. Bunney. The biological basis of an antidepressant response to sleep deprivation and relapse: Review and hypothesis. *American Journal of Psychiatry* 1990; 1:14–21.

21. G-Y. Hu and J. Storm. Excitatory amino acids acting on metabotropic glutamate receptors broaden the action potential in hippocampal neurons. *Brain Research* 1991; 568:339–344.

22. S. Avissar and G. Schreiber. The involvement of guanine nucleotide binding proteins in the pathogenesis and treatment of affective disorders. *Biological Psychiatry* 1992; 31:435–459.

23. D. Ebert, H. Feistel, and A. Barocka. Effects of sleep deprivation on the limbic system and the frontal lobes in affective disorders: A study with Tc-99m-HMPAO SPECT. *Psychiatry Research: Neuroimaging* 1992; 40:247–251.

24. B. Parry, S. Berga, N. Mostofi, et al. Morning versus evening bright light treatment of late luteal phase dysphoric disorder. *American Journal of Psychiatry* 1989; 146:1215–1217.

25. D. Avery, A. Khan, S. Dager, et al. Bright light treatment of winter depression: Morning vs evening light. *Acta Psychiatrica Scandinavica* 1990; 82:335–338.

26. E. Richelson. Pharmacology of antidepressants—Characteristics of the ideal drug. *Mayo Clinic Proceedings* 1994; 69:1069–1081. Certain drugs block the reuptake system which normally removes serotonin from the synapse. This increases the effective levels of ST in the synapse. The drugs are called "selective ST re-uptake inhibitors."

27. S. Starkstein, R. Robinson, and T. Price. Comparison of cortical and subcortical lesions in the production of post stroke mood disorders. *Brain* 1987; 110:1045–1059.

28. A. House, M. Dennis, C. Warlow, et al. Mood disorders after stroke and their relation to lesion location. *Brain* 1990; 113:1113–1129.

29. W. Drevets and M. Raichle. Positron emission tomographic imaging studies of human emotional disorders. In *The Cognitive Neurosciences*, ed. M. Gazzaniga. Cambridge, Mass., The MIT Press, 1995; 1153–1164.

30. W. Drevets, J. Price, J. Simpson, Jr., et al. Subgenual prefrontal cortex abnormalities in mood disorders. *Nature* 1997; 386:824–827.

31. A. Damasio. Towards a neuropathology of emotion and mood. *Nature* 1997; 386:769–770.

32. H. Stewart. *A Chime of Windbells*. Rutland, Vt., Tuttle, 1969, 185.

Chapter 141   Operational Differences between Absorption and Insight-Wisdom

1. R. Sperry. *Science and Moral Priority*. New York, Columbia University Press, 1983, 71.

2. P. Venables and M. Christie. *Research in Psychophysiology*. London, Wiley, 1975, v.

Chapter 142   Reflections on Kensho, Personal, and Neurological

1. D. Suzuki. *Sengai the Zen Master*. London, Faber & Faber, 1971.

2. H. Dumoulin. *Christianity Meets Buddhism*. LaSalle, Ill., Open Court, 1974.

3. D. Tranel and A. Damasio. Knowledge without awareness: An autonomic index of facial recognition by prosopagnostics. *Science* 1985; 228:1453–1454. At present, the autonomic skin test results in themselves would not separate a disorder at the simpler, more reflexive early level of recognition from a disorder farther down at the output level.

4. J. Hyvarinen. *The Parietal Cortex of Monkey and Man*. Berlin, Springer-Verlag, 1982.

5. M. Rizzo and D. Robin. Simultanagnosia. *Neurology* 1990; 40:447–455. The shorter term for this disorder is *simultagnosia*. The functions of the brain are, of course, not highly localized, but depend rather on countless connections among different modules and systems. Therefore, for the record, I want to state clearly the following qualification: to describe the *dys*function that occurs after an isolated site in the brain is damaged is not the same as to specify in any final way what its *normal* function is or what its *amplified* function might be.

6. M. Gentilini, P. Nichelli, and R. Schoenhuber. Assessment of attention in mild head injury. In *Mild Head Injury*, eds. H. Levin, H. Eisenberg, and A. Benton. New York, Oxford University Press, 1989, 163–175. By definition, diffuse injuries to the brain serve no useful purpose *if* one is trying to localize functions to a particular site.

7. C. Ricci and C. Blundo. Perception of ambiguous figures after focal brain lesions. *Neuropsychologia* 1990; 28:1163–1173.

8. L. Miller. Impulsivity, risk-taking, and the ability to synthesize fragmented information after frontal lobectomy. *Neuropsychologia* 1992; 30:69–79.

9. D. Paré and M. Steriade. The reticular thalamic nucleus projects to the contralateral dorsal thalamus in macaque monkey. *Neuroscience Letters* 1993; 154:96–100.

10. R. Emerson. *Essays by Ralph Waldo Emerson; from Self-Reliance*. New York, Perennial Library, Harper & Row, 1926, 50.

11. J. Campbell. *The Masks of God: Oriental Mythology*. New York, Viking, 1962, 428.

12. P. Haskel. *Bankei Zen*. New York, Grove Press, 1984, 125–132.

13. A. Maslow. The "core-religious" or "transcendent" experience. In *The Highest State of Consciousness*, ed. J. White. Garden City, N.Y., Anchor/Doubleday, 1972, 352–364.

14. Two subtle components are implicit in this "don't intervene" message. One is that some potential "habit energy" of a previously active self seems (if only indirectly) to be off in a covert compartment. The other is that this vaguely inferred (i) is also being gently reminded to *avoid* doing something. Is the mere inference of an illusory self giving rise to an "avoid meddling" impulse? If so, then one might hypothesize that such an advisory component of nonintervention would drop out when the same person underwent successively deeper episodes of kensho.

15. N. Waddell, trans. and ed. *The Unborn: The Life and Teaching of Zen Master Bankei, 1622–1693*. San Francisco, North Point Press, 1984.

16. Q-P. Ma, Y-S. Shi, and J-S. Han. Naloxone blocks opioid peptide release in n. accumbens and amygdala elicited by morphine injected into periaqueductal gray. *Brain Research Bulletin* 1992; 28:351–354.

17. S. Mullen and W. Penfield. Illusions of comparative interpretation and emotion. *Archives of Neurology and Psychiatry* 1959; 81:269–284.

18. Myokyo-ni [I. Schloegl]. *Gentling the Bull. The Ten Bull Pictures. A Spiritual Journey.* London, Zen Centre, n.d.

Chapter 143   Selective Mechanisms Underlying Kensho

1. Thomas Henry Huxley, quoted in I. Asimov and J. Shulman, eds., *Isaac Asimov's Book of Science and Nature Quotations.* New York, Weidenfeld & Nicolson, 1988, 277.

2. R. Devaney. Chaotic explosions in simple dynamical systems. In *The Ubiquity of Chaos*, ed. S. Krasner. Washington, D.C., American Association for the Advancement of Science, 1990, 1–9.

3. D. Zaidel. Hemi-field asymmetries in memory for incongruous scenes. *Cortex* 1988; 24:231–244.

4. F. Wilson and E. Rolls. Neuronal responses related to the novelty and familiarity of visual stimuli in the substantia innominata, diagonal band of Broca and periventricular region of the primate basal forebrain. *Experimental Brain Research* 1990; 80:104–120.

5. D. Suzuki. *Essays in Zen Buddhism.* First Series. New York, Grove Press, 1949, 249.

6. M. Okawa, M. Matousek, and I. Petersen. Spontaneous vigilance fluctuations in the daytime. *Psychophysiology* 1984; 21:207–211. Our peaks of vigilance recur every 60 to 110 minutes, not exactly every 90 minutes.

7. M. Steriade, F. Amzica, and O. Contreras. Synchronization of fast (30–40 Hz) spontaneous cortical rhythms during brain activation. *Journal of Neuroscience* 1996; 16:392–417. This recent paper makes the point that fast rhythms can, in fact, be synchronized, and that they can also be coherent within a relatively limited *local* area of cortex. Hence, it is not accurate to assume that all low voltage fast-wave activities are necessarily *de*synchronized. In keeping with all the long-established semantic conventions, and to avoid further confusion, I have retained the term "D-sleep" to describe that active sleep state accompanied by low voltage fast-wave forms.

8. R. Bucke. *Cosmic Consciousness.* Secaucus, N.J., Citadel, 1973, 8.

9. O. Sacks. *Awakenings.* Garden City, N.Y., Doubleday, 1974. Later adapted into a motion picture.

10. *Ibid.,* 202.

11. S. Starkey. Melatonin and 5-hydroxytryptamine phase advance the rat circadian clock by activation of nitric oxide synthesis. *Neuroscience Letters* 1996; 211:199–202. Humans respond to light and dark differently than do rats. Therefore, we need further studies—in primates—to clarify which of the several messenger molecules is the most effective stimulus for shifting our clock at different hours of our circadian cycle.

12. M. Lewis, M. Mishkin, E. Bragin, et al. Opiate receptor gradients in monkey cerebral cortex: Correspondence with sensory processing hierarchies. *Science* 1981; 211:1166–1169.

13. S. Wise and M. Herkenham. Opiate receptor distribution in the cerebral cortex of the rhesus monkey. *Science* 1982; 218:387–388.

14. Potential examples of this mechanism are to be found in the later phases of near-death experiences, in the terminal deathbed experiences, and in some of the unusual experiences under general anesthesia (see chapter 104).

15. T. Hirai and E. Jones. Distribution of tachykinin and enkephalin-immunoreactive fibers in the human thalamus. *Brain Research. Brain Research Reviews* 1989; 14:35–52.

16. Once β-endorphin is released, nitric oxide can further enhance its analgesic and possibly other effects. See L. Tseng, J. Xu, and G. Pieper. Increase of nitric oxide production by L-arginine potentiates I.C.V. administered β-endorphin-induced antinociception in the mouse. *European Journal of Pharmacology* 1992; 212:301–303.

17. T. Barreca, C. Siani, R. Franceschini, et al. Diurnal β-endorphin changes in human cerebrospinal fluid. *Life Sciences* 1986; 38:2263–2267. The fluid samples were obtained from the third ventricle next to the hypothalamus.

18. H. Thoreau. *Walden.* 1854; Princeton, N.J., Princeton University Press, 1989.

19. Clearly, much remains to be learned about how the shallower and deeper levels of meditation influence the peaks and valleys of *all* the messenger molecules and receptors in the brain.

20. J. Austin. *Chase, Chance and Creativity. The Lucky Art of Novelty.* New York, Columbia University Press, 1978, 161.

21. On rare occasions, a person may drop off to sleep at night and then awaken the next morning already in a momentary state of "no-self." See A. Faraday. A psychology of no-self. *Noetic Sciences Review* 1994; spring:17–19.

22. R. Bucke, *Cosmic Consciousness*, 68.

Chapter 145   The State of Ultimate Pure Being

1. D. Suzuki and W. King. Conversations with D.T. Suzuki. *The Eastern Buddhist.* New Series 1988; 21(spring):84.

2. C. Chang, ed. *Original Teachings of Chan Buddhism*, rev. ed. New York, Grove Press, 1982, 13.

3. This is not to overlook the fact that rare "transpersonal" experiences of "primordial" states, which some persons describe using the word "ultimate," may occur late in the course of exposures to psychedelic drugs, as noted in chapter 139.

4. Thich Nhat Hanh. *Peace Is Every Step.* New York, Bantam, 1991.

5. G. Jordan. LSD and mystical experiences. In *The Highest State of Consciousness*, ed. J. White. Garden City, N.Y., Anchor/Doubleday, 1972, 278–294.

6. J. Cleary and T. Cleary. *The Blue Cliff Record*, vol. 1. Boulder, Col., Shambhala, 1978, 1.

7. Among the early Indian Buddhist schools, the total cessation or experience was termed *nirodh,* and the cessation of awareness was given the name *nirvana.* See D. Goleman. The Buddha on meditation and states of consciousness. Pt. I: The teachings. *Journal of Transpersonal Psychology* 1972; 4:1–44.

8. F. Merrell-Wolff. *The Philosophy of Consciousness Without an Object.* New York, Julian Press, 1973.

9. G. Welbon. *The Buddhist Nirvana and Its Western Interpreters.* Chicago, University of Chicago Press, 1968.

10. C. Naranjo. Meditation and psychosomatic health. In *Dimensions in Wholestic Healing*, eds. H. Otto and J. Knight. Chicago, Nelson Hall, 1979, 253–265.

11. Reserved for chapter 148 is a discussion of how the state of Pure Being relates to the sequence of pictures in the series of the bull and the herdsman.

12. R. Aitken and D. Steindl-Rast. *The Ground We Share.* Liguori, Mo., Triumph Books, 1994, 125. The quoted term came from an earlier poem by Gerald Manley Hopkins.

Chapter 146   The Power of Silence

1. Walt Whitman, quoted in C. Curtis and F. Greenslet, eds., *The Practical Cogitator.* Boston, Houghton Mifflin, 1953, 497.

2. R. Sasaki. *The Record of Lin-Chi.* Kyoto, Japan, Institute for Zen Studies, 1975, 1.

3. D. Suzuki. *Essays in Zen Buddhism.* First Series. London, Rider, 1949, 261.

4. H. Smith. *Forgotten Truth. The Primordial Tradition.* New York, Harper & Row, 1976. This *mu* is not to be confused with the *Mu* of Zen.

5. Hu Shih. The development of Zen Buddhism in China. In *Anthology of Zen*, ed. W. Briggs. New York, Grove Press, 1961, 7–30. Master Tao-sheng played a leading role in founding the school of sudden enlightenment in China.

6. T. Leggett. *The Second Zen Reader.* Rutland, Vt., Tuttle, 1988, 175.

7. R. Emerson. The over-soul. In *Emerson's Essays.* New York, Perennial Library, Harper & Row, 1926, 200.

8. Leggett, *op. cit.* 184. The tale is oddly reminiscent of a Groucho Marx riposte.

9. H. Maezumi and B. Glassman. *The Hazy Moon of Enlightenment.* Los Angeles, Center Publications, 1977, 69–74.

10. I discovered this sentence, without citation, in a newspaper. In a handwritten, illustrated personal communication of August 1992, Marceau explains that he is still searching for the source of his quotation. There has not been a word from him since.

11. A. Greeley. *The Sociology of the Paranormal. A Reconnaissance.* Sage Research Paper, vol. 3, series 90-023. Beverly Hills, Calif.

12. Gallup Opinion Index Report no. 145, 53–55, 1977–78.

13. A. Watts. This is it. In *The Highest State of Consciousness,* ed. J. White. Garden City, N.Y., Anchor/(Doubleday), 1972, 436–451.

14. Empirically, meditation appears to reduce the drive to chatter in many persons. Further studies are indicated to see how much reduced verbalizations may relate to the kind of relative or absolute reduction of left hemispheric verbal language functions that may be observed in a PET scan (see figure 12 and color plate).

15. J. Campbell. *Power of Myth.* New York, Doubleday, 1988, 98.

16. It is reasonable to consider that the same kinds of events which help finally dissolve the self would also spill over to involve adjacent circuits which mediate the sense of hearing. The way that enkephalin terminals supply the hearing pathway in the brain stem is one example.

17. W. Hess and H. Fischer. Brain and consciousness: A discussion about the function of the brain. *Perspectives in Biology and Medicine* 1973; 17:109–118.

Chapter 147   Beyond Sudden States of Enlightenment

1. P. Haskel. *Bankei Zen.* New York, Grove Press, 1984, 125–132.

2. *The Teaching of Buddha.* Tokyo, Bukkyo Dendo Kyokai, 1966, 59. Words attributed to the Buddha may have originated in his followers.

3. W. James. *The Varieties of Religious Experience.* New York, Mentor/New American, 1958.

4. P. Teilhard de Chardin. *The Phenomenon of Man,* trans. B. Wall. New York, Harper Bros., 1959, 261.

5. D. Suzuki. *The Zen Doctrine of No-Mind.* New York, Weiser, 1969, 27.

6. L. Nordstrom. Mysticism without transcendence: Reflections on liberation and emptiness. *Philosophy East and West* 1981; 31:89–95.

Chapter 148   The Exceptional Stage of Ongoing Enlightened Traits

1. T. Cleary. *Sayings and Doings of Pai-Chang.* Los Angeles, Center Publications, 1978, 81.

2. D. Suzuki. *Essays in Zen Buddhism.* First Series. New York, Grove Press, 1949, 223.

3. H. -J. Kim. *Dogen Kigen—Mystical Realist.* Tucson, University of Arizona Press, 1975, 67–68. Kim concludes that at this point, the liberated person can both negate and subsume any distinctions between self and other.

4. K. Sekida. *Zen Training. Methods and Philosophy.* New York, Weatherhill, 1975, 234–235. Sekida also uses the same term, "positive samadhi," to describe the more common everyday varieties of short-lasting effortless high-level performance. Currently, athletes speak of this as playing "in the zone."

5. N. Waddell. *The Unborn: The Life and Teaching of Zen Master Bankei 1622–1693.* San Francisco, North Point Press, 1984, 132–133.

6. P. Reps. *Zen Flesh, Zen Bones.* Rutland, Vt., Tuttle, 1971, 22.

7. I. Miura and R. Sasaki. *The Zen Koan: Its History and Use in Rinzai Zen.* New York, Harcourt Brace & World, 58. Hakuin cautions that only the resolute monk who passes every koan hurdle arrives at this stage.

8. Myokyo-ni [Irmgard Schloegl]. *Gentling the Bull. The Ten Bull Pictures. A Spiritual Journey.* London, Zen Centre, n.d.

9. From one of the many excellent gathas by Robert Aitken in his book, *The Dragon Who Never Sleeps.* Berkeley, Calif., Parallax Press, 1992.

Chapter 149   Simplicity and Stability

1. M. Fischer, in M. Strauss, ed., *Familiar Medical Quotations*. Boston, Little, Brown, 56.
2. R. Emerson. The over-soul. In *The Complete Writings of Ralph Waldo Emerson*. New York, Wise, 1929, 207.
3. I. Schloegl. *The Wisdom of the Zen Masters*. London, Sheldon Press, 1975, 18.
4. D. Suzuki. *Studies in Zen*. New York, Delta, 1955, 38.
5. A. Maslow. The "core-religious" or "transcendent" experience. In *The Highest State of Consciousness*, ed. J. White. Garden City, N.Y., Anchor/Doubleday, 1972, 352–364.
6. R. Emerson. *Emerson's Essays*. New York, Perennial Library. Harper & Row, 1926, 202–208.
7. H. Stewart. *A Net of Fireflies. Japanese Haiku and Haiku Paintings*. Rutland, Vt., Tuttle, 1960, 126–127.
8. J. Ruysbroeck, in J. Cohen and J.-F. Phipps, eds., *The Common Experience*. London, Rider, 1979, 100.
9. It is typical of D.T. Suzuki that in later years he used to joke that the word really translated as "great stupidity." See A. Irwin Switzer III. *D.T. Suzuki; A Biography*. London, The Buddhist Society, 1985, 12.
10. R. Sasaki. Zen, a religion. In *Anthology of Zen*, ed. W. Briggs. New York, Grove Press, 1961, 111–121.
11. D. Anthony, B. Ecker, and K. Wilber. *Spiritual Choices. The Problems of Recognizing Authentic Paths to Inner Transformation*. New York, Paragon House, 1987, 349.

Chapter 150   An Ethical Base of Zen?

1. P. Yampolsky. *The Platform Sutra of the Sixth Patriarch*. New York, Columbia University Press, 1967.
2. R. Tsunoda, W. de Barry, and D. Keene. *Sources of Japanese Traditions*. New York, Columbia University Press, 1958, 242.
3. A. Maslow. New introduction: Religions, values, and peak-experiences (New edition). *Journal of Transpersonal Psychology* 1970; 2:83–90.
4. A. Maslow. The "core-religious" or "transcendent" experience. In *The Highest State of Consciousness*, ed. J. White. Garden City, N.Y., Anchor/Doubleday, 1972, 352–364.
5. I. Miura and R. Sasaki. *Zen Dust. The History of the Koan and Koan Study in Rinzai (Lin-Chi) Zen*. Kyoto, The First Zen Institute of America in Japan, 1966, 74.
6. Wong Mon-lam. *The Sutra of Wei Lang* (Hui-neng). London, Luzac, 1944, 124.
7. W. Wordsworth. Prelude II, 130, quoted in R. Blyth, *Zen in English Literature and Oriental Classics*. Tokyo, Hokuseido Press, 1942, 417.
8. R. Aitken. *The Mind of Clover. Essays in Zen Buddhist Ethics*. San Francisco, North Point Press, 1984, 155.
9. Z. Shibayama. *Zen Comments on the Mumonkun*. New York, Harper & Row, 1974, 70.
10. *Ibid.*, 67.
11. R. Pirsig. *Zen and the Art of Motorcycle Maintenance*. New York, Bantam, 1974, 288.
12. F. Massimini, M. Csikszentmihalyi, and M. Carli. The monitoring of optimal experience. *Journal of Nervous and Mental Disease* 1987; 175:545–549.
13. S. Radhakrishnan. *The Principal Upanishads*. London, Allen & Unwin, 1953, 106.
14. M. Hoffman. Is altruism part of human nature? *Journal of Personality and Social Psychology* 1981; 40:121–137.
15. A. Watts. Psychotherapy and liberation. In *The Highest State of Consciousness*, ed. J. White. Garden City, N.Y., Anchor/Doubleday, 1972, 195–203.

Chapter 151   Compassion, the Native Virtue

1. D. Suzuki. *Studies in the Lankavatara Sutra*. London, Routledge & Kegan Paul, 1930, 297.
2. A. Petrie. *Individuality in Pain and Suffering*, 2nd ed. Chicago, University of Chicago Press, 1978.

3. M. Hunt. *The Compassionate Beast*. New York, Morrow, 1990, 13.

4. K. Gibran. *The Prophet*. New York, Knopf, 1968, 97.

5. N. Kobori. The ripening persimmon. An interview with Kobori Nanrei Roshi. *Parabola* 1985; 10:72–79.

6. W. James. *The Principles of Psychology*, vol. 2. New York, Holt, 1918, 369.

7. Myokyo-ni [Irmgard Schloegl]. *Gentling the Bull. The Ten Bull Pictures. A Spiritual Journey*. London, Zen Centre, n.d.

8. Y. Toyokura. Neurology in art and literature. A bibliography. *Neurological Medicine (Tokyo)* 1991; 35:91–112.

9. R. Thurman. Edicts of Asoka. In *The Path of Compassion. Writings on Socially Engaged Buddhism*, ed. F. Eppsteiner. Berkeley, Calif., Parallax Press, 1988, 111–119.

10. A. Kotler. Editor's introduction. In Thich Nhat Hanh. *Peace is Every Step*. New York, Bantam, ix–xv. The quotation is from page 57.

11. M. Hunt, *op. cit.*, 50.

12. *Ibid.*, 204.

13. W. Damon. *The Moral Child*. New York, Free Press, 1988, 31–50.

14. T. Lesh. Zen meditation and the development of empathy in counselors. In *Biofeedback and Self-Control*, ed. J. Komiya. Chicago, Aldine-Atherton, 1970, 113–148.

15. F. Eppsteiner, in *The Path of Compassion. Writing on Socially Engaged Buddhism*, ed. F. Eppsteiner. Berkeley, Calif., Parallax Press, 1988, 57.

16. R. Masunaga. *A Primer of Soto Zen*. Honolulu, East-West Center Press, 1971, 106–107. At first, to Western eyes, the multiple arms of Avalokiteshvara seem bizarre. What they symbolize, however, are the many skillful means—*upaya*—which this bodhisattva of compassion uses to help all beings.

17. A. Einstein. *New York Times*, 29 March 1972,

18. J. Campbell. *Power of Myth*. New York, Doubleday, 1988, 22.

Chapter 152   Etching In and Out

1. G. Globus. Potential contribution of meditation to neuroscience. In *Meditation: Classic and Contemporary Perspectives*, eds. D. Shapiro and R. Walsh. New York, Aldine, 1984, 681–685.

2. J. Olney. Excitatory amino acids and neuropsychiatric disorders. *Biological Psychiatry* 1989; 26:505–525.

3. P. McGeer, J. Eccles, and E. McGeer. *Molecular Neurobiology of the Mammalian Brain*. New York, Plenum Press, 1978, 190.

4. W. Nauta and M. Feirtag. *Fundamental Neuroanatomy*. New York, W.H. Freeman, 1986.

5. R. Auer and B. Siesjö. Biological differences between ischemia, hypoglycemia, and epilepsy. *Annals of Neurology* 1988; 24:699–707.

6. R. Albin and J. Greenamyre. Alternative excitotoxic hypotheses. *Neurology* 1992; 42:733–738. The current system for naming these amino acid receptors is based on the particular agonist molecule which best excites them: NMDA, kainate, or quisqualate.

7. J. Olney, J. Labruyere, J. Collins, et al. D-Aminophosphonovalerate is 100-fold more powerful than D-alphaaminoadipate in blocking *N*-methylaspartate neurotoxicity. *Brain Research* 1981; 221:207–210.

8. S. Watson and H. Akil. Opioid peptides and related substances: Immunocytochemistry. In *Neurosecretion and Brain Peptides*, eds. J. Martin, S. Reichlin, and K. Bick. New York, Raven Press, 1981, 77–86.

9. A. Farooqui and L. Horrocks. Excitatory amino acid receptors, neural membrane phospholipid metabolism and neurological disorders. *Brain Research. Brain Research Reviews* 1991; 16:171–191.

10. S. Rothman, J. Thurston, and R. Hauhart. Delayed neurotoxicity of excitatory amino acids in vitro. *Neurosciences* 1987; 22:471–480.

11. M. Okazaki, P. Aitken, and J. Nadler. Mossy fiber lesion reduces the probability that kainic acid will provoke CA3 hippocampal pyramidal cell bursting. *Brain Research* 1988; 440:352–356.

12. J. Vicedomini and J. Nadler. Stimulation-induced status epilepticus: Role of the hippocampal mossy fibers in the seizures and associated neuropathology. *Brain Research* 1990; 512:70–74.

13. B. Rogers, M. Barnes, C. Mitchell, et al. Functional deficits after sustained stimulation of the perforant path. *Brain Research* 1989; 493:41–50.

14. B. Stein and R. Sapolsky. Chemical adrenalectomy reduces hippocampal damage induced by kainic acid. *Brain Research* 1988; 473:175–180.

15. H. Fujikura, H. Kato, S. Hakano, et al. A serotonin S_2 antagonist, naftidrofuryl, exhibited a protective effect on ischemic neuronal damage in the gerbil. *Brain Research* 1989; 494:387–390.

16. In contrast, the activation of ST_{1A} receptors exerts a protective effect against excitoxic cell death. See N. Akaike and T. Shirasaki. Modulation of NMDA receptors in isolated rat CNS neurons by the competitive and noncompetitive drugs and 5-HT. In *Vision, Memory and the Temporal Lobe,* E. Iwai and M. Mishkin. New York, Elsevier, 1990, 417–420.

17. A. Cheramy, R. Romo, and J. Glowinski. Role of corticostriatal glutamatergic neurons in the presynaptic control of dopamine release. In *Neurotransmitter Interactions in the Basal Ganglia,* eds. M. Sandler, C. Feuerstein, B. Scatton, et al. New York, Raven Press, 1987, 133–131.

18. M. Christie, P. Rowe, and P. Beart. Effect of excitotoxin lesions in the medial prefrontal cortex on cortical and subcortical catecholamine turnover in the rat. *Journal of Neurochemistry* 1986; 47:1593–1597.

19. D. Stevens and C. Cotman. Excitatory amino acid antagonists depress transmission in hippocampal projections to the lateral septum. *Brain Research* 1986; 382:437–440.

20. H. Moises and J. Walker. Electrophysiological effects of dynorphin peptides on hippocampal pyramidal cells in rat. *European Journal of Pharmacology* 1985; 108:85–98.

21. K. Stevens, G. Shiotsu, and L. Stein. Hippocampal μ receptors mediate opioid reinforcement in the CA3 region. *Brain Research* 1991; 545:8–16.

22. R. Caudle and L. Isaac. Intrathecal dynorphin (1–13) results in an irreversible loss of the tail-flick reflex in rats. *Brain Research* 1987, 435:1 6.

23. Again, for contrast, the process of cell death can be shaped in the other direction. Injections of certain morphine-like opiates do stop some of the nerve cell damage caused by excitotoxic amino acids. Thus, dextromethorphan and dextrorphan act either by blocking the amino acid receptor itself or the special calcium ion channel linked to it. See C. Carpenter, S. Marks, D. Watson, et al. Dextromethorphan and dextrorphan as calcium channel antagonists. *Brain Research* 1988; 439:372–375.

24. A. Freese, K. Swartz, M. During, et al. Kynurenine metabolites of tryptophan: Implications for neurologic diseases. *Neurology* 1990; 40:691–695.

25. A. McGregor and J. Herbert. Differential effects of excitotoxic basolateral and corticomedial lesions of the amygdala on the behavioral and endocrine responses to either sexual or aggression-promoting stimuli in the male rat. *Brain Research* 1992; 574:9–20.

26. M. Morgan, L. Romanski, and J. LeDoux. Extinction of emotional learning: Contribution of medial prefrontal cortex. *Neuroscience Letters* 1993; 163:109–113. The interactions in this general region are complex. Their psychophysiology needs to be studied carefully in primates and correlated with the most recent neuroimaging and autopsy techniques applicable to humans. See chapter 140.

27. A technical term, *apoptosis,* is applied to the set of cellular mechanisms that evolve slowly, activate processes intrinsic to the nerve cell, and lead ultimately to its death. These have been called "suicide" mechanisms. See chapter 153, reference 5.

28. Researchers will appreciate that self-appointed subjects are *not* the best ones for this postmortem study. The few genuine sages must be tracked down, verified, studied repeatedly during life, and then convinced to sign up for an autopsy, in advance.

29. In neurology such lesions are called nuclear, and internuclear, respectively.

30. G. Riedel. Function of metabotropic glutamate receptors in learning and memory. *Trends in Neurosciences* 1996; 19:219–244.

Chapter 153   Aging in the Brain

1. P. Haskel. *Bankei Zen.* New York, Grove Press, 1984, 125–132.
2. J. Hackett. *The Zen Haiku and Other Zen Poems of J.W. Hackett.* Tokyo, Japan Publications, 1983, 51.
3. C. Jung. *Two Essays on Analytical Psychology.* Bollinger Series 20. New York, Pantheon, 1953, 60, 177. Jung believed that personal development after the age of 35 proceeded through steps which finally reconciled the opposites.
4. *Ibid.*, 74.
5. R. Pittman, J. Mills, A. DiBenedetto, et al. Neuronal cell death: Searching for the smoking gun. *Current Opinion in Neurobiology* 1994; 4:87–94.
6. J. Austin, E. Connole, D. Kett, et al. Studies in aging of the brain V. Reduced norepinephrine, dopamine and cyclic AMP in rat brain with advancing age. *Age* 1978; 1:121–124.
7. M. Mattson. Neurotransmitters in the regulation of neuronal cytoarchitecture. *Brain Research. Brain Research Reviews* 1988; 13:179–199.
8. S. Zola-Morgan, L. Squire, and G. Amaral. Human amnesia and the medial temporal region: Enduring memory impairment following a bilateral lesion limited to field CA1 of the hippocampus. *Journal of Neuroscience* 1986; 6:2950–2967.
9. M. West and H. Gunderson. Unbiased stereological estimation of the numbers of neurons in the human hippocampus. *Journal of Comparative Neurology* 1990; 296:1–22.
10. J. Eccles. Mechanisms of learning in complex systems. In *Handbook of Physiology.* Sec. 1, *The Nervous System,* vol. 5, pt. 1., eds. V. Mountcastle, F. Plum, and S. Geiger. Bethesda, Md., American Physiological Society, 1987, 137–167.
11. C. Houser, J. Miyashiro, B. Swartz, et al. Altered patterns of dynorphin immunoreactivity suggest mossy fiber reorganization in human hippocampal epilepsy. *Journal of Neuroscience* 1990; 10:267–282. Some of these mossy fibers could then be able to pulse dynorphin into the hippocampal circuitry as it reorganizes. See T. Sutula, G. Cascino, J. Cavozos, et al. Mossy fiber synaptic reorganization in the epileptic human temporal lobe. *Annals of Neurology* 1989; 26:321–330.
12. G. Battaglia, A. Norman, and I. Creese. Differential serotonin 2 receptor recovery in mature and senescent rat brain after irreversible receptor modification: Effect of chronic receptor treatment. *Journal of Pharmacology and Experimental Therapeutics* 1987; 243:69–75.
13. S. Dewey, N. Volkow, J. Logan, et al. Age-related decreases in muscarinic cholinergic receptor binding in the human brain measured with positron emission tomography (PET). *Journal of Neuroscience Research* 1990; 27:569–575.
14. J. Rinne, P. Lönnberg, and P. Marjamaki. Age-dependent decline in human brain dopamine D_1 and D_2 receptors. *Brain Research* 1990; 508:349–352.
15. J. DeKeyser, G. Ebinger, and G. Vauquelin. Age-related changes in the human nigrostriatal dopaminergic system. *Annals of Neurology* 1990; 27:157–161.
16. P. McBride, H. Tierney, M. DeMeo, et al. Effects of age and gender on CNS serotonergic responsivity in normal adults. *Biological Psychiatry* 1990; 27:1143–1155.
17. B. Lawlor, T. Sunderland, J. Hill, et al. Evidence for a decline with age in behavioral responsivity to the serotonin agonist, м-chlorophenylpiperazine, in healthy human subjects. *Psychiatry Research* 1989; 29:1–10.
18. W. McEntee and T. Crook. Age-associated memory impairment. A role for catecholamines. *Neurology* 1990; 40:526–530.
19. P. Coleman and D. Flood. Dendritic proliferation in the ageing brain as a compensatory repair mechanism. *Progress in Brain Research* 1986; 70:227–237.
20. R. Sekuler and C. Owsley. The spatial vision of older humans. *In Aging and Human Visual Function,* eds. R. Sekuler, D. Kline, and K. Dismukes. New York, Liss, 1982, 185–202.
21. A. Maslow. *Religions, Values and Peak-Experiences.* New York, Viking, 1970.
22. B. Roberts. *The Experience of No-Self: A Contemplative Journey.* Sunspot, N.M., Iroquois House, 1982, 194.
23. A. Storr. *Solitude. A Return to the Self.* New York, Ballantine, 1988.

Chapter 154   The Celebration of Nature

1. A variation on the same old story cited in C. Jung. *Psychology and Religion: West and East,* 2nd ed., vol. 11. Bollingen Series 20. Princeton, N.J., Princeton University Press, 1969, 539.
2. R. Blyth. *Zen in English Literature and Oriental Classics.* Tokyo, Hokuseido Press, 1942, 418.
3. D. Suzuki. *Studies in Zen.* New York, Delta, 1955, 188.
4. M. Laski. *Ecstasy, a Study of Some Secular and Religious Experiences.* New York, Greenwood, 1968, 190.
5. A. Greeley. *The Sociology of the Paranormal. A Reconnaissance.* Sage Research Paper, vol. 3, series 90-023. Beverly Hills, Calif. 1975.
6. R. Ulrich, R. Simons, B. Losito, et al. Stress recovery during exposure to natural and urban environments. *Journal of Environmental Psychology* 11:201–230.
7. Zeno of Citium (334–262 B.C.) held that the wise man will do his duty, based on his knowing what nature requires.
8. R. Emerson. Spiritual laws, In *Essays by Ralph Waldo Emerson.* New York, Harper & Row, 1951, 93–94.
9. T. Leggett. *Zen and the Ways.* Boulder, Colo., Shambhala, 1978, 61. Daikaku was born in China, and lived from 1203 to 1268.

Chapter 155   Expressing Zen in Action

1. Thomas Henry Huxley, in G. Seldes, *The Great Quotations.* New York, Pocket Books, 1967, 3.
2. Sun Yat-sen, in G. Seldes, *The Great Quotations,* New York, Pocket Books, 1967, 4.
3. P. Wienpahl. *The Matter of Zen.* London, George Allen & Unwin, 1965, 124.
4. T. Leggett. *Zen and the Ways.* Boulder, Colo., Shambhala, 1978, 117.
5. S. Omori and K. Terayama. *Zen and the Art of Calligraphy,* trans. J. Stevens. London, Routledge & Kegan Paul, 1978, 11–16.
6. For example, my former colleagues in Kyoto have found what happens when acetylcholine acts on its muscarinic receptors on *presynaptic* terminals. Here, ACH inhibits impulses from flowing on to the next cell. See A. Akaike, M. Sasa, and S. Takaori. Muscarinic inhibition as a dominant role in cholinergic regulation of transmission in the caudate nucleus. *Journal of Pharmacology and Experimental Therapeutics* 1988; 246:1129–1136.
7. D. Suzuki and W. King. Conversations with D.T. Suzuki. *The Eastern Buddhist* New Series 1988; 21(spring):82–100.
8. J. Stein. The control of movement. In *Functions of the Brain,* ed. C. Coen. Oxford, Clarendon Press, 1985, 67–97.
9. Taken together, the two large basal ganglia called the caudate and putamen constitute the *dorsal striatum* (see figure 7). They have many interconnections with the frontal cortex. These interactions provide vital avenues for delaying and inhibiting some of our older patterned responses. On the other hand, when certain positive, reinforcing stimuli enter this same frontal-striatal system, the balance tips toward newer response tendencies, ones which are part of the new *learning* process. (See N. White. Reward or reinforcement: What's the difference? *Neuroscience and Biobehavioral Reviews* 1989; 13:181–186.) In contrast, the *ventral striatum* includes the region around the nucleus accumbens (the nucleus "leaning" against the septum). Here, rewarding stimuli appear to encourage motivation, drive, and other forward-moving approach behaviors. The mesolimbic dopamine system delivers an important supply of DA to energize the outer shell of this nucleus accumbens, whereas the nigrostriatal system supplies DA to nerve cells reaching its inner core. See A. Deutch and D. Cameron. Pharmacological characterization of dopamine systems in the nucleus accumbens core and shell. *Neuroscience* 1992; 46:49–56.
10. W. Nauta and M. Feirtag. *Fundamental Neuroanatomy.* New York, W.H. Freeman, 1986.
11. O. Creutzfeldt. Diversification and synthesis of sensory systems across the cortical link. In *Advances in Physiological Sciences.* Vol. 16, *Sensory Functions,* eds. E. Grastyan and P. Molnar. Hungary, Pergamon, 1981, 17–34.

12. The primary motor cortex lies just in front of the central fissure (see figure 2). It contains the giant-sized Betz cells. Not depicted as such are two other motoric regions which lie, successively, in front of it. One is the smaller supplementary motor cortex. It helps initiate and govern motor sequences. Some of these sequences are both more internally inspired and bilateral in nature. The second is the large premotor cortex. It extends forward to the frontal association cortex, and works intimately with its sensory partner, the parietal cortex. See S. Wise. The nonprimary motor cortex and its role in the cerebral control of movement. In *Dynamic Aspects of Neocortical Function*, eds. G. Edelman, W. Gall, and W. Cowan. New York, Wiley, 1984, 525–555.

13. M. Shahani. Visual input and the motor system in man. In *Brain Mechanisms in Memory and Learning: From the Single Neuron to Man*, ed. M. Brazier. New York, Raven Press, 1979, 345–349.

14. D. Suzuki. *Zen and Japanese Culture*. Bollingen Series 64. Princeton, N.J., Princeton University Press, 1973.

15. K. Heilman and T. Vanden Abell. Right hemisphere dominance for attention: The mechanisms underlying hemispheric asymmetries of inattention (neglect). *Neurology* 1980; 30:327–330. See also references 13 and 14 in chapter 62.

16. There are several kinds of event-related negative cortical potentials. Various degrees of *intention* enter into the tasks that are currently being used to study them. The different potentials include (a) the contingent negative variation (an expectancy wave); (b) the particular kind of readiness potential which is related to the subject's intention to carry out a brief *voluntary act*; (c) what might be termed an ongoing monitoring potential. This is related to the series of quasi-voluntary controls that subjects keep adding as their limb continues to move toward a target.

17. J. Adler and J. Sifft. Alpha EEG and simple reaction time. *Perceptual and Motor Skills* 1981; 52:306.

18. V. Castiello, Paulignan, and M. Jeannerod. Temporal dissociation of motor responses and subjective awareness. *Brain* 1991; 114:2639–2655.

19. B. Libet, C. Gleason, E. Wright, et al. Time of conscious intention to act in relation to onset of cerebral activity (readiness potential). *Brain* 1983; 106:623–642.

20. H. Jokeit and S. Makeig. Different event-related patterns of gamma-band power in brain waves of fast- and slow-reacting subjects. *Proceedings of the National Academy of Sciences of the United States of America* 1994; 91:6339–6343.

21. R. Näätänen. The inverted-U relationship between activation and performance: A critical review. In *Attention and Performance IV*, ed. S. Kornblum. New York, Academic Press, 1973, 155–174.

22. M. Maezumi and B. Glassman. *The Hazy Moon of Enlightenment*. Los Angeles, Center Publications, 1977, 69–74.

23. K. Shibuki and D. Okada. Endogenous nitric oxide release required for long term synaptic depression in the cerebellum. *Nature* 1991; 349:326–328. The glutamate receptors being described in this chapter 155 are of the NMDA type.

24. J. Grafman, I. Litvan, S. Massaquoi, et al. Cognitive planning deficit in patients with cerebellar atrophy. *Neurology* 1992; 42:1493–1496.

25. M. Ito. Long-term depression. *Annual Review of Neuroscience* 1989; 12:85–102.

Chapter 156   The Other Side of Zen

1. R. Blyth. *Zen and Zen Classics*, vol. 1. Tokyo, Hokuseido Press, 1972, 122–123.

2. C. Jung. *Psychology and Religion. West and East*, vol. 11. Bollingen Series 20. New York, Pantheon, 1958, 507.

3. C. Vogel, R. Albin, and J. Albers. Lotus footdrop: Sciatic neuropathy in the thigh. *Neurology* 1991; 41:605–606. Humans are built differently. No one meditation posture fits all. In the early years, it is advisable to conform and endure. At present, for sesshin, this aging author now spares his knees, alternating between a 6-inch cushion on a 12-inch stool, and sitting Burmese-style with both ankles on the pad and the left leg in front.

4. W. Johnston. *The Still Point. Reflections on Zen and Christian Mysticism.* New York, Fordham University Press, 1970, 108.
5. H. Welch. *The Buddhist Revival in China.* Cambridge, Mass., Harvard University Press, 1968, 253.
6. R. Blyth. *Zen in English Literature and Oriental Classics.* Tokyo, Hokuseido Press, 1942, 352.
7. M. Roth and J. Stevens. *Zen Guide.* New York, Weatherhill, 1985, xviii.
8. E. Becker. *Zen: A Rational Critique.* New York, Norton, 1961, 124.
9. C. Grof and S. Grof. *The Stormy Search for the Self.* Los Angeles, Tarcher, 1990.
10. H. Thoreau. *Walden.* 1854; Princeton, N.J., Princeton University Press, 1989.
11. K. Wilber. The Spectrum Model. In *Spiritual Choices. The Problems of Recognizing Authentic Paths to Inner Transformation,* eds. D. Anthony, B. Ecker, and K. Wilber. New York, Paragon House, 1987, 237–260.
12. S. Radhakrishnan. *The Principal Upanishads.* New York, Harper, 1953, 145.
13. K. Kraft. *Zen. Tradition and Transition.* New York, Grove Press, 1988.

Chapter 157　Still-Evolving Brains in Still-Evolving Societies

1. K. Lorenz, in M. Strauss, ed., *Familiar Medical Quotations.* Boston, Little, Brown, 1968, 163.
2. P. Teilhard de Chardin. *The Phenomenon of Man.* New York, Harper & Row, 1965, 254–268. (Italics are the author's.)
3. The time scale will be foreshortened for many Americans. Forty-seven percent of them believe that only in the last 10,000 years did God create man. (Gallup poll taken in 1991, cited in the *Denver Post,* 25 April 1992.)
4. J. Venter, U. de Porzio, D. Robinson, et al. Evolution of neurotransmitter receptor systems. *Progress in Neurobiology* 1988; 30:105–169.
5. R. Dixon, B. Kobilka, D. Strader, et al. Cloning of the gene and cDNA for mammalian β-adrenergic receptor and homology with rhodopsin. *Nature* 1986; 321:75–79.
6. L. Gilbert, W. Combest, W. Smith, et al. Neuropeptides, second messengers and insect molting. *Bioessays* 1988; 8:153–156.
7. S. Stanley. *Extinction.* New York, Scientific American Library, 1987.
8. R. Lewontin. The Evolution of cognition. In *Thinking, an Invitation to Cognitive Science,* vol. 3, eds. D. Osherson and E. Smith. Cambridge, Mass., The MIT Press, 1990, 229–246.
9. E. Armstrong. Evolution of the brain. In *The Human Nervous System,* ed. G. Paxinos. San Diego, Academic Press, 1990, 1–16. Many kinds of selection pressures are still in operation. It would be a mistake to focus on the mere fact that the *gross* brain weight of humans today *seems* about the same. Countless subtle inherited changes in the brain's chemical anatomy and physiological complexity may have taken place during the past 80,000 years or so. Brains have had to cope with such hazardous developments as battle-axes, gunpowder, fast automobiles, etc.
10. Senate Committee on Judiciary. 102nd Cong., 1991.
11. The genetic option in the following six sentences was composed in 1994 before seeing the movie *Little Buddha.* It is a less complicated option than the novel approach used to clone "Dolly" the sheep, as reported in 1997. It also allows the child to profit from the genetic diversity of both parents.
12. In medicine, currently, the DNA and enzyme screening techniques tend to be used chiefly to select *out* undesired defects. This particular futurist scenario is not one which our century can be comfortable with. But the underlying point is straightforward: similar screening principles might someday be used to select *in* those desired traits that had already been linked to biological markers.

Chapter 158　Commentary on the Trait Change of Ongoing Enlightenment

1. P. Haskel. *Bankei Zen.* New York, Grove Press, 1984, 125–132.
2. K. Gibran. *The Prophet.* New York, Knopf, 1968, 85.
3. Henri Bergson, from *Creative Evolution,* in *The Home Book of Quotations,* ed. B. Stevenson. New York, Crown, 1967.

4. E. DiGiusto and N. Bond. Imagery and the autonomic nervous system: Some methodological issues. *Perceptual and Motor Skills* 1979; 48:427–438.

5. A. Colby and W. Damon. *Some Do Care: Contemporary Lives of Moral Commitment.* New York, Free Press, 1992.

6. A glaring exception is nonintervention, a subtle quality described in chapter 142.

7. Colby and Damon, *op. cit.,* 70–71.

8. *Ibid.,* 167.

9. *Ibid.,* 311.

10. R. Phillips, B. Malamut, J. Bachevalier, et al. Dissociation of the effects of inferior temporal and limbic lesions on object discrimination learning with 24-h intertrial intervals. *Behavioral Brain Research* 1988; 27:99–107.

11. J. Wu. *The Golden Age of Zen.* Taipei, Taiwan, United Publishing Center, 1975. Distributed by Paragon Book Gallery. New York City.

In Closing

1. A. de Saint-Exupéry. *Wartime Writings 1939–1944.* New York, Harcourt Brace Jovanovich, 1986.

2. J. Campbell. *The Masks of God: Oriental Mythology.* New York, Viking, 1962, 280.

3. A. Toga and J. Mazziota. *Brain Mapping: The Methods.* San Diego, Academic Press, 1996. Information needs to be integrated in three dimensions using several of the cited methods.

4. Present address for correspondence: 2445 Moscow Mountain Road, Moscow ID, 83843–9132.

Appendix A   Introduction to the *Heart Sutra*

1. C. Chung-yuan. *Original Teachings of Chán Buddhism.* New York, Vintage, 1971, 35.

2. T. Leggett. *The Second Zen Reader.* Rutland, Vt., Tuttle, 1988, 15–16.

3. I. Schloegl. *Zen Traces* 1982; 4(March):4–11.

Appendix B   Selections from *Afirmation of Faith in Mind*

1. D. Suzuki. *Essays in Zen Buddhism.* First Series. New York, Grove Press, 1949, 196–201.

2. R. Blyth. *Zen and Zen Classics,* vol. 1. Tokyo, Hokuseido Press, 1972, 100–103.

3. P. Kapleau. *Zen: Dawn in the West.* Garden City, N.Y., Anchor Press, 1980, 184–189.

Source Notes

I wish to express my appreciation to the following authors, their copyright owners, and their publishers for permission to reprint excerpts from their copyrighted works, as indicated here and as specified further in the reference pages:

University of Chicago Press, for the excerpt from Norman Maclean's *A River Runs Through It*, 1976, p. 61. James W. Hackett, for three haiku, selected from his *The Zen Haiku and Other Poems of J. W. Hackett*. Tokyo, Japan Publications, 1983. Distributed in the United States by Kodansha International, through Harper & Row, 10 E. 53rd St. New York, NY 10022.

Hunter House, for numerous citations to the work by Stanislav Grof in his *LSD Psychotherapy*, originally published in 1980. (The publishers state that the 1994 edition can be ordered from them at P.O. Box 2914 Alameda, CA 94501, or by calling 1-800-266-5592).

Nelson-Hall Publishers, for permission to cite quotations from a chapter by S. Grof, entitled "Varieties of Transpersonal Experiences: Observations from LSD Psychotherapy," pp. 311–345, in the book edited by S. Dean *Psychiatry and Mysticism* (1975).

W. W. Norton, for verses in A. R. Ammon's poem, "Gravelly Run," from *The Selected Poems, Expanded Edition*, copyright 1986.

Scribner, a division of Simon and Schuster, for the description by Charles Lindbergh, selected from *The Spirit of St. Louis*; original copyright renewed 1981 by Anne Morrow Lindbergh.

The James Thurber Literary Estate, for the quotation about eating, used by special permission of Rosemary Thurber.

Charles E. Tuttle Co., for the description of the Zen prototype person by Harold Stewart, taken from his book, *A Net of Fireflies*; and also for his translation of the haiku, by Shoha, about the faint scent of plum blossoms.

Portions of several chapters appeared in an earlier form in the journals indicated below, and are used herein by permission. Chapters 7, 8, 9, and 32 appeared in *The Eastern Buddhist* 1991; 24(2): 69–97. Chapters 124, 125, and 126 appeared in *Ultimate Reality and Meaning* 1992; 15(1): 60–76. Chapter 146 appeared in *The Theosophist* 1996; 118(3): 117–120, published by The Theosophical Publishing House, Adyar, Madras, 600 020, India.

The epigraphs appearing at the beginning of each part are taken from the following sources:

Front: A. Einstein. In *The Great Quotations*, ed. G. Seldes. New York, Pocket Books, 1967, 816. H. Thoreau. in *Isaac Asimov's Book of Science and Nature Quotations*, eds. I. Asimov and J. Shulman. New York, Weidenfeld and Nicholson, 1988, 276.

Part I: J. VanRuysbroeck. In *Mysticism*, ed. E. Underhill. New York, Dutton, 1961, 334.

Part II: J. Donne. *Holy Sonnets*. Source uncited.

Part III: I. Pavlov. In Asimov and Shulman, ibid., 258.

Part IV: C. Jung. *Psychology and Religion: West and East.* Bollingen Series 20. New York, Pantheon, 1958, 544.

Part V: J. Burroughs. *The Light of Day.* Boston, Houghton Mifflin, 1900. 63.

Part VI: D. Suzuki. *Studies in Zen.* New York, Dell, 1955, 136.

Part VII: Huang-po. In *The Zen Teaching of Huang Po on the Transmission of Mind*, ed. J. Blofeld. New York, Grove, 1958, 92.

Part VIII: Master Dogen. In *Dogen Kigen—Mystical Realist*, H.-J. Kim. Tucson, University of Arizona Press, 1975, 133.

Index

Comic perspective, 414
Commandments, 74, 525
Commissures, 362
Compassion, 47, 64, 461 678, 680, 727
  mudra of, 649–650
  responsibility inherent in, 650–653
Comprehension (keynote of kensho), 496
  (table), 591, 617, 622
Computers, 156, 393, 396
Conditioning, 332–334, 347, 522, 621, 622
  drugs and, 222, 328–329
  to intervals of time, 561–562
  unlearning and, 329–331, 621
Confucianism, 62, 144, 681
Conscience, 522
Consciousness, 280, 281, 325, 380, 431, 458,
  479, 517, 592, 605–606, 652, 653
  alternate states of, 305–311, 323, 464, 624,
  688
  daily variation in, 339, 340(fig)
  destabilization of, 308–309
  development of meanings within, 522–525
  fields within (schematic), 476(fig), 477(fig),
  602, 610(fig)
  heightening, 266, 267
  "opening up and restructuring," 298–299
  ordinary, 295–298, 300(table), 320
  states of, 4, 299–305(tables), 769
  theories for "transcendent," 182, 184
  theory for "emptiness" of, 287
Controlled Substances Act of 1970, 427
Corpus callosum, 151(fig), 358, 359, 360
Cortex, 161, 163–164, 503–504, 518
  "athalamic," 264, 763, 802
Corticosterone, 238–239
Corticotropin-releasing factor (CRF), 212,
  237–238, 464, 506, 590
Cortisol, 239, 349, 588
Cravings, 173–174, 424, 461
Creativity, 63, 258, 621
CRF. See Corticotropin-releasing factor
Crying, 349, 404, 416, 612
Cyclic adenosine monophosphate (cAMP),
  193, 204, 568, 587
  production of, 224–225
Cyclic guanosine monophosphate (cGMP),
  412, 676, 794

DA. See Dopamine
Daigu, 453
Daikaku, 499, 667
Daily life practice (Shugyo), 23, 141, 336, 692
Daito Kokushi, 60, 117, 274, 275
Daitoku-ji, 10, 60

Daiun Harada-roshi, 578
Dalai Lama (Tenzin Gyatso), 334, 350
Damage (caution against making functional
  interpretations based solely on), 162, 172,
  176, 735, 813
Darwin, Charles, 349, 392, 393–394, 415, 416,
  444, 450, 685
Davidson, J., 78, 288
Davy, Humphrey, 407–408, 409, 411
Deafness (transient, in absorption), 500
Death, attitudes toward, 448–450, 569
Death of nerve cell. See Excitotoxins
  apoptosis and, 819
Deathbed experiences, 447–448, 449–450,
  451–452
Deautomatization, 281
Declaration of a Global Ethic by Parliament of
  Worlds' Religions, 356–357
Deconditioning, 329, 333–334
Defeat, 230–231
Defensive behaviors, 40, 233
Deikman, Arthur, 25, 34, 281
Déjà vu, 251, 252
Delusions, 380, 398, 652
Dendrites, 86, 87, 152, 153(fig), 154, 159, 662
Dentate nucleus, 676
Depersonalization, 49
Depression, 459, 615
  biological cycles and, 587–588
  and meditation, 584–585
  and sleep deprivation, 341, 342, 586–587
  treatment of, 585–586
Deprivation, 100. See also by type
Derealization, 49
Desires, 74
Desynchronized sleep (D-sleep), 81, 90, 106,
  166, 202, 207, 212, 227, 312, 313, 315, 340,
  341–342, 406, 413, 462–463, 623, 772
  awakening from, 343–344
  dreams in, 323, 382
  LSD and, 422–423, 464
  functional changes during, 316–320
  and lucid dreams, 326, 327
  and rapid eye movements (REM), 320–322
Desynchronization, desynchrony, 181–182,
  462–463
  not all fast rhythms are desynchronized,
  737, 814
Diazepam (Valium), 237, 262, 568
Diencephalon, 361
Diffuseness, 128
Disinhibition, 255, 462, 676
Dispassion, 128, 129, 652
Distributed functions, 393, 394, 602